AF616269

Clinical Aspects of Immunology

CLINICAL ASPECTS OF IMMUNOLOGY

EDITED BY

P.J.LACHMANN
ScD FRCP PRCPath FRS
Sheila Joan Smith Professor of Immunology
and Honorary Director of MRC Molecular Immunopathology Unit
University of Cambridge, UK

SIR KEITH PETERS
MD(Hon) MB FRCP FRCPath
Regius Professor of Physic
University of Cambridge School of Clinical Medicine
Addenbrooke's Hospital, Cambridge, UK

F.S.ROSEN
MD
James L. Gamble Professor of Pediatrics
Harvard Medical School, Boston, USA

M.J.WALPORT
PhD FRCP MRCPath
Professor of Rheumatology
Royal Postgraduate Medical School
Hammersmith Hospital, London, UK

IN THREE VOLUMES
VOLUME 3

FIFTH EDITION

BOSTON
BLACKWELL SCIENTIFIC PUBLICATIONS
OXFORD LONDON EDINBURGH
MELBOURNE PARIS BERLIN VIENNA

Editorial offices:
238 Main Street, Cambridge
Massachusetts 02142, USA
Osney Mead, Oxford OX2 0EL, England
25 John Street, London WC1N 2BL
England
23 Ainslie Place, Edinburgh EH3 6AJ
Scotland
54 University Street, Carlton
Victoria 3053, Australia

Other Editorial Offices:
Librairie Arnette SA
2, rue Casimir-Delavigne
75006 Paris
France

Blackwell Wissenschafts-Verlag
Meinekestrasse 4
D-1000 Berlin 15
Germany

Blackwell MZV
Feldgasse 13
A-1238 Wien
Austria

First published 1963
Revised reprint 1964
Second edition 1968
Third edition 1975
Fourth edition 1982
Fifth edition 1993

Set by Setrite Typesetters, Hong Kong
Printed and bound in the USA
by The Maple-Vail Book
Manufacturing Group, New York

93 94 95 96 5 4 3 2 1

DISTRIBUTORS

USA
Blackwell Scientific Publications, Inc.
238 Main Street
Cambridge, Massachusetts 02142
(*Orders*: Tel: 617 876-7000
800 759-6102)

Canada
Times Mirror Professional Publishing, Ltd
130 Flaska Drive
Markham, Ontario L6G 1B8
(*Orders*: Tel: 416 470-6739
800 268-4178)

Australia
Blackwell Scientific Publications Pty Ltd
54 University Street
Carlton, Victoria 3053
(*Orders*: Tel: 03 347-5552)

Outside North America and Australia
Marston Book Services Ltd
PO Box 87
Oxford OX2 0DT
(*Orders*: Tel: 0865 791155
Fax: 0865 791927
Telex: 837515)

Library of Congress
Cataloguing-in-Publication Data

Clinical aspects of immunology/
edited by P.J. Lachmann ... [*et al.*].
—5th ed.
p. cm.
Includes bibliographical references and index.
ISBN 0-86542-297-4
1. Clinical immunology. 2. Immunology.
I. Lachmann, P.F. (Peter Julius)
[DNLM: 1. Hypersensitivity. 2. Immunity.
WD 300 C641]
RC582.C52 1993
616.07'9—dc20
DNLM/DLC
for Library of Congress

Contents

List of Contributors

C.L.Anderson MD, *Department of Internal Medicine, The Ohio State University College of Medicine, Columbus, USA*

B.M.Ansell MB ChB, FRCP, MRCS, *Consultant Rheumatologist, Stoke Poges, UK*

M.A.Arnaout MD, *Director, Leukocyte Biology and Inflammation Program, Associate Physician, Renal Unit and Department of Medicine, Massachusetts General Hospital, Charlestown and Associate Professor of Medicine, Harvard Medical School, Boston, USA*

J.-F.Bach MD, DSc, *Professor and Director, Département d'Immunologie Clinique, Hospital Necker, Paris, France*

J.I.Bell DM, FRCP, *Nuffield Professor of Clinical Medicine, John Radcliffe Hospital, Oxford, UK*

R.M.Bernstein MA, MD, FRCP, *Consultant Rheumatologist, Manchester Royal Infirmary, University of Manchester, UK*

K.Berzins PhD, *Associate Professor, Department of Immunology, Stockholm University, Stockholm, Sweden*

J.M.Blackwell PhD, *Glaxo Professor of Molecular Parasitology, Departments of Pathology and Medicine, University of Cambridge, UK*

E.Bonifacio PhD, *Lecturer, Department of Immunology, London Hospital Medical College, UK*

L.K.Borysiewicz MB, PhD, FRCP, *Professor of Medicine, University of Wales College of Medicine, Cardiff, UK*

G.F.Bottazzo MD, FRCP, FRCPath, *Professor of Immunology and Clinical Immunology, Department of Immunology, London Hospital Medical College, UK*

D.L.Brown MD, FRCPath, *Consultant Immunologist, Addenbrooke's Hospital, Cambridge, UK*

A.E.Butterworth MB BChir, PhD, *Medical Research Council External Scientific Staff and Honorary Reader in Medical Parasitology, University of Cambridge, UK*

Sir Roy Calne MA, MS, FRCS, FRS, *Professor of Surgery, Department of Surgery, University of Cambridge Clinical School, Addenbrooke's Hospital, Cambridge, UK*

T.A.Calvelli PhD, *Associate Professor, Departments of Pediatrics, Microbiology and Immunology, Albert Einstein College of Medicine, Bronx, USA*

R.D.Campbell BSc, PhD, *Senior Scientist, MRC Immunochemistry Unit, Department of Biochemistry, University of Oxford, UK*

D.A.Carson MD, *Professor, Department of Medicine, University of California, San Diego, USA*

R.K.Chandra OC, MD, PhD, DSc(Hon), DPhil(Hon), FRCPC, *Professor of Pediatrics, Medicine and Biochemistry, Memorial University of Newfoundland and Director, WHO Center for Nutritional Immunology, St. John's, Newfoundland, Canada*

T.A.Chatila MD, *Assistant Professor of Pediatrics, Harvard Medical School, Division of Immunology, The Children's Hospital, Boston, USA*

P.M.S.Clark PhD, MRCPath, *Principal Biochemist, Addenbrooke's Hospital, Cambridge, UK*

S.C.Clark PhD, *Vice President, Discovery Research, Genetics Institute Inc., Cambridge, USA*

J.Cohen MB BS, MSc, FRCP, *Professor and Director of Department of Infectious Diseases and Bacteriology and Honorary Consultant Physician, Royal Postgraduate Medical School, Hammersmith Hospital, London, UK*

P.J.Cole BSc, MB BS, FRCP, MRCS, *Professor, National Heart and Lung Institute, Brompton Hospital, London, UK*

D.H.Conrad PhD, *Department of Microbiology and Immunology, Medical College of Virginia, Richmond, USA*

A.Cooke BSc, DPhil, *Lecturer in Immunology, Department of Pathology, University of Cambridge, UK*

R.S.Cotran MD, *F.B. Mallory Professor of Pathology, Harvard Medical School, and Chairman, Department of Pathology, Brigham and Women's Hospital, Boston, USA*

C.A.Dinarello MD, *Professor of Medicine and Pediatrics, Tufts University School of Medicine, New England Medical Center, Boston, USA*

W.F.Doe MSc, FRACP, FRCP, *Professor of Medicine and Clinical Science, John Curtin School of Medical Research, Australian National University, Canberra, Australia*

R.M.du Bois MA, MD, FRCP, *Consultant Physician, Royal Brompton National Heart & Lung Hospital and Honorary Senior Lecturer, National Heart & Lung Institute, London, UK*

I.Dunham BA, DPhil, *Postdoctoral Research Fellow, Paediatric Research Unit, Guy's Hospital, London, UK*

A.L.W.F.Eddleston DM, FRCP, *Professor of Liver Immunology, Institute of Liver Studies, King's College School of Medicine and Dentistry, London, UK*

G.I.Evan MA, PhD, *Senior Scientist, Imperial Cancer Research Fund Laboratories, London, UK*

P.W.Ewan MB, FRCP, MRCPath, *MRC Clinical Scientist and Honorary Consultant in Allergy and Clinical Immunology, MRC Molecular Immunopathology Unit, University of Cambridge School of Clinical Medicine and Addenbrooke's Hospital, UK*

J.M.Farrant MD, MRCP, *Wellcome Clinical Research Fellow, Institute of Liver Studies, King's College School of Medicine and Dentistry, London, UK*

A.J.Frew MA, MD, MB BChir, MRCP, *Senior Lecturer, Department of University Medicine, Southampton General Hospital, UK*

R.S.Geha MD, *Professor of Pediatrics, Harvard Medical School, and Chief, Division of Immunology, The Children's Hospital, Boston, USA*

I.Gigli MD, *Professor of Medicine and Chief, Division of Dermatology, University of California, San Diego, USA*

S.Gordon MB ChB, PhD, *Glaxo Professor of Cellular Pathology, Sir William Dunn School of Pathology, University of Oxford, UK*

C.D.Gregory PhD, *Senior Lecturer, Department of Immunology, University of Birmingham Medical School, UK*

E.C.Guinan MD, *Assistant Professor of Pediatrics, Division of Pediatric Oncology, Dana–Farber Cancer Institute, Harvard Medical School, Boston, USA*

A.G.Hadley BSc, DPhil, *Manager, Antibody Function Laboratory, International Blood Group Reference Laboratory, Bristol, UK*

C.N.Hales MD, PhD, FRCP, FRCPath, FRS, *Professor and Head of Department of Clinical Biochemistry, Addenbrooke's Hospital, Cambridge, UK*

F.C.Hay BTech, PhD, *Professor of Immunology, and Head of Department of Cellular and Molecular Sciences,*

P.G.Hellewell PhD, *Senior Lecturer, Department of Applied Pharmacology, National Heart & Lung Institute, London, UK*

B.Henderson BSc, PhD, *Senior Lecturer in Biochemistry, Institute of Dental Surgery, University of London, UK*

P.M.Henson PhD, *Professor of Pathology and Medicine, National Jewish Center for Immunology and Respiratory Medicine, Denver, USA*

G.A.Higgs BSc, PhD, *Head of Inflammation Biology, Celltech Ltd, Slough, UK*

T.Hirano MD, PhD, *Professor, Division of Molecular Oncology, Biomedical Research Centre, Osaka University Medical School, Japan*

S.T.Holgate MD, DSc, FRCP, *MRC Clinical Professor of Immunopharmacology, Medicine 1, Southampton General Hospital, UK*

N.Holmes PhD, *Division of Immunology, Department of Pathology, University of Cambridge, UK*

J.Hopkins BSc, PhD, MIBiol, *Senior Lecturer in Veterinary Pathology, Royal (Dick) School of Veterinary Studies, University of Edinburgh, UK*

N.C.Hughes-Jones DM, PhD, FRCP, FRS, *Honorary Member, Scientific Staff, MRC Molecular Immunopathology Unit, MRC Centre, Cambridge, UK*

The Late J.H.Humphrey FRS, *Latterly of the Department of Immunology, Royal Postgraduate Medical School, London, UK*

G.Husby MD, *Professor of Rheumatology, Department of Rheumatology, The University of Tromsø, Norway*

J.Ivanyi MD, PhD, *Director of MRC Tuberculosis and Related Infections Unit, Hammersmith Hospital, London, UK*

H.H.Jabara *Chief Technologist, The Children's Hospital, Boston, USA*

N.D.James BSc, MRCP, FRCR, *Lecturer in Oncology, Ludwig Institute for Cancer Research, St. Mary's Hospital Medical School, London, UK*

E.Jenkinson BSc, PhD, *Department of Anatomy, University of Birmingham Medical School, UK*

J.P.Johnson PhD, *Senior Scientist, Institute for Immunology, University of Munich, Republic of Germany*

P.M.Johnson MA, PhD, DSc, MRCPath, *Professor of Immunology, University of Liverpool, UK*

R.B.Johnston, Jr MD, *Adjunct Professor of Pediatrics, Yale University School of Medicine, New Haven, USA*

D.L.Kasper MD, *William Ellery Channing Professor of Medicine, Harvard Medical School, Co-Director, Channing Laboratory, Brigham and Women's Hospital, and Chief, Division of Infectious Diseases, Beth Israel Hospital, Boston, USA*

A.B.Kay PhD, DSc, FRCP, *Professor and Director, Department of Allergy and Clinical Immunology, National Heart & Lung Institute, London, UK*

D.M.Kenney PhD, *Assistant Professor of Pediatrics, Harvard Medical School and Investigator, The Center for Blood Research, Boston, USA*

T.Kishimoto MD, PhD, *Professor, Department of Internal Medicine III, Osaka University Medical School, Japan*

G.G.B.Klaus PhD, MS, BVSc, *Laboratory of Cellular Immunology, National Institute for Medical Research, London, UK*

S.C.Knight PhD, FIBiol, *Head, Antigen Presentation Research Group, MRC Clinical Research Centre, Harrow, UK*

R.R.Kretschmer MD, FAAP, FAAAI, *Head, Division of Immunology, Unidad de Investigación Biomédica CMN-IMSS and Subdivisión de Medicina Experimental Universidad Nacional Autónoma de Mexico, Mexico DF*

P.J.Lachmann ScD, FRCP, PRCPath, FRS, *Sheila Joan Smith Professor of Immunology and Honorary Director of MRC Molecular Immunopathology Unit, MRC Centre, Cambridge, UK*

R.I.Lechler PhD, FRCP, *Professor of Molecular Immunology and Honorary Consultant in Medicine, Department of Immunology, Royal Postgraduate Medical School, Hammersmith Hospital, London, UK*

T.H.Lee MD, MRCPath, FRCP, *Professor of Allergy and Allied Respiratory Disorders, Guy's Hospital, London, UK*

P.F.Lehmann MA, MSc, PhD, *Associate Professor of Microbiology, Medical College of Ohio, Toledo, USA*

T.Lehner MD, BDS, PhD (Hon), FRCPath, FDS RDS, *Head, Division of Immunology, United Medical and Dental Schools of Guy's and St. Thomas's Hospitals, London, UK*

M.H.Lessof MA, MD, FRCP, *Emeritus Professor of Medicine, United Schools of Guy's and St. Thomas's Hospitals, London, UK*

C.M.Lockwood MB BChir, FRCP, *Wellcome Reader in the School of Clinical Medicine, University of Cambridge, Addenbrooke's Hospital, Cambridge, UK*

T.T.MacDonald PhD, MRCPath, *Reader in Gut Immunology and Wellcome Senior Lecturer, Department of Paediatric Gastroenterology, St. Bartholomew's Hospital, London, UK*

I.C.M.MacLennan MB BS, PhD, MRCP, FRCPath, *Head of Department of Immunology, University of Birmingham Medical School, UK*

P.D.Mason BSc, MRCP, *Squibb Lecturer in Renal Medicine, Department of Medicine, Royal Postgraduate Medical School, Hammersmith Hospital, London, UK*

I.McConnell MA, PhD, BVMS, MRCVS, MRCPath, FRSE, *Professor of Veterinary Pathology, Royal (Dick) School of Veterinary Studies, University of Edinburgh, UK*

I.G.McFarlane PhD, MRCPath, *Consultant Biochemist, Institute of Liver Studies, King's College School of Medicine and Dentistry, London, UK*

A.M.McGregor MA, MD, FRCP, *Professor of Medicine, King's College School of Medicine, London, UK*

A.J.McMichael PhD, MB BChir, MRCP, FRS, *MRC Clinical Research Professor of Immunology, Institute of Molecular Medicine, University of Oxford, UK*

P.A.R.Meyer MA, MB BChir, MRCP, *Wellcome Research Fellow, Department of Ophthalmology, Addenbrooke's Hospital, Cambridge, UK*

N.A.Mitchison BSc, DPhil, FRS, *Scientific Director, Deutsches Rheuma — Forschungszentrum Berlin, Republic of Germany*

S.Moncada PhD, DSc, *Research Director, Wellcome Research Laboratories, Beckenham, UK*

P.J.Morris PhD, FRCS, FACS(Hon), FRACS *Nuffield Professor of Surgery, University of Oxford, UK*

J.B.Natvig MD, PhD, *Professor, Institute of Immunology and Rheumatology, University of Oslo, Norway*

P.E.Newburger MD, *Associate Professor of Pediatrics and Molecular Genetics/Microbiology, Department of Pediatrics, University of Massachusetts Medical School, Worcester, USA*

A.Newman Taylor MSc, FRCP, FFOM, *Consultant Physician, Royal Brompton National Heart & Lung Hospital and Honorary Senior Lecturer, National Heart & Lung Institute, London, UK*

J.Newsom-Davis MA, MD, FRCP, FRS, *Professor of Clinical Neurology, Neurosciences Group, Institute of Molecular Medicine, University of Oxford, John Radcliffe Hospital, Oxford, UK*

G.J.V.Nossal MD, PhD, FRCP, FRS, *Director, The Walter and Eliza Hall Institute of Medical Research, Melbourne, Australia*

D.B.G.Oliveira PhD, MRCP, *Lister Institute Research Fellow and Honorary Consultant Physician, Department of Medicine, University of Cambridge School of Clinical Medicine, Addenbrooke's Hospital, Cambridge, UK*

W.H.Ouwehand MD, PhD, *Consultant Haematologist, Lecturer in Transfusion Medicine, Division of Transfusion Medicine, University of Cambridge, UK*

M.J.Owen BA, PhD, *Principal Scientist, Imperial Cancer Research Fund, Lincoln's Inn Fields, London, UK*

J.L.Pace PhD, *Research Associate Professor, Departments of Pathology/Oncology and Microbiology/Molecular Genetics/Immunology, Wilkinson Laboratory for Cancer Research, University of Kansas Medical Center, Kansas City, USA*

D.C.Parker PhD, *Professor, Department of Molecular Genetics and Microbiology, University of Massachusetts Medical School, Worcester, USA*

D.M.V.Parrott PhD, DSc, FRS(Edin), *Visiting Professor, Department of Paediatric Gastroenterology, St. Bartholomew's Hospital, London, UK*

T.W.Pearson PhD, *Professor, Department of Biochemistry and Microbiology, University of Victoria, Canada*

P.Perlmann PhD, *Professor Emeritus, Department of Immunology, Stockholm University, Sweden*

D.K.Peters MD(Hon), MB FRCP, FRCPath, *Regius Professor of Physic, University of Cambridge School of Clinical Medicine, Addenbrooke's Hospital, Cambridge, UK*

E.R.Pettipher BSc, PhD, *Senior Research Scientist, Pfizer Central Research, Groton, USA*

A.J.Pinching DPhil, FRCP, *Louis Freedman Professor of Immunology, Medical College of St. Bartholomew's Hospital, London, UK*

T.A.E.Platts-Mills MD, PhD, FRCP, *Oscar Swineford Jr. Professor of Medicine and Microbiology, and Head, Division of Allergy and Clinical Immunology, University of Virginia, Charlotsville, USA*

J.H.L.Playfair MB BChir, DSc, PhD, *Professor of Immunology, University College Medical School, London, UK*

J.S.Pober MD, PhD, *Professor of Pathology, Immunobiology and Biology, and Director, Molecular Cardiobiology, Boyer Center for Molecular Medicine, Yale University School of Medicine, New Haven, USA*

E.R.Podack MD, *Professor of Microbiology, Immunology and Oncology, Department of Microbiology and Immunology, University of Miami School of Medicine, USA*

R.Pujol-Borrell MD, PhD, *Associate Professor of Immunology, Hospital Universitari Germans Trias I, Barcelona, Spain*

C.D.Pusey MSc, FRCP, *Reader in Renal Medicine and Honorary Consultant Physician, Department of Medicine, Royal Postgraduate Medical School, Hammersmith Hospital, London, UK*

T.H.Rabbitts BSc, PhD, FRS, *Joint Head of Protein and Nucleic Acid Division, MRC Laboratory of Molecular Biology, Cambridge, UK*

A.J.Rees MSc, FRCP, *Professor of Nephrology, Department of Medicine, Royal Postgraduate Medical School, Hammersmith Hospital, London, UK*

J.R.Regueiro PhD, *Senior Registrar, Department of Immunology, Hospital 12 de Octubre, Madrid, Spain*

G.Reimer MD, *Assistant Professor (Privatdozent) of Dermatology, University of Erlangen-Nürnberg, Republic of Germany*

G.Riethmüller MD, *Director, Institute for Immunology, University of Munich, Republic of Germany*

A.B.Rickinson PhD, *Head of Department of Cancer Studies, Cancer Research Campaign Laboratories, The Medical School, University of Birmingham, UK*

F.S.Rosen MD, *James L. Gamble Professor of Pediatrics, Harvard Medical School, Boston, USA*

G.D.Ross PhD, *Professor and Chairman, Department of Microbiology and Immunology, University of Louisville, USA*

A.Rubinstein MD, *Professor, Departments of Pediatrics, Microbiology and Immunology, Albert Einstein College of Medicine, Bronx, USA*

C.O.S.Savage PhD, MRCP, *Clinical Scientist and Honorary Consultant Physician, Clinical Research Centre, Northwick Park Hospital, Harrow, UK*

L.B.Schwartz MD, PhD, *Charles and Evelyn Thomas Professor of Medicine, Medical College of Virginia, Virginia Commonwealth University, Richmond, USA*

J.P.Scott MD, *Associate Professor, Mayo Clinic, Rochester, USA*

M.Seligmann MD, FRCPath, *Professor of Immunology and Head of Department of Immunohaematology, Hospital Saint-Louis, Paris, France*

D.W.Shaw MD, *Clinical Fellow, Division of Dermatology, Department of Medicine, University of California, San Diego, USA*

M.J.Sicklick MD, *Department of Pediatrics, Albert Einstein College of Medicine, Bronx, USA*

K.Sikora MA, PhD, FRCP, FRCR, *Department of Clinical Oncology, Royal Postgraduate Medical School, Hammersmith Hospital, London, UK*

G.J.Silverman MD, *Assistant Professor, Division of Rheumatology, Department of Medicine, University of California, San Diego, USA*

J.G.P.Sissons MD, FRCP, *Professor of Medicine, University of Cambridge School of Clinical Medicine, UK*

The Late T.F.Slater MSc, PhD, DSc, MD(Hon), D.Univ(Paris), *Latterly Professor of Biochemistry, Brunel University, Uxbridge, UK*

T.A.Springer PhD, *Latham Family Professor, Harvard Medical School, Boston, USA*

C.J.F.Spry DPhil, FRCP, FRCPath, *British Heart Foundation Professor of Cardiovascular Immunology, St. George's Hospital Medical School, London, UK*

G.T.Stevenson MD, DPhil, *Professor of Immunochemistry, University of Southampton, UK*

R.Storb MD, *Professor of Medicine, University of Washington and Member, Fred Hutchinson Cancer Research Center, Washington, USA*

T.B.Strom MD, DSc(Hon), *Professor of Medicine, Harvard Medical School and Head, Division of Immunology, Beth Israel Hospital, Boston, USA*

Q.A.Summers MB BS, FRACP, *Research Fellow, Medicine 1, Southampton General Hospital, UK*

E.M.Tan MD, *W.M. Keck Autoimmune Disease Center, The Scripps Research Institute, La Jolla, USA*

C.Terhorst PhD, *Chief, Division of Immunology, Beth Israel Hospital, Harvard Medical School, Boston, USA*

H.C.Thomas BSc, PhD, FRCP, FRCPath, *Professor of Medicine, St. Mary's Hospital Medical School, Imperial College of Science, Technology and Medicine, University of London, UK*

J.Trowsdale PhD, *Head, Human Immunogenetics Laboratory, Imperial Cancer Research Fund, Lincoln's Inn Fields, London, UK*

M.W.Turner DSc(Med), FRCPath, *Professor of Molecular Immunology, Institute of Child Health, University of London, UK*

E.R.Unanue MD, *Professor and Chairman, Department of Pathology, Washington University School of Medicine, St. Louis, USA*

H.Valdimarsson MD, FRCPath, *Professor and Chairman, Department of Immunology, Landspitalinn, The National University Hospital, Reykjavik, Iceland*

P.J.W.Venables MD, MRCP, *Senior Lecturer in Rheumatology, Kennedy Institute of Rheumatology, London, UK*

D.Vercelli MD, *Assistant Professor of Pediatrics, Harvard Medical School, Boston, USA*

A.C.Vincent MB BS, MSc, MRCPath, *University Lecturer in Clinical Neoroimmunology, Neurosciences Group, Institute of Molecular Medicine, University of Oxford, John Radcliffe Hospital, Oxford, UK*

M.Wahlgren MD, PhD, *Associate Professor, Department of Immunology, Stockholm University, Sweden*

B.H.Waksman MD, *Adjunct Professor of Pathology, New York University and Visiting Scientist in Neurology, Harvard University, Boston, USA*

H.Waldmann FRS, *Kay Kendall Professor of Therapeutic Immunology, University of Cambridge, UK*

T.A.Waldmann MD, *Chief, Metabolism Branch, National Cancer Institute, National Institute of Health, Bethesda, USA*

J.Wallwork MB ChB, FRCS Ed, *Consultant Cardiothoracic Surgeon, Department of Cardiothoracic Surgery, Papworth Hospital, Cambridge, UK*

M.J.Walport PhD, FRCP, MRCPath, *Professor of Rheumatology, Royal Postgraduate Medical School, Hammersmith Hospital, London, UK*

S.Ward PhD, *Assistant Professor, Department of Microbiology, The University of Texas Southwestern Medical Center at Dallas, USA*

J.A.Warner PhD, *Lecturer in Allergy and Immunology, Child Health, University of Southampton, Southampton General Hospital, UK*

J.O.Warner MD, FRCP, DCH, *Professor of Child Health, University of Southampton, Southampton General Hospital, UK*

A.H.Waters PhD, FRCP, FRCPath, *Head of Department of Haematology, St. Bartholomew's Hospital and Medical College, London, UK*

R.J.Wedgwood MD, *Professor Emeritus, Department of Pediatrics, University of Washington, USA*

A.P.Weetman MD, FRCP, *Professor of Medicine, University of Sheffield Clinical Sciences Centre, Northern General Hospital, Sheffield, UK*

M.R.Wessels MD, *Assistant Professor of Medicine, Harvard Medical School, Associate Physician, Channing Laboratory, Brigham and Women's Hospital and Associate Physician, Division of Infectious Diseases, Beth Israel Hospital, Boston, USA*

J.R.W.Wilkinson MD, MRCP, *Lecturer in Medicine, University of Southampton, UK*

H.N.A.Willcox MA, MB BChir, PhD, *University Research Lecturer, Neurosciences Group, Institute of Molecular Medicine, University of Oxford, John Radcliffe Hospital, Oxford, UK*

R.C.Williams Jr MD, *Eminent Scholar, Marcia Whitney Schott Chair in Rheumatoid Arthritis, Department of Medicine, University of Florida School of Medicine, Gainesville, USA*

G.Winter PhD, FRS, *Member, MRC Laboratory of Molecular Biology, Cambridge, UK*

R.P.Witherspoon MD, *Associate Professor of Medicine, University of Washington and Associate Member, Fred Hutchinson Cancer Research Center, Washington, USA*

P.Woo PhD, FRCP, *Head, Section of Molecular Rheumatology, Clinical Research Centre, Northwick Park Hospital, Harrow, UK*

K.J.Wood PhD, *University Lecturer in Immunology, Royal Postgraduate Medical School, Hammersmith Hospital, London, UK*

Preface to the Fifth Edition

Eleven years have gone by since the Fourth Edition of *Clinical Aspects* was published. These years have seen no slackening in the rate of progress of immunology or of its clinical aspects and the book has again required major restructuring and almost total rewriting. For this task two further editors have been recruited and Peter Lachmann and Keith Peters warmly welcome Fred Rosen, from the Center for Blood Research at Harvard University, and Mark Walport, from the Royal Postgraduate Medical School, as co-editors. Together with an American editor we have for this edition recruited authors from further afield, particularly from the United States, but also from Australia, Canada, France, Germany, Iceland, Japan, Mexico, Norway and Sweden. The book has again grown substantially. This edition has 109 chapters compared with the 64 of the Fourth Edition. The editors have discovered that as the number of authors increases linearly the difficulty of obtaining chapters on time rises exponentially and we are only too aware that this edition has had a longer incubation period than we had either hoped or expected. Nevertheless, with the help of contributors in updating their chapters, we are confident that the book is a timely overview of the subject for the rest of the millennium.

The editors would like to express their sincere thanks to those contributors to the Fourth Edition who are not contributing this time. We would also like to welcome all those contributing to this edition for the first time.

We were greatly saddened by the death of several of the contributors to the Fourth Edition: Ed Franklin, Mavis Gunter, John Humphrey, Henry Kunkel and Tony Waterson. All are a sadly felt loss to immunology, to medicine and to this book. The chapter written in the Fourth Edition by Gerry Klaus and John Humphrey has been revised for this edition by Gerry Klaus alone and is published as a tribute to John. We were also greatly saddened by the death of one of the contributors to this edition, Trevor Slater, while the book was in press. Trevor was a major British authority on oxygen radicals and a wonderfully enthusiastic scientist.

The new layout of the book reflects the great changes that have occurred in immunology in the past 10 years. There are new chapters on newly characterized molecules: adhesion molecules, Fc receptors and various cytokines. The mystery of the T cell receptors has now been solved and their genes are considered alongside those for immunoglobulins which they closely resemble. Understanding of the complement system has expanded to such an extent that there are now two additional chapters on complement receptors and complement deficiencies. Antigens have been joined by superantigens. The new techniques section contains chapters on molecular biology and on transgenic animals as well as on antibody engineering; and monoclonal antibody therapy has advanced to the stage where it is well worthy of its own chapter. Allergy is promoted to having its own section as is connective tissue disease, immunodeficiency and the acquired immune deficiency syndrome. The AIDS epidemic is indeed the greatest change that has occurred in the clinical aspects of immunology. The organ-specific section contains similar chapter titles to earlier editions but the contents reflect the great changes that have occurred with changes in the basic science.

P.J.L., D.K.P.
F.S.R., M.J.W.

Section 9
Immunology of Infection

73: Overview: Parasitism and Immunity

J.H.L. Playfair

Parasitism and immunity

It might not strike the desperate physician battling for the life of a pneumonic plague, Lassa fever or cerebral malaria victim that parasitism is an ancient and in most cases respectable way of life. At its best, the host–parasite balance is certainly more harmonious than the other food-sharing relationship — that between predator and prey. There are more species of parasite on earth than of free-living animals and there is probably no free-living animal that does not harbour at least one parasite. Parasitologists sometimes distinguish among mutualism, where both partners benefit, commensalism, where only one benefits, and parasitism where one benefits and the other suffers, but these distinctions are by no means hard and fast. What we can say is that the parasite needs the host more than vice versa, and this is why it is often useful, in attempting to understand the host–parasite relationship in particular cases, to consider the matter from the viewpoint of the parasite.

The first self-evident conclusion is that no successful parasite can afford to kill or enfeeble its host, at least not to the extent of limiting its own survival and spread. Parasite growth cannot therefore be permitted to continue indefinitely. At a crude level, the supply of essential metabolites or of space will impose limitations on parasite numbers, but there is a far more subtle means for the parasite to achieve the same end, namely to take advantage of host immunity. It is a sobering thought that, while we see our highly sophisticated immune system as an evolutionary adaptation against parasites, a successful parasite might see just the opposite — a convenient arrangement by which, at no great cost to itself, it can be assured of living room in a healthy mobile host.

In this chapter, therefore, equal emphasis will be placed on adaptations by both host and parasite in arriving at the various kinds of host–parasite balance which will be described in more detail in the following chapters.

The parasite, 1

Classes of parasite

For the purposes of this discussion, parasites will be considered as belonging to five major categories: viruses, bacteria, fungi, protozoa and helminths (worms).

The popular restriction of the word to the two latter groups, with the further implication that 'parasite' diseases are mainly tropical, has no real appeal to the immunologist since, as will be seen, it is usually the entry, habitat, mode of spread and evasion strategies of the parasite that dictate whether and how successfully immunity develops, and these cut across all taxonomic barriers. A sixth group, the parasitic insects, will be considered here mainly in their capacity as vectors.

Entry and habitat

Some parasites can obtain their nutritional requirements without actually entering the tissues of their host: staphylococci or dermatophytes on the skin, *Streptococcus mutans* on the teeth, *Candida* in the mouth and lactobacilli or amoebae in the intestine are examples. It does not follow that these cannot cause disease, because they may release toxins that can enter and damage cells (e.g. diphtheria). Nor can it be assumed that they are out of reach of the immune system: lysozyme in tears and IgA in the gut are two well-known protective factors that act externally to the body.

Most medically important parasites, however, have adapted to an existence within the body, either intracellularly or in the extracellular spaces, and this means that they must break through the outer layers of skin or mucous membranes. Five routes are available (see Table 73.1): (i) Wounds and burns allow entry of organisms, including those that normally colonize the skin (e.g. staphylococci) but also free-living ones (e.g. *Clostridium tetani*). Such parasites are then in an environment to which they may not be well adapted, a situation that often leads to severe disease. (ii) Some bacteria, fungi and protozoa, and all viruses, gain entry to cells by first attaching via specific receptor–receptor interaction. This clearly requires a high degree of adaptation by the parasite, and may considerably restrict the range of host species available to it. It also constitutes a vulnerable stage for parasite survival because of the effectiveness of specific antibody in blocking attachment. (iii) Some bacteria (e.g. cholera), protozoa such as *Entamoeba*, and worms such as the

Table 73.1. Routes of microbial entry

Site of entry	Method of entry	Examples
Skin	Wounds, burns	*Staphylococcus* *Streptococcus* Tetanus
	Insect bites	Malaria, trypanosomiasis, typhus, yellow fever
	Direct penetration	Schistosomiasis
Nose and throat	Attach to cells	Adenovirus
	Attach to teeth	*Streptococcus mutans*
Respiratory tract	Receptor on epithelium	Influenza
	Mucus/ciliary defects	*Bordetella pertussis*
Gut	Attach and penetrate	*Salmonella* Poliomyelitis
	Attach without penetration	Cholera *Giardia* Hookworm
Genitourinary tract	Attach to epithelium	*Neisseria gonorrhoeae*

cercarial stage of the schistosome can damage skin or mucous surfaces by their enzymatic secretions; in most cases there is a previous attachment stage as well. (iv) Other organisms allow themselves to be ingested by phagocytic cells but have evolved mechanisms for avoiding destruction: these include bacteria (e.g. mycobacteria), fungi (e.g. *Histoplasma*) and protozoa (e.g. *Leishmania*) and such infections, regardless of the class of organism, have a number of features in common. (v) Finally there are the organisms that make use of biting insects, solving simultaneously the problems of skin penetration and spread over large distances. In return for these advantages, they must modify their life cycle for two very different modes of existence — an extraordinary feat of adaptation.

Multiplication and spread

An alarming feature of most parasites, from the host's viewpoint, is their capacity for rapid multiplication. It is not necessary to be exposed to a large number of viral particles, staphylococci, or African trypanosomes — to give three particularly fast-growing examples — in order for a heavy infection to result. With helminth infections, on the other hand, no multiplication occurs in the host and the density of infection is exactly proportional to the degree of exposure. Between these extremes are a variety of more slowly dividing organisms, of which the tubercle bacillus and the spirochaete are representative. Growth rates become particularly important when an antibody response is involved, since B lymphocytes cannot divide more than about once per day, so that the production of sufficient antibody to opsonize, for example, a population of *Streptococcus pneumoniae*, with a doubling time of 20 minutes, constitutes a literal race against time.

The extent to which a parasite spreads from the site of entry is also of great significance for the effectiveness of immunity. A rhinovirus spreading directly from cell to cell may be susceptible to mechanisms that kill the cell (e.g. cytotoxic T cells) or prevent viral replication in it (e.g. interferon) but antibody will be ineffective. The malaria parasite, which is free in the blood for two stages of a few minutes each (the sporozoite and merozoite) is potentially susceptible to antibody, but high concentrations and high affinity will be needed to reach every organism in such a brief time. The spread of polio virus to the central nervous system (CNS) via the blood can be prevented by preexistent antibody, but is too rapid to induce a *de novo* antibody response, while at the other extreme the spread of rabies to the CNS via nerves is slow enough to give time for vaccination after exposure to confer protection. Spread may be relatively passive, as when bacteria are swept into a lymphatic or a blood-sucking insect injects organisms directly into the blood, or it may be actively promoted by microbial secretions: staphylococci and streptococci are particularly rich in enzymes that damage or dissolve connective tissue.

The host, 1: natural immunity

Apart from the simple physical barrier of intact epithelium, keratin, fur, etc., a variety of secreted factors protect against infection, particularly bacterial. Fatty acids in sebaceous secretions, HCl in the stomach, lactic acid in the vagina, mucus in the respiratory tract and lysozyme in tears, saliva and plasma all help to keep bacterial numbers down. Evolution of constitutive defences of this kind is evidently limited by the need to avoid damage to host tissues.

Complement

The role of the complement system in infection can be easily judged by the effect of specific deficiencies (see Chapter 67), but its importance can be undervalued if one considers only the natural parasites of a particular host which must, by definition, have adapted either to avoid triggering the complement cascade or to escape the consequences. The finding that blood trypanosomes of human origin fail to survive in birds because they activate the alternative pathway (Kierszenbaum *et al.* 1976) gives a hint of the potential of this system. It is worth remembering that an individual host species is only susceptible to infection by a tiny proportion of the available parasites: for example there are over 8000 species of parasitic protozoa but only about 20 of these survive in humans (Cohen 1974).

Interferons and other cytokines

The interferons (IFN) represent an interesting halfway stage between natural and adaptive immunity, being produced in response to, and effective against, viral infection but without any of the fine specificity associated with 'true' adaptive responses by lymphocytes. The demonstration that tumour necrosis factor (TNF) also has antiviral activity (Wong and Goeddel 1986), while IFN-β2 is predominantly a B cell differentiation factor (now known as interleukin 6 (IL-6), plus the evidence that IFN-γ has effects on almost all components of the immune system, emphasizes the fact that the name by which a cytokine is generally known is not necessarily a good guide to its real function. Almost all the available cytokines have now been shown to have an effect on one infection or another, but when studied closely these effects almost invariably turn out to be indirect ones, frequently involving the activation of macrophages or other cells to enhance their own killing mechanisms (see 'Cell-mediated immunity', below).

Phagocytic cells and their killing mechanisms

Phagocytosis represents the oldest defence mechanism, traceable back to the first cellular organisms (Weir *et al.* 1981), and much of the power of complement and antibody lies in their ability to enhance it, which is why deficiencies of neutrophils, of C3 and of antibody produce somewhat similar clinical effects (see Chapters 66–68). Ironically, the ways in which phagocytic cells recognize micro-organisms in the absence of complement or antibody are still far from clear, though a role for sugar–lectin interactions is emerging as an important general mechanism: the lectin may be on the microbe (e.g. bacterial pili and fimbriae) or on the phagocytic cell (e.g. the mannose, galactose and fucose 'receptors' on macrophages) (Ofek and Sharon 1988). The encounter between bacteria and phagocytes perfectly illustrates the delicate balance of forces at play in any established host–parasite system. Thus the bacterial capsule inhibits direct attachment to phagocytes, but antibody to the (usually polysaccharide) capsule allows attachment via Fc receptors. In turn bacteria can produce molecules that immobilize antibody (e.g. staphylococcal protein A) or cleave it (e.g. gonococcal proteases). Again phagocytes are attracted by bacterial products (e.g. *N*-formyl-L-methionyl-L-leucyl-phenylalanine (FMLP), but bacterial coagulase hinders their progress while other enzymes kill the phagocyte. If phagocytosis is nevertheless successful, most bacteria will be killed and digested (see below), but some can avoid killing (e.g. mycobacteria) and others, though killed, cannot be fully digested (e.g. peptidoglycan of streptococcal cell walls).

Intracellular killing mechanisms have been particularly well studied for staphylococci and some fungi in neutrophils, and are conventionally classified as oxidative and non-oxidative. Oxidative killing requires a supply of oxygen and an intact membrane nicotinamide adenine dinucleotide phosphate (NADPH) oxidase (absent in chronic granulomatous disease): there is considerable controversy over the precise role of the various reactive oxygen intermediates (ROI) such as superoxide (O_2), hydrogen peroxide (H_2O_2), hydroxyl radical (OH) and singlet oxygen (O) (see Chapter 20), and it is probable that different micro-organisms are susceptible to different intermediates, and others to the acidification of pH that accompanies the oxygen burst. It has recently become clear that ROI can also be active in extracellular killing, although very high local concentrations are required in order to overcome the inhibitory effects of antioxidants such as catalase. This can be achieved by the formation of a contact zone between the secretory cell and its target (Seim and Espevik 1983). Macrophages appear to produce ROI in the same way as neutrophils (Nathan 1983), but they usually lack the myeloperoxidase which catalyses the toxic reaction between H_2O_2 and halides. Production of ROI by both types of cell can be enhanced by cytokines — particularly TNF in the case of neutrophils and IFN-γ for macrophages (Nathan 1987). It is still not clear whether killing of antibody-coated target cells (antibody-dependent cell-mediated cytotoxicity (ADCC)) operates via the oxidative pathway, but some stimuli, e.g. immune complexes, appear to be able to inhibit ADCC by monocytes while enhancing the non-specific lysis of non-antibody-coated target cells, which is predominantly oxidative (Geffner *et al.* 1987). The effectiveness of oxidative killing depends on whether the parasite in question can defend itself, as many bacteria, protozoa and worms can by catalase and other antioxidants (Babior 1978; Callahan *et al.* 1988). There is also evidence that some antiparasitic drugs owe their action partly to synergy with oxidative processes (Krungkrai and Yuthavong 1987). It has recently become clear that reactive nitrogen intermediates,

Table 73.2. Some non-oxidative killing mechanisms. Reviews in Nathan (1983), Gabay (1988) and Lachmann (1987).

Host component	Effective against
Complement	Bacteria (Gram-negative) Trypanosomes, *Leishmania* *Entamoeba*
Lysozyme	Bacteria (Gram-positive)
Interferon	Viruses, ?malaria
Tumour necrosis factor	Viruses, bacteria, malaria
C-reactive protein	Bacteria
Cationic proteins	
Neutrophil: defensins	Bacteria, fungi
cathepsin G	Bacteria, fungi
BPI	Bacteria, (Gram-negative)
Eosinophil: ECP	Worms, malaria
Lactoferrin	Bacteria, yeasts
Polyamines, heparin	Malaria
Arginase	Schistosomes
Lipids: HDL	Trypanosomes
oxidized LDL	Malaria

BPI = bactericidal/permeability binding protein; HDL = high-density lipoprotein; LDL = low-density lipoprotein.

particularly nitric oxide (NO) are powerfully toxic to intracellular parasites such as Toxoplasma and Leishmania. Nitric oxide is characteristically produced by macrophages stimulated by IFN-γ or TNF (Liew and Cox 1991).

Non-oxidative killing is less well understood, though a number of highly toxic proteins have been isolated from eosinophils, neutrophils and macrophages (see Table 73.2). The danger inherent in the secretion of such toxic molecules is well illustrated by the myocarditis of the hyper-eosinophilic syndrome, in which blood levels of eosinophil cationic protein (ECP) can reach up to 30 times the normal level (Wassom *et al.* 1981). Nevertheless, ECP is also highly toxic to helminths (Spry 1985) and blood-stage malaria parasites (Waters *et al.* 1987), and may play a valuable role when focused on the right target.

Natural and other killer cells

A variety of other cells have been shown to kill micro-organisms *in vitro*, though the proof that such killing occurs *in vivo* is usually lacking. These include natural killer (NK) cells, basophils and platelets. Natural killer cells have been shown, by depletion experiments, to control hepatitis, vaccinia and cytomegalovirus levels in mice, but appeared not to affect lymphocytic choriomeningitis virus (Bukowski *et al.* 1983). Some of the antiviral effects of IFN-γ could therefore be secondary to its effect on NK cells. In addition, there is evidence that NK cells themselves can produce IFN-γ, representing a more rapid but less specific response than that provided by T cells (Bancroft *et al.* 1987). The role of basophils (Wakelin 1978) and platelets (Damonneville *et al.* 1988) appears to be mainly confined to helminth infections.

The parasite, 2: direct tissue damage

The concept of disease implies some element of tissue damage or functional impairment, and is by no means synonymous with parasitization. Indeed, tissue damage is frequently the consequence of over-enthusiastic immune reactions (see 'Immunopathology', below). Nevertheless, some tissue damage is the direct result of infection, the two major causes being intracellular organisms, especially viruses, that destroy their host cell and extracellular organisms, predominantly bacteria, that secrete toxins. In the latter case it is important to distinguish between toxins that directly attack cells, such as the exotoxins of staphylococci, tetanus, cholera, etc., and the endotoxins which trigger cells to release normal products but in excessive amount, as lipopolysaccharide (LPS) does in causing macrophages to release IL-1 and TNF. The latter will be considered below (see 'Immunopathology').

The host, 2: adaptive immunity

There is considerable evidence that adaptive (that is, lymphocyte-based) immunity developed in response to the threat from parasitic organisms. The immunoglobulin germline gene repertoire appears to be biased towards specificities corresponding to common bacterial antigens (Perlmutter *et al.* 1985), while the T cell receptor system favours the recognition of small foreign peptides of intracellular origin (Townsend 1987). Correspondingly, deficiencies affecting B cells show up predominantly with extracellular bacterial and fungal infections, and those affecting T cells with viral and intracellular bacterial, fungal or protozoal infections (see Chapter 66). We must conclude that whatever their advantage to the parasite and notwithstanding the very real dangers of immunopathology, adaptive immune mechanisms are of overall benefit to the host too.

Antibody

Germ-free animals are essentially agammaglobulinaemic, but 2–3 weeks' healthy sojourn in the average animal house are sufficient to raise serum immunoglobulin (Ig) to normal levels. Much of this is presumably against normal commensal organisms and underlines the point that lymphocyte receptors recognize shape and not virulence, which is a problem in terms of avoiding self-reactivity but an inestimable boon when it comes to anticipating novel microbial antigens — an ever-present need, as will be seen (see 'Antigenic variation', below).

The effectiveness of an antibody response, given a susceptible infection, depends on three principal features: (i) how much is made and how fast; (ii) its specificity, which for a given antigen is closely related to affinity; and (iii) isotype and the ability to switch. These are worth considering separately, but it will be seen that they share a common feature, namely a central role for T cells.

AMOUNT OF ANTIBODY

The example of lobar pneumonia already quoted emphasizes the importance of a speedy antibody response. Genetic factors probably come to bear here, because in mice it has been possible to select for large or small primary antibody responses irrespective of specificity (Biozzi *et al*. 1979). At least 10 genes were found to be involved and major histocompatibility complex (MHC) type played only a minor role. The 'high antibody' line of mice were more resistant than the 'low' line to *Trypanosoma cruzi*, and responded better to vaccines against a murine malaria and against rabies. On the other hand the 'low' line, in which some macrophage functions are enhanced, showed greater resistance to *Salmonella*, *Brucella*, *Yersinia*, mycobacteria and *Schistosoma mansoni*. It is important to stress that this quantitative antigen-independent difference in antibody responsiveness is quite distinct from the all-or-nothing MHC-related 'Ir gene' phenomenon, which is restricted to small peptides and has become a major concern in the design of peptide vaccines (Zanetti *et al*. 1987). A third level of genetic differences, the immunoglobulin V gene repertoire itself, probably contributes relatively little during normal responses (but see below).

SPECIFICITY AND AFFINITY

In general, high-affinity antibody is more biologically effective than low (Alhstedt *et al*. 1974), and there is evidence, again from mouse experiments, that affinity and its maturation is genetically controlled in a manner unrelated to the overall amount made (Steward *et al*. 1986). One striking correlation is between low affinity and the incidence of chronic immune complex disease (Devey *et al*. 1984). In a study of antibody responses to tetanus toxoid in humans, considerable differences between individuals were found; unexpectedly, low affinity correlated with high levels of the IgG-4 subclass (Devey *et al*. 1985). The role of T cells in both affinity maturation and isotype switching may provide the link (Mayer *et al*. 1985), and the two abnormalities are found together in certain diseases such as rheumatoid arthritis (Devey *et al*. 1987).

ISOTYPES AND SWITCHING

The existence of different heavy-chain constant-region genes in tandem on the same chromosome is a wonderfully elegant way of allowing successive Ig isotypes, with different biological activities but with the same antigen specificity, to be brought to bear on an infectious organism. With the exception of some T cell-independent antigens which induce only IgM, responses restricted to a single isotype are rare, but the proportions of the various isotypes are very different with different types of antigen. Several mechanisms contribute to this. For example the tendency for antigens given orally to induce IgA may be due to the fact that gut-associated T helper cells selectively stimulate IgA-bearing B cells (Teale and Abraham 1987). In mice there is growing evidence for at least two subpopulations of CD4 +ve helper cells, each with a tendency to secrete different cytokines; thus the Th2 population, which secretes IL-4 and IL-5, seems to particularly help IgE antibody and, interestingly, eosinophil production and differentiation as well (Bottomly 1988). It is tempting to speculate that helminth antigens would favour the stimulation of this type of T cell. However, it must be added that the evidence for these CD4 +ve T cell subsets in man is still controversial (Paliard *et al.* 1988).

In most cases, however, the reason for isotype preferences is unknown, though they are very striking, particularly among the subclasses of IgG. In bacterial infection, antibodies to protein antigens tend to be predominantly IgG-1 and to polysaccharide antigens IgG-2; the generally poor responses of children to organisms with polysaccharide capsules are associated with the late development of IgG-2 (and IgG-4) responses (Hammarstrom and Edvard Smith 1986a). Viral infections, on the other hand, induce preferentially IgG-1 and IgG-3, and seldom IgG-2 (Skvaril 1986), while in helminth infections IgG-4 and IgG-3 are strikingly prominent, as is Ig-E (Catty *et al.* 1986). There is evidence that IgG-4 production requires an intact classical complement pathway (Bird and Lachmann 1988). As a general rule the responses to vaccination reflect the same subclass preferences as mentioned above for infection (Hammarstrom and Edvard Smith 1986b).

Surprisingly, allotypic variants in the IgG heavy chain and kappa light chain also have an effect on response and/or susceptibility to certain infections; this has been shown for tetanus toxoid, bacterial polysaccharides and *Salmonella*. It is not known whether this reflects biologically significant differences in the constant regions or a linkage with particular variable genes (Whittingham and Propert 1986).

ANTIBODY-DEPENDENT EFFECTOR MECHANISMS

The effectiveness of antibody also depends, of course, on the parasite concerned and its susceptibility to the available effector mechanisms. Most vulnerable of all are those organisms that need to attach to a specific receptor in order to enter their target cell, since in most cases antibody binding to the corresponding parasite antigen will block entry; this is the basis of many attempts to identify antigens as vaccine candidates. However, the opposite can also occur as in the case of dengue and some other viruses infecting macrophages, which they enter more readily in the presence of low levels of antibody, thanks to macrophage Fc receptors (Halstead 1979). A similar paradox has been encountered with certain malarial anti-gamete antibodies which enhance transmission, presumably by facilitating some stage of sexual development in the mosquito.

Antibodies against toxins represent another comparatively straightforward protective mechanism whose effectiveness, being based on the physical presence of the immunoglobulin molecule, is not isotype-dependent. Other direct actions of antibody include the immobilization of motile organisms; in the case of bacterial flagella, the larger IgM molecule is the most effective, which is in keeping with the fact that the major flagellar protein is a T-independent antigen. But for the majority of its useful effects antibody relies on complement or phagocytic cells, or both, to finish off the parasite. These are powerful systems when activated, with considerable potential for damaging host tissue (see 'Immunopathology', below) and it is interesting that the genes for the IgG subclasses with the least complement-activating and opsonizing activity (G-2 and G-4) lie 3′ to G-1 and G-3 so that isotype switching tends to occur away from the potentially immunopathological subclasses. In the same way, the association of high levels of specific IgG-4 antibodies with prolonged exposure to antigen, as is seen in chronic helminth infections, may be an attempt to block IgE-mediated hypersensitivity reactions (Ottesen *et al.* 1985). Modulation of the immune response in this way takes us into the realm of immunosuppression, which will be discussed later (see below).

Phagocytic cells exhibit important differences in their activity against antibody-coated parasites. Thus, neutrophils are highly effective against the general run of bacteria and fungi, while the resident macrophages of the liver, the Kupffer cells, appear to lack oxygen-dependent antimicrobial activity, e.g. against *Listeria* infection, for which recruitment of a new population of blood monocytes is needed. It has been suggested that Kupffer cells have matured beyond the microbicidal state — perhaps, again, to diminish the danger of pathological host damage (Ding and Nathan 1988).

The role of eosinophils in infectious disease has undergone some revision in recent years: rather than being predominantly 'anti-inflammatory' cells as was thought, it appears that their major useful purpose may be to destroy parasites (and perhaps tumours), though this carries with it the usual danger of host tissue damage (Spry 1985).

Cell-mediated immunity

Implicit in the concept of cell-mediated immunity (CMI) is the idea that T cell functions evolved in response to intracellular parasites, which are generally speaking inaccessible to antibody. The two principal types of CMI are further specialized to deal with (i) organisms residing in cells such as macrophages that could, if sufficiently activated, kill them and (ii) organisms residing in cells with no antimicrobial capacity. The latter, for the most part viruses, require cytotoxicity to be applied from outside, plus a receptor system that can detect any infected cell: the CD8 +ve cytotoxic T cell with its recognition of small foreign peptides attached to Class I MHC molecules fulfils this requirement. In the case of intrinsically cytotoxic host cells a more restricted recognition is needed, coupled to the ability to secrete cytokines appropriate to the function to be activated, and this is provided by the CD4 +ve T cell—Class II MHC system, which operates against bacterial, fungal and protozoal infections of the macrophage.

There are, however, some exceptions to this tidy scheme, principally involving non-viral infections of cells other than macrophages. Examples are the killing of Schwann cells infected with *Mycobacterium leprae* (Chiplunkar *et al.* 1986), of lymphocytes containing the protozoon *Theileria parva* (Morrison *et al.* 1986), and of liver cells containing malaria schizonts (Schofield *et al.* 1987); in all these cases CD8 +ve T cells are the normal effectors, though cytotoxicity by CD4 +ve T cells can sometimes be demonstrated too, as it can for some viruses (Braakman *et al.* 1987). The possibility that lysed macrophages might release and disseminate viable parasites will be considered along with the other pathological complications of CMI (see below).

The final effector mechanisms of CMI are largely unknown. Recent evidence that CD8 +ve T cells kill their target by the insertion of perforins (Young and Cohn 1986) has been challenged as a generalization (Clark 1988), while the study of macrophage activation by T cells is currently aimed principally at cataloguing the effects of cytokines, alone and in combination — a very necessary process which has revealed many unexpected activities but does not lead directly to an understanding of the antimicrobial mechanisms. With he exception of an inhibitory effect of TNF on mouse trypanosomes *in vitro* (Kongshavn and Ghadirian 1988), no case has emerged of direct microbial killing by recognized cytokines. Rather, their effects are secondary to the switching on of latent intracellular mechanisms such as antiviral 2′-5′-A synthetase (IFNs, TNF) or the oxygen or nitrogen burst (IFNs, TNF, colony-stimulating factors (CSFs)).

The parasite, 3: survival strategies

Any parasite confronted by the battery of natural and adaptive defences discussed above would soon come to grief if it did not have counter-defences of its own. It follows that parasitic organisms of medical importance must have evolved strategies for survival at least long enough to permit spread to another host, and indeed in most cases they are sufficient to prevent elimination altogether. It could also be safely predicted that the survival strategy of an individual species of parasite will be tailored to the host immune component from which it is most in danger, and that there must be at least as many survival strategies as there are defence mechanisms. However, they can conveniently be considered in three categories: (i) attempts to conceal the presence of the parasite; (ii) attempts to confuse the immune system by antigenic variation; and (iii) attempts to suppress immunity.

Concealment

The ultimate parasite survival strategy would be residence in a cell without microbial properties, insensitive to cytokine activation and with no surface MHC antigens, and some parasites do achieve this, or very nearly — notably the slow viruses in brain cells. In cases where the host cell normally does express MHC antigens, a parasite may attempt to down-regulate these, as happens with *Leishmania* (Reiner *et al.* 1987). When the host cell is a macrophage, the best strategy appears to be to resist the killing mechanisms, either by escaping from phagosome to cytoplasm (e.g. *Leishmania*), preventing lysosomes fusing with the phagosome (e.g. *Toxoplasma*) or evolving an indestructible cell wall (e.g. mycobacteria).

Extracellular parasites must of course adopt a different approach. The bacterial capsule may be regarded as a form of concealment of bacterial surface molecules from receptors on phagocytes, though this advantage is lost once anticapsular antibody is made. Antigenic mimicry (Table 73.3) represents another theoretically ideal strategy, but the chances of the parasite surface exclusively imitating host-like molecules must be remote in the extreme, and it is hard to be convinced that well-known examples such as streptococci (cardiac muscle), *Yersinia* (human leucocyte antigen (HLA-B27) and the spirochaete serve very much purpose in prolonging parasite survival, though they are sometimes very potent in inducing autoimmunity (see below). More recently, however, Damian, a strong early proponent of molecular mimicry as a genuine parasite survival mechanism, has suggested that carbohydrate rather than protein epitopes are likely to be the easiest to mimic, since only a few glycosyl transferases need to be held in common by parasite and host (Damian 1987). Curiously, it has also emerged that proteins with a high degree of cross-reactivity between species, such as the heat-shock (or 'stress') proteins of bacteria, are nevertheless strong immunogens (Young *et al.* 1987), suggesting that 'near-mimicry' is not a particularly good way to avoid immunity.

An alternative solution to the same problem is camouflage by the uptake of host molecules, and here the worms, with their relatively slow surface turnover, have achieved some notable successes — the classic example being the schistosome which less than a week after invasion is virtually covered with host-derived glycolipids, MHC molecules, non-specific Ig, etc., and no longer reacts with antiparasitic antibody (Smithers and Doenhoff 1982). Another helminth, *Echinococcus*, goes even further in this direction and makes for itself a (hydatid) cyst of host material, inside which a large colony of worms can survive even though the host circulation contains highly potent antibodies (Williams 1982). Only the surgeon's knife can interrupt this near-perfect state of parasitism.

Table 73.3. Some examples of parasite–host mimicry

Parasite	Host molecule
Bacteria	
Streptococcus	Heart
Klebsiella	HLA-B27
Mycobacterium tuberculosis	65 kD heat-shock protein
Neisseria meningitidis B capsule	Embryonic brain
Protozoa	
Malaria	Thymosin α-1
Trypanosoma cruzi	Heart, nerve
Helminths	
Schistosoma	Glutathione transferase

Antigenic variation

Organisms with an extracellular phase are normally susceptible to antibody-mediated attack by complement, phagocytic cells, etc., and if they are rapidly dividing, like most viruses and bacteria, continuous camouflage by host material would be extremely difficult to achieve. An alternative is to vary the antigens recognized by antibody, so that no population of antibodies remains effective for very long. This requires either devoting a considerable amount of the genome to genes for different surface antigens, as the African trypanosome does, or encouraging mutation of immunodominant antigens or recombination between similar parasites: the influenza virus uses both the latter devices. The speed with which antigenic variation occurs will considerably influence the outcome. With the trypanosomes, variant follows variant at a few days' interval and, since there are at least 1000 variants available, the antibody response eventually cannot keep pace (Vickerman and Barry 1982). With influenza it is rather a question of year-to-year variation, so that immunity built up against one epidemic is useless against the next, at least as regards the antibody response, though the cytotoxic T cells appear to be much less affected. With bacteria such as salmonellae and streptococci and viruses such as the adenoviruses, antigenic variation over long time spans has led to the coexistence of multiple stable variants (or 'serotypes'), to each of which a host must become immune; a similar diversity is thought to explain the slow development of effective immunity against malaria (Anders 1986).

Antigenic variation clearly poses great problems for the host, but it is not always an ideal solution for the parasite, which runs the risk of overwhelming the host — as happens in trypanosomiasis (sleeping sickness) and occasionally on a pandemic scale with influenza. Such parasites cannot be regarded as well adapted to man and are presumably still in a process of evolution.

Immunosuppression

This is one of the most enigmatic and most debated aspects of infectious disease. Some of the strategies employed by bacteria against antibody molecules, complement and phagocytic cells have already been mentioned, and the list could be lengthened to include virtually all parasites. In this section attention will be focused on the somewhat more subtle ways in which parasites can sabotage adaptive immune responses. Few of these are fully understood, but it is possible to distinguish various levels at which they may operate, namely antigen presentation, cytokines and lymphocytes themselves. The extent to which these are interlinked can be best appreciated by a consideration of the suppressor T cell.

THE SUPPRESSOR T CELL

No entity in modern immunology arouses such passions as the innocent-sounding suppressor T cell. Originally postulated to explain high-dose tolerance (Gershon and Kondo 1970), it was soon adopted by students of allergy (Ishizaka 1984) and autoimmunity (Cooke and Lydyard 1981) to provide a framework for understanding — or at least discussing — self-tolerance, autoimmune disease and hypersensitivity. As the correlation grew between suppressive effects, I-J antigens and the CD8 +ve T cell subset, numerous models of infectious disease were naturally scrutinized for evidence that T cells of this type were responsible for failure to eliminate parasites or to prevent immunopathology, in many cases with positive results, as will be seen. But, at the same time, the breakthrough in cloning T cells and their receptors, coupled with the failure to find I-J genes in the MHC, brought with them a scepticism as to whether suppressor T cells, as a discrete lineage, existed at all, since with one possible exception (Modlin *et al.* 1987) T clones have turned out to be of helper or cytotoxic type.

Some of this scepticism may be exaggerated. For example, while CD4 +ve and CD8 +ve cells certainly have very different overall effects in their classical roles as 'helper' and 'cytotoxic' cells, at the level of cytokine production there is considerable overlap. Both types of T cell can secrete IFN-γ, which has suppressive effects in many situations, particularly against antibody production, and also transforming growth factor β (TGF-β) one of the most suppressive cytokines yet discovered (Kehrl *et al.* 1986). In any case, most cytokines can be stimulatory or inhibitory depending on circumstances, so the concept of a helper and/or suppressor cell is not so unthinkable as it once was. It has also been pointed out that a 'classical' cytotoxic cell could act as a suppressor, for instance by killing antigen-presenting cells (Braakman *et al.* 1987).

The link with the MHC is also more complex than at first appeared. I-J is now thought of as related to anti-self T cell receptors rather than the MHC itself (Murphy 1987) but an interesting association has been noted between T cell functions and the I region genes in the mouse: I-A and I-E. Mice which lack the ability to express I-E tend to be resistant to certain parasites, notably nematode worms (Wassom *et al.* 1987). Such mice apparently lack the ability to generate suppressor T cells in certain systems. Furthermore treatment with monoclonal anti-I-E antibodies enhanced the resistance of mice to *Leishmania donovani*, while anti-I-A reduced it, which is the result that would be expected if T helper cells responded to I-A and T suppressor cells to I-E (Blackwell and Roberts 1987). Experiments of this kind support the concept that suppressor cells are a separate entity, responsible for the disease progression in some cases. The differential involvement of I-A and I-E might also favour the idea that different parasite antigens or epitopes induce help and suppression, for which the experimental justification comes mostly from the study of the lysozyme molecule (Benjamin *et al.* 1984). If this idea is right, it is tremendously important because it offers perhaps the only real promise of vaccines that improve on nature, for example by exclusively inducing help in situations requiring large amounts of antibody, or suppression in diseases where immunopathology is the dominant problem. It is of course also possible that the selection of I-A or I-E is not a function of the antigen but of the presenting cell, in which case the technique of vaccination becomes all-important. A case in point may be the effect of IFN-γ (Knop *et al.* 1984) and IL-2 (Malkovsky *et al.* 1985) in inhibiting the induction of suppressor T cells; both of these molecules have been shown to have powerful adjuvant activity in experimental vaccination models (Playfair and De Souza 1987; Weinberg and Merigan 1988).

Even without adding further examples, I think the point has been made that suppressor T cells could account for a great many of the phenomena encountered by parasite immunologists. However, the most satisfying of models may survive only until a better hypothesis turns up, and it remains perfectly possible that all the T suppressor cell effects ever reported will eventually be explained in some other way. Allusion has already been made to the idea that switching of antihelminth antibody from the IgE to the IgG4 isotype may be useful in diminishing hypersensitivity; a T cell that induced this switch in an experimental model where hypersensitivity was the read-out might well be classified as a suppressor cell. A particularly thought-provoking example is the association between disease progression in murine leishmaniasis and excessive IL-3 production by T cells (Lelchuk *et al.* 1988), which could be interpreted in 'suppressor' language but can also be explained (more convincingly in my view) as an expansionary effect on the host cell in which the parasite grows best, in this case a newly recruited macrophage with limited cytotoxic capacity. If this is the true mechanism, are the IL-3 producing T cells suppressors? And, if so, what are they suppressing, apart from recovery? It might in the long run be more useful to speak of 'T health' and 'T disease' cells, whose phenotype may be different in different conditions.

OTHER SUPPRESSIVE MECHANISMS

T cells are by no means the only potentially suppressive elements in the immune system. Frequently immunosuppression is secondary to macrophage activation and mainly due to prostaglandin secretion. Indeed it seems to be a general rule that over-activity of the natural immune system is accompanied by some degree of adaptive immune suppression: the Biozzi mice already referred to are an example where this tendency is genetically in-built, but many normal animals subjected to prolonged macrophage activation, as for example during blood-stage malaria (Weidanz 1982), develop quite severe immunosuppression, affecting both antibody and cell-mediated responses. Suppression of this kind is, of course, non-antigen-specific, and can be of clinical significance, as in the case of patients with mild malaria whose response to bacterial polysaccharide vaccines is impaired as long as they are parasitaemic (Williamson and Greenwood 1978). Interference with the cytokine network can also lead to severe unresponsiveness, and here IL-2 seems to be particularly susceptible: an IL-2 inhibitor has been found in murine malaria (Lelchuk and Playfair 1985), and a reduction of IL-2 receptors in patients infected with *Trypanosoma cruzi* (Beltz *et al.* 1988). It is likely that many more such examples will come to light.

We cannot leave this topic without a mention of the viruses that infect lymphocytes and/or macrophages themselves and thus erode the very heart of the immune system. These are numerous and of varying significance (Table 73.4), and, while measles and cytomegalovirus (CMV), for instance, can cause quite prolonged non-specific immunosuppression, they have been put in the shade by human immunodeficiency virus (HIV), whose combination of receptor system (CD4) and antigenic variation makes it, of all parasites, the one against which the immune system is most utterly impotent. It is indeed fortunate for the human race that its method of spread is (as yet) relatively inefficient.

Table 73.4. Persistence of micro-organisms within cells of the immune system

Cells	Examples
Lymphocytes	
T	HIV (CD4 +ve only)
	Measles
	Adenovirus
	Mumps
	Varicella–zoster
	Rubella
B	Epstein–Barr virus
	Theileria parva
Macrophages	HIV, CMV
	Rubella
	Dengue
	Tuberculosis, leprosy
	Salmonella typhi, Brucella
	Leishmania
	Toxoplasma
	Trypanosoma cruzi
	Histoplasma
	Rickettsia

Finally it is worth asking the question: is immunosuppression really useful to the parasite? There are plenty of instances where immunosuppression by one parasite favours the growth of others, as HIV does for pneumocystis, etc., and malaria may for Epstein–Barr virus (EBV) (Facer and Playfair 1989). But, since the parasites that thrive best in immunosuppressed hosts (the opportunists, see below) are often unable to control their growth in the absence of immunity, leading to a mutually unsatisfactory lethal outcome, generalized immunosuppression would not seem particularly beneficial for the parasite that initiated it, and can probably best be regarded as an evolutionary accident.

The host, 3: immunopathology

It has been known for nearly 100 years that immune responses to infectious organisms could cause the symptoms of disease; indeed delayed hypersensitivity was originally known as 'bacterial allergy' to distinguish it from anaphylactic reactions to simple proteins. Thanks to the vision of Gell and Coombs (Coombs and Gell 1975), we subsequently acquired a classification of immunopathological responses into four types, each of which includes examples due to infectious agents (Table 73.5). On the whole this classification has stood the test of time remarkably well, but when considering infectious disease two additional aspects are worth bearing in mind: the pathological role of the cytokine network and the special problems of autoimmunity.

Cytokines

Endotoxin (or 'Gram-negative') shock is perhaps the best-known example of a severe body-wide pathological process initiated by a parasite product. It is generally attributed to activation of complement, mainly by the alternative pathway, leading to a neutrophil-mediated attack on vascular endothelium in the lungs and elsewhere (Hammerschmidt 1987). What was somewhat unexpected was the demonstration that all, or most, of the symptoms could be prevented by antibodies against a single cytokine — TNF (Tracey *et al.*

Table 73.5. Hypersensitivity reactions in infectious disease

		Example
Type 1	IgE +ve mast cells	*Ascaris* (lung) Hydatid cyst
Type 2	Autoantibodies	*Mycoplasma* Streptococcal myocarditis *Trypanosoma cruzi*
Type 3	1 Immune complexes, polymorphonuclear leucocytes, complement	*Streptococcus* Erythema nodosum Glomerulonephritis Meningococcus Hepatitis B Quartan malaria Fungal allergic alveolitis
	2 DIC	Septicaemia
Type 4	T cells and macrophages	Tuberculosis granuloma Tuberculoid leprosy Schistosome egg granuloma *T. cruzi*?
Cytokine over-production	(TNF, IL-1)	Gram-negative bacteria (LPS) Staphylococci (TSSTI) Mycobacteria (leucocyte adhesion molecule) Yeast Malaria (exoantigens)

1987). This observation serves as a model for the study of other shock-inducing molecules, e.g. from staphylococci (Jupin *et al.* 1988), malaria parasites (Bate *et al.* 1988), etc., and also of the involvement of other cytokines such as IL-1 and IFN-γ (Billiau 1988). At the very least, it seems likely that monoclonal antibodies to these and other cytokines will be tried in a variety of life-threatening complications of infection. Time will tell which combinations of disease and antibody go best together.

Autoimmunity

While the tissue-damaging mechanisms of autoimmune disease are in general no different from those responsible for destroying infectious organisms, the loss of self-tolerance itself during some infections but not others deserves separate consideration. Polyclonal activation (Dziarski 1988), antigenic mimicry (Ebringer 1983), aberrrant MHC expression (Botazzo *et al.* 1986) and the idiotype network (Cooke *et al.* 1983) have all been invoked, but there does not seem to be, and probably never will be, a single all-embracing explanation (Roitt 1984).

A particular category of autoantibodies — those which stimulate or block hormone receptors — have been admitted into the Gell and Coombs classification as type 5.

Hypersensitivity

The examples in Table 73.5 for the most part speak for themselves but, as always, it is interesting to speculate whether host or parasite benefits most from these reactions. In the case of type 1 responses to worms, one can imagine that local inflammation is one of the only ways to dislodge an intestinal worm, but an *Ascaris*-induced asthmatic attack does not seem to benefit either partner. Type 4 hypersensitivities often reflect an especially difficult dilemma: whether to mount a tissue-destructive cell-mediated response in order to eliminate intracellular organisms, or to damp it down and let them survive. The two ends of the leprosy 'spectrum' — tuberculoid and lepromatous — represent two approaches by the immune system, neither of them particularly satisfactory. A beautiful illustration of the problem is the granulomatous response to the eggs of *Schistosoma mansoni* in the liver: normal mice (and people) die of portal hypertension from the cirrhosis; T-deprived mice die of liver failure from necrosis by the egg enzymes (Lucas *et al.* 1980). The only way for the host to avoid this impasse is to deal with the infection at an earlier stage.

Host–parasite balance

Returning to our opening theme, we can say that no successful parasite will allow itself to be too rapidly eliminated, or to destroy its host. Having reviewed some of the strategies available to both partners, we are in a better position to understand the variations in what might be termed the 'parasite–host contract'. It is hard to speak of a 'standard' relationship here, but perhaps we are accustomed to thinking of the common childhood viruses as coming closest: high transmission enables the virus to spread within the community despite a rapid and complete elimination in the individual host. Only a vigorous vaccination campaign can upset this stable relationship. Such an arrangement would clearly not suit the malaria parasite, where transmission depends on a mosquito vector whose movements are not totally predictable, and this presumably explains why in this disease almost everyone is a carrier: if they were not, the disease would die out. Hepatitis B would come somewhere between the two, a few carriers being enough to maintain the level in the community.

Like other contracts, the host–parasite balance comes to prominence when one side departs from the rules. A host that becomes immunodeficient, for whatever reason, will fail to control the growth of parasites, including some that normally cause no trouble at all; these are the opportunists, most of which have been all too little studied hitherto, since they were not thought of as serious pathogens. In the same way, a parasite of one host species may occasionally visit another species with which it has not continuously co-evolved; the resulting zoonotic infection is likely to be unusually severe since the host's immune system, for all its repertoires, receptors and networks, is taken by surprise.

References

Alhstedt S., Holmgren, J. and Hanson, L.A. (1974). Protective capacity of antibodies against *E. coli* O antigen with special reference to the avidity. *Int. Arch. Allergy* **46**, 470.

Anders, R.F. (1986). Multiple cross-reactivities amongst antigens of *Plasmodium falciparum* impair the development of protective immunity against malaria. *Parasite Immunol.* **8**, 529–39.

Babior, B.M. (1978). Oxygen-dependent microbial killing by phagocytes. *N. Engl. J. Med.* **298**, 659–725.

Bancroft, G.J., Schreiber, R.D., Bosma, G.C. Bosma, M.J. and Unanue, E.R. (1987). A T cell independent mechanism of macrophage activation by interferon-γ *J. Immunol.* **139**, 1104–7.

Bate, C.A.W., Taverne, J. and Playfair, J.H.L. (1988). Malarial parasites induce tumour necrosis factor production by macrophages. *Immunology* **64**, 227–31.

Beltz, L.A., Sztein, M.B. and Kierszenbaum, F. (1988). Novel mechanism for *Trypanosoma cruzi*-induced suppression of human lymphocytes: inhibition of IL-2 receptor expression. *J. Immunol.* **141**, 289–94.

Benjamin, D.C., Berzofsky, J.A., East, I.J. *et al.* (1984). The antigenic structure of proteins: a reappraisal. *Ann. Rev. Immunol.* **2**, 67–101.

Billiau, A. (1988). Gamma-interferon: the match that lights the fire? *Immunol. Today* **9**, 37–40.

Biozzi, G., Mouton, D., Santanna, O.A. *et al.* (1979). Genetics of immunoresponsiveness to natural antigens in the mouse. *Cur. Topics Microbiol. Immunol.* **85**, 31–98.

Bird, P. and Lachmann, P.J. (1988). The regulation of IgG subclass production in man: low serum IgG4 in inherited deficiencies of the classical pathway of C3 activation. *Eur. J. Immunol.* **18**, 1217–22.

Blackwell, J.M. and Roberts, M.B. (1987). Immunomodulation of murine visceral leishmaniasis by administration of monoclonal anti-Ia antibodies: differential effects of anti-I-A vs. anti-I-E antibodies. *Eur. J. Immunol.* **17**, 1669–72.

Bottazzo, G.F., Todd, I., Mirakian, R., Belfiore, A. and Pujol-Borrell, R. (1986) Organ-specific autoimmunity: a 1986 overview. *Immunol. Rev.* **94**, 137–69.

Bottomly, K., (1988). A functional dichotomy in CD4+ T lymphocytes. *Immunol. Today* **9**, 268–74.

Braakman, E., Rotteveel, F.T.M., Van Bleek, G., Van Seventer, G.A. and Lucas, C.J. (1987). Are MHC Class II-restricted cytotoxic T lymphocytes important? *Immunol. Today* **8**, 265–7.

Bukowski, J.F., Woda, B.A., Habu, S., Okumura, K. and Welsh, R.M. (1983). Natural killer cell depletion enhances virus synthesis and virus-induced hepatitis *in vivo*. *J. Immunol.* **131**, 1531–8.

Callahan, H.L., Crouch, R.K. and James, E.R. (1988). Helminth anti-oxidant enzymes: a protective mechanism against host oxidants? *Parasitol. Today* **4**, 218–25.

Catty, D., Jassim, A., Hassan, K. and Raykundalia, C. (1986). IgG subclasses in parasitic infestations. *Monog. Allergy* **19**, 144–55.

Chiplunkar, S., De Libero, G. and Kaufmann, S.E. (1986). *Mycobacterium leprae*- specific Lyt-2+ T lymphocytes with cytolytic activıty. *Infect. Immunity* **54**, 793–7.

Clark, W.R. (1988). Perforin — a primary or auxiliary lytic mechanism? *Immunol. Today* **9**, 101–4.

Cohen, S. (1974). The immune response to parasites. In *Parasites in the Immunised Host: Mechanisms of Survival*, ed. R. Porter and J. Knight, CIBA Foundation Symposium 25, Elsevier/North-Holland, Amsterdam.

Cooke, A. and Lydyard, P.M. (1981). The role of T cells in autoimmune diseases. *Pathol. Res. Pract.* **171**, 173–96.

Cooke, A., Lydyard, P.M. and Roitt, I.M. (1983). Mechanisms of autoimmunity: a role for cross-reactive idiotypes. *Immunol. Today* **4**, 170–5.

Coombs, R.R.A. and Gell, P.G.H. (1975). Classification of allergic reactions responsible for clinical hypersensitivity and disease. In *Clinical Aspects of Immunology*, 3rd edn, eds P.G.H. Gell, R.R.A. Coombs and P.J. Lachmann, pp. 761–81. Blackwell Scientific Publications, Oxford.

Damian, R.T. (1987). Molecular mimicry revisited. *Parasitol. Today* **3**, 263–6.

Damonneville, M., Wietzerbin, J., Pancre, V. *et al.* (1988). Recombinant tumour necrosis factors mediate platelet cytotoxicity to *Schistosoma mansoni* larvae. *J. Immunol.* **140**, 3962–5.

Devey, M.E., Bleasdale, K.M., Stanley, C. and Steward, M.W. (1984). Failure of affinity maturation leads to increased susceptibility to immune complex glomerulonephritis. *Immunology* **52**, 377.

Devey, M.E., Bleasdale, K.M., French, M.A.H. and Harrison, G. (1985). The IgG4 subclass is associated with low affinity antibody response to tetanus toxoid in man. *Immunology* **55**, 565–7.

Devey, M.E., Bleasdale, K.M. and Isenberg, D.A. (1987). Antibody affinity and IgG subclass of responses to tetanus toxoid in patients with rheumatoid arthritis and systemic lupus erythematosus. *Clin. Exp. Immunol.* **68**, 562–9.

Ding, A. and Nathan, C. (1988). Analysis of the non-functional respiratory burst in murine Kupffer cells. *J. Exp. Med.* **167**, 1154–70.

Dziarski, R. (1988). Autoimmunity: polyclonal activation or antigen induction? *Immunol. Today* **9**, 340–2.

Ebringer, A. (1983). The cross-tolerance hypothesis, HLA-B27 and ankylosing spondylitis. *Br. J. Rheumatol.* **22** (suppl. 2), 53–66.

Facer, C.A. and Playfair, J.H.L. (1989). Malaria, Epstein–Barr virus, and the genesis of lymphomas. *Adv. Cancer Res.* **53**, 33–72.

Gabay, J.E. (1988). Microbicidal mechanisms of phagocytes. *Curr. Opinion Immunol.* **1**, 36–40.

Geffner, J.R., Giordano, M., Serebrinsky, G. and Isturiz, M. (1987). The role of reactive oxygen intermediates in non-specific monocyte cytotoxicity induced by immune complexes. *Clin. Exp. Immunol.* **67**, 646–54.

Gershon, R.K. and Kondo, K. (1970). Cell interactions in the induction of tolerance. *Immunology* **18**, 723–37.

Halstead, S.B. (1979). *In vivo* enhancement of dengue virus infection in rhesus monkeys by passively transferred antibody. *J. Infect. Dis.* **140**, 527–33.

Hammerschmidt, D.E. (1987). Activation of complement and granulocytes in shock. In *Complement in Health and Disease*, ed. K. Whaley, MTP Press, Lancaster.

Hammarstrom, L. and Edvard Smith, C.I., (1986a). IgG subclasses in bacterial infections *Monog. Allergy* **19**, 122–33.

Hammarstrom, L., and Edvard Smith, C.I. (1986b). IgG subclass changes in response to vaccination. *Monog. Allergy* **19**, 241–52.

Ishizaka, K. (1984). Regulation of IgE synthesis. *Ann. Rev. Immunol.* **2**, 159–82.

Jupin, C., Anderson, S., Damias, C., Alouf, J.E. and Parant, M.

(1988). Toxic shock syndrome toxin 1 as an inducer of human tumour necrosis factors and γ interferon. *J. Exp. Med.* **167**, 752–61.

Kehrl, J.H., Wakefield, L.M., Roberts, A.B. *et al.* (1986). Production of transforming growth factor β by human T lymphocytes and its potential in the regulation of T cell growth. *J. Exp. Med.* **163**, 1037–50.

Kierszenbaum, F., Ivanyi, J. and Budzko, D.B. (1976). Mechanisms of natural resistance to trypanosomal infection: role of complement in avian resistance to *Trypanosoma cruzi* infection. *Immunology* **30**, 1–6.

Knop, J., Stremmer, R., Taborski, V., Freitag, W., De Maeyer-Guignard, J., and Macher, E. (1984). Inhibition of the T suppressor circuit of DTH by IFN. *J. Immunol.* **133**, 2412–16.

Kongshavn, P.A.L. and Ghadirian, E. (1988). Enhancing and suppressive effects of tumour necrosis factor/cachectin on growth of *Trypanosoma musculi*. *Parasite Immunol.* **10**, 581–8.

Krungkrai, S.R. and Yuthavong, Y. (1987). The anti-malarial action on *Plasmodium falciparum* of qinghaosu and artestunate in combination with agents which modulate oxidant stress. *Trans. Roy. Soc. Trop. Med. Hyg.* **81**, 710–14.

Lachmann, P.J. (1987). Plugs, burns and poisons. *Bioassays* **7**, 223–9.

Lelchuk, R. and Playfair, J.H.L. (1985). Serum IL-2 inhibitor in mice. I. Increase during infection. *Immunology* **56**, 113–18.

Lelchuk, R., Graveley, R. and Liew, F.Y. (1988). Susceptibility to murine cutaneous leishmaniasis with the capacity to generate interleukin 3 in response to leishmania antigen *in vitro*. *Cell. Immunol.* **111**, 66–76.

Liew, F.Y. and Cox, F.E.G. (1991). Nonspecific defence mechanisms: the role of nitric oxide. *Parasitology Today* **7**, A17–A21.

Lucas, S., Musallam, R., Bain, J., Hassonah, O., Bickle, Q. and Doenhoff, M. (1980). The pathological effects of immunosuppression of *Schistosoma mansoni*-infected mice, with particular reference to survival and hepatotoxicity after thymectomy and treatment with antithymocyte serum, and treatment with hydrocortisone acetate. *Trans. Roy. Soc. Trop. Med. Hyg.* **74**, 633–43.

Malkovsky, M., Medawar, P.H., Thatcher, D.R. *et al.* (1985). Acquired immunological tolerance of foreign cells is impaired by recombinant interleukin 2 or vitamin A acetate. *Proc. Nat. Acad. Sci. (USA)* **82**, 536–8.

Mayer, L., Posnett, D.N. and Kunkel, H.G. (1985). Human malignant T cells capable of inducing an immunoglobulin class switch. *J. Exp. Med.* **161**, 134.

Modlin, R.L., Brenner, M.B., Krangel, M.S., Duby, A.D. and Bloom, B.R. (1987). T-cell receptors of human suppressor cells. *Nature* **329**, 541–5.

Morrison, W.I., Goddeeris, B.M., Teale, A.J., Baldwin, C.L., Bensaid, A. and Ellis, J. (1986). Cell-mediated immune responses of cattle to *Theileria parva*. *Immunol. Today* **7**, 211–13.

Murphy, D.B. (1987). The I-J puzzle. *Ann. Rev. Immunol.* **5**, 407–27.

Nathan, C.F. (1983). Mechanisms of macrophage anti-microbial activity. *Trans. Roy. Soc. Trop. Med. Hyg.* **77**, 620–30.

Nathan, C.F. (1987). Secretory products of macrophages. *J. Clin. Invest.* **79**, 319–26.

Ofek, I. and Sharon, N. (1988). Lectinophagocytosis: a molecular mechanism of recognition between cell surface sugars and lectins in the phagocytosis of bacteria. *Infect. Immunity* **56**, 539–47.

Ottesen, E.A., Skvaril, F., Tripathy, S.P., Poindexter, R.W. and Hussain, R. (1985). Prominence of IgG4 in the IgG antibody response to human filariasis. *J. Immunol.* **134**, 2707–12.

Paliard, X., Malefijt, R. de W., Yssel, H. *et al.* (1988). Simultaneous production of IL-2, IL-4 and IFNγ by activated human CD4+ and CD8+ T cell clones. *J. Immunol.* **141**, 849–55.

Perlmutter, R., Berson, B., Griffin, J.A. and Hood, L. (1985). Diversity in the germline antibody repertoire: molecular evolution of the T15 V_H gene family. *J. Exp. Med.* **162**, 1998–2016.

Playfair, J.H.L. and de Souza, J.B. (1987). Recombinant gamma interferon is a potent adjuvant for a malaria vaccine in mice. *Clin. Exp. Immunol.* **67**, 5–10.

Reiner, N.E., Ng, W. and McMaster, W.R. (1987). Parasite-accessory cell interactions in murine leishmaniasis. II. *Leishmania donovani* suppresses macrophage expression of Class I and Class II major histocompatibility complex gene products. *J. Immunol.* **138**, 1926–32.

Roitt, I.M. (1984). Prevailing theories in autoimmune disorders. *Triangle* **23**, 67–76.

Schofield, L., Villaquiran, J., Ferreira, J., Schellekens, H., Nussenzweig, R. and Nussenzweig, V. (1987). γ-Interferon, CD8+ T cells and antibodies required for immunity to malaria sporozoites. *Nature* **330**, 664–6.

Seim, S. and Espevik, T. (1983). *J. Reticuloendothelial Soc.* **33**, 417–28.

Skvaril, F. (1986). IgG subclasses in viral infections. *Monog. Allergy* **19**, 134–43.

Smithers, S.R. and Doenhoff, M.J. (1982). Schistosomiasis. In *Immunology of Parasitic Infections*, ed. S. Cohen and K.S. Warren, pp. 527–607, Blackwell Scientific Publications, Oxford.

Spry, C.J.F. (1985). Synthesis and secretion of eosinophil granule substances. *Immunol. Today* **6**, 332–5.

Steward, M.W., Stanley, C. and Furlong, M.D. (1986). Antibody affinity maturation in selectively bred high and low affinity mice. *Eur. J. Immunol.* **16**, 59–63.

Teale, J.M. and Abraham, K.M. (1987). The regulaton of antibody class expression. *Immunol. Today* **8**, 122–6.

Townsend, A.R.M. (1987). Recognition of influenza virus proteins by cytotoxic T lymphocytes. *Immunol. Res.* **6**, 80–100.

Tracey, K.J., Fong, Y., Hesse, D.G. *et al.* (1987). Anti-cachectin/TNF monoclonal antibodies prevent septic shock during lethal bacteraemia. *Nature* **330**, 662–4.

Vickerman, K. and Barry, J.D. (1982). African trypanosomiasis. In *Immunology of Parasitic Infections*, ed. S. Cohen and K.S. Warren, pp. 204–60, Blackwell Scientific Publications, Oxford.

Wakelin, D. (1978). Immunity to intestinal parasites. *Nature* **273**, 617–20.

Wassom, D.L., Loegering, D.A., Solley, G.O. *et al.* (1981). Elevated serum levels of the eosinophil granule major basic protein in patients with eosinophilia. *J. Clin. Invest.* **67**, 651–61.

Wassom, D.L., Krco, C.J. and David, C.S. (1987). I-E expression and susceptibility to parasite infection. *Immunol. Today* **8**, 39–43.

Waters, L.S., Taverne, J., Tai, P.-C., Spry, C.J.F., Targett, G.A.T. and Playfair, J.H.L. (1987). Killing of *Plasmodium falciparum* by eosinophil secretory products. *Infect. Immunity* **55**,

877–81.

Weidanz, W.P. (1982). Malaria and alterations in immune reactivity. *Br. Med. Bull.* **38** (2), 167–71.

Weinberg, A. and Merigan, T.C. (1988). Recombinant interleukin-2 as an adjuvant for vaccine induced protection: immunisation of guinea pigs with herpes simplex virus subunit vaccines. *J. Immunol.* **140**, 294–9.

Weir, D.M., Glass, E. and Stewart, J. (1981). Recognition, adherence and phagocytosis. *Ann. Immunol. (Inst. Pasteur)* **132D**, 131–49.

Whittingham, S. and Propert, D.N. (1986). Gm and Km allotypes, immune response and disease susceptibility. *Monog. Allergy* **19**, 52–70.

Williams, J.F. (1982). Cestode infections. In *Immunology of Parasitic Infections*, ed. S. Cohen & K.S. Warren, pp. 676–714, Blackwell Scientific Publications, Oxford.

Williamson, W.A. and Greenwood, B.M. (1978). Impairment of the immune response to vaccination after acute malaria. *Lancet* **i**, 1328–9.

Wong, G.H.W. and Goeddel, D.V. (1986). Tumour necrosis factors α and β inhibit virus replication and synergize with interferons. *Nature (London)* **323**, 819–22.

Young, D.B., Ivanyi, J., Cox, J.H. and Lamb, J.R. (1987). The 65KDa antigen of mycobacteria — a common bacterial protein? *Immunol. Today* **8**, 215–19.

Young, J.D.E. and Cohn, Z.A. (1986). Cell-mediated killing: a common mechanism? *Cell* **46**, 641–2.

Zanetti, M., Sercarz, E. and Salk, J. (1987). The immunology of new generation vaccines. *Immunol. Today* **8**, 18–25.

74: Immunity to Extracellular Bacteria

M.R. Wessels and D.L. Kasper

We live in continuous close contact with a large variety of bacterial species, many of which have the potential, under certain circumstances, to cause invasive infection. That clinically evident bacterial infections are not more common is testimony to the remarkable degree of protection afforded by the interplay of multiple levels of immune defence in the immunocompetent host. Conversely, the predictable development of life-threatening bacterial infection in patients with major defects in epithelial or mucosal integrity, in humoral immune factors or in phagocyte function demonstrates the essential role of each level of immune defence in protecting the host against bacterial infection. Non-specific physicochemical barriers are an important first line of defence. Patients with severe burns are at high risk for development of bacterial infection because of the breach in skin integrity. Normal secretions of mucosal surfaces may physically remove organisms and, in many cases, exert an antibacterial effect. Disruption of the normal mucociliary clearance of bacteria from the tracheobronchial tree may contribute to the recurrent bronchopulmonary infections in patients with cystic fibrosis. The low pH of gastric juice effectively kills many bacteria, serving as an important defence against enteric pathogens. The oral inoculum required to produce *Salmonella* gastroenteritis in human volunteers is lowered dramatically if gastric acidity is first neutralized. Colonization of the skin, the oro- and nasopharynx and the gastrointestinal tract with commensal flora may also act as a non-specific defence mechanism by preventing more pathogenic bacteria from finding a niche in or on the host.

Immune defence against bacteria which succeed in surmounting these non-specific barriers depends largely on humoral immune factors, i.e. complement and antibody, and on phagocytes. While a predominant role for one or more of these systems has been described for immunity to certain infections, in many, if not most, cases there is significant interplay between the various arms of the immune system (Table 74.1). None the less, it is useful to consider each system separately in analysing the role of complement, antibody and phagocytic leucocytes in immunity to extracellular bacteria. A distinction has been made between the immune response to bacterial pathogens traditionally considered to be extracellular pathogens, e.g. pyogenic organisms such as staphylococci and streptococci, most enteric Gram-negative bacilli, versus those thought to be intracellular pathogens, e.g. *Brucella* spp., *Listeria monocytogenes* and mycobacteria. Complement, specific antibodies

Table 74.1. Levels of immune defence against extracellular bacteria

Immune effector system	Mechanism(s) of action	Examples of defects
Skin and mucosal surfaces	Physical barrier	Severe burns: systemic invasion by colonizing bacteria
Mucosal secretions	Washing action pH Antibacterial enzymes Secretory IgA	Cystic fibrosis: recurrent respiratory tract infections Gastric achlorhydria: increased susceptibility to *Salmonella* infection
Humoral immunity		
Complement	Direct bacterial killing (serum bactericidal reaction) Opsonization	Deficiency of terminal C′ components: recurrent disseminated *Neisseria* infections
Antibody	Prevention of adherence Neutralization of toxins Direct killing (synergistic with C′) Opsonization (synergistic with C′)	Deficiency of specific antibody: *Haemophilus influenzae* bacteraemia in a non-immune child
Phagocytic leucocytes		
Circulating phagocytes	Phagocytosis Secretion of microbicidal factors	Granulocytopenia following cancer chemotherapy: bacteraemia from colonizing flora
Reticuloendothelial system	Early clearance of blood-borne organisms	Post-splenectomy sepsis: fulminant bacteraemia with encapsulated bacteria

and phagocytic leucocytes are the primary immune effector systems involved in defence against extracellular pathogens, while T lymphocytes and macrophages play an important role in immunity to intracellular organisms. This discussion will focus on the mechanisms of immunity of primary importance for extracellular pathogens, recognizing that immune mechanisms classically considered relevant only to intracellular pathogens may also play a significant role for certain organisms.

The role of complement

The complement system plays a major part in defending the host against bacterial infection. In the non-immune host, activation of the complement cascade by molecules on the bacterial surface is the first step in clearance of the organisms from the blood. Activation of complement leads to bacterial killing by two basic mechanisms: (i) by direct lysis, the serum bactericidal reaction, or (ii) by opsonization for ingestion and killing by phagocytes. In addition, activation of the complement system results in the generation of chemotactic peptides, primarily C5a, which bind to circulating phagocytes, resulting in activation of cellular microbicidal systems and chemotaxis of circulating phagocytic cells along a gradient of chemoattractant fragments to the site of inflammation (Chenoweth and Hugli 1978). The fate of bacterial organisms reaching the bloodstream is determined to a large extent by the degree to which the bacterial surface promotes activation of the complement cascade, and effective deposition of the C5b–9 membrane attack complex and/or opsonic fragments, primarily C3b.

Complement activation by bacteria

The complement system may be activated by bacterial surfaces through several different mechanisms. Early models of complement activation on erythrocytes indicated that antibody binding was required for activation via the classical pathway, while the alternative pathway could be activated independent of antibody. While this general model applies to the majority of situations in which bacteria activate complement, more recent studies have shown that, under certain circumstances, bacterial cells or purified constituent molecules may directly activate the classical pathway, without a requirement for antibody. In addition, binding of antibody to the bacterial surface may not only activate the classical pathway, but also facilitate alternative pathway activation. Several different molecules on bacterial surfaces have been shown to play a role in complement activation. Depending on the relationship of these constituents to other bacterial surface components, and the presence or absence of antibody, activation of the complement cascade at the bacterial surface is frequently the critical step leading to clearance of an invading micro-organism.

Lipopolysaccharide, or LPS, is a major constituent of the outer membrane of Gram-negative bacteria. Lipopolysaccharide is made up of a lipid moiety, lipid A, covalently linked to a core polysaccharide containing 2-keto-3-deoxyoctonoate (KDO) and heptose residues. These parts of the LPS structure are relatively constant among most Gram-negative organisms (Luderitz *et al.* 1984). In addition, 'smooth' strains have LPS to which an O-polysaccharide or oligosaccharide side-chain is attached to the core polysaccharide (Fig. 74.1). Variation in the composition of the O side-chain is responsible for antigenic differences between the LPS of different Gram-negative organisms (Kaufmann 1966; Luderitz *et al.* 1966). Lipopolysaccharide from a variety of Gram-negative bacteria has been shown to activate complement via the alternative pathway, without a requirement for specific antibody (Pillemer *et al.* 1955; Joiner *et al.* 1984). The efficiency of LPS as an activator of the alternative pathway may be related to the experimental observation that C3b bound to LPS has a low affinity for the regulatory protein factor H relative to that for factor B (Pangburn *et al.* 1980). Therefore, inactivation of C3b is inefficient, favouring the formation of the C3 convertase C3bBb, leading to amplification of alternative pathway activation. It is also clear that rough organisms, that is, those bearing LPS lacking O side-chains, are capable of complement activation via the classical pathway, in the absence of antibody (Cooper and Morrison 1978; Clas and Loos 1981).

Gram-positive bacteria lack an outer membrane and do not have LPS. However, other surface molecules on these organisms may activate complement. Peptidoglycan, the major component of Gram-positive cell walls, is a complex polysaccharide–peptide consisting of polysaccharide chains of alternating β(1→4)-linked residues of *N*-acetyl-glucosamine and *N*-acetylmuramic aid, joined by cross-linking peptide side-chains. This polymer is probably responsible for the ability of Gram-positive cell walls to activate the alternative pathway in the absence of antibody (Winkelstein and Tomasz 1977; Wilkinson *et al.* 1979; Verbrugh *et al.* 1980). Much like the situation with LPS activation of the alternative pathway, C3b bound to the cell wall of pneumococci has a greater affinity for factor B than for factor H, leading to efficient formation of C3bBb (Brown *et al.* 1983a). Thus, in both Gram-negative and Gram-positive bacteria, the ability of surface molecules to activate the alternative pathway is related to relative affinity of bound C3b for factor B (resulting in amplification of alternative pathway activation) versus factor H (leading to down-regulation of alternative pathway activation).

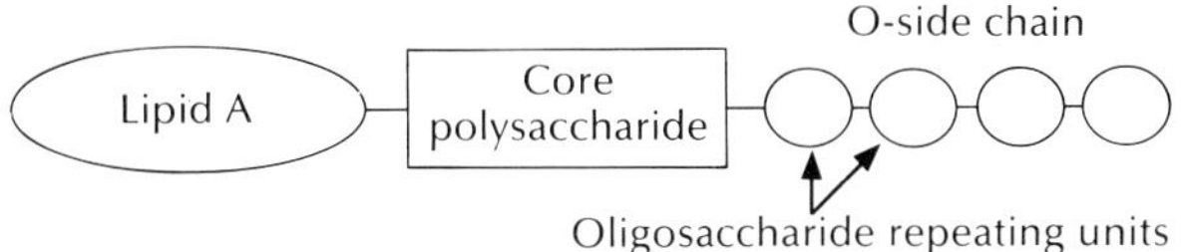

Fig. 74.1. Schematic diagram of the general structure of LPS on Gram-negative bacteria. 'Smooth' forms of LPS contain O side-chains of multiple oligosaccharide repeating units. 'Rough' forms of LPS contain lipid A and core polysaccharide, but lack O side-chains.

Since the alternative pathway is readily activated by these ubiquitous components of both Gram-negative outer membranes (LPS) and Gram-positive cell walls (peptidoglycan), it is not surprising that a number of important bacterial pathogens mask these structures with other surface molecules, presumably as a means to evade complement-mediated clearance by the host. *Streptococcus pyogenes* strains bearing large amounts of M protein on their cell surfaces are relatively resistant to opsonophagocytic killing (Lancefield 1962). Horstmann *et al.* (1988) have shown that M protein binds factor H, suggesting that the antiphagocytic effect may be due to inhibition of complement activation on this basis. In addition, the presence of M protein on the cell surface may prevent complement components bound to the bacterial cell wall from interacting with complement receptors on phagocytes (Weis *et al.* 1985). Surface proteins of other bacteria may serve a similar function.

The presence of a polysaccharide capsule around both Gram-positive and Gram-negative organisms may also play an important role in inhibiting complement activation. The nine-carbon sugar acid, *N*-acetyl-neuraminic acid, or sialic acid, is present as a prominent residue in the capsular polysaccharides of several important bacterial pathogens including groups B and C *Neisseria meningitidis, Escherichia coli* K1 and group B *Streptococcus* (Kasper *et al.* 1973; Jennings *et al.* 1977, 1983a, b; Wessels *et al.* 1987a). The presence of surface-associated sialic acid has been shown to inhibit complement activation by sheep erythrocytes, and other particles, and it is likely that sialic acid-containing bacterial capsules function in this capacity to protect the organism from complement-mediated lysis or opsonophagocytosis (Fig. 74.2; Van Dijk *et al.* 1977; Fearon 1978; Pangburn and Muller-Eberhard 1978). Evidence supporting this hypothesis has been obtained from studies of type III group B *Streptococcus*. Intact organisms of type III group B *Streptococcus* failed to activate the alternative pathway in the absence of anticapsular antibody; removal of the sialic acid residues from the polysaccharide side-chains of the bacterial capsule converted the organisms into efficient activators of the alternative pathway (Edwards *et al.* 1982). Resistance of encapsulated pneumococci to phagocytosis may be related to the observation that C3b bound to the pneumococcal capsule has a low affinity for factor B; therefore, the competing reaction of bound C3b with the inhibitory protein factor H is favoured, and the C3b convertase C3bBb is not generated to a sufficient extent to support efficient alternative pathway activation.

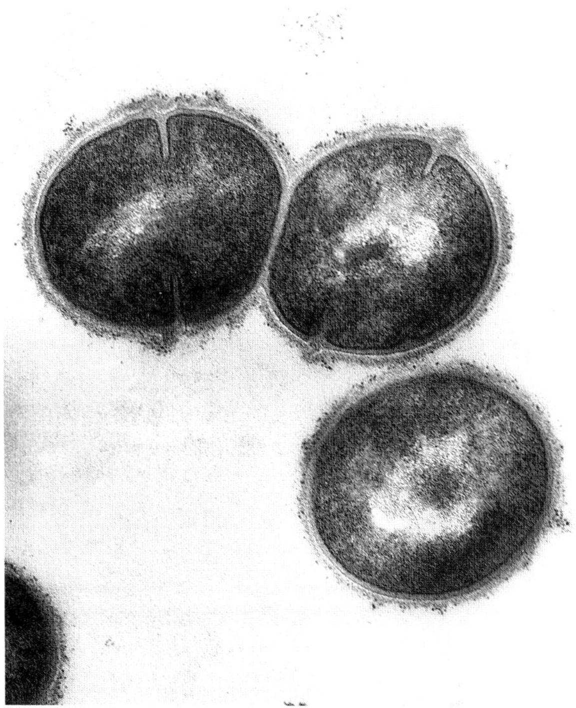

Fig. 74.2. Capsular polysaccharide of group B *Streptococcus*. Electron micrograph of organisms of group B *Streptococcus* following incubation with anticapsular antibody and ferritin-labelled anti-IgG. An irregular layer of capsular polysaccharide is visible exterior to the cell wall, decorated by ferritin particles (× 12 880).

Complement-mediated bactericidal and bacteriolytic action

Gram-negative bacteria may be killed, and often lysed, by fresh serum, a process known as the serum bactericidal reaction (Taylor 1983). This serum bactericidal reaction depends on the deposition on the bacterial outer membrane of the terminal complement component membrane attack complex, consisting of fragments C5b–9 (Joiner *et al.* 1985). The C5b–9 complex appears to insert into the outer membrane (Feingold *et al.* 1968). In the presence of normal serum, the loss of integrity of the outer membrane permits access of serum lysozyme to the bacterial cell wall. Lysozyme catalyses the digestion of peptidoglycan, the major cell wall structural polymer, leading to dissolution of the cell wall and bacterial cell lysis (Inoue *et al.* 1959). The observation that Gram-negative organisms may be killed but not lysed in lysozyme-depleted serum suggests that the C5b–9 complex may breach the inner membrane as well. The importance of the terminal complement components in the serum bactericidal reaction is illustrated by the clinical observation that patients with deficiencies in C6, C7, or C8 may suffer recurrent episodes of bacteraemia with *Neisseria meningitidis* and *N. gonorrhoeae* (Lee *et al.* 1978; Nicholson and Lepow 1979; see also Chapter 67). Gram-positive bacteria are resistant to direct complement-mediated lysis, presumably because of the greater thickness and rigidity of the Gram-positive cell wall.

Smooth strains of Gram-negative bacteria, those producing an LPS core which is highly substituted with O-specific side-chains, are generally more resistant to antibody-independent killing by

Table 74.2. Bacterial mechanisms to resist complement mediated killing

Bacterial property	Effect on C′ mediated killing
Rigid cell wall (Gram-positive bacteria)	Resists direct lysis
'Smooth' LPS	Promotes ineffective binding of C3b to O-side chains, rather than to outer membrane
Capsular polysaccharide	Steric interference with access of phagocyte C3 receptors to C3b bound to bacterial surface
	Inhibition of alternative pathway activation (sialic acid containing capsules)

serum than are rough isolates (Table 74.2). This difference appears to be due, in part, to the capacity of rough strains to directly activate the classical pathway of complement, in the absence of antibody (Cooper and Morrison 1978). Evidence for such a mechanism has been reported in studies of *E. coli* J5, a rough mutant strain deficient in galactose-4-epimerase, rendering this strain incapable of adding O-specific side-chains to its LPS. The J5 strain demonstrated antibody-independent activation of the classical pathway, resulting in effective bacterial killing, while the smooth parent *E. coli* strain from which J5 was derived was not killed by this mechanism (Betz and Isleker 1981). Thus, the more efficient killing of rough strains in serum may reflect the additional activation of the classical pathway by such strains.

While both smooth and rough strains may be killed via activation of the alternative pathway, smooth strains tend to be relatively resistant. This difference between serum-sensitive and serum-resistant strains appears to depend not on the capacity of their cell surfaces to activate the alternative pathway, but rather on the ability of the bound complement components to generate the deposition of the C5b−9 membrane attack complex on the bacterial outer membrane (Binns *et al.* 1982; Joiner *et al.* 1982a, b). In a serum-resistant strain of *Salmonella*, C3b was preferentially deposited on LPS molecules with long O-polysaccharide side-chains (Joiner *et al.* 1986). In contrast to C3b deposited on the outer membrane, these molecules tended to dissociate and be released from the bacterial cell rather than leading to productive insertion of the membrane attack complex into the outer membrane. This observation is consistent with the hypothesis that the membrane attack complex must be formed in close physical proximity to the outer membrane in order for effective killing; those complexes formed in association with C3b bound to structures extending relatively far from the cell surface may be sterically prevented from interacting with the outer membrane.

Complement-mediated opsonophagocytosis

Complement plays a major role in opsonizing bacterial pathogens for phagocytosis by fixed mononuclear phagocytes in the liver and spleen, and by circulating phagocytes in the form of macrophages and granulocytes, primarily neutrophils. Experiments in guinea-pigs depleted of complement by treatment with cobra venom factor indicated that an intact complement system was required for efficient bloodstream clearance of *Streptococcus pneumoniae*, even in the presence of anticapsular antibody. Furthermore, in animals with an intact complement system, the site of bacterial clearance was shifted, with relatively more organisms being cleared by the liver than by the spleen. This effect was more marked in the presence of antibody (Brown *et al.* 1983b). Similarly, hepatic clearance of *Salmonella typhimurium in vitro* has been shown to depend on complement-mediated opsonization (Friedman and Moon 1980).

Circulating phagocytic cells also have receptors for C3b, and these cells are able to phagocytose micro-organisms previously opsonized with C3b (Fearon 1980; Beller *et al.* 1982; Arnaut *et al.* 1983). For certain bacteria, bound C3b appears to be a sufficient signal for phagocytosis by resting neutrophils and monocytes, while phagocytosis of other bacteria requires a second signal, in the form of bound immunoglobulin G (IgG), fibronectin or other undefined activators of the phagocyte. In addition, the site of complement deposition on the bacterial surface in relation to other structures such as surface proteins and capsular polysaccharides is an important determinant of the efficiency of complement-mediated phagocytosis. Thus, for example, C3b bound to the cell wall of an organism may be ineffective as an opsonin if it is shielded from phagocyte complement receptors by a thick polysaccharide capsule. Evidence for such a mechanism has been reported for complement-mediated opsonization of pneumococci; C3b deposited on the cell wall failed to promote phagocytosis, while C3b fixed to the polysaccharide capsule via the interaction with anticapsular antibody led to efficient opsonophagocytosis of the organisms (Brown *et al.* 1983a).

Experiments with other Gram-positive organisms such as *Streptococcus pneumoniae* and *Staphylococcus aureus* have indicated that bacterial capsules may not prevent the deposition of complement components on the subcapsular bacterial surface; however, the presence of the capsule appears to prevent interaction of the bound fragments with complement receptors on phagocytes, presumably by steric interference with access of the phagocyte complement receptors to the opsonic fragments bound to the cell wall of the bacterium (Wilkinson *et al.* 1979; Winkelstein *et al.* 1980; Brown *et al.* 1983b). In the case of *S. aureus*, Lee *et al.* (1987) showed that capsule-deficient mutants derived from a heavily encapsulated, virulent strain were sensitive to phagocytic killing by leucocytes and non-immune serum, while the wild-type strain was resistant.

The role of antibody (Table 74.3)

The complement system is the mainstay of humoral immune defence against extracellular bacteria in the immunologically naïve host. However, the complement system alone is inadequate for efficient killing or opsonization of a number of organisms which are pathogens of man. Clearance of these bacteria requires the participation of the other major arm of the humoral immune system, specific antibodies. In addition, the clearance of complement-sensitive bacteria may also be greatly enhanced by the synergistic action of antibodies with complement components in promoting direct lysis or opsonophagocytosis.

Table 74.3. Actions of antibodies in defence against extracellular bacteria

Mechanism of action	Examples
Prevention of adherence	Salivary IgA prevents attachment of oral streptococci
Neutralization of toxins	Diphtheria, tetanus
Bacterial lysis (in concert with C′ system)	Anti-LPS antibodies
Opsonization for phagocytosis	Antibodies against pneumococcal capsular polysaccharide

Antibodies may also play a role in preventing bacterial attachment. The initial phase of bacterial invasion involves adherence of the organism to an epithelial surface. This attachment is mediated by the interaction of specific molecules on the bacterial surface with receptor molecules on host epithelial cells. Antibodies directed against antigens on the bacterial surface may block attachment, thereby preventing infection. Uropathogenic *E. coli*, for example, must adhere to the mucous membranes of the genitourinary tract in order to produce urinary tract infection (O'Hanley *et al.* 1985). Attachment is mediated by lectin-like proteins, or adhesins, which bind to specific sugar residues of host epithelial cell glycolipids. The adhesin proteins are located on the ends of hairlike structures called pili, which project from the bacterial surface (Lund *et al.* 1987; Moch *et al.* 1987). Adhesins recognize receptor oligosaccharides not only on epithelial cells, but also as soluble compounds present in the secretions bathing the mucosal surface. The presence of soluble receptor molecules in secretions may serve as a host defence mechanism by binding to the adhesin proteins, thereby preventing their interaction with receptors on epithelial cells. Such a role has been suggested for mannose-containing Tamm–Horsfall uromucoids in binding to and preventing attachment of *E. coli* bearing mannose-binding pili (O'Hanley *et al.* 1985). In addition, specific antibodies may play a role in interfering with bacterial adherence to epithelial surfaces. For example, antibodies directed against the binding region of the adhesin molecule of another type of pili, those that recognize the galactose β(1→4)galactose disaccharide, have been shown to block adherence of uropathogenic *E. coli*, and to prevent experimental pyelonephritis in animals (Schmidt *et al.* 1988).

Antibodies of the IgA class are particularly important in defending the host against bacterial invasion at mucosal surfaces. These antibodies are synthesized by plasma cells at the mucosal surface, then linked to secretory component, a protein produced by mucosal epithelial cells. Secretory IgA antibodies are quite specifically localized, in terms of their distribution on mucosal surfaces at different body sites. Thus, salivary IgA has been shown to prevent attachment of oral streptococci to the buccal mucosa, while IgA antibodies in the gut play an important role in preventing the attachment of diarrhoeal pathogens such as *Vibrio cholerae*. The mechanism by which secretory IgA prevents bacterial attachment or invasion is not clear; secretory IgA antibodies do not promote opsonophagocytosis directly, or by activation of the alternative or classical pathways of complement. They may function by binding to bacterial surface antigens which mediate adherence, thereby blocking bacterial attachment. A number of pathogenic bacteria elaborate enzymes which have proteolytic activity against IgA antibodies, presumably an adaptation to allow the organism to overcome local immunity. Such IgA proteases have been demonstrated for *Neisseria gonorrhoeae, Haemophilus influenzae*, oral streptococci involved in formation of dental plaque, and others (Plaut *et al*. 1975; Killian *et al*. 1979).

Antibodies also play an important role in host defence against extracellular products of pathogenic bacteria. Thus, antibodies against diphtheria or tetanus toxins constitute the basic immunological protection mechanism against these diseases, by binding to the toxins and preventing their pathological effects on target host cells. Effective use has been made of this phenomenon in prevention of these two diseases through immunization with modified (detoxified) forms of diphtheria and tetanus toxins to elicit antibodies which neutralize the native toxins.

Perhaps the most important function of antibacterial antibodies is their capacity to bind specifically to bacterial surface antigens, thereby facilitating complement activation and bacterial killing through direct lysis or by opsonophagocytosis. Rough strains of Gram-negative bacteria, those lacking LPS O side-chains, are typically serum-sensitive; that is, their surfaces directly activate the alternative pathway of complement, resulting in deposition of lytic and opsonic complement components on the bacterial outer membrane, and bacterial killing. Smooth strains, those having LPS O side-chains, are often serum resistant, and fail to effectively activate the complement cascade directly. Clearance of serum-resistant strains of Gram-negative bacteria requires specific antibody. Binding of LPS-specific antibody to the surface of a smooth strain results in activation of the classical pathway and efficient deposition of opsonic complement components. As Gram-positive organisms are not lysed directly in serum, defence against encapsulated Gram-positive pathogens depends upon the synergistic action of antibody and complement for efficient opsonophagocytic killing. While neutrophils and macrophages have receptors for the Fc portion of IgG, phagocytosis of bacteria coated with antibody is slow in comparison with that for organisms opsonized by both IgG and C3b. Both the isotype and subclass of an antibody may influence its opsonic function. Phagocytic cells have receptors for IgG and IgA, but not for IgM. Immunoglobulin M class antibodies, however, are more efficient activators of complement when bound to the bacterial surface, as a single molecule of bound IgM can activate complement while two or more IgG molecules are required (Borsos and Rapp 1965). Immunoglobulin G1 and IgG3 antibodies bound to bacterial cells can activate complement via the classical pathway, antibodies of these subclasses also bind more tightly to phagocytic cell IgG receptors than do IgG2 and IgG4 antibodies (Alexander *et al*. 1978).

As mentioned above in the context of complement activation, the presence of a polysaccharide capsule may make a bacterial pathogen a poor activator of the complement cascade. The capsule may also interfere with bacterial clearance by sterically interfering with the interaction of phagocyte Fc receptors with antibodies bound to the bacterial cell wall. Therefore, antibodies directed against cell wall antigens are often ineffective as opsonins for encapsulated bacteria, despite their ability to bind to the organisms. In contrast, antibodies directed against the capsular polysaccharide are capable of fixing complement and promoting efficient opsonophagocytosis. Specific anticapsular antibodies play an important role in immunity to encapsulated Gram-negative pathogens such as *Neisseria meningitidis* and *Haemophilus influenzae*, and to Gram-positive species such as *Streptococcus pneumoniae* and group B *Streptococcus* (Goldschneider *et al*. 1969; Robbins *et al*. 1973; Baker *et al*. 1977; Austrian 1981).

A large number of bacterial capsular polysaccharides have been purified and used as vaccines (Robbins 1978; Jennings 1983). The efficacy of polysaccharides as immunogens has been variable; certain polysaccharides reliably elicit protective levels of antibody in a high proportion of recipients, while others are poor immunogens. Small differences in chemical structure may result in vastly different immunogenicity. For example, the group C meningococcal polysaccharide, a homopolymer of α(2→9)-linked sialic acid residues, is immunogenic in over 90% of adult subjects (Gotschlich *et al.* 1969). In contrast, the group B meningococcal polysaccharide, an α(2→8)-linked sialic acid homopolymer, is non-immunogenic (Wyle *et al.* 1972; Kasper *et al.* 1973). The remarkable structural specificity of these immune responses may reflect a self-tolerance mechanism, as α(2→8)-linked sialyl-oligosaccharides are present as cell surface epitopes of human neural cell adhesion molecules (Edelman 1985). It is likely that bacteria evolved capsular polysaccharide structures resembling mammalian oligosaccharides as a means of escaping immune detection. Our understanding of antibody recognition of polysaccharide antigens is based largely on the studies of Kabat and co-workers, who, beginning in the 1950s, carried out a series of experiments using a dextran–antidextran model. These investigators found that the epitope recognized by antidextran antibodies was a relatively simple one: the binding of antidextran antibodies to high-molecular-weight dextran could be completely inhibited by homologous oligosaccharides of six or seven sugar residues (Kabat 1961; Sharon *et al.* 1982). It might be anticipated, then, that bacterial polysaccharides having structural similarity to host oligosaccharides would not be recognized because of self-tolerance. None the less, many bacterial polysaccharides are immunogenic despite striking similarity between their repeating unit structures and the structure of oligosaccharide determinants of human glycoproteins or glycolipids. Recent studies of antibody binding to the capsular polysaccharides of pathogenic bacteria may explain this apparent paradox. Studies of antibody binding to the capsular polysaccharides of type III group B *Streptococcus* and of type 14 *Streptococcus pneumoniae* and similar experiments on the capsule of *Neisseria meningitidis* group B suggest that the anticapsular antibodies against each of these polysaccharides recognize a conformational epitope, which is expressed only in high-molecular-weight polymers of the antigen and not in short-chain oligosaccharides such as those present on host glycoproteins or glycolipids (Wessels *et al.* 1987b; Kabat *et al.* 1988; Wessels and Kasper 1989). Proteins on the bacterial surface may also serve as antigenic targets for antibodies. For example, antibodies directed against the M proteins of group A *Streptococcus*, in concert with complement components, effectively opsonize these organisms for phagocytosis by neutrophils (Hirst and Lancefield 1939; Beachey *et al.* 1979).

The role of other plasma proteins

In addition to antibodies and the proteins of the complement system, certain other plasma proteins may play a role in opsonizing bacteria for ingestion and killing by host phagocytes. C-reactive protein is a 115 000 dalton protein which binds with high affinity to phosphorylcholine, a major constituent of pneumococcal cell walls (McCarty 1982). The interaction of C-reactive protein with pneumococci results in activation of the classical pathway of complement, and appears to provide some degree of protection against experimental challenge with pneumococcal organisms in mice (Claus *et al.* 1977; Mold *et al.* 1981; Yother *et al.* 1982). Another plasma protein which may act as an opsonin is fibronectin. This 440 000 dalton glycoprotein binds to many, but not all, bacterial pathogens and also to monocytes and macrophages, suggesting that it may serve an opsonic function (Bevilacque *et al.* 1981; Myhre and Kuusela 1983). The importance to host defence of fibronectin binding to microorganisms *in vivo* remains to be determined. Several recent reports have described lectin-like mannose-binding proteins, first from the serum of rabbits, and subsequently from humans (Kawasaki *et al.* 1978, 1983). Though their amino acid sequences are not homologous, the overall structure of the human mannose-binding protein is similar to that of C1q, with a globular carbohydrate-binding domain and a collagen-like domain (Ezekowitz *et al.* 1988). Evidence has been presented suggesting that mannose-binding protein may play an opsonic role by binding to microbial surfaces rich in mannose and perhaps other carbohydrate residues (Kuhlman *et al.* 1989). For further discussion of mannose binding protein and its ability to activate complement see Chapter 67.

The role of phagocytic leucocytes

While certain Gram-negative bacteria may be killed directly by complement-mediated lysis, phagocytic leucocytes represent the major effector system for killing organisms which gain entry into the bloodstream or host tissues. Circulating neutrophils and monocytes and fixed macrophages of the reticuloendothelial system are the cells primarily responsible for the phagocytic killing of bacteria. Monocytes and macrophages, like neutrophils, possess membrane receptors for the Fc portion of IgG and for C3b (Unkeless 1977; Lane *et al.* 1980). Macrophages also have lectin-like receptors which recognize mannose residues and other sugars present on microbial surfaces and may facilitate phagocytosis (Berton and Gordon 1983; Sung *et al.* 1983). They are able to ingest micro-organisms, but their phagocytic ability is less efficient than that of neutrophils, and they lack some of the bactericidal systems present in neutrophils. Mononuclear phagocytes also play an important role in initiating the immune response by degrading and processing bacterial antigens for presentation to lymphoid cells. A major function of the reticuloendothelial system in host defence against extracellular bacteria is the initial rapid clearance of blood-borne micro-organisms. Early studies on bloodstream clearance of bacteria showed a prompt decrease in the number of circulating organisms during the first few hours after injection in experimental animals. Avirulent strains were cleared completely during this period, while more virulent strains showed an initial decrease in density, followed by proliferation and either death of the animal or subsequent decrease in bacterial number and eventual clearance (Rogers 1960). In experimental pneumococcal bacteraemia, the initial clearance phase has been shown to be due to removal of the organisms from the bloodstream by fixed mononuclear phagocytes, primarily in the liver and spleen (Brown *et al.* 1981). Complement appears to play an important role in this process, as complement depletion impairs clearance and results in a shift in the site of clearance, with relatively more organisms being cleared in the spleen rather than the liver. In immune animals, the presence of antibody results in increased clearance and a shift in the site of clearance to the liver (Brown *et al.* 1983b). These observations may explain why asplenic patients occasionally develop overwhelming sepsis from pneumococcal bacteraemia: in the absence of specific antibodies, the spleen plays a critical role in removing the organisms from the bloodstream.

Defence against extracellular bacteria which escape clearance by the reticuloendothelial system depends largely on circulating granulocytes. Neutrophils which encounter microbial particles may have phagocytosis stimulated directly by surface contact with the micro-organism. The presence of bound IgG and C3b on the surface of the organism, however, greatly enhances phagocytosis (Scribner and Fahrney 1976; Malbran *et al.* 1987). These opsonic ligands bind to specific receptors for the Fc portion of IgG or to C3 receptors on the neutrophil cell membrane. Contact of the phagocyte with the microbial surface triggers cyclic adenosine monophosphate (cAMP) production and degranulation, while the neutrophil cell membrane invaginates and surrounds the bacterial particle to form a phagolysosome (Zucker-Franklin and Hirsch 1964; Pryzwansky *et al.* 1979, 1981; MacRae *et al.* 1980). Stimulation of the neutrophil metabolic burst activates a series of oxygen-dependent and oxygen-independent microbicidal systems, resulting in killing of the ingested bacteria. The metabolic burst is accompanied by an increase in O_2 uptake by the neutrophil, and production of superoxide anion (O_2^-), which undergoes rapid dismutation to H_2O_2. The generation of reduced oxygen intermediates and H_2O_2 are responsible for the O_2-dependent antimicrobial mechanism. Degranulation of both specific and azurophilic granules in the region of the phagolysosome makes available the O_2-dependent myeloperoxidase system, as well as O_2-independent antimicrobial systems including lysozyme, lactoferrin, glycosidases and proteases, all of which have antibacterial properties (Leffell and Spitznagel 1975; Rest *et al.* 1978; Spitznagel 1983).

Certain surface molecules of extracellular bacteria appear to represent adaptations enabling the organisms to resist phagocytosis. As has been discussed above capsular polysaccharides of several species of bacteria have been shown to inhibit complement activation. The ability of bacterial capsules to inhibit complement activation or to prevent access of bound C3b to C3 receptors on the phagocytes seem to be the factors primarily responsible for the antiphagocytic property of the surface macromolecules. Proteins on the bacterial surface may also interfere with opsonophagocytosis. M protein on the surface of group A streptococci appears to inhibit phagocytosis, perhaps on the basis of the failure of this antigen to activate the alternative pathway of complement, and by preventing access of phagocyte receptors to opsonins bound to the bacterial surface. Protein A, found on the surface of many *Staphylococcus aureus* strains, binds the Fc portion of IgG. Protein A-rich strains are relatively resistant to opsonization in normal serum, suggesting that protein A-bound IgG may sterically block access of C3b to the bacterial surface (Peterson *et al.* 1977).

In addition to the strategies evolved by bacteria to evade attachment and ingestion by phagocytes, certain pathogens produce enzymes or other products which may help the organism resist being killed after being ingested by the phagocyte. For example, the production of catalase by organisms like staphylococci may play a role in protecting the organism from the myeloperoxidase–hydrogen peroxide antimicrobial system of the neutrophil (Mandell 1975). In general, however, those organisms considered to be extracellular pathogens are readily killed, once ingested by neutrophils or monocyte/macrophages, in contrast to intracellular pathogens, which may survive inside phagocytes.

T lymphocytes in immunity to extracellular bacteria

The preceding discussion has focused on complement, antibody and phagocytic leucocytes as the principal immune effector systems involved in host defence against extracellular bacteria, while cell-mediated immunity, involving T lymphocytes and monocyte/macrophages generally has been considered to be operative against intracellular pathogens, i.e. viruses, mycobacteria and certain intracellular bacteria such as *Listeria monocytogenes* and *Salmonella typhi*. While this distinction is useful in describing specific patterns of immune response, recent studies have suggested that cell-mediated immunity may also play a role in host defence against certain bacterial pathogens generally thought of as extracellular bacteria. Onderdonk, Kasper and co-workers have shown that specific immunity against *Bacteroides fragilis* may be transferred from immune to naïve mice by passive immunization with splenic T lymphocytes, or with a cell-free lysate of the T cells (Onderdonk *et al.* 1982; Zaleznik *et al.* 1985). This T cell factor protected naïve mice from development of intra-abdominal abscesses after intraperitoneal challenge with *B. fragilis*, but did not protect against challenge with other bacteria, suggesting an antigen-specific effect. The nature of this immune T cell factor or the mechanism by which it mediates an antibacterial effect has not been determined. Markham *et al.* have demonstrated a role for T cells in immunity to *Pseudomonas aeruginosa*. In the *Pseudomonas* model, T cell factor(s) elicited by immunization of mice with capsular polysaccharide appear to mediate direct bacterial killing (Markham *et al.* 1985). Thus, at least for certain extracellular bacteria, T cells appear to play a role in immunity.

References

Alexander, M.D., Andrews, J.A., Leslie, R.G. and Wood N.J. (1978). The binding of human and guinea pig IgG subclasses to homologous monocyte and macrophage receptors. *Immunology* **35**, 115–23.

Arnaut, M.A., Todd, R.F., Danan, N., Melamed, J., Schlossman, S.F. and Colten, H.R. (1983). Inhibition of phagocytosis of complement C3 or immunoglobulin G-coated particles and of C3bi binding by monoclonal antibodies to a monocyte–granulocyte membrane glycoprotein (Mo 1). *J. Clin. Invest.* **72**, 171–9.

Austrian, R. (1981). Some observations on the *Pneumococcus* and on the current status of pneumococcal disease and its prevention. *Rev. Infect. Dis.* **3** (suppl.), S1–S17.

Baker, C.J., Kasper, D.L., Tager, I.B. *et al.* (1977). Quantitative determination of antibody to capsular polysaccharides in infection with type III strains group B *Streptococcus*. *J. Clin. Invest.* **59**, 810–18.

Beachey, E.H., Stollerman, G.H., Johnson, R.H., Ofek, I. and Bisno, A.L. (1979). Human immune response to immunization with a structurally defined polypeptide fragment of streptococcal M protein. *J. Exp. Med.* **150**, 862–77.

Beller, D.I., Springer, T.A. and Schreiber, R.D. (1982). Anti-Mac-1 selectively inhibits the mouse and human type three complement receptor. *J. Exp. Med.* **156**, 1000–9.

Berton, G. and Gordon, S. (1983). Modulation of macrophage mannosyl-specific receptors by cultivation on immobilised zymosan: effects on superoxide-anion release and phagocytosis. *Immunology* **49**, 705–15.

Betz, S.J. and Isleker, H. (1981). Antibody-independent interactions between *Escherichia coli* J5 and human complement components. *J. Immunol.* **127**, 1748–54.

Bevilacque, M.P., Amrani, D., Mosesson, M.W. and Bianco, C. (1981). Receptors for cold insoluble globulin (plasma fibronectin) on human monocytes. *J. Exp. Med.* **153**, 42–60.

Binns, M.W., Mayden, J. and Levin, R.P. (1982). Further characterization of complement resistance conferred on *Escherichia coli* by the plasmid genes traT of R100 and iss of Col-V, I-K94. *Infect. Immunity* **35**, 654–9.

Borsos, T. and Rapp, H.J. (1965). Hemolysin titration based on fixation of the activated first component of complement: evidence that one molecule of hemolysin suffices to sensitize an erythrocyte. *J. Immunol.* **95**, 559–66.

Brown, E.J., Hosea, S.W. and Frank, M.M. (1981). The role

of complement in the localization of pneumococci in the splanchnic reticuloendothelial system during experimental bacteremia. *J. Immunol.* **126**, 2230–5.

Brown, E.J., Joiner, K., Gaither, T., Hammer, C. and Frank, M.M. (1983a). The interaction of C3b bound to pneumococci with factor H, factor I and properdin factor B of the human complement system. *J. Immunol.* **131**, 409–15.

Brown, E.J., Hosea, S.W. and Frank, M.M. (1983b). The role of antibody and complement in the reticuloendothelial clearance of pneumococci from the bloodstream. *Rev. Infect. Dis.* **5** (S4), S797–S805.

Chenoweth, D.E. and Hugli, T.E. (1978). Demonstration of specific C5a receptors on intact human polymorphonuclear leukocytes. *Proc. Nat. Acad. Sci. (USA)* **75**, 3943–7.

Clas, F. and Loos, M. (1981). Antibody-independent binding of the first component of complement (C1) and its subcomponent C1q to the S and R forms of *Salmonella minnesota*. *Infect. Immunity* **31**, 1138–44.

Claus, D.R., Siegel, J., Petras, K., Osmand, A.P. and Gewurz, H. (1977). Interaction of C-reactive protein with the first component of human complement. *J. Immunol.* **119**, 187–92.

Cooper, N.R. and Morrison, D.C. (1978). Binding and activation of the first component of human complement by the lipid A region of lipopolysaccharides. *J. Immunol.* **120**, 1862–9.

Edelman, G.M. (1985). Cell adhesion and the molecular processes of morphogenesis. *Ann. Rev. Biochem.* **54**, 135–69.

Edwards, M.S., Kasper, D.L., Jennings, H.J., Baker, C.J. and Nicholson-Weller, A. (1982). Capsular sialic acid prevents activation of the alternative complement pathway by type III, group B streptococci. *J. Immunol.* **128**, 1278–83.

Ezekowitz, R.A.B., Day, L. and Herman, G. (1988). A human mannose-binding protein is an acute phase reactant that shares sequence homology with other vertebrate lectins. *J. Exp. Med.* **167**, 1034–46.

Fearon, D.T. (1978). Regulation by membrane sialic acid of B1H-dependent decay–dissociation of amplification C3 convertase of the alternative complement pathway. *Proc. Nat. Acad. Sci. (USA)* **75**, 1971–5.

Fearon, D.T. (1980). Identification of the membrane glycoprotein that is the C3b receptor of the human erythrocyte, polymorphonuclear leukocyte, B lymphocyte, and monocyte. *J. Exp. Med.* **152**, 20–30.

Feingold, D.S., Goldman, J.N. and Kuritz, H.M. (1968). Locus of the lethal event in the serum bactericidal reaction. *J. Bacteriol.* **96**, 2127–31.

Friedman, R.L. and Moon, R.J. (1980). Role of Kupffer cells, complement and specific antibody in the bactericidal activities of perfused livers. *Infect. Immunity* **29**, 152–7.

Goldschneider, I., Gotschlich, E.C. and Artenstein, M.S. (1969). Human immunity to the meningococcus, I. The role of humoral antibodies. *J. Exp. Med.* **129**, 1307–26.

Gotschlich, E.C., Goldschneider, I. and Artenstein, M.S. (1969). Human immunity to the meningococcus. IV. Immunogenicity of the group A and group C meningococcus in human volunteers. *J. Exp. Med.* **129**, 1367–84.

Hirst, G.K. and Lancefield, R.C. (1939). Antigenic properties of the type-specific substances derived from group A hemolytic streptococci. *J. Exp. Med.* **69**, 425–45.

Horstmann, R.D., Sievertsen, H.J., Knobloch, J. and Fischetti, V.A. (1988). Antiphagocytic activity of streptococcal M protein: selective binding of complement control protein factor H. *Proc. Nat. Acad. Sci. (USA)* **85**, 1657–61.

Inoue, K., Tanigawa, Y., Takubo, M., Satani, M. and Amano, T. (1959). Quantitative studies on immune bacteriolysis. II. The role of lysozyme in immune bacteriolysis. *Biken J.* **2**, 1–20.

Jennings, H.J. (1983). Capsular polysaccharides as human vaccines. *Adv. Carbohydr. Chem. Biochem.* **41**, 155–208.

Jennings, H.J., Bhattacharjee, A.K., Bundle, D.R., Kenny, C.P., Martin, A. and Smith, I.C.P. (1977). Structure of the capsular polysaccharides of *Neisseria meningitidis* as determined by ^{13}C-nuclear magnetic resonance spectroscopy. *J. Infect. Dis.* **136** (suppl.), 78–83.

Jennings, H.J., Katzenellenbogen, E., Lugowski, C. and Kasper, D.L. (1983a). Structure of the native polysaccharide antigens of type Ia and type Ib group B *Streptococcus. Biochemistry (USA)* **22**, 1258–63.

Jennings, H.J., Rosell, K.-G. and Kasper, D.L. (1983b). Structural determination of the capsular polysaccharide antigen of type II group B *Streptococcus. J. Biol. Chem.* **258**, 1793–8.

Joiner, K.A., Hammer, C.H., Brown, E.J., Cole, R.J. and Frank, M.M. (1982a). Studies on the mechanism of bacterial resistance to complement-mediated killing. I. Terminal complement components are deposited and released from *Salmonella minnesota* S218 without causing bacterial death. *J. Exp. Med.* **155**, 797–808.

Joiner, K.A., Hammer, C.H., Brown, E.J. and Frank, M.M. (1982b). Studies on the mechanism of bacterial resistance to complement-mediated killing. II. C8 and C9 release C5b67 from the surface of *Salmonella minnesota* S218 because the terminal complex does not insert into the bacterial outer membrane. *J. Exp. Med.* **155**, 809–19.

Joiner, K.A., Goldman, R., Schmetz, M. *et al.* (1984). A quantitative analysis of C3 binding to O-antigen capsule, lipopolysaccharide, and outer membrane protein of *E. coli* 0111B4. *J. Immunol.* **132**, 369–75.

Joiner, K.A., Schmetz, M.A., Sanders, M.E., Murray, T.G., Hammer, C.H. and Dourmashkin, R. (1985). Multimeric complement component C9 is necessary for killing of *Escherichia coli* J5 by terminal attack complex C5b–9. *Proc. Nat. Acad. Sci. (USA)* **82**, 4808–12.

Joiner, K.A., Grossman, N., Schmetz, M. and Leive, L. (1986). C3 binds preferentially to long-chain lipopolysaccharide during alternative pathway activation by *Salmonella montevideo*. *J. Immunol.* **136**, 710–15.

Kabat, E.A. (1961). Inhibition reactions. In *Experimental Immunochemistry*, 2nd edn, ed. E.A. Kabat and M.M. Mayer, pp. 241–67, Charles C. Thomas, Springfield, Illinois.

Kabat, E.A., Liao, J., Osserman, E.F., Gamian, A., Michon, F. and Jennings, H.J. (1988). The epitope associated with the binding of the capsular polysaccharide of group B meningococcus and of *Escherichia coli* K1 to a human monoclonal macroglobulin, IgM^{NOV}. *J. Exp. Med.* **168**, 699–711.

Kasper, D.L., Winkelhake, J.L., Zollinger, W.D., Brandt, B.L. and Artenstein, M.S. (1973). Immunochemical similarity between polysaccharide antigens of *Escherichia coli* O7:K1(L):NM and group B *Neisseria meningitidis*. *J. Immunol.* **110**, 262–8.

Kaufmann, F. (1966). *The Bacteriology of Enterobacteriaceae*. Williams & Wilkins, Baltimore.

Kawasaki, N., Kawasaki, T. and Yamashura, I. (1983). Isolation and characterization of a mannose-binding protein from human serum. *J. Biochem.* **94**, 937–47.

Kawasaki, T., Eton, R. and Yamashura, I. (1978). Isolation and characterization of a mannose-binding protein from rabbit liver. *Biochem. Biophys. Res. Commun.* **81**, 1018–24.

Killian, M., Mestecky, J. and Schrohenloher, R.E. (1979). Pathogenic species of the genus *Haemophilus* and *Streptococcus pneumoniae* produce immunoglobulin A1 protease. *Infect. Immunity* **26**, 143–9.

Kuhlman, M., Joiner, K. and Ezekowitz, R.A. (1989). The human mannose-binding protein functions as an opsonin. *J. Exp. Med.* **169**, 1733–45.

Lancefield, R.C. (1962). Current knowledge of type-specific M antigen of group A streptococci. *J. Immunol.* **89**, 307–13.

Lane, B.C., Kan-Mitchell, J., Mithcell, M.S. and Cooper, S.M. (1980). Structural evidence for distinct IgG subclass-specific Fc receptors on mouse peritoneal macrophages. *J. Exp. Med.* **152**, 1147–61.

Lee, J.C., Betley, M.J., Hopkins, C.A., Perez, N.E. and Pier, G.B. (1987). Virulence studies, in mice, of transposon-induced mutants of *Staphylococcus aureus* differing in capsule size. *J. Infect. Dis.* **156**, 741–50.

Lee, T.J., Utsinger, P.D., Snyderman, R., Yount, W.J. and Sparling, P.F. (1978). Familial deficiency of the seventh component of complement associated with recurrent bacteremic infections due to *Neisseria*. *J. Infect. Dis.* **138**, 359–68.

Leffell, M.S. and Spitznagel, J.K. (1975). Fate of human lactoferrin and myeloperoxidase in phagocytizing human neutrophils: effects of immunoglobulin G subclasses and immune complexes coated on latex beads. *Infect. Immunity* **12**, 813–20.

Luderitz, O., Staub, A.M. and Westphal, O. (1966). Immunochemistry of O and R antigens of *Salmonella* and related *Enterobacteriaceae*. *Bacteriol. Rev.* **30**, 192–255.

Luderitz, O., Tanamoto, K., Galanos, C. *et al.* (1984). Lipopolysaccharides: structural principles and biologic activities. *Rev. Infect. Dis.* **6**, 428–31.

Lund, B., Lindberg, F., Marklund, B.I. and Normark, S. (1987). The pap O protein is the α-D-galactopyranosyl (1→4)-β-D-galactopyranose-binding adhesin of uropathogenic *Escherichia coli*. *Proc. Nat. Acad. Sci. (USA)* **84**, 5898–902.

McCarty, M. (1982). Historical perspectives on C-reactive protein, in C-reactive protein and the plasma protein response to tissue injury. *Ann. NY Acad. Sci.* **389**, 1–10.

MacRae, E.K., Pryzwansky, K.B., Cooney, M.H. and Spitznagel, J.K. (1980). Scanning electron microscopic observations of early stages of phagocytosis of *E. coli* by human neutrophils. *Cell Tissue Res.* **209**, 65–70.

Malbran, A., Frank, M.M. and Fries, L.F. (1987). Interactions of monomeric IgG bearing covalently bound C3b with polymorphonuclear leucocytes. *Immunology* **61**, 15–20.

Mandell, G.L. (1975). Catalase, superoxide dismutase, and virulence of *Staphylococcus aureus*. *In vitro* and *in vivo* studies with emphasis on staphylococcal–leukocyte interaction. *J. Clin. Invest.* **55**, 561–6.

Markham, R.B., Pier, G.B., Goelliner, J.J. and Mizel, S.B. (1985). *In vitro* T cell-mediated killing of *Pseudomonas aeruginosa* II: the role of macrophages and T cell subsets in T cell killing. *J. Immunol.* **134**, 4112–17.

Moch, T., Hoschützky, H., Hacker, J., Kröncke, K.D. and Jann, K. (1987). Isolation and characterization of the α-sialyl-β-2,3-galactosyl-specific adhesin from fimbriated *Escherichia coli*. *Proc. Nat. Acad. Sci. (USA)* **84**, 3462–6.

Mold, C., Nakayama, S., Holzer, T.J., Gewurz, H. and Du Clos, T.W. (1981). C-reactive protein is protective against *Streptococcus pneumoniae* infections in mice. *J. Exp. Med.* **154**, 1703–8.

Myhre, E.B. and Kuusela, P. (1983). Binding of human fibronectin to group A, C and G streptococci. *Infect. Immunity* **40**, 29–34.

Nicholson, A. and Lepow, I.H. (1979). Host defense against *Neisseria meningitidis* requires a complement dependent bactericidal activity. *Science* **205**, 298–9.

O'Hanley, P., Lark, D., Falkow, S. and Schoolnik, G. (1985). Molecular basis of *Escherichia coli* colonization of the upper urinary tract in BALB/c- mice. *J. Clin. Invest.* **75**, 347–60.

Onderdonk, A.B., Markham, R.B., Zaleznik, D.F., Cisneros, R.L. and Kasper, D.L. (1982). Evidence for T cell-dependent immunity to *Bacteroides fragilis* in an intraabdominal abscess model. *J. Clin. Invest.* **69**, 9–16.

Pangburn, M.K. and Muller-Eberhard, H.J. (1978). Complement C3 convertase: cell surface restriction of B1H control and generation of restriction on neuraminidase-treated cells. *Proc. Nat. Acad. Sci. (USA)* **75**, 2416–20.

Pangburn, M.K., Morrison, D.C., Schreiber, R.D. and Muller-Eberhard, H.J. (1980). Activation of the alternative complement pathway: recognition of surface structures on activators by bound C3b. *J. Immunol.* **124**, 977–82.

Peterson, P.K., Verhoef, J., Sabath, L.K. and Quie, P.G. (1977). Effect of protein A on staphylococcal opsonization. *Infect. Immunity* **15**, 760–4.

Pillemer, L., Schoenberg, M.D., Blum, L. and Wurz, L. (1955). Properdin system and immunity. II. Interaction of the properdin system with polysaccharides. *Science* **122**, 545–9.

Plaut, A.G., Gilbert, J.V., Artenstein, M.S. and Capra, J.D. (1975). *Neisseria gonorrhoeae* and *Neisseria meningitidis*: extracellular enzyme cleaves human immunoglobulin A. *Science* **190**, 1103–5.

Pryzwansky, K.B., MacRae, E.K., Spitznagel, J.K. and Cooney, M.H. (1979). Early degranulation of human neutrophils: immunocytochemical studies of surface and intracellular phagocytic events. *Cell* **18**, 1025–33.

Pryzwansky, K.B., Steiner, A.L., Spitznagel, J.K. and Kaspoor, C.L. (1981). Compartmentalization of cyclic AMP during phagocytosis by human neutrophilic granulocytes. *Science* **211**, 407–10.

Rest, R.F., Cooney, M.H. and Spitznagel, J.K. (1978). Bactericidal activity of specific and azurophil granules from human neutrophils: studies with outer membrane mutants of *Salmonella typhimurium* LT-2. *Infect. Immunity* **19**, 131–7.

Robbins, J.B. (1978). Vaccines for the prevention of encapsulated bacterial diseases: current status, problems and prospects for the future. *Immunochemistry* **15**, 839–54.

Robbins, J.B., Parke, J.C., Jr, Schneerson, R. and Whisnant, J.K. (1973). Quantitative measurement of 'natural' and immunization-induced *Haemophilus influenzae* type b capsular polysaccharide antibodies. *Pediatr. Res.* **7**, 103–10.

Rogers, D.E. (1960). Host mechanisms which act to remove bacteria from the bloodstream. *Bacteriol. Rev.* **24**, 50–66.

Schmidt, M.A., O'Hanley, P., Lark, D. and Schoolnik, G.K. (1988). Synthetic peptides corresponding to protective epitopes of *Escherichia coli* digalactoside-binding pilin prevent infection in a murine pyelonephritis model. *Proc. Nat. Acad. Sci. (USA)* **85**, 1247–51.

Scribner, D.J. and Fahrney, D. (1976). Neutrophil receptors for

IgG and complement: their roles in the attachment and ingestion phases of phagocytosis. *J. Immunol.* **116**, 892–7.

Sharon, E., Kabat, E.A. and Morrison, S.L. (1982). Immunochemical characterization of binding sites of hybridoma antibodies specific for α(1→6) linked dextran. *Mol. Immunol.* **19**, 375–88.

Spitznagel, J.K. (1983). Microbial interactions with neutrophils. *Rev. Infect. Dis.* 5 (S4), S806–S822.

Sung, S.S., Nelson, R.S. and Silverstein, S.C. (1983). Yeast mannan inhibit binding and phagocytosis of zymosan by mouse peritoneal macrophages. *J. Cell Biol.* **96**, 160–6.

Taylor, P.W. (1983). Bactericidal and bacteriolytic activity of serum against gram-negative bacteria. *Microbiol. Rev.* **47**, 46–83.

Unkeless, J.C. (1977). The presence of two Fc receptors on mouse macrophages: evidence from a variant cell line and differential trypsin sensitivity. *J. Exp. Med.* **145**, 931–45.

Van Dijk, W.C., Verbrugh, H.A., van der Tol, M.E., Peters, R. and Verhoef, J. (1977). Role of *Escherichia coli* K capsular antigens during complement activation, C3 fixation and opsonization. *Infect. Immunity* **25**, 603–9.

Verbrugh, H.A., Van Dijk, W.C., Peters, R. *et al.* (1980). Opsonic recognition of staphylococci mediated by cell wall peptidoglycan: antibody independent activation of human complement and opsonic activity of peptidoglycan antibodies. *J. Immunol.* **124**, 1167–73.

Weis, J.J., Law, S.K., Levine, R.P. and Cleary, P.P. (1985). Resistance to phagocytosis by group A streptococci: failure of deposited complement opsonins to interact with cellular receptors. *J. Immunol.* **134**, 500–5.

Wessels, M.R. and Kasper, D.L. (1989). Antibody recognition of the type 14 pneumococcal capsule: evidence for a conformational epitope in a neutral polysaccharide. *J. Exp. Med.* **169**, 2121–31.

Wessels, M.R., Pozsgay, V., Kasper, D.L. and Jennings, H.J. (1987a). Structure and immunochemistry of an oligosaccharide repeating unit of the capsular polysaccharide of type III group B *Streptococcus*: a revised structure for the type III group B streptococcal polysaccharide antigen. *J. Biol. Chem.* **262**, 8262–7.

Wessels, M.R., Muños, A. and Kasper, D.L. (1987b). A model of high-affinity antibody binding to type III group B *Streptococcus* capsular polysaccharide. *Proc. Nat. Acad. Sci. (USA)* **84**, 9170–4.

Wilkinson, B.J., Sisson, S.P., Kim, Y. and Peterson, P.K. (1979). Localization of the third component of complement on the cell wall of encapsulated *Staphylococcus aureus*: implications for the mechanisms of resistance to phagocytosis. *Infect. Immunity* **26**, 1159–63.

Winkelstein, J.A. and Tomasz, A. (1977). Activation of the alternative pathway by pneumococcal cell walls. *J. Immunol.* **118**, 451–4.

Winkelstein, J.A., Abramanovitz, A.S., Tomasz, A. (1980). Activation of C3 via the alternative complement pathway results in fixation of C3b to the pneumococcal cell wall. *J. Immunol.* **24**, 2502–6.

Wyle, F.A., Artenstein, M.S., Brandt, B.L. *et al.* (1972). Immunogenic responses of man to group B meningococcal polysaccharide vaccines. *J. Infect. Dis.* **126**, 514–22.

Yother, J., Volanakis, J.E., Briles, D.E. (1982). Human C-reactive protein is protective against fatal *Streptococcus pneumoniae* infections in mice. *J. Immunol.* **128**, 2374–5.

Zaleznik, D.F., Finberg, R.W., Shapiro, M.E., Onderdonk, A.B. and Kasper, D.L. (1985). A soluble suppressor T cell factor protects against experimental intraabdominal abscesses. *J. Clin. Invest.* **75**, 1023–7.

Zucker-Franklin, D. and Hirsch, J.G. (1964). Electron microscope studies on the degranulation of rabbit peritoneal leukocytes during phagocytosis. *J. Exp. Med.* **120**, 569–75.

75: Gram-negative Shock

J. Cohen

Clinical aspects

Shock is a familiar concept to clinicians but it is difficult to define. It is best thought of as a syndrome due to prolonged tissue hypoperfusion, and is characterized by hypotension, hypoxia, oliguria and microvascular abnormalities. Shock can result from severe haemorrhage, from major cardiovascular insults such as myocardial infarction and pulmonary embolus, from anaphylaxis and as a complication of serious sepsis. Traditionally, 'septic shock' has been used as a synonym for shock associated with Gram-negative bacteraemia, even though many organisms can induce a shock-like state (Table 75.1). Indeed, it is now becoming clear that in many of these infections the underlying mechanisms are remarkably similar, irrespective of whether the inciting cause is bacterial, viral or protozoal. Nevertheless, it is Gram-negative shock which has been studied most intensively and will be the subject of this chapter.

Epidemiological studies from the UK and elsewhere show that Gram-negative organisms account for approximately half of all bacteraemic isolates (Bryan *et al.* 1983; Eliasen *et al.* 1986; Forgacs *et al.* 1986; Ispahani *et al.* 1987). Of these, *Escherichia coli* constitute about 50%, *Haemophilus influenzae* and *Pseudomonas aeruginosa* represent 5–10% each, and the remainder are a variety of common coliform bacteria. The overall mortality associated with Gram-negative bacteraemia is of the order of 20%, but this figure is influenced by factors such as age, the nature of the underlying disease, the use of appropriate antibiotics and the presence of shock (Kreger *et al.* 1980). The true incidence of shock is uncertain; as noted above,

Table 75.1. Infections that may cause a syndrome of septic shock

Gram-negative bacteria	Coliforms, e.g. *Escherichia coli*; *Pseudomonas aeruginosa*; cholera; typhoid; plague
Gram-positive bacteria	*Staphylococcus aureus*; *Clostridia*; *Streptococcus pneumoniae*; diphtheria
Spirochaetes	Syphilis; relapsing fever; Jarisch–Herxheimer reaction
Rickettsia	Rocky Mountain spotted fever; louse-borne typhus
Viruses	Haemorrhagic fevers; Coxsackie B
Fungi	*Candida* spp.; *Aspergillus*?
Parasites	Malaria; trypanosomiasis

there is no universally accepted definition, and it will depend a good deal on the nature of the patient population and the institution at which the study was done. However, most series report an incidence of 20–40%, and in these patients the mortality is 75% or more. It is of note that this figure has changed little during the last 20 years, despite the introduction of intensive care units and many new and 'more powerful' antibiotics (Sanford 1985).

Conventional management of the shocked patient includes the use of oxygen and broad-spectrum antibiotics, fluid replacement and, if necessary, inotropes. This treatment, while valuable, is limited because it does little to prevent the toxin-mediated injury which underlies the syndrome of Gram-negative shock. The toxin concerned is endotoxin (also called lipopolysaccharide, LPS), and in recent years much has been learnt of its biochemistry and its role in initiating septic shock.

Endotoxin

Biochemistry

The endotoxin molecule is situated in the outer part of the cell wall of Gram-negative bacteria, external to the peptidoglycan layer which provides the mechanical rigidity of the cell (Fig. 75.1). Endotoxin has three components (Fig. 75.2). The outermost, the O-specific polysaccharide, consists of repeating units of polysaccharides, each comprising between three and five sugar residues. Their sugar composition and linkage patterns differ from strain to strain, the details having been the subject of intense investigation (Jann and Jann 1984). The reasons for this interest are threefold: firstly, the precise configuration of the O chain confers serotypic specificity upon a particular strain, and is the basis of the taxonomic identification of many common Gram-negative bacteria (the Kaufmann–White scheme). Secondly, antibodies to the O chain provide type-specific protection in animal models of infection (see below).

Internal to the O chain is the core region, a hetero-oligosaccharide which is itself divided into two components. The outer core contains common sugars such as D-glucose, D-galactose, and *N*-acetyl-D-glucosamine. In contrast, in the inner core there are two unusual sugars, heptose and KDO (3-deoxy-D-*manno*-2-octulosonic acid), as well as charged residues such as phosphate and ethanolamine. Whereas there are many hundreds of different O chains, the structure of the core is more conserved; all *Salmonella* species, for instance, have the same core structure, and amongst *E. coli* there are just six minor variations.

A number of cell wall-deficient mutant strains of Gram-negative bacteria have been important tools in studying host responses to endotoxin. These strains have lost the entire O side-chain and varying parts of the core. They are known as rough, or R, strains because of their colonial morphology on agar; they look dry and wrinkled in contrast to the smooth, glistening appearance of the intact parent strain. Rough mutants are labelled Ra to Re depending on the extent of the deletion (Fig. 75.3)

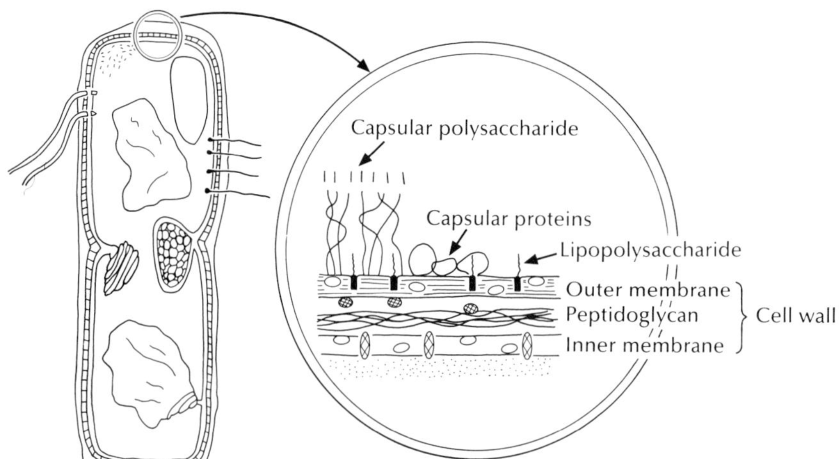

Fig. 75.1. The general structure of endotoxin in relation to the bacterial cell wall.

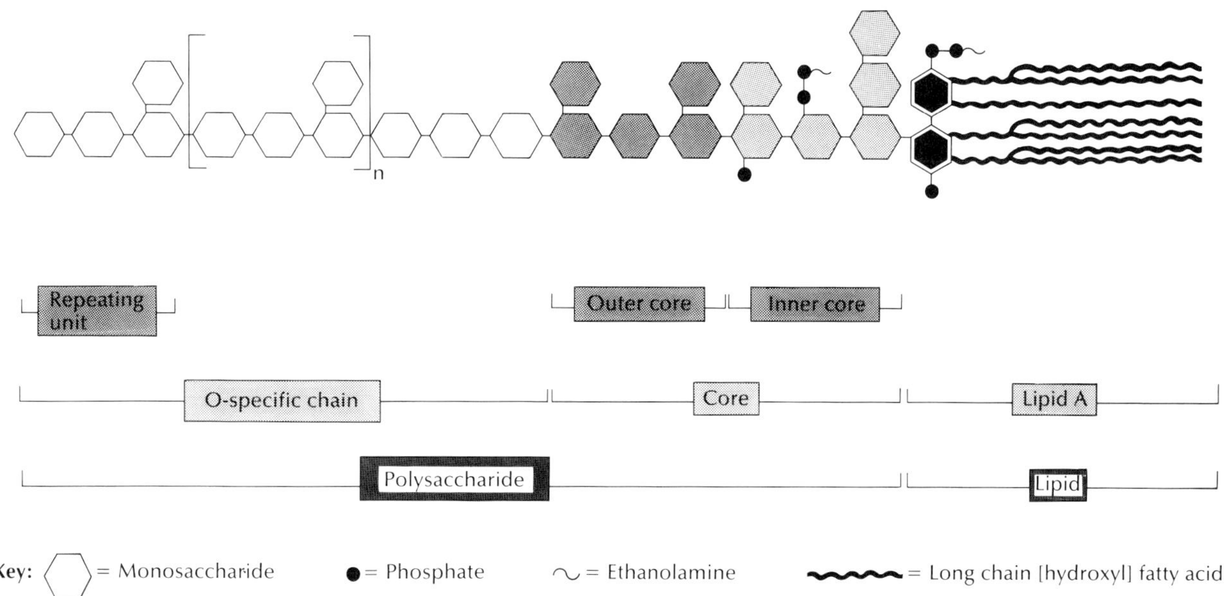

Fig. 75.2. The biochemical structure of endotoxin (lipopolysaccharide), illustrating its tripartite nature.

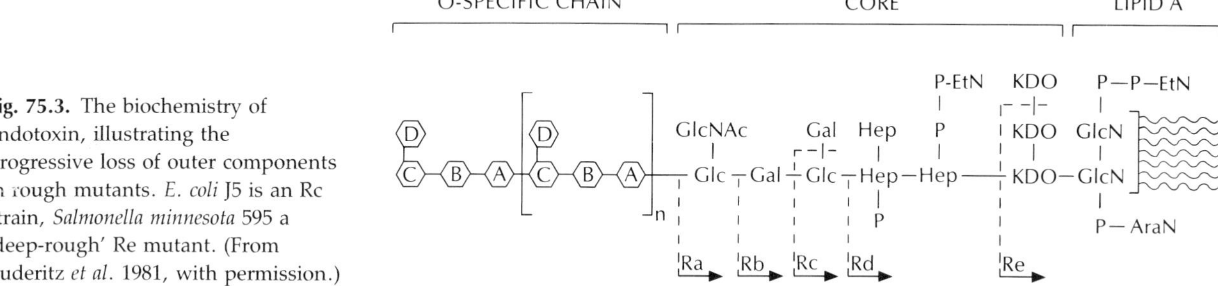

Fig. 75.3. The biochemistry of endotoxin, illustrating the progressive loss of outer components in rough mutants. *E. coli* J5 is an Rc strain, *Salmonella minnesota* 595 a 'deep-rough' Re mutant. (From Luderitz *et al.* 1981, with permission.)

Two such strains have been studied extensively, *E. coli* J5 (Rc) and *Salmonella minnesota* R595 (Re) (see below).

The innermost domain of endotoxin is lipid A. It is a β-1.6-linked D-glucosamine carrying two phosphoryl groups. This hydrophilic backbone is substituted by at least five acyl residues, of which at least one must be a 3-acyloxyacyl group. This model of the structure of lipid A was first developed from conventional biochemical studies, but has recently been confirmed by its complete *de novo* biosynthesis (Rietschel *et al.* 1987). Studies of both natural and synthetic lipid A have shown that it is the site of virtually all the biological properties attributed to endotoxin, and experiments with several precursor molecules have given some insight into structure–function relationships (Brade *et al.* 1988). It is particularly interesting that lipid A is highly conserved amongst Gram-negative bacteria, explaining why the clinical features of Gram-negative shock are the same, irrespective of whether the infection is due to *E. coli* or *Pseudomonas aeruginosa*.

Immunology

A comprehensive account of the immunology of endotoxin is beyond the scope of this chapter. The following section describes those aspects that have particular relevance to septic shock.

IMMUNOGENETICS

The fact that strains of mice differed in their response to endotoxin was first noted more than 40 years ago, but work on the genetic control of endotoxin responsiveness had to wait till 20 years later when it was shown that C3H/HeJ mice were highly resistant to endotoxin lethality (Sultzer 1968). Classical genetic studies indicated that this resistance was attributable to a single, autosomal dominant gene (now designated *Lps*) located on chromosome 4. Hence C3H/HeJ mice carry the defective allele, Lps^d.

The consequences of bearing the defective allele are considerably broader than simply resistance to mortality; virtually every biological response to endotoxin is modified. These responses include the induction of inflammation, tumour necrosis, tolerance, adjuvanticity and so on. A curious observation is that C3H/HeJ mice have an increased susceptibility to infection with live Gram-negative bacteria, probably a reflection of the fact that the Lps^d gene confers a much wider abnormality in immune responsiveness than simply resistance to endotoxin (Michalek *et al*. 1980)

The consequences of bearing the Lps^d gene are not yet known in detail. Nevertheless it is clear that the defect in C3H/HeJ mice is a failure to respond in particular to the lipid A component of endotoxin. Proposed mechanisms include a failure to process lipid A into a suitable form (Vogel *et al*. 1984) and/or an inability to recognize it at the cell membrane.

EFFECTS ON LYMPHORETICULAR CELLS

Intravenous injection of endotoxin induces a lymphopenia which persists for about 5 hours in man and rather longer in rats. No particular subset of cells is particularly susceptible (Cohen *et al*. 1987). *In vitro*, all three cell types — B cells, T cells and macrophages — can be affected by endotoxin to a varying degree. The most unambiguous effects are on B cells, which undergo antigen-independent proliferative and differentiation responses upon exposure to endotoxin (Morrison and Ryan 1979). The fact that endotoxin is a polyclonal B cell activator needs to be remembered when interpreting serological responses in ill patients; unexpectedly high titres in diagnostic tests may simply be a non-specific response to gut-derived endotoxin.

The interaction of endotoxin with T cells is more complex; studies in C3H/HeJ mice have been particularly helpful in demonstrating that LPS-induced adjuvanticity is T cell-dependent (Michalek *et al*. 1980), and both Mita *et al*. (1982) and Vogel *et al*. (1982) have shown that endotoxin is directly mitogenic for a small proportion of splenic T cells. Perhaps of greater practical importance is the finding that B cells stimulated with tiny doses of endotoxin can have a marked effect on T cell proliferation (Forbes *et al*. 1975); an interaction of this kind has been proposed as the basis for the role of endotoxin in the graft-versus-host reaction (Moore *et al*. 1987).

Macrophages activated by endotoxin are altered both morphologically and functionally, and the consequences are profound. Monokine production, prostaglandin secretion, glucose metabolism, phagocytosis and tumour cytotoxicity are all affected (Morrison and Ryan 1979). Interestingly, high concentrations of LPS are toxic to macrophages; cells from C3H/HeJ mice are resistant to this effect.

EFFECTS ON NEUTROPHILS

That endotoxin exerts an effect on neutrophils is apparent from the profound neutropenia that follows within an hour of the intravenous injection of LPS. This neutropenia is due largely to leucoagglutination and margination of the circulating pool, and is transient; it is followed within 2–3 hours by a neutrophilia caused by both increased myelopoiesis and release of granulocytes from the marrow (Proctor 1985).

Endotoxin can also influence many of the functional properties of neutrophils. The generation of the complement fragment C5a (see below) is probably the major mechanism influencing chemotaxis, although there is some evidence to suggest that there is an additional, complement-independent mechanism dependent on release of lactoferrin (Oseas *et al*. 1981). Confusingly, endotoxin can also directly inhibit chemotaxis, as well as stimulating adherence (Wilson 1985). Of the other major properties of neutrophils, phagocytosis is probably uninfluenced by LPS, while the effects on bactericidal activity are complex. There is no direct evidence that endotoxin causes lysosomal degranulation; however, several metabolic processes are enhanced. Nitroblue tetrazolium dye reduction is increased, as is hexose monophosphate shunt activity. Demonstration of enhanced production of reactive oxygen intermediates is dependent on the experimental conditions, and requires the cells to be adherent (Wilson 1985). The confusing and at times contradictory results that are obtained when neutrophils are studied in isolation illustrates the difficulty of extrapolating these findings to the *in vivo* situation of inflammation, in which humoral factors — notably complement, interleukin 1 (IL-1) and tumour necrosis factor — play a dominant role (see below and Movat *et al.* 1987).

An additional interaction between neutrophils and endotoxin, which has only recently been identified, concerns a 50 kD (rabbit) or 60 kD (human) protein called bactericidal/permeability binding protein (BPI). It is tightly bound to the membranes of myeloperoxidase containing primary granules, binds avidly to LPS and rapidly kills Gram-negative bacteria. Sequence data revealed marked homology with an acute-phase protein called LBP (lipopolysaccharide-binding protein), and suggested that there may be a family of such proteins involved in host defences against Gram-negative infection (Tobias *et al.* 1988).

COMPLEMENT

In a series of experiments using LPS of defined biochemical structure, Galanos *et al.* (1971), Morrison and Kline (1977) and others showed that endotoxin could activate complement by three different mechanisms, namely: antibody-independent activation of C1 by lipid A, direct activation of the alternative pathway by core glycolipid, and antibody-dependent classical pathway activation by the O polysaccharide.

There is little doubt that septic shock is accompanied by complement activation; it is less clear if this activation is a requirement for the development of any or all of the pathological features of shock (McPhaden and Whaley 1985). McCabe (1973) has shown that, in man, serum complement levels correlate with outcome from shock but data from experimental animals have produced somewhat conflicting results. Spink *et al.* (1964) carried out important early work in dogs which established a relationship between lethality and the degree of hypocomplementaemia. Later studies used dogs complement-depleted with cobra venom factor (CVF). From *et al.* (1970) found that this had a modest effect on LPS-induced hypotension but no effect on mortality. Experiments in C6-deficient rabbits have given divergent results: Brown and Lachmann (1971) finding the complement deficient animals partially protected, and Johnson and Ward (1971) the reverse. In C4-deficient guinea pigs, May *et al.* (1972) indicated that complement might actually be protective — the complement-intact animals had a lower mortality. In contrast, in dogs Garner *et al.* (1974) demonstrated a marked protective effect of complement depletion. Such apparently conflicting results may be explained in part on the basis of interspecies differences, but it is likely that it also accurately reflects a rather complex situation in which the net effect of complement depletion can indeed vary in different experimental conditions. See also Chapter 67 for further discussion on complement deficiencies and endotoxin shock.

A related area in which complement appears to play a critical role is that of acute lung injury (adult respiratory distress syndrome, ARDS). This syndrome is a common accompaniment to septic shock; injury is mediated by free oxygen radicals and is dependent on both complement and neutrophils, and endotoxin is a potent inducer of injury (Meyrick 1986; Till and Ward 1986; Worthen *et al.* 1986).

TOLERANCE

The use of the term tolerance in relation to endotoxin requires some explanation, since it is used in two rather separate ways. Firstly, endotoxin can influence conventional immunological tolerance. Claman (1963) first showed that, in mice, endotoxin could abrogate the development of tolerance to a foreign antigen, in this case bovine γ-globulin. Others have reported similar results (reviewed in Morrison and Ryan 1979), although the cellular basis of this response remains elusive. Another facet of 'classical' tolerance is the ability to generate antibodies against self, and Fournie *et al.* (1974) have reported that mice injected with deoxyribonucleic acid (DNA) and endotoxin produced enhanced levels of anti-DNA.

The second application of tolerance is in relation to endotoxin itself. It has been known for a long time that responses to most of the biological properties of endotoxin (pyrogenicity, lethality, tumour necrosis, etc.) decrease progressively upon repeated administration of suitably timed doses of LPS. Endotoxin tolerance develops in two stages. Early-phase tolerance develops within a few hours of the challenge and lasts no more than 48 hours. It is independent of the source of the endotoxin, i.e. it is dependent on lipid A (Egawa *et al.* 1984). In contrast, late-phase tolerance begins on the fourth or fifth day, is transferable with serum and demonstrates marked O specificity (Johnston and Greisman 1985). Endotoxin tolerance has been of importance for two reasons: it underlies attempts to develop immunotherapeutic approaches to septic shock (see below), and it has caused considerable difficulties in interpreting the results of experimental studies of shock, since even tiny amounts of endotoxin contaminating, say, a monoclonal antibody can induce tolerance and hence 'spurious' protection (Woods *et al.* 1987).

Immunopathology

The general aspects of immune responses to Gram-negative bacteria are considered in Chapter 74; the following section is concerned specifically with host defences to LPS and the mechanisms of endotoxin-induced shock.

Host defences against endotoxin

Several different detoxification mechanisms have evolved to deal with the removal of the small amount of endotoxin that periodically leaks into the circulation from the gut.

A bolus injection of endotoxin is cleared from the circulation in two phases, the first lasting 15–60 minutes and accounting for about 50% of the injected dose. This is accompanied by the appearance of endotoxin in the cells of the fixed reticuloendothelial system, primarily liver and spleen. (A small amount is found in lung and kidneys; none enters the brain.) Endotoxin is processed in Kupffer cells and passes to hepatocytes and then to the bile ducts to be excreted via the gut. In hepatic failure, endotoxin overflow into the systemic circulation becomes an important consideration (Liehr 1980). In contrast, the liver plays a less important role in the detoxification of massive amounts of endotoxin, as occurs in septic shock. This is because the inevitable hypotension causes shunting of blood away from the splanchnic bed.

The second, slow phase of elimination lasts many hours, and is attributable to binding of LPS to high-density lipoproteins (HDL) (Tobias *et al.* 1985), which act as scavengers. In addition serum seems to possess other proteins and/or enzymes with the ability to bind endotoxin. These include the LPS-binding proteins LBP and BPI (see above), but others are poorly characterized (Skarnes 1985). The final important component of host defence is antibody.

The role of antibody

Several studies have found that antibody titres to various components of Gram-negative bacteria are correlated with outcome from septicaemia. Zinner and McCabe (1976) showed that the presence of a high titre of immunoglobulin G (IgG) antibody to the O-specific side-chain of the infecting strain significantly reduced the incidence of shock and death. Furthermore both these workers and others (Pollack *et al.* 1983) found that antibody to core glycolipid also conferred protection; such antibody is of course not type-specific but is directed against the common endotoxin core, and should in theory be effective irrespective of the infecting strain.

The nature of the protection afforded by these antibodies is complex. Anti-O antibodies will induce complement-mediated lysis, but only in serum-sensitive isolates; since most bacteraemic strains are serum-resistant (Roantree and Rantz 1960), this is probably not an important mechanism at least in so far as septic shock is concerned. Anti-O antibodies are, however, effective opsonins (Young *et al.* 1975; Pudifin *et al.* 1985), but the role of anti-core antibodies in opsonization is less clear; most investigators agree that, at best, they are only weakly active (Young *et al.* 1975; Vreede *et al.* 1986). The means by which anti-core antibodies appear to protect experimental animals from shock and death (see below) is controversial. The most favoured hypothesis is that they act as antitoxins, binding to and neutralizing the biologically active LPS core, a concept that is supported by the fact that IgM antibodies are the most effective (McCutchan and Ziegler 1983). For this to be true it requires that the antibodies gain access to the core structures which are normally concealed beneath the O side-chain (Fig. 75.2), or that they act on free endotoxin released during cell division or by the action of antibiotics (Andersen and Solberg 1978; Cohen and McConnell 1986). More recent experiments using monoclonal antibodies to core determinants have produced conflicting results (see below), and it is still unclear whether the protection observed by some with anti-core antibodies is indeed due to a specific immunological mechanism.

Mediators of endotoxicity

The complex pathological events that occur in septic shock are not caused by endotoxin *per se*, but rather by a series of mediators, each of which contributes some part of the overall clinical picture. Many such mediators have been identified: they include arachidonic acid metabolites, components of the coagulation cascade, endorphins and complement (Table 75.2). A detailed description of the part played by each is beyond the scope of this chapter; further information is available in the references given in the table. In general, although there is evidence that these mediator systems are indeed activated in septic shock, none are alone responsible for all the clinical features, and in many cases attempts to intervene with neutralizing or blocking agents have not been successful.

From the point of view of the immunologist, the greatest interest has been in the part played by lymphokines as mediators of shock. The more familiar function of lymphokines in immunoregulation is well established (see Chapters 14–17), but it has become clear that they are also closely involved in several of the pathological aspects of shock. Most attention has focused on tumour necrosis factor (TNF, also called cachectin).

Adoptive transfer experiments with endotoxin-resistant C3H/HeJ mice and the congenic sensitive C3H/HeN strain had implicated macrophages as the source of this resistance. It was known that macrophages produced copious amounts of TNF in response to endotoxin, and Beutler and co-workers suggested that TNF might be a mediator of endotoxin lethality. They showed that mice could be protected from LPS-induced injury by a polyclonal antibody to murine TNF (Beutler *et al.* 1985), and that mice given TNF in appropriate doses developed shock and tissue injury similar to that seen after endotoxin (Tracey *et al.* 1986). Subsequently the *in vivo* effects of TNF and its relationship to endotoxin-induced injury were described in more detail (Remick *et al.* 1987; Mathison *et al.* 1988), confirming that TNF does indeed appear to mediate many of the metabolic, haematological and pathological features of septic shock. Extending these findings to man, Michie and co-workers showed that when endotoxin was given to healthy volunteers the onset of symptoms coincided with the appearance of TNF in the circulation (Michie *et al.* 1988), and several studies have shown that serum TNF levels are elevated in patients with Gram-negative septicaemia (Waage *et al.* 1987; Girardin *et al.* 1988).

Table 75.2. Mediators of septic shock

Mediators	Reference
Complement	McPhaden and Whaley 1985
Cytokines	See text
Endorphins	Faden and Holaday 1980
Platelet-activating factor	Braquet *et al.* 1987
Prostaglandins	Jacobs 1985
Reactive oxygen intermediates	Cochrane 1985
Coagulation cascade	Coleman 1987

However, the idea that TNF was perhaps the single, primary mediator of endotoxin-induced injury proved to be over-optimistic. The close and frequently overlapping properties of TNF and the other monokines, especially IL-1 (Le and Vilcek 1987), extends to their role in shock. As well as IL-1 (Okusawa *et al.* 1988), there is evidence that interferon gamma (IFN-γ) (Kawasaki *et al.* 1987) and IL-2 (Chong 1987; Weyand *et al.* 1987) also participate, and it is likely that others, notably IL-6, will also be implicated. There are also some curious inconsistencies in the 'TNF hypothesis'. Rothstein and Schreiber (1988) have shown that TNF alone was of low toxicity for normal mice, but caused lethal shock if given with nanogram amounts of endotoxin. In a fascinating experiment, Kiener *et al.* (1988) used monophosphoryl lipid A (MPL), a non-toxic derivative of lipid A, and showed that, while both compounds induced macrophages to produce the same amount of TNF, the animals challenged with MPL survived while those given lipid A died.

In summary, endotoxin acts through mediators, of which there are many. Lymphokines, and especially TNF, are a critical component of the host response, but no single mediator appears to be solely responsible for all of the pathological features of septic shock.

Immunotherapy

Neutralization of endotoxin

The biochemical conservation of the structure of endotoxin suggested to several investigators the possibility of using neutralizing antibodies as treatment for septic shock. One strategy has been to make a polyclonal antibody in horses against a pool of common O antigens (Lachman *et al.* 1984). However, most work has been directed at the common core structure of endotoxin. This approach was made possible by taking advantage of cell wall-deficient mutants of Gram-negative bacteria in which endotoxin (LPS) was exposed on the cell surface. Two strains in particular were used, an Rc mutant of *E. coli* 0111 : B5 called the J5 strain, and an Re mutant of *Salmonella minnesota*, R595. It was reasoned that by immunizing rabbits with these bacteria it should be possible to make an antibody which could react with — and neutralize — endotoxin from any infecting strain. In a series of experiments, it was shown that these antibodies could protect experimental animals from challenge with LPS or live organisms, either the homologous immunizing strain or, most persuasively, a heterologous strain (Ziegler *et al.* 1973a, b). Further, anti-core antisera protected animals in both the dermal and generalized Shwartzmann phenomenon (Braude and Douglas 1972).

Based on these observations a clinical trial was done in which a human antiserum was made in volunteers immunized with boiled *E. coli* J5. In a large double-blind study, patients in septic shock received the J5 antiserum or preimmune serum as control, in addition to standard treatment (Ziegler *et al.* 1982). The results were impressive: in 212 bacteraemic patients the mortality in the J5 group was 22% compared with 39% in the controls. Moreover, in a subset of those with severe shock, the figures were 44% (J5) and 77% (controls). In a later study the same material was evaluated for prophylaxis, with the same favourable outcome (Baumgartner *et al.* 1985). One area for concern, though, was the subsequent finding that the protection seen in the J5-treated groups could not be attributed to higher antibody levels in the patients or the material given, leading to questions about the mechanism of the protection.

While these results were encouraging it was clearly impractical to use immunized volunteers as a regular source of antiserum. One way round this would be to use intravenous immunoglobulin (IVIG). Conventional IVIG contains measurable amounts of antibody to endotoxin (Stoll *et al.* 1987), but limited experience suggests that it is ineffective in shock (Baumgartner and Glauser 1987; Cohen 1988). An alternative is hyperimmune globulin, selected on the basis of high antibody titres to endotoxin core determinants, but a well-conducted study found that this too was of no benefit (Calandra *et al.* 1988). It is possible that the failure of IVIG (which is mostly IgG) reflects the importance of IgM as an antitoxin (see above).

Monoclonal antibodies were another means of ensuring adequate supplies, and large numbers of both murine and human monoclonals were produced. Despite the fact that many of these antibodies appeared to bind endotoxin *in vitro*, the results from animal protection studies have been variable, some antibodies giving protection, others not (Teng *et al.* 1985; Appelmelk *et al.* 1988; Dunn 1988; Greisman and Johnston 1988). This, taken with the failure of the IVIG studies and the worries surrounding the clinical studies, has led some to question the whole basis of the anti-endotoxin hypothesis (Ziegler 1988). Nevertheless, large scale clinical trials with monoclonal antibodies to endotoxin core have been done, and the results reported recently (Gorelick *et al.* 1990, Ziegler *et al.* 1991). Although both studies showed some benefit it was only seen in subgroups of patients, and doubts remain about the mode of action and clinical indications for these reagents (Cohen and Glauser 1991).

Neutralization of cytokines

The possible therapeutic role of antibodies to cytokines is still in its infancy, and most interest has centred on TNF. The experiments of Beutler *et al.* (1985) showed that mice could be protected from LPS by a polyclonal antiserum given before the challenge, and this was taken a step further when Tracey *et al.* (1987) demonstrated that Fab fragments of a murine monoclonal antibody against human recombinant TNF protected baboons from *E. coli*-induced shock. Here again benefit was shown only if the antibody was given before the challenge. However, using different antibodies, others have shown protection from *E. coli*-induced shock in mice (Silva *et al.* 1990) and LPS-induced injury in primates (Exley *et al.* 1989) with antibody given up to 45 minutes after challenge, indicating that clinical use could be feasible.

An attractive aspect of anti-TNF (rather than anti-endotoxin) is that it might be effective in infections due to Gram-positive as well as Gram-negative organisms, since at least in some cases the mediator systems seem to be the same (Yamamoto *et al.* 1986; Jupin *et al.* 1988). One of the concerns in using anti-TNF in man is the unknown effect of neutralizing a protein which under normal circumstances participates in host defences against infection (Parant *et al.* 1987). Nevertheless clinical trials have now begun (Exley *et al.* 1990) and it remains to be seen if the promise of therapeutic benefit in the short term outweighs the theoretical disadvantages.

References

Andersen, B.M. and Solberg, O. (1978). Liberation of endotoxin during growth of *Neisseria meningitidis* in chemically-defined medium. *Acta Pathol. Microbiol. Scand.* **86**, 275–81.

Appelmelk, B.J., Verweij-Van Vught, A.M., Maaskant, J.J. *et al.* (1988). Production and characterisation of mouse monoclonal antibodies reacting with the lipopolysaccharide core region of gram-negative bacilli. *J. Med. Microbiol.* **26**, 107–14.

Baumgartner, J.-D. and Glauser, M.P. (1987). Controversies in the use of passive immunotherapy for bacterial infections in the critically ill patient. *Rev. Infect. Dis.* **9**, 194–205.

Baumgartner, J.-D., Glauser, M.P., McCutchan, J.A. *et al.* (1985). Prevention of gram-negative shock and death in surgical patients by antibody to endotoxin core glycolipid. *Lancet* **ii**, 59–63.

Beutler, B., Milsark, I.W. and Cerami, A. (1985). Passive immunization against cachectin/tumor necrosis factor protects mice from lethal effect of endotoxin. *Science* **229**, 869–71.

Brade, H., Brade, L. and Rietschel, E.T. (1988). Structure–activity relationships of bacterial lipopolysaccharides (endotoxins). *Zentralbl. Bakteriol. Hyg. A* **268**, 151–79.

Braquet, P., Touqui, L., Shen, T.Y. and Vargaftig, B.B. (1987). Perspectives in platelet-activating factor research. *Pharmacol. Rev.* **39**, 98–137.

Braude, A.I. and Douglas, H. (1972). Passive immunization against the local Shwartzmann reaction. *J. Immunol.* **108**, 505–12.

Brown, D.L. and Lachmann, P.J. (1971). The behaviour of complement and platelets in lethal endotoxin shock in rabbits. *Int. Arch. Allergy Appl. Immunol.* **34**, 193.

Bryan, C.S., Reynolds, K.L. and Brenner, E.R. (1983). Analysis of 1,186 episodes of gram-negative bacteremia in non-university hospitals: the effects of antimicrobial therapy. *Rev. Infect. Dis.* **5**, 629–38.

Calandra, T., Glauser, M.P., Schellekens, J. *et al.* (1988). Treatment of gram-negative septic shock with human IgG antibody to *Escherichia coli* J5: a prospective double-blind randomized trial. *J. Infect. Dis.* **158**, 312–19.

Chong, K.-T. (1987). Prophylactic administration of interleukin-2 protects mice from lethal challenge with Gram-negative bacteria. *Infect. Immunity* **55**, 668–73.

Claman, H.N. (1963). Tolerance to a protein antigen in adult mice and the effect of nonspecific factors. *J. Immunol.* **91**, 833–9.

Cochrane, C.G. (1985). The contact system in septic shock. In *Pathophysiology of Endotoxin*, ed. L.B. Hinshaw, pp. 286–98, Elsevier, Amsterdam.

Cohen, J. (1988). Intravenous immunoglobulin (IVIG) for gram negative infection: a critical review. *J. Hosp. Infect.* **12** (suppl. D), 47–54.

Cohen, J. and McConnell, J.S. (1986). Release of endotoxin from bacteria exposed to ciprofloxacin and its prevention with Polymyxin B. *Eur. J. Clin. Microbiol.* **5**, 13–17.

Cohen J. and Glauser M.P. (1991). Septic shock: treatment. *Lancet* **338**, 736–9.

Cohen, J., Faulkner, L., Bowman, C., Green, C. and Aslam, M. (1987). The effect of endotoxin on peripheral blood lymphocytes in the rat. *J. Clin. Lab. Immunol.* **23**, 175–7

Coleman, R.W. (1987). The role of plasma proteases in septic shock. *N. Engl. J. Med.* **320**, 1207–9.

Dunn, D.L. (1988). Antibody immunotherapy of gram-negative bacterial sepsis in an immunosuppressed animal model. *Transplantation* **45**, 424–9.

Egawa, K., Yoshida, M., Sakaino, R. and Kasai, N. (1984). Hepatic drug-metabolizing enzyme system and endotoxin tolerance: structural requirement of LPS in induction of an early tolerance. *Microbiol. Immunol.* **28**, 1181–90.

Eliasen, K., Nielsen, P.B. and Espersen, F. (1986). A one-year survey of nosocomial bacteraemia at a Danish university hospital. *J. Hyg. (Cambridge)* **97**, 471–8.

Exley, A.R., Buurman, W., Bodmer, M. and Cohen, J. (1989). Monoclonal antibody to recombinant human tumour necrosis factor in the treatment and prophylaxis of endotoxic shock in Cynomolgus monkeys. *Clin. Sci.* **76**, 50.

Exley, A.R., Cohen, J., Buurman, W.A. *et al.* (1990) Monoclonal antibody to TNF in severe septic shock. *Lancet* **335**, 1275–7.

Faden, A.I. and Holaday, J.W. (1980). Experimental endotoxin shock: the pathophysiologic function of endorphins and treatment with opiate antagonists. *J. Infect. Dis.* **142**, 229–38.

Forbes, J.T., Nakao, Y. and Smith, R.T. (1975). T mitogens trigger LPS responsiveness in mouse thymus cells. *J. Immunol.* **114**, 1004–7.

Forgacs, I.C., Eykyn, S.J. and Bradley, R.D. (1986). Serious infection in the intensive therapy unit: a 15 year study of bacteraemia. *Quart. J. Med.* **60**, 773–9.

Fournie, G.J., Lambert, P.H. and Miescher, P.A. (1974). Release of DNA in circulating blood and induction of anti-DNA antibodies after injection of bacterial lipopolysaccharides. *J. Exp. Med.* **140**, 1189–206.

From, A.H., Gewurz, H., Gruniger, R.P., Pickering, R.J. and Spink, W.W. (1970). Complement in endotoxin shock: effect of complement depletion on the early hypotensive phase. *Infect. Immunity* **2**, 38–41.

Galanos, C., Riethschel, E.T., Luderitz, O. and Westphal, O. (1971), Interaction of lipopolysaccharides and lipid A with complement. *Eur. J. Biochem.* **19**, 143–52.

Garner, R., Chater, B.V. and Brown, D.L. (1974). The role of complement in endotoxin shock and disseminated intravascular coagulation: experimental observations in the dog. *Br. J. Haematol.* **28**, 393–401.

Gorelick, K., Scannan, P.J., Hannigan, J., Wedel, N. and Ackerman, S.K. (1990). Randomised placebo-controlled study of E5 monoclonal antiendotoxin antibody. In *Therapeutic Monoclonal Antibodies* eds C.A. Borrebaeck and J.W. Larrick, pp. 253–61, Stockton Press, New York.

Girardin, E., Grau, G., Dayer, J.-M., Roux-Lombard, P. and Lambert, P.-H. (1988). Tumor necrosis factor and interleukin-1 in the serum of children with severe infectious purpura. *N. Engl. J. Med.* **319**, 397–400.

Greisman, S.E. and Johnston, C.A. (1988). Failure of antisera to J5 and R595 rough mutants to reduce endotoxemic lethality. *J. Infect. Dis.* **157**, 54–64.

Ispahani, P., Pearson, N.J. and Greenwood, D. (1987). An analysis of community and hospital-acquired bacteraemia in a large teaching hospital in the United Kingdom. *Quart. J. Med.* **63**. 427–40.

Jacobs, E.R. (1985). Overview of mediators affecting pulmonary and systemic vascular changes in endotoxemia. In *Pathophysiology of Endotoxin*, ed. L.B. Hinshaw, pp. 1–15, Elsevier, Amsterdam.

Jann, K. and Jann, B. (1984). Structure and biosynthesis of O-antigens. In *Chemistry of Endotoxin*, ed. E.T. Rietschel, pp. 138–86 Elsevier, Amsterdam.

Johnston, C.A. and Greisman S.E. (1985). Mechanisms of endotoxin tolerance. In *Pathophysiology of Endotoxin*, ed. L.B. Hinshaw, pp. 359–402, Elsevier, Amsterdam.

Johnson, K.J. and Ward, P.A. (1971). Protective function of C6 in rabbits treated with bacterial endotoxin. *J. Immunol.* **106**, 1225–7.

Jupin, C., Anderson, S., Damais, C., Alouf, J.E. and Parant, M. (1988). Toxic shock syndrome toxin 1 as an inducer of human tumor necrosis factors and gamma interferon. *J. Exp. Med.* **167**, 752–61.

Kawasaki, H., Moriyama, M. and Tanaka, A. (1987). Augmentation of endotoxin fever by recombinant human beta interferon in rabbits. *Infect. Immunity* **55**, 1121–5.

Kiener, P.A., Marek, F., Rodgers, G., Lin, P.-F., Warr, G. and Desiderio, J. (1988), Induction of tumor necrosis factor, IFN-gamma, and acute lethality in mice by toxic and non-toxic forms of lipid A. *J. Immunol.* **141**, 870–4.

Kreger, B.E., Craven, D.E. and McCabe, W.R. (1980). Gram-negative bacteremia, IV. Re-evaluation of clinical features and treatment in 612 patients. *Am J. Med.* **68**, 344–55.

Lachman, E., Pitsoe, S.B. and Gaffin, S.L. (1984). Anti-lipopolysaccharide immunotherapy in management of septic shock of obstetric and gynaecological origin. *Lancet* **i**, 981–3.

Le, J. and Vilcek, J. (1987). Tumor necrosis factor and interleukin 1: cytokines with multiple overlapping biological activities. *Lab. Invest.* **56**, 234–48.

Liehr, H. (1980). Endotoxemia in liver disease. In *The Reticuloendothelial System and the Pathogenesis of Liver Disease*, ed. H. Liehr and M. Grun pp. 325–36, Elsevier, Amsterdam.

Luderitz, O., Galanos, C. and Rietschel, E. (1981). Endotoxins of Gram negative bacteria. *Pharmacol. Ther.* **15**, 383–402.

McCabe, W.R. (1973). Serum complement levels in bacteremia due to gram negative organisms. *N. Engl. J. Med.* **288**, 21–3.

McCutchan, J.A. and Ziegler, E.J. (1983). Treatment with anti-gram-negative antibodies. *Lancet* **ii**, 802–3.

McPhaden, A.R. and Whaley, K. (1985). The complement system in sepsis and trauma. *Br. Med. Bull.* **41**, 281–6.

Mathison, J.C., Wolfson, E. and Ulevitch, R.J. (1988). Participation of tumor necrosis factor in the mediation of gram negative bacterial lipopolysaccharide-induced injury in rabbits. *J. Clin. Invest.* **81**, 1925–37.

May, J.E., Kane, M.A. and Frank, M.M. (1972). Host defense against bacterial endotoxemia. Contribution of the early and late components of complement to detoxification. *J. Immunol.* **109**, 893–5.

Meyrick, B.O. (1986). Endotoxin-mediated pulmonary endothelial cell injury. *Fed. Proc.* **45**, 19–24.

Michalek, S.M., Moore, R.N., McGhee, J.R. Rosenstreich, D.L. and Mergenhagen, S.E. (1980). The primary role of lymphoreticular cells in the mediation of host responses to bacterial endotoxin. *J. Infect. Dis.* **141**, 55–63.

Michie, H.R., Manogue, K.R., Spriggs, D.R. *et al.* (1988). Detection of circulating tumor necrosis factor after endotoxin administration. *N. Engl. J. Med.* **318**, 1481–6.

Mita, A., Ohta, H. and Mita, T. (1982). Induction of splenic T cell proliferation by lipid A in mice immunised with sheep red blood cells. *J. Immunol.* **128**, 1709–11.

Moore, R.H., Lampert, I.A., Chia, Y., Aber, V.R. and Cohen, J. (1987). Effect of immunisation with *Escherichia coli* J5 on graft-versus-host disease induced by minor histocompatibility antigens in mice. *Transplantation* **44**, 249–53.

Morrison, D.C. and Kline, L.F. (1977). Activation of the classical and properdin pathways of complement by bacterial lipopolysaccharides. *J. Immunol.* **118**, 362–8.

Morrison, D.C. and Ryan, J.L. (1979). Bacterial endotoxins and host immune responses. *Adv. Immunol.* **28**, 293–378.

Movat, H.Z., Cybulsky, M.I., Colditz, I.G., Chan, M.K. and Dinarello, C.A. (1987). Acute inflammation in gram-negative infection: endotoxin, interleukin 1, tumor necrosis factor and neutrophils. *Fed. Proc.* **46**, 97–104.

Okusawa, S., Gelfland, J.A., Ikejima, T., Connolly, R.J. and Dinarello, C.A. (1988). Interleukin 1 induces a shock-like state in rabbits: synergism with tumor necrosis factor and the effect of cyclooxygenase inhibition. *J. Clin. Invest.* **81**, 1162–72.

Oseas, R., Yang, H.-H., Baehner, R.L. and Boxer, C.A. (1981). Lactoferrin: a promoter of polymorphonuclear leukocyte adhesiveness. *Blood* **57**, 939–45.

Parant, M., Parant, F., Vinit, M.-A and Chedid, L. (1987). Protective effect of recombinant human tumor necrosis factor against bacterial and fungal experimental infections. *Comptes Rendus Acad. Sci. Paris, Sér. III* **304**, 1–4.

Pollack, M., Huang, A.I., Prescot, R.K. *et al.* (1983). Enhanced survival in *Pseudomonas aeruginosa* septicemia associated with high levels of circulating antibody to *Escherichia coli* endotoxin core. *J. Clin. Invest.* **72**, 1874–81.

Proctor, R.A. (1985). Effects of endotoxins on neutrophils. In *Cellular Biology of Endotoxin*, ed. L.J. Berry, pp. 244–59, Elsevier, Amsterdam.

Pudifin, D., L'Hoste, I., Duursma, J. and Garrin, S.L. (1985). Opsonisaton of Gram-negative bacteria by anti-lipopolysaccharide antibodies. *Lancet* **ii**, 1009–10.

Remick, D.G., Kunkel, R.G., Larrick, J.W., and Kunkel, S.L. (1987). Acute *in vivo* effects of human recombinant tumor necrosis factor. *Lab. Invest.* **56**, 583–90.

Rietschel, E.T., Brade, L., Brandenburg, K. *et al.* (1987). Chemical structure and biologic activity of bacterial and synthetic lipid A. *Rev. Infect. Dis.* **9**, S527–S536.

Roantree, R.J. and Rantz, L.A (1960). A study of the relationship of the normal bactericidal activity of human serum to bacterial infection. *J. Clin. Invest.* **39**, 72–81.

Rothstein, J.L. and Schreiber, H. (1988). Synergy between tumor necrosis factor and bacterial products cause hemorrhagic necrosis and lethal shock in normal mice. *Proc. Nat. Acad. Sci. (USA)* **85**, 607–11.

Sanford, J.P. (1985). Epidemiology and overview of the problem. In *Septic Shock*, ed. R.K. Root and M.A. Sande, pp. 1–12, Churchill Livingstone, New York.

Silva, A.T., Bayston, K.F. and Cohen, J. (1989). Prophylactic and therapeutic effect of a monoclonal antibody to tumour necrosis factor in experimental gram negative shock. *J. Infect. Dis.* **162**, 421–7.

Skarnes, R.C. (1985). *In vivo* distribution and detoxification of endotoxins. In *Cellular Biology of Endotoxin*, ed. L.J. Berry, pp. 56–81, Elsevier, Amsterdam.

Spink, W.W., Davis, R.B., Potter, R. and Chartrand, S. (1964). The initial stage of canine endotoxin shock as an expression of anaphylactic shock: studies on complement titers and plasma histamine concentrations. *J. Clin. Invest.* **43**, 696–704.

Stoll, B.J., Pollack, M. and Hooper, J.A. (1987). Antibodies to endotoxin core determinants in normal subjects and in immune globulins for intravenous use. *Serodiagnosis Immunother.* **1**, 21–31.

Sultzer, B.M. (1968). Genetic control of leucocyte responses to endotoxin. *Nature* **219**, 1253–4.

Teng, N.H., Kaplan, H.S., Hebert, J.M. *et al.* (1985). Protection against gram-negative bacteremia and endotoxemia with human monoclonal IgM antibodies. *Proc. Nat. Acad. Sci. (USA)* **82**, 1790–4.

Till, G.O. and Ward, P.A. (1986). Systemic complement activation and acute lung injury. *Fed. Proc.* **45**, 13–18.

Tobias, P.S., McAdam, K.P., Soldau, K. and Ulevitch, R.J. (1985). Control of lipopolysaccharide–high-density lipoprotein interactions by an acute phase reactant in human serum. *Infect. Immun.* **50**, 73–6.

Tobias, P.S., Mathison, J.C. and Ulevitch, R.J. (1988). A family of lipopolysaccharide binding proteins involved in responses to Gram-negative sepsis. *J. Biol. Chem.* **263**, 13479–81.

Tracey, K.J., Beutler, B., Lowry, S.F. *et al.* (1986). Shock and tissue injury induced by recombinant human cachectin. *Science* **234**, 470–4.

Tracey, K.J., Fong, Y., Hesse, D.G. *et al.* (1987). Anti-cachectin/TNF monoclonal antibodies prevent septic shock during lethal bacteraemia. *Nature* **330**, 662–4.

Vogel, S.N., Weedon, L.L., Wahl, I.M. and Rosenstreich, D.L. (1982). BCG-induced enhancement of endotoxin sensitivity in C3H/HeJ mice. II. T cell modulation of macrophage sensitivity to LPS *in vitro*. *Immunobiology* **160**, 479–93.

Vogel, S.N., Madonna, G.S., Wahl, L.M. and Rick, P.D. (1984). *In vitro* stimulation of C3H/HeJ B cells and macrophages by a lipid A precursor molecule derived from *Salmonella typhimurium*. *J. Immunol.* **132**, 347–53.

Vreede, R.W., Marcelis, J.H. and Verhoef, J. (1986). Antibodies raised against rough mutants of *Escherichia coli* and *Salmonella* strains are opsonic only in the presence of complement. *Infect. Immun.* **52**, 892–6.

Waage, A., Halstensen, A. and Espevik, T. (1987). Association between tumour necrosis factor in serum and fatal outcome in patients with meningococcal disease. *Lancet* **i**, 355–7.

Weyand, C., Goronzy, J., Fathman, C.G. and O'Hanley, P. (1987). Administration *in vivo* of recombinant interleukin 2 protects mice against septic death. *J. Clin. Invest.* **79**, 1756–63.

Wilson, M.E. (1985). Effects of bacterial endotoxins on neutrophil function. *Rev. Infect. Dis.* **7**, 404–18.

Woods, J.P., Black, J.R., Barritt, D.S., Connell, T.D. and Cannon, J.G. (1987). Resistance to meningococcemia apparently conferred by anti-H.8 monoclonal antibody is due to contaminating endotoxin and not to specific immunoprotection. *Infect. Immun.* **55**, 1927–8.

Worthen, G.S., Haslett, C., Smedly, L.A. *et al.* (1986). Lung vascular injury induced by chemotactic factors: enhancement by bacterial endotoxins. *Fed. Proc.* **45**, 7–12.

Yamamoto, A., Nagamuta, M., Usami, H. *et al.* (1986). Release of tumor necrosis factor (TNF) into mouse peritoneal fluids by OK-432, a streptococcal protein. *Immunopharmacology* **11**, 79–86.

Young, L.S. Stevens, P. and Ingram, J. (1975). Functional role of antibody against 'core' glycolipid of Enterobacteriaceae. *J. Clin. Invest.* **56**, 850–61.

Ziegler, E.J. (1988). Protective antibody to endotoxin core: the emperor's new clothes? *J. Infect. Dis.* **158**, 286–90.

Ziegler, E.J., Douglas, H. and Braude, A.I. (1973a). Human antiserum for prevention of the local Shwartzmann reaction and death from bacterial lipopolysaccharides. *J. Clin. Invest.* **52**, 3236–8.

Ziegler, E.J., Douglas, H., Sherman, J.E., Davis, C.E. and Braude, A.I. (1973b). Treatment of *E. coli* and *Klebsiella* bacteremia in agranulocytic animals with antiserum to a UDP-GAL epimerase-deficient mutant. *J. Immunol.* **111**, 433–8.

Ziegler, E.J., Fischer, C.J., Jr., Sprung, C. *et al.* (1991). Treatment of Gram negative bacteremia and septic shock with HA-1A human monoclonal antibody against endotoxin. *N. Engl. J. Med.* **324**, 429–36.

Ziegler, E.J., McCutchan, J.A., Fierer, J. *et al.* (1982). Treatment of gram-negative bacteremia and shock with human antiserum to a mutant *Escherichia coli*. *N. Engl. J. Med.* **307**, 1225–30.

Zinner, S.H. and McCabe, W.R. (1976). Effects of IgM and IgG antibody in patients with bacteremia due to gram negative bacilli. *J. Infect. Dis.* **133**, 37–45.

76: Infections with Intracellular Bacteria

J. Ivanyi

Diseases caused by intracellular bacteria involve complex interactions between bacterial organisms and the infected host. The outcome of these interactions, occurring at the time of the entrance of bacilli to host cells and during and following intracellular multiplication, is integral to the ways in which the bacilli escape host defence reactions as well as to the mechanisms leading to tissue pathology. At each of these levels, immunological responses of the infected host decide between a self-healing or pathogenic outcome and may also determine several of the clinical manifestations of disease. Intracellular bacteria are the aetiological agents for human diseases of considerable importance: tuberculosis and leprosy each affect about 10 million people world-wide with high mortality or suffering devastating chronic illness. Atypical mycobacterioses are currently some of the infections most strongly associated with the acquired immune deficiency syndrome (AIDS). Trachoma afflicts about 500 million people and the sexually transmitted chlamydial infections are a frequent cause of female infertility and neonatal illness. Salmonellosis remains a major enteric infection of adults and neonates in Third World countries.

The immunological study of this subject has been orientated essentially towards the following aspects:

1 Interaction of the pathogen with host target cells. This includes the molecular biology and the study of structural determinants of virulence. They have been related to the entry, replication and persistence of bacteria in host cells. The biochemistry and genetic study of macrophage function have been essential parts of the analysis.

2 Mechanisms of the pathogenesis of disease. Special attention has been given to the role of lymphokines and monokines in inflammatory cellular reactions and tissue pathology.

3 Mechanisms of protective immunity. Major advances in the definition of individual antigens has enabled the systematic analysis of the effective constituents with prospects for subunit vaccine development. Intensive research is aimed at the role of T cell subsets, their specificity and genetic restriction.

4 Immunodiagnostic applications are being advanced by the analysis of the species specificity of immunodominant antigenic epitopes.

The investigation of mycobacterial diseases has been the most extensive area whereas the study of other intracellular bacterial infections has recorded only more recent, although impressively rapid, progress. Whilst antituberculous resistance 'serves as a paradigm of a purely cell-mediated immune response' (Collins 1979), protection by antibodies may play a significant role in salmonellosis, in brucellosis and in rickettsial and chlamydial infections.

Tuberculosis

Pathogenesis

Mycobacterium tuberculosis is transmitted by inhalation of airborne particles ('droplet nuclei'), which settle usually in the base of the lungs. Following multiplication, the organisms spread via hilar lymph nodes and haematogenously to any tissue, but most commonly to the lung apices. T cell-mediated immunity is demonstrable by the delayed-type hypersensitivity (DTH) skin reaction to tuberculin 6–8 weeks post-infection and the local granulomatous reaction can contain the spread of infection. In most individuals, this leads to self-healing but, in infants and young children, dissemination of infection can cause primary tuberculosis, characterized by hilar, mediastinal and cervical lymphadenitis, usually without pulmonary cavities. Consequently, only low levels of bacilli are present in bronchial secretion and sputum.

Secondary tuberculosis with typical cavitary pathology, representing the majority of adult disease, results from the reactivation of dormant bacilli which had spread during primary infection to the apices of the lungs or other organs (Stead 1967). This is known to occur most frequently in young adults, in the elderly or in the postpartum period. Both innate resistance and T cell-mediated immunity initially restrain the infection but probably fail to kill off certain organisms, which then persist in a latent metabolic state for several years in host tissues. However, the nature of the failure in immunological mechanisms resulting in recrudescence of bacterial growth is poorly understood. Experimental studies demonstrated reactivation of persistent bacilli by hydrocortisone following chemotherapy or after the natural course of infection (Rees 1954; Lovik and Closs 1984). Recent studies which showed greater relapse of Bacillus Calmette–Guérin (BCG) infection in mice that were sensitized 3 weeks previously than in freshly infected animals suggested that mycobacterial reactivation may even be aggravated by host T cell immunity (Cox and Ivanyi 1988).

Lung lesions consisting of macrophage, epithelioid cell and lymphocyte infiltration progress to tubercle formation and undergo a caseous type of necrosis followed by either calcification and sclerosis or liquefaction of the necrotic tissue. The typical lung cavity, consisting of a necrotic zone surrounded by a capsule, is the ideal site for the multiplication of massive numbers of tubercle bacilli. Similar lesions may develop in other organs but lymph node tubercles have limited caseation with few bacteria whilst small lesions occur in miliary tuberculosis and in tuberculous meningitis.

Granuloma formation in tuberculous infections is associated with T cell-dependent recruitment of bone marrow-derived macrophages. Activated macrophages are the source of interleukin 1 (IL-1), which stimulates amyloid A synthesis in the liver (McAdam *et al.* 1983), and also of hydrolytic enzymes, which through liquefaction of the caseous centres of tuberculous lesions cause the cavitation. The latter process was found to be amplified in rabbits by prior BCG sensitization (Yamamura 1958), thus indicating a distinct pathogenic role of T cell-mediated 'hypersensitivity' in tuberculosis. Although tuberculous granulomas initially have the beneficial function of containing the spread of infection in the body, they seem to be inefficient in bactericidal activity and allow the survival of persistent bacilli.

Tuberculosis is associated with human immunodeficiency virus (HIV) infection, particularly in populations with a high prevalence of tuberculous exposure. Intravenous drug abusers in Western countries and populations of several countries in Africa are at especially high risk. The clinical manifestations are atypical, often disseminated to organs other than the lungs, the latter with hilar or mediastinal lymphadenopathy and localized to middle or lower lobes without cavitation.

Immune repertoire

The analysis of antigenic constituents of tubercle bacilli has advanced greatly in recent years (see Ivanyi *et al.* 1988b). Using monoclonal antibodies, species-specific epitopes were identified on 38 kD and 14 kD protein antigens. On the other hand, a 65 kD antigen, representing a heat-shock protein of conserved structure, contains numerous epitopes cross-reactive with other bacteria. In view of their pronounced immunogenicity, it was proposed that stress proteins could play a special role in the host response during mycobacterial infection in terms of either protective immunity or pathogenic interactions (Young *et al.* 1988). This could result from the recognition of different antigenic determinants whereby the response to the conserved self-like sequences could induce autoimmune reactions with associated pathology during chronic mycobacterial infection.

Analysis of T cell clones from BCG-vaccinated healthy subjects identified some epitopes which are specific for the *M. tuberculosis* complex (i.e. including *M. bovis*), but the majority of clones were cross-reactive with other species of mycobacteria (Mustafa *et al.* 1986b). CD4 T cell clones obtained from tuberculosis patients were specific for 19 and 65 kD antigens (Oftung *et al.* 1987). On the other hand CD8 clones from the pleural effusion of tuberculosis patients were directed to either 71 or 100 kD antigens, thus indicating that the immunodominant repertoires may be different for the CD4 and CD8 cells respectively (Rees *et al.* 1989).

Serological studies using either a monoclonal-based competition test or enzyme-linked immunosorbent assay (ELISA) with purified antigens have examined the immunodominant specificities in pulmonary tuberculosis (Ivanyi *et al.* 1988a; Jackett *et al.* 1988). Sputum-positive patients were identified best on the basis of raised antibody titres to the 38 kD antigen whereas sputum-negative patients were better discriminated from controls on the basis of anti-19 kD antibody levels. The antibody repertoire was analysed also in child tuberculosis but in the majority only low titres were found (Bothamley *et al.* 1988). In tuberculous meningitis, antibodies in the cerebrospinal fluid are directed mainly towards the lipoarabinomannan cell wall antigen (Chandramuki *et al.* 1989). It is of interest that sensitized healthy individuals showed the most pronounced serological response to the 14 kD antigen. In general, these results suggest that distinct antibody specificities are stimulated in various stages of infection or types of tuberculosis.

Protective immunity

Phagocytosis of bacteria is generally followed by phagosome–lysosome fusion, making possible the antimicrobial action of lysosomal enzymes. Although inhibition of fusion by tubercle bacilli was considered to be a virulence factor, it is also known that tubercle bacilli coated with antibody allow the formation of phagolysosomes and yet replicate intracellularly while in contact with lysosomal contents (Hart *et al.* 1987).

Experimental studies have established the mandatory role of T cells in acquired resistance to infection with tubercle bacilli (see Collins 1979; Ivanyi 1986). Protection can be transferred adoptively by lymphocytes but not by serum from immunized donors whilst T cell-deficient mice show enhanced susceptibility to infection. However, the two most commonly used T cell tests, namely the skin DTH reaction and the *in vitro* T cell proliferative assay in response to antigens within bacterial extracts, do not reflect the degree of host protection. Paradoxically, these tests are perhaps more representative of 'hypersensitivity' reactions, which are also involved in the pathogenesis of tissue destruction. Whilst it is not known whether protection is mediated by a population of T cells of certain specificity or lymphokine-secreting phenotype, the fact remains that none of the available T cell assays is yet suitable to determine the degree of protection in individuals who were immunized either through infection or BCG vaccination.

The study of the mechanisms of protective immunity in experimental models suggested the importance of the interaction between T cells and macrophages. Three stages can be identified in this relationship:

1 Macrophages harbouring the bacteria act as antigen-processing cells which present the respective antigenic epitopes to corresponding T cells. Hence, this stage is antigen-specific and major histocompatibility complex (MHC)-restricted.
2 T cells proliferate and secrete various lymphokines, some of which are targeted to bind and to activate macrophages. Interferon gamma (IFN-γ) is the main mediator of tuberculocidal activity.
3 Activated macrophages have enhanced bactericidal activity to intracellular parasites as part of their generally increased metabolic activities.

The killing of intracellular parasites was previously attributed to reactive oxygen metabolites, namely to the production of H_2O_2, which can be stimulated by IFN-γ. In contrast, Kaufmann and Flesch (1988) have recently suggested that the tuberculostatic activity of mouse macrophages is independent of reactive oxygen metabolites on the basis that phagocytosis of *M. bovis* by activated macrophages did not induce an oxidative burst and that the tuberculostatic activity of macrophages was not reversed by several scavengers of oxygen metabolites.

Currently there is a debate about the relative contribution of T lymphocyte subsets to antituberculous protective immunity. Whilst CD4 cells could be the main source of IFN-γ as the representative macrophage-activating factor, recent experimental studies also suggested a role for CD8 cells. This was shown through interference with adoptive immunity by anti-CD8 antibody, as demonstrated by the increased bacterial counts in mice which had been ablated of CD8 cells or of the tuberculostatic activity of Lyt-2+ve T cell lines (Hussein *et al*. 1987; Orme 1987; Kaufmann and Flesch 1988). CD8 cells could lyse in a Class I MHC-restricted way the over-infected 'refractory' macrophages and release their bacterial content for attack by newly recruited macrophages from bone marrow with fresh bactericidal activity. Alternatively, CD8 cells could mediate protection by a non-cognate (non-MHC-restricted) mechanism involving humoral mediators targeted at macrophages.

Present evidence suggests that induction of protective immunity to tuberculosis requires the inoculation of a live attenuated mycobacterium, e.g. *M. bovis* strain BCG. Vaccination in man is well established in many countries but the degree of protection as determined in several controlled trials was found to be variable (ten Dam 1984). The most valuable is probably the alleviation of the most severe forms of disease in children by neonatal vaccination (Curtis *et al*. 1984; Tidjani *et al*. 1986). The latter procedure is therefore the recommended policy 'for all newborns or young children in high-risk countries and areas' (WHO Tuberculosis Control Programme 1986).

Genetic aspects

Population studies typing for human leucocyte antigen (HLA) Class I alleles reported only weak associations which did not seem to be consistent whilst typing for HLA Class II specificities has been showing more promising results. Preferential transmission of DR2 was reported in offspring with pulmonary tuberculosis when compared with healthy offspring from both diseased and healthy parents (Singh *et al*. 1983). In another population study, HLA-DR2 and DQwl were positively associated and DQw3 was negatively associated with pulmonary tuberculosis (Bothamley *et al*. 1989). In the same study, HLA-DR2 was found to be associated with high antibody levels of patients to the 38 kD protein antigen of *M. tuberculosis*. The possible relationship between immune responses to this antigen and pathogenic mechanisms has been suggested on the basis of the linked association between the frequency of disease and the immune responsiveness with HLA-DR2. Conceivably, individuals with the high antibody response phenotype could have developed disease as a result of impaired or actively suppressed protective T cell immunity to the 38 kD antigen. In other studies, the DR4 haplotype was associated with high DTH responsiveness to a mycobacterial extract (Ottenhof *et al*. 1986). However, a relationship of this genetic factor to tuberculosis was not established. Furthermore, the role of non-HLA genes has also been implicated (Shields *et al*. 1987). Multifactorial genetic elements including the H-2 locus are known to play a role in the outcome of tuberculous infection in inbred strains of mice (Adu *et al*. 1983; Closs *et al*. 1983; Buschman *et al*. 1988). An innate resistance gene (Bcg) on chromosome 1 which is targeted on macrophage function controls the early stage of infection with BCG (Buschman *et al*. 1988) whereas the Igh locus has been shown to control the extent of granuloma formation and macrophage activation in response to stimulation by BCG cell walls (Callis *et al.* 1983).

Atypical mycobacterioses

The designation atypical mycobacterioses is used mainly for infections with members of the *M. avium–intracellulare-scrofulaceum* (MAIS) complex. These mycobacteria exist in the natural environment and can be isolated from mucosal secretions of clinically healthy subjects. It is assumed that silent infections originate from inhalation and ingestion of infected aerosols and water rather than from infected persons. *Mycobacterium avium–intracellulare–scrofulaceum* organisms are considerably less virulent than tubercle bacilli and become pathogenic in immunocompromised hosts, namely in association with HIV infection, cancer chemotherapy and chronic or terminal lung or renal disease (Collins 1988). Generally MAIS infections are very difficult to treat due to their high degree of drug resistance. The incidence of AIDS-associated mycobacterioses is currently rising in Western countries and they represent an important clinical and epidemiological problem. Whilst tuberculosis may precede AIDS, infections with the much less virulent MAIS occur later when immunodeficiency has fully developed (Pinching 1987).

The clinical presentation and chest radiology of MAIS infections is atypical, with sputum culture often negative. The diagnosis is often confirmed by positive culture of blood, bone marrow, faeces or rectal biopsy (Kiehn *et al.* 1985). The diagnostic aspect is important when considering that as many as 50% of AIDS patients in the United States were reported to be infected with MAIS (see Collins 1988). It is not yet understood why the infection in AIDS patients is restricted to three (1, 4 or 8) serotypes with rare occurrence of the other 28 serotypes which are found in immunocompromised patients undergoing cancer or transplant chemotherapy.

The mechanisms which determine the differences in the virulence of tubercle bacilli and MAIS are essentially unknown. However, it is of interest that human monocytes take up more MAIS than *M. tuberculosis* organisms upon incubation *in vitro* and that only the former uptake is strongly C3-dependent (Swartz *et al.* 1988). Whilst the pathogenicity of MAIS in mice is generally low, a few of the several existing serotypes have been found relatively more virulent. The initial bacterial growth in mice is under genetic control by the innate resistance Bcg gene (Goto *et al.* 1984). Virulent strains have a flat translucent form whereas avirulent strains are of domed opaque morphology. However, the virulence grade of MAIS strains in mice does not parallel the incidence frequencies in AIDS patients. In mice, T cell depletion potentiates the growth of the virulent strains only, suggesting that avirulent organisms are eliminated merely by the non-immune macrophage-mediated innate resistance of the host (Collins 1988). Acquired resistance to infection with at least certain virulent strains of *M. avium* in mice seems to be less than that observed against *M. tuberculosis* (Takashima and Collins 1988). This was interpreted to be due to greater resistance to killing by macrophages rather than a lower degree of immunization.

Johne's and Crohn's disease

Johne's disease in ruminants and Crohn's disease in man are similar chronic granulomatous diseases of the bowel affecting principally the ileum and colon. The mycobacterial aetiology is generally accepted for Johne's but disputed for Crohn's disease (Morgan 1987). The causative organism, *M. paratuberculosis*, closely related to the *M. avium* complex but non-pathogenic for birds, has a characteristic dependence on the iron-chelating factor mycobactin for *in vitro* growth. The pathogenic role of hypersensitivity in Johne's disease was proposed on the basis of findings that clinical signs linked with DTH occurred after oral infection of sheep and declined following 'desensitization' by the intravenous injection of a soluble extract from *M. paratuberculosis* (Merkal *et al.* 1968, 1970). The dispute in respect of Crohn's disease relates mainly to the outcome of isolation of mycobacteria from the affected intestinal tissue. There is convincing evidence that some isolates are definitely *M. paratuberculosis* (McFadden *et al.* 1987). However, in another study other mycobacterial species (e.g. *M. kansasii* and *M. fortuitum* complex) were also regularly isolated not only from Crohn's disease but also from ulcerative colitis and from non-inflammatory bowel disease patients (Graham *et al.* 1987). The favoured hypothesis of these authors, that the disease could be due to 'an abnormal immune response to a common antigen', deserves more intensive immunological investigation for the future.

Leprosy

Clinical spectrum

Tuberculoid leprosy displays pronounced T cell immunity with low antibody levels whereas the lepromatous form of the disease (LL) is characterized by T cell anergy and high antibody levels to *M. leprae*. Apart from these polar forms, certain patients are classified as 'borderline' with manifestations which combine to a variable degree the features from each end of the spectrum (Ridley and Jopling 1966). Progressive temporal deterioration from the reactive tuberculoid to the anergic lepromatous form (i.e. downgrading) is a characteristic natural evolution of the disease. There are major geographical differences in the relative distribution of patients within the spectrum of disease, the lepromatous form being common in Asia whilst the tuberculoid disease is the prevailing form in most African countries. 'Upgrading' of the disease reflects a change from the lepromatous to the tuberculoid form within borderline categories. The acute 'reversal' inflammatory reaction (type I) has only occasional spontaneous occurrence but results more commonly from abrupt reduction of viable bacteria during chemotherapy. The clinically most aggravating aspects are due to the neuritis which is probably due to the infiltration of nerves with T lymphocytes. Another reactional syndrome (type II), erythema nodosum leprosum (ENL), which occurs in about half of LL patients, may involve the pathogenic role of immune complexes formed at increased levels in the blood and also deposited within lesions (Ridley and Ridley 1983).

Histopathology

Schwann cells of unmyelinated fibres are the predilective site for intracellular *M. leprae* infection. Mycobacterial antigens have been localized in Schwann cells, in macrophages and extracellularly, but without a clear relationship to neurological manifestations. Granulomas, representing the essential form of tissue pathology, differ in their organization between the polar forms of the disease. Lepromatous-type granulomas contain randomly assorted undifferentiated histiocytic 'foamy' cells with abundant bacilli, few lymphocytes and no epithelioid or giant cells. Tuberculoid-type granulomas are composed of epithelioid cells, giant cells and many lymphocytes, but few *M. leprae* bacilli whilst ENL is characterized by neutrophilic and increased lymphocytic infiltration of granulomas. Polar forms of leprosy differ in the representation of T cell subsets: the CD4 population predominates in tuberculoid lesions (CD4/CD8 = 1.9) whereas the CD8 population predominates in lepromatous lesions (CD4/CD8 = 0.6) (Modlin and Rea 1988). It is of interest that these ratios are characteristic only of the leprosy lesions and are not reflected in cell counts in the peripheral blood. There are also distinct differences in the cellular organization of granulomas. In tuberculoid granulomas CD4 cells are associated with macrophages in the core of the granuloma and CD8 cells prevail at the mantle surrounding the granuloma, whilst in lepromatous lesions these cells are admixed. CD4 cells of the 4B4 phenotype (helper/inducer) are predominant in tuberculoid lesions whilst 2H4 phenotype cells (supressor/inducer) are more frequent in lepromatous lesions. Analysis of macrophage subpopulations showed that interdigitating cells and mature macrophages were localized to the periphery of granulomas (Collings *et al*. 1985). T lymphocytes in lepromatous lesions are deficient in IL-2 production but normal in their display of the IL-2 receptor (Tac), indicating their prior stimulation with antigen and/or IL-1 and that they might respond to exogenously supplied IL-2.

Immune repertoire

Species-specific determinants of *M. leprae* identified by monoclonal antibodies are represented by the terminal trisaccharide of phenolic glycolipid I (Gaylord and Brennan 1987) and by epitopes on protein antigens of 65, 36, 35, 28, 18 and 12 kD (see Ivanyi *et al*. 1988b). Serological studies suggested that the phenolic glycolipid I and 35 kD protein species-specific epitopes are the most immunodominant in patients with LL (Ivanyi *et al*. 1988a). In tuberculoid leprosy, antibody levels are not significantly elevated in the majority of patients when compared with healthy individuals in endemic regions. Therefore, the application of serology in leprosy control is of potential interest for the differential diagnosis between multi- and paucibacillary disease and for the more reliable choice of multi-drug chemotherapy. Prospective epidemiological studies, currently in progress, are aiming to evaluate the potential prognostic value of serological surveys in endemically infected populations.

The specificity of T cells has been analysed using fractions separated by sodium dodecyl sulphate (SDS) polyacrylamide gel electrophoresis from the soluble extract of *M. leprae*. By this technique, the most frequent stimulatory antigens were found in the 65, 35 and 20–10 kD region both in leprosy patients and in healthy household contacts (Mendez-Samperio *et al.* 1988). Analysis of T cell clones revealed the immunogenicity of epitopes of various degrees of cross-reactivity with other mycobacterial species. *M. leprae*-specific T cell epitopes were identified on the 18, 36 and 65 kD protein antigens (Mustafa *et al.* 1986a; van Schooten *et al.* 1988). These determinants are of further interest for the development of a specific skin test and their production as synthetic peptides seems feasible.

Genetic aspects

Several studies examined the possible association between HLA type and susceptibility or clinical form of leprosy (de Vries *et al.*, 1988). Human leucocyte antigen Class II MHC alleles are associated either with a particular form of leprosy or with the magnitude of immune response to *M. leprae* antigens. In this context, HLA-DQ1 and DR2 have been found associated with the occurrence of the lepromatous disease, and DR3 with enhanced T cell immunity to *M. leprae* antigens in tuberculoid patients. Recent detailed analysis of T cell specificities to one mycobacterial protein (65 kD) indicates that the selection of epitopes is restricted by several HLA-DR genes. Thus, preferential, genetically regulated, responsiveness to distinct antigenic epitopes may in effect be responsible for the protective or pathogenic interactions in the infected host.

Anergy

The main immunological feature of LL is the lack of adequate T cell immunity to *M. leprae*. This is demonstrable as a failure to give a DTH skin reaction or *in vitro* proliferation of peripheral blood lymphocytes to a soluble extract from *M. leprae* (leprosin). Although a certain proportion of patients are also anergic to tuberculin, the majority of LL patients do respond to it, despite the considerable cross-reactivity with several antigens of *M. leprae*. This apparent loss of response to the common epitopes led to the search for *M. leprae*-specific constituents which may stimulate suppressor T cells with regulatory immunopathogenic function. CD8 lymphocytes from lepromatous but not from tuberculoid or control subjects were shown to act as suppressor cells with specificity for the phenolic glycolipid of *M. leprae* (Bloom and Mehra 1984). Other investigators, however, found 'suppressor' cell activity to be expressed even more in tuberculoid leprosy and without distinct specificity (Rea 1983). Moreover, depletion of CD8 cells failed to restore CD4 proliferative reactions to *M. leprae*, indicating a deletion or a defect of the CD4 cell population (Bach *et al.* 1983). Subsequently, attempts were made to restore the responsiveness by supplementing the cultures of LL T cells with exogenous IL-2. Variable results were obtained but it appears that reversal of the specific anergy was achieved only in a minority of cases (Nogueira *et al.* 1983). Another mechanism for anergy could be the 'refractory' status of accessory cells. This could have a basis in competition for antigen-presenting function between antigens binding to the same MHC-coded Class II molecules. Alternatively, poorly degradable polysaccharide or glycolipid constituents may persist in tissues for long periods after the killing and disintegration of *M. leprae*. In this context it is of interest that arabinomannan and lipoarabinomannan are inhibitory for antigen processing of native protein antigens (Moreno *et al.* 1988).

Listeriosis

Listeria monocytogenes is a Gram-positive bacterium of low pathogenicity for humans with rarely apparent manifestation of infection but causing more severe outbreaks of disease in sheep and cattle. Human disease has various manifestations from general symptoms, lymphadenitis and abortion to severe illness in congenitally infected neonates and in immunocompromised patients; the latter groups often present as meningitis. Little is known about the immunology of human listeriosis while extensive experimental studies in mice have shown the organism to be a facultative intracellular parasite which evokes T cell-mediated host resistance. *Listeria monocytogenes* grows in mice mainly within resident macrophages of the spleen and liver while activated macrophages recruited from blood monocytes are bactericidal (North 1970). Moreover, the organisms can also invade and grow in several types of non-phagocytic cells. The main virulence factor in mice is a sulphhydryl-activated haemolysin related to streptolysin O. Pathogenicity was thought to be due to lysis of the phagolysosomal membrane, releasing the bacteria to the cytoplasm (Geoffroy *et al.* 1987). However, on the basis of experiments which failed to show a direct relationship between cytolytic activity *in vitro* and the degree of virulence it was suggested that the haemolysin may exert its role as a regulatory multifunctional molecule rather than by its lytic activity (Kathariou *et al.* 1988). Mutant strains (produced using conjugative transposons) defective in haemolysin production are avirulent in mice and fail to multiply in mouse macrophages and fibroblasts (Portnoy *et al.* 1988). However, non-haemolytic mutants do still grow in human cell lines, suggesting that the haemolysin may not be an essential virulence factor for man.

Innate host resistance of mice is expressed within 24–48 hours of intravenous infection. Analysis of inbred strains initially suggested genetic control by a single non-H-2 gene designated Lr but subsequent studies showed the effector role of C5 and also the contribution of more than one genetic locus (see Blackwell 1988). Resistance mediated by bone marrow-derived cells is abrogated with as little as 200 rad γ irradiation. On the basis of studies of radiation bone marrow chimeras it appears that the resistance phenotype is determined by an influx of monocytes to the host site of infection (Stevenson *et al.* 1981).

Potent and long-lasting acquired resistance to *Listeria* infection is T cell-mediated. *Listeria*-specific T cells produce IFN-γ and other lymphokines which recruit and activate macrophages for bactericidal activity within 2–3 days of infection (Buchmeier and Schreiber 1985; Lepay *et al.* 1985). It seems that intracellular growth of virulent bacteria is an absolute prerequisite for the induction of protective immunity (Berche *et al.* 1987). This cannot be substituted by repeated injections of even very high doses of dead bacteria. Thus, antigenic load is not the critical factor but the mechanism by which replication of bacilli induces the protective T cell response is not understood.

The precise role and interaction between T cell subsets and macrophages in the murine protective immunity to *Listeria* infection is a subject of controversy. Injection of cloned L3T4 +ve (CD4) T cells was shown to be protective against challenge infection involving IFN-γ release as the mediator of protection (Magee and Wing 1988). Although these results strongly suggest a direct effector role for L3T4 +ve cells, other experiments attributed the main effector function to Lyt-2 +ve cells (Mielke *et al.* 1988). Selective T cell depletion with monoclonal antibodies showed that DTH to listerial antigen was abolished by anti-L3T4 whereas immune elimination of viable bacilli from spleens was inhibited by anti-Lyt-2 antibody only. These results are corroborated by the earlier finding that protection from *Listeria* infection is H-2 Class I MHC-restricted (Cheers and Sandrin 1983) and by the demonstration of specific cytolysis of *L. monocytogenes*-infected cells by Lyt-2 cell lines (De Libero and Kaufmann 1986). Moreover, the role of Lyt-2 (CD4) cells in protection could also explain the apparently paradoxical observation of enhanced protection to infection by the injection of anti-I-A monoclonal antibody (Kurlander and Jones 1987). While distinct functions can be allocated to the L3T4 +ve and Lyt-2 +ve cells, both subsets contribute to granuloma formation and it is likely that, whenever the Lyt-2 subset is quantitatively limiting, its function could be augmented by L3T4 T cell-secreted IL-2.

Legionellosis

Legionella pneumophila, a Gram-negative facultative intracellular pathogen, is the causative agent of Legionnaires' disease. The organism is resistant to killing by opsonizing serum antibodies. It multiplies in human monocytes and macrophages following entry by coiling phagocytosis within distinctive replicative phagosomes which are inhibited from acidification and fusion with lysosomes. These characteristics are mandatory for virulence, since avirulent mutants which are bound and ingested by monocytes fail to multiply intracellularly (Horwitz 1987). Coiling phagocytosis represents the process in which monocyte pseudopods coil around the organism as it is internalized. The phagocytosis of *L. pneumophila* has been shown to be mediated by CR3 and CR1 complement receptors and not by Fc receptors (Payne and Horwitz 1987). It was suggested that this route of entry, perhaps also shared by other intracellular pathogens, could enable the organisms to avoid exposure to metabolites of the oxidative burst.

The antigens of *L. pneumophila* have been analysed by the Western blot technique with rabbit and human antisera (Sampson *et al.* 1986). Sera from culture-confirmed patients react most frequently (78%) with a 58 kD antigen common to all tested *Legionella* strains whereas responses to the strain-specific 14 and 25 kD bands were less frequent. The immunodominance and also the persistence of response indicate the usefulness of the common antigen for serodiagnosis.

Protective immunity in Legionnaires' disease can be attributed primarily to T cell-mediated reactions. There is also compelling evidence that IFN-γ produced by the sensitized cells is the single factor capable of activating human alveolar macrophages to inhibit the intracellular multiplication of *L. pneumophila* (Nash *et al.* 1988). The predominant role of T cell-mediated protection was demonstrated also in guinea-pigs, which are considerably more susceptible to *L. pneumophila* infection than mice (Breiman and Horwitz 1987; Yamamoto *et al.* 1987). Infected guinea pigs acquire resistance to subsequent challenge and bacterial multiplication is suppressed by supernatants from mitogen stimulated cells but not by opsonization with immune serum. In addition to persistence in macrophages, it was found that tumour necrosis factor (TNF) augments the killing of *L. pneumophila* by polymorphonuclear leucocytes (PMN) and that *in vivo* treatment with TNF resulted in protection of mice from mortality (Blanchard *et al.* 1988). The killing of *Legionella* by TNF-activated PMN cells could represent the effector phase of the immune resistance involving T cell-secreted IFN-γ in the induction of TNF production by macrophages.

Brucellosis

Brucellosis is a chronic disease in man with variable severity and undulating fever, contracted usually through contact with diseased cattle or other farm animals. The infectious agents, *Brucella abortus*, *B. melitensis* and *B. suis*, are facultative intracellular bacteria. Studies on the nature of protective immunity have largely been performed in mouse experimental models. In common with other intracellular pathogens, protection is mediated mainly by T cells and activated macrophages (Cheers 1984). Moreover, evidence for the role of humoral immunity was obtained by passive transfer with polyclonal and monoclonal antibodies (Montaraz *et al.* 1986). The protective monoclonal antibodies injected 4 hours prior to intraperitoneal live challenge were specific for the O polysaccharide expressed on the surface of *B. abortus* whereas antibodies to the porin antigen failed to confer protection. Subsequent experiments showed that active immunization with porin–lipopolysaccharide (LPS) complexes induced as good protection as the living attenuated *B. abortus* 19 vaccine (Winter *et al.* 1988). This study also confirmed that protection is conferred by antibodies to the O polysaccharide and not to the porin protein. Whether the porin–LPS vaccine gives protection of sufficiently long duration has yet to be established.

Immunological assays have been used for the diagnosis of brucellosis. While skin testing for DTH reactions is unreliable, antibody levels represented by both immunoglobulin M (IgM) and IgG classes and demonstrable by routine agglutination or complement fixation are valuable for the initial diagnosis of disease. In the chronic phase, relapse is accompanied in most cases by a selective increase of IgG antibody titres (Pellicer *et al.* 1988).

Chlamydial infections

Major human diseases caused by *Chlamydia trachomatis* are the chronic ocular infection, trachoma, and sexually transmitted infections. Although chlamydiae are sensitive to common antibiotics, they persist as latent drug-resistant intracellular organisms in the infected host. Therefore, the role of immunological mechanisms which control the host responses to this obligate intracellular bacterium remain of considerable interest (Levitt and Barol 1987).

The intracellular multiplication of *C. trachomatis* occurs initially in mucosal epithelial cells and later in macrophages or fibroblasts. Following entry by active endocytosis, phagolysosome fusion is inhibited and chlamydiae multiply in cytoplasmic inclusions, followed by exocytosis or cell lysis and reinfection of new cells (Todd and Caldwell 1985). The chlamydial developmental cycle alternates between the infectious extracellular 'elementary body' and the intracellular non-infectious metabolically active 'reticulate body'. Transition between the replicative stage and latency of the organism is affected by the nutrient and growth activity of host cells. The mechanisms of entry and cytopathogenicity, however, vary considerably when studied in several cell lines of diverse histogenetic origin (see Lamont and Nichols 1981).

Local mucosal infection in humans and experimental animals with *Chlamydia* leads to T cell immunity expressed by DTH and lymphocyte stimulation *in vitro* (see Lamont and Nichols 1981). Protection from challenge in mice can be adoptively transferred by T cells but the effector mechanisms mediated by lymphokines, such as IFN-γ, seem to be rather inefficient, resulting only in bacteriostasis, thus permitting persistent intracellular infection (Byrne *et al.* 1986).

Several earlier studies indicated a protective function for serum and secretory antibodies (Monnickendam and Pearce 1983; Williams *et al.* 1984). The study of monoclonal antibodies has been directed to a major outer membrane protein which is of principal structural and functional importance for the organism. An antibody to a species-specific epitope of this antigen was shown to neutralize the infectivity of chlamydiae *in vitro* (Peeling *et al.* 1984) while a serovar-specific antibody neutralized the infection for monkey eyes (Zhang *et al.* 1987). The species- and the several serovar-specific domains of this molecule have been localized at the level of peptide sequences (Baehr *et al.* 1988; Conlan *et al.* 1988). Serovar-specific epitopes are known to be the most immunodominant also in the course of natural infection whereas the species-specific domains are poorly immunogenic in the native antigen. The latter responses could be augmented with the use of appropriate synthetic peptides, which are of interest as a prospective vaccine. In the immediate future monoclonal antibodies to the outer membrane protein represent promising culture-independent diagnostic assays of high specificity and sensitivity (Tam *et al.* 1984; Stephens *et al.* 1988). In addition a genus-specific monoclonal antibody directed to *Chlamydia* lipopolysaccharide was shown to be diagnostically valuable (Mearns *et al.* 1988).

Chlamydial infections in infants lead to polyclonal B cell stimulation which is associated with an increase in the number of B cells and with hypergammaglobulinaemia (see Levitt and Barol 1987). This effect is demonstrable also *in vitro*, using purified human or mouse B cells. Specific antibody levels in mice injected with *C. trachomatis* are initially elevated, followed later by a suppressed response. The polyclonal immunomodulatory effects could also influence the outcome of homologous or other coinciding local infections.

Rickettsial infections

The diseases Rocky Mountain spotted fever, boutonneuse fever and rickettsial pox are caused by the obligate intracellular bacteria *Rickettsia rickettsii*, *R. conorii* and *R. akari* respectively. Together with *R. typhi* and *R. tsutsugamushi*, which causes scrub typhus, they represent the 'spotted fever group' of the genus *Rickettsia*. Serological evidence suggests a high prevalence of unapparent infection with *R. conorii* and the incidence of boutonneuse fever in some countries appears to be rising. The immunological study of rickettsial infection has been pursued almost exclusively in mouse experimental models. The protective immune response to these infections is T cell-mediated and convalescent animals are resistant to rechallenge (Kenyon and Pedersen 1980). Analysis of the specificity of mouse T cell hybridomas showed the existence of various cross-reactive and species-specific antigenic determinants but those responsible for protective immunity are not known. Moreover, the factors responsible for the virulence of spotted fever group rickettsiae have not as yet been identified. Monoclonal antibodies to a closely related pair of *R. rickettsii* strains with high or low virulence identified unique epitopes on two surface proteins (Anacker *et al.* 1986) whilst another monoclonal antibody directed to surface proteins (120 kD) protected mice from lethal challenge infection (Feng *et al.* 1987).

The outcome of intraperitoneal infection with *R. tsutsugamushi* is genetically controlled (Groves *et al.* 1980). The fulminant lethal infection in susceptible C3H/HeDub mice produces a mononuclear peritoneal exudate of greater magnitude than in resistant C3H/RV mice but with a lower content of Ia-bearing cells (Jerrels 1983). Suppression of Ia expression could be due to humoral mediators such as α-fetoprotein, prostaglandins or corticosteroids. Interferon gamma is an important defence factor in rickettsial infection since neutralizing IFN-γ *in vivo* with monoclonal antibody converts completely resistant mice into mice that are susceptible to *R. conorii* infection (Li *et al.* 1987), and recombinant mouse IFN-γ has been shown to be inhibitory for the intracellular growth of *Rickettsia* in cultured fibroblasts (Turco and Winkler 1983). However, IFN-γ levels and their time course do not parallel protection, suggesting that other mechanisms also participate in the anti-rickettsial resistance.

Salmonellosis

There are many different serotypes of pathogenic salmonellae and the invasive strains are facultative intracellular parasites. The determinants of virulence remain unknown, with the exception of a cryptic plasmid (Baird *et al.* 1985). The primary targets of natural infection with pathogenic salmonellae are the epithelial mucosal cells of the gut. However, they are merely the entry route to regional lymph nodes, with subsequent bacteraemia and multiplication within host macrophages. Inbred mice infected with *Salmonella typhimurium* can be characterized as either susceptible or resistant on the basis of viable bacterial counts in organs. This natural resistance, without participation of T cells, is controlled by an autosomal dominant gene (Ity) located on chromosone 1 (Blackwell 1988). The expression of natural resistance is mediated by resident macrophages through their bactericidal handling of the organisms or by the recruitment of monocytes from bone marrow. Moreover, corresponding differences in intracellular killing were observed for blood granulocytes (van Dissell *et al.* 1985).

Subsequent immunological reactions are mediated by T cells along the lines applicable to other intracellular bacteria. Thus, infection with avirulent *S. enteritidis* will protect mice against challenge with virulent *S. typhimurium* (Davies and Kotlarski 1976). Particularly effective protection against 1000 × 50% lethal infection lasting at least 7 months was imparted by the *aro*A −ve mutant SL3235 strain of *S. typhimurium* in hypersusceptible C3H/HeJ mice (Killar and Eisenstein 1985). It is surprising that adoptive transfer of protection in this system could not be achieved with purified T cells but only with an adherent cell fraction enriched in macrophages. The authors considered suppressor T cells or genetic factors, but a full explanation for this puzzling loss of adoptive immunity is as yet unknown.

The auxotrophic attenuated *Salmonella* strains are also potential vaccine carriers of heterologous antigens. This could be particularly attractive for other intracellular pathogens, most of which, in common with salmonellae, fail to protect as killed vaccines. *S. typhimurium* strains with a deleted *aro*A gene (Hoiseth and Stocker 1981) lack enzymes involved in the synthesis of chorismic acid, which is essential for the pathway of aromatic compounds and eventually nucleotide synthesis. As this pathway is not available in mammalian cells, the growth of *aro*A −ve strains is attenuated *in vivo*. Persistence of viable organisms for a significant period is a prerequisite for effective vaccination. However, persistence alone does not appear to be sufficient because persisting strains with an additional purine mutation become ineffective as vaccines (O'Callaghan *et al.* 1988).

Antibody levels to various antigens of salmonellae in humans with typhoid correlate with previous infection but not with protection. However, convincing evidence of antibody-mediated protection was presented in mouse experimental models. Rabbit antisera to porins representing a 37–45 kD fraction of outer membrane proteins of *S. typhi* protected 100% of 100 times 50% lethal dose (LD_{50})-challenged mice (Isibasi *et al.* 1988). Even better protection was achieved following active immunization in mice challenged intraperitoneally with bacteria in mucin. However the question remains open is about the degree of antibody-mediated protection following natural parenteral infection. Outer membrane proteins which also confer considerable cross-immunity between various strains of salmonellae might be protective even for different Gram-negative bacteria in view of their extensive structural homology (Fujio 1987). Furthermore, optimal immunity could be induced by porins complexed with polysaccharides, which provide the adjuvant function (Svenson *et al.* 1979; Kussi *et al.* 1981).

Yersinia infections

Yersinia enterocolitica and *Y. pseudotuberculosis* can cause mesenteric lymphadenitis with various gastrointestinal symptoms in children and adults. In addition, *Yersinia* infections are related to the subsequent development of reactive arthritis syndromes (Toivanen *et al.* 1985). These species of yersiniae, like the salmonellae, invade intestinal epithelial cells to gain access to macrophages, where they multiply and from which they may disseminate throughout the body. The genetic study of virulence suggested the role of *yop* plasmid-encoded outer membrane proteins, the expression of which is enhanced at the transcriptional level by higher temperature and low calcium concentration (Bolin and Wolf-Watz 1988). This virulence factor is responsible for the inhibition of phagocytosis in infected macrophages (Rosqvist *et al.* 1988). The adherence and invasion of epithelial cells is due to a 10 kD surface protein which is coded by the *inv* chromosomal gene with target tissue specificity controlled by another *ail* locus (Miller and Falkow 1988). The *inv* invasin expression is higher in *Y. pseudotuberculosis* grown at 28°C than at 37°C but this is apparently controlled by other loci because the expression of the *inv* gene fused with lac Z in *Escherichia coli* is not temperature-regulated (Isberg *et al.* 1988).

Specific protection against challenge in outbred mice (Simonet *et al.* 1985) was achieved by immunization with a non-virulent strain of *Y. pseudotuberculosis*, which did not persist in tissues, suggesting that protective immunity can be induced by antigens not encoded by the virulence plasmid. Another study demonstrated passive protection by rabbit antiserum directed against the V antigen of yersiniae (Une and Brubaker 1984). The study of genetic factors of resistance to *Y. enterocolitica* infections showed that C57Bl/b mice were 1000-fold more resistant than four other tested strains (Hancock *et al.* 1986). This strain difference does not match with the Ity innate resistance gene. Instead, the differences were found to be due to T cell-mediated immunity operating probably within ileal Peyer's patches.

The immunological analysis of *Yersinia*-triggered reactive arthritis is of considerable interest because the findings could be applicable also to reactive arthritides triggered by other microorganisms (Toivanen *et al.* 1985). The characteristic features of these patients are represented by association with HLA-B27, milder diarrhoea in the initial phase, elevated anti-*Yersinia* serum IgG and secretory IgA antibodies and weaker *in vitro* lymphocyte responses to *Yersinia* and to other Gram-negative enteric bacteria. The pathogenesis of this type of arthritis was tentatively attributed to an initial failure of defence against the infection followed by persistence of intracellular bacteria which trigger 'apparently futile and perhaps harmful' antibody production (Toivanen *et al.* 1985).

Tularaemia

Tularaemia is a typical zoonosis, largely tick-borne, transmitted usually during the handling of infected animals and manifested by prolonged fever, glandular swelling and skin lesions. The causative organism, *Francisella tularensis*, is a Gram-negative facultative intracellular bacterium. Immunological research on the experimental infection of mice with an attenuated strain has been addressed to the study of genetic restriction of adoptive immunity. The transfer of protection by splenic T cells between H-2 congenic B10 strains was found to be restricted by the I-A and not by the K or D regions of the H-2 complex (Anthony and Kongshavn 1988). Relating these data to the relative contribution of CD4 and CD8 cells to protective immunity against intracellular bacteria, the authors assume that CD4 cells may be protective in the early stage of infection whereas CD8 cells might be effective in late stages of infection.

References

Adu, H.O., Curtis, J. and Turk, J.L. (1983). Role of the major histocompatibility complex in resistance and granuloma formation in response to *Mycobacterium lepraemurium* infection. *Infect. Immunity* **40**, 720–5.

Anacker, R.L., List, R.L., Mann, R.E. and Wiedbrauk, D.L. (1986). Antigenic heterogeneity in high- and low-virulence strains of *Rickettsia rickettsii* revealed by monoclonal antibodies. *Infect. Immunity* **51**, 653–60.

Anthony, L.S.D. and Kongshavn, P.A.L. (1988). H-2 restriction in acquired cell-mediated immunity to infection with *Francisella tularensis* LVS. *Infect. Immunity* **56**, 452–6.

Bach, M.A., Wallack, D., Flaguel, B. and Cottenot, F. (1983). *In vitro* proliferative responses to *M. leprae* and PPD of isolated T cell subsets from leprosy patients. *Clin. Exp. Immunol.* **52**, 107–14.

Baehr, W., Zhang, Y.-X., Joseph, T. *et al.* (1988). Mapping antigenic domains expressed by *Chlamydia trachomatis* major outer membrane protein genes. *Proc. Nat. Acad. Sci. (USA)* **85**, 4000–4.

Baird, G.D., Manning, E.J. and Jones, P.W. (1985). Evidence for related virulence sequences in plasmids of *Salmonella dublin* and *Salmonella typhimurium*. *J. Gen. Microbiol.* **131**, 1815–20.

Berche, P., Gaillard, J.-L. and Sansonetti, P.J. (1987). Intracellular growth of *Listeria monocytogenes* as a prerequisite for *in vivo* induction of T cell-mediated immunity. *J. Immunol.* **138** (7), 2266–71.

Blackwell, J.M. (1988). Bacterial infections. In *Genetics of Resistance to Bacterial and Parasitic Infection*, Ed. D. Wakelin, and J.M. Blackwell, pp. 63–101, Taylor & Francis, London.

Blanchard, D.K., Djeu, J.Y., Klein, T.W., Friedman, H. and Stewart, II, W.E. (1988). Protective effects of tumour necrosis factor in experimental *Legionella pneumophila* infections of mice via activation of PMN function. *J. Leukocyte Biol.* **43**, 429–35.

Bloom, B.R. and Mehra, V. (1984). Immunological unresponsiveness in leprosy. *Immunol. Rev.* **80**, 5–25.

Bolin, I. and Wolf-Watz, H. (1988). The virulence plasmid encoded Yop2b protein of *Yersinia pseudotuberculosis* is a virulence determinant regulated by calcium and temperature at transcriptional level. *Mol. Microbiol.* **2**, 237–45.

Bothamley, G., Udani, P., Rudd, R., Festenstein, F. and Ivanyi, J. (1988). Antibody levels in smear-positive and smear-negative thoracic tuberculosis of adults and children. *Eur. J. Clin. Microbiol. Infect. Dis.* **7**, 639–46.

Bothamley, G.H., Beck, J.S., Schreuder, G.M.T. *et al.* (1989). Association of tuberculosis and *M. tuberculosis* specific antibody levels with HLA. *J. Infect. Dis.* **159**, 549–55.

Breiman, R.F. and Horwitz, M.A. (1987). Guinea pigs sublethally infected with aerosolized *Legionella pneumophila* develop humoral and cell-mediated immune responses and are protected against lethal aerosol challenge. *J. Exp. Med.* **164**, 799–811.

Buchmeier, N.A. and Schreiber, R.D. (1985). Requirement of endogenous interferon-gamma production for resolution of *Listeria monocytogenes* infection. *Proc. Nat. Acad. Sci. (USA)* **82**, 7404–10.

Buschman, E., Apt, A.S., Nickonenko, B.V., Moroz, A.M., Averbakh, M.H. and Skamene, E. (1988). Genetic aspects of innate resistance and acquired immunity to mycobacteria in inbred mice. *Springer Semin. Immunopathol.* **10**, 319–36.

Byrne, G.I., Lehmann, L.K. and Landry, G.J. (1986). Induction of tryptophan catabolism is the mechanism for gamma interferon-mediated inhibition of intracellular *Chlamydia psittaci* replication in T24 cells. *Infect. Immunity* **53**, 347–51.

Callis, A.H., Schrier, D.J., David, C. and Moore, V.L. (1983). Immunogenetics of BCG induced anergy in mice controlled by Igh and H-2 linked genes. *Immunology* **49**, 609–16.

Chandramuki, A., Bothamley, G.H., Brennan, P.J. and Ivanyi, J. (1989). Antibody levels to defined antigens of *Mycobacterium tuberculosis* in tuberculous meningitis. *J. Clin. Microbiol.* **17**, 821–5.

Cheers, C. (1984). Pathogenesis and cellular immunity in experimental murine brucellosis. *Dev. Biol. Stand.* **56**, 237–46.

Cheers, C. and Sandrin, M.S. (1983). Restriction in adoptive transfer of resistance to *Listeria monocytogenes*. II. Use of congenic and mutant mice show transfer to be H-2K restricted. *Cell. Immunol.* **78**, 199–205.

Closs, O., Lovik, M., Wigzell, H. and Taylor, B. (1983). H-2-linked gene(s) influence the granulomatous reaction to viable *M. lepraemurium* in the mouse. *Scand. J. Immunol.* **18**, 59–63.

Collings, L.A., Tidman, N. and Poulter, L.W. (1985). Quantitation of HLA-DR expression by cells involved in the skin lesions of tuberculoid and lepromatous leprosy. *Clin. Exp. Immunol.* **61**, 58.

Collins, F.M. (1979). Cellular antimicrobial immunity. *Crit. Rev. Microbiol.* **7**, 27–91.

Collins, F.M. (1988). AIDS-related mycobacterial disease. *Springer Semin. Immunopathol.* **10**, 375–91.

Conlan, J.W., Clarke, I.N. and Ward, M.E. (1988). Epitope mapping with solid-phase peptides: identification of type-, subspecies-, species- and genus-reactive antibody binding domains on the major outer membrane protein of *Chlamydia trachomatis*. *Mol. Microbiol.* **2** (5), 673–9.

Cox, J.H. and Ivanyi, J.H. (1988). The role of host factors for the chemotherapy of BCG infection in inbred strains of mice. *APMIS* **96**, 927–32.

Curtis, H.M., Leck, I. and Bamford, F.N. (1984). Incidence of childhood tuberculosis after neonatal BCG vaccination. *Lancet* **i**, 145–8.

Davies, R. and Kotlarski, I. (1976). The role of thymus-derived cells in immunity to *Salmonella* infection. *Aust. J. Exp. Biol. Med. Sci.* **54**, 221–36.

De Libero, G. and Kaufmann, S.H.E. (1986). Antigen-specific Lyt-2^+ cytolytic T lymphocytes from mice infected with the intracellular bacterium *Listeria monocytogenes*. *J. Immunol.* **137**, 2688–94.

de Vries, R.R.P., Ottenhoff, T.H.M. and van Schooten, W.C.A. (1988). Human leukocyte antigen (HLA) and mycobacterial disease. *Springer Semin. Immunopathol.* **10**, 319–36.

Feng, H.M., Walker, D.H. and Wang, J.G. (1987). Analysis of T-cell-dependent and independent antigens of *Rickettsia conorii* with monoclonal antibodies. *Infect. Immunity* **55**, 7–15.

Fujio, Y. (1987). DNA and amino acid sequences of outer membrane proteins and lipoproteins. In *Bacterial Outer Membranes as Model Systems*, ed. M. Inouye, pp. 419–32, John Wiley, New York.

Gaylord, H. and Brennan, P.J. (1987). Leprosy and the leprosy bacillus: recent developments in characterization of antigens and immunology of the disease. *Ann. Rev. Microbiol.* **41**, 645–75.

Geoffroy, C., Gaillard, J.L., Alouf, J.E. and Berche, P. (1987). Purification, characterization and toxicity of the sulfhydryl-activated hemolysin listeriolysin O from *Listeria monocytogenes*. *Infect. Immunity* **55**, 1641–50.

Goto, Y., Nakamura, R.M., Takahashi, H. and Tokunaga, T. (1984). Genetic control of resistance to *Mycobacterium* intracellulare infection in mice. *Infect. Immunity* **46**, 135–40.

Graham, D.Y., Markesich, D.C. and Yoshimura, H.H. (1987). Mycobacteria and inflammatory bowel disease: results of culture. *Gastroenterology* **92**, 436–42.

Groves, M.G., Rosenstreich, D.L., Taylor, B.A. and Osterman, J.V. (1980). Host defenses in experimental scrub typhus: mapping the gene that controls natural resistance in mice. *J. Immunol.* **125**, 1359–99.

Hancock, G.E., Schaedler, R.W. and MacDonald, T.T. (1986). *Yersinia enterocolitica* infection in resistant and susceptible strains of mice. *Infect. Immunity* **53**, 26–31.

Hart, P.D'A., Young, M.R., Gordon, A.H. and Sullivan, K.H. (1987). Inhibition of phagosome–lysosome fusion in macrophages by certain mycobacteria can be explained by inhibition of lysosomal movements observed after phagocytosis. *J. Exp. Med.* **166**, 933–44.

Hoiseth, S.K. and Stocker, B.A.D. (1981). Aromatic-dependent *Salmonella typhimurium* are non-virulent and are effective live vaccines. *Nature (London)* **241**, 238–9.

Horwitz, M.A. (1987). Characterization of avirulent mutant *Legionella pneumophila* that survive but do not multiply within human monocytes. *J. Exp. Med.* **166**, 1310–28.

Hussein, S., Curtis, J., Griffiths, D. and Turk, J.L. (1987). Study of DTH and resistance in *Mycobacterium lepraemurium* infection using a T-cell line isolated from mice infected with *Mycobacterium bovis* (BCG). *Cell. Immunol.* **105**, 423–36.

Isberg, R.R., Swain, A. and Falkow, S. (1988). Analysis of expression and thermoregulation of the *Yersinia pseudotuberculosis inv* gene with hybrid proteins. *Infect. Immunity* **56**, 2133–8.

Isibasi, A., Ortiz, V., Vargas, M. *et al.* (1988). Protection against *Salmonella typhi* infection in mice after immunization with outer membrane proteins isolated from *Salmonella typhi* 9,12,d,Vi. *Infect. Immunity* **56**, 2953–9.

Ivanyi, J. (1986). Pathogenic and protective interactions in mycobacterial infections. *Clin. Immunol. Allergy* **6**, 127–57.

Ivanyi, J., Bothamley, G.H. and Jackett, P.S. (1988a). Immunodiagnostic assays for tuberculosis and leprosy. *Br. Med. Bull.* **44**, 635–49.

Ivanyi, J., Sharp, K., Jackett, P. and Bothamley, G. (1988b). Immunological study of the defined constituents of *Mycobacteria*. *Springer Semin. Immunopathol.* **10**, 279–300.

Jackett, P.S., Bothamley, G.H., Batra, H.V., Mistry, A., Young, D.B. and Ivanyi, J. (1988). Specificity of antibodies to immunodominant mycobacterial antigens in pulmonary tuberculosis. *J. Clin. Microbiol.* **26**, 2313–18.

Jerrels, T.R. (1983). Association of an inflammatory I region-associated antigen-positive macrophage influx and genetic resistance of inbred mice to *Rickettsia tsutsugamushi*. *Infect. Immunity* **42**, 549–57.

Kathariou, S., Rocourt, J., Hof, H. and Goebel, W. (1988). Levels of *Listeria monocytogenes* Hemolysin are not directly proportional to virulence in experimental infections of mice. *Infect. Immunity* **56**, 534–6.

Kaufmann, S.H.E. and Flesch, I.E.A. (1988). The role of T cell–macrophage interactions in tuberculosis. *Springer Semin. Immunopathol.* **10**, 337–58.

Kenyon, R.H. and Pedersen, C.E. Jr., (1980). Immune responses to *Rickettsia akari* infection in congenitally athymic nude mice. *Infect. Immunity* **28**, 310–13.

Kiehn, T.E., Edwards, F.F. and Brannon, R. (1985). Infections caused by *M. avium*-complex in immunocompromized patients: diagnosis by blood culture and fecal examination, antimicrobial susceptibility test and morphological and serological characteristics. *J. Clin. Microbiol.* **21**, 168–77.

Killar, L.M. and Eisenstein, T.K. (1985). Immunity to *Salmonella typhimurium* infection in C3H/HeJ and C3H/HeNCr1BR mice: studies with an aromatic-dependent live *S. typhimurium* strain as a vaccine. *Infect. Immunity* **47**, 605–12.

Kurlander, R.J. and Jones, F. (1987). The effects of an anti-I-A^b antibody on murine host resistance to *Listeria monocytogenes*. *J. Immunol.* **138**, 2679–86.

Kussi, N., Nurminen, M., Saxen, H. and Makela, P.H. (1981). Immunization with major outer membrane protein (porin) preparations in experimental murine salmonellosis: effect of lipopolysaccharide. *Infect. Immunity* **34**, 328–32.

Lamont, H.C. and Nichols, R.L. (1981). Immunology of chlamydial infections. In *Immunology of Human Infection*, ed. A.J. Nahmias and R.J. O'Reilly, pp. 441–7, Plenum, New York.

Lepay, D.A., Steinman, R.M., Nathan, C.F., Murray, H.W. and Cohn, Z.A. (1985). Liver macrophages in murine listerosis: cell-mediated immunity is correlated with an influx of macrophages capable of generating reactive oxygen intermediates. *J. Exp. Med.* **161**, 1503–12.

Levitt, D. and Barol, J. (1987). The immunobiology of *Chlamydia*. *Immunol. Today* **8**, 246–51.

Li, H., Jerrels, T.R., Spitalny, G.L. and Walker, D.H. (1987). Gamma interferon as a crucial host defense against *Rickettsia conorii in vivo*. *Infect. Immunity* **55**, 1252–5.

Lovik, M. and Closs, O. (1984). Survival of *Mycobacterium lepraemurium* in C67BL mice after acquired protective immunity. *Clin. Exp. Immunol.* **57**, 115–22.

McAdam, K.P.W.J., Foss, N.T., Garcia, C. *et al.* (1983). Amloidosis and the serum amyloid. A protein response to muramyl dipeptide analogs and different mycobacterial species. *Infect. Immunity* **39**, 1147–54.

McFadden, J.J., Butcher, P.D., Chiodini, R. and Hermon-Taylor, J. (1987). Crohn's disease-isolated mycobacteria are identical to *Mycobacterium paratuberculosis*, as determined by DNA probes that distinguish between mycobacterial species. *J. Clin. Microbiol.* **25**, 796–801.

Magee, D.M. and Wing, E.J. (1988). Cloned L3T4$^+$ T lymphocytes protect mice against *Listeria monocytes* by secreting IFN-γ. *J. Immunol.* **141**, 3203–7.

Mearns, G., Richmond, S.J. and Storey, C. (1988). Sensitive immune dot blot test for diagnosis of *Chlamydia trachomatis* infection. *J. Clin. Microbiol.* **26**, 1810–13.

Mendez-Samperio, P., Lamb, J., Bothamley, G., Stanley, P., Ellis, C. and Ivanyi, J. (1989). Molecular study of the T cell repertoire in family contacts and patients with leprosy. *J. Immunol.* **142**, 3599–604.

Merkal, R.S., Larsen, A.B., Kopecky, K.E. *et al.* (1968). Experimental paratuberculosis in sheep after oral, intratracheal or intravenous inoculation: serological and intradermal tests. *Am. J. Vet. Res.* **29**, 963–9.

Merkal, R.S., Kopecky, K.E., Larsen, A.B. and Ness, R.B. (1970). Immunologic mechanisms in bovine paratuberculosis. *Am. J. Vet. Res.* **31**, 475–85.

Mielke, M.E.A., Ehlers, S. and Hahn, H. (1988). T-cell subsets in delayed-type hypersensitivity, protection, and granuloma formation in primary and secondary *Listeria* infection in mice: superior role of Lyt-2$^+$ cells in acquired immunity. *Infect. Immunity* **56**, 1920–5.

Miller, V.L. and Falkow, S. (1988). Evidence for two genetic loci in *Yersinia enterocolitica* that can promote invasion of epithelial cells. *Infect. Immunity* **56**, 1242–8.

Modlin, R.L. and Rea, T.H. (1988). Immunopathology of leprosy granulomas. *Springer Semin. Immunopathol.* **10**, 359–74.

Monnickendam, M.A. and Pearce, J.H. (1983). Immune responses and chlamydial infections. *Br. Med. Bull.* **39**, 187–93.

Montaraz, J.A., Winter, A.J., Hunter, D.M., Sdowa, B.A., Wu, A.M. and Adams, L.G. (1986). Protection against *Brucella abortus* in mice with O-polysaccharide-specific monoclonal antibodies. *Infect. Immunity* **51**, 961–3.

Moreno, C., Mehlert, A. and Lamb, J. (1988). The inhibitory effects of mycobacterial lipoarabinomannan and polysaccharides upon polyclonal and monoclonal human T cell proliferation. *Clin. Exp. Immunol.* **74**, 206–10.

Morgan, K.L. (1987). Johne's and Crohn's chronic inflammatory bowel diseases of infectious aetiology? *Lancet* **i**, 1017–19.

Mustafa, A.S., Gill, H.K., Nerland, A. *et al.* (1986a). Human T cell clones recognise a major *M. leprae* protein antigen expressed in *E. coli*. *Nature* **319**, 63–6.

Mustafa, A.S., Kvalheim, G., Degre, M. and Godal, T. (1986b). *Mycobacterium bovis* BCG-induced human T cell clones from BCG-vaccinated healthy subjects: antigen specificity and lymphokine production. *Infect. Immunity* **53**, 491–7.

Nash, T.W., Libby, D.M. and Horwitz, M.A. (1988). IFN-γ-activated human alveolar macrophages inhibit the intracellular multiplication of *Legionella pneumophila*. *J. Immunol.* **140**, 3978–81.

Nogueira, N., Kaplan, G., Levy, E. *et al.* (1983). Defective gamma interferon production in leprosy: reversal with antigen and IL-2. *J. Exp. Med.* **158**, 2165–70.

North, R.J. (1970). The relative importance of blood monocytes and fixed macrophages to the expression of cell-mediated immunity to infection. *J. Exp. Med.* **132**, 521–34.

O'Callaghan, D., Maskell, D., Liew, F.Y., Easmon, C.S.F. and Dougan, G. (1988). Characterization of aromatic- and purine-dependent *Salmonella typhimurium*: attenuation, persistence, and ability to induce protective immunity in BALB/c mice. *Infect. Immunity* **56**, 419–23.

Oftung, F., Mustafa, A.S., Husson, R., Young, R.A. and Godal, T. (1987). Human T cell clones recognise two abundant *Mycobacterium tuberculosis* protein antigens expressed in *Escherichia coli*. *J. Immunol.* **138**, 927–31.

Orme, I.M. (1987). The kinetics of emergence and loss of mediator T lymphocytes acquired in response to infection with *Mycobacterium tuberculosis*. *J. Immunol* **138**, 293–8.

Ottenhoff, T.H.M., Torres, P., De Las Aguas, J.T. *et al.* (1986). Evidence for an HLA-DR4-associated immune-response gene for *Mycobacterium tuberculosis*. *Lancet* **ii**, 310–13.

Payne, N.R. and Horwitz, M.A. (1987). Phagocytosis of *Legionella pneumophila* is mediated by human monocyte complement receptors. *J. Exp. Med.* **166**, 1377–89.

Peeling, R., Maclean, I.W. and Brunham, R.C. (1984). *In vitro* neutralization of *Chlamydia trachomatis* with monoclonal antibody to an epitope on the major outer membrane protein. *Infect. Immunity* **46**, 484–8.

Pellicer, T., Ariza, J., Foz, A., Pallares, R. and Gudiol, F. (1988). Specific antibodies detected during relapse of human brucellosis. *J. Infect. Dis.* **157**, 918–24.

Pinching, A.J. (1987). Acquired immune deficiency syndrome: with special reference to tuberculosis. *Tubercle* **68**, 65–9.

Portnoy, D.A., Jacks, P.S. and Hinrichs, D.J. (1988). Role of hemolysin for the intracellular growth of *Listeria monocytogenes*. *J. Exp. Med.* **167**, 1459–71.

Rea, T.H. (1983). Suppressor cell activity and phenotypes in the blood or tissues of patients with leprosy. *Clin. Exp. Immunol.* **54**, 323–38.

Rees, A., Scoging, A., Mehlert, A., Young, D.B. and Ivanyi, J. (1989). Specificity of proliferative response of human CD8 clones to mycobacterial antigens. *Eur. J. Immunol.* **18**, 1881–7.

Rees, R.J.W. (1954). Some experimental approaches to the tuberculosis problem. *Br. Med. Bull.* **10**, (2), 104–8.

Ridley, D.S. and Jopling, W.H. (1966). Classification of leprosy according to immunity: a five-group system. *Int. J. Leprosy* **34**, 255–73.

Ridley, M.J. and Ridley, D.S. (1983). The immunopathology of erythema nodosum leprosum: the role of extravascular complexes. *Leprosy Rev.* **54**, 95–107.

Rosqvist, R., Bolin, I. and Wolf-Watz, H. (1988). Inhibition of phagocytosis in *Yersinia pseudotuberculosis*: a virulence plasmid-encoded ability involving the Yop2b protein. *Infect. Immunity* **56**, 2139–43.

Sampson, J.S., Plikaytis, B.B. and Wilkinson, H.W. (1986). Immunologic response of patients with legionellosis against major protein-containing antigens of *Legionella pneumophila* serogroup 1 as shown by immunoblot analysis. *J. Clin. Microbiol.* **23**, 92–9.

Shields, E.D., Russell, D.A., Perlonk-Vanco, M.A. (1987). Genetic epidemiology of the susceptibility to leprosy. *J. Clin. Invest.* **79**, 1139–43.

Simonet, M., Berche, P., Mazigh, D. and Veron, M. (1985). Protection against *Yersinia* infection induced by non-virulence-plasmid-encoded antigens. *J. Med. Microbiol.* **20**, 225–31.

Singh, S.P.N., Mehra, N.K., Dingley, H.B., Pande, J.N. and Vaidya, M.C. (1983). Human leukocyte antigen (HLA)-linked control of susceptibility to pulmonary tuberculosis and association with HLA-DR types. *J. Infect. Dis.* **148**, 676–81.

Stead, W.W. (1967). Pathogenesis of a first episode of chronic pulmonary tuberculosis in man: recrudescence of residuals of the primary infection or exogenous reinfection? *Am. Rev. Respir. Dis.* **95**, 729–45.

Stephens, R.S., Wagar, E.A. and Schoolnik, G.K. (1988). High-resolution mapping of serovar-specific and common antigenic determinants of the major outer membrane protein of *Chlamydia Trachomatis*. *J. Exp. Med.* **167**, 817–31.

Stevenson, M.M., Kongshavn, P.A.L. and Skamene, E. (1981). Genetic linkage of resistance to *Listeria monocytogenes* with macrophage inflammatory responses. *J. Immunol.* **127**, 402–7.

Svenson, S.B., Nurminen, M. and Lindberg, A.A. (1979). Artificial *Salmonella* vaccines: O-antigenic oligosaccharide-protein conjugates induce protection against infection with *Salmonella typhimurium*. *Infect. Immunity* **25**, 863–72.

Swartz, R.P., Naai, D., Vogel, C.-W. and Yeager, H., Jr. (1988). Differences in uptake of mycobacteria by human monocytes: a role for complement. *Infect. Immunity* **56**, 2223–7.

Takashima, T. and Collins, F.M. (1988). T-cell-mediated immunity in persistent *Mycobacterium intracellulare* infections in mice. *Infect. Immunity* **56**, 2782–7.

Tam, M.R., Stamm, W.E., Hansfield, H.H. *et al.* (1984). Culture-independent diagnosis of *Chlamydia trachomatis* using monoclonal antibodies. *N. Engl. J. Med.* **310**, 1146–50.

ten Dam, H.G. (1984). Research on BCG vaccination. *Adv. Tuberculosis Res.* **21**, 79–106.

Tidjani, O., Amedome, A. and ten Dam, H.G. (1986). The protective effect of BCG vaccination of the newborn against childhood tuberculosis in an African community. *Tubercle* **67**, 269–81.

Todd, W.J. and Caldwell, H.D. (1985). The interaction of *Chlamydia trachomatis* with host cells: ultrastructural studies of the mechanism of release of a biovar II strain from HeLa 229 cells. *J. Infect. Dis.* **151**, 1037–44.

Toivanen, A., Granfors, K., Lahesmaa-Rantala, R., Leino, R., Stahlberg, T. and Vuento, R. (1985). Pathogenesis of *Yersinia*-triggered reactive arthritis: immunological, microbiological, and clinical aspects. *Immunol. Rev.* **86**, 47–70.

Turco, J. and Winkler, H.H. (1983). Cloned mouse interferon-gamma inhibits the growth of *Rickettsia prowazekii* in cultured mouse fibroblasts. *J. Exp. Med.* **258**, 2159–64.

Une, T. and Brubaker, R.R. (1984). Roles of V antigen in promoting virulence and immunity in yersiniae. *J. Immunol.* **133**, 2226–30.

van Dissel, J.T., Stikkelbroeck, J.J.M., Sluiter, W., Leijh, P.C.J. and van Furth, R. (1985). Course of an intraperitoneal inflammation during a *Salmonella typhimurium* infection in *Salmonella*-resistant CBA and *Salmonella*-susceptible C57BL/10 mice. In *Genetic Control of Host Resistance to Infection and Malignancy*, ed. E. Skamene, pp. 245–55, Alan R. Liss, New York.

van Schooten, W.C.A., Ottenhoff, T.H.M., Klatser, P.R., Thole, J., De Vries, R.R.P. and Kolk, A.H.J. (1988). T cell epitopes on the 36K and 65K *Mycobacterium leprae* antigens defined by human T cell clones. *Eur. J. Immunol.* **18**, 849–54.

WHO Tuberculosis Control Programme (1986). Efficacy of infant BCG immunization. *Weekly Epidemiol. Rec.* **61**, 213–20.

Williams, D.M., Schachter, J., Weiner, M.H. and Grubbs, B. (1984). Antibody in host defense against mouse pneumonitis agent (murine *Chlamydia trachomatis*). *Infect. Immunity* **45**, 674–8.

Winter, A.J., Rowe, G.E., Duncan, J.R. *et al.* (1988). Effectiveness of natural and synthetic complexes of porin and O polysaccharide as vaccines against *Brucella abortus* in mice. *Infect. Immunity* **56**, 2808–17.

Yamamoto, Y., Klein, T.W., Newton, C.A., Widen, R. and Friedman H. (1987). Differential growth of *Legionella pneumophila* in guinea pig versus mouse macrophage cultures. *Infect. Immunity* **55**, 1369–74.

Yamamura, Y. (1958). The pathogenesis of tuberculous cavities. *Adv. Tuberculosis Res.* **9**, 13–23.

Young, D.B., Mehlert, A., Bal, V., Mendez-Samperio, P., Ivanyi, J. and Lamb, J.R. (1988). Stress proteins and the immune response to mycobacteria — antigens as virulence factors? *Antonie van Leeuwenhoek* **54**, 431–9.

Zhang, Y.-X., Stewart, S., Joseph, T., Taylor, H.R. and Caldwell, H.D. (1987). Protective monoclonal antibodies recognize epitopes located on the major outer membrane protein of *Chlamydia trachomatis*. *J. Immunol.* **138**, 575–81.

77: Viruses

J.G.P. Sissons and L.K. Borysiewicz

Introduction

Viruses have long been used as experimental tools by immunologists, and the study of the immune response to viruses has contributed much to our understanding of basic immunological mechanisms — especially of the mechanism by which non-self determinants on cells are recognized. This experimental attention viruses have received is a reflection of the driving role they have played in the evolution of the immune system. However, there are, of course, important practical and clinical reasons for attempting to understand the immunology of virus infections — these include the needs for rational design of vaccines and for understanding the pathogenesis of human virus diseases.

Viruses as antigens

Classification

A full classification of animal viruses is beyond the scope of this chapter — there are accounts elsewhere (Murphy and Kingsbury 1990). Viruses range in size from small ribonucleic acid (RNA) viruses coding for a single protein and incapable of independent replication (such as hepatitis delta virus), to the large and complex deoxyribonucleic acid (DNA) viruses such as the herpes- or poxviruses, whose genomes encode in the region of 200 proteins, including most of the enzymes needed for their replication. Viruses are conventionally classified (by the International Committee on Taxonomy of Viruses) into families, genera and species. This classification depends on nucleic acid type, the presence or absence of an envelope, the genome replication strategy, whether the genome is positive- or negative-sense, and whether the genome is segmented or not. The families containing human and animal viruses and some of their characteristics are given in Table 77.1.

Structure

An increasing amount of information is becoming available on the fine structure of viruses. Several small viruses have now been studied at molecular resolution by X-ray crystallography — poliovirus and foot-and-mouth disease virus (FMDV) are examples particularly relevant to virus immunology (Hogle *et al.* 1987; Acharya *et al.* 1989; and see below). Isolated proteins of more complex viruses have also been analysed by X-ray diffraction — in the case of the influenza virus haemagglutinin (HA), this has enabled the epitopes recognized by antibodies to be precisely located on the molecule (Wiley and Skehel 1987). The consequence of binding of antibody on conformational structure can be studied and the effect on virus receptor interactions analysed.

The structure of the membranes of enveloped viruses and of the glycoproteins they contain has also been studied extensively. These membrane glycoproteins found in enveloped viruses are processed, glycosylated and exported to the plasma membrane of infected cells by the same mechanisms as the endogenous cellular glycoproteins — indeed, viruses were used as probes to first elucidate the normal cellular pathways for processing glycoproteins. Viral glycoproteins have attracted much attention because of their importance in receptor binding and as targets for neutralizing antibody. It was formerly thought that, because of their location on the cell surface, they were the target for all immunological recognition including T cells: it is now clear that this is not the case and that T cells recognize determinants from intracellular proteins equally well.

Replication

A brief description is given of the replicative cycle of viruses, stressing those points relevant to the immunology of virus infection. The cycle can be divided into a number of distinct stages as follows.

VIRUS BINDING AND ENTRY

Some viruses bind to specific protein receptors on the plasma membrane, the distribution of which may be a major determinant of the cellular tropism of the virus. Examples are the use of CD4 by the glycoprotein 120 (gp120) of human immunodeficiency virus (HIV) and of the CR2 complement receptor by gp340 of Epstein–Barr virus (EBV) (see Chapter 78). CD4 is a member of the immunoglobulin (Ig) superfamily of molecules and recent evidence has implicated other members of this family as receptors for picornaviruses. Intercellular adhesion molecule (ICAM)-1 (whose endogenous ligand is the lymphocyte integrin, lymphocyte function-associated antigen (LFA)-1) appears to be the cellular receptor for rhinoviruses, and the poliovirus receptor has recently been isolated and shown to be another, but hitherto unidentified, member of the Ig superfamily (Greve *et al.* 1989; Mendelsohn *et al.* 1989; Staunton *et al.* 1989; Racaniello 1990). However, both these members of the Ig superfamily are widely distributed on a number of cell types, and the differing tropisms of rhinoviruses and polioviruses cannot be explained on the distribution of their receptors alone.

Influenza virus binds to sialic acid on cell membrane glycoproteins and glycolipids. The receptor-binding domain is a shallow pocket near the top of the globular heads of the HA and the three-dimensional structure of its interaction with sialic acid has been determined (Wiley and Skehel 1987). For most viruses, receptors, remain to be defined, whether particular carbohydrate groups (such as sialic acid for influenza virus) or specific cell surface proteins.

Cells may still be permissive for replication even if they lack receptors, as shown by their ability to support replication following transfection of viral nucleic acid. To enter the intracellular environment, viruses must cross a lipid membrane, penetration of which is an energy-dependent process. Viruses which bind to membrane receptors are endocytosed via coated pits into the endosomal compartment. Following this, the virus fuses with the endosomal membrane and is translocated into the cytoplasm. For example, in the case of influenza, the HA undergoes pH-dependent cleavage into two components, allowing it to act as a fusion protein. Some viruses can bypass the requirement

Table 77.1. Examples of human and animal pathogenic viruses

Virus family	Genome	Envelope	Individual agents	Clinical syndromes
Picornaviruses				
(entero)	ssRNA (+)	−	Poliovirus	Poliomyelitis
			Coxsackie viruses	Pericarditis/Bornholm
			Echoviruses	Gastroenteritis
			Hepatitis A	Infectious hepatitis
(cardio)				
(rhino)			Rhinoviruses (1−89)	Common cold
(aptho)			Foot-and-mouth virus	Foot-and-mouth disease (cattle)
Calciviruses	ssRNA (+)	−	Norwalk agent	Gastroenteritis
Togaviruses	ssRNA (+)	+	Alphaviruses	Haemorrhagic fever viruses
			Flaviviruses	
			Yellow fever	Yellow fever
			Dengue	Dengue fever
			Rubella	German measles
Coronaviruses	ssRNA (+)	+		Common cold/URTI
Paramyxoviruses	ssRNA (−)	+	Parainfluenza (1−4)	Common cold/URTI
			Measles	Measles
			Respiratory syncytial virus	Childhood bronchiolitis
Rhabdoviruses	ssRNA (−)	+	Rabies	Rabies
Orthomyxoviruses	ssRNA (−)	+	Influenza A, B and C	URTI
Bunyaviruses	ssRNA (−)	+	Phlebovirus	Sandfly fever
Arenaviruses	ssRNA (−)	+	Lassa Junin/Machupo	Lassa fever etc.
			LCMV	Asymptomatic/encephalitis
Retroviruses	ssRNA (−)	+	HTLV I and II	T cell lymphoma
			HTLV III	AIDS
Reoviruses	dsRNA (+/−)	−	Rotavirus	Gastroenteritis
			Reovirus 1, 2 and 3	Encephalitis (mice)
Poxviruses	dsDNA	+	Smallpox/vaccinia	
			Orf	
			Molluscum contagiosum	
Herpesviruses	dsDNA	+	Herpes simplex 1 and 2	Cold sores
			VZV	Chicken pox/zoster
			Cytomegalovirus	Infectious mononucleosis
			EBV	(IM)/pneumonitis
				IM/Burkitt's lymphoma
Adenoviruses	dsDNA	−	Human adenoviruses (1−37)	URTI
Papovaviruses	dsDNA	−	BK/JC viruses	Multifocal leucoencephalopathy
Hepadnaviruses	dsDNA	+	Hepatitis B	Serum hepatitis
Parvoviruses	ssDNA	−		Erythema infectiosum

ssRNA = single stranded ribonucleic acid; dsRNA = double stranded ribonucleic acid; URTI = upper respiratory tract infection.

for endocytosis by fusing directly with the cell membrane by the action of a specific fusion glycoprotein inserted into the viral envelope (e.g. Sendai virus, measles virus).

REPLICATION

Virus penetration is followed by uncoating, release of the virus genome and virus replication.

All viruses have to generate a messenger RNA (mRNA) that can be recognized by the cell's translational machinery but they adopt very different strategies to achieve this end. Viral genomes differ widely in structure — they may be RNA or DNA and segmented or non-segmented — and the general strategy of virus replication differs with respect to the nature of the virus genome and its site of replication within the cell. Replication of single-stranded RNA viruses depends on the RNA configuration. In positive-stranded viruses the viral RNA is in the appropriate configuration to serve as a direct template for translation of viral proteins. These then transcribe the genome into the reactive configuration for further transcription of progeny virus RNA in the positive configuration.

If the RNA is in the 'wrong' configuration to direct translation, as in negative-stranded viruses, a transcriptase enzyme packaged within the virion transcribes the negative genome to positive mRNA. Under the control of proteins translated from this mRNA, a full-length positive copy of the genome is made which serves as a template for progeny negative-stranded virus RNA. In the case of the retroviruses, the genomic RNA is transcribed into double-stranded DNA by the virus reverse transriptase. This DNA is then integrated into the host cell DNA, from which progeny RNA can be transcribed (Weiss 1985).

Double-stranded DNA viruses can use host cell transcriptional enzymes. Papovaviruses, adenoviruses and herpesviruses undergo two or three cycles of regulated transcription, with expression of non-structural gene products. These are required for genome replication and structural protein synthesis (Roizman and Sears 1990). Poxviruses replicate within the cytoplasm, with transcription occurring in the core of the virion. Parvoviruses are often defective, requiring the presence of helper viruses. Hepatitis B virus (HBV) has a unique replication cycle: reverse transcriptase activity is associated with the viral DNA polymerase, and this transcribes genomic DNA from an RNA intermediate. Integration of viral DNA into chromosomal DNA (although it may sometimes occur) is not an essential feature of hepadnavirus replication — as it is in retroviruses, to which they bear some similarity.

Thus, viruses encode a number of proteins required to direct synthesis of viral products, in addition to coding for virus structural proteins. These non-structural proteins are expressed in various cell compartments, including the cell surface, and immune responses can be directed against them as well as against structural proteins.

ASSEMBLY AND RELEASE

Virus capsid assembly varies among individual viruses but involves aggregation of the structural proteins into a thermodynamically stable structure in the cell (Harrison 1990).

Virus release from infected cells is achieved by one of two mechanisms. Non-enveloped viruses, such as polio, accumulate within the cytoplasm; host cell macromolecular synthesis is inhibited, the cell disrupted and virus released (Rueckert 1990).

Enveloped viruses, however, bud from the surface of infected cells. Virus glycoproteins are inserted into the host cell membrane and displace normal host cell membrane glycoproteins. The virus capsid proteins interact with the cytoplasmic portion of the inserted viral glycoprotein and the virus is encased within the membrane, which is then extruded from the cell surface (Wiley and Skehel 1990). Variations of this are observed: herpesvirus acquire their envelope from the nuclear membrane, not the cell surface, and are released in vesicles (Roizman and Sears 1990). This method of virus release requires cell integrity to be maintained late into the infection, and the effect of enveloped virus infection on host cell macromolecular synthesis is in consequence often subtle and selective.

Antigenic variation

One particular feature of viruses as antigens deserves special emphasis — the ability of some viruses to exhibit antigenic variation. This is to a large extent a reflection of the replicative strategy of those particular viruses which show this phenomenon, and which leads to their genomic variation. Firstly, the intrinsic mutation rate may be high. Positive-strand RNA viruses are dependent on the viral RNA polymerase, which has a high error rate for transcription (1 in 10^4 base pairs read) (Holland *et al.* 1982). In the absence of a proof-reading or repair system as applies to DNA, these errors are rapidly compounded and transmitted to progeny particles — thereby maintaining high evolution rates and a high level of antigenic variation in these viruses.

Another example is influenza virus, which has a segmented (negative-strand) RNA genome which can undergo genetic mixing with other strains of the virus — including avian and animal strains — to produce 'reassortants'. This process leads to 'antigenic shift', when the haemagglutinin gene changes abruptly due to incorporation of the HA from a different strain into an existing human strain. The more gradually operating phenomenon of 'antigenic drift' is produced by variation in the amino acids situated on projecting loops around the receptor-binding pocket on the HA molecule, which are the target for neutralizing antibody — the amino acids in the floor of the pocket being highly conserved (Wiley and Skehel 1987).

The lentiretroviruses also exhibit great genomic diversity, so that multiple different sequence variants may be found in a single persistently infected host (Meyerhans *et al.* 1989). In their case this diversity results from multiple single-point nucleotide substitutions as a result of copying errors by the viral reverse transcriptase. In the case of the env gene of HIV this results in antigenic variation in the envelope protein, which is an important target for neutralizing antibody. Such antigenic variants may then be subjected to a degree of *in vivo* selection because of their failure to be neutralized by pre-existing antibody (Albert *et al.* 1990). The question also arises of whether, in the case of HIV, 'escape mutants' may emerge which are not recognized by cytotoxic T lymphocytes (CTL) (Phillips *et al.* 1990). The resultant continual emergence of new antigenic variants is probably a contributory factor in the pathogenesis of the lentiretroviruses and has been best documented in equine infectious anaemia and visna virus infection in sheep (Clements *et al.* 1988).

Latent and persistent infection

The term persistence is applied to those viruses which persist in the host following acute primary infection, usually for the lifetime of the host. For many such viruses persistence is an invariable concomitant of their replicative cycle (e.g. the retroviruses); for others it depends on the cell type the virus infects, undergoing lytic replication in some cells and being latent in others (e.g. the herpesviruses). Some other viruses only infrequently establish persistent infection and it is not an essential facet of their replication (e.g. measles virus, hepatitis B virus). Some viruses replicate at a low level during persistence (e.g. EBV) whereas others exhibit classical latency (e.g. herpes simplex virus (HSV)) in which no, or very limited, transcription takes place and there is no virus replication; latent virus may reactivate under the influence of various stimuli. The molecular events involved in persistence and latency are complex and not completely elucidated — for instance, it is likely that latency depends in large part on transcriptional control of the virus exerted by the presence or absence of specific cellular nucleic acid-binding proteins. The extent of virus gene expression during persistence is variable — there may be expression of a limited set of genes essential to maintain persistence with a block to transcription of later genes coding for structural proteins of the virus and factors needed for replication. The state of the viral genome during persistence is also crucial to understanding its mechanism: for instance, retroviruses integrate their proviral DNA into chromosomal DNA, and EBV DNA is maintained as episomes during its non-lytic infection in B cells (see Ahmed and Stevens (1990) for further details on persistent viruses).

Persistent infections are controlled in large part by the immune response in the normal host and tend to produce disease principally in the clinical setting of immunosuppression. This relationship with the immune response may be complex; it is worth noting that the cellular sites of persistent virus infection frequently include cells which may be less accessible to the immune system, such as epithelial or neuronal cells and the cells of the immune system itself.

Immunologically non-specific resistance

Host resistance to virus infections may be classified into several distinct phases (Janeway 1989; Table 77.2). There are a number of important mechanisms of non-specific immunity which operate before the generation of specific humoral and cellular antiviral immunity.

Interferons (see also Chapter 17)

The interferons (IFNs) were all originally described for their antiviral effect, but are now recognized to

Table 77.2. Host defence against viral infection — three phases

Phase	Characteristics	Mechanisms
Immediate (<4 h)	Non-specific, innate No memory No specific T cells	Natural killer cells Lack of cell receptors
Early (4–96 h)	Non-specific inducible No memory No specific T cells	Interferons (IFN) α and β IFN-activated NK cells
Late (> 96 h)	Specific, inducible Memory Specific T cells	Specific antibody Cytotoxic T cells

have many other actions — in particular, antiproliferative and 'immunomodulatory' ones. Three types of IFN are recognized: α, β and γ. There are about 14 IFN-α genes, two or more IFN-β genes (IFN-β2 is now synonymous with interleukin (IL)-6 — see below) and one IFN-γ gene. Interferon-γ is released by activated T cells and is really better regarded as a lymphokine (and would perhaps be better named as an interleukin). It is the major macrophage-activating factor, and macrophage activation by IFN-γ appears to be important in the resolution of protozoal diseases and intracellular bacterial infections.

Although for some IFNs it seems now to be a subsidiary part of their actions, their antiviral effect is undoubtedly significant *in vivo*. For instance, animals treated with antibody to interferon experience much more severe virus diseases. Viruses are the most effective inducers of IFNs — RNA viruses rather more so than DNA viruses — but double-stranded RNAs and synthetic polyribonucleotides are also effective. It has long been established that IFNs induce the antiviral state by a mechanism that involves binding to receptors on the cell surface (which for IFN-α and β is a glycoprotein encoded on human chromosome 21) and the induction of new protein synthesis. However, despite a great deal of work, there is no consensus on the precise basis for the resistance to virus infection induced by IFNs: in many cases the translation of virus-specific mRNAs is inhibited but for other viruses IFNs may also interfere with penetration and uncoating. Although the levels of 2,5-oligoandenylate synthetase and of a protein kinase increase markedly in IFN-treated cells, intensive studies of both these enzyme systems have failed to implicate them definitively in the induction of the antiviral state (Joklik 1990).

The administration of pharmacological doses of recombinant IFNs to patients has shown that they cause fever and malaise in recipients — effects which may be dose-limiting. This suggests that they may be responsible for these same symptoms during natural infection, although IL-1 and tumour necrosis factor (TNF) can also produce fever.

Tumour necrosis factor itself also has an antiviral effect: the mechanism is less studied than, and probably different from, that of IFN, although the antiviral effects of both cytokines are synergistic. Tumour necrosis factor has been reported to inhibit the replication of DNA and RNA viruses, but it can also lyse cells infected with some viruses (vesicular stomatitis and adenoviruses — Wong and Goeddel 1986).

Natural killer cells

Natural killer (NK) cells are the subject of a separate chapter in this volume (Chapter 31). For the purposes of discussion here, they are defined as cytolytic lymphocytes which are non-T cells (without a rearranged T cell receptor gene) and which, in humans, possess the CD3 −ve, CD16 +ve phenotype. Natural killer cell cytotoxicity is not major histocompatibility complex (MHC)-restricted and is relatively easy to assay *in vitro* compared with CTL assays. Many virus-infected (and tumour-derived) target cells show increased susceptibility to NK cell lysis, but the molecular basis for this is unclear. The NK cell 'receptor' is as yet unidentified and so are the recognition molecules on their target cells. However, virus proteins expressed on the cell surface do not appear to be recognition structures. Whilst NK cells show spontaneous cytotoxicity, their lytic activity is enhanced by IFNs, so that they may be regarded as having inducible function. Interferon pretreatment also renders non-infected target cells less susceptible to lysis by NK cells. However, the enhanced susceptibility to NK lysis shown by virus-infected cells is not mediated by IFN; it presumably depends on a virus-induced alteration in the expression of some unidentified membrane structure. There is evidence for an inverse correlation between the surface expression of Class I MHC molecules and susceptibility to NK cell lysis. Consistent with this are the observations that IFNs increase Class I MHC expression (possibly explaining their protection effect on uninfected cells) and that several viruses may decrease Class I MHC expression (Welsh and Vargas-Cortes 1991).

Although they may have other roles, accumulating evidence suggests that NK cells are of importance in natural resistance to viral infections. In mice depletion of NK cells (with antibody to the glycolipid asialo-GM1) results in much more severe infection with murine cytomegalovirus (MCMV) and death from lethal hepatitis. Beige mice, which have a defect in NK cell function, show the same phenomenon. In both cases adoptive transfer of cloned NK cells reverses this propensity to severe infection. However, resistance to other viruses, such as lymphocytic choriomeningitis virus (LCMV), is unimpaired in these models, suggesting that viruses may differ in the extent to which resolution of infection depends on NK lysis (Bukowski *et al.* 1985). There is inevitably less information in humans. However, a single patient has been reported who lacked functional NK cells and circulating CD16 +ve cells, and who suffered from recurrent herpesvirus infections (Biron *et al.* 1989). On the other hand, children with deficiency of the adhesion protein LFA-1 do not show increased susceptibility to virus infections, despite having markedly impaired function of all cytotoxic lymphocytes (including NK cells).

There is increased NK cell activity, assessed by *in vitro* assays, during acute virus infections in humans, although the precise phenotype of the effector cell is not always completely characterized, which necessitates caution in interpreting results. For instance, during primary infection with EBV in normal subjects, there is increased non-MHC-restricted cytotoxicity in the peripheral blood, but this seems to be mediated predominantly by cells which are CD3 +ve than by 'true' phenotypic NK cells as defined above (Strang and Rickinson 1987).

'Innate' genetically mediated resistance

There is evidence for additional mechanisms of non-immunological resistance to specific virus infections in experimental animals, which are genetically determined. One such piece of evidence comes from the study of MCMV infection, where resistance maps to a gene designated CMV-1, which, although H2-linked, is not an H2 or other known immunologically active molecule (Grundy *et al.* 1981; Lawson *et al.* 1988). The relevance to human virus infection remains to be determined — particularly when the gene confers resistance to virus challenge only by somewhat unusual routes, such as intraperitoneal challenge in the case of CMV-1. Obviously such genes would be much more difficult to identify in humans.

Immune response to viruses

The specific immune response to viruses has been extensively studied. Here we deal first with general aspects before going on to discuss the immune response to particular viruses (the immunology of EBV and HIV is dealt with in Chapters 78 and 71).

Antibody

The induction of the antibody response to viruses is essentially similar to that for other protein antigens, and it is mainly effector aspects which are discussed here.

All Ig isotypes — IgM, IgG and IgA — can be produced in response to virus infection, depending on whether infection is primary and on the site of infection, i.e. whether mucosal or parenteral. It is generally accepted that the principal mechanism by which antibody interferes with virus infection is by 'neutralization' of virions. This effect is produced principally by direct binding of antibody to epitopes on viral proteins which are involved in mediating attachment to receptors on the target cell surface. Thus, although all proteins encoded by a given virus are theoretically capable of eliciting an antibody response, it is antibody to the surface proteins on the virion (which are usually also present on the surface of virus-infected cells) that are of particular importance in effective immunity. Furthermore, although most linear peptides derived from the primary sequence of a protein are capable of eliciting an antibody response following immunization with peptides, it is antibody directed to epitopes accessible on the surface of the folded protein which appear to be protective *in vivo*. Such epitopes may be conformational rather than strictly linear, composed of 15–20 amino acids in a discontinuous array in the linear sequence (Laver *et al*. 1990).

Direct blocking by antibody of determinants which bind to virus receptors may not be the only way in which they cause neutralization. In the case of poliovirus, antibody binding may result in a conformational change in the virion which prevents its binding to its receptor or uncoating after its entry into the cell (Thomas *et al*. 1986; Rueckert 1990). Complement may enhance neutralization of viruses by antibody. Another possible effector mechanism which may be activated by antibody is antibody-dependent cell-mediated cytotoxicity (ADCC). The human effector cells for ADCC are CD16 +ve lymphocytes and are identical to NK cells. Whilst a wide range of virus-infected cells have been shown to be susceptible to ADCC *in vitro*, the *in vivo* significance of ADCC remains unclear (Sissons and Oldstone 1980).

Immunoglobulin A antibody is important in neutralizing virus on mucosal surfaces: secretory IgA is induced by those viruses whose primary route of entry is through the respiratory or gastrointestinal tract. It is probably important that the same route is used for vaccines against these viruses so that an appropriate IgA response is induced, as shown by the experience with the live and killed polio vaccines (Dhar and Ogra 1985; and see below).

Complement

Complement is activated via the classical pathway by antibody bound to virus; the resultant deposition of C3b may aid the clearance of virus by opsonization. Those viruses which possess a lipid envelope may be susceptible to complement-mediated membrane damage produced by C5b–9. It seems likely that complement will act principally against viruses in the fluid phase in blood; however, there is some evidence that complement may also lyse virus-infected cells. Cells infected with EBV or measles can activate the alternative pathway of complement activation and the presence of antibody enhances this activation and facilitates lysis. Whether complement plays any necessary role *in vivo* in clearing virus-infected cells — certainly outside the circulation — is perhaps doubtful. In particular, all observations to date indicate that human complement deficiency states are not associated with any undue propensity to severe virus infections (Sissons 1987).

Virus-specific T cells

HELPER T CELLS

Helper T (T_h) cells recognize processed peptides derived from viral proteins and presented to them by antigen-presenting cells (APC) — principally dendritic cells, macrophages and B cells. Helper T cells are generally restricted in their recognition of peptides by Class II MHC molecules and in humans are CD4 +ve. Virus-specific T_h clones have been studied in some detail *in vitro* — particularly for influenza. For influenza provision of help is cross-reactive and may also be in other viruses. At the peptide level it is clear that the peptides predominantly recognized by T_h cells are not necessarily the same as those recognized by antibody. Thus peptides throughout the influenza virus HA molecule may be recognized by T_h cells, in contrast to the predominantly conformational epitopes, or clustering of peptides on exposed surfaces of the molecule, which are recognized by antibody (Burt *et al*. 1989). Helper T cells provide help in the form of cytokines/growth factors such as IL-2, IL-4 and αIFN, and CD4 +ve cells may also act as effector cells mediating delayed-type hypersensitivity (DTH) or cytotoxicity.

SUPPRESSOR T CELLS

Suppressor T (T_s) cells have been studied in experimental virus systems, where a population of T cells which suppress Class II MHC-restricted DTH in murine influenza and in HSV infection has been described. It has been suggested that they may limit the tissue damage which virus-specific DTH cells may potentially cause (Ada *et al*. 1981; Nash 1990). In humans, active infection with certain viruses (herpesviruses — EBV, cytomegalovirus (CMV) and HSV — in particular) is associated with increased numbers of CD8 +ve cells in peripheral blood, and with suppression of lectin-induced Ig synthesis *in vitro*. However, whether these CD8 +ve cells play any role in the pathogenesis of these virus infections *in vivo* is unknown (Schooley *et al*. 1983).

CYTOTOXIC T CELLS

Class I MHC-restricted virus-specific cytotoxic T (T_c) cells have been extensively studied in virus systems, ever since the first description of their MHC restriction in the context of murine LCMV infection (see Zinkernagel and Doherty 1979). Class II MHC-restricted virus-specific CD4 +ve cells may also be cytotoxic — although when all lectin-induced cytotoxic cells from human peripheral blood lymphocytes (PBL) are analysed in limiting dilution the majority (90%) are CD8 +ve (Moretta *et al*. 1989). Virus-specific T_c cells recognize viral proteins as processed peptides bound to MHC molecules. In general, endogenous synthesis of viral proteins within the cell is required for association of their peptides with Class I MHC molecules to occur in the endoplasmic reticulum, whereas exogenous viral proteins are processed through the endosomal pathway, and associate with Class II MHC molecules. The induction of virus-specific T_c cell memory requires presentation of peptide associated with Class I MHC, but the evidence suggests that this presentation can occur on any Class I MHC-bearing cell — and not just on specialized APC (Townsend 1987).

The possible role of T_c cells expressing the γδ T cell receptor in virus infections has received very little study at the time of writing. One study has suggested they may be involved in the late clearance of influenza from the lungs of infected mice (Carding *et al*. 1990). Their very different distribution in mice, where they are localized to epithelial surfaces in normal animals (which does not appear to be the case in humans), makes extrapolation to human virus infections difficult.

The role of the immune response in virus clearance *in vivo*

How do these individual components of the immune response act *in vivo* to clear virus infections? Evidence derives both from experimental models and from human immunodeficiencies.

Experimental models

The study of experimental models of virus infection has contributed a great deal of the information which underpins this whole field, much of it probably applicable to human virus infections. They offer opportunities which are not possible in clinical studies — in particular, the use of adoptive transfer or subset deletion to analyse the role of individual components of the immune response in clearing infection, or to study pathogenesis. Only a few key examples are referred to here.

There have been relatively few studies of the adoptive transfer of antibody in experimental virus infections. There is evidence to suggest that it plays a particular role in recovery from toga-, picorna- and papovavirus infection in mice, although the protective effect appears to depend on the additional presence of macrophages in some cases (Zisman *et al*. 1971; Mims *et al*. 1991).

Many studies have examined the protective effects of virus-specific T cells in experimental virus infections. In murine influenza infection it has been shown that adoptively transferred CD8 +ve virus-specific T_c cells clear virus from the lungs, whereas CD4 +ve Class II MHC-restricted T cells mediating DTH may increase mortality (Ada *et al*. 1981). In apparent contrast, in experimental murine herpes simplex infection CD4 +ve DTH cells exert a protective effect during primary infection (Nash *et al*. 1985). In MCMV infection the majority of T_c cells present during persistent infection are CD8 +ve T_c cells directed against the MCMV major immediate early protein — this population is protective on adoptive transfer (Reddehase *et al*. 1987). In LCMV infection virus-specific T_c cells clear virus from the brain of adult infected mice, apparently without causing major cell death — but when adoptively transferred to chronic LCMV carrier mice they cause cerebral damage and death (Buchmeier *et al*. 1980; and see below).

Virus infections in immunodeficiencies

Although it is important to document the immune responses which occur in human virus infections, this in itself will not determine which elements of the response are critical in recovery from infection. However, some answer to this question may be found from examining virus infections which occur in human immunodeficiency states.

ANTIBODY DEFICIENCY

Antibody deficiency is in general associated with a propensity to bacterial infection and relatively little excess virus infection compared with T cell deficiencies, but there are important specific exceptions. Boys with X-linked agammaglobulinaemia are at risk of unusually severe illness with enteroviruses; there is a greatly increased risk of paralytic poliomyelitis following polio immunization, and of chronic or recurrent meningoencephalitis and myositis due to echovirus. Chronic rotavirus infection is also described. The enterovirus infections respond at least partly to Ig replacement and it seems reasonable to infer that antibody is particularly important in clearing these infections (Webster 1984). Virus infections are not a particular problem in common variable immunodeficiency or in the isolated deficiencies of individual Ig isotypes.

COMPLEMENT COMPONENT DEFICIENCIES

Complement component deficiencies are associated with recurrent bacterial infections or, for C1–C4 deficiency, with chronic immune complex disease, and these patients do not appear to be unduly prone to severe virus infections (Sissons 1987).

SEVERE COMBINED IMMUNODEFICIENCY DISEASES

Severe combined immunodeficiency diseases (SCID), in which both cellular and humoral immunity are severely impaired, are characterized clinically by severe infections with all pathogens including viruses. Severe combined immunodeficiency diseases are of diverse aetiology (see Chapter 66). One particular autosomal recessive form is characterized by an inability to express Class II MHC molecules on any cells ('SCID with Class II MHC deficiency'). Infections with viruses are a particular problem in this group of patients, whose T cells are unable to present antigen normally and who cannot mount DTH reactions (de Preval *et al.* 1988).

T CELL DEFICIENCIES

T cell deficiencies, such as the third and fourth pharyngeal pouch (Di George) syndrome, are associated with overwhelming viral (as well as mycobacterial and fungal) infections. Measles, vaccinia and the herpesviruses are the most frequent viruses which cause problems (Rosen *et al.* 1984).

It may thus be deduced that T cells are especially requisite for the normal resolution of virus infections, and that this is unlikely to be a consequence of their providing help for antibody production to T-dependent antigens (as most virus infections are not seen to excess in Ig deficiency). It is presumably rather a result of failure to generate effector T cells capable of eliminating virus-infected cells.

The potential importance of NK cells should also be remembered. As mentioned above, a single patient deficient in functional and phenotypic NK cells has been reported — and presented with severe and chronic herpesvirus infections (Biron *et al.* 1989). However, patients with LFA-1 deficiency and impaired function of all cytotoxic lymphocytes do not have an increased propensity to virus infection.

ACQUIRED IMMUNODEFICIENCY

Acquired immunodeficiencies associated with T cell defects, whether from iatrogenic drug-induced immunosuppression or from acquired immune deficiency syndrome (AIDS), is also associated with an increased incidence of virus infections — especially with reactivation and dissemination of endogenous persistent viruses, and severe primary infection with viruses transmitted by an allograft or by blood products. With prolonged immunosuppression the risk of virally induced tumours, particularly EBV-associated lymphomas, rises significantly.

However, the frequency and clinical severity of these infections does vary between the different types of organ transplantation and AIDS. For instance, severe CMV pneumonitis is a particular problem in bone marrow and in heart/lung transplantation but is less common in renal transplantation and in AIDS. In contrast, CMV retinitis affects 10–15% of patients with AIDS, but is uncommon in allograft recipients (Rubin 1990).

It has been shown that there is a reduced precursor frequency of virus-specific T cells for EBV and CMV in allograft recipients, which is presumably a factor predisposing to severe infection (Rickinson *et al.* 1985). The much more global immunosuppression in AIDS, affecting macrophages and APC as well as T cells, is probably responsible for the comparatively greater frequency and severity of virus infections. Nevertheless, factors specific to the type of organ graft seem likely to play some part — such as the viruses which may be transmitted by the graft itself, or the type of immunosuppression used and the efficacy of immunological reconstitution following bone marrow transplantation. These issues are further addressed in Chapter 46 and Section 10.

Induction of immunity by vaccines and immunotherapy

An alternative way of gaining insight into the nature of protective immunity is to analyse the immune responses induced by effective vaccines and the efficacy of 'immunotherapy' such as passive transfer of antibody.

The immune response to vaccines is usually assessed by measuring the neutralizing antibodies they induce, and it is assumed these are responsible for the observed protective effect. Indeed, this is probably a correct assumption in large part. However, some vaccines have been shown to be capable of inducing effector T cells — in particular, live virus vaccines or those employing live virus vectors. In experimental animals recombinant vaccinia virus vectors readily induce effector T cells against the foreign viral genes they express and it has been shown that for some viruses (such as MCMV) immunity may depend on the induced CTL rather than on antibody; at present we simply do not have enough information to know if this is true for any human virus infection.

Passive transfer of antiviral antibody has been used clinically to protect subjects at particular risk of acquiring certain virus infections, and can clearly provide some degree of protection in these situations. Examples include the prophylaxis of varicella in immunocompromised children (Straus *et al.* 1988), primary human CMV infection in seronegative organ allograft recipients (Snydman 1990) and neotal acquisition of maternal HBV infection (Beasley *et al.* 1983). In all these cases there is evidence from controlled trials of a protective effect, and it can thus be inferred that antibody alone can provide protection against primary infection. There are, perhaps not surprisingly, no examples of adoptive immunotherapy with human virus-specific T cells; although some groups are interested in this approach, it is difficult to imagine that the preparation of specific effector T cells *in vitro* will be a realistic routine therapeutic option.

Human virus infections

Analysing the relative protective role of the different components of the immune response to viruses in humans is obviously difficult and relies on inferences from the induction of immunity by natural infection or by vaccination and observing the consequences of immunodeficiency.

The measurement of antibody to viruses is relatively straightforward. The assessment of T cell responses presents rather more problems. As a rule only the peripheral blood compartment can be sampled (compared with spleen, lymph nodes and infected tissues in experimental animals). Secondary *in vitro* stimulation must usually be used to obtain a sufficient number of activated T cells for experiments; this risks selectively expanding T cells unrepresentative of the population *in vivo*, and functional assessment may be difficult — for instance, cytotoxicity cannot easily be assayed for viruses such as hepatitis B and papilloma, for which there are no tissue culture systems and DTH cannot be measured *in vitro*. Despite these difficulties some information is available for a number of human virus infections as discussed below.

Influenza

Influenza is one of the best studied acute virus infections of humans. Humoral immunity to influenza is subtype-specific, the subtypes being characterized by the HA and neuraminidase (N). The internal proteins of the virion — the nucleoprotein (NP) and matrix (M) protein — are highly conserved between subtypes; antigenic shift involves the acquisition of new HA or N genes by the reassortment between viruses, and antigenic drift mutations in those regions of the HA and N glycoproteins which interact with antibody (Wiley and Skehel 1987; Burt *et al.* 1989). Presence of antibody to the HA and N of a particular subtype correlates with immunity to that influenza subtype, and there is good reason to suppose antibody is the principal mediator of resistance to reinfection. Passive transfer of monoclonal antibody to HA or N protects mice from challenge, whereas antibody to M or NP does not.

However, influenza-specific T_c cells are also subtype-specific and can be demonstrated during the recovery phase of infection. Both NP and HA subtype-specific T_c cells can be shown, thereby providing cross-reactivity between serologically different HA and N strains. The ability to generate an influenza-specific T_c cell response from seropositive human donors, by secondary *in vitro* stimulation, wanes with time following the last natural exposure to the virus (McMichael *et al.* 1983).

In mice both NP- and HA-specific T_c cells can produce protection in adoptive transfer experiments — cross-reactive protection in the case of NP-specific T_c cells (Townsend 1987). The main role of the T_c cell response seems to be to clear established infection, with the evidence suggesting it is less important in resistance to reinfection.

Measles

Measles virus infection is initiated by infection of respiratory epithelium, but during the immediately following phase of viraemia the virus is present in lymphocytes and monocytes. There is lymphopenia at this point, and it is a long-standing observation that measles has a suppressive effect on *in vivo* and *in vitro* T cell responses (K. von Pirquet having first observed that children with measles lost tuberculin skin reactivity), which persists for several weeks after recovery from the clinical syndrome. Measles virus infects both B and T cells but only replicates in them when they are activated — *in vitro* proliferative responses are suppressed for a corresponding period to the loss of skin tests (Whittle *et al.* 1978; McChesney and Oldstone 1987). Measles is followed by lifelong immunity: maternal antibody provides immunity in the first 6 months of life, but the lesson from immunodeficiency states is that it is T cell deficiencies which are particularly associated with severe measles, and that the T cell response is crucially important in resolution of infection. It is, however, interesting to note that the typical morbilliform rash is not seen in T-cell-deficient subjects with measles, suggesting the rash is T-cell-mediated. Antibody to both the viral HA and fusion glycoproteins is required for immunity. Inactivated measles vaccine, which lacked antigenic F protein, was associated with the syndrome of atypical measles in the recipients when they subsequently encountered wild-type measles virus; severe lung involvement is characteristic of this syndrome, and appears to be immunopathologically mediated with features of an Arthus reaction. Measles has been shown to be associated with the induction of specific T_c cells as well as antibody; however, the bulk of memory T_c cells, at least as studied *in vitro* as T cell lines and clones, are CD4 +ve rather than CD8 +ve in phenotype, and show specificity for the internal N protein as well as HA (Jacobson *et al.* 1987).

Interest has centred on the association of measles with central nervous system (CNS) disease. Post-infectious measles encephalitis occurs in about 1:1000 cases and is demyelinating in type; it is thought to have an autoimmune basis but this has not been formally proven. In immunocompromised patients measles can also produce a progressive direct infectious encephalitis. However, especial interest has been aroused by subacute sclerosing panencephalitis (SSPE) — a rare (1:100 000) complication which usually occurs 6–8 years after acute measles virus infection and is characterized by an inexorably progressive course to death. Neuronal cells are packed with virus nucleocapsids but it is very difficult to recover infectious virus from the brain. The present view is that defective virus, with deletions in the envelope genes which prevent virus budding and release from the cell, is responsible for the syndrome. Affected children have very high titres of measles antibody, and virus persisting in their lymphocytes, but, although it was formerly suggested that aberrant immune responses might be a causal factor, this now appears less likely (Norrby and Oxman 1990).

MUMPS

Mumps — another paramyxovirus — is associated with the presence of mumps virus-specific T_c cells in the cerebrospinal fluid of children with meningoencephalitis, but here it has been suggested that they may play an immunopathogenic role, being responsible for the production of the CNS inflammation (Kreth *et al*. 1982). Certainly mumps is not associated with severe disease in the immunosuppressed patient and its resolution would seem by inference to be less dependent on effector T cell immunity than is measles.

Picornaviruses

These 27 nm, non-enveloped, single, positive-strand RNA viruses are widely prevalent pathogens of man. They are classified into four families: enteroviruses (comprising the three polioviruses, Coxsackie A and B viruses, echoviruses and numbered enteroviruses including hepatitis A), apthoviruses (including FMDV), rhinoviruses (100+ serotypes of the common cold virus) and cardioviruses (mostly murine). The virus genome is translated into a single polyprotein which is cleaved by virus proteases into four capsid and size non-structural proteins. *In vitro* these viruses are usually cytolytic, down-regulating host cell protein synthesis. Their tissue tropism is partly determined by specific receptor–ligand interactions (see above), the virus receptor being formed by a groove or 'canyon' identified in the capsid structure of the virion by X-ray crystallography.

Natural infection with an enterovirus such as polio results in local replication in intestinal epithelial cells, particularly those overlying Peyer's patches, and adjacent lymphoid tissue. This is followed by a viraemic phase, at which point the infection is halted in the majority of individuals, with the development of a type-specific neutralizing antibody response. These antibodies recognize variable regions of the major coat proteins of the virus, VP1–VP3. The neutralizing sites have been mapped, using monoclonal antibody escape mutants, and are found adjacent to the receptor-binding groove and at the vertices of the pentamers forming the capsid of the virion. It is unlikely that the virus is 'neutralized' by steric hindrance with receptor binding. Only two antibody molecules need bind each virion to achieve neutralization. It is more likely that antibody alters the capsid structure to block uncoating or cross-links pentamers on the virion.

In a small proportion of infected subjects, virus disseminates to the meninges and the nervous system. Transmission is probably vascular, although neuronal spread occurs within the CNS. These neurotropic viruses differ genomically from vaccine strains but the mutation is in the 5′ non-coding region (position 472) of the genome, rather than the capsid proteins. Thus pathogenicity is not totally explained by differential virus tropism at the level of receptor–ligand interaction.

The importance of neutralizing antibody in host protection is underlined by the susceptibility of X-linked agammaglobulinaemic subjects to enteroviral meningitis, which is ameliorated by passively transferred intrathecal Ig. However, efficient generation of anti-picornaviral antibody is entirely dependent on a T_h response. Peptide-specific responses to the FMDV 'loop' (VP1 141–160) can be induced in H-2^d mice only if a 'foreign' T cell epitope is linked to the peptide. Furthermore, the 'help' was B cell clone-specific, as neutralizing antibodies were observed with some but not all T cell epitopes used.

Even if neutralizing antibody is of paramount importance in host protection against these viruses, other effector T cell responses are also generated. Hepatitis A-specific CTL have been identified and isolated from liver biopsies, suggesting that some of the liver injury consequent on this infection may be immunopathologically mediated (Vallbracht *et al*. 1989).

Herpesviruses

Immunity to this important group of viruses has been extensively studied in animal models and in humans. However, their structural complexity — they may encode up to 200 proteins in the case of CMV — makes them less than ideal as model systems, compared with structurally simpler viruses such as influenza. Gene expression of these viruses is under complex regulation: during the full replicative cycle there is a temporally regulated sequence of expression of groups of genes designated immediate early (IE or α), early (or β) and late (or γ). In general the first two groups encode mainly non-structural proteins, whereas the late genes encode the structural proteins of the virion. However, during persistent infection and latency, gene expression from herpesviruses may be very limited, depending on the cell type, to certain genes — usually IE genes — with functions crucial to the maintenance of latency or persistence. Epstein–Barr virus gene expression during non-lytic persistence in B cells is limited to a set of genes necessary for episomal maintenance, analogous to the IE genes (see Chapter 78).

HERPES SIMPLEX VIRUS

The primary site of latency of the alphaherpesviruses, HSV and varicella–zoster virus (VZV), is in neurones. It is not known whether latently infected nerve cells are susceptible to immunological recognition but this seems unlikely. On reactivation virus is transported down the axon and replicates in epithelial cells adjacent to the nerve ending to produce a herpetic lesion. Clearly reactivation occurs despite the presence of antibody, and most efforts to implicate defects in human host immunity with HSV reactivation have centred on analysing T cell responses against HSV antigens or infected cells *in vitro*. Proliferative responses increase following reactivation episodes. Herpes simplex virus-specific T_c cells can also be generated *in vitro* from PBL and their specificity for glycoproteins shown. A decrease in IFN-α production and in NK cell activity has been reported in the prodrome preceding appearance of the lesions (Cunningham and Merigan 1983). However, the causal relationship of any of these responses to reactivation or to its containment remains unclear. Non-immunological and physical factors clearly play a part in reactivation, in addition to any immunological ones; indeed, it is striking that the most severe type of HSV disease — HSV encephalitis — usually occurs in apparently immunocompetent patients and is rare in AIDS.

VARICELLA–ZOSTER VIRUS

Varicella–zoster virus reactivation usually occurs in elderly and immunosuppressed subjects. Again, T cell immunity appears crucial to maintain the virus–host relationship. Varicella–zoster virus-specific T_c cells can be shown in normal seropositive subjects, with specificity for glycoproteins at least (Hickling *et al.* 1987). Passive transfer of antibody (zoster immune globulin (ZIG)) is moderately effective in reducing the incidence of severe primary disease in the immunosuppressed but has little effect after reactivation (Straus *et al.* 1988).

CYTOMEGALOVIRUS

Cytomegalovirus causes particular clinical problems in immunosuppressed organ transplant recipients and patients with AIDS. As mentioned above, work on MCMV has shown that a major population of T_c cells are directed against IE proteins during persistent infection; T_c cells against the major IE protein can transfer resistance, and vaccination of mice with a recombinant vaccinia virus expressing this protein protects them from lethal challenge (Reddehase *et al.* 1987). In asymptomatic humans there is also a rather high precursor frequency of memory T_c cells directed against the human CMV major IE protein in a majority of seropositive subjects, accounting for up to 60% of all CMV-specific T_c cells in some subjects (Borysiewicz *et al.* 1988). It has also been reported that T_c cells can be directly detected in the blood of bone marrow transplant recipients with active CMV infection and that their presence correlates with survival. The assumption is that CMV-specific T_c cells may provide a surveillance mechanism capable of recognizing infected cells at an early stage of the virus cycle.

In the absence (at least until recently) of effective chemotherapy, CMV immune globulin has been used to treat CMV disease, but on its own there is no clear evidence of benefit (it may have some adjunctive effect with ganciclovir in CMV pneumonitis). In contrast, there is evidence that it may reduce the incidence of severe primary CMV disease when given prophylactically to seronegative organ allograft recipients (Snydan 1990) — which accords with the view that antibody is principally of use to prevent primary infection or limit viraemia.

Hepatitis B virus

Hepatitis B virus is the prototype member of the hepadnaviruses (analogous viruses are found in woodchucks, ground squirrels, ducks and other animals) and is the causative agent of hepatitis B. The hepadnaviruses have small circular, partially single-stranded DNA genomes, with the longer negative strand being about 3 kb. They have a unique strategy of replication which involves the production of new negative-strand, closed, circular viral DNA from an RNA intermediate by reverse transcription; this is packaged into the virion and the positive strand of DNA is then synthesized. This suggests a common ancestry with the retroviruses; however, in addition to the differences above, hepadnaviruses do not integrate into host chromosomal DNA of necessity as do retroviruses. Nevertheless, integration may occur in association with persistent infection, which follows about 10% of cases of acute HBV infection. Detailed discussion of the biology of HBV is available elsewhere; it is discussed here for its interesting immunological aspects.

Acute infection is associated with the production of antibody to the virus-encoded proteins — surface (HBs) antigen, core (HBc) antigen and e antigen — and anti-HBc and anti-HBs persist after recovery. Anti-HBs is the main neutralizing antibody, and the induction of anti-HBs with HBV vaccine made from HBs antigen is associated with protection. Many of the extrahepatic manifestations of HBV infection are probably mediated by immune complexes of anti-HBs/HBs antigen — including the arthritis, rash and glomerulonephritis. Persistent infection is characterized by the persistence of HBs antigen without anti-HBs, and by anti-HBc; persistence of e antigen correlates with high infectivity of serum. Particular interest centres on the mechanism of liver injury in persistent HBV infection, which it is suggested may result from HBV-specific CTL lysing virus-infected hepatocytes. Formal proof of this hypothesis is made difficult by the absence of any tissue culture system for HBV, which limits *in vitro* experiments. However, CTL apparently recognizing determinants in HBc antigen and e antigen have been described in the peripheral blood of patients with chronic liver disease. Infiltrating CD8 cells can be shown in the liver, and there is some evidence that they are HBV-specific T_c cells (Mondelli *et al.* 1982; Barnaba *et al.* 1989): immunosuppression ameliorates HBV-associated chronic active hepatitis. Administration of IFN-α to chronic HBV carriers results in the disappearance of markers of HBV replication in about a third of cases. It is suggested that at least part of the mechanism for this effect is the induction of Class I MHC expression on hepatocytes (which normally express only a low amount) by IFN, rendering them susceptible to lysis by T_c cells. In fact, IFN administration is often accompanied by transient evidence of worsening liver function, which could be consistent with hepatocyte damage due to cytotoxic effector cells. In support of this concept, it has recently been shown that in transgenic mice in which HBV envelope protein is expressed in the liver, HBV envelope-specific CD8 +ve CTL can produce liver injury *in vivo* (Moriyama *et al.* 1990).

Virus immunopathology

It is now well appreciated that the immune response against viruses can be responsible for tissue damage and may have a pathogenic effect as well as a protective one (Sissons and Borysiewicz 1985). Virus immunopathology has been particularly well studied in certain experimental models, such as LCMV infection of mice (Buchmeier *et al.* 1980; Oehen *et al.* 1991); human examples may exist but are rather harder to prove. In addition to the antiviral immune response directly or indirectly producing pathology, viruses may infect immunocompetent cells and induce ineffective or aberrant immune responses. These two broad areas of pathogenic interaction between viruses and the immune system are considered below (and see Table 77.3).

Immunopathology induced by the antiviral immune response

ANTIBODY

Antibody can in some circumstances facilitate virus infection of cells which express Fc receptors. This phenomenon, named antibody-dependent enhancement, was first described for dengue virus. When non-neutralizing antibody against dengue virus is added to the virus in the presence of macrophages, the virus replicates to much higher titres; this results from antibody–virus complexes binding to Fc receptors and entering the macrophages by receptor-mediated endocytosis, in addition to the normal route of entry. This *in vitro* phenomenon has been adduced as a possible factor in the pathogenesis of the dengue shock syndrome (DSS). Subjects at risk of DSS are those who have experienced previous infection and then acquire a second infection with a different serotype of dengue virus. It is hypothesized that non-neutralizing antibody from the first infection may mediate enhancement with more widespread infection of macrophages, consequent mediator release and shock (Halstead 1988). A similar mechanism has

Table 77.3. Examples of *in vivo* immunopathology consequent on the immune response to viruses

Mechanism	Virus	Host	Comment
Inappropriate production of antibody	Dengue	Man	Non-neutralizing antibody-enhanced replication in macrophages
	RSV	Man	Killed vaccine-enhanced bronchiolitis following natural infection
	Measles	Man	Killed vaccine-enhanced disease following natural or live vaccine exposure
Immune complex disease	Hepatitis B	Man	Associated with arthralgia, rash, glomerulonephritis and polyarteritis nodosa
	Aleutian disease	Mink	Immune complex disease with glomerulonephritis
	LCMV	Mouse	Immune complex disease with glomerulonephritis — severity is dependent on strain
	LDH virus	Mouse	Less severe than LCMV — low incidence of nephritis
	Infectious anaemia virus	Horse	Immune complex disease related to antigen — antigenic variation in viral glycoproteins within the individual host
	Infectious peritonitis virus	Cat	Circulating immune complexes and disseminated intravascular coagulation (DIC)
T-cell-mediated	Hepatitis B (HBV)	Man	Liver injury in persistent HBV infection mediated by antiviral T cells?
	Measles	Man	Rash of measles dependent on T cell response
	Mumps	Man	Possible meningoencephalitis
	LCMV	Mouse	Fatal meningoencephalitis following intracerebral injection
	Influenza	Mouse	T cells mediating delayed hypersensitivity may enhance pneumonia
	Coxsackie	Mouse	Chronic cardiomyopathy ameliorated by T cell depletion
Enhanced mediator release	Dengue	Man	Haemorrhagic syndrome due to procoagulant release by infected macrophages

LDH = lactic dehydrogenase.

been described *in vitro* for other flaviviruses and C3b may also produce a similar enhancement effect through the CR3 receptor on the macrophage (Cardosa *et al.* 1983).

Antibody can also be involved in the development of virus-induced immune complex disease. There are well-described animal models of chronic immune complex disease induced by persistent virus infections. These include the glomerulonephritis associated with LCMV infection and with lactic dehydrogenase virus in mice, and with Aleutian disease in mink, which is caused by persistent parvovirus infection (Buchmeier *et al.* 1980; Porter *et al.* 1980). The arthralgias and rash associated with many acute human virus infections may have an immune complex basis (for instance, with HBV infection). Clear evidence for an association between persistent human virus infections and chronic immune complex disease is harder to find. There is an association between persistent HBV infection and membranous glomerulonephritis but an immune complex causation has not been formally shown (Hirose *et al.* 1984). The mechanism underlying the association between rubella and parvoviruses and arthritis has again not been clearly proved, although an immune complex aetiology is plausible.

T CELLS

T cells may also mediate tissue injury. The ability of virus-specific T_c cells to produce tissue damage has been best characterized in the LCMV model. Here, infection with LCMV by the intracerebral route in immunosuppressed or neonatal mice results in survival; adoptive transfer of LCMV-specific T_c cells to these animals or intracerebral infection in the immunocompetent adult mouse results in their death from cerebral oedema (Buchmeier *et al.* 1980). T cells mediating DTH may produce injury in the lung in murine influenza infection; adoptive transfer of virus-specific Class II MHC-restricted T cells results in the earlier death of infected mice (Ada *et al.* 1981). Analogies to these experimental examples in human virus infections are inevitably more speculative. The liver injury associated with chronic HBV infection may be mediated by virus-specific T_c cells and is discussed above. It has been proposed that the virus-specific T_c cells detectable in the cerebrospinal fluid (CSF) during mumps meningitis may be tissue-damaging, but this is even more speculative.

VIRUS-INDUCED CYTOKINE RELEASE

It now seems likely that the pathogenesis of certain bacterial and parasitic diseases may be due in part to the release of cytokines, such as TNF in endotoxin shock and severe malaria. Do viruses also produce pathogenic effects by inducing the release of cytokines? It seems plausible that this sort of mechanism might underlie the viral haemmorrhagic fevers, such as Lassa, or the dengue shock syndrome, but there are no studies as yet to test this. Some viruses may induce cytokine release as a facet of their normal replicative cycle; for instance, EBV may induce the release of autocrine B cell growth factors which facilitate the growth of EBV-immortalized B cells (Swendeman and Thorley-Lawson 1987).

Virus infection of immunocompetent cells

Some viruses also produce direct pathogenic effects both via and on the immune system by infecting immunocompetent cells, often with consequent effects on their function. Those viruses which establish persistent infection seem frequently to infect, and persist in, cells of the immune system. Lymphocytes and monocytes undergo activation and differentiation from a resting state in response to external signals, and the induction of virus gene transcription (which depends in part on cellular transcriptional factors) is frequently linked to the associated changes in transcription of cellular genes. Each of the major classes of immunocompetent cells may be infected by particular viruses.

T CELLS

Human immunodeficiency virus is dealt with elsewhere (Chapter 70). The first human retrovirus to be described, human T cell lymphotrophic virus (HTLV)-1, also infects CD4+ve T cells, and is causally associated with adult T cell leukaemia and tropical spastic paraparesis. Human T cell lymphotrophic virus 1 is transforming rather than lytic, and this may be related to the induction of IL-2 receptor expression in consequence of *trans*-activation of cellular genes by the 'tax' *trans*-activator protein of the virus (Cross *et al.* 1987).

The most recently described herpesvirus, human herpesvirus 6 (HHV-6), also infects human T cell lines *in vitro* and probably persists in T cells. Apart from producing the clinical syndrome of roseola infantum on primary infection in children, HHV-6 has not been causally associated with illness; nor has any definite functional effect on T cells been attributed to the virus (Lopez and Honess 1990).

In acute measles infection measles virus has been demonstrated in T cells, and impairment of T cell responses can be shown and may be clinically significant (Whittle *et al.* 1978).

B CELLS

Epstein–Barr virus, the principal human virus whose biology is intimately linked with the B cell, is covered in Chapter 78.

MONOCYTES/MACROPHAGES

Human monocytes can be infected with a number of different viruses; their capacity to migrate to tissues and acquire a different activated phenotype (as tissue macrophages) makes them an important route by which viruses could disseminate and reactivate at local tissue sites, including the nervous system. They probably play an important role in the pathogenesis of retrovirus infections for these reasons, as shown experimentally for visna virus (Narayan and Clements 1990).

Of the herpesviruses human CMV is carried in monocytes. The virus can be detected by polymerase chain reaction (PCR) in the monocytes of all carriers, although they do not produce infectious virus. However, *in vitro* infection of monocyte lines does not result in virus gene expression, but induction of differentiation (by phorbol esters) results in transcriptional activation of human CMV immediate early genes (Shelbourn *et al*. 1989).

Virus evasion of the immune response

There is recent evidence from several *in vitro* systems that viruses can modulate the expression of cell surface molecules involved in the induction and effector components of the immune response. This can have clear functional consequences *in vitro*, although it remains to be seen whether the same applies *in vivo*.

Adenovirus can down-regulate the amount of Class I MHC molecules on the cell surface, to the point where the infected cell can no longer be recognized by adenovirus-specific T_c cells. This effect is mediated by a specific adenovirus gene product (encoded in the E3 region), which is responsible for the retention of Class I MHC molecules in the endoplasmic reticulum (Burgert and Kwist 1985). Human CMV infection is also associated with a 10-fold reduction in Class I MHC expression, accompanied by an apparent abrogation of the ability of the cell to present other exogenous antigens (such as other viruses) in the context of Class I MHC. This appears more likely to be a post-transcriptionally mediated effect (Borysiewicz *et al*. 1991).

It is now appreciated that a range of adhesion molecules, in addition to the T cell receptor interaction with antigen plus MHC, are important in target–effector cell binding and recognition. These include the interactions between ICAM-1 and LFA-1 and between LFA-3 and CD2. Further recent work indicates that expression of these adhesion molecules can be modulated by viruses: EBV transformation may be associated with reduced expression of LFA-1 — Burkitt's lymphoma lines which show this are resistant to lysis by EBV-specific T_c cells (Inghirami *et al*. 1990); CMV can induce an increase in surface expression of ICAM-1 — which, together with the down-regulation of Class I MHC, could relate to the increased susceptibility to NK cell lysis shown by CMV-infected cells (Borysiewicz *et al*. 1991).

Another intriguing aspect is the recognition that some viral genomes code for proteins with homologies to human proteins involved in the immune response. Vaccinia virus is particularly striking, with homologous genes to those for the IL-2 receptor, serpins and complement proteins; the vaccinia protein with homology to the C4-binding protein can inhibit the classical pathway of complement activation (Traktman 1990). Herpes simplex virus has a glycoprotein (gC) which acts as a C3b receptor. Cytomegalovirus has a glycoprotein which is homologous to the Class I MHC heavy chain, although whether and how it has any pathogenic function remains to be seen (Beck and Barrell 1988). Epstein–Barr virus possesses a gene (BCRF1) with homology to a cytokine synthesis inhibitory factor (IL-10) produced by murine TH2 cells, and with similar functional activity (Moore *et al*. 1990). The pathogenic significance of most of these homologous genes remains to be assessed, but the degree of homology and their retention by the virus suggests they may be 'captured' cellular genes conferring some selective advantage on the virus.

Viruses and autoimmunity

There are several potential mechanisms by which viruses could induce autoimune responses. These include: polyclonal activation of B cells, production of anti-idiotypic antibodies against antiviral antibodies (the anti-idiotype might then simulate a viral protein and bind to cell surface receptors), and 'molecular mimicry', where viral epitopes shared with host antigens result in cross-reactive antibody or T cells (Oldstone 1987). Animal models for all these mechanisms exist, but none of them have been unequivocally shown to operate in humans. Other possible mechanisms can also be envisaged, such as viral interference with normal suppressor cell regulation, but are still more speculative (Borysiewicz 1991).

Conclusion

A better understanding of immunity to virus infections might be expected to have clinical consequences in two main ways: by aiding vaccine design and application, and by throwing light on the pathogenesis of virus diseases and hence possibly their therapy.

Vaccine design

It is a striking fact that nearly all successful vaccines against viruses have been designed empirically and developed using animal models. In the light of all the new knowledge, it should be possible to approach vaccine design in a more rational way — especially for subunit vaccines. This is of course being done and peptide and recombinant vector-based vaccines have been used in animals; however, their development and application to humans are proving slower than anticipated principally because of concerns over their safety (for live virus vectors) or their likely efficacy and the relative lack of good adjuvants (for peptides). It is, for example, salutary that (at the time of writing) the only vaccine clearly shown to prevent simian immunodeficiency virus (SIV) infection (the simian model for HIV infection) is whole inactivated virus — a technology first used 50 years ago. The most effective subunit vaccine currently in use is the hepatitis B vaccine, consisting of HBV surface antigen. However, it is noteworthy that a proportion of subjects fail to make a good anti-HBs response to the vaccine; this has been shown to correlate with homozygosity for the extended MHC haplotype, B8, SC01, DR3, suggesting genetic non-responsiveness in those individuals (Alper *et al*. 1989). It may be anticipated that other subunit vaccines will reveal similar genetic non-responders.

Nevertheless, particularly for the more complex persistent viruses, a thorough knowledge of their immunology and immunopathogenesis seems likely to eventually benefit vaccine design.

There is a clear precedent for the possibility that vaccines may cause adverse reactions by virtue of the immune responses they induce. The killed vaccine against respiratory syncytial virus (RSV) was associated with more severe illness in vaccinees than controls when they subsequently encountered the wild-type virus; so too was the killed measles vaccine. This was associated with failure of these vaccines to produce antibody to the F protein of the viruses. Possible explanations for this phenomenon include the development of an Arthus reaction or the involvement of DTH (Kim *et al*. 1976). Recent work on the LCMV model, using recombinant vaccinia viruses expression LCMV genes as vaccines, has shown that some recombinant vaccines can also enhance the severity of disease (Oehen *et al*. 1991).

Understanding pathogenesis

Increased understanding of exactly how viruses produce disease (which of course involves more than just understanding their immunology) could aid recognition of a viral aetiology in diseases whose cause is currently unknown. Again this seems particularly so for persistent virus infections. For instance, the recognition of the spectrum of disease produced by animal lentiretrovirus infection, from arthritis to CNS disease, raises the possibility of a similar aetiology for analogous human diseases. Greater understanding of their pathogenesis may also lead to a more rational approach to the therapy of persistent virus infections, as well as to their prevention.

References

Acharya, R., Fry, E., Stuart, D., Fox, G., Rowlands, D. and Brown, F. (1989). The three-dimensional structure of foot-and-mouth disease virus at 2.9 A resolution. *Nature* **337**, 709–16.

Ada, G.L., Leung, K.-N. and Ertl, H. (1981). An analysis of effector T cell generation and function in mice exposed to influenza A or Sendai viruses. *Immunol. Rev.* **58**, 5–24.

Ahmed, R. and Stevens, J.G. (1990). Viral persistence. In *Virology*, ed. B.N. Fields and D.M. Knipe, pp. 241–66, Raven Press, New York.

Albert, J., Abrahamsson, B., Nagy, K. *et al*. (1990). Rapid development of isolate-specific neutralising antibodies after primary HIV-1 infection and consequent emergence of virus variants which resist neutralisation by autologous sera. *AIDS* **4**, 107–12.

Alper, C.A., Kruskall, M.S., Marcus-Bagley, D. *et al*. (1989). Genetic prediction of nonresponse to hepatitis B vaccine. *N. Engl. J. Med.* **321**, 708–12.

Barnaba, V., Franco, A., Alberti, A., Balsano, C., Benvenuto, R. and Balsano, F. (1989) Recognition of hepatitis B virus envelope proteins by liver infiltrating T lymphocytes in chronic HBV infection. *J. Immunol.* **143**, 2650–5.

Beasley, R.P., Hwang, L.-Y., Stevens, C.E. *et al*. (1983). Efficacy of hepatitis B immune globulin for prevention of perinatal transmission of the hepatitis virus carrier state. *Hepatology* **3**, 135–41.

Beck, S. and Barrell, B.G. (1988). Human cytomegalovirus

encodes a glycoprotein homologous to MHC class 1 antigens. *Nature* **331**, 269–72.

Biron, C.A., Byron, K.S. and Sullivan, J.S. (1989). Severe herpes virus infections in an adolescent without natural killer cells. *N. Engl. J. Med.* **320**, 1731–5.

Borysiewicz, L.K. (1991). Virus infection and autoimmunity. *Autoimmunity* (in press).

Borysiewicz, L.K., Hickling, J.K., Graham, S. *et al.* (1988). Human cytomegalovirus specific cytotoxic T cells — relative frequency of stage specific CTL recognising the 72 kDa immediate early protein and glycoprotein B expressed by recombinant vaccinia viruses. *J. Exp. Med.* **168**, 919–31.

Borysiewicz, L.K., Wronska, D., McMichael, A.J. and Minson, A.C. (1991). Inhibition of antigen presentation and MHC class I expression by human cytomegalovirus (submitted for publication).

Buchmeier, M.J., Welsh, R.M., Dutko, F.J. and Oldstone, M.B.A. (1980). The virology and immunobiology of lymphocytic choriomeningitis virus infection. *Adv. Immunol.* **30**, 275–331.

Bukowski, J.F., Warner, J.F., Dennert, G. and Welsh, R.M. (1985). Adoptive transfer studies demonstrating the antiviral effects of NK cells *in vivo*. *J. Exp. Med.* **161**, 40–52.

Burgert, H.-G. and Kvist, S. (1985). An adenovirus type 2 glycoprotein blocks cell surface expression of human histocompatibility class 1 antigens. *Cell* **41**, 987–97.

Burt, D.S., Mills, K.H.G., Skehel, J.J. and Thomas, D.B. (1989). Diversity of the class II restricted T cell repertoire for influenza haemagglutination and antigenic drift. *J. Exp. Med.* **170**, 383–97.

Carding, S.R., Allen, W., Kyes, S., Haydey, A., Bottomly, K. and Doherty, P.L. (1990). Late dominance of the inflammatory process in murine influenza by gamma/delta$^+$ T cells. *J. Exp. Med.* **172**, 1225–31.

Cardosa, M.J., Porterfield, J.S. and Gordon, S. (1983). Complement receptor mediates enhanced flavivirus replication in macrophages. *J. Exp. Med.* **158**, 258–63.

Clements, J.E., Godovin, S.L., Montelero, R.C. and Narayan, O. (1988). Antigenic variation in lentiviral diseases. *Ann. Rev. Immunol.* **6**, 139–59.

Cross, S.L., Feinberg, M.B., Wolf, J.B., Holbrook, N.J., Wong-Staal, F. and Leonard, W.J. (1987). Regulation of the human interleukin-2 receptor α chain promoter: activation of a nonfunctional promoter by the transactivator gene of HTLV-1. *Cell* **49**, 47–56.

Cunningham, A.L. and Merigan, T.C. (1983). Alpha interferon production appears to predict time of recurrence of herpes labialis. *J. Immunol.* **130**, 2397–400.

de Preval, C., Hadem, M.R. and Mach, B. (1988). Regulation of genes for HLA class II antigens in cell lines from patients with severe combined immunodeficiency. *N. Engl. J. Med.* **318**, 1295–300.

Dhar, R. and Ogra, P.L. (1985). Local immune responses. *Br. Med. Bull.* **41**, 27–33.

Greve, J.M., Davis, G., Meyer, A.M. *et al.* (1989). The major human rhinovirus receptor is ICAM-1. *Cell* **56**, 839–47.

Grundy, J.E., McKenzie, J.S. and Stanley, N.F. (1981). Influence of H2 and non-H2 genes on resistance to murine cytomegalovirus infection. *Infection and Immunity* **32**, 277–86.

Halstead, S.B. (1988). Pathogenesis of dengue: challenges to molecular biology. *Science* **237**, 1210–12.

Harrison, S.C. (1990). Principles of virus structure. In *Virology* ed. B.N. Fields and D.M. Knipe, pp. 37–62, Raven Press, New York.

Hickling, J.K., Borysiewicz, L.K. and Sissons, J.G.P. (1987). Varicella zoster virus specific cytotoxic T lymphocytes (Tc): detection and frequency analysis of HLA class I restricted Tc in human peripheral blood. *J. Virol.* **61**, 3463–9.

Hirose, H., Udo, K., Kojima, M. *et al.* (1984). Deposition of hepatitis B e antigen in membranous glomerulonephritis: identification by $F(ab)_2$ fragments of monoclonal antibody. *Kidney Int.* **26**, 338–41.

Hogle, J.M., Chow, M. and Filman, D.J. (1987). The structure of poliovirus. *Sci. Am.* **256**, 42–9.

Holland, J., Spindler, K., Horodyski, F., Grabam, E., Nichol, S. and Van de Pol, S. (1982). Rapid evolution of RNA genomes. *Science* **215**, 1577–85.

Inghirami, G., Grignani, F., Sternas, L., Lombardi, L., Knowles, D.M. and Dalla-Favera, R. (1990). Down-regulation of LFA-1 adhesion receptors by C-*myc* oncogene in human B lymphoblastoid cells. *Science* **250**, 682–6.

Jacobson, S., Rose, J.W., Flerlage, M.L., McFarlin, D.E. and McFarland, H.F. (1987). Induction of measles virus specific cytotoxic T cells by purified measles virus nucleocapsid and haemagglutinin polypeptides. *Viral Immunol.* **1**, 153–62.

Janeway, C.A. (1989). Natural killer cells: a primitive immune system. *Nature* **341**, 108.

Joklik, W.K. (1990). Interferons. In *Virology*, ed. B.N. Fields and D.M. Knipe, pp. 383–410, Raven Press, New York.

Kim, H.W., Leikin, S.L., Arrobio, J.O., Brandt, C.D., Channock, R.M. and Parrott, R.H. (1976). Cell mediated immunity to respiratory syncytial virus infection induced by inactivated vaccine or by injection. *Pediatr. Res.* **10**, 75–8.

Kreth, H.W., Kress, L., Kress, H.G., Ott, H.F. and Eckert, G. (1982). Demonstration of primary cytotoxic T cells in venous blood and cerebrospinal fluid of children with mumps meningitis. *J. Immunol.* **128**, 2411–15.

Laver, W.G., Air, G.M., Webster, R.G. and Smith-Gill, S.J. (1990). Epitopes on protein antigens: misconceptions and realities. *Cell* **61**, 553–6.

Lawson, C.M., Grundy, J.E. and Shellam, G.R. (1988). Antibody responses to murine cytomegalovirus in genetically resistant and susceptible strains of mice. *J. Gen. Virol.* **69**, 1987–98.

Lopez, C. and Honess, R.W. (1990). Human herpesvirus 6. In *Virology*, ed. B.N. Fields and D.M. Knipe, pp. 2055–62, Raven Press, New York.

McChesney, M.B. and Oldstone, M.B.A. (1987). Viruses perturb lymphocyte functions: selected principles characterising virus induced immunosuppression. *Ann. Rev. Immunol.* **5**, 279–304.

McMichael, A.J., Gotch, F.M., Noble, G.R. and Beare, P.A. (1983). Cytotoxic T cell immunity to influenza. *N. Engl. J. Med.* **309**, 13–17.

Mendelsohn, C.L., Wimmer, E. and Racaniello, V.R. (1989). Cellular receptor for poliovirus: molecular cloning, nucleotide sequence, and expression of a new member of the immunoglobulin superfamily. *Cell* **56**, 855–65.

Meyerhans, A., Cheynier, R., Albert, J. *et al.* (1989). Temporal fluctuations in HIV quasispecies *in vivo* are not reflected by sequential HIV isolations. *Cell* **58**, 901–10.

Mims, C.A., White, D.O. and Borysiewicz, L.K. (1984 and 1991).

Viral Pathogenesis and Immunology. Blackwell Scientific Publications, Oxford (in press).

Mondelli, M., Mieli Vezgni, G., Alberti, A. *et al.* (1982). Specificity of T lymphocyte cytotoxicity to autologous hepatocytes in chronic HBV infection. *J. Immunol.* **129**, 2273–8.

Moore, K.W., Vieira, P., Fiorentino, D.F., Trounstine, M.L., Khan, T.A. and Mosmann, T.R. (1990). Homology of cytokine synthesis inhibitor factor (IL-10) to the Epstein–Barr virus gene BCRFI. *Science* **248**, 1230–7.

Moretta, A., Pantaleo, G., Moretta, L., Cerottini, J.-C. and Mingari, M.C. (1989). Direct demonstration of the clonogenic potential of every human peripheral blood T-cell: clonal analysis of HLA-DR expression and cytolytic activity. *J. Exp. Med.* **157**: 743–54.

Moriyama, T., Guilhot, S., Klopchin, K. *et al.* (1990). Immunobiology and pathogenesis of hepatocellular injury in hepatitis B virus transgenic mice. *Science* **248**, 361–4.

Murphy, F.A. and Kingsbury, D.W. (1990). Virus taxonomy. In *Virology*, ed. B.N. Fields and D.M. Knipe, pp. 9–36, Raven Press, New York.

Narayan, O. and Clements, J.E. (1990). Lentiviruses. In *Virology*, ed. B.N. Fields, and D.M. Knipe, pp. 1571–89, Raven Press, New York.

Nash, A.A., Leung, K.-N. & Wildy, P. (1985). The T-cell-mediated immune response of mice to herpes simplex virus. In *The Herpes Viruses*, ed. B. Roizman and C. Lopez, vol. IV, pp. 87–102, Plenum Publishing Corporation.

Norrby, E. and Oxman, M.N. (1990). Measles virus. In *Virology*, ed. B.N. Fields and D.M. Knipe, pp. 1013–44, Raven Press, New York.

Oehen, S., Hengartner, H. and Zinkernagel, R.M. (1991). Vaccination for disease. *Science* **251**, 195–8.

Oldstone, M.B.A. (1987). Molecular mimicry and autoimmune disease. *Cell* **50**, 819–20.

Philips, R.E., Rowland-Jones, S., Nixon, D.F. *et al.* (1991). Human immunodeficiency virus genetic variation that can escape cytotoxic T cell recognition. *Nature* **354**, 435–9.

Porter, D.D., Larsen, A.E. and Porter, H.G. (1980). Aleutian disease ot mink. *Adv. Immunol.* 29, 261.

Racaniello, V.R. (1990). Picornaviruses: cell receptors for picornaviruses. *Curr. Topics Microbiol. Immunol.* **161**, 1–22.

Reddehase, M.J., Mutter, U., Munch, K., Buhring, K.-H. and Koszinowski, U.H. (1987). CD8-positive T lymphocytes specific for murine cytomegalovirus immediate early antigens mediate protective immunity. *J. Virol.* **61**, 3102–8.

Rickinson, A.B., Yao, Q.Y. and Wallace, L.E. (1985). Epstein–Barr virus as a model of virus–host interactions. *Br. Med. Bull.* **41**, 75–9.

Roizman, B. and Sears, A.E. (1990). Herpes simplex viruses and their replication. In *Virology*, ed. B.N. Fields and D.M. Knipe, ch. 65, pp. 1795–841, Raven Press, New York.

Rosen, F.S., Cooper, M.D. and Wedgwood, R.J.P. (1984). The primary immunodeficiencies. *N. Engl. J. Med.* **311**, 300–10.

Rubin, R.H. (1990). Cytomegalovirus infections — epidemiology, diagnosis and treatment strategies. *Rev. Infect. Dis.* **12**, S973–S1229.

Rueckert, R.R. (1990). Picornaviridae and their replication. In *Virology*, ed. B.N. Fields and D.M. Knipe, ch. 20, pp. 507–48, Raven Press, New York.

Schooley, R.T., Hirsch, M.S., Colvin, R.B., *et al.* (1983). Association of herpesvirus infections with T-lymphocyte subset alterations, glomerulopathy, and opportunistic infections after renal transplantation. *N. Engl. J. Med.* **308**, 307–13.

Shelbourn, S.L., Kothari, S., Sissons, J.G.P. and Sinclair, J.H. (1989). Repression of human cytomegalovirus gene expression associated with a novel immediate early regulatory region binding factor. *Nucleic Acids Res.* **17**, 9165–71.

Sissons, J.G.P. (1987). Complement and viruses. In *Complement in Health and Disease*, ed. K. Whaley, pp. 255–66. MTP Press, Lancaster.

Sissons, J.G.P. and Borysiewicz, L.K. (1985). Virus immunopathology. *Br. Med. Bull.* **41**, 24–40.

Sissons, J.G.P. and Oldstone, M.B.A. (1980). The antibody mediated destruction of virus infected cells. *Adv. Immunol.* **29**, 209– 60.

Snydman, D.R. (1990). Cytomegalovirus immunoglobulins in the prevention and treatment of cytomegalovirus disease. *Rev. Infect. Dis.* **12**, S839–S848.

Staunton, D.E., Merluzzi, V.J., Rothlein, R., Barton, R., Marlin, S.D. and Springer, T.A. (1989). A cell adhesion molecule, ICAM-1, is the major surface receptor for rhinoviruses. *Cell* **56**, 849–53.

Strang, G. and Rickinson, A.B. (1987). Multiple HLA class 1-dependent cytotoxicities constitute the 'non-HLA-restricted' response in infectious mononucleosis. *Eur. J. Immunol.* **17**, 1007–13.

Straus, S.E., Osborne, J.M. and Inchanspe, G. (1988). Varicella–zoster virus infections — natural history, treatment and prevention. *Ann. Intern. Med.* **108**, 221–37.

Swendeman, S. and Thorley-Lawson, D.A. (1987). The activation antigen BLAST-2, when shed, is an autocrine growth factor for normal and transformed B cells. *EMBO J.* **6**, 1637–42.

Thomas, A.A., Vrizsen, M.R. and Boeye, A. (1986). Relationship between poliovirus neutralisation and aggregation. *J. Virol.* **59**, 479–85.

Townsend, A.R.M. (1987). Recognition of influenza proteins by cytotoxic T cells. *Immunol. Res.* **6**, 80–100.

Traktman, P. (1990). Poxviruses: an emerging portrait of biological strategy. *Cell* **62**, 621–6.

Vallbracht, A., Maier, K., Stierhof, Y.D., Wiedemann, K.H., Fietmig, B. and Fleischer, B. (1989). Liver derived cytotoxic T cells in hepatitis A virus infection. *J. Infect. Dis.* **160**, 209–17.

Webster, A.D.B. (1984). Echovirus disease in hypogammaglobulinaemia patients. *Clin Rheum. Dis.* **10**, 189–203.

Weiss, R. (1985). Human T-cell retroviruses. In *RNA Tumour Viruses*, ed. R. Weiss, N. Teich, H. Varmus and J. Coffin, vol. II, pp. 405–86. Cold Spring Harbor.

Welsh, R.M. and Vargas-Cortes, M. (1991) Regulation and role of natural killer cells in virus infections. In *The Natural Immune System*, ed. C.E. Lewis and J.O'D. McGhee. Oxford University Press (in press).

Whittle, H.C., Dossetor, J., Odinlojn, S.A., Bryceson, A.D.M. and Greenwood, B.M. (1978). Cell mediated immunity during natural measles infection. *J. Clin. Invest.* **62**, 678–84.

Wiley, D.C. and Skehel, J.J. (1987). The structure and function of the haemagglutinin membrane glycoprotein of influenza virus. *Ann. Rev. Biochem.* **56**, 365–94.

Wiley, D.C. and Skehel, J.J. (1990). Viral membranes. In *Virology*, ed. B.N. Fields and D.M. Knipe, ch. 4, pp. 63–85, Raven

Press, New York.

Wong, G.H.W. and Goeddel, D. (1986). Tumour necrosis factors α and β inhibit virus replication and synergise with interferons. *Nature* **323**, 819–22.

Zinkernagel, R.M. and Doherty, P.L. (1979). MHC restricted cytotoxic T cells: studies on the biological role of polymorphic major transplantation antigens determining T cell restriction specificity, function and responsiveness. *Adv. Immunol.* **27**, 51–177.

Zisman, B., Wheelock, E.F. and Allison, A.C. (1971). Role of macrophages and antibody in resistance of mice against yellow fever viruses. *J. Immunol.* **107**, 236–43.

78: Immunology of Epstein–Barr Virus Infection

A.B. Rickinson and C.D. Gregory

Introduction

There are several reasons why Epstein–Barr virus (EBV), one of the six known human herpesviruses, warrants special attention in a textbook devoted to the clinical aspects of immunology. Firstly, the virus preferentially infects B lymphocytes and has the capacity to activate resting B cells into the proliferating lymphoblastoid state. Secondly, there are at least two important clinical conditions which are consequent upon EBV-induced B cell activation *in vivo* — one a self-limiting lymphoproliferative disease, infectious mononucleosis (IM), which is induced by primary EBV infection and associated with an unusually vigorous T-cell-mediated response to EBV-activated B cells, the other a progressive B lymphoproliferative disease which occurs in EBV-infected individuals whose cell-mediated immune system is severely compromised. In addition, the virus is strongly linked to two human tumours, endemic Burkitt's lymphoma (BL) and undifferentiated nasopharyngeal carcinoma (NPC), and it is interesting to question whether host immune responses capable of detecting normal EBV-infected cells also have the capacity to recognize such EBV +ve malignant cell populations.

Before discussing what is known about the immunological aspects of EBV infection, we shall briefly review the viral antigens which are expressed in the virus's two principal habitats *in vivo*. These habitats are the B lymphoid system, where the infection appears to be largely non-productive with limited virus gene expression, and stratified pharyngeal epithelium (and possibly other epithelial sites), where the virus replicates fully in a cell differentiation-dependent manner.

Epstein–Barr virus infection of B cells: identity of the virus's 'latent cycle' antigens

The essential details of the *in vitro* interaction between EBV and resting human B cells are presented diagrammatically in Fig. 78.1. Virus entry into B cells occurs through a specific interaction

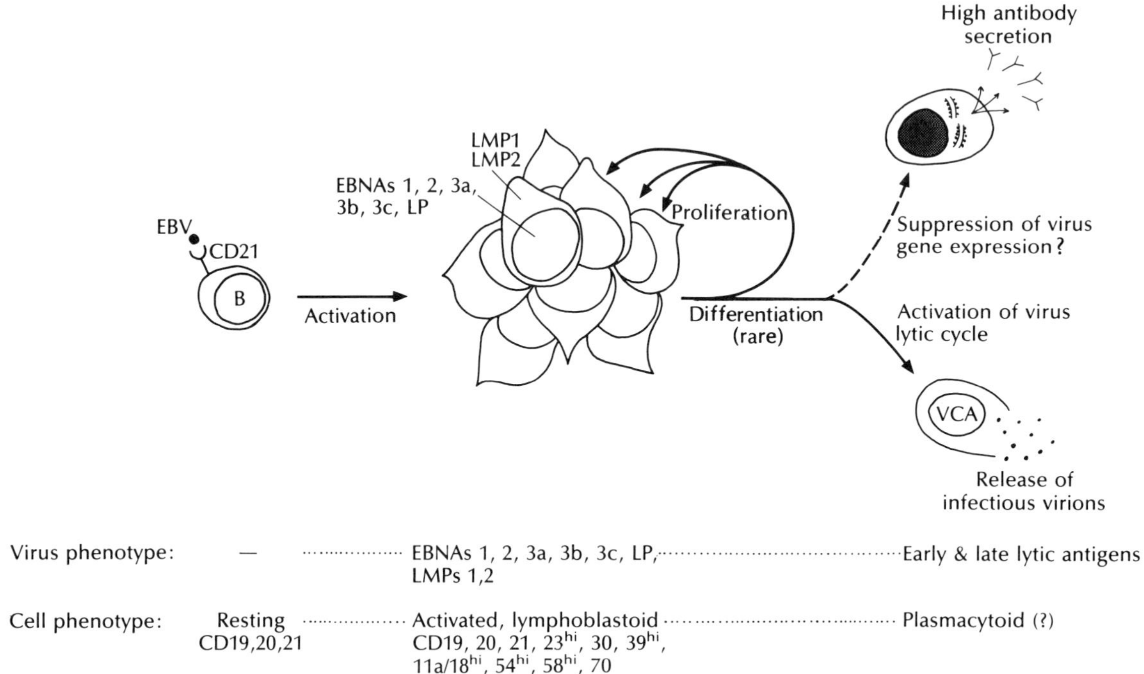

Fig. 78.1. Diagrammatic representation of the *in vitro* interaction between EBV and resting human B cells. Virus infection of resting cells via the EBV receptor molecule CD21 is followed by expression of a limited number of EBV-coded proteins ('latent' gene products), leading to activation of cells to the proliferating lymphoblastoid state. Major changes in the cell surface phenotype occur with marked up-regulation of a number of cellular activation antigens (CD23, CD30, CD39, CD70) and adhesion molecules (CD11a/CD18, CD54, CD58) from the very low or undetectable levels of these proteins on the resting B cell membrane. Occasional cells within the lymphoblastoid cell line cease proliferation and move either into virus lytic cycle, leading to cell death and release of infectious virions, or towards a more plasmacytoid stage of differentiation with increased immunoglobulin production. The controls governing lytic cycle entry and plasmacytoid differentiation are not so far understood.

between the major viral envelope glycoprotein (GP340) and a cell surface glycoprotein, the C3d receptor (CD21, CR2), whose expression is generally held to be restricted to the B lymphocyte lineage (Cooper *et al*, 1988). Since GP340 contains a peptide sequence identical to the CR2-binding domain of the C3d molecule, this suggests that the virus's initial interaction with CR2 occurs through the same binding site as the natural ligand (Nemerow *et al*. 1989). Following this initial binding the virus appears to be internalized via the B cell's endocytic pathway, delivery of the nucleocapsid into the cell cytoplasm being dependent on an endocytic membrane fusion event in which a second viral envelope glycoprotein, GP85, may play a role. Initiation of the infection ultimately requires delivery of the virus nucleocapsid to the cell nucleus, and release of the virus genome.

In the B cell environment, EBV usually expresses only a limited number of viral proteins. These 'latent cycle' products include six nuclear antigens (EBNAs 1, 2, 3a, 3b, 3c and LP) and two latent membrane proteins LMP-1 and LMP-2 (Farrell 1989; Kieff and Liebowitz 1990). The overall pattern of EBV latent gene expression is illustrated in Fig. 78.2. The latent proteins identified here are of considerable interest since it is through their coordinate action that the resting B cell is both activated into the cell cycle and subsequently maintained in the proliferating lymphoblastoid state. All eight latent proteins remain constitutively expressed in the EBV-transformed lymphoblastoid cell lines (LCLs) which arise with great efficiency following EBV infection of resting human B cells *in vitro*.

The six EBNAs are antigenically distinct and, as illustrated in Fig. 78.3(a), are detectable as proteins of unique size when protein extracts from an EBV-transformed B cell line are separated by polyacrylamide gel electrophoresis (PAGE) and then immunoblotted with a polyspecific human serum. The EBNAs can also be detected by immunofluor-

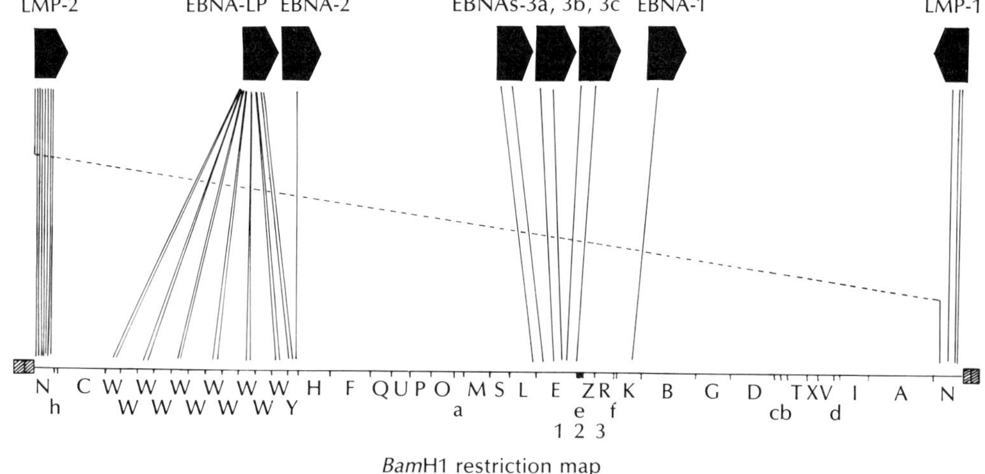

Fig. 78.2. Diagrammatic representation of the EBV genome (*Bam*HI restriction map of the B95.8 strain genome) showing the location of the exons encoding the latent proteins constitutively expressed in EBV-transformed lymphoblastoid cell lines. Expression of all six EBNA messenger ribonucleic acids (mRNAs) is co-ordinately controlled via one of two promoter regions in the *Bam*HI C and W regions of the viral genome; expression of the two LMP mRNAs is separately controlled from promoter regions in the *Bam*HI N region and, for LMP-2 mRNA, expression requires prior circularization of the genome.

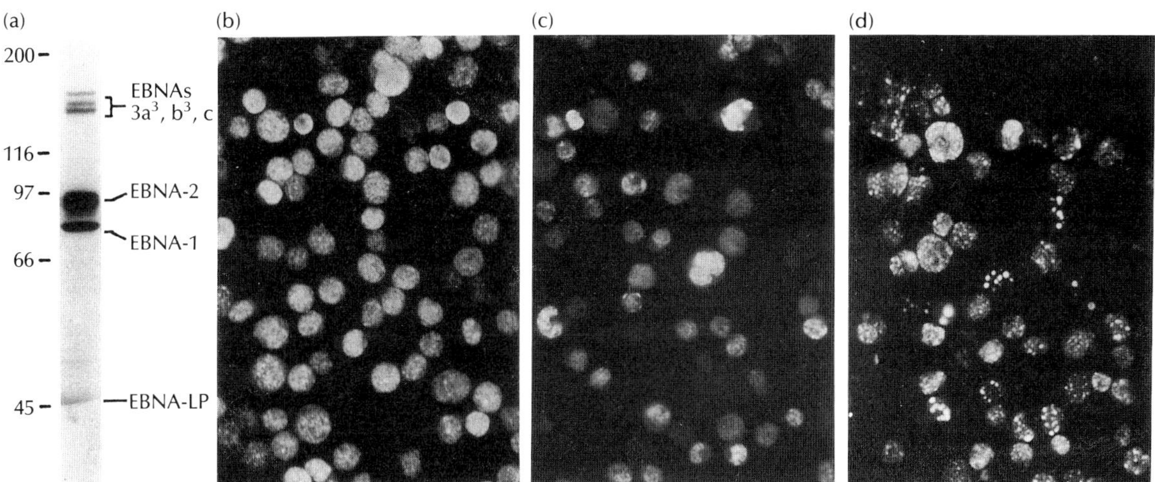

Fig. 78.3. (a) Immunoblot of protein extracts from a latently infected EBV-transformed LCL probed with a polyspecific human serum containing antibodies to EBNAs 1, 2, 3a and 3c. (b) Immunofluorescence staining of an EBV-transformed LCL with a monospecific human serum with reactivity against EBNA-1. (c) Immunofluorescence staining of an EBV-transformed LCL with a monoclonal antibody against EBNA-2. (d) Immunofluorescence staining of an EBV-transformed LCL with a monoclonal antibody against EBNA-LP.

escence-staining of EBV-transformed cell smears, using a sensitive anticomplement-enhanced assay. Staining with monospecific or monoclonal antibody preparations in fact shows that the individual EBNAs have different distributions within the nucleus; thus EBNA-1 staining is fine and granular and extends throughout the nuclear area (Fig. 78.3(b)) EBNA-2 staining spares nucleoli (Fig. 78.3(c)), whilst EBNA-LP staining is located in distinct globules (Fig. 78.3(d)). The particular conditions established for the original anti-EBNA immunofluorescence test (Reedman and Klein 1973) tend to favour the detection of antibodies to EBNA-1 but it should be borne in mind when screening human sera that reactivities to other EBNAs can also contribute to the observed staining.

In many respects the process of virus-induced B cell activation illustrated in Fig. 78.1 resembles that which can be initiated in the B cell by physiological signals, i.e. by cognate antigen and T-cell-derived factors. A similar pattern of cell surface changes is induced in both situations, with increased expression of several cellular 'activation' antigens (CD23, CD30 and CD39 are good examples) and of the cellular adhesion molecules — lymphocyte function-associated antigen (LFA)-1 (CD11a/CD18), intercellular adhesion molecule (ICAM)-1 (CD54) and LFA-3 (CD58). The important differences between the two systems are: (i) that antigen-driven activation is dependent upon T cell help whereas virus-driven activation is not; and (ii) that the antigen-driven activation of resting B cells to the lymphoblastoid state is transient, progressing either to plasma cell formation or back to the resting phase, whereas EBV-infected B cells become permanently 'locked' in the proliferating lymphoblastoid state. Note that virus-induced changes in the cell surface phenotype, particularly the enhanced adhesion molecule profile, are important because they influence how accessible EBV-infected B cells are to cell-mediated immune responses (see later).

The EBV–B cell interaction as described above is essentially non-productive; limited virus gene expression causes virus-induced cell growth without leading to full virus replication. In fact, this type of interaction is not completely stable and many *in vitro*-transformed LCLs will at any one time contain a small proportion of cells (usually <1%) which have recently entered virus productive cycle and which are therefore destined to die with the release of infectious progeny virions into the culture supernatant. Preliminary evidence suggests that this spontaneous movement from latent into lytic cycle is dependent upon a change in the degree of differentiation of the infected cell, possibly from the lymphoblastoid to an early plasmacytoid state. Another possible outcome is for the infected B cell to move into full plasmacytoid differentiation with loss of proliferative capacity but without entry into lytic cycle. The controls governing entry into these separate pathways from the proliferating lymphoblastoid state are still not understood. The cell differentiation dependence of EBV–host cell interactions is even more clearly illustrated when one examines the behaviour of the virus in its other major target tissue, stratified epithelium.

Epstein–Barr virus infection of epithelial cells: identity of the virus's 'lytic cycle' antigens

In contrast to the ease with which EBV–B cell interactions can be studied in the laboratory, it has not been possible to reproduce the epithelial cell infection efficiently *in vitro*. Our knowledge of the virus 'lytic cycle' antigens therefore comes mainly from work on the semi-permissive B cell lines described above and, more recently, from direct examination of EBV-infected epithelial cells *in vivo*. Full virus replication in an epithelial environment was first suggested by the detection of late viral antigens in desquamating epithelial cells isolated from the buccal fluid of IM patients, i.e. individuals undergoing primary EBV infection (Sixbey *et al.* 1984). Indeed, such replication appears to persist, usually at a low level, throughout the lifelong virus carrier state. However, the clearest indication of the permissive nature of the epithelial cell infection has come from EBV carriers in which the virus–host balance has been altered as a result of T cell impairment. Thus the oral 'hairy' leucoplakia (OHL) which frequently develops on the lateral borders of the tongue of acquired immune deficiency syndrome (AIDS) patients is now recognized to be an EBV-associated lesion, with complete virus replication occurring in the differentiating outer layers of stratified lingual epithelial cells (Greenspan *et al.* 1985). Figure 78.4 presents a section through an OHL lesion; there is general thickening of the lingual epithelium but no gross disturbance of normal squamous epithelial differentiation. *In situ* hybridization with a radio-labelled EBV deoxyribonucleic acid (DNA) probe (from the BamHIW repeat region of the virus genome) gives a strong signal in the outer, more differentiated, half of the epithelium, indicating the location of lytically infected cells. The permissiveness of epithelium for EBV is therefore closely linked to ordered squamous cell differentiation, and the difficulty of reproducing this differentiation faithfully *in vitro* probably underlies the inability of cultured epithelium to support complete virus replication.

Three groups of EBV lytic cycle antigens have been defined by immunofluorescence staining of cell smears from semi-permissive B cell lines, using human sera (Henle, G. and Henle 1979). These groups of antigens, and available data on the

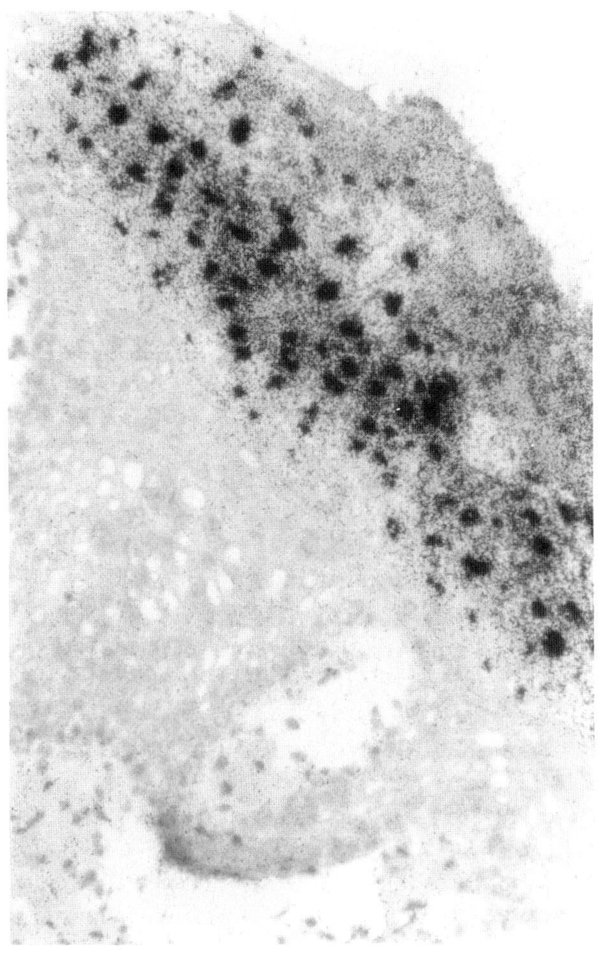

Fig. 78.4. Section through an oral hairy leucoplakia lesion showing detection of replicating EBV genomes (i.e. lytically infected cells) by *in situ* hybridization with a radiolabelled probe from the BamHI W region of the viral genome. Full virus replication is restricted to the outer more differentiated half of the squamous epithelium.

identity of their individual components, are shown in Table 78.1. The early antigen (EA) complex has been divided into diffuse (D) and restricted (R) components on the basis of differential sensitivity to methanol fixation and of intracellular location. These two subgroups of non-structural virus-coded proteins are expressed in cells early in the lytic cycle, before the initiation of viral DNA replication, and at least three individual components of the EA(D) group and two of the EA(R) group have now been identified. Likewise two of the major late antigenic complexes, the virus capsid antigen (VCA) and membrane antigen (MA), are also being dissected into a number of separate components. Of the four viral envelope glycoproteins now thought to be present in mature virions, GP340 is by far the most abundant species and is the major target for the virus-neutralizing antibody response in man; neutralization via anti-GP85 antibodies has also been demonstrated.

It is important to stress that EBV, a large herpesvirus with a genome of >170 kbp, has the capacity to encode at least 50 to 100 individual proteins (Farrell 1989; Kieff and Liebowitz 1990). Conventional immunofluorescence assays used in the diagnostic laboratory to detect 'anti-EBNA', 'anti-EA' or 'anti-VCA' activity in patients' sera will therefore each be measuring the summation of antibody reactivities against a number of separate viral proteins. This need not detract from the usefulness of such assays, as long as it is recognized that in particularly important cases additional techniques, such as immunoblotting or enzyme-linked immunosorbent assay (ELISA) against individual EBV proteins expressed from recombinant vectors, will be required to obtain a more accurate profile of the anti-EBV antibodies in patients' sera. Figure 78.5 illustrates the point by showing immunoblots of protein extracts from a semi-permissive EBV-transformed B cell line (expressing both latent and lytic cycle antigens) probed with four different sera (HS1–4) from EBV-immune individuals. All four sera gave 'anti-EBNA' reactivity by conventional immunofluorescence, yet by immunoblotting they showed distinct patterns of reactivity against EBNA-1 alone (HS1), EBNAs 1 and 2 (HS2) or EBNAs 1, 2 and 3a, b, c (HS3 and HS4). In addition, HS4 showed strong reactivity against the 50–55 kD BMRF1 protein component of the EA(D) complex.

Immune response to primary Epstein–Barr virus infection

In most societies primary infection occurs within the first few years of life and is generally asymptomatic. In the West, however, primary infection is often delayed until adolescence or later and up to 50% of such cases show clinical symptoms of infectious mononucleosis – malaise, fever, pharyngitis, lymphadenopathy and/or hepatosplenomegaly (Henle, W. and Henle, 1979). Our understanding of the virological and immunological events of the primary infection comes almost entirely from the study of IM patients. It is questionable whether this is an accurate, albeit

Table 78.1. Antigenic components of the early antigen, virus capsid antigen and membrane antigen complexes

Complex	Characteristics Location Fixation	Components	
		Size[a]	Reading frame[b]
EA(D)	Early, non-structural proteins Nuclear and/or cytoplasmic Acetone/methanol-fixed cells	p50–55 p44 p70–90	BMRF1 BSLF2 + BMLF1 BHLF1
EA(R)	Early, non-structural proteins Cytoplasmic Acetone-fixed cells	p85 p17	? BHRF1
VCA	Late, structural or non-structural proteins Nuclear and/or cytoplasmic Acetone-fixed cells	p150 GP110	BcLF1 BALF4
MA	Late, virus envelope proteins Plasma membrane Viable cells	GP350/220 GP85 GP78/55 GP35	BLLF1 BXLF2 BILF2 BDLF3

a Apparent size from mobility on sodium dodecyl sulphate polyacrylamide gel electrophoresis (SDS-PAGE) of protein (p) or glycoprotein (GP).
b Open reading frame in B95.8 virus genomic sequence which encodes the antigen in question, e.g. BMRF1 is *Bam*HI fragment M, rightward reading frame 1 (Baer *et al.* 1984).

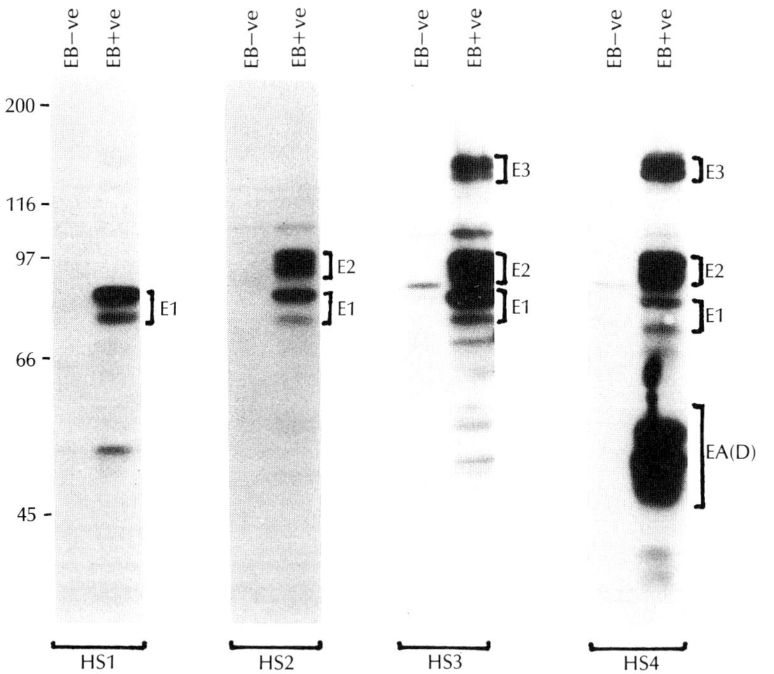

Fig. 78.5. Immunoblots of protein extracts from an EBV −ve control cell line and from an EBV-transformed LCL having the majority of cells latently infected and a small number of cells in lytic cycle. Sera from four different healthy EBV-infected individuals (HS 1, 2, 3, 4) were used to probe the same paired cell extracts; the four sera show different antibody reactivities with respect to the latent cycle antigens, EBNAs 1, 2, 3a, 3b and 3c, and to the lytic cycle EA(D) antigen.

exaggerated, reflection of the pattern of events which occurs during asymptomatic primary infection or whether the two situations are qualitatively as well as quantitatively distinct.

The antigenic challenge in IM is thought to come from EBV lytic cycle proteins expressed in productively infected oropharyngeal epithelium and from EBV latent cycle proteins expressed in infected B lymphocytes. Infectious virus, detectable in cord blood lymphocyte transformation assays, is shed at high titre into the oropharynx of acute IM patients whilst the presence of circulating virus-infected B cells is apparent from the 'spontaneous' transformation of the patients' leucocytes into EBV-positive LCLs when the cells are placed in culture without the addition of exogenous virus. The assumption is that oropharyngeal epithelium is the primary site of infection for EBV, an orally transmitted agent, and that progeny virions produced at this site subsequently enter circulating B cells, thereby generalizing the infection throughout the body (see Fig. 78.7).

Primary humoral response

The prodromal period for IM is of the order of 40 days and by the time of onset of clinical symptoms immunoglobulin M (IgM) and IgG serum antibody responses to VCA are already detectable in immunofluorescence assays. Antibodies to EA (predominantly EA(D)) and MA are also present at this time, presumably of both IgM and IgG classes although most serological surveys have only assayed IgG. The general pattern of responses during and after the clinical course of IM is illustrated in Fig. 78.6. The precise antigenic specificities being recognized in these conventional immunofluorescence assays have not yet been fully determined by further analysis using immunoblotting or ELISA but there clearly are antigenic preferences which distinguish the acute and convalescent antibody profiles. Thus anti-MA reactivity is preferentially due to anti-GP85 antibodies in acute IM sera (Pearson *et al.* 1979) and the lack of strong anti-GP340 reactivity probably explains why virus-neutralizing antibody titres are comparatively low at this stage.

One of the most interesting features of IM sera is the unusual spectrum of reactivity against latent cycle antigens, most particularly the EBNAs. It has been known for some time that anti-EBNA testing, using the conventional anticomplement immunofluorescence assay and the EBV-positive Raji cell line as a source of antigen, does not reveal detectable antibody reactivity in IM sera until some weeks/months into the convalescent period (Henle, G. and Henle 1979: Henle, W. and Henle 1979; see also Fig. 78.6). This reflects the fact that

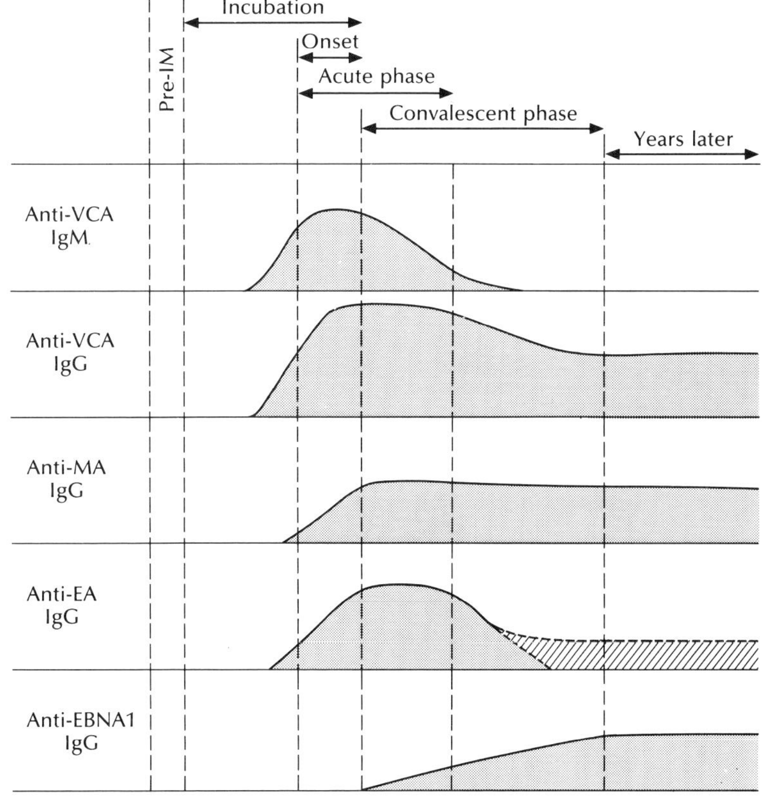

Fig. 78.6. Diagrammatic representation of anti-EBV antibody responses during and after a primary EBV infection accompanied by infectious mononucleosis (adopted from Henle, G. and Henle 1979). By the time clinical symptoms appear, anti-VCA, anti-MA and anti-EA antibodies are already detectable but may subsequently increase in titre during the acute phase of the disease. During convalescence, anti-VCA IgM antibodies disappear whilst anti-VCA IgG and anti-MA IgG titres stabilize; anti-EA IgG antibodies either disappear during convalescence or stabilize at low levels. Anti-EBNA-1 antibodies, detectable by anti-complement immunofluorescence staining, usually do not appear until the convalescent phase and then rise to a stable level.

the assay preferentially detects the IgG anti-EBNA-1 antibody response which develops late following primary infection. Immunoblotting has more recently revealed a strong IgM anti-EBNA-1 response in IM sera, the dominant immunogenic epitope being the gly–ala co-polymer repeat region in the central domain of the EBNA-1 molecule (Rhodes *et al.* 1987). Indeed, cross-reactive recognition of certain cellular proteins with related gly–ala repeats explains some, but by no means all, of the autoimmune reactivities in IM sera. More recent immunoblotting and immunofluorescence assays (using target cells selectively expressing either EBNA-1 or EBNA-2 after gene transfection) has shown that the IgG response to EBNA-2 peaks much earlier than the corresponding anti-EBNA-1 response, so that the differential between these two reactivities is a useful index of the progression of a primary EBV infection (Henle *et al.* 1987).

Auto- and heterophile antibodies of IgM class are another characteristic feature of IM sera, and the presence of one particular heterophile antibody detected in the Paul–Bunnell test can be taken as firm evidence of a primary EBV-related mononucleosis (and excludes similar, though rarer, syndromes induced by cytomegalovirus or toxoplasma infection). Not all cases of EBV-induced IM give positive Paul–Bunnell tests, however, 'false negatives' being particularly prevalent amongst the increasing number of IM patients now found in the pre-adolescent age-group. Unequivocal identification of EBV-induced IM therefore requires the detection of EBV-specific antibodies (usually anti-VCA) of the IgM class.

Primary cell-mediated response

One of the principal diagnostic features of IM is the presence of elevated numbers of 'atypical lymphocytes' both in the circulation and infiltrating many tissues (but excluding bone marrow). The majority of these atypical cells are not EBV-infected B lymphocytes but lymphoblasts of thymic origin (Sheldon *et al.* 1973) with CD8 +ve T cells predominant (Reinherz *et al.* 1980). This is a key finding, being the first indication that the lymphoproliferation seen in IM is not all directly EBV-driven; indeed, much of it represents an unusually vigorous cell-mediated immune response to infection with this B lymphotropic agent.

The functional analysis of this T cell response suggests that it is composed of several complex reactivities. One important feature is the presence of a broad-ranging suppressor T cell activity (Reinherz *et al.* 1980); thus mononuclear cell preparations from IM blood respond very poorly to antigen- or mitogen-induced stimulation *in vitro* and the IM T cell fraction is even capable of efficiently suppressing the response of normal mononuclear cells to such stimuli. This 'pan-suppression' which is evident in *in vitro* assays may also explain why IM patients are transiently unresponsive in conventional *in vivo* tests of cell-mediated immune function.

A second unusual feature of IM T cell populations is their ability, after being depleted of all conventional natural killer (NK) cell activity by removal of CD16 +ve cells, to lyse both the autologous EBV-transformed LCL and several allogeneic, human leucocyte antigen (HLA)-mismatched LCLs in short-term cytotoxicity assays. This observation (Svedmyr and Jondal 1975) is of some historical interest since IM was the first clinical situation in which the human cytotoxic T cell response to a natural pathogen could be analysed for evidence of major histocompatibility complex (MHC) restriction, and the immediate inference was that restriction did not occur! In fact, more recent work (Strang and Rickinson 1987) has shown that lysis of the autologous LCL is indeed carried out by activated CD8 +ve cytotoxic T cells which are both EBV-specific and HLA Class I MHC antigen-restricted in their function (i.e. exactly the reactivity which is subsequently established in the T cell memory of lifelong virus carriers). The cytotoxic reactivities detectable against allogeneic HLA-mismatched LCLs are mediated by other components within the CD8 +ve T cell pool which appear to be coincidentally expanded *in vivo* alongside the true virus-specific response; their reactivity against particular allogeneic LCL targets seems to reflect fortuitous cross-recognition involving HLA Class I MHC molecules as alloantigens. The true antigenic specificity of these 'coincidentally expanded' T cell clones remains obscure. They may have entirely irrelevant reactivities and therefore play no effective role in the control of the infection; alternatively they could be part of an as yet undisclosed cytotoxic response to EBV lytic cycle antigens whose specific reactivity would not have been revealed in the assays carried out to date using the latently infected autologous LCL as an *in vitro* target.

A summary diagram of the virological and immunological events of IM is presented in Fig. 78.7; note that this is almost certainly an over-simplification of what is an extremely complex situation. Infectious mononucleosis is a disease accompanied by profound regulatory disturbance of the immune system, in which both humoral and cell-mediated arms of the immune response are polyclonally activated and where only a fraction of the responses are demonstrably EBV-specific. It is not certain why such exaggerated responses occur. However, direct EBV-driven B cell activation represents one way in which inappropriate (auto/heterophile) antibody-producing clones might be expanded, whilst the highly immunogenic nature of the EBV-transformed lymphoblastoid cell might explain why a generalized proliferation of such cells could elicit such a vigorous T cell response. As to the pathogenesis of the disease, the coincidence of the onset of disease symptoms with the appearance of circulating T lymphocytosis strongly suggests that the clinical symptoms of IM are immunopathological in nature (Svedmyr *et al.* 1984).

Recently there has been much interest in cases of 'chronic mononucleosis' where, following primary EBV infection, IM-like symptoms either

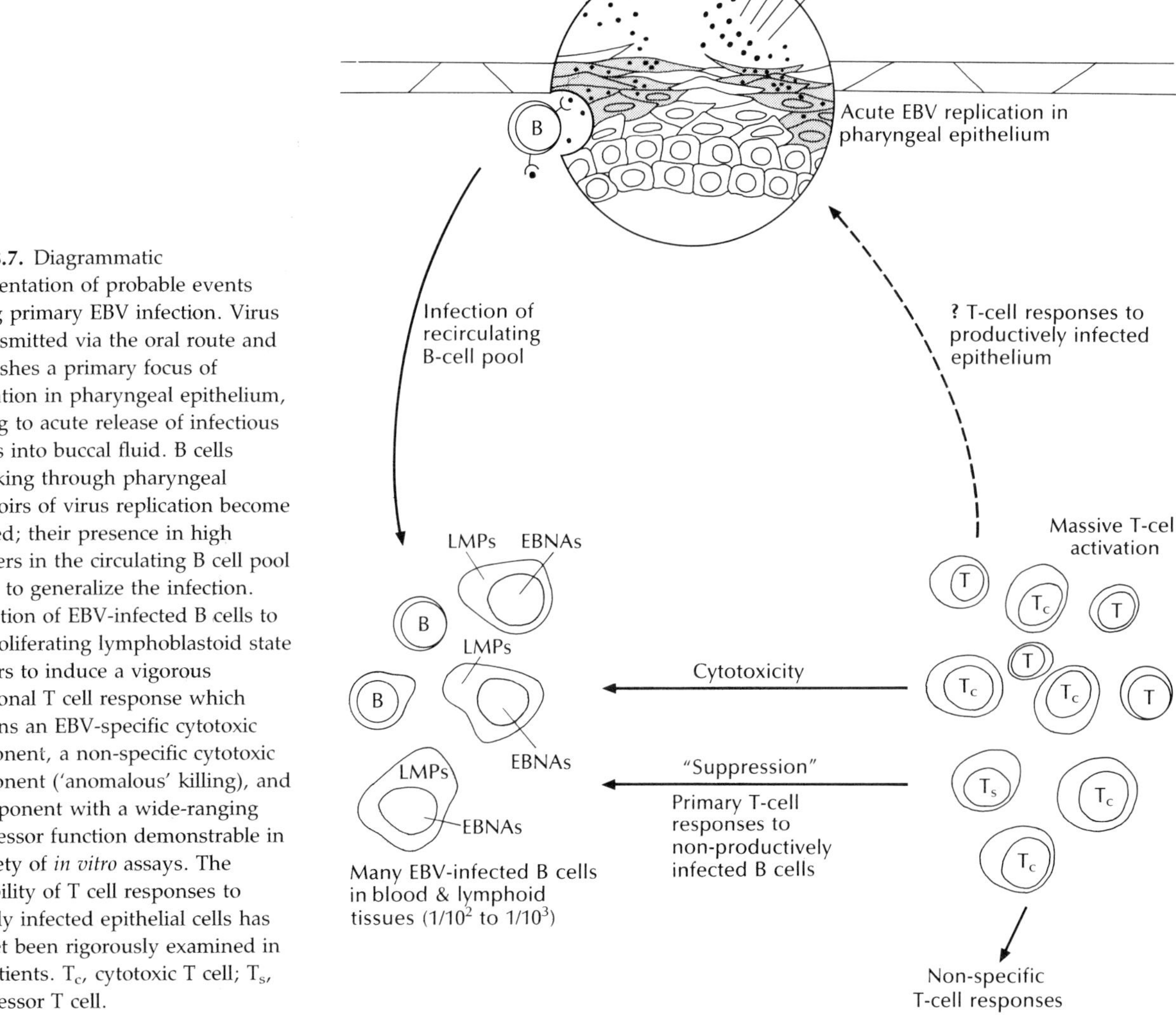

Fig. 78.7. Diagrammatic representation of probable events during primary EBV infection. Virus is transmitted via the oral route and establishes a primary focus of replication in pharyngeal epithelium, leading to acute release of infectious virions into buccal fluid. B cells trafficking through pharyngeal reservoirs of virus replication become infected; their presence in high numbers in the circulating B cell pool serves to generalize the infection. Activation of EBV-infected B cells to the proliferating lymphoblastoid state appears to induce a vigorous polyclonal T cell response which contains an EBV-specific cytotoxic component, a non-specific cytotoxic component ('anomalous' killing), and a component with a wide-ranging suppressor function demonstrable in a variety of *in vitro* assays. The possibility of T cell responses to lytically infected epithelial cells has not yet been rigorously examined in IM patients. T_c, cytotoxic T cell; T_s, suppressor T cell.

persist or recur frequently over a period of years. True cases of EBV-induced chronic IM do exist but they are quite rare; to date, one of the best diagnostic criteria identifying such cases is the continuing absence of IgG anti-EBNA-1 antibodies in the presence of strong anti-VCA, anti-EA and often anti-EBNA-2 responses (Henle *et al.* 1987). Most reported cases of 'post-viral fatigue syndrome' (a poorly defined condition having certain features in common with true chronic mononucleosis) have no documented link with a primary EBV infection, do not fulfil the above serological criteria and have no relationship to EBV.

Immune response to persistent Epstein–Barr virus infection

Primary infection, whether subclinical or associated with IM, always leads to the establishment of a lifelong virus carrier state. Recent studies suggest that EBV can be found in both epithelial and lymphoid habitats even in the long-term virus carrier, albeit at much lower levels than in IM patients. Continued low-grade virus replication in the oropharynx must be occurring to account for the presence of transforming virus at low titre in buccal fluid, whilst the continued presence of virus-infected circulating B cells is clear from the capacity of cultured leucocytes to give rise to LCLs by spontaneous outgrowth. Both lytic and latent cycle antigens continue to be expressed *in vivo* therefore, and this persistent antigenic challenge serves to maintain both humoral and cellular immune responses at stable levels for life (see Fig. 78.9).

Persistent humoral response

In the vast majority of cases resolution of the acute phase of primary infection is followed over the next few months by a gradual change in the serological profile to that characteristic of the healthy virus carrier (Henle, W. and Henle 1979). These changes are illustrated diagrammatically in Fig. 78.6. Thus IgM antibodies (virus-specific as well as heterophile and autoreactive) disappear whilst IgG antibodies to VCA and MA (now including both anti-GP340 and anti-GP85 reactivities) reach stable levels; anti-EA antibodies, assayed by immunofluorescence, either stabilize at relatively low titres or fall below the level of detection. Perhaps the most important of the serological reactivities to lytic cycle antigens are the anti-GP340 antibodies of the IgG class since these are known to have potent virus-neutralizing activity (Thorley-Lawson and Geilinger 1980), thus preventing the spread of cell-free virus *in vivo*, and can also mediate antibody-dependent cellular cytotoxicity against lytically infected cells through binding to GP340 expressed on the cell membrane (Pearson *et al.* 1979).

The gradual appearance of anti-EBNA antibody reactivity in the sera of convalescent IM patients, detected using the standard anticomplement immunofluorescence assay, largely reflects the delayed development of IgG antibody responses to EBNA-1. After primary infection, all healthy virus carriers maintain stable levels of IgG anti-EBNA-1 antibodies, detectable not only by immunofluorescence but also by immunoblotting. On the other hand, IgG antibodies to other EBNA species (EBNA 2, 3a, 3b, 3c and LP) are detectable in only a proportion of healthy carriers, differences between individual carriers in respect of their anti-EBNA reactivities remaining relatively stable with time (see Fig. 78.5). It is interesting that the best-characterized antibody responses against latent cycle proteins of EBV should be against the virus-coded intranuclear antigens; the stability of these anti-EBNA responses suggests that latently infected EBNA +ve cells are continually being destroyed *in vivo*, with concomitant release of the intranuclear EBV antigens providing a constant antigenic stimulus.

Persistent cell-mediated response

The availability of an *in vitro* system to study EBV-induced B cell growth transformation has been a considerable advantage in identifying cell-mediated immune controls which might interrupt the B cell infection. Initial studies (Thorley-Lawson *et al.* 1977) indicated that the events of transformation could be delayed at an early stage (that is, before entry of infected cells into the cell cycle) if autologous T cells were added back to the EBV-infected B cell population soon after the latter's exposure to virus. This effect, seen in cultures from all adult donors whether or not these individuals had been naturally infected with EBV, has been variously ascribed to the antiviral actions of interferons (α and γ) released from the cultured

T cells. Perhaps the most important inference from such experimental findings is that *in vivo* the EBV-B cell interaction may be sensitive to control by T-cell-derived cytokines. This could be a very important means of control if such cytokines were able to inhibit EBV gene expression in infected cells *in vivo* for longer periods than have been observed in the *in vitro* model system.

A second important means of control apparent from *in vitro* studies is that mediated by virus-specific cytotoxic T cells (CTLs). Thus it was shown that EBV-infected cultures of peripheral blood lymphocytes from seronegative adult donors (i.e. individuals not yet naturally infected with EBV) gave rise to LCLs within 3–4 weeks (Fig. 78.8(a), (b)), whereas in the corresponding cultures from seropositive donors foci of activated B cells appearing within 7–10 days (Fig. 78.8(c)) were subsequently destroyed by a T-cell mediated mechanism (Fig. 78.8(d)). This 'regression' of B cell outgrowth was brought about by virus-specific CTLs (predominantly CD8 +ve and HLA Class I MHC antigen-restricted) which had been reactivated *in vitro* from memory T cells present in the circulation of the seropositive donors (Rickinson 1986). A simple limiting dilution assay allowed the strength of regression (i.e. the frequency of EBV-specific memory T cells) to be titrated and, just as with serum antibody titrations, prospective studies have emphasized the stability of memory T cell numbers in the blood of individual donors. Furthermore, it is possible to follow convalescent IM patients and monitor the gradual development of the memory T cell response to a steady-state level which is thereafter stably maintained.

With the development of EBV-specific CD8 +ve CTL cell lines and clones expanded in interleukin 2 (IL-2)-conditioned medium, work has concen-

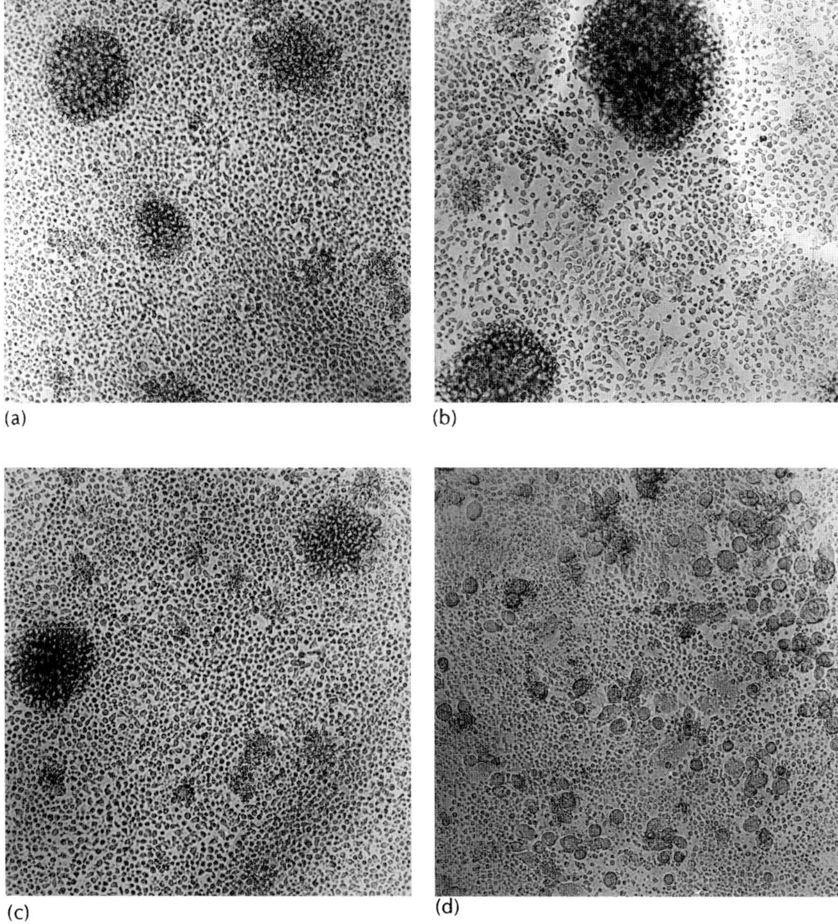

Fig. 78.8. Photomicrographs illustrating the appearance of T-cell-mediated regression of EBV-infected B cell outgrowth *in vitro*, and its dependence upon the EBV immune status of the individual donor. Blood mononuclear cell cultures from an EBV-non-immune donor 10 days (a) and 4 weeks (b) after exposure to a high-titre preparation of B95.8 strain EBV; outgrowth of EBV-transformed B cells occurs undisturbed by T cells co-resident in the culture. Blood mononuclear cell cultures from an EBV-immune donor, likewise exposed to B95.8 strain EBV *in vitro*, show an initial growth of EBV-transformed B cells at 10 days (c); thereafter the cells are destroyed by a virus-specific cytotoxic T cell response occurring *in vitro*, leading to a regression of B cell outgrowth and degeneration of the culture at 4 weeks (d).

trated on identifying the target structures which the CTL response recognizes. It was originally postulated that recognition was through an EBV-coded 'lymphocyte-detected membrane antigen (LYDMA)' which was constitutively expressed on all *in vitro* transformed LCLs, i.e. a novel latent cycle antigen found on the cell membrane. In fact, the seminal work of recent years on the influenza virus system has made it clear that MHC-restricted CTL recognition does not involve viral proteins in their native form but small peptide fragments derived from viral antigens by intracellular proteolytic cleavage and presented as an MHC antigen/peptide on the cell surface for interaction with the T cell receptor (Townsend *et al.* 1986). In the wake of this finding, it became clear that recognition in the EBV system might be mediated via peptides derived from any one of the eight latent cycle antigens, quite irrespective of the native location of these viral proteins in the transformed cell. The precise identity of the immunogenic peptide must depend upon the identity of the HLA Class I MHC molecule with which it complexes, i.e. there are at least as many 'LYDMAs' as there are HLA Class I MHC antigens. Recent work has indeed identified individual EBV-specific CTL responses, each restricted through a different HLA Class I MHC molecule, where the immunogenic peptides appear to be derived from different latent cycle antigens, namely EBNA-2, EBNA-3a and LMP-1. This is an important advance in our understanding of EBV immunity, but much more work needs to be done before the picture is complete. In the influenza virus system, it is worth noting that most human CTL responses appear to be directed against peptide epitopes derived from just two or three of the 10 viral antigens expressed in infected cells. Whether a subset of EBV latent cycle antigens likewise preferentially provides the target peptides for CTL recognition is an important issue which remains to be resolved.

Another illuminating facet of EBV-specific CTL recognition is the crucial role played by cell adhesion pathways in facilitating the initial contact between effector and target cells. These cell–cell contacts, involving LFA-1 and CD2 molecules on the effector cell and their respective ligands ICAM-1 and LFA-3 on the target cell, appear to facilitate immunologically-specific recognition occurring subsequently through the T cell receptor pathway (Shaw *et al.* 1986; see also Chapter 11). The accessibility of an EBV-infected B cell to immune recognition is therefore critically dependent not just upon its expression of the relevant viral target antigens but also upon its level of cellular ICAM-1 and LFA-3 expression. As described earlier, EBV-induced B cell activation is accompanied by a dramatic up-regulation of these adhesion molecules from the minimal levels present on resting B cells (see Fig. 78.1) and recent evidence suggests that one particular virus latent cycle antigen, LMP-1, is responsible for inducing this change in the adhesion molecule profile. During the EBV infection of B cells, therefore, the timing of LMP expression (which lags behind that of the EBNA proteins) is of particular importance in determining the cells' accessibility to T cell surveillance mechanisms.

Figure 78.9 presents a summary diagram of possible interactions involved in virus persistence in the immunocompetent host. The CTL surveillance system described above is obviously one important feature of immune control over the infection in B cells. Whether virus replication in epithelium is also controlled by CTL responses is an open question. There is as yet no firm evidence that the latent cycle proteins are ever expressed in an epithelial environment; thus immune control of the epithelial infection is more likely to be achieved through T cells specific for processed forms of lytic cycle antigens. Analysis of this question is still in its infancy and no CTL preparations specific for lytically infected targets have yet been described. Some progress is being made, however, on proliferative CD4+ve T cell responses with specificity for virus structural antigens; thus HLA Class II MHC antigen-restricted clones specific for GP340 have been isolated from immune donors. One possible role for such T cells *in vivo* would be to induce inflammatory responses at sites of virus replication through lymphokine release; such release would depend upon the specific recognition of processed antigen on local antigen presenting cells.

Failures of immunological control

X-linked lymphoproliferative syndrome/fatal infectious mononucleosis

Purtilo and colleagues first described a rare X-linked immunodeficiency characterized in the

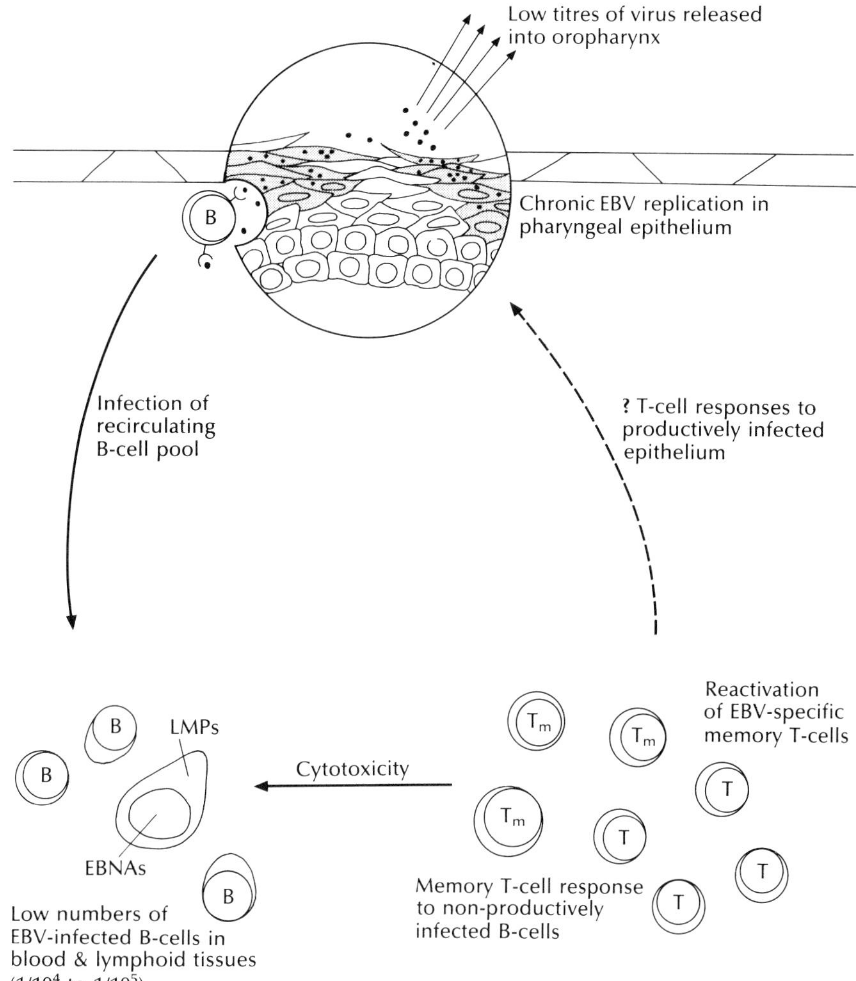

Fig. 78.9. Diagrammatic representation of probable events during persistent EBV infection. Low-grade virus replication occurs in pharyngeal epithelium, leading to chronic release of infectious virions into buccal fluid. Such chronic replication probably serves to maintain low numbers of infected B cells in the recirculating pool, although the extent to which such new recruitment occurs is not clear. Occasional activation of EBV-infected B cells to the proliferating lymphoblastoid state remains a feature of the virus carrier state, but outgrowth of such infected B cells is controlled by EBV-specific cytotoxic T cells reactivated from the memory cell pool. T cell responses against lytically infected epithelial cells may also be maintained in virus carriers, but their existence remains to be properly documented. T_m, memory T cell.

majority of affected male children by a failure to survive primary EBV infection (Purtilo *et al.* 1985). Some two-thirds of such boys die within 2–3 weeks of their infection from an unusually severe IM-like disease characterized by EBV-induced B cell activation, widespread polyclonal T cell activation and what appears to be the immunopathological destruction of internal organs, such as liver, spleen and thymus. The precise nature of the immune defect is still not understood. Anti-EBV antibody responses are generally impaired during the acute phase of the disease, and even in long-term survivors, but this is probably a consequence of some more basic immune regulatory dysfunction and not a sufficient explanation *per se* for the host's extreme sensitivity to EBV. The fact that many survivors suffer either hypogammaglobulinaemia or aplastic anaemia reinforces the view that X-linked lymphoproliferative syndrome lies at the extreme end of the IM disease spectrum, since severe cases of IM in immunologically competent individuals can produce similar complications.

It is to be hoped that identification of the precise genetic defect underlying X-linked lymphoproliferative syndrome (Skare *et al.* 1987) will help to elucidate the pathogenesis of the EBV-induced disease. There is certainly still much to learn about the immunological and virological events which occur following primary EBV infection in such patients. Rare non-familial cases of fatal IM appear to follow a similar clinical course. In both these situations the disease often appears to be immunopathological in nature, perhaps reflecting a failure to control (rather than a failure to initiate) the virus-induced cell-mediated response.

'Post-transplant' lymphoma/lymphoproliferative disease of the immunocompromised host

Severe impairment of the T cell system, whether congenital (as in the Wiskott–Aldrich syndrome) or induced by immunosuppressive agents (as in allograft recipients or AIDS patients), is accompanied by a greatly increased risk of EBV +ve lymphoproliferative disease (Purtilo and Klein 1981). Multiple foci of EBV-infected B cells, each focus consisting of one or more cell clones, appear in lymphoid tissue and grow progressively to kill the host if left unchecked. Recent studies have shown that the form of infection seen in these lymphoproliferative lesions *in vivo* is indistinguishable from that which exists in EBV-transformed LCLs *in vitro*; that is, the cells are expressing the full spectrum of EBV latent cycle antigens and also display the characteristic B lymphoblastoid cell surface phenotype with high expression of cellular activation antigens and adhesion molecules (Young *et al.* 1989). Figure 78.10 shows frozen sections of such a lymphoproliferative lesion stained with monoclonal antibodies to EBNA-2 (Fig. 78.10(a)) and to LMP-1 (Fig. 78.10(b)); the tumour cells are clearly positive for both EBV latent proteins.

These findings suggest that such EBV +ve B cells have been allowed to expand *in vivo* because of the lack of any effective T cell control. Furthermore, one would predict that the proliferating LCL-like cells would still be sensitive to immune recognition should T cell function be restored. This indeed seems to be the case since, in allograft recipients, reduction of the immunosuppressive therapy and consequent recovery of T cell responsiveness is followed by regression of the EBV +ve lesions (Starzl *et al.* 1984).

Many features of this disease — its oligoclonal nature, the absence of any specific chromosomal changes in the proliferating cells, the typical histology with areas of 'geographical necrosis' and the capacity for regression — precisely mirror the fatal lymphoproliferative disease which is induced by EBV on experimental infection of cotton-top tamarins (Cleary *et al.* 1985). One concludes that EBV is the primary, perhaps the sole, driving-force behind these fatal lymphoproliferations in the natural host just as it is in the animal model. Note that the human disease can progress from oligo- to monoclonality but there is as yet no indication that this involves any specific second step in the pathogenic sequence. It may simply reflect dominance by the fastest-growing EBV +ve B cell clone *in vivo* (see Rowe *et al.* 1991), exactly as can occur *in vitro* during the establishment of an EBV-transformed LCL.

Endemic Burkitt's lymphoma

Compared with the direct role played by the virus in the 'post-transplant' lymphomas described above, EBV's relationship with endemic BL is much more complex. Infection with EBV here

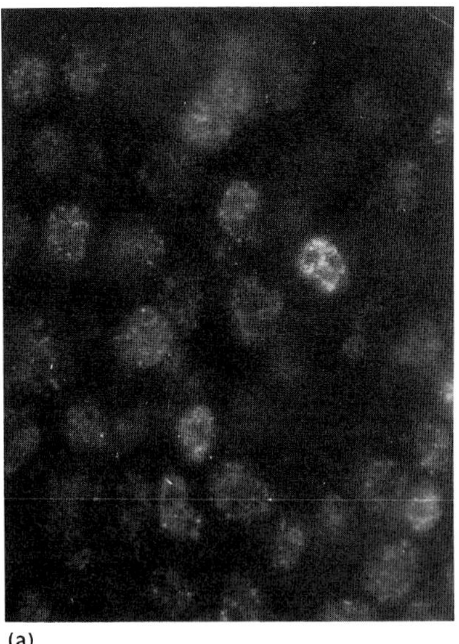
(a)

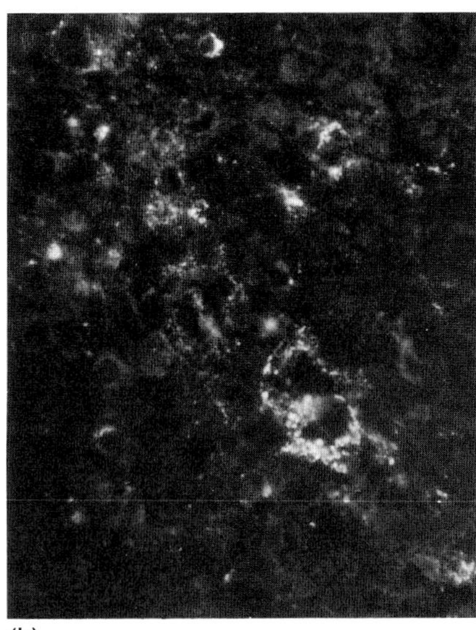
(b)

Fig. 78.10. Frozen sections through a lymphoproliferative lesion which arose in an immunosuppressed allograft recipient. Positive immunofluorescence staining with monoclonal antibodies specific (a) for EBNA-2 and (b) for LMP-1 indicates the LCL-like nature of EBV gene expression in the lymphoma cells.

seems to be just one step in a larger chain of events culminating in the malignant conversion of a single target B cell; the tumour arises as a monoclonal population of cells derived from that single malignant progenitor.

The endemic form of BL is that seen in equatorial regions of Africa and New Guinea, where the disease is the most common cancer of childhood. Here the geographical distribution of the tumour exactly parallels that of holoendemic *Plasmodium falciparum* malaria, suggesting that some feature of the chronic parasitic infection facilitates the oncogenic process. Epstein–Barr virus shows a striking association with endemic BL in that essentially all such malignancies are EBV genome +ve (Lenoir 1986). The consistency of this association argues against the presence of the virus merely as an opportunistic passenger and in favour of an aetiological relationship between virus and tumour. This is not to say that EBV alone is sufficient to cause BL development. Clearly this is not the case since a crucial second step in BL pathogenesis involves a chromosomal translocation which leads to deregulated expression of the cellular proto-oncogene c-myc (Lenoir 1986).

Endemic BL is frequently held up as a paradigm of multi-step carcinogenesis in man and readers are referred to several interesting reviews which discuss possible sequences of events leading to outgrowth of the EBV +ve tumour (Klein 1987; Lenoir and Bornkamm 1987; Magrath 1990). The point of immediate relevance in the present context is whether these EBV +ve malignant B cells are subject to the same T-cell-mediated immune controls *in vivo* as are the EBV-infected LCL-like cells which are continually arising and being destroyed in healthy virus carriers. In fact, studies with paired BL/LCL cell lines (the BL line derived from the tumour biopsy cells, the LCL generated by virus-induced transformation of the same patient's normal B cells) have made it clear that the EBV +ve tumour cells are *not* sensitive to recognition by virus-specific CTL effectors (Rooney *et al*. 1985). More recent work has shown that such tumour cell 'escape' from T cell surveillance reflects both the special nature of the EBV infection in BL cells and the particular cell surface phenotype which these cells display. Thus EBV expression in endemic BL biopsy cells is restricted to just a subset of those latent cycle antigens routinely found in LCL cells; to date only one of the latent cycle antigens, EBNA-1, has been detected (Rowe *et al*. 1987). Many of the target proteins providing epitopes for virus-specific T cell recognition are therefore not present in BL cells. Furthermore, endemic BL cells express, at the most, only very low levels of the cellular adhesion molecules (in particular, ICAM-1 and LFA-3) upon which efficient effector–target cell interactions depend (Gregory *et al*. 1988). This also favours the relative inaccessibility of the tumour to immune T cell control.

Conclusion

Epstein–Barr virus is therefore associated with a whole spectrum of benign and malignant lymphoproliferations and the analysis of these conditions has provided some interesting insights into the life style of a B lymphotropic agent and the impact which such an agent can make on the immune system. The recent identification of an epithelial lesion, OHL, as a focus of lytic EBV infection and the long-standing association between the virus and an epithelial malignancy, NPC, emphasize the need to understand how EBV is perceived by the immune response in its epithelial as well as its lymphoid habitat. This is likely to be an important focus of research in the future progress of EBV immunology.

References

Baer, R., Bankier, A.T., Biggin, M.D. *et al*. (1984) DNA sequence and expression of the B95-8 Epstein–Barr virus genome. *Nature* **310**, 207–11.

Cleary, M.L., Epstein, M.A., Finerty, S. *et al*. (1985). Individual tumours of multifocal Epstein–Barr virus-induced malignant lymphomas in tamarins arise from different B-cell clones. *Science* **228**, 722–4.

Cooper, N.R., Moore, M.D. and Nemerow, G.R. (1988). Immunobiology of CR2, the B lymphocyte receptor for Epstein–Barr virus and the C3d complement fragment. *Ann. Rev. Immunol.* **6**, 85–113.

Farrell, P. (1989). The Epstein–Barr virus genome. In *Advances in Viral Oncology*, ed. G. Klein, vol. VIII, pp. 103–32, Raven Press, New York.

Greenspan, J.S., Greenspan, D., Lennette, E.T. *et al*. (1985). Replication of Epstein–Barr virus within the epithelial cells of oral 'hairy' leukoplakia, an AIDS-associated lesion. *N. Engl. J. Med.* **313**, 1564–71.

Gregory, C.D., Murray, R.J., Edwards, C.F. and Rickinson, A.B. (1988). Down regulation of cell adhesion molecules LFA-3 and ICAM-1 in Epstein–Barr virus-positive Burkitt's lymphoma underlies tumour cell escape from virus-specific T cell surveillance. *J. Exp. Med.* **167**, 1811–24.

Henle, G. and Henle, W. (1979). The virus as the etiologic agent of infectious mononucleosis. In *The Epstein–Barr Virus*, ed. M.A. Epstein and B.G. Achong, pp. 298–320, Springer-Verlag, Berlin, Heidelberg, New York.

Henle, W. and Henle, G. (1979). Seroepidemiology of the virus. In *The Epstein–Barr Virus*, ed. M.A. Epstein and B.G. Achong, pp. 61–78, Springer-Verlag, Berlin, Heidelberg, New York.

Henle, W., Henle, G., Andersson, J. *et al.* (1987). Antibody responses to Epstein–Barr virus-determined nuclear antigen (EBNA)-1 and EBNA 2 in acute and chronic Epstein–Barr virus infection. *Proc. Nat. Acad. Sci. (USA)* **84**, 570–4.

Kieff, E. and Liebowitz, D. (1990). Epstein–Barr virus and its replication. In *Virology*, ed. B.N. Fields, D.M. Knipe *et al.*, pp. 1889–920, Raven Press, New York.

Klein, G. (1987). In defense of the 'old' Burkitt lymphoma scenario. In *Advances in Viral Oncology*, ed. G. Klein, vol. VII, pp. 207–11, Raven Press, New York.

Lenoir, G.M. (1986). Role of the virus, chromosomal translocations and cellular oncogenes in the aetiology of Burkitt's lymphoma. In *The Epstein–Barr Virus: Recent Advances*, ed. M.A. Epstein and B.G. Achong, pp. 183–205, William Heinemann Medical Books, London.

Lenoir, G.M. and Bornkamm, G.W. (1987). Burkitt's lymphoma, a human cancer model for the study of the multistep development of cancer: proposal for a new scenario. In *Advances in Viral Oncology*, ed. G. Klein, vol. VI, pp. 173–206. Raven Press, New York.

Magrath, I. (1990). The pathogenesis of Burkitt's lymphoma. *Adv. Cancer Res.* **55**, 133–270.

Nemerow, G.R., Houghton, R.A., Moore, M.D. and Cooper, N.R. (1989). Identification of an epitope in the major envelope protein of Epstein–Barr virus that mediates viral binding to the B lymphocyte EBV receptor (CR2). *Cell* **56**, 369–77.

Pearson, G.R., Qualtière, L.F., Klein, G., Norin, T. and Bal, I.S. (1979). Epstein–Barr virus-specific antibody-dependent cellular cytotoxicity in patients with Burkitt's lymphoma. *Int. J. Cancer* **24**: 402–6.

Purtilo, D.T. and Klein, G. (eds.) (1981). Symposium on Epstein–Barr virus-induced lymphoproliferative diseases in immunodeficient patients. *Cancer Res.* **41**, 4209–304.

Purtilo, D.T., Tatsumi, E., Manolov, Y. *et al.* (1985). Epstein–Barr virus as an etiological agent in the pathogenesis of lymphoproliferative and aproliferative diseases in immune deficient patients. *Int. Rev. Exp. Pathol.* **27**, 114–83.

Reedman, B.M. and Klein, G. (1973). Cellular localisation of an Epstein–Barr virus (EBV)-associated complement-fixing antigen in producer and non-producer lymphoblastoid cell lines. *Int. J. Cancer* **11**, 599–620.

Reinherz, E.L., O'Brien, C., Rosenthal, P. and Schlossman, S.F. (1980). The cellular basis for viral-induced immunodeficiency: analysis by monoclonal antibodies. *J. Immunol.* **125**, 1269–74.

Rhodes, G., Rumpold, H., Kurki, P., Patrick, K.M., Carson, D.A. and Vaughan, J.H. (1987). Autoantibodies in infectious mononucleosis have specificity for the glycine–alanine repeating region of the Epstein–Barr virus nuclear antigen. *J. Exp. Med.* **165**, 1026–40.

Rickinson, A.B. (1986). Cellular immunological responses to the virus infection. In *The Epstein–Barr Virus: Recent Advances*, ed. M.A. Epstein and B.G. Achong, pp. 75–125, William Heinemann Medical Books, London.

Rooney, C.M., Rowe, M., Wallace, L.E. and Rickinson, A.B. (1985). Epstein–Barr virus-positive Burkitt's lymphoma cells not recognised by virus-specific T cell surveillance. *Nature* **317**, 629–31.

Rowe, M., Rowe, D.T., Gregory, C.D. *et al.* (1987). Differences in B cell growth phenotype reflect novel patterns of Epstein–Barr virus latent gene expression in Burkitt's lymphoma cells. *EMBO J.* **6**, 2743–51.

Rowe, M., Young, L.S., Crocker, J., Stokes, H., Henderson, S. and Rickinson, A.B. (1991). Epstein–Barr virus (EBV)-associated lymphoproliferative disease in the SCID mouse model: implications for the pathogenesis of EBV-positive lymphomas in man. *J. Exp. Med.* **173**, 147–58.

Shaw, S., Luce, G.E.G., Quinoner, R., Gress, R.E., Springer, T.A. and Sanders, M.E. (1986). Two antigen-independent adhesion pathways used by human cytotoxic T cell clones. *Nature* **323**, 262–4.

Sheldon, P.J., Papamichail, M., Hemsted, E.H. and Holborow E.J. (1973). Thymic origin of atypical lymphoid cells in infectious mononucleosis. *Lancet* **i**, 1153–5.

Sixbey, J.W., Nedrud, J.G., Raab-Traub, N., Hanes, R.A. and Pagano, J.S. (1984). Epstein–Barr virus replication in oropharyngeal epithelial cells. *N. Engl. J. Med.* **310**, 1225–30.

Skare, J.C., Milunsky, A., Byron, K.S. and Sullivan, J.L. (1987). Mapping the X-linked lymphoproliferative syndrome. *Proc. Nat. Acad. Sci. (USA)* **84**, 2015–18.

Starzl, T.E., Nalesnik, M.A., Porter, K.A. *et al.* (1984). Reversibility of lymphomas and lymphoproliferative lesions developing under cyclosporin A-steroid therapy. *Lancet* **i**, 583–7.

Strang, G. and Rickinson, A.B. (1987). Multiple HLA class I-dependent cytotoxicities constitute the non-HLA-restricted response in infectious mononucleosis. *Eur. J. Immunol.* **17**, 1007–13.

Svedmyr, E. and Jondal, M. (1975). Cytotoxic effector cells specific for B cell lines transformed by Epstein–Barr virus are present in patients with infectious mononucleosis. *Proc. Nat. Acad. Sci. (USA)* **72**, 1622–6.

Svedmyr, E., Ernberg, I., Seeley, J. *et al.* (1984). Viroologic, immunologic, and clinical observations on a patient during the incubation, acute, and convalescent phases of infectious mononucleosis. *Clin. Immunol. Immunopathol.* **30**, 437–50.

Thorley-Lawson, D.A. and Geilinger, K. (1980). Monoclonal antibodies against the major glycoprotein (GP 350/220) of Epstein–Barr virus neutralise infectivity. *Proc. Nat. Acad. Sci. (USA)* **77**, 5307–11.

Thorley-Lawson, D.A., Chess, L. and Strominger, J.L. (1977). Suppression of *in vitro* Epstein–Barr virus infection: a new role for adult human T lymphocytes. *J. Exp. Med.* **146** 495–508.

Townsend, A.R.M., Rothbard, J., Gotch, F.M., Bahadur, G., Wraith, D. and McMichael, A.J. (1986). The epitopes of influenza nucleoprotein recognised by cytotoxic T lymphocytes can be defined with short synthetic peptides. *Cell* **44**, 959–68.

Young, L.S., Alfieri, C., Hennessy, K. *et al.* (1989). Epstein–Barr virus transformation-associated genes are expressed in tissues from patients with EBV lymphoproliferative disease. *N. Engl. J. Med.* **321** 1080–5.

79: Malaria

P. Perlmann, K. Berzins and M. Wahlgren

Malaria: the disease and the parasite

Out of 123 malarial species only four naturally infect man (*Plasmodium falciparum*, *P. vivax*, *P. ovale*, *P. malariae*). Three other Plasmodiidae (*P. cynomolgi*, *P. knowlesi*, *P. simium*) can be transmitted to man, although extremely rarely, and when occurring these are usually laboratory infections. The early symptoms of malaria infections are fever, headache and malaise, in non-endemic areas frequently mistaken as due to viral infection. The fever pattern later follows the characteristic syndrome of three stages, cold, hot and sweating, which occur every second (*P. falciparum*, *P. vivax*, *P. ovale*) or third (*P. malariae*) day. *Plasmodium ovale* and *P. malariae* cause relatively mild forms of malaria. The malaise during *P. vivax* is usually worse than during *P. falciparum* infections. However, while *P. vivax* rarely kills its host, *P. falciparum* is responsible for several million deaths each year. Cerebral malaria is one of the most serious forms of the disease.

Malarial infections were until recently prevalent in both temperate and tropical areas of the world. Today, 300–400 million individuals are infected each year, but the transmission is confined mainly to tropical and subtropical areas of the southern hemisphere (Fig. 79.1). During the 1960s and 1970s there was a dramatic return of the disease. Insecticide resistance of the *Anopheles* vector and drug resistance of the parasite are considered to be important contributing factors.

The frequencies of malaria infections vary dramatically between different parts of Asia, Africa and the Americas. Factors influencing transmission are environmental, such as temperature and rainfall, or socio-economic, such as migration and economic status. Genetic factors are also of importance; thus, the high frequencies of certain genetically determined haemoglobinopathies (i.e. sickle-haemoglobin, thalassaemias) or enzyme deficiencies (glucose-6-phosphate dehydrogenase

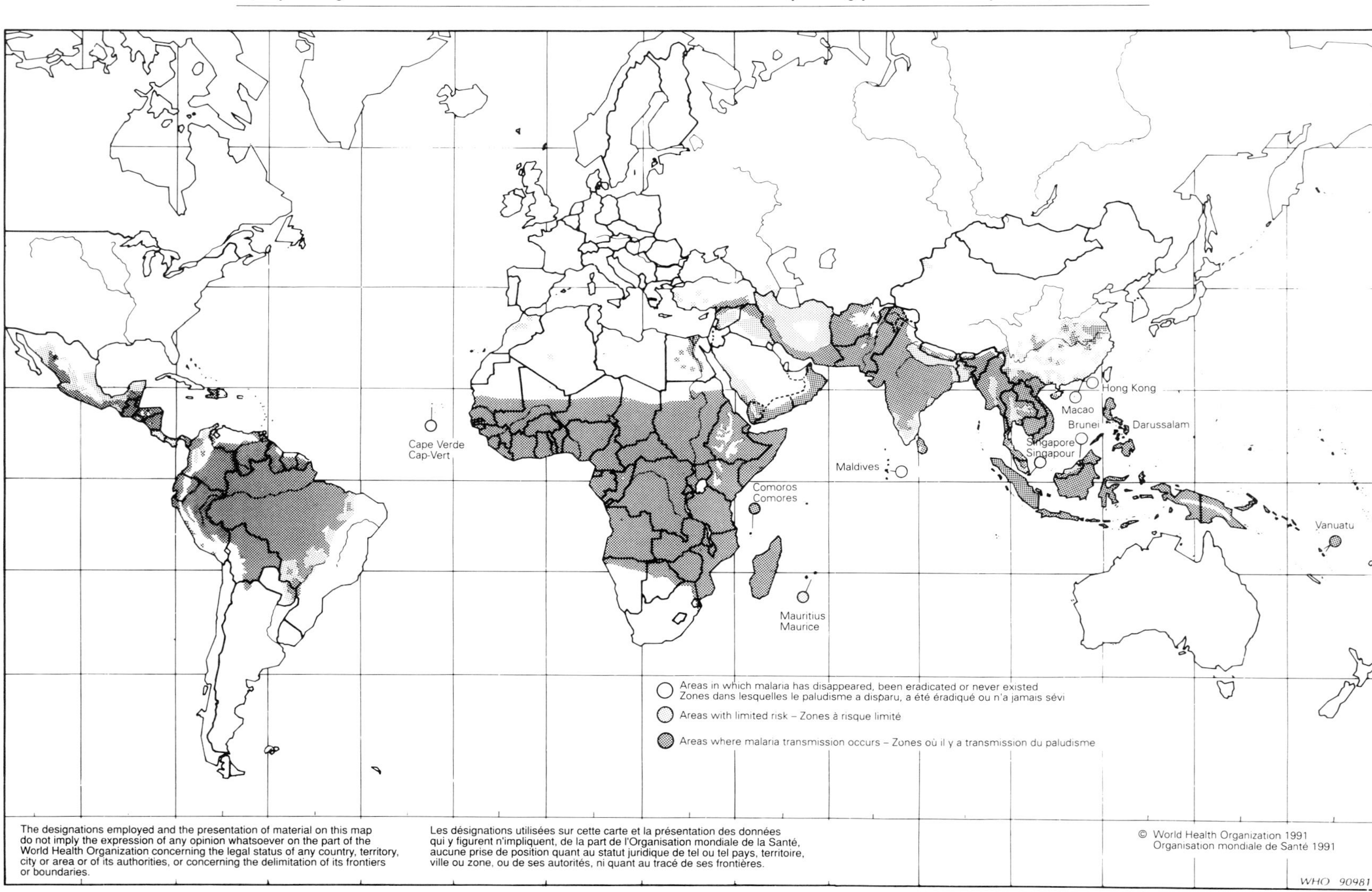

Fig. 79.1. Epidemiological assessment of the status of malaria. From World Health Organization (1991).

(G-6-PD)) in areas where malaria is or has been endemic are believed to be because the heterozygotes for these anomalies are relatively resistant to *P. falciparum* malaria. Similarly, it has been suggested that a relative insusceptibility to *P. vivax* in blacks of West Africa is due to the rarity of the Duffy blood group determinant (Miller *et al.* 1976).

Malaria is called epidemic when the incidence rapidly rises above the usual level, while it is called endemic when there is a constant measurable incidence of natural transmission over several years. The prevalence in a community can be scored by estimating the proportion of infants and children who have enlarged spleens (spleen rate).

The opinion that malaria parasites were spread by bad air (*mala aria*, Italian) from marshes (*palus*, Latin) gave the disease its name malaria or *paludisme/paludismo*. However, in 1847, Meckel found 'protoplasmic masses' in the blood of malaria-infected individuals and later, in 1880, Laveran fully described the malaria parasites (including exflagellation) and understood that the parasites were the cause of the disease. The mosquito transmission was later described by Ross, Bignami, Grassi and Bastianelli (reviewed by Wernsdorfer 1980). Only female anopheline mosquitoes carry the infective plasmodiidae, (sporozoites), which are injected into the bloodstream with the saliva, while taking a blood meal. The sporozoites travel with the circulation and within a few minutes bind to and enter the liver cells (Fig. 79.2). Here they undergo mitotic division (exoerythrocytic cycle) and a single sporozoite can sometimes multiply into 30 000 merozoites. While some of the parasites remain in the liver (hypnozoites, *P. vivax*, *P. ovale*), others break the cells within a week or two (*P. falciparum*), while longer incubation times (2–4 weeks) precede the appearance of *P. vivax*, *P. ovale* or *P. malariae* parasites in the blood. The merozoites invade the red blood cells and are now called rings (immature trophozoites). They increase into mature tropho-

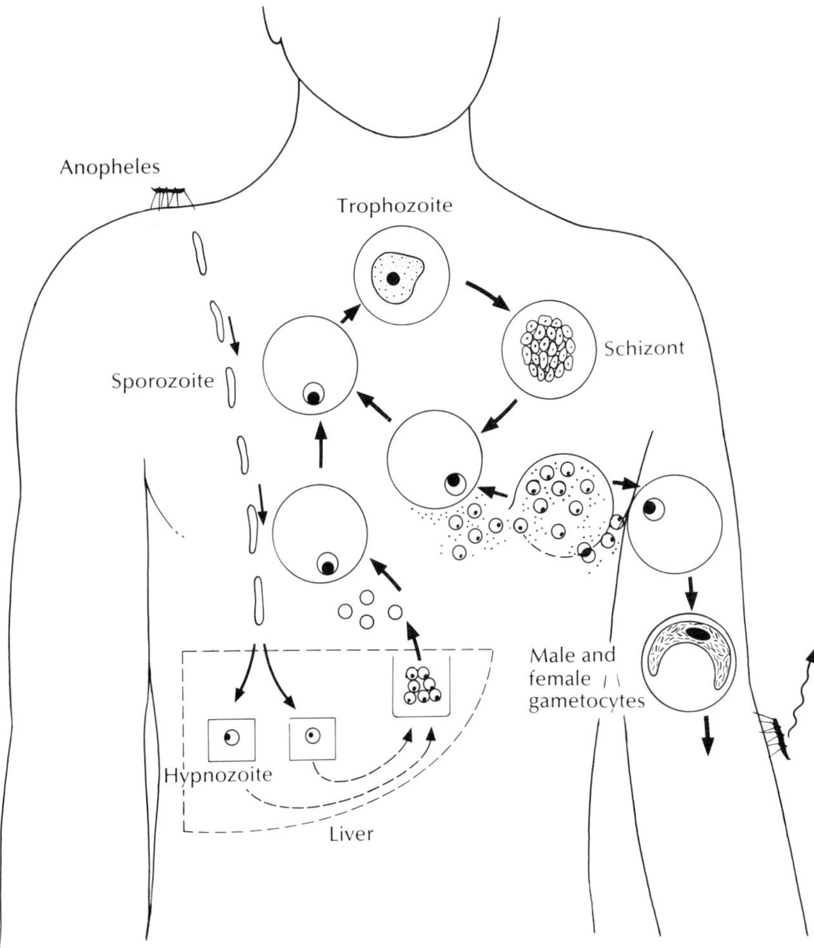

Fig. 79.2. Life cycle of malaria in man.

zoites and later undergo mitotic division into schizonts, containing up to 32 merozoites (*P. falciparum*). This erythrocytic part of the life cycle is completed after 48 (*P. falciparum*, *P. vivax*, *P. ovale*) or 72 (*P. malariae*) hours by the release of merozoites from rupturing schizonts and the invasion of fresh erythrocytes (Fig. 79.2). Not all parasites continue development into asexual-stage parasites (trophozoites, schizonts); some transform into male or female gametocytes (sexual stages). These intraerythrocytic, sexual stages are present in the peripheral circulation and are the transmissible forms of the parasites, taken up into the mosquito gut during a blood meal. Here the male gametocytes exflagellate and fuse with female gametes, and the zygotes transform into ookinetes. The sporozoite is the ultimate developmental stage in the mosquito, invading the salivary glands (and other tissues) from which they will be injected into the next host (Fig. 79.2).

Acquired malaria immunity

General

Although clinical immunity to plasmodial infection can be acquired, this requires repeated infections and takes many years. Moreover, acquired immunity, resulting in apparently complete clinical protection, is rarely, if ever, sterile. Thus, individuals who live in highly endemic malarious areas and develop no disease in spite of repeated reinfections almost always have low-grade parasitaemias in their blood. In addition, acquired immunity is not long-lasting and requires constant exposure to the parasite in order to be maintained. Therefore, fully protected immune individuals who move to a non-endemic area usually lose their immune protection within a few years.

These features of acquired malaria immunity reflect the long-standing adaptation of the parasite to the vertebrate host and its immune system. One of the important characteristics of this adaptation is the genetic diversity of many of the parasite's major immunogens, giving rise to potentially protective immune responses (see below). This intraspecies diversity is believed to be one of the major reasons for the slow development of an efficient immune protection. A second major factor is the effect of the parasite on immune regulation, an effect responsible for immunosuppression in acute infection, poor immunological memory, autoimmune reactivity and a variety of immunopathological phenomena (see below).

In addition to being species-specific, naturally acquired immunity is essentially stage-specific, reflecting the fact that the major immunogens which the different life cycle stages of the parasite present to the immune system are antigenically distinct molecules. Plasmodia causing malaria have been found in a large number of vertebrates. In general, the various vertebrates are infected by different plasmodial species, indicating a high degree of specificity in the host–parasite interaction.

Mouse malaria models

Several of the plasmodial species naturally infecting rodents have been adapted to laboratory mice. Since mice are not the natural hosts for these parasites, the course and outcome of these laboratory infections may be different from what is seen in the natural hosts. In spite of this, these mouse models have been invaluable for the elucidation of the mechanisms of antiplasmodial immune responses, in particular, of the relative protective (or pathogenic) roles of the T and B cell systems (Del Giudice *et al.* 1988b; Weidanz and Long, 1988). The two major reasons accounting for this are: (i) the possibility of studying infection in mice which are T- or B-cell-deficient either congenically or through experimental manipulation; and (ii) the existence of many plasmodial species or strains differing in their capacities to give rise to predominantly T- or B-cell-dependent immune responses. In the following a few examples may serve to illustrate the importance of these models.

Similarly to what has been seen in the human *P. falciparum* system, vaccination of mice with irradiated sporozoites (*P. berghei*) induces immunity against sporozoite infection (Nussenzweig *et al.* 1969). Mice may also be protected by monoclonal antibodies to epitopes occurring in the repeated amino acid sequences of their circumsporozoite (CS) protein, the immunodominant protein which covers the surface of the sporozoite in all plasmodial species (Yoshida *et al.* 1980). It was thought for some time that anti-CS protein antibodies, by preventing penetration of the sporozoites into the liver cells, would be sufficient to induce protective sporozoite immunity. However, protection from sporozoite infection has also been shown to include T-cell-dependent but antibody-independent effector mechanisms which prevent development of the sporozoite in the infected liver cells. These mechanisms, which certainly play a major role in naturally acquired sporozoite immunity, appear to involve both interferon gamma (IFN-γ), released from antigen-activated T cells and inhibiting parasite growth, and the specific cytotoxicity of CD8 +ve T cells to infected liver cells (see below).

Not unexpectedly, the mouse malaria models also show that T cells play a crucial role in immunity to the asexual blood stages of the parasite, both by regulating antibody production and by mediating an antibody-independent parasite control. Although perhaps over-simplified, it may be said that antibodies are usually important for the control of parasite loads in acute infection while T cells are necessary for both induction and maintenance of immunity. However, there is a large variation in T or B cell requirements, depending on the plasmodial species or strain, the maturity of the red blood cells which they infect preferentially (reticulocytes vs. normocytes) and the genetic constitution of the mice (Jayawardena 1981; Long 1988). Two extreme examples are *P. yoelii* (27X), which is non-lethal in normal mice but lethal in their B-cell-deprived littermates, and *P. chabaudi adami*, where B-cell-deficient mice resolve acute infection as well as normal mice. More recent studies have thrown further light on the protective mechanism involved in these systems. In the *P. yoelii* model, antibodies to an epitope in the C terminus of a 230 kD glycoprotein (Py230) homologous to Pf195, the major merozoite surface antigen of *P. falciparum* (see below), appear to play an important role in protective immunity (Burns *et al*. 1988). In contrast, in the *P. chabaudi adami* model, specific immunity could be obtained by adoptive transfer into nude mice of *P. chabaudi*-specific T cell lines or even an interleukin 2 (IL-2)/IFN-γ-producing clone of L3T4 +ve (= CD4 +ve) phenotype (Brake *et al*. 1988) (Fig. 79.3). Although the parasite antigen involved is not known, the finding that a T cell clone of restricted specificity can efficiently protect is of considerable interest. These results also provide additional evidence to earlier results indicating that CD4 +ve cells are important in the defence against blood-stage infections (Jayawardena *et al*. 1982). In *P. chabaudi chabaudi* infection, it has now also been shown that CD4 +ve T cells of the IFN-γ/IL-2-producing type (Th1) play a crucial role during the initial phase of a protective immune response, while IL-4/IL-5-producing CD4 +ve T cells of the helper type (Th2), together with antibodies, are important during later phases (Langhorne 1990).

Acquired immunity in humans

The pace at which immunity develops in humans is intimately related to the level of malarial endemicity in the area in which the individual resides (Molineaux and Gramiccia 1980; Björkman *et al*. 1987). In certain highly endemic areas with perennial transmission (e.g. Papua New Guinea, Liberia) about 5 years are needed to develop protective immunity. In less endemic areas as much as 10–15 years of exposure may be needed to acquire protection.

The infant born of an immune mother living in a highly endemic area, although bitten by infected mosquitoes each week, is protected against malaria during the first 6 months of life due to transferred maternal immunity. Severe and deadly *P. falciparum* infections occur at high frequency during the rest of the first 2 years of life. By this age the child has developed some resistance to infection and falls ill with fever and malaise but rarely with severe forms of the disease. Children of 5 years or more, residing in highly endemic areas, remain largely asymptomatic although carrying the infective parasites in the blood (a state of immunity called premunition). In the children parasite densities are high until the age of 2, whereafter they successively fall with the acquisition of immunity (Fig. 79.4(a)). Circulating parasites are virtually absent from the blood of 15-year-olds. The size of the spleen is the largest in 3–4-year-old children, whereafter it regresses in size (Fig. 79.4(a)).

The levels of total immunoglobulin M (IgM)/IgG increase as a child who lives under endemic conditions gets older and reach about four times the concentrations found in Caucasians (IgM 3.5–4 g/l; IgG 35–40 g/l) (Fig. 79.4(b), (c); McGregor 1974; Björkman 1985). However, only a fraction of all serum antibodies are specific for the parasites, and autoantibodies are frequent in the sera of malaria-exposed individuals (Table 79.1).

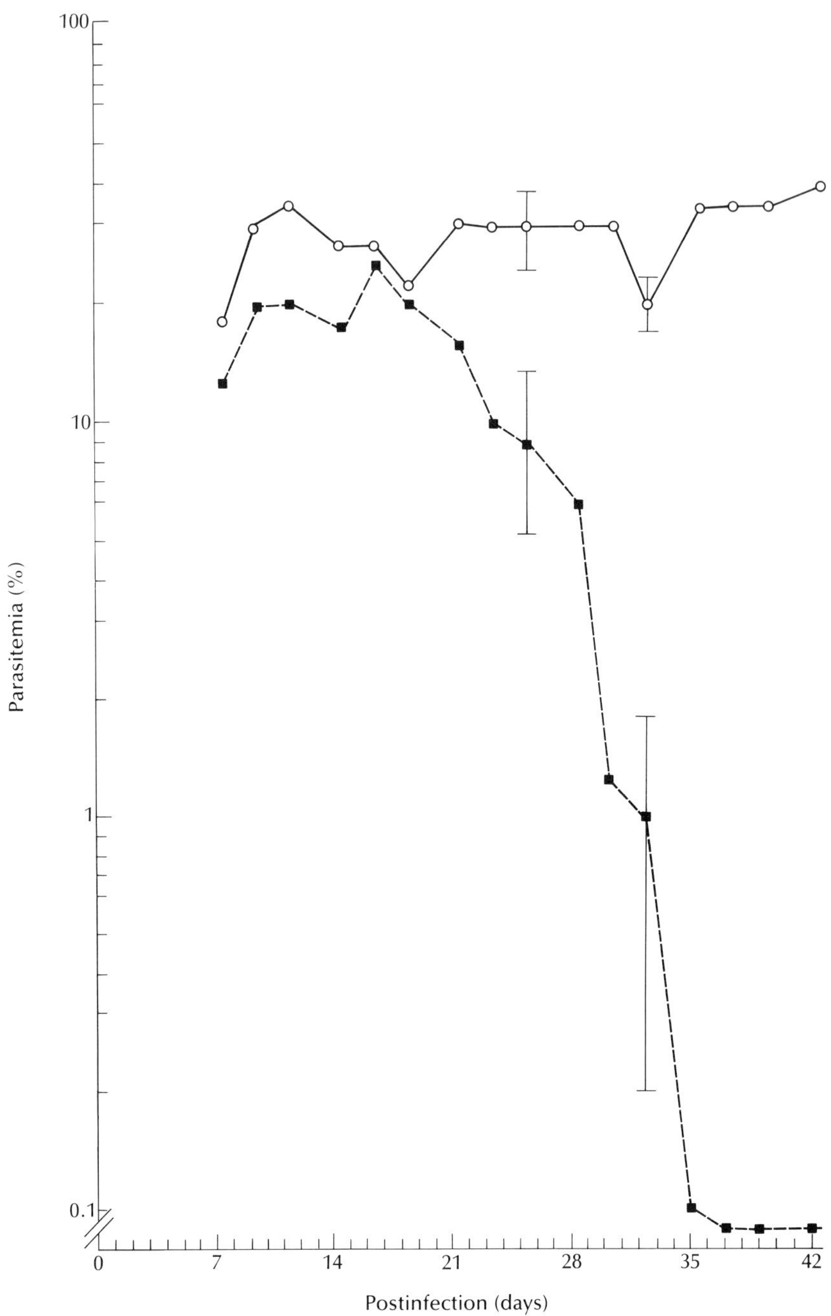

Fig. 79.3. Adoptive transfer of a protective T cell clone into athymic nude mice infected with *P. chabaudi adami*. Recipient *nu/nu* mice received cloned T cells intravenously, control *nu/nu* mice received no cells. From Weidanz and Long (1988).

Antimalaria antibody levels to asexual parasites (indirect immunofluorescence assay (IFA), enzyme-linked immunosorbent assay (ELISA)) of IgM, IgG and IgG-2 isotypes usually rise in parallel with age and acquisition of clinical immunity while IgG-1, IgG-3 and IgG-4 show a more complex pattern (McGregor 1974; Cornille-Brögger *et al.* 1978; Wahlgren *et al.* 1986b). On the average, the expression of different isotypes in individual sera appears to reflect a sequential downstream (5′ to 3′) activation of the corresponding Igh-C genes in *P. falciparum*-specific B cell clones (Wahlgren *et al.* 1986c).

Several parasite molecules involved in the formation of protective immunity have been identified during the last ten years (see below). T cell

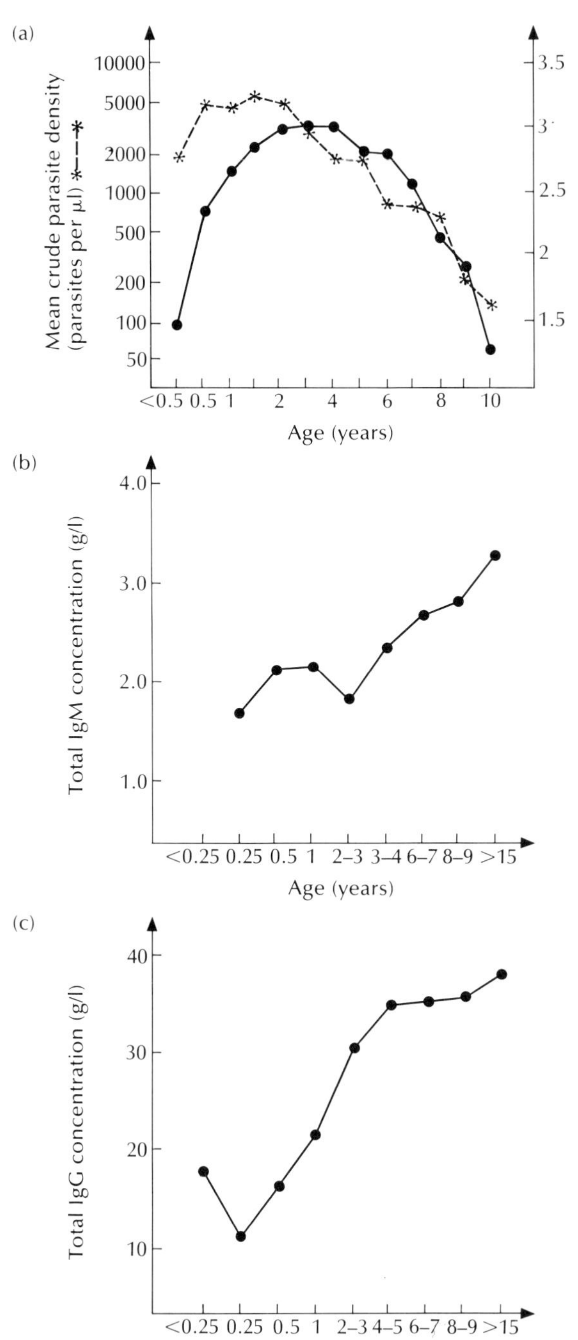

Fig. 79.4. (a) Mean parasite density (–*–*–) and mean spleen size (–●–●–) in relation to age in a highly endemic area of Liberia. (b) and (c) Mean concentrations of total IgM (a) and IgG (b) in relation to age in residents in a highly endemic area of Liberia. Modified from Björkman (1985).

proliferative responses and antibody levels to these antigens have been measured in populations living in endemic areas. Thus, when sera were assayed for antibodies to a restricted number of parasite antigens (mainly the non-polymorphic antigen Pf155/RESA, ring- infected erythrocyte surface antigen) (Perlmann *et al*. 1984) in the membrane of infected erythrocytes, the frequency of positive sera as well as the antibody titres rose in parallel with age, development of clinical immunity and exposure (Wahlgren *et al*. 1986b; Deloron *et al*. 1987; Nguyen-Dinh *et al*. 1987; Högh *et al*. 1991). Adults living under identical conditions of high perennial transmission show either a strong or a weak antibody response to Pf155/RESA and the antibody response (or lack of it) is remarkably stable over several years, suggesting that the differences between individuals are of genetic origin (Björkman *et al*. 1990; Petersen *et al*. 1990). In areas where transmission is seasonal, antibody titres to Pf155/RESA decrease during the dry seasons (Perlmann *et al*. 1989). The T cell proliferative capacity, as measured by ^{3}H-thymidine incorporation and IFN-γ production, does not show any such seasonal variation (Troye-Blomberg *et al*. 1989).

S antigens are another group of asexual but highly polymorphic blood-stage antigens (see below) to which the antibody titres increase with age and level of immunity (Wilson *et al*. 1969; Forsyth *et al*. 1988). However, the IgG response to a cloned S antigen (FC27) in a Papua New Guinean population clearly varied over a period of two years, apparently reflecting a variation in exposure to this serotype. Thus, elimination of a serotype from a parasite population in a community could presumably be the result of serotype-specific immunity (Forsyth *et al*. 1988). The antibody levels to the major protein on sporozoites (CS protein) increase with age when tested with human sera from a rural area of Tanzania and from other malaria endemic areas. Antibodies which can inhibit sporozoite invasion *in vitro* of hepatocytes similarly increase with age (Del Giudice *et al*. 1988a; Hollingdale 1988).

Malarial antigens and humoral immune responses

General

With the complex life cycle of the malaria parasite it presents a large number of antigens to the immune system of the host. Although certain antigenic epitopes or antigens are shared between sporozoites, exoerythrocytic (liver) stages, asexual

Table 79.1. Antoantibodies in malaria-infected subjects

Anti-erythrocyte (haemagglutinin)	Kano *et al.* 1968
Anti-erythrocyte	Rosenberg *et al.* 1973
Anti-erythrocyte	Wahlgren *et al.* 1983
Anti-cytoskeletal	Mortazavi-Milani *et al.* 1984
Anti-erythrocyte (spectrin, 4.1)	Berzins *et al.* 1983
Anti-tubulin	Howard *et al.* 1987
Anti-smooth muscle	Boonpucknavig and Ekapanyakul 1984
Anti-mitochondria	Boonpucknavig and Ekapanyakul 1984
Anti-T	Zouali *et al.* 1982
Anti-ribonucleoprotein	Zouali *et al.* 1986
Anti-lymphocyte	de Souza and Playfair, 1983
Anti-immunoglobulin	Greenwood *et al.* 1971
Anti-single-stranded DNA	Adu *et al.* 1982
Anti-nuclear	Daniel Ribeiro *et al.* 1984

blood stages and gametocytes (Bianco *et al.* 1988; Szarfman *et al.* 1988), the antigens involved in parasite-neutralizing immune responses are essentially stage-specific. In attempts to identify antigens involved in protective immunity, the genes of a large number of *P. falciparum* antigens have been cloned and sequenced. A common feature of many genes coding for *P. falciparum* proteins, either transported into an intracellular organelle or exported outside the parasitophorous vacuole, is a 5′ miniexon possessing a region coding for sequences with relatively high basic amino acid content terminated by a hydrophobic core segment (Fig. 79.5; Kemp *et al.* 1987). This is thought to represent signal sequences, the presence of which in the final protein is not known.

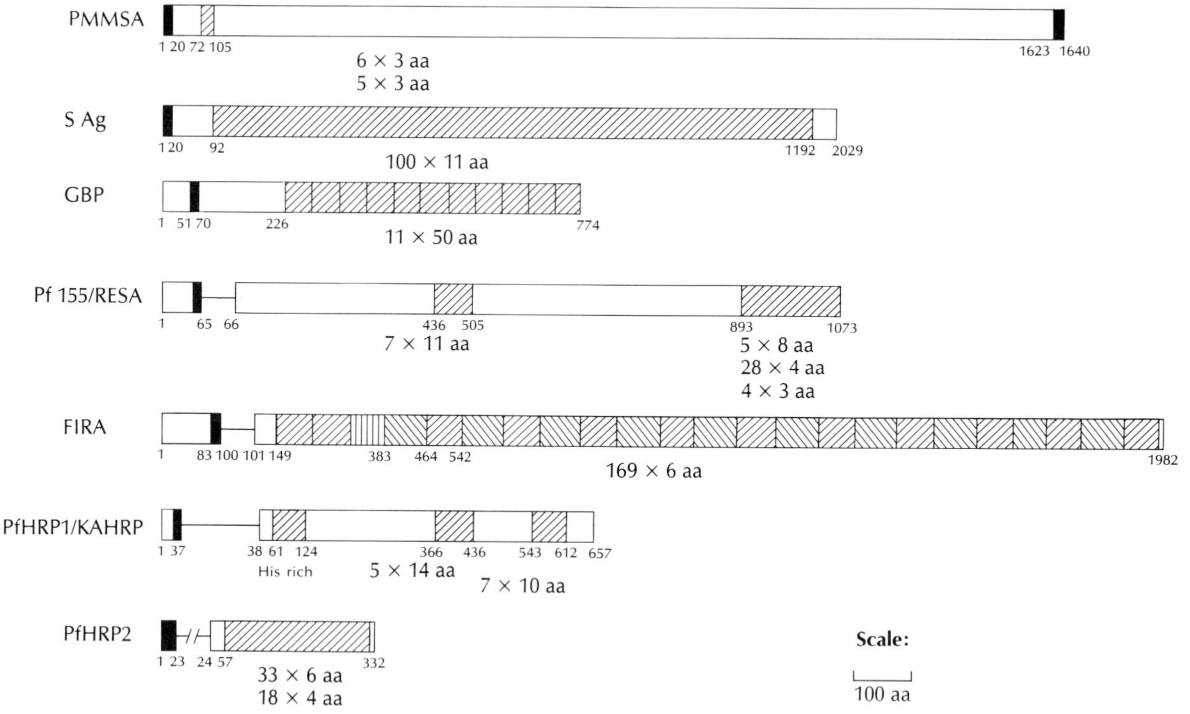

Fig. 79.5. Structure of genes for blood-stage antigens. The boxed regions represent exons and the lines represent introns. Filled segments represent hydrophobic segments of signal sequences and, for the PMMSA, a C-terminal anchor segment. Hatched areas represent repetitive regions, and the number and size (aa) of repeats is shown below each molecule. The numbers represent amino acid positions. Modified from Kemp *et al.* (1987).

The deduced amino acid sequences of the gene products have revealed other peculiar characteristics among the malarial antigens (Kemp *et al.* 1987; Anders *et al.* 1988).

Firstly, many of the antigens contain regions of tandemly repeated short amino acid sequences, which are often also immunodominant (Anders *et al.* 1988). Figure 79.5 gives some examples of how the repeat regions may appear in different *P. falciparum* antigens (see also Figs 79.6, 79.7 and 79.8 below). While the repeat region constitutes only a small part of some antigens, it covers the major part of the sequence of other antigens. Two or several repeat regions with related sequences appear within certain antigens. In some antigens the repeat sequence varies between different strains of the parasite, causing antigenic polymorphism. Different degrees of degeneration in the repeat sequences may occur but in some antigens the repeats are relatively conserved. In these latter antigens (e.g. CS protein and Pf155/RESA (see below)), the conserved repeats suggest a considerable selective pressure for sequences of vital importance for the parasite. Several *P. falciparum* antigens, encoded by distinct genes, have repeat regions containing closely related antigenic determinants, causing extensive antigenic cross-reactions (Anders 1986; Mattei *et al.* 1989; Udomsangpetch *et al.* 1989b). This might reflect a mechanism whereby the parasite evades the immune attack by the host either by absorption of antibodies on antigens non-essential for the survival of the parasite or by induction of antibodies of low affinity which are inefficient in parasite neutralization (Anders 1986).

Secondly, the sequence of several antigens is dominated by one or two amino acids. Thus, the asexual blood stages of *P. falciparum* contain a group of histidine-rich antigens (Howard 1988) and a group of asparagine-rich antigens (Wahlgren *et al.* 1986a) as well as antigens rich in glutamic acid (Triglia *et al.* 1988), serine (Bzik *et al.* 1988) or alanine (Stahl *et al.* 1985) residues. The genetic and functional basis and the immunological implications of these structural properties are not known.

Pre-erythrocytic stages

Although the sporozoites introduced into the bloodstream by a mosquito bite are relatively few and are exposed to the immune system for only a short period of time, they may evoke a stage-specific immune response. A large proportion of adult individuals living in areas of endemic malaria develop antibodies against the sporozoites, as detected by immunofluorescence or CS precipitation (Nardin *et al.* 1979; Tapchaisri *et al.* 1983; Druilhe *et al.* 1986), and longitudinal studies showed that the levels of anti-sporozoite antibodies persisted over several years in the absence of reinfection (Druilhe *et al.* 1986). However, children from the corresponding areas were either negative or showed low reactivity in these assays, indicating a slow build-up of the anti-sporozoite antibody levels. Recent prospective studies revealed that the serum levels of anti-sporozoite antibodies appear not to correlate with protection (Hoffman *et al.* 1987). Nevertheless, it has been known for a long time that immunization of volunteers with sporozoites by bites from irradiated mosquitoes induces a protective immunity against challenge with live sporozoites (Clyde *et al.* 1973; Rieckmann *et al.* 1974). The protection was species-specific in that *P. falciparum* sporozoites protected against *P. falciparum* challenge but not against *P. vivax* challenge and vice versa. The protection was efficient against challenge with various geographical isolates and strains, indicating no antigenic diversity in the crucial epitopes (Clyde *et al.* 1973; McCarthy and Clyde 1977). Furthermore, when individuals immune to sporozoites were challenged with asexual blood-stage parasites, they were fully susceptible to infection, demonstrating the stage specificity of the sporozoite-induced immunity. The mechanism of this protective immunity is not known in detail, but appears to comprise both antibody-mediated and cell-mediated components (see below).

SPOROZOITES

The antibody response to sporozoites is mainly but not exclusively (Hollingdale *et al.* 1990) directed against one single antigen, the CS protein, which covers the entire surface of the sporozoites. Recently a second sporozoite surface antigen, SSP2, was identified in several malarial species (Hedstrom *et al.* 1990). Vaccination experiments in mice with CS protein and SSP2 from *P. yoelii* showed that while either antigen by itself only induced partial protection against a *P. yoelii* sporozoite challenge, mice immunized with both antigens were fully protected (Khusmith *et al.* 1991).

The CS proteins of many different malarial species have been identified and all show similar structural and biosynthetic properties (Santoro *et al.* 1983). Thus, all are of molecular weights between 40 and 60 kD (*P. falciparum* 58 kD and *P. vivax* 45 kD) with intracellular precursor proteins of between 5 and 10 kD higher molecular weight. The homology between CS proteins is also reflected by antigenic cross-reactivities between the proteins of some species (Nussenzweig and Nussenzweig 1988).

The basis for the immunological characteristics of CS proteins became evident when their primary structures were deduced from their gene sequences. A schematic representation of the CS protein structure is shown in Fig. 79.6 as exemplified by the *P. falciparum* protein. The proteins are dominated by a large central region of tandemly repeated amino acid sequences comprising up to 50% of the molecule. These repeats differ in length and amino acid sequence between different species of malaria. The *P. falciparum* repeat region is formed by units of the four amino acids Asn–Ala–Asn–Pro (NANP in one letter code) repeated about 40 times. A few repeat units have the variant sequence Asn–Val–Asp–Pro (NVDP). The immunodominant repeat region of the *P. vivax* CS protein is composed of the nonapeptide unit Gly–Asp–Arg–Ala–Asp–Gly–Gln–Pro–Ala (McCutchan *et al.* 1985). Different strains within these species have different numbers of repeats, causing a size polymorphism of the protein. The *P. falciparum* CS protein contains two regions of well-conserved sequences (RI and RII) which show a high degree of homology with regions in the *P. knowlesi* and *P. vivax* CS proteins (McCutchan *et al.* 1985). The RI region seems to be involved in the binding of the sporozoite to hepatocytes, as a synthetic peptide corresponding to the sequence of this region specifically bound to surface proteins of a hepatoma cell line, and antibodies against this peptide inhibited sporozoite invasion into these cells (Aley *et al* 1986). The RII region shows a high degree of sequence homology with human thrombospondin (Kobayashi *et al.* 1986), as well as with properdin and the terminal complement components (Goundis and Reid 1988; Robson *et al.* 1988), and might be involved in the evasion of the parasite from complement-mediated defence mechanisms by the host.

A further characteristic of the CS proteins is the presence of regions rich in charged amino acids, which may contain α-helical structures (Dame *et al.* 1984). One such charged region flanks the repeat region N-terminally and includes the RI region, and similarly the sequences flanking both sides of the RII region are rich in charged amino acids (Fig. 79.6). Sequence variations observed between CS proteins of different *P. falciparum* strains have been mapped within these charged regions of the molecule (de la Cruz *et al.* 1987). Importantly, the few immunodominant T cell epitopes of the *P. falciparum* CS protein appear to be located in these polymorphic regions (see below).

The immunodominant epitopes of the *P. falciparum* CS protein are contained within the NANP repeat region, with a minimal epitope comprising three such tetramers. Both monoclonal and polyclonal antibodies to these epitopes induce the CS precipitation reaction *in vitro* (Nardin *et al.* 1982; Zavala *et al.* 1985), which is thought to indicate antibodies with sporozoite-neutralizing capacity. Such antibodies also inhibit the invasion of sporozoites into hepatoma cells *in vitro* (Zavala

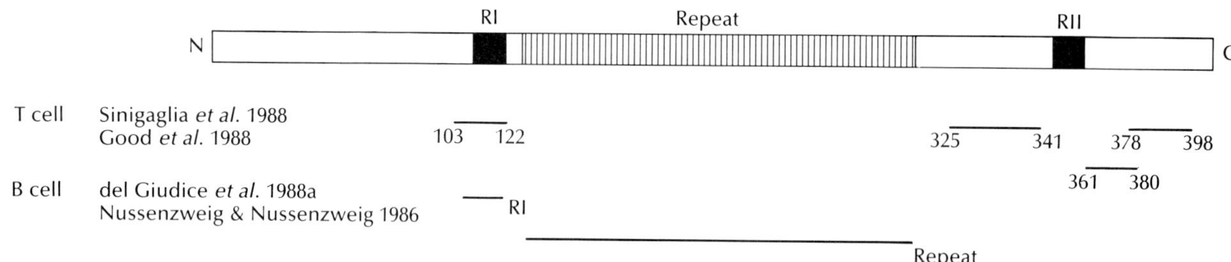

Fig. 79.6. Structure of the gene coding for the *P. falciparum* circumsporozoite protein. Dominant T and B cell reactive sites are indicated. Figures denote amino acid positions in the protein. RI and RII represent regions of conserved sequences. See text for further explanations.

et al. 1985). The synthetic peptide $(NANP)_3$ could block almost all reactivity of human antibodies with sporozoites, indicating that the antibodies recognized mainly linear epitopes in the CS protein repeat region (Nussenzweig and Nussenzweig 1986). Most antibodies elicited by immunization of rabbits or mice with peptides containing NANP repeats also reacted with the native CS protein.

In a recent study the RI region of the *P. falciparum* CS protein was also identified as immunogenic (Del Giudice *et al.* 1988a). Using a synthetic peptide corresponding to the sequence of the RI region, antibodies were detected in human sera from a malaria endemic area. The majority of these sera also contained antibodies to the NANP repetitive epitopes. The significance of the RI antibodies with regard to protective immunity is not known.

LIVER STAGES

When the sporozoite has entered a hepatocyte, it still carries CS protein, and reactivity with anti-CS antibodies is sustained up to 48 hours after invasion (Hollingdale 1988), by which time the parasite has started to acquire antigens reactive with antibodies to asexual blood stages (Szarfman *et al.* 1988). However, liver stage-specific antigens also appear which are immunogenic in natural infections (Druilhe *et al.* 1984). The gene of one liver stage-specific antigen was recently cloned and shown to encode an antigen containing an immunodominant region of tandemly repeated sequences of 17 amino acids (Guerin-Marchand *et al.* 1987; Hollingdale *et al.* 1990). Liver stage-specific antigens on the surface of infected hepatocytes have not as yet been identified and their significance as targets for protective immunity is unclear (Mazier *et al.* 1988).

Asexual blood stages

While the immune response to sporozoites is largely directed towards the CS-protein, the asexual blood stages give rise to a very polyspecific response involving a large number of different antigens during different phases of the erythrocytic cycle. A part of the protective immunity against these stages of *P. falciparum* is mediated by antibodies, as demonstrated in the classical passive transfer experiments by Cohen *et al.* (1961) and McGregor *et al.* (1963) (see below). Similarly, protection against *P. falciparum* challenge was obtained in *Aotus* monkeys by passive transfer of human IgG from immune individuals (Diggs *et al.* 1972). The mechanism of this protection and the specificity of the antibodies active in this context is unknown. Among the antigens believed to be relevant for protective immunity, two main categories have been studied most extensively: firstly, merozoite antigens including antigens present on the merozoite surface and, secondly, antigens expressed on the surface of infected erythrocytes.

MEROZOITE SURFACE ANTIGENS

The invasion of merozoites into erythrocytes is a multi-step process involving binding of the merozoite to the erythrocyte surface, reorientation of the apical end of the merozoite, containing the rhoptry organelles, towards the erythrocyte and, finally, entrance into the erythrocyte by invagination of the erythrocyte membrane. The molecular events in this invasion process are unknown but it is thought that material expelled from the rhoptries initiates the invagination and provides the material needed for the parasitophorous vacuole membrane.

Antibodies to merozoite surface antigens may mediate obstruction of the erythrocytic life cycle of the parasite, either by killing the merozoites or by blocking merozoite invasion into erythrocytes. Five or six major and several minor polypeptides have been localized to the merozoite surface and four of these are derived from one precursor protein, PMMSA (precursor to major merozoite surface antigens) or Pf195 (Heidrich 1988). The PMMSA, which is the major schizont glycoprotein, varies in size between different strains of *P. falciparum* (180–200 kD) and may in its intact form interact with human erythrocytes in a sialic acid-dependent binding (Perkins and Rocco 1988). In association with schizont rupture and merozoite release, the PMMSA is fragmented into smaller, defined, merozoite surface polypeptides (Holder 1988). A single 19 kD fragment remains on the parasite during erythrocyte invasion and is the target of invasion inhibiting antibodies (Blackman *et al.* 1990). The gene of the PMMSA of several *P. falciparum* strains has been cloned and sequenced and found to consist of strain-variable

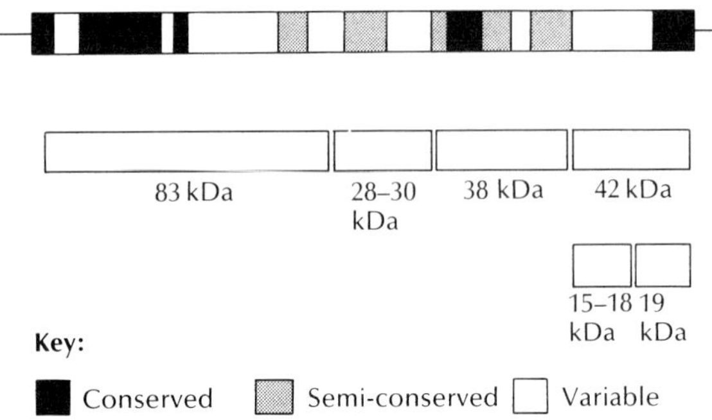

Fig. 79.7. Location of regions of structural diversity in the *P. falciparum* PMMSA antigen based on comparison between sequences of the antigen from four different parasite strains. The location in the protein sequence of the merozoite-associated processing fragments of PMMSA is indicated. From Holder (1988).

sequences separated by conserved or semiconserved sequences (Tanabe *et al.* 1987; Holder 1988) (Fig. 79.7). Variation in sequences occur both within a region of tandemly repeated tetrapeptide sequences and in regions with no repeats. The polymorphism of PMMSA falls into two distinct types, suggesting that the antigen is encoded by dimorphic alleles (Tanabe *et al.* 1987).

Antibodies to PMMSA have been demonstrated in individuals living in areas where malaria is highly endemic (Schmidt-Ullrich *et al.* 1986; Holder 1988) but no apparent correlation was seen with clinical immunity (Wahlgren *et al.* 1986b). The potential role of PMMSA in protective immunity is, however, indicated by vaccination experiments in a mouse model system as well as by the capacity of antibodies to PMMSA to inhibit merozoite reinvasion *in vitro* (Holder 1988; Long 1988). Consequently, intact PMMSA or polypeptides containing sequences from different regions of PMMSA have been used in vaccination trials in monkeys and shown to provide partial protection to *P. falciparum* challenge (Perrin *et al.* 1984; Cheung *et al.* 1986; Patarroyo *et al.* 1987; Holder *et al.* 1988). Siddiqui *et al.* (1987) obtained complete protection of *Aotus* monkeys against challenge with the homologous *P. falciparum* strain by immunization with a purified PMMSA preparation (see also Fig. 79.17), and serum from these monkeys was shown to inhibit *in vitro* growth of the same parasite strain (Hui and Siddiqui 1987). Sequences from conserved regions of PMMSA were also included in the first trial in humans with a subunit with a blood-stage vaccine (Patarroyo *et al.* 1988).

Several merozoite surface antigens not related to PMMSA have been described and include the acidic–basic repeat antigen (ABRA) with an M_r of ~100 kD (Stahl *et al.* 1986; Weber *et al.* 1988) and merozoite surface antigen 2 (MSA-2), a structurally and antigenically diverse glycoprotein with an M_r of 46–53 kD (Smythe *et al.* 1988, 1990; Clark *et al.* 1989). Assays of antibody responses to the latter antigen among individuals in Papua New Guinea showed that the great majority had such antibodies and there was an age-dependent increase both in their prevalence and titres (R.F. Anders unpublished data). Furthermore, monoclonal antibodies to this antigen inhibited merozoite invasion in a strain-restricted manner (Clark *et al.* 1989).

INTRACELLULAR MEROZOITE ANTIGENS

A large number of antigens have been localized by means of immunofluorescence or immunoelectron microscopy to the rhoptries or micronemes in the apical complex of *P. falciparum* merozoites. These include among others an 82/41 kD protein complex (Bushell *et al.* 1988), a 140/130/105 kD protein complex (Cooper *et al.* 1988) and a 110 kD protein (Sam-Yellowe *et al.* 1988), as well as a 155 kD antigen (Brown *et al.* 1985; Uni *et al.* 1987). The latter antigen was, however, with improved analysis recently localized to dense granules, another type of organelle in the apical part of the merozoites (Aikawa *et al.* 1990). The presumed role of the rhoptry material in the merozoite invasion process makes these antigens possible targets for protective antibodies. In accordance with this, monoclonal antibodies to some of the rhoptry antigens have been shown to inhibit merozoite invasion *in vitro* (Perrin *et al.* 1981; Cooper *et al.* 1988). Although the dense granules release their contents into the parasitophorous vacuole space only after merozoite entry (Torii *et al.* 1989), antibodies to the 155 kD antigen are also efficient inhibitors of merozoite invasion (Berzins *et al.* 1986; Ruangjirachuporn *et al.* 1988; Perlmann *et al.* 1989).

Immunization of monkeys with an affinity-purified preparation of the 41 kD antigen induced a marked degree of protection against challenge with *P. falciparum* parasites (Perrin *et al.* 1988). The

Table 79.2. Some characteristics of *Plasmodium falciparum* antigens associated with the infected erythrocyte membrane

Antigen	Molecular weight	Surface exposure	Cytoskeletal association	Repeats	Possible function
PfEMP2/MESA	250–280	–	4.1	+	?
PfEMP1	~300	+	?	?	Binding to endothelial cells?
Ag332	>500	+	?	Extensive	Binding to endothelial cells?
Pf155/RESA	155	–	+	+	Merozoite invasion?
Pf110	110	–	+	?	Merozoite invasion?
HRP1/KAHRP	80–120	–	+	+	Knob formation
HRP2	65–85	Secreted	–	+	?
Transferrin R	93; 102	+	?	?	Transferrin binding

gene for this antigen has recently been cloned and sequenced, revealing that the antigen is highly conserved in several different parasite isolates and does not contain any tandemly repeated sequences (Certa *et al.* 1988). The antigen displayed a high degree of homology with the glycolytic enzyme aldolase from vertebrates and also exhibited this enzymatic activity. Establishment of the degree of antigenic cross-reactivity between the parasite and human enzymes will determine the suitability of this antigen as a vaccine component.

The 155 kD protein present in dense granules, designated Pf155/RESA, is, like PMMSA, one of the most studied asexual blood-stage antigens. The antigen is deposited in the erythrocyte membrane during or shortly after merozoite invasion and may be detected in this location in erythrocytes containing early stages (rings and early trophozoites) of the parasite, using a modified indirect immunofluorescence assay involving a fixation step as well as air-drying (Perlmann *et al.* 1984). The protein Pf155/RESA is not exposed on the outside of the infected erythrocyte membrane (Perlmann *et al.* 1984) but seems to be associated with the erythrocyte cytoskeleton intracellularly (Brown *et al.* 1985) (Table 79.2). A similar location in infected erythrocytes was reported for the M_r 110 kD rhoptry antigen (Sam-Yellowe *et al.* 1988). A *P. chabaudi* antigen of M_r 105 kD sharing a number of physical and immunological characteristics with Pf155/RESA has similarly been identified in the membrane of infected erythrocytes (Gabriel *et al.* 1986). Molecules similar to Pf155/RESA have also been described in erythrocytes infected with *P. fragile* (Nguyen-Dinh *et al.* 1988) and *P. yoelii* (Murakami and Tanabe 1985).

The complete gene and protein sequences of Pf155/RESA are known (Favaloro *et al.* 1986). The antigen contains two regions of tandemly repeated amino acid sequences, one in the carboxy terminus (3′ repeat region) and one in the middle of the antigen (5′ repeat region) (Fig. 79.8). These regions are immunodominant and no strain- or isolate-associated antigenic diversity was detected in the antigen (Perlmann *et al.* 1987). However, the number of C-terminal repeats may vary in different isolates and a short sequence adjacent (upstream) of this region has been found to be dimorphic,

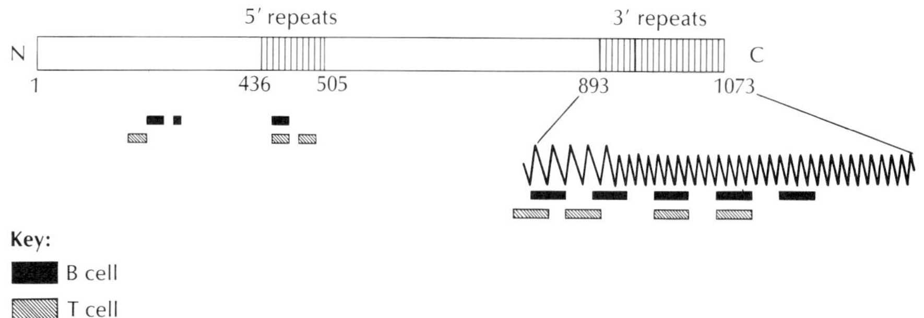

Fig. 79.8. Schematic representation of the location of some important B cell and T cell epitopes in Pf155/RESA. B cell epitopes: Anders (1986); Berzins *et al.* (1986); Perlmann *et al.* (1986); Anders *et al.* (1988). T cell epitopes: Kabilan *et al.* (1988); Rzepczyk *et al.* (1988); Troye-Blomberg *et al.* (1988, 1989).

indicating that the Pf155/RESA gene exists in at least two allelic forms (Åslund 1990). Furthermore, a variant of the *P. falciparum* strain FCR3 was described which lacks Pf155/RESA (Cappai *et al.* 1989).

Antibodies to Pf155/RESA are found at elevated levels in sera from immune individuals and from patients with repeated *P. falciparum* infections but at low incidence in patients with primary infections. Cross-sectional studies of African children living in highly endemic areas with perennial transmission suggested that the appearance of antibodies to Pf155/RESA is correlated with the acquisition of clinical immunity (Wahlgren *et al.* 1986b). A significant fraction of these antibodies reacts with linear epitopes formed by different amino acid sequences located in the 3′ or 5′ repeat blocks (Perlmann *et al.* 1989) and these anti-repeat antibodies show an unusually high capacity to inhibit merozoite invasion *in vitro* (Berzins *et al.* 1986; Perlmann *et al.* 1986). More direct evidence for Pf155/RESA being involved in protective immunity comes from vaccination trials in *Aotus* monkeys, where immunization with fusion proteins containing the repeat regions of the antigen induced partial protection against *P. falciparum* challenge (Collins *et al.* 1986). However, in recent vaccination trials conducted by the same investigators with Pf155/RESA, little or no protection was obtained, which may be explained by differences in immunization protocols and immunogens used (Collins *et al.* 1991; Pye *et al.* 1991).

ANTIGENS ON THE SURFACE OF INFECTED ERYTHROCYTES

Along with parasite maturation within the erythrocyte, parasite-associated changes occur in the host cell membrane. The presence of several parasite-derived proteins has been demonstrated in the membrane of erythrocytes infected with late-stage parasites (Table 79.2; Hommel and Semoff 1988; see also Howard 1988). In contrast to the above-mentioned rhoptry antigens of 110 and 155 kD, which are deposited in the erythrocyte membrane during merozoite invasion, these antigens are synthesized by the intracellular parasite and are transported through the erythrocyte cytoplasm to the erythrocyte membrane (Table 79.2; Howard 1988).

Using *P. falciparum*-immune squirrel-monkey serum, Hommel *et al.* (1983) demonstrated parasite-specific antigenic determinants on host erythrocytes. These antigens were modulated by the presence or absence of the spleen and by immune pressure. Parasites isolated during secondary and recrudescent peaks expressed erythrocyte-associated surface antigens different from those expressed by parasites isolated during the primary infection. Six variant antigenic types distinct from the original population were identified. This study indicated that *P. falciparum* may use antigenic variation as a means of evading the host immune defence.

By means of an antibody-mediated agglutination assay, Marsh and Howard (1986) demonstrated antigenic diversity of infected erythrocyte surface antigens in Gambian children naturally infected with *P. falciparum*. Serum from 10 children in the convalescent stage of malaria infection reacted with infected cells from the same child but generally not with infected cells from other children. In contrast, sera from adult Gambians often reacted with the surface of infected cells from all of the children, indicating that the surface antigens contain both diverse and conserved epitopes.

A typical feature in *P. falciparum* is the appearance of knob-like protrusions on erythrocytes infected with late-stage parasites. These carry parasite-derived antigenic material (Kilejian 1979) and may also expose modified antigenic host cell epitopes (Winograd and Sherman 1989). Parasite maturation beyond the trophozoite stage is not usually seen in the peripheral blood of patients infected with *P. falciparum*, despite high parasitaemias. This sequestration of the parasites has been suggested to be due to specific adhesion of infected erythrocytes to the walls of capillaries and post-capillary venules (Trager *et al.* 1966). It has been suggested that the knob-like protrusions are sites of interaction with the vascular endothelium (Luse and Miller 1971; Hommel and Semoff 1988). An assay for analysis of the cytoadherence of infected erythrocytes *in vitro* has been developed, using certain melanoma cell lines or endothelial cells (Fig. 79.9(a)) (Udeinya *et al.* 1985). Three parasite-derived proteins have been identified as associated with the knobs: HRP1/KAHRP (histidine-rich protein 1/knob-associated histidine rich protein), PfEMP1 (erythrocyte membrane protein 1) and PfEMP2 (also designated MESA (mature parasite-infected erythrocyte surface antigen)) (Howard 1988). The proteins HRP1

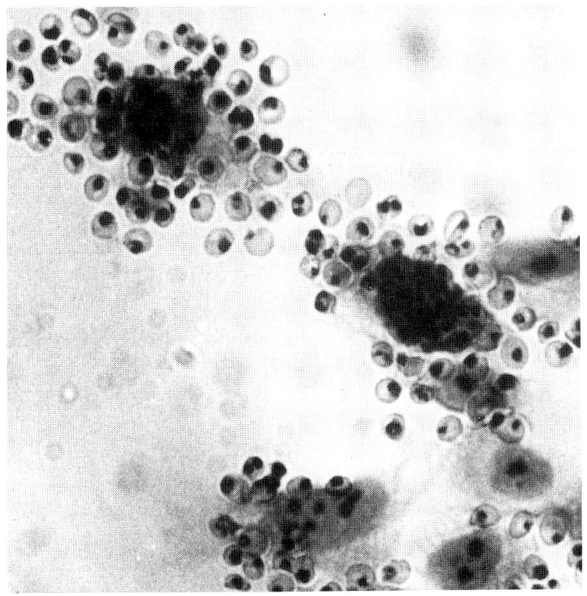

(a)

(b)

Fig. 79.9. (a) Cytoadherence of *P. falciparum*-infected erythrocytes to melanoma cells. Melanoma cells expressing receptors for infected erythrocytes are used as a substitute for endothelial cells due to difficulties in growing the latter cells *in vitro*; see also Udenyia *et al.* 1985 and Udomsangpetch *et al.* (1989a). (b) Erythrocytes infected with asexual *P. falciparum* malaria parasites bind uninfected erythrocytes in spontaneous rosette formation; see also Udomsangpetch *et al.* (1989c) and Wahlgren *et al.* (1989).

and PfEMP2 are located in association with the cytoskeleton on the cytoplasmic phase of the erythrocyte membrane and are thought to constitute the electron-dense material observed underneath the knobs by electron microscopy (Howard 1988). While the presence of HRP1 is believed to be restricted to knob-forming parasites, PfEMP2 is also present in parasites which have lost their knobs after long-term *in vitro* cultivation (Howard 1988). The protein PfEMP1 is a strain-specific and size-polymorphic high-molecular-weight antigen (220–350 kD), which is restricted to knobby parasites and is exposed on the erythrocyte surface at the knobs (Leech *et al.* 1984; Magowan *et al.* 1988). This antigen is implicated as responsible for cytoadherence either directly or by being very closely associated with another as yet unidentified functional molecule (Howard 1988). However, recently the binding of infected erythrocytes to endothelial cells was also found to take place in the absence of knobs (Biggs *et al.* 1989; Udomsangpetch *et al.* 1989a) and the binding of both knobby and knobless cells could be inhibited by a human monoclonal antibody specific for a surface-located antigen, Ag332 (Mattei *et al.* 1989; Udomsangpetch *et al.* 1989a), which might be related to PfEMP1. A significant cross-reaction of this monoclonal with another high-molecular-weight antigen of 260 kD in the erythrocyte membrane, adds this antigen also to the list of possible cytoadherence molecules.

A recently discovered feature of *P. falciparum*-infected erythrocytes is the binding to their surface of uninfected red blood cells, leading to spontaneous rosette formation (Fig. 79.9(b)) (Wahlgren 1986; Handunnetti *et al.* 1989; Udomsangpetch *et al.* 1989c). Spontaneous rosetting is found to a variable extent among both parasites grown *in vitro* for many years and parasites obtained directly from patients. Inhibition experiments with different antibodies indicate that the molecule(s) involved in rosetting are distinct from those involved in cytoadherence (Udomsangpetch *et al.* 1989c). Furthermore, a cloned rosetting parasite failed to bind to endothelial cells and cytoadherent parasites did not rosette, indicating that these are two distinct phenomena involving different molecular mechanisms. Although the rosetting parasites were knobless and the antigen has been claimed to be knob-associated, antibodies to HRP1/KAHRP (Kilejian 1979; Taylor *et al.* 1987) of *P. falciparum* inhibit rosetting but do not interfere with endothelial binding (Carlson *et al.* 1990a). This is of particular interest as anti-HRP1 antibodies have also been found to strongly stain the basement membrane in brain capillaries of cerebral malaria patients (Igarishi *et al.* 1987). As both cytoadherence and rosetting are phenomena apparently associated with parasite sequestration (David *et al.* 1988) in the infected host (*P. falciparum*, *P. chabaudi*, *P. fragile*), it is possible that both phenomena are also involved in the pathology of cerebral malaria.

OTHER ANTIGENS

The S antigens form a family of heat-stable, soluble *P. falciparum* antigens synthesized late in the erythrocytic cycle and then transported into the parasitophorous vacuole. After rupture of the erythrocytes the antigens are found in the plasma or in the culture supernatant *in vitro*. The S antigens exhibit an extensive serological diversity and constitute stable markers for serotyping *P. falciparum* isolates (Wilson 1980). The S antigens are dominated by a central immunodominant region of tandemly repeated amino acid sequences (Fig. 79.5) which differ in length, number and sequence between different parasite isolates and form the basis for their antigenic diversity (Brown *et al.* 1987).

Several *P. falciparum* merozoite-associated antigens with high asparagine content have recently been cloned and characterized: asparagine-rich protein, ARP (Stahl *et al.* 1986), clustered asparagine-rich protein, CARP (Wahlgren *et al.* 1986a) and Ag10b (Franzén *et al.* 1989). The protein CARP shows no apparent antigenic or sequential diversity and probably plays a role in merozoite invasion as monoclonal antibodies inhibit invasion *in vitro* of several different strains of parasites (Wahlgren *et al.* 1986a). Monoclonal antibodies to Ag10b similarly inhibit merozoite invasion but in an isolate-specific manner. Interestingly, yet another monoclonal antibody to Ag10b was found to dose-dependently enhance reinvasion of erythrocytes and also to induce a more rapid maturation of intraerythrocytic parasites in all isolates tested (Franzén *et al.* 1989).

Heat-shock proteins (HSP) are a group of proteins which have awakened great interest in several parasite systems due to their constitutive expression in large amounts and their potential immunological implications (Newport *et al.* 1988). *Plasmodium falciparum* possesses at least five different genes in the HSP-70 family, two of which have been cloned and sequenced. One of the proteins (PfHSP-70-1) contains a region of tandemly repeated tetrapeptide sequences which is probably immunodominant (Bianco *et al.* 1986) while the other protein (PfHSP-70-2) lacks such repeats. Although the malarial HSPs show high homology with mammalian HSPs and PfHSP-70-2 also with mammalian glucose-regulated proteins and immunoglobulin heavy chain-binding proteins (Mattei *et al.* 1988), they are highly immunogenic and could thus give rise to autoimmune responses with possible pathological consequences. Interestingly, the carboxy terminal sequence of PfHSP-70-2 shows a significant resemblance to the putative hepatocyte-binding domain RI of the CS protein (Fig. 79.6) (Peterson *et al.* 1988). Thus, this HSP may either induce antibodies which inhibit sporozoite invasion into hepatocytes, and thereby prevent superinfection of the host, or absorb sporozoite invasion inhibitory antibodies directed against the RI region of the CS protein.

Sexual stages

Parasite-neutralizing immune responses acting on the sexual stages of the malaria parasite do not change the course of the disease in the host but prevent transmission of the parasite through mosquitoes to new hosts. Transmission-blocking immunity may act in the mosquito gut on gametes, preventing fertilization, or on zygotes, preventing the development of fertilized zygotes (Carter *et al.* 1988). While antibodies against antigens present on the surface of gametes are formed during natural infections, antibodies against zygotes may be induced by experimental immunization as the zygote antigens are not present or are poorly expressed in the blood forms (Carter *et al.* 1989).

Studies of transmission blocking immunity involve a membrane feeding device in which infected erythrocytes are mixed with the antibodies to be studied, and then fed to mosquitoes. The mosquitoes are later dissected for counting of the number of oocysts in the midguts and transmission blocking activities are reflected by decreased numbers of infected mosquitoes and decreased numbers of oocysts per gut (Carter *et al.* 1988). Transmission-blocking immunity against *P. vivax* develops in humans already during primary infections and is boosted by subsequent infections (Mendis *et al.* 1987). However, when the concentration of these antibodies is decreased either with time after infection or by dilution, they may instead cause a drastic enhancement of oocyst numbers (Peiris *et al.* 1988). The same shift from inhibition to enhancement may be achieved with certain monoclonal antibodies, indicating that it is strictly concentration-dependent (Peiris *et al.* 1988). The relevance of naturally occurring transmission-blocking immunity in controlling malaria incidence was indicated during recent epidemics of *P. vivax* malaria in Sri Lanka (de Zoysa *et al.* 1988).

Using monoclonal antibodies, putative target antigens for transmission-blocking immunity have been identified on the surface of *P. falciparum* gametes (Meuwissen and Ponnudurai 1988). A complex consisting of a 230 kD protein and a doublet of hydrophobic glycoproteins of 48/45 kD appears on gametes and remains on the zygote surface for a few hours after fertilization. These proteins are then replaced on the zygote and ookinete surface by a lipoglycoprotein of 25 kD. The gene for this latter protein has been cloned and sequenced and shown to contain four tandemly repeated epidermal growth factor (EGF)-like domains (Kaslow *et al.* 1988).

Analysis of the antibody response to these antigens in human sera from Papua New Guinea, where *P. falciparum* transmission is intense, showed that no antibodies were present to the 25 kD zygote surface protein (Carter *et al.* 1989). While antibodies to certain intracellular gamete-specific proteins occurred with high frequency, the antibody response to the gamete surface proteins of 230 and 48/45 kD was variable and independent of the general antibody response to gametes, indicating a genetic restriction, possibly involving the major histocompatibility complex (MHC), in the immune response to the latter proteins. An MHC-restricted antibody response to these proteins was also obtained in different strains of H-2 congenic mice (Good *et al.* 1988b).

Plasmodium falciparum gametocytes contain an antigen which appears to be identical or very similar to the merozoite antigen Pf155/RESA (Masuda *et al.* 1986). Immunoelectron microscopic studies suggest that during gametogenesis the antigen moves from the parasite to the erythrocyte membrane and may have an important function in membrane disruption, resulting in the release of the gametes (Quakyi *et al.* 1989).

Cellular responses in malaria infection

General

Plasmodia induce a large variety of immune responses in the infected host. While some of these are protective, others may be counter-productive, by helping the parasite to evade the immune response, or may be harmful to the host, by giving rise to immunopathological reactions. In this section, we will focus on some of the cellular mechanisms involved in the human antiplasmodial immune responses and, in particular, point to some of the reactions believed to be implicated in protection towards the different life cycle stages of the parasite. However, as the knowledge of human antiplasmodial immunity is incomplete in comparison with that of experimental malaria, we will also refer to some of the animal work rendering valid information about what is going on in human malaria. For a more complete discussion of immune mechanisms in animal malaria, see Jayawardena (1981) and Weidanz and Long (1988).

Relative role of antibodies and T cells

As discussed above, plasmodial infection induces a large variety of parasite-specific antibodies and both the number and levels of antibodies to the different life cycle stages increase significantly upon repeated exposure. As is to be expected, there is no clear-cut correlation between total anti-malaria antibodies and protective immunity in general. Nevertheless, as long as 30 years ago, transfer of immune IgG in the human *P. falciparum* system was shown to have curative effects in Gambian children and to give rise to a certain protection (Cohen *et al.* 1961; McGregor *et al.* 1963) (Fig. 79.10). There is a large body of evidence from different animal systems indicating that antibodies are important for clearance of parasite loads (Deans and Cohen 1983; Weidanz and Long 1988) and this is certainly also true for the human malarias. However, a more solid proof of this requires studies of antibody responses to defined epitopes of well-characterized antigens and such studies have only just begun. Studies of mouse malaria models also indicate that the protective importance of antibodies relative to that of antibody-independent T cell responses varies among different plasmodial species (see above) and this may also have to be

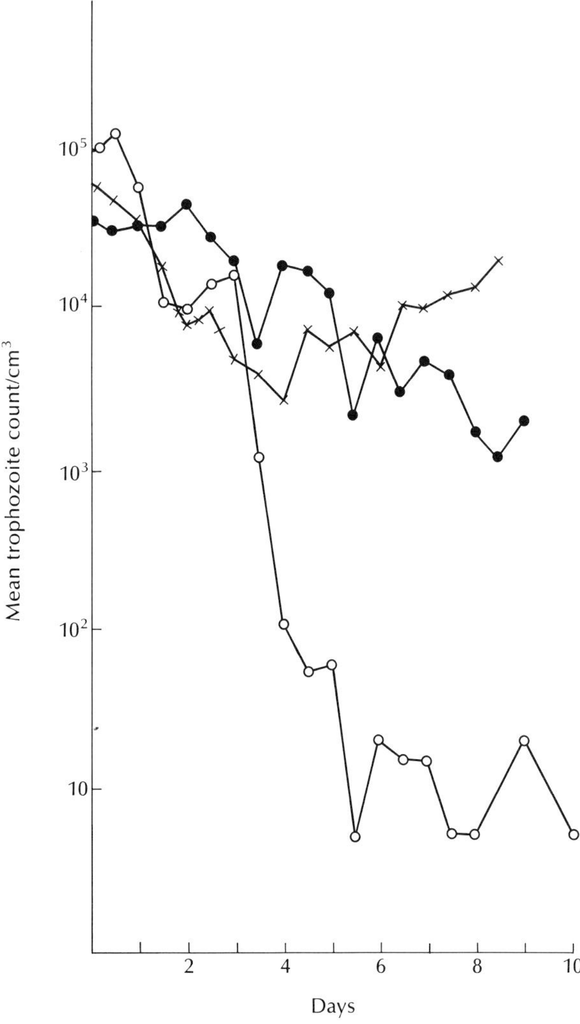

Fig. 79.10. The effect of gammaglobulin injection of children with acute *P. falciparum* malaria. The treated children received either γ-globulin prepared from blood donors in Great Britain or γ-globulin prepared from Gambian adults. Modified from Cohen *et al.* (1961).

taken into account for establishing the relative role of antibodies in the different human malaria systems.

Even in those experimental malaria systems in which the protective importance of antibodies is well established, it was early recognized that maintenance of immunity is under T cell control (Chen *et al.* 1977). In general, protective antimalarial antibodies are of T cell dependent isotypes and their production requires an intact and functioning T cell system (Troye-Blomberg and Perlmann 1988; Weidanz and Long 1988). Furthermore, T cells also control the antibody-independent effector systems involved in antiplasmodial immunity, systems including non-lymphoid effector cells and probably T effector cells as well. Therefore, the key role of the T cell system in acquired malaria immunity will be the focus of the following discussion.

Deficiencies in immune regulation and immunosuppression

As in other infectious diseases, a large number of irregular immune responses are a hallmark of acute plasmodial infection. One of the characteristics of *P. falciparum* infection is B cell hyper-reactivity, resulting in hypergammaglobulinaemia (Cohen *et al.* 1961) and multiple autoantibody production (see Table 79.1 above; Marsh and Greenwood 1986). B cell hyper-reactivity in *P. falciparum* malaria may be associated with depressed specific responses to antigens such as tetanus toxoid, *Salmonella typhi* or meningococcal vaccine (Greenwood 1984).

B cell hyper-reactivity is believed to reflect polyclonal B cell activation by non-specific 'mitogens' acting as polyclonal B or T cell activators (Greenwood 1974; Rosenberg 1978). However, it should be recalled that an overload of specific antigens also induces T-cell-dependent polyclonal B cell activation (Kabilan *et al.* 1987). A good illustration of deficiencies in T-cell-dependent B cell control in malaria is the failure of T cells from acutely *P. falciparum*-infected individuals to prevent the abnormal proliferation of Epstein–Barr virus (EBV)-infected B cells, a phenomenon which has been implicated in the association of malaria with Burkitt's lymphoma in certain areas of Africa (Whittle *et al.* 1984).

Taken together, available data suggest that most of the irregularities observed at the B cell level in acute malaria infection reflect deficiencies in T cell control. Studies both of T cell reactivities in *in vivo* experimental malaria systems (Jayawardena 1981; Weidanz and Long 1988) and of human lymphocytes *in vitro* fully support this view. Thus, numerous studies have reported on alterations in both size and composition of the pool of T cells found in the circulation in acute malaria infection, including a decrease in the ratio of CD4+ve/CD8+ve cells and a significant rise of T-cells bearing the γ/δ-receptor (Ho *et al.* 1990). It has also been claimed that the frequently observed decrease in the number of circulating T cells reflects the effect of T-cell-specific autoantibodies. However, redistribution of cells to the spleen or elsewhere (Kumararatne *et al.* 1987) may be a more likely explanation and the clinical significance of the changes found in the blood is uncertain (Troye-Blomberg and Perlmann 1988). In any event, there is convincing evidence that the proliferative response of T cells to certain antigens as well as mitogens is severely suppressed in patients with acute infection. When T cells from acute patients are exposed to crude or partially purified plasmodial antigen *in vitro*, they do not respond with either proliferation or IFN-γ release although the same preparations may induce strong responses in T cells from immune donors or from convalescent patients (Troye-Blomberg *et al.* 1984, 1987; Riley *et al.* 1988a, b) (Fig. 79.11). However, some defined *P. falciparum* antigens induce normal responses also in T cells from acutely ill patients (Bygbjerg *et al.* 1985; Troye-Blomberg *et al.* 1987), suggesting that the suppression induced by crude preparations is antigen-specific.

The mechanisms of malaria-induced suppression in acutely ill patients are poorly understood. They have been shown to involve deficiencies in both IL-2 production and expression of cell-bound IL-2 receptors, accompanied by elevated levels of soluble IL-2 receptors in acute sera. The defect could not be abolished by addition of either IL-1 or IL-2 and was not due to suppressor cells of monocyte/macrophage type (Troye-Blomberg *et al.* 1987; Ho *et al.* 1988). Similar observations have also been made in murine malaria models (Lelchuk *et al.* 1984; Lelchuk and Playfair 1985). However, the factors responsible for the down-regulation described in these examples remain to be established. Moreover, there are good reasons to believe that immunosuppression in acute malaria infection is multifactorial, including both antigen-specific and non-specific mechanisms and the generation of suppressor cells (Russo and Weidanz 1988; Weidanz and Long 1988). As

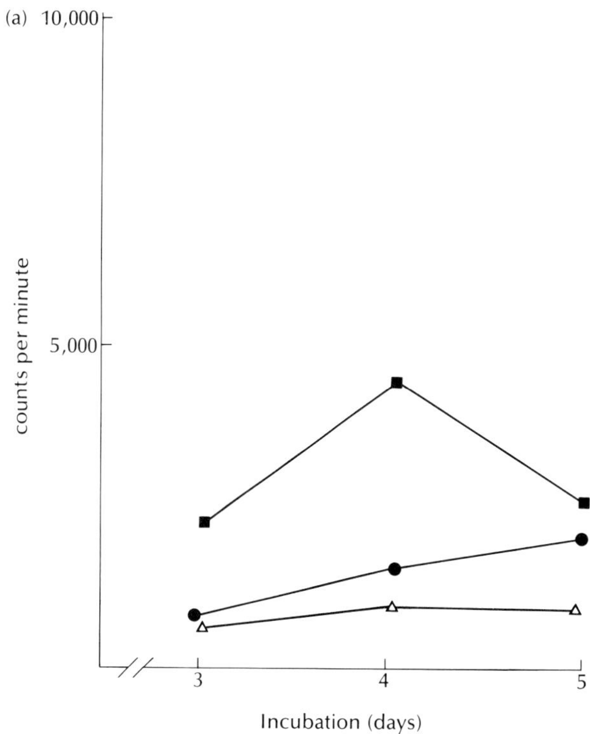

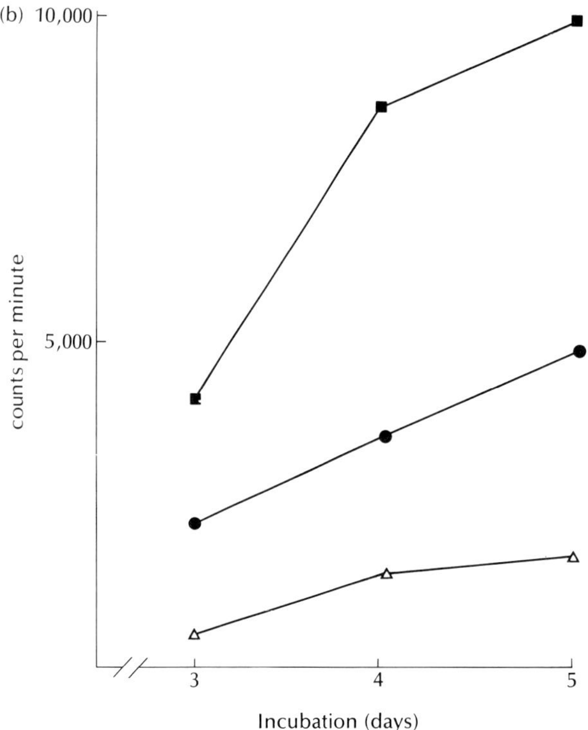

Fig. 79.11. ^{3}H-thymidine incorporation in T cells of an acutely infected *P. falciparum* patient (a) and a clinically immune donor (b). The lymphocytes were stimulated with aliquots of the same preparation of either *P. falciparum* or RBC ghost antigen. From Troye-Blomberg and Perlmann (1988).

immunosuppression is assumed to be partly responsible for the slow development of protective immunity in malaria, further elucidation of these mechanisms is highly desirable.

T cell activation and epitope mapping

Exploration of T cell responses in humans rests on *in vitro* experimentation, mostly performed with lymphocytes from the peripheral blood. In spite of their obvious limitations, these procedures are now providing important information on the activity and function of the human T cell system in the acquisition of antiplasmodial immunity.

Exposure of human T cells from immune donors to crude malarial antigen results in proliferation and lymphokine release. Although the use of poorly defined antigens has sometimes made it difficult to distinguish antigen-specific from polyclonal responses, the existence of specific responses and their changes in different phases of the disease is well established (Troye-Blomberg and Perlmann 1988). As with humoral immunity, the development of methods for continuous culturing of *P. falciparum* (Trager and Jensen 1976) and, in particular, the cloning and large-scale production of defined plasmodial antigens have also led to rapid advances in the field of cellular immunity. An important contributing factor — a cellular corollary to the monoclonal antibodies — has been the access to plasmodia-specific T cell lines and clones which permit studies of fine specificity, MHC restriction and possible function of various T cell epitopes. T cell clones specific for antigens from either asexual blood stages, gametes or the CS protein from sporozoites of *P. falciparum* have been described (Sinigaglia and Pink 1985; Chizzolini and Perrin 1986; Good *et al.* 1987a,b; Guttinger *et al.* 1988; Sinigaglia *et al.* 1988a). Such clones were generated by stimulation of lymphocytes with either intact antigens or synthetic peptides and were obtained both from donors primed to *P. falciparum* through natural infection and from donors with no previous malaria experience. This latter alternative is of practical importance for delineating T-cell-activating sequences in individual antigens but does not automatically tell whether or not the corresponding epitope is also involved in immune responses induced by natural infection or vaccination. The majority of T cell clones investigated thus far are of helper/inducer (CD4 +ve) phenotype and their response to antigen stimulation has been shown to be restricted by Class II MHC restriction elements.

Both T cell clones and unselected T cell populations from *P. falciparum*-primed donors have been utilized to map various plasmodial antigens for T-cell-activating epitopes, using fusion proteins or synthetic peptides as stimulants presented by autologous or MHC-matched antigen-presenting cells. Investigation of two of the major vaccine candidate antigens from the asexual blood stages, PMMSA/Pf195 and Pf155/RESA (see above), has led to the delineation of immunodominant T cell epitopes in each of these. For PMMSA, T-cell-activating sites have been localized to a non-polymorphic stretch in the amino terminal region, which also contains B cell epitopes. Some PMMSA-specific clones raised from donors not previously exposed to the parasite also responded to infected erythrocytes, suggesting that the corresponding epitope should also be immunogenic in natural infection (Crisanti *et al.* 1988; Sinigaglia *et al.* 1988c). The antigen Pf155/RESA has been mapped for T cell epitopes by stimulating lymphocytes from immune African donors with synthetic peptides (Table 79.3). The strongest and most frequent responses (≈40%) were obtained with peptides corresponding to conserved sequences in the two amino acid repeat regions of the molecule (Fig. 79.8 and see above), indicating that they represented T cell epitopes which were immunodominant in nature. Thus far, two epitopes, of different sequences and probably restricted by different Class II MHC elements, have been defined (Kabilan *et al.* 1988; Rzepczyk *et al.* 1988; Troye-Blomberg *et al.* 1989). A Class II MHC restriction to Ia^k and Ia^d was also found when either peptides corresponding to the repeat sequences of Pf155/RESA or the entire polypeptide expressed in vaccinia virus were used to immunize congenic mice (Lew *et al.* 1989).

More extensive studies have been performed with the *P. falciparum* CS protein, which has been mapped in its entire length (see above). Immunization of congenic mice indicated that this protein contains very few immunodominant T cell epitopes, restricted by different H-2 Class II MHC elements (Del Giudice *et al.* 1986; Good *et al.* 1986; Togna *et al.* 1986; Dontfraid *et al.* 1988). While one of these sites was localized in the central amino acid repeat region, which also contains its im-

Table 79.3. T cell proliferation or interferon gamma secretion of T cells when incubated with synthetic peptides[a]

Sequence of peptide[b]	Proliferation (% responders)	Interferon-γ (% responders)
N-terminal sequences		
EKVDNLGRSGGDIIK (176–190)	10	17
Repeats		
TVAEEHVEEPTVAEE (484–498)	40	23
C-terminal sequences		
LKKLSSIMERYAGGK (834–848)	16	8
IVGYIMHGISTINTEMK (862–878)	29	29
Repeats		
EENVEHDAEENVEENV (925–940)	39	35
EENVEENVEENVEENV (944–959)	28	16
YDEENVEEHDEEYDE (1059–1073)	41	31

Source: modified from Troye-Blomberg *et al.* (1989).
a The cells, obtained from malaria-infected donors, were incubated with synthetic peptides corresponding to short sequences of Pf155/RESA.
b Residue number, according to Favaloro *et al.* (1986), in parentheses.

munodominant B cell epitopes, a few T helper cell-activating sites were found outside the repeat region. The most prominent of these sites, located ~40 amino acids downstream, does not appear to be B cell reactive and has been shown to contain two T cell epitopes, each under different Class II MHC restriction. Moreover, this region, which is polymorphic and thus different in different *P. falciparum* strains (de la Cruz *et al.* 1987, 1988), also contains at least one Class I MHC-restricted T cell epitope seen by CS protein-specific cytotoxic T cells (CD8 +ve) (Good *et al.* 1988a, b). *In vitro* stimulation of T cells from either malaria-primed or naïve donors indicated that the polymorphic CS protein regions containing T cell epitopes reactive with murine lymphocytes were also the immunodominant T-cell-reactive regions in the human system (Good *et al.* 1988c; Sinigaglia *et al.* 1988a). The fact that the CS protein and probably also other plasmodial antigens (Good *et al.* 1988b) have a limited number of dominant T cell epitopes and that these are located in polymorphic regions of the molecule (Lockyer *et al.* 1989) explains their poor immunogenicity and raises a number of important issues regarding their usefulness as vaccine immunogens. However, further studies are needed to settle this, particularly since major population differences in T cell responses to the CS protein have been reported (Zevering *et al.* 1990). Moreover, an additional T helper epitope which obviously lacks Class II MHC restriction has recently been identified in a non-polymorphic region close to the C terminus of the *P. falciparum* CS protein (Guttinger *et al.* 1988; Sinigaglia *et al.* 1988b).

Mechanisms involved in parasite control by the immune system

Proliferation of T lymphocytes *in vitro* provides important information as to the immunogenicity of a foreign antigen. It also reflects the degree of priming and the existence of immunological memory in individuals previously exposed to the parasite. Important as this may be, it says close to nothing regarding the biological significance of a given response. Although available evidence indicates beyond reasonable doubt that T cells play a pivotal role in acquired malaria immunity, the mechanisms by which they do this are incompletely understood.

Assessment of the biological significance of a cellular response requires performance of functional tests. Thus, the possible helper effect of T cells can easily be studied in T–B co-operation systems *in vitro*. Using such a system in combination with *in vivo* experiments in a mouse malaria model (*P. chabaudi*), Pearson *et al.* (1983) obtained a good correlation between antibodies produced *in vitro* and their capacity to control challenge infection *in vivo*. In a human *P. falciparum* system, it has recently been shown that stimulation of

T cells with Pf155/RESA can induce *in vitro* production of specific IgG antibodies in cells from Pf155/RESA-seropositive donors (Kabilan *et al.* 1987; Troye-Blomberg *et al.* 1987). Since some of the immunodominant T helper cell-activating epitopes are already known (Kabilan *et al.* 1988; Troye-Blomberg *et al.* 1988, 1989), further experiments should make it possible to relate T cell specificity to that of the B cells with which they co-operate. Such experiments should provide a basis for the construction of vaccine immunogens. In many experimental malarias investigated, the importance of CD4 +ve rather than CD8 +ve cells for control of the erythrocytic stages of the parasite is well established (Süss *et al.* 1988; Weidanz and Long 1988; Kumar *et al.* 1989) (Fig. 79.12). However, the phenotypic and functional characterization of the CD4 +ve cells involved require further exploration. This is important since it is likely that the cells amplifying antibody production (i.e. Th2 cells) are not the same as those regulating the antibody-independent immune responses (i.e. Th1 cells). The sequential appearance of such cells (Th1 followed by Th2) during the development of protective immunity has been seen in C57Bl6 mice infected with *P. chabaudi chabaudi* (Langhorne 1989). In the mouse *P. chabaudi adami* system, T cell clones which provide antibody-independent protection upon transfer appear to be of the IL-2/IFN-γ-producing Th1 type (Cavacini *et al.* 1986; Brake *et al.* 1988).

It is assumed that CD4 +ve cells are equally important in the regulation of the human immune response to the blood stages of the parasite. Attempts to define the nature and function of CD4 +ve cells involved in different phases of infection or immunity are only just beginning. Studies of the cellular regulation in human malaria have focused on the appearance of various cytokines either in supernatants of antigen-activated T cells or in the serum of malaria patients. However, as the different cytokines have many different functions and form a closely interacting network but only a few of these factors have been investigated in malaria, knowledge of their role in this infection is scarce. Thus, as mentioned above, IL-2 production appears to be down-regulated (independently of IL-1) in acute disease (Troye-Blomberg *et al.* 1987; Ho *et al.* 1988). Those CD4 +ve T cells that express IL-4 rather than IFN-γ appear to be associated with T-cell-dependent antibody production (Troye-Blomberg *et al.* 1990) but little is known about other lymphokines such as IL-6, which is produced in large amounts during blood-stage infection (Kern *et al.* 1989).

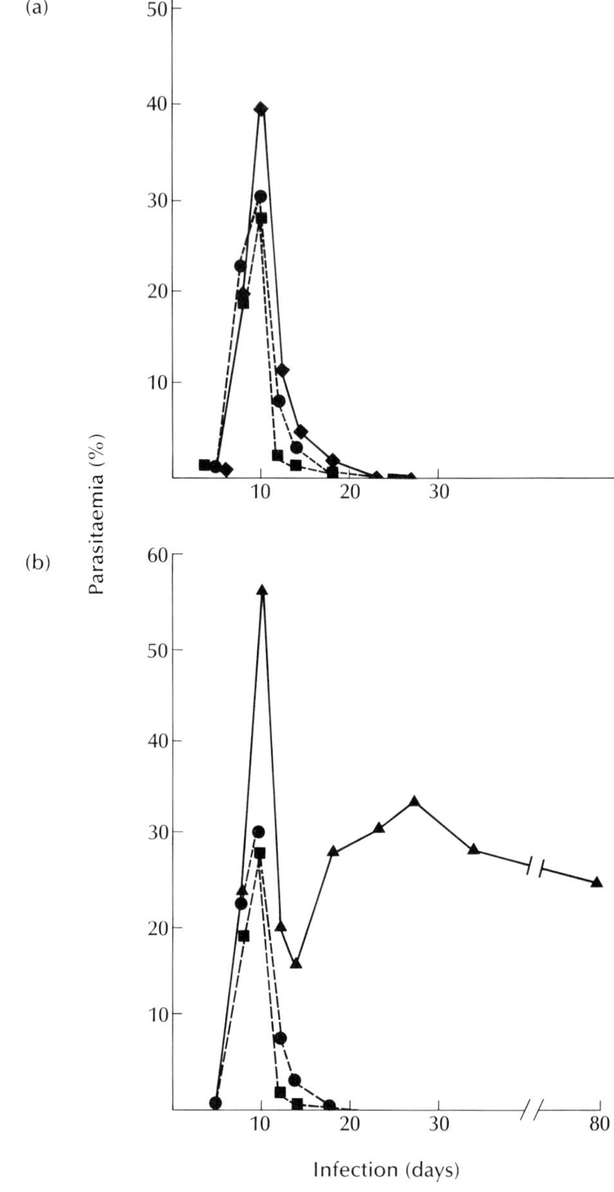

Fig. 79.12. Course of infection of *P. chabaudi* in mice depleted of different T cell populations by treatment *in vivo* with antibodies. (a) Mice treated with anti-CD8 antibodies; (b) mice treated with anti-CD4 antibodies. Controls were treated with PBS or an irrelevant antibody. Modified from Süss *et al.* (1988).

More information is available regarding the induction of interferons by the parasite. Work on interferons and their possible role in experimental malaria has been reviewed by Allison and Eugui 1983; Troye-Blomberg and Perlmann 1988; Weidanz and Long 1988. Recent work in human malaria has concentrated on IFN-γ. Exposure *in vitro* of blood T lymphocytes from *P. falciparum*-primed individuals to either crude or defined antigens from the blood stages of the parasite results in significant release of this lymphokine (Riley *et al.* 1988a; Troye-Blomberg and Perlmann 1988; Kabilan *et al.* 1990), a release which appears to correlate with the donors' degree of clinical immunity (Troye-Blomberg *et al.* 1987). Importantly, when such lymphocytes were stimulated with either the antigen Pf155/RESA or short synthetic peptides corresponding to its immunodominant T cell epitopes, there was no clear-cut correlation in individual donors between proliferation (^{3}H-thymidine incorporation) and IFN-γ release, indicating that the two phenomena are partially independent processes, perhaps occurring in different cells (Kabilan *et al.* 1988; Riley *et al.* 1988b; Troye-Blomberg *et al.* 1989). In any event, these observations are of practical importance since they show that several parameters of T cell activation should be analysed to obtain a reliable measure of the frequency of cells primed to a given epitope in a T cell preparation.

Interferon-γ has many functions, including either enhancement or depression of B lymphocytes, increase of expression of Class II MHC and macrophage activation. It appears to be one of the factors important for the induction of cell-mediated resistance to the parasite (Shear *et al.* 1989; Stevenson *et al.* 1990). Activated macrophages as well as other effector cells such as neutrophils (Kharazmi *et al.* 1987) are known to be involved in this resistance by generating products toxic to the parasites. Important in this context is the generation of reactive oxygen intermediates which subject intraerythrocytic parasites to oxidant stress (Allison and Eugui 1983; Clark and Hunt 1983; Ockenhouse *et al.* 1984; Descamps-Latscha *et al.* 1987; Malhotra *et al.* 1988; Nnalue and Friedman 1988). However, other macrophage-derived products acting via different mechanisms may also inhibit the growth of intraerythrocytic parasites (Rzepczyk *et al.* 1984).

Another primarily macrophage-derived factor which has recently given rise to much interest in malaria is tumour necrosis factor (TNF)/cachectin. Tumour necrosis factor is found at elevated levels in the plasma of malaria patients as well as in culture supernatants of their mononuclear cells stimulated with endotoxin or parasitized erythrocytes (Scuderi *et al.* 1986; Kwiatkowski *et al.* 1989). Although TNF appears to be a main factor in the causation of fever and pathology in severe malaria (Clark *et al.* 1987b; Grau *et al.* 1987; see also below), it is also known to be involved in parasite suppression (Clark 1987; Taverne *et al.* 1987; Stevenson and Ghadirian 1989). Tumour necrosis factor, which is part of a network of interacting cytokines, does not directly kill the parasites. Its parasiticidal effects may include priming of effector cells and involve generation of C-reactive protein (Pied *et al.* 1989), reactive oxygen intermediates or lipid peroxidation (Clark *et al.* 1987a, c; Larrick *et al.* 1987; Rockett *et al.* 1988).

The preceding discussion of immune mechanisms controlling parasite growth and survival has concentrated on the asexual blood stages. Until recently, antibodies have been considered as the main factors controlling the pre-erythrocytic stages of plasmodia, by preventing sporozoite penetration into liver cells but also by inhibiting intrahepatocytic development (Mazier *et al.* 1986). However, recent studies indicate that cellular mechanisms play a major role in the defence against sporozoite infection (Fig. 79.13), particularly as it appears that antibodies which are inhibitory at high concentration may enhance sporozoite penetration into liver cells at lower concentration (cited in Mazier *et al.* 1988). Animal experiments indicate that T cells of CD8 +ve phenotype are of major importance in the control of the preerythrocytic stages (Schofield *et al.* 1987;

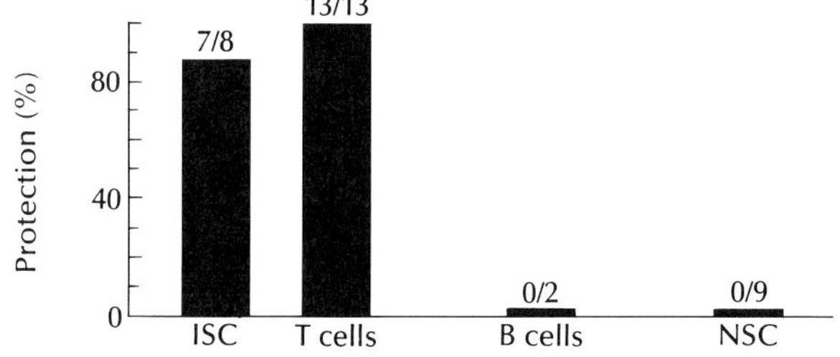

Fig. 79.13. Adoptive transfer of immunity to sporozoite challenge. Recipient mice received immune spleen cells (ISC), T cells, B cells, or normal spleen cells (NSC). Modified from Egan *et al.* (1987).

Weiss *et al.* 1988). Activation of these T cells is believed to be brought about by parasite antigens expressed on the surface of infected hepatocytes. Although the CS protein may be a major candidate, the involvement of liver or erythrocytic stage-specific antigens is not excluded (Mazier *et al.* 1988). Circumsporozoite protein-specific CD8 +ve T cells have indeed been shown specifically to kill cells such as transfected fibroblasts or infected hepatocytes expressing the homologous CS protein (Kumar *et al.* 1988; Weiss *et al.* 1990). Passive transfer into mice of cloned CD8 +ve T cells specific for CS protein from *Plasmodium berghei* has also been shown to confer protection against challenge infection with that parasite (Romero *et al.* 1989). However, it is not known whether cell-mediated cytotoxicity or IFN-γ, generated by antigen-activated T cells, is the major factor in the control of intracellular sporozoite development. This development is inhibited both *in vivo* and *in vitro* by IFN-γ. The target for IFN-γ-mediated inhibition appears to be the infected hepatocyte rather than the parasite itself (Ferreira *et al.* 1986; Maheshwari *et al.* 1986; Vergara *et al.* 1987) (Fig. 79.14). In addition to this direct parasiticidal effect, which is not observed in the erythrocytic stages, IFN-γ may also act through activation of macrophages and other effector cells which have been seen to kill intrahepatocytic parasites by a phagocytic pathway (Meis and Verhave 1988). Other cytokines involved in cell-mediated control of liver-stage development are IL-1 (Mellouk *et al.* 1987) and IL-6 (Helle *et al.* 1988) as well as TNF, which acts, in part, by inducing liver cells to produce C-reactive protein (Pied *et al.* 1989; Mazier *et al.* 1990).

Antibodies to antigens of the sexual stages of the malaria parasite induce transmission-blocking immunity by inhibiting fertilization or post-fertilization development (reviewed by Targett 1988). However, low concentrations of inhibitory antibodies have been shown to enhance gametocyte infectivity (Ponnudurai *et al.* 1987; Peiris *et al.* 1988) and cell-mediated mechanisms may be important for inhibition. This is supported by the finding of a CD4 +ve T-cell-dependent transmission-blocking immunity in a murine malaria system, induced by vaccination with microgametes (Harte *et al.* 1985) and by the induction of T cell proliferation and IFN-γ release *in vitro* by *P. falciparum* gamete antigens in a human system (Good *et al.* 1987b).

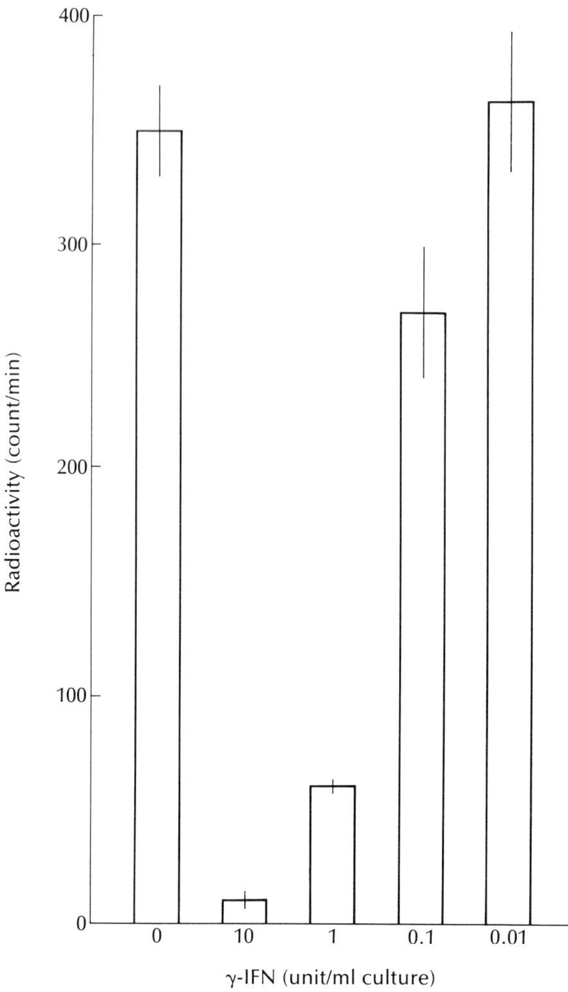

Fig. 79.14. *In vitro* inhibition by IFN-γ of *P. berghei* development in human hepatoma cells. Modified from Ferreira *et al.* (1986).

Severe malaria and immunopathology

Cerebral malaria

Since cerebral malaria is the leading cause of mortality in *P. falciparum* infection, the elucidation of the underlying mechanism(s) has been the objective of many investigations. The recent definition by the World Health Organization (WHO) (1986) was 'severe and complicated malaria, frequently of sudden onset with a convulsion followed by unrousable coma'. This clearly restricts the definition so as not to include minor metrological symptoms frequent in subjects with *P. falciparum* malaria. However, in practice any degree of impaired consciousness could indicate severe cerebral involvement and a potentially fatal course. At autopsy cerebral oedema and small petechial (or ring) haemorrhages are seen, concentrated in the white matter of the cerebral hemispheres. Microscopically, large numbers of infected and uninfected erythrocytes in small venules and capillaries and blockage of the vessels are typical findings (McPherson *et al.* 1985; Aikawa, 1988). Moreover, in a controlled study little or no extravascular inflammation was found and leucocytes were absent within and outside cerebral vessels (McPherson *et al.* 1985). The strongest correlation found between vascular pathology and cerebral malaria was the tightness of packing of red blood cells in the vessels, 'where it is quite clear that cerebral malaria patients have a higher average density of packing and considerably larger proportion of tightly packed vessels' (McPherson *et al.* 1985).

Parasite maturation beyond the trophozoite stage is not usually seen in the peripheral blood of patients infected with *P. falciparum* malaria, despite high parasitaemias. The morphological and molecular basis of this sequestration, reflecting adhesion of infected erythrocytes to capillaries and post-capillary venules has been discussed above. Another phenomenon which may be particularly important in the context of cerebral malaria is the capacity of certain *P. falciparum*-infected erythrocytes to bind uninfected red blood cells to their surface (spontaneous rosette formation, see above; Wahlgren 1986; Handunnetti *et al.* 1989; Udomsangpetch *et al.* 1989c) (Fig. 79.15). Although adhesion of the infected erythrocytes to the endothelium probably plays a pathophysiological role in cerebral malaria, rosetting may be most important as being responsible for the formation of aggregates of parasitized and non-parasitized erythrocytes which obstruct cerebral capillaries (Wahlgren *et al.* 1989; Kaul *et al.* 1991). Recently it was found that all *P. falciparum* isolates obtained from Gambian children with cerebral malaria were able to form rosettes, while those from children with mild forms of the disease either did not form rosettes or had a significantly lower rosetting rate (Carlson *et al.* 1990b). Also, plasma of children with cerebral malaria lacked anti-rosetting activity while plasma of children with mild disease were frequently able to disrupt rosettes *in vitro* (Carlson *et al.* 1990b).

An important role of monokines and lymphokines in human cerebral malaria has been suggested (Clark 1987; Grau *et al.* 1988; see also above). Tumor necrosis factor/cachectin is thought to induce increased vascular permeability and shock in patients with severe Gram-negative septicaemia as bacterial endotoxins activate monocytes to release TNF. Yet other effects of TNF are production of fever, hypoglycaemia, pulmonary neutrophil margination, liver damage, elevated blood lactate and acute renal tubular necrosis, all symptoms seen in patients with severe malaria (Phillips and Warrell 1986; Kwiatkowski 1989; Kwiatkowski *et al.* 1989). In experimental malaria systems, increased permeability of the blood–brain barrier has been described (Maegraith and Fletcher 1972). Interestingly, injection of *P. berghei*-infected mice with cyclosporin A or antibodies to granulocyte–macrophage colony-stimulating factor (GM-CSF) and IL-3 prevents both the severe neurological findings and excessive TNF release in the serum, indicating T cell involvement in these animal models (Grau *et al.* 1987, 1988). Plugging of the cerebral vessels with infected and uninfected erythrocytes is, however, not found in this murine malaria model. Moreover, in the human system

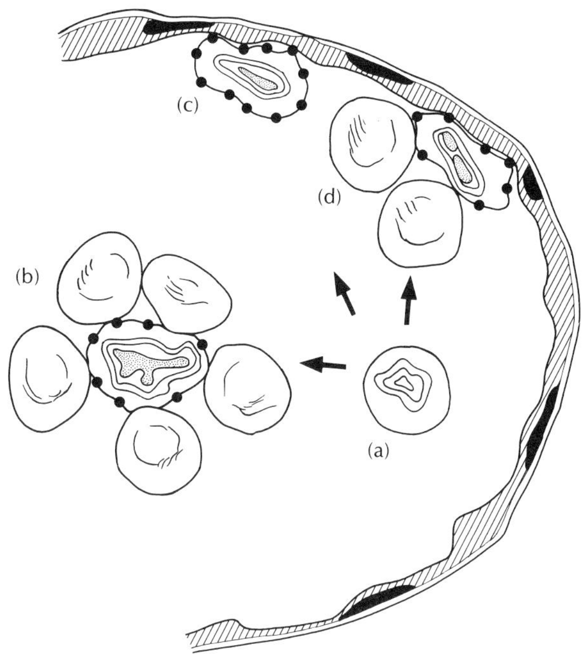

Fig. 79.15. Possible mechanisms for sequestration of *P. falciparum*-infected erythrocytes in a venule or capillary. (a) Immature infected erythrocytes circulate in the peripheral blood; early trophozoites express surface antigens which mediate (b) spontaneous rosette formation or (c) binding to the endothelial lining of the vessels or (d) both.

there is no increase in the permeability of the blood–brain barrier (Phillips and Warrell 1986), although children with malaria have increased levels of circulating TNF (Kwiatkowski *et al.* 1990). Compared with children with uncomplicated malaria, mean plasma TNF levels are twice as high in cerebral malaria survivors and 10 times as high in fatal cases (Kwiatkowski *et al.* 1990). In humans with cerebral malaria TNF might act by upregulating the number of vascular (endothelial) receptor structures, such as intercellular adhesion molecule (ICAM)-1, to which infected erythrocytes can bind. Polyclonally activated or malaria-specific T cells could further enhance TNF secretion or directly activate endothelial cells through IFN-γ or leucotriene release (Clark 1987). The deposition of immune complexes in cerebral vessels has been described but does not seem to be a major factor in the formation of cerebral pathology (Phillips and Warrell 1986; Aikawa 1988). Similarly, disseminated intravascular coagulation might be present in some individuals with cerebral malaria, but this is not a general finding (Phillips and Warrell 1986).

Anaemia and other complications

Common findings in malaria-infected individuals are anaemia, low haematocrit and dyserythropoietic changes of the bone marrow. Folic acid deficiency may also be present. The anaemia can to some extent be explained by the hypersplenism seen in malaria subjects and the large numbers of erythrocytes destroyed by the rupture of malaria-infected cells. In addition, the survival of normal erythrocytes is reduced in malaria (Seed and Kreier 1980; Marsh and Greenwood 1986). There may be an increased consumption by infected erythrocytes of ferrous ions, as parasite-induced transferrin receptors are present at the infected erythrocyte surface (Haldar *et al.* 1986; Rodriguez and Jungery 1986).

Complement, immune complexes, antigens and antibodies bind to the erythrocyte surface in *P. falciparum*-infected individuals. Anti-erythrocyte autoantibodies are found in experimental malaria and in the serum of human malaria patients (see Table 79.1 above). Moreover, children from malarious areas frequently display positive Coombs' test, indicating a correlation with the presence of anaemia (Facer 1980). Antimalarial antibodies directed to surface-located parasite antigens could also be of importance (Howard 1988). Similarly, parasite antigens bound to uninfected erythrocytes, such as the erythrocyte-binding antigens (Camus and Hadley 1985; Miller *et al.* 1988), might induce direct or indirect destruction of erythrocytes. The activation of neutrophil granulocytes, monocytes and other phagocytic cells by cytokines (IFN-γ, TNF) and/or through binding of erythrocyte surface-associated IgG, immune complexes and complement may be instrumental in the increased destruction of erythrocytes in malaria-infected subjects (Marsh and Greenwood 1986; Clark 1987).

Chronic glomerular lesions can develop in *P. malariae*-infected individuals. This is frequently complicated by a nephrotic syndrome that is poorly responsive to antimalarials or corticosteroids (Manson-Bahr and Bell 1988). The deposition of circulating immune complexes is believed to be involved in the causation of these complications (Marsh and Greenwood 1986). Similarly, acute glomerular lesions have been described both in human (*P. malariae*, *P. falciparum*) and experimental malaria.

Massive enlargement of the spleen is common in children with malaria. Although, in immune adults this is frequently due to kala-azar or schistosomiasis, splenomegaly seen in this age-group may also be due to chronic malaria (tropical splenomegaly syndrome, TSS). Individual, possibly hereditary, factors seem to be involved. Anaemia, leucopenia and thrombocytopenia are common. Both specific antimalarial antibodies and total IgM/IgG are elevated but there is a marked overproduction of IgM. The aetiology of the disease is not clear but it has been suggested to be due to a defect in the suppressor T cell population, which controls B cell activation (Fakunle and Greenwood 1976; Piessens *et al.* 1985). The tropical splenomegaly syndrome frequently responds to prolonged antimalarial treatment.

Burkitt's lymphoma, a non-Hodgkin's lymphoma, originating from EBV +ve B cells, is frequently found in children living in areas where malaria is highly endemic (Papua New Guinea, Africa). T cells obtained from children with acute malaria are unable to normally inhibit the spontaneous outgrowth of EBV-infected B cells *in vitro*. As the geographical distribution of the disease corresponds closely to that of malaria, it has been suggested that malaria plays a role in the tumour development (Burkitt 1970; Whittle *et al.* 1984; see also above).

Diagnosis

A number of diagnostic tests are available for the detection of antimalarial antibodies, malaria parasites, malarial antigens or malaria ribonucleic/deoxyribonucleic acid (RNA/DNA) (World Health Organization 1988). Microscopic examination of blood smears, however, remains the method of choice for the diagnosis. Although both effective and efficient, the microscopic diagnosis has disadvantages, as continuous microscopy leads to fatigue and consequently errors. The microscope is expensive, needs careful maintenance and requires competent operators. Thus, there is a need for alternative diagnostic methods which are cheap, simple and reliable.

Spot hybridization with DNA probes has been successfully applied in the diagnosis of malaria infections. In a current assay for detection of *P. falciparum* parasites, a DNA probe containing 21 base pair repeats is utilized (Franzén *et al.* 1984). The sensitivity approaches the level of the light microscope and the assay has already been used in epidemiological studies (Holmberg *et al.* 1987). Deoxyribonucleic acid probes for drug resistance and other phenotypic characteristics of malaria parasites are being developed. In other attempts to diagnose malaria the visualization of parasite RNA/DNA using fluorescent nucleotide-binding drugs (acridine orange) is being tried (Rickman *et al.* 1989).

Malaria parasites or parasite antigens can be quantitated by means of ELISA or radio immunoassay, (World Health Organization 1988). The two basic concepts have been either direct detection of soluble antigens in the patient's serum or inhibition of antibody binding by blood or solubilized infected erythrocytes. The inhibition assay using polyclonal antibodies is a sensitive diagnostic method. The use of defined antibody preparations (affinity-purified polyclonal or monoclonal antibodies) has also been reported but with lower detection rate. However, soluble antigens from asexual *P. falciparum* parasites can be detected in sera by ELISA with monoclonal antibodies to the antigens (World Health Organization 1988). Enzyme-linked immunosorbent assays based on the detection of the CS protein in infected mosquitoes have been developed and are being evaluated in epidemiological studies (Zavala *et al.* 1982; World Health Organization 1988).

Serological tests that detect antibodies to the parasite have been used extensively during the last 30 years. Here, the oldest is the indirect haemagglutination assay, where soluble malarial antigens are used to coat tanned red blood cells (RBCs). Although the haemagglutination assay is simple and rapid, it is of relatively low sensitivity and favours detection of antibodies of the IgM class. Among the more sensitive techniques, the IFA, using air-dried or air-dried and acetone-fixed crude parasite material, has been used extensively in serological studies. This conventional IFA detects antibody binding to a large number of parasite antigens located internally or associated with the surface of infected erythrocytes (Fig. 79.16). Detection of antibody binding reflects experience of malaria, but says little about the clinical immune status of the individual. A modification of the IFA, erythrocyte membrane immunofluorescence (EMIF), merely detects antigens located at the infected erythrocyte surface (Fig. 79.17). The significance of this method lies in the restricted specificity of the antibodies which it detects (Perlmann *et al.* 1984). The EMIF uses glutaraldehyde-fixed and air-dried monolayers of ring-infected RBCs, a procedure which limits antibody binding to the surface of infected erythrocytes (Fig. 79.16). In several cross-sectional studies a positive relationship has been established between EMIF titres and the acquisition of clinical immunity (Wahlgren *et al.* 1986b; Nguyen-Dinh *et al.* 1987). For quantitative studies this assay has also been developed as a cell ELISA (Perlmann *et al.* 1984; Deloron *et al.* 1987).

Enzyme-linked immunosorbent assays and RIA have long been used to detect antibodies to crude soluble infected erythrocyte extracts (World Health Organization 1988). Well-defined solid-phase antigens (synthetic peptides, fusion proteins) and assays detecting different IgM/IgG isotypes have also been developed (Wahlgren *et al.* 1986). Synthetic peptides corresponding to repeated sequences of Pf155/RESA, CS protein, PMMSA, S antigens and others are presently being evaluated in 'epitope-specific' epidemiological studies (Forsyth *et al.* 1988; Björkman *et al.* 1990; Petersen *et al.* 1989; Srivastava *et al.* 1989; see also above).

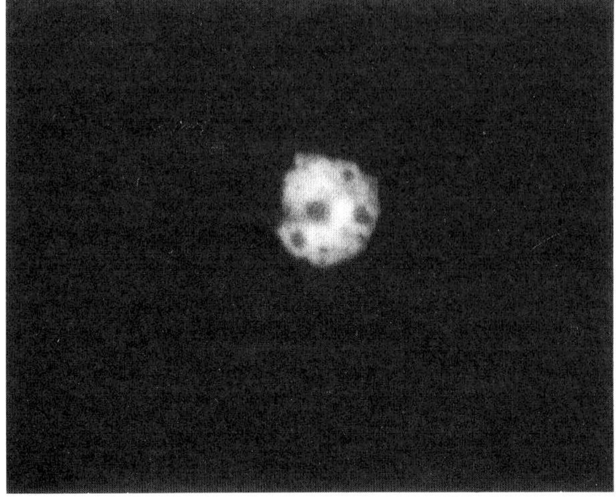

(a)

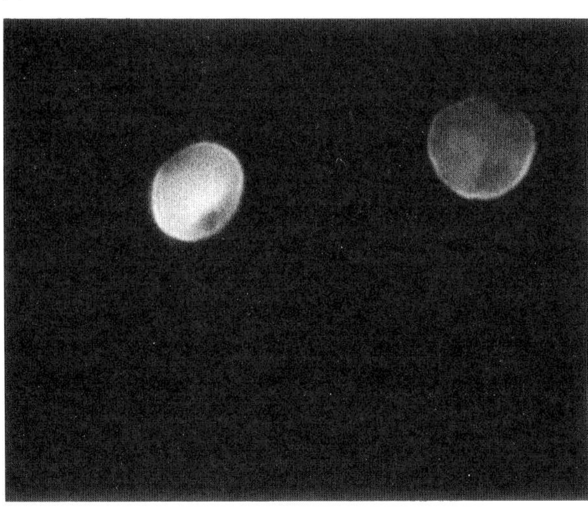

(b)

Fig. 79.16. Indirect immunofluorescence with human sera and *P. falciparum*-infected erythrocytes. (a) Conventional immunofluorescence staining of the entire infected erythrocyte using air-dried late-stage infected erythrocytes. (b) Erythrocyte membrane immunofluorescence (EMIF), using ring-stage infected erythrocytes that have been glutaraldehyde-fixed and air-dried. See also Perlmann *et al.* (1984).

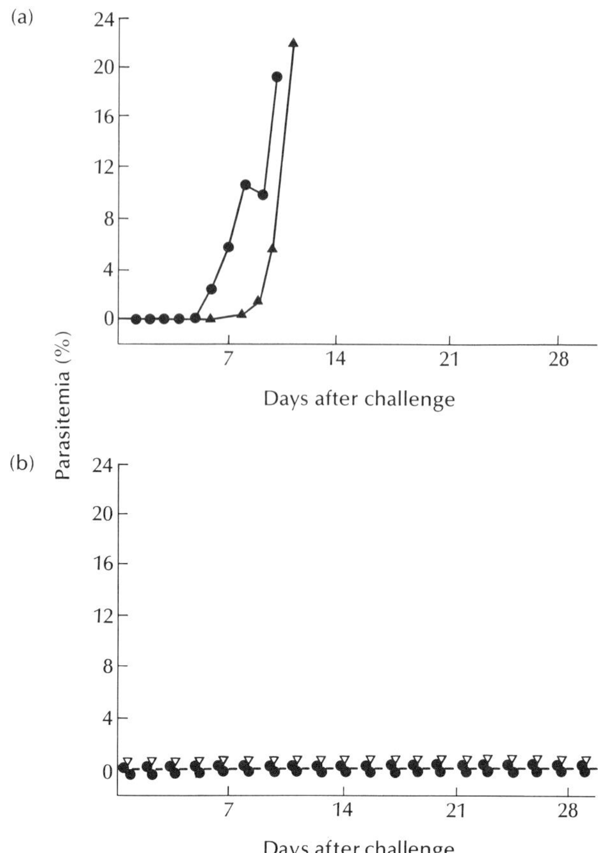

Fig. 79.17. Course of *P. falciparum* infection in vaccinated *Aotus* monkeys. (a) Unimmunized control monkeys which were drug treated to prevent death. (b) Monkeys immunized with PMMSA antigen were completely protected, and no patent parasitaemia was detected over a 60-day period. Modified from Siddiqui *et al.* (1987).

Vaccines

Attempts to control malaria after World War II were initially quite successful. However, during the 1960s and 1970s, there was a dramatic return of the disease. Although this return has many complicated causes, the rapid spread of insecticide resistance in the *Anopheles* vector and drug resistance in the parasites are considered to be important contributing factors. For this reason, vaccine development has emerged as a research goal of highest priority in malaria immunology.

As discussed in the preceding sections, acquired immunity to malaria is both species- and stage-specific. Accordingly, three different types of vaccines are currently being developed. Most of the work done until now deals with *P. falciparum* but work on *P. vivax* is rapidly catching up.

The three types of vaccine under construction and testing are: (i) sporozoite vaccines, expected to prevent infection and the development of the parasite in the liver; (ii) vaccines to the asexual blood stages of the parasite, expected to prevent disease or at least to decrease its morbidity and mortality; and (iii) vaccines to the parasite's sexual stages, expected to block transmission from the vertebrate host to the mosquito. The latter vaccine has no effect on the infected patient but is believed to be an important complementary tool for controlling the spread of malaria and, not least, the development of drug-resistant variants (Miller *et al*. 1986).

As it is not presently feasible to culture parasites in sufficient amounts, malaria vaccines will not be based on the use of killed or attenuated whole organisms. Rather, they will be subunit vaccines in which the immunogens are defined antigens or fragments thereof, produced by peptide synthesis or recombinant DNA technology. Some of the problems inherent in this methodology will be discussed in the following paragraphs.

As reviewed in the preceding sections and by Nussenzweig and Nussenzweig (1986, 1988), there is good evidence that immunization of either animals or human volunteers with irradiated sporozoites may induce complete or partial protection against infection. The recognition of the fact that the repeat sequences of the CS protein are the immunodominant structures seen by neutralizing antibodies has led to several attempts to use these sequences as vaccine immunogens in humans. Three clinical trials with a *P. falciparum* sporozoite vaccine in small groups of volunteers have been published until now. In two, the vaccine immunogen was a trimer of the CS protein tetra-amino acid repeat Asn–Ala–Asn–Pro (see above), coupled to tetanus toxoid as the carrier (Herrington *et al*. 1987; Etlinger *et al*. 1988a). In the other, it was a gene construct (R32 tet32), consisting of 32 repeats with a 32 amino acid tail encoded by the vector (Ballou *et al*. 1987). In all three trials vaccinees developed antibodies which were both peptide- and sporozoite-specific and also gave some positive responses in lymphocyte proliferation tests. However, the responses were generally weak, and partial or complete protection to subsequent sporozoite challenge was obtained only in a few individuals.

Although these results indicate that synthetic immunogens containing very short amino acid sequences of the natural parasite antigen may induce protection, it is obvious that they were not sufficient to constitute the basis for a vaccine. Subsequently, it was argued that improvement of the antibody response induced by vaccination would be a prerequisite for improved protection. A new vaccine formulation was used in which the gene construct R32 tet32 (see above) was incorporated into liposomes containing monophosphoryl lipid A as adjuvant. With this vaccine, which was low in toxicity and pyrogenicity, very high anti-sporozoite antibody titres were obtained both in monkeys and in human volunteers (Richards *et al*. 1989; Alving and Richards 1990). However, there is as yet no evidence for improved protection. In view of the importance of the T cell system for sporozoite immunity (see above) it can be questioned if such modifications which do not take T cell responses into consideration will ever give satisfactory results. Inclusion of T cell epitopes on a foreign carrier protein in the immunogen has several disadvantages (Etlinger *et al*. 1988a, b). To obtain a long-lasting antibody response which can be boosted by repeated natural infections, the vaccine immunogen should contain T helper cell epitopes derived from the parasite, preferably the CS protein itself. Moreover, as antibody-independent cell-mediated immunity appears to be crucial for inhibition of parasite development in the liver, an efficient sporozoite vaccine should also contain T cell epitopes capable of sensitizing CD4+ve as well as CD8+ve effector cells (see above). As it has been claimed that the CS protein contains only a few T cell epitopes and that the most dominant ones are located in a polymorphic region of the molecule (de la Cruz *et al*. 1988), it may be necessary to include several of these variants or even T-cell-activating epitopes from other parasite antigens in order to overcome MHC restriction and to induce satisfactory responses in the majority of vaccinees. The recently described T helper epitope which lacks obvious MHC restriction may also be of interest in this context (Sinigaglia and Pink 1990).

Development of vaccines against the asexual blood stages ('merozoite vaccines') has focused on antigens involved in erythrocyte invasion or sequestration of infected erythrocytes, i.e. parasite antigens on the surface of merozoites or infected erythrocytes or antigens released at schizont burst (see above). As described above, many of these antigens display a considerable strain diversity, which obviously hampers their use as vaccine immunogens. However, they also contain structures which are both conserved and immunogenic in humans. Purified antigens, gene constructs and synthetic peptides have been used in vaccination trials in monkeys and have given partial or, in some instances, complete protection (e.g. Siddiqui *et al*. 1987) (Fig. 79.17). For a comprehensive review of this field see Perrin *et al*. (1988). Thus far, only one trial (phase I and II) in human volunteers has been reported (Patarroyo *et al.* 1988). These authors obtained complete protection or delayed onset of parasitaemia after challenge with infected erythrocytes by vaccinating with synthetic polymers of short sequences from three different blood-stage antigens as well as from the CS protein. The results are of considerable interest, although it is not known which of the sequences included in the vaccine were actually inducing protection since there was no correlation between antibody or T cell responses on the one hand and protection of the vaccinees on the other hand. The exact and optimal composition of the immunogen, the longevity of protection and its possible boosting by subsequent infections also require further investigation.

Transmission-blocking immunity has been shown to be boosted by natural infection in human malaria, particularly *P. vivax* (Mendis *et al.* 1987) and can be induced in experimental animals by vaccination with sexual stages of the parasite. For *P. falciparum*, several different antigens expressed on gametocytes or zygotes have been identified as targets of transmission-blocking immunity (see above) but their immunogenicity in man, MHC restriction and variability require further exploration (Good *et al.* 1988b; Carter *et al.* 1989). A promising candidate for a transmission-blocking vaccine appears to be a protein called Pfs25, which is expressed on zygotes and oökinetes (Kaslow 1990).

In conclusion, although there are no efficient malaria vaccines at hand, this is a rapidly advancing field and several clinical trials will take place in the next few years. Although efforts up to now have focused on monovalent vaccines, the final vaccines will certainly be polyvalent. The complicated epidemiology of malaria will require vaccines containing immunogens protecting against both sporozoite infection and blood-stage development. Moreover, since vaccination may induce antigen loss or variation (Klotz *et al.* 1987), an efficient vaccine should probably contain epitopes derived from several blood-stage antigens. A major problem which remains to be resolved is the formulation of the vaccines. Attempts to construct live vaccines by oral immunization of mice with a recombinant and attenuated *Salmonella typhimurium* vector transformed with the CS protein gene from the rodent parasite *P. berghei* have given promising results. These mice developed an antibody-independent but CD8 +ve T-cell-dependent immunity which gave protection against sporozoite challenge (Sadoff *et al.* 1988; Aggarwal *et al.* 1990). Efforts are also being made to use recombinant vaccinia or herpes simplex virus as a vector for mono- or polyvalent malaria vaccines (Edwards *et al.* 1988; von Brunn *et al.* 1988). For vaccines based on the use of synthetic peptides a 'multiple antigen peptide system' (MAP) has recently been designed to overcome the requirement of foreign carriers (Tam 1988). It consists of an oligolysine core carrying several (usually eight) branching arms containing the antigenic epitopes. Multiple antigen peptide systems based on tandemly arranged T and B cell epitopes from the CS protein of *P. berghei* have been shown to elicit both high antibody titres and efficient protection against sporozoite challenge in immunized mice (Tam *et al.* 1990). Another problem to be resolved concerns adjuvanticity of the immunogens as Freund's complete adjuvant, which has been used successfully in many animal trials, cannot be used in humans. Therefore, attempts are now being made to improve immunogenicity and delivery by adding hydrophobic tails to the malaria antigens or inserting them into proteosomes or liposomes (Lowell *et al.* 1988; Richards *et al.* 1988, 1989) or by targeting the antigen by conjugation with antibodies to the antigen-presenting cells (Barber and Carayanniotis 1988). Although promising results have been obtained from several of these approaches, their usefulness in human vaccines remains to be explored.

References

Adu, D., Williams, D.G., Quakyi, I.A. *et al.* (1982). Anti-ssDNA and antinuclear antibodies in human malaria. *Clin. Exp. Immunol.* **49**, 310–16.

Aggarwal, A., Kumar, S., Jaffe, R., Hone, D., Gross, M. and Sadoff, J. (1990). Oral *Salmonella*: malaria circumsporozoite recombinants induce specific $CD8^+$ cytotoxic T cells. *J. Exp. Med.* **172**, 1083–90.

Aikawa, M. (1988). Human cerebral malaria. *Am. J. Trop. Med. Hyg.* **39**, 3–10.

Aikawa, M., Torii, M., Sjölander, A., Berzins, K., Perlmann, P. and Miller, L.H. (1990). Pf155/RESA antigen is localized in dense granules of *Plasmodium falciparum* merozoites. *Exp. Parasitol.* **71**, 326–9.

Aley, S.B., Bates, M.D., Tam, J.P. and Hollingdale, M.R. (1986). Synthetic peptides from the circumsporozoite proteins of *Plasmodium falciparum* and *Plasmodium knowlesi* recognize the human hepatoma cell line HepG2-A16 *in vitro*. *J. Exp. Med.* **164**, 1915–22.

Allison, A.C. and Eugui, E.M. (1983). The role of cell-mediated immune responses in resistance to malaria, with special reference to oxidant stress. *Ann. Rev. Immunol.* **1**, 361–92.

Alving, C.R. and Richards, R.L. (1990). Liposomes containing lipid A: a potent nontoxic adjuvant for a human malaria sporozoite vaccine. *Immunol. Lett.* **25**, 275–9.

Anders, R.F. (1986). Multiple cross-reactivities amongst antigens of *Plasmodium falciparum* impair the development of protective immunity against malaria. *Parasite Immunol.* **8**, 529–39.

Anders, R.F., Coppel, R.L., Brown, G.V. and Kemp, D.J. (1988). Antigens with repeated amino acid sequences from the asexual blood stages of *Plasmodium falciparum*. *Prog. Allergy* **41**, 148–72.

Åslund, L. (1990). Identification of structures important for diagnosis and prophylaxis of malarial infections. Thesis, Uppsala University. ISBN 91-554-2624-7.

Ballou, W.R., Hoffman, S.L., Sherwood, J.A. *et al.* (1987). Safety and efficacy of a recombinant DNA *Plasmodium falciparum* sporozoite vaccine. *Lancet* **i**, 1276–81.

Barber, B.H. and Carayanniotis, G. (1988). Antigen delivery by immunotargeting: a possibility for adjuvant free vaccines? In *Technological Advances in Vaccine Development*, ed. L. Lasky, pp. 471–81, Alan R. Liss, New York.

Berzins, K., Wahlgren, M. and Perlmann, P. (1983). Studies on the specificity of anti-erythrocyte antibodies in the serum of patients with malaria. *Clin. Exp. Immunol.* **54**, 313–18.

Berzins, K., Perlmann, H., Wåhlin, B. *et al.* (1986). Rabbit and human antibodies to a repeated amino acid sequence of a *Plasmodium falciparum* antigen, Pf155, react with the native protein and inhibit merozoite invasion. *Proc. Nat. Acad. Sci. (USA)* **83**, 1065–9.

Bianco, A.E., Favaloro, J.M., Burkot, T.R. *et al.* (1986). A repetitive antigen of *Plasmodium falciparum* that is homologous to heat shock protein 70 of *Drosophila melanogaster*. *Proc. Nat. Acad. Sci. (USA)* **83**, 8713–17.

Bianco, A.E., Crewther, P.E., Coppel, R.L. *et al.* (1988). Patterns of antigen expression in asexual blood stages and gametocytes of *Plasmodium falciparum*. *Am. J. Trop. Med. Hyg.* **38**, 258–67.

Biggs, B.A., Culvenor, J.G., Ng, J.S., Kemp, D.J. and Brown, G.V. (1989). *Plasmodium falciparum*: cytoadherence of a knobless clone. *Exp. Parasitol.* **69**, 189–97.

Björkman, A. (1985). Malaria epidemiology, drug protection and drug susceptibility in a holoendemic area of Liberia. Thesis, Karolinska Institutet, Stockholm.

Björkman, A., Hanson, A.P., Brohult, J. *et al.* (1987). Yekepa project in Liberia. In *Proceedings of the Conference on Malaria in Africa*, ed. A.A. Buck, pp. 185–95, American Institute of Biological Sciences, Washington.

Björkman, A., Perlmann, H., Petersen, E. *et al.* (1990). Consecutive determinations of seroreactivities to Pf155/RESA antigen and to its different repetitive sequences in adult men from a holoendemic area of Liberia. *Parasite Immunol.* **12**, 115–23.

Blackman, M.J., Heidrich, H.-G., Donachie, S., McBride, J.S. and Holder, A.A. (1990). A single fragment of a malaria merozoite surface protein remains on the parasite during red cell invasion and is the target of invasion-inhibiting antibodies. *J. Exp. Med.* **172**, 379–82.

Boonpucknavig, S. and Ekapanyakul, G. (1984). Autoantibodies in sera of Thai patients with *Plasmodium falciparum* infection. *Clin. Exp. Immunol.* **58**, 77–82.

Brake, D.A., Long, C.A. and Weidanz, W.P. (1988). Adoptive protection against *Plasmodium chabaudi adami* malaria in athymic nude mice by a cloned T cell line. *J. Immunol.* **140**, 1989–93.

Brown, G.V., Culvenor, J.G., Crewther, P.E. *et al.* (1985). Localization of the ring-infected erythrocyte surface antigen (RESA) of *Plasmodium falciparum* in merozoites and ring-infected erythrocytes. *J. Exp. Med.* **162**, 774–9.

Brown, H., Kemp, D.J., Barzaga, N., Brown, G.V., Anders, R.F. and Coppel, R.L. (1987). Sequence variation in S-antigen genes of *Plasmodium falciparum*. *Mol. Biol. Med.* **4**, 365–76.

Burkitt, D.P. (1970). Geographical distribution. In *Burkitt's Lymphoma*, ed. D.P. Burkitt and D.H. Wright, pp. 186–97, Livingstone, Edinburgh.

Burns, J.M., Daly, T.M., Vaidya, A.B. and Long, C.A. (1988). The 3′ portion of the gene for a *Plasmodium yoelli* merozoite surface antigen encodes the epitope recognized by a protective monoclonal antibody. *Proc. Nat. Acad. Sci. (USA)* **85**, 602–6.

Bushell, G.R., Ingram, L.T., Fardoulys, C.A. and Cooper, J.A. (1988). An antigenic complex in the rhoptries of *Plasmodium falciparum*. *Mol. Biochem. Parasitol.* **28**, 105–12.

Bygbjerg, I.C., Jepsen, S., Theander, T.G. and Ödum, N. (1985). Specific proliferative response of human lymphocytes to purified soluble antigens from *Plasmodium falciparum in vitro* cultures and antigens from malaria patients' sera. *Clin. Exp. Immunol.* **59**, 421–6.

Bzik, D.J., Li, W., Horii, T. and Inselburg, J. (1988). Amino acid sequence of the serine-repeat antigen (SERA) of *Plasmodium falciparum* determined from cloned cDNA. *Mol. Biochem. Parasitol.* **30**, 279–88.

Camus, D. and Hadley, T.J. (1985). A *Plasmodium falciparum* antigen that binds to host erythrocytes and merozoites. *Science* **230**, 553–6.

Cappai, R., van Schravendijk, M.-R., Anders, R.F. *et al.* (1989). Expression of the RESA gene in *Plasmodium falciparum* isolate FCR3 is prevented by a subtelomeric deletion. *Mol. Cell. Biol.* **9**, 3584–7.

Carlson, J., Holmquist, G., Taylor, D.W., Perlmann, P. and Wahlgren, M. (1990a). Antibodies to histidine-rich protein (PfHRP1) disrupt spontaneously formed *Plasmodium falciparum* erythrocyte rosettes. *Proc. Nat. Acad. Sci. (USA)* **87**, 2511–15.

Carlson, J., Helmby, H., Hill, A.V.S., Brewster, D., Greenwood, B.M. and Wahlgren, M. (1990b). Human cerebral malaria: association with erythrocyte rosetting and lack of anti-rosetting antibodies. *Lancet* **336**, 1457–60.

Carter, R., Kumar, N., Quakyi, I.A. *et al.* (1988). Immunity to sexual stages of malaria parasites. *Prog. Allergy* **41**, 193–214.

Carter, R., Graves, P.M., Quakyi, I.A. and Good, M.F. (1989). Restricted or absent immune responses in human populations to *Plasmodium falciparum* gamete antigens that are targets of malaria transmission blocking antibodies. *J. Exp. Med.* **169**, 135–47.

Cavacini, L.A., Long, C.A. and Weidanz, W.P. (1986). T-cell immunity in murine malaria: adoptive transfer of resistance to *Plasmodium chabaudi adami* in nude mice with splenic T cells. *Infect. Immunity* **52**, 637–43.

Certa, U., Ghersa, P., Döbeli, H. *et al.* (1988). Aldolase activity of a *Plasmodium falciparum* protein with protective properties. *Science* **240**, 1036–8.

Chen, D.H., Tigelaar, R.E. and Weinbaum, F.I. (1977). Immunity to sporozoite-induced malaria infection in mice. I. The effect of immunization of T and B cell-deficient mice. *J. Immunol.* **118**, 1322–7.

Cheung, A., Leban, J., Shaw, A.R. *et al.* (1986). Immunization with synthetic peptides of a *Plasmodium falciparum* surface antigen induces antimerozoite antibodies. *Proc. Nat. Acad. Sci. (USA)* **83**, 8328–32.

Chizzolini, C. and Perrin, L. (1986). Antigen-specific and MHC-restricted *Plasmodium falciparum* induced human T lymphocyte clones. *J. Immunol.* **137**, 1022–8.

Clark, I.A. (1987). Cell-mediated immunity in protection and pathology of malaria. *Parasitol. Today* **3**, 300–5.

Clark, I.A. and Hunt, N.H. (1983). Evidence for reactive oxygen intermediates causing hemolysis and parasite death in malaria. *Infect. Immunity* **39**, 1–6.

Clark, I.A., Butcher, G.A., Buffinton, G.D., Hunt, N.H. and Cowden, W.B. (1987a). Toxicity of certain products of lipid peroxidation to the human malaria parasite *Plasmodium falciparum*. *Biochem. Pharmacol.* **36**, 543–6.

Clark, I.A., Cowden, W.B., Butcher, G.A. and Hunt, N.H. (1987b). Possible roles of tumor necrosis factor in the pathology of malaria. *Am. J. Pathol.* **129**, 192–9.

Clark, I.A., Hunt, N.H., Butcher, G.A. and Cowden, W.B. (1987c). Inhibition of murine malaria (*Plasmodium chabaudi*) *in vivo* by recombinant interferon-γ or tumor necrosis factor, and its enhancement by butylated hydroxyanisole. *J. Immunol.* **139**, 3493–6.

Clark, J.T., Donachie, S., Anand, R., Wilson, C.F., Heidrich, H.-G. and McBride, J.S. (1989). 46–53 Kilodalton glycoprotein from the surface of *Plasmodium falciparum* merozoites. *Mol. Biochem. Parasitol.* **32**, 15–24.

Clyde, D.F., McCarthy, V.C., Miller, R.M. and Hornick, R.B. (1973). Specificity of protection of man against sporozoite-induced falciparum malaria. *Am. J. Med. Sci.* **266**, 398–403.

Cohen, S., McGregor, I.A. and Carrington, S. (1961). Gamma-globulin and acquired immunity to human malaria. *Nature (London)* **192**, 733–7.

Collins, W.E., Anders, R.F., Pappaioanou, M. *et al.* (1986). Immunization of *Aotus* monkeys with recombinant proteins of an erythrocyte surface antigen of *Plasmodium falciparum*. *Nature (London)* **323**, 259–62.

Collins, W.E., Anders, R.F., Ruebush, T.K. *et al.* (1991). Immunization of owl monkeys with the ring-infected erythrocyte surface antigen of *Plasmodium falciparum*. *Am. J. Trop. Med. Hyg.* **44**, 34–41.

Cooper, J.A., Ingram, L.T., Bushell, G.R. *et al.* (1988). The 140/130/105 kilodalton protein complex in the rhoptries of *Plasmodium falciparum* consists of discrete polypeptides. *Mol. Biochem. Parasitol.* **29**, 251–60.

Cornille-Brögger, R., Mathews, H.M., Storey, J., Askhar, T.S., Brögger, S. and Molineaux, L. (1978). Changing patterns in the humoral immune response to malaria before, during and after the application of control measures: a longitudinal study in the West African savanna. *Bull. WHO* **56**, 579–600.

Crisanti, A., Müller, H.-M., Hilbich, C. *et al.* (1988). Epitopes recognized by human T-cells map within the conserved part of the GP190 of *P. falciparum*. *Science* **240**, 1324–6.

Dame, J.B., Williams, J.L., McCutchan, T.F. *et al.* (1984). Structure of the gene encoding the immunodominant surface antigen on the sporozoite of the human malaria parasite *Plasmodium falciparum*. *Science* **225**, 593–9.

Daniel Ribeiro, C.T., de Roquefeuil, S., Druilhe, P. *et al.* (1984). Abnormal anti-single stranded (ss) DNA activity in sera from *Plasmodium falciparum* infected individuals. *Trans. Roy. Soc. Trop. Med. Hyg.* **78**, 742–6.

David, P.H., Handunetti, S.M., Leech, J.H., Gamage, P. and Mendis, K.N. (1988). Rosetting: a new cytoadherence property of malaria-infected erythrocytes. *Am. J. Trop. Med. Hyg.* **38**, 289–97.

Deans, J.A. and Cohen, S. (1983). Immunology of malaria. *Ann. Rev. Microbiol.* **37**, 25–49.

de la Cruz, V.F., Lal, A.A. and McCutchan, T.F. (1987). Sequence variation in putative functional domains of the circumsporozoite protein of *Plasmodium falciparum*: implications for vaccine development. *J. Biol. Chem.* **262**, 11935–9.

de la Cruz, V.F., Maloy, W.L., Miller, L.H., Lal, A.A., Good, M.F. and McCutchan, T.F. (1988). Lack of cross-reactivity between variant T cell determinants from malaria circumsporozoite protein. *J. Immunol.* **141**, 2456–60.

Del Giudice, G., Cooper, J.A., Merino, J. *et al.* (1986). The antibody response in mice to carrier-free synthetic polymers of *Plasmodium falciparum* circumsporozoite repetitive epitope is I-A^b-restricted: possible implications for malaria vaccines. *J. Immunol.* **137**, 2952–5.

Del Giudice, G., Cheng, Q., Mazier, D. *et al.* (1988a). Immunogenicity of a non-repetitive sequence of *Plasmodium falciparum* circumsporozoite protein in man and mice. *Immunology* **63**, 187–91.

Del Giudice, G., Grau, G.E. and Lambert, P.-H. (1988b). Host responsiveness to malaria epitopes and immunopathology. *Prog. Allergy* **41**, 288–333.

Deloron, P., Le Bras, J., Savel, J. and Coulaud, J.P. (1987). Antibodies to the Pf155 antigen of *Plasmodium falciparum*: measurement by cell-ELISA and correlation with expected immune protection. *Am. J. Trop. Med. Hyg.* **37**, 22–6.

Descamps-Latscha, B., Lunel-Fabiani, F., Karabinis, A. and Druihle, P. (1987). Generation of reactive oxygen species in whole blood from patients with acute falciparum malaria. *Parasite Immunol.* **9**, 275–9.

de Souza, J.B. and Playfair, J.H.L. (1983). Antilymphocyte autoantibody in lethal mouse malaria and its suppression by non-lethal malaria. *Parasite Immunol.* **5**, 257–65.

de Zoysa, A.P.K., Herath, P.R.J., Abhayawardana, T.A., Padmalal, U.K.G.K. and Mendis, K.N. (1988). Modulation of human malaria transmission by anti-gamete transmission blocking immunity. *Trans. Roy. Soc. Trop. Med. Hyg.* **82**, 548–53.

Diggs, C.L., Wellde, B.T., Anderson, J.S., Weber, R.M. and Rodriguez, E. (1972). The protective effect of African human immunoglobulin G in *Aotus trivirgatus* infected with Asian *Plasmodium falciparum*. *Proc. Helminthol. Soc. Washington* **39**, 449–56.

Dontfraid, F., Cochran, M.A., Pombo, D. *et al.* (1988). Human and murine CD4 T cell epitopes map to the same region of the malaria circumsporozoite protein: limited immunogenicity of sporozoites and circumsporozoite protein. *Mol. Biol. Med.* **5**, 185–196.

Druilhe, P., Puebla, R.M., Miltgen, F., Perrin, L. and Gentilini, M. (1984). Species- and stage-specific antigens in exoerythrocytic stages of *Plasmodium falciparum*. *Am. J. Trop. Med. Hyg.* **33**, 336–41.

Druilhe, P., Pradier, O., Marc, J.-P., Miltgen, F., Mazier, D. and Parent, G. (1986). Levels of antibodies to *Plasmodium falciparum* sporozoite surface antigens reflect malaria transmission rates and are persistent in the absence of reinfection. *Infect. Immunity* **53**, 393–7.

Edwards, S.J., Triglia, T., Sheppard, M. and Langford, C.J. (1988). *Plasmodium falciparum* antigens in recombinant HSV-1. In *Technological Advances in Vaccine Development*, ed. L. Lasky, pp. 223–34, Alan R. Liss, New York.

Egan, J.E., Weber, J.L., Ballou, W.R. *et al.* (1987). Efficacy of murine malaria sporozoite vaccines: implications for human vaccine development. *Science* **236**, 453–6.

Etlinger, H.M., Felix, A.M., Gillesen, D. *et al.* (1988a). Assessment in humans of a synthetic peptide-based vaccine against the sporozoite stage of the human malaria parasite, *Plasmodium falciparum*. *J. Immunol.* **140**, 626–33.

Etlinger, H.M., Heimer, E.P., Trzeciak, A., Felix, A.M. and Gillessen, D. (1988b). Assessment in mice of a synthetic peptide-based vaccine against the sporozoite stage of the human malaria parasite, *P. falciparum*. *Immunology* **64**, 551–8.

Facer, C.A. (1980). Direct antiglobulin reactions in Gambian children with *P. falciparum* malaria. III. Expression of IgG subclass determinants and genetic markers and association with anaemia. *Clin. Exp. Immunol.* **41**, 81–90.

Fakunle, Y.M. and Greenwood, B.M. (1976). Metabolism of IgM in the tropical splenomegaly syndrome. *Trans. Roy. Soc. Trop. Med. Hyg.* **70**, 346–8.

Favaloro, J.M., Coppel, R.L., Corcoran, L.M. *et al.* (1986). Structure of the RESA gene of *Plasmodium falciparum*. *Nucleic Acids Res.* **14**, 8265–77.

Ferreira, A., Schofield, L., Enea, V. *et al.* (1986). Inhibition of development of exoerythrocytic forms of malaria parasites by γ-interferon. *Science* **232**, 881–4.

Forsyth, K.P., Anders, R.F., Kemp, D.J. and Alpers, M.P. (1988). New approaches to the serotypic analysis of the epidemiology of *Plasmodium falciparum*. *Phil. Trans. Roy. Soc. (London) B* **321**, 485–93.

Franzén, L., Westin, G., Shabo, R. *et al.* (1984). Analysis of clinical specimens by hybridisation with probe containing repetitive DNA from *Plasmodium falciparum*: a novel approach to malaria diagnosis. *Lancet* **i**, 525–8.

Franzén, L., Wåhlin, B., Wahlgren, M. *et al.* (1989). Enhancement or inhibition of *Plasmodium falciparum* erythrocyte reinvasion *in vitro* by antibodies to an asparagine rich protein. *Mol. Biochem. Parasitol.* **32**, 201–12.

Gabriel, J.A., Holmquist, G., Perlmann, H., Berzins, K., Wigzell, H. and Perlmann, P. (1986). Identification of a *Plasmodium chabaudi* antigen present in the membrane of ring stage infected erythrocytes. *Mol. Biochem. Parasitol.* **20**, 67–75.

Good, M.F., Berzofsky, J.A., Maloy, W.L. *et al.* (1986). Genetic control of the immune response in mice to a *Plasmodium falciparum* sporozoite vaccine: widespread nonresponsiveness to single malaria T epitope in highly repetitive vaccine. *J. Exp. Med.* **164**, 655–60.

Good, M.F., Maloy, W.L., Lunde, M.N. *et al.* (1987a). Construction of synthetic immunogen: use of new T-helper epitope on malaria circumsporozoite protein. *Science* **235**, 1059–62.

Good, M.F., Quakyi, I.A., Saul, A., Berzofsky, J.A., Carter, R. and Miller, L.H. (1987b). Human T clones reactive to the sexual stages of *Plasmodium falciparum* malaria: high frequency of gamete-reactive T cells in peripheral blood from nonexposed donors. *J. Immunol.* **138**, 306–11.

Good, M.F., Berzofsky, J.A. and Miller, L.H. (1988a). The T cell response to the malaria circumsporozoite protein: an immunological approach to vaccine development. *Ann. Rev. Immunol.* **6**, 663–88.

Good, M.F., Miller, L.H., Kumar, S. *et al.* (1988b). Limited immunological recognition of critical malaria vaccine candidate antigens. *Science* **242**, 574–7.

Good, M.F., Pombo, D., Quakyi, I.A. *et al.* (1988c). Human T-cell recognition of the circumsporozoite protein of *Plasmodium falciparum*: immunodominant T-cell domains map to the polymorphic regions of the molecule. *Proc. Nat. Acad. Sci. (USA)* **85**, 1199–203.

Goundis, D. and Reid, K.B.M. (1988). Properdin, the terminal complement components, thrombospondin and the circumsporozoite protein of malaria parasites contain similar sequence motifs. *Nature (London)* **335**, 82–5.

Grau, G.E., Fajardo, L.F., Piguet, P.-F., Allet, B., Lambert, P.-H. and Vassali, P. (1987). Tumor necrosis factor (cachectin) as an essential mediator in murine cerebral malaria. *Science* **237**, 1210–12.

Grau, G.E., Kindler, V., Piguet, P.-F., Lambert, P.-H. and Vassalli, P. (1988). Prevention of experimental cerebral malaria by anticytokine antibodies: interleukin 3 and granulocyte macrophage colony-stimulating factor are intermediates in increased tumor necrosis factor production and macrophage accumulation. *J. Exp. Med.* **168**, 1499–504.

Greenwood, B.M. (1974). Possible role of a B-cell mitogen in hypergammaglobulinaemia in malaria and trypanosomiasis. *Lancet* **i**, 435–6.

Greenwood, B.M. (1984). Immunosuppression in malaria and trypanosomiasis. In *Parasites in the Immunized Host: Mechanisms of Survival*. Ciba Foundation Symposia No. 25, pp. 137–46.

Greenwood, B.M., Muller, A.S. and Valkenburg, H.A. (1971). Rheumatoid factor in Nigerian sera. *Clin. Exp. Immunol.* **8**, 161–73.

Guerin-Marchand, C., Druilhe, P., Galey, B. *et al.* (1987). A liver-stage-specific antigen of *Plasmodium falciparum* characterized by gene cloning. *Nature (London)* **329**, 164–7.

Guttinger, M., Caspers, P., Takacs, B. *et al.* (1988). Human T cells recognize polymorphic and non-polymorphic regions of the *Plasmodium falciparum* circumsporozoite protein. *EMBO J.* **7**, 2555–8.

Haldar, K., Henderson, C.L. and Cross, G.A.M. (1986). Indentification of the parasite transferrin receptor of *Plasmodium falciparum*-infected erythrocytes and its acylation via 1,2-diacyl-*sn*-glycerol. *Proc. Nat. Acad. Sci. (USA)* **83**, 8565–9.

Handunnetti, S.M., David, P.H., Perera, K.L.R.L. and Mendis, K.N. (1989). Uninfected erythrocytes form 'rosettes' around *Plasmodium falciparum* infected erythrocytes. *Am. J. Trop. Med. Hyg.* **40**, 115–18.

Harte, P.G., Rogers, N. and Targett, G.A.T. (1985). Role of T cells in preventing transmission of rodent malaria. *Immunology* **56**, 1–7.

Hedstrom, R.C., Campbell, J.R., Leef, M.L. *et al.* (1990). A malaria sporozoite surface antigen distinct from the circumsporozoite protein. *Bull. WHO* **68**, 152–7.

Heidrich, H.-G. (1988). Isolation and functional characterization of *Plasmodium falciparum* merozoite antigens. *Biol. Cell* **64**, 205–14.

Helle, M., Brakenhoff, J.P.J., De Groot, E.R. and Aarden, L.A. (1988). Interleukin 6 is involved in interleukin 1-induced activities. *Eur. J. Immunol.* **18**, 957–9.

Herrington, D.A., Clyde, D.F., Losonsky, G. *et al.* (1987). Safety and immunogenicity in man of a synthetic peptide malaria vaccine against *Plasmodium falciparum* sporozoites. *Nature (London)* **328**, 257–9.

Ho, M., Webster, H.K., Green, B., Looareesuwan, S., Kongchareon, S. and White, N.J. (1988). Defective production of and response to IL-2 in acute human falciparum malaria. *J. Immunol.* **141**, 2755–9.

Ho, M., Webster, H.K., Tongtawe, P., Pattanapanyasat, K. and Weidanz, W.P. (1990). Increased γδ T cells in acute *Plasmodium falciparum* malaria. *Immunol. Lett.* **25**, 139–42.

Hoffman, S.L., Oster, C.N., Plowe, C.V. *et al.* (1987). Naturally acquired antibodies to sporozoites do not prevent malaria: vaccine development implications. *Science* **237**, 639–42.

Hogh, B., Marbiah, N.T., Petersen, E. *et al.* (1991). A longitudinal study of seroreactivities to *Plasmodium falciparum* antigens in infants and children living in a holoendemic area of Liberia. *Am. J. Trop. Med. Hyg.* **44**, 191–200.

Holder, A.A. (1988). The precursor to major merozoite surface antigens: structure and role in immunity. *Prog. Allergy* **41**, 72–97.

Holder, A.A., Freeman, R.R. and Nicholls, S.C. (1988). Immunization against *Plasmodium falciparum* with recombinant polypeptides produced in *Escherichia coli*. *Parasite Immunol.* **10**, 607–17.

Hollingdale, M.R. (1988). Biology and immunology of sporozoite invasion of liver cells and exoerythrocytic development of malaria parasites. *Prog. Allergy* **41**, 15–48.

Hollingdale, M.R., Aikawa, M., Atkinson, C.T. *et al.* (1990). Non-CS pre-erythrocytic protective antigens. *Immunol. Lett.* **25**, 71–6.

Holmberg, M., Shenton, F.C., Franzén, L. *et al.* (1987). Use of a DNA hybridization assay for the detection of *Plasmodium falciparum* in field trials. *Am. J. Trop. Med. Hyg.* **37**, 230–4.

Hommel, M. and Semoff, S. (1988). Expression and function of erythrocyte-associated surface antigens in malaria. *Biol. Cell* **64**, 183–203.

Hommel, M., David, P.H. and Oligino, L.D. (1983). Surface alterations of erythrocytes in *Plasmodium falciparum* malaria: antigenic variation, antigenic diversity, and the role of the spleen. *J. Exp. Med.* **157**, 1137–48.

Howard, M.K., Gull, K. and Miles, M.A. (1987). Antibodies to tubulin in patients with parasitic infections. *Clin. Exp. Immunol.* **68**, 78–85.

Howard, R.J. (1988). Malaria proteins at the membrane of *Plasmodium falciparum*-infected erythrocytes and their involvement in cytoadherence to endothelial cells. *Prog. Allergy* **41**, 98–147.

Hui, G.S.N. and Siddiqui, W.A. (1987). Serum from Pf195 protected *Aotus* monkeys inhibit *Plasmodium falciparum* growth *in vitro*. *Exp. Parasitol.* **64**, 519–22.

Igarishi, I., Oo, M.M., Stanley, H., Reese, R. and Aikawa, M. (1987). Knob antigen deposition in cerebral malaria. *Am. J. Trop. Med.* **37**, 511–15.

Jayawardena, A.N. (1981). Immune responses to malaria. In *Parasitic Diseases*, ed. J.M. Mansfield, vol. I, pp. 85–136, Marcel Dekker, New York and Basle.

Jayawardena, A.N., Murphy, D.B., Janeway, C.A. and Gershon, R.K. (1982). T cell-mediated immunity in malaria. I. The Ly phenotype of T cells mediating resistance to *Plasmodium yoelii*. *J. Immunol.* **129**, 377–81.

Kabilan, L., Troye-Blomberg, M., Patarroyo, M.E., Björkman, A. and Perlmann, P. (1987). Regulation of the immune response in *Plasmodium falciparum* malaria. IV. T cell dependent production of immunoglobulin and anti-*P. falciparum* antibodies *in vitro*. *Clin. Exp. Immunol.* **68**, 288–97.

Kabilan, L., Troye-Blomberg, M., Perlmann, H. *et al.* (1988). T-cell epitopes in Pf155/RESA, a major candidate for a *Plasmodium falciparum* malaria vaccine. *Proc. Nat. Acad. Sci. (USA)* **85**, 5659–63.

Kabilàn, L., Troye-Blomberg, M., Andersson, G. *et al.* (1990). Number of cells from *Plasmodium falciparum*-immune donors that produce gamma interferon *in vitro* in response to Pf155/RESA, a malaria vaccine candidate antigen. *Infect. Immunity* **58**, 2989–94.

Kano, K., McGregor, I.A. and Milgrom, F. (1968). Hemagglutinins in sera of Africans of Gambia. *Proc. Soc. Exp. Biol.* **129**, 849–53.

Kaslow, D.C. (1990). Immunogenicity of *Plasmodium falciparum* sexual stage antigens: implications for the design of transmission blocking vaccine. *Immunol. Lett.* **25**, 83–6.

Kaslow, D.C., Quakyi, I.A., Syin, C. *et al.* (1988). A vaccine candidate from the sexual stage of human malaria that contains EGF-like domains. *Nature (London)* **333**, 74–6.

Kaul, D.K., Roth, E.F., Nagel, R.L., Howard, R.J. and Handunnetti, S.M. (1991). Rosetting of *Plasmodium falciparum*-infected red blood cells with uninfected red blood cells enhances microvascular obstruction under flow conditions. *Blood* **78**, 812–9.

Kemp, D.J., Coppel, R.L. and Anders, R.F. (1987). Repetitive proteins and genes of malaria. *Ann. Rev. Microbiol.* **41**, 181–201.

Kern, P., Hemmer, C.J., Van Damme, J., Gruss, H.J. and Dietrich, M. (1989). Elevated tumor necrosis factor alpha and interleukin-6 serum levels as markers for complicated *Plasmodium falciparum* malaria. *Am. J. Med.* **87**, 139–43.

Kharazmi, A., Jepsen, S. and Andersen, B.J. (1987). Generation of reactive oxygen radicals by human phagocytic cells activated by *Plasmodium falciparum*. *Scand. J. Immunol.* **25**, 335–41.

Khusmith, S., Charoenvit, Y., Kumar, S., Sedegah, M., Beaudoin, R.L. and Hoffman, S.L. (1991). Protection against malaria by vaccination with sporozoite surface protein 2 plus CS protein. *Nature* **252**, 715–18.

Kilejian, A. (1979). Characterisation of a protein correlated with the production of knob-like protrusions on membranes of erythrocytes infected with *Plasmodium falciparum*. *Proc. Nat. Acad. Sci. (USA)* **76**, 4650–3.

Klotz, F.W., Hudson, D.E., Coon, H.G. and Miller, L.H. (1987). Vaccination-induced variation in the 140 kD merozoite surface antigen of *Plasmodium knowlesi* malaria. *J. Exp. Med.* **165**,

359–67.

Kobayashi, S., Eden-McCutchan, F., Framson, P. and Bornstein, P. (1986). Partial amino acid sequence of human thrombospondin as determined by analysis of cDNA clones: homology to malarial circumsporozoite proteins. *Biochemistry* **25**, 8418–25.

Kumar, S., Miller, L.H., Quakyi, I.A. *et al.* (1988). Cytotoxic T cells specific for the circumsporozoite protein of *Plasmodium falciparum*. *Nature (London)* **334**, 258–60.

Kumar, S., Good, M.F., Dontfraid, F., Vinetz, J.M. and Miller, L.H. (1989). Interdependence of CD4$^+$ T cells and malarial spleen in immunity to *Plasmodium vinckei vinckei*: relevance to vaccine development. *J. Immunol.* **143**, 2017–23.

Kumararatne, D.S., Phillips, R.S., Sinclair, D., Parrott, M.V.D. and Forrester, J.B. (1987). Lymphocyte migration in murine malaria during the primary patent parasitaemia of *Plasmodium chabaudi* infections. *Clin. Exp. Immunol.* **68**, 65–77.

Kwiatkowski, D. (1989). Febrile temperatures can synchronize the growth of *Plasmodium falciparum in vitro*. *J. Exp. Med.* **169**, 357–61.

Kwiatkowski, D., Cannon, J.G., Manogue, K.R., Cerami, A., Dinarello, C.A. and Greenwood, B.M. (1989). Tumour necrosis factor production in *Falciparum* malaria and its association with schizont rupture. *Clin. Exp. Immunol.* **77**, 361–6.

Kwiatkowski, D., Hill, A.V.S., Sambou, I. *et al.* (1990). TNF concentration in fatal cerebral, non-fatal cerebral, and uncomplicated *Plasmodium falciparum* malaria. *Lancet* **336**, 1201–4.

Langhorne, J. (1989). The role of CD4$^+$ T-cells in the immune response to *Plasmodium chabaudi*. *Parasitol. Today* **5**, 362–4.

Larrick, J.W., Graham, D., Toy, K., Sin, L.S., Senyk, G. and Fendly, B.M. (1987). Recombinant tumor necrosis factor causes activation of human granulocytes. *Blood* **69**, 640–4.

Leech, J.H., Barnwell, J.W., Miller, L.H. and Howard, R.J. (1984). Identification of a strain-specific malarial antigen exposed on the surface of *Plasmodium falciparum*-infected erythrocytes. *J. Exp. Med.* **159**, 1567–75.

Lelchuk, R. and Playfair, J.H.L. (1985). Serum IL-2 inhibitor in mice. I. Increase during infection. *Immunology* **56**, 113–18.

Lelchuk, R., Rose, G. and Playfair, J.H.L. (1984). Changes in the capacity of macrophages and T cells to produce interleukins during murine malaria infection. *Cell. Immunol.* **84**, 253–63.

Lew, A.M., Langford, C.J., Pye, D., Edwards, S., Corcoran, L. and Anders, R.F. (1989). Class II restriction in mice to the malaria candidate vaccine ring infected erythrocyte surface antigen (RESA) as synthetic peptides or as expressed in recombinant vaccinia. *J. Immunol.* **142**, 4012–16.

Lockyer, M.J., Marsh, K. and Newbold, C.I. (1989). Wild isolates of *Plasmodium falciparum* show extensive polymorphism in T cell epitopes of the circumsporozoite protein. *Mol. Biochem. Parasitol.* **37**, 275–80.

Long, C.A. (1988). Immunity to murine malaria parasites. In *The Biology of Parasitism*, ed. P.T. Englund and A. Sher, pp. 233–48, Alan R. Liss, New York.

Lowell, G.H., Ballou, W.R., Smith, L.F., Wirtz, R.A., Zollinger, W.D. and Hockmeyer, W.T. (1988). Proteosome-lipopetide vaccines: enhancement of immunogenicity for malaria CS peptides. *Science* **240**, 800–2.

Luse, S.A. and Miller, L.H. (1971). *Plasmodium falciparum* malaria: ultrastructure of parasitized erythrocytes in cardiac vessels. *Am. J. Trop. Med. Hyg.* **20**, 650–5.

McCarthy, V. and Clyde, D. (1977). *Plasmodium vivax*: correlation of circumsporozoite precipitation (CSP) reaction with sporozoite-induced protective immunity in man. *Exp. Parasitol.* **41**, 167–71.

McCutchan, T.F., Lal, A.A., de la Cruz, V.F. *et al.* (1985). Sequence of the immunodominant epitope for the surface protein on sporozoites of *Plasmodium vivax*. *Science* **230**, 1381–3.

McGregor, I.A. (1974). Mechanisms of acquired immunity and epidemiological patterns of antibody responses in malaria in man. *Bull. WHO* **50**, 259–66.

McGregor, I.A., Carrington, S.C. and Cohen, S. (1963). Treatment of East African *Plasmodium falciparum* malaria with West African human gamma-globulin. *Trans. Roy. Soc. Trop. Med. Hyg.* **57**, 170–5.

McPherson, G.G., Warrell, M.J., White, N.J., Looareesuwan, S. and Warrell, D.A. (1985). Human cerebral malaria: a quantitative ultrastructural analysis of parasitized erythrocyte sequestration. *Am. J. Pathol.* **119**, 385–401.

Maegraith, B.G. and Fletcher, A. (1972). The pathogenesis of mammalian malaria. *Adv. Parasitol.* **10**, 49–75.

Magowan, C., Wollish, W., Anderson, L. and Leech, J. (1988). Cytoadherence by *Plasmodium falciparum*-infected erythrocytes is correlated with the expression of a family of variable proteins on infected erythrocytes. *J. Exp. Med.* **168**, 1307–20.

Maheshwari, R.K., Czarniecki, C.W., Dutta, G.P., Puri, S.K., Dhawan, B.N. and Friedman, R.M. (1986). Recombinant human gamma interferon inhibits simian malaria. *Infect. Immunity* **53**, 628–30.

Malhotra, K., Salmon, D., Le Bras, J. and Vilde, J.L. (1988). Susceptibility of *Plasmodium falciparum* to a peroxidase-mediated oxygen-dependent microbicidal system. *Infect. Immunity* **56**, 3305–9.

Manson-Bahr, P.E.C. and Bell, D.P. (eds.) (1987). *Manson's Tropical Diseases*, 19th edn, Baillière, Tindall, London.

Marsh, K. and Greenwood, B.M. (1986). The immunopathology of malaria. In *Clinics in Tropical Medicine and Communicable Diseases*, ed. G.T. Strickland, pp. 91–125, W.B. Saunders, Philadelphia.

Marsh, K. and Howard, R.J. (1986). Antigens induced on erythrocytes by *P. falciparum*: expression of diverse and conserved determinants. *Science* **231**, 150–3.

Masuda, A., Zavala, F., Nussenzweig, V. and Nussenzweig, R.S. (1986). Monoclonal anti-gametocyte antibodies identify an antigen present in all blood stages of *Plasmodium falciparum*. *Mol. Biochem. Parasitol.* **19**, 213–22.

Mattei, D., Ozaki, L.S. and Pereira da Silva, L. (1988). A *Plasmodium falciparum* gene encoding a heat shock-like antigen related to the rat 78 kd glucose-regulated protein. *Nucleic Acids Res.* **16**, 5204.

Mattei, D., Berzins, K., Wahlgren, M. *et al.* (1989). Cross-reactive determinants present on different *Plasmodium falciparum* antigens. *Parasite Immunol.* **11**, 15–30.

Mazier, D., Mellouk, S., Beaudoin, R.L. *et al.* (1986). Effect of antibodies to recombinant and synthetic peptides on *P. falciparum* sporozoites *in vitro*. *Science* **231**, 156–9.

Mazier, D., Miltgen, F., Nudelman, S. *et al.* (1988). Pre-erythrocytic stages of plasmodia: role of specific and non-specific factors. *Biol. Cell* **64**, 165–72,

Mazier, D., Rénia, L., Nussler, A. *et al.* (1990). Hepatic phase of malaria is the target of cellular mechanisms induced by the previous and the subsequent stages: a crucial role for liver nonparenchymal cells. *Immunol. Lett.* **25**, 65–70.

Meis, J.F.G.M. and Verhave, J.P. (1988). Exoerythrocytic development of malaria parasites. *Adv. Parasitol.* **27**, 1–66.

Mellouk, S., Maheshwari, R.K., Rhodes-Feuillette, A. *et al.* (1987). Inhibitory activity of interferons and interleukin 1 on the development of *Plasmodium falciparum* in human hepatocyte cultures. *J. Immunol.* **139**, 4192–5.

Mendis, K.N., Munesinghe, Y.D., de Silva, Y.N.Y., Keragalla, I. and Carter, R. (1987). Malaria transmission-blocking immunity induced by natural infections of *Plasmodium vivax* in humans. *Infect. Immunity* **55**, 369–72.

Meuwissen, J.H.E.T. and Ponnudurai, T. (1988). Biology and biochemistry of sexual and sporogenic stages of *Plasmodium falciparum*: a review. *Biol. Cell* **64**, 245–49.

Miller, L.H., Mason, S.J., Clyde, D.F. and McGinniss, M.H. (1976). The resistance factor to *Plasmodium vivax* in blacks: the Duffy-blood-group genotype, FyFy. *N. Engl. J. Med.* **295**, 302–4.

Miller, L.H., Howard, R.J., Carter, R., Good, M.F., Nussenzweig, V. and Nussenzweig, R.S. (1986). Research toward malaria vaccines. *Science* **234**, 1349–56.

Miller, L.H., Hudson, D. and Haynes, J.D. (1988). Identification of *Plasmodium knowlesi* erythrocyte binding proteins. *Mol. Biochem. Parasitol.* **31**, 217–22.

Molineaux, L. and Gramiccia, G. (1980). *The Garki Project: Research on the Epidemiology and Control of Malaria in the Sudan Savanna of West Africa*, WHO, Geneva.

Mortazavi-Milani, S.M., Badakere, S.S. and Holborow, E.J. (1984). Antibody to intermediate filaments of the cytoskeleton in the sera of patients with acute malaria. *Clin. Exp. Immunol.* **55**, 177–82.

Murakami, K. and Tanabe, K. (1985). An antigen of *Plasmodium yoelii* that translocates into the mouse erythrocyte membrane upon entry into the host cell. *J. Cell. Sci.* **73**, 311–20.

Nardin, E.H., Nussenzweig, R.S., McGregor, I.A. and Bryan, J.H. (1979). Antibodies to sporozoites: their frequent occurrence in individuals living in an area of hyperendemic malaria. *Science* **206**, 597–9.

Nardin, E.H., Nussenzweig, V., Nussenzweig, R.S. *et al.* (1982). Circumsporozoite proteins of human malaria parasites *Plasmodium falciparum* and *Plasmodium vivax*. *J. Exp. Med.* **156**, 20–30.

Newport, G., Culpepper, J. and Agabian, N. (1988). Parasite heat-shock proteins. *Parasitol. Today* **4**, 306–12.

Nguyen-Dinh, P., Berzins, K., Collins, W.E., Wahlgren, M., Udomsangpetch, R. and Perlmann, P. (1987). Antibodies to Pf155, a major antigen of *Plasmodium falciparum*: longitudinal studies in humans. *Am. J. Trop. Med. Hyg.* **37**, 501–5.

Nguyen-Dinh, P., Deloron, P.L., Barber, A.M. and Collins, W.E. (1988). *Plasmodium fragile*: detection of a ring-infected erythrocyte surface antigen (RESA). *Exp. Parasitol.* **65**, 119–24.

Nnalue, N.A. and Friedman, M.J. (1988). Evidence for a neutrophil-mediated protective response in malaria. *Parasite Immunol.* **10**, 47–58.

Nussenzweig, R., Vanderberg, J. and Most, H. (1969). Protective immunity produced by the injection of X-irradiated sporozoites of *Plasmodium berghei*. IV. Dose response, specificity and humoral immunity. *Military Med.* **134**, 1176–82.

Nussenzweig, V. and Nussenzweig, R. (1986). Development of a sporozoite malaria vaccine. *Am. J. Trop. Med. Hyg.* **35**, 678–88.

Nussenzweig, V. and Nussenzweig, R.S. (1988). Sporozoite malaria vaccines. In *The Biology of Parasitism*, ed. P.T. Englund and A. Sher, pp. 183–99, Alan R. Liss, New York.

Ockenhouse, C.F., Schulman, S. and Shear, H.L. (1984). Induction of crisis forms in the human malaria parasite *Plasmodium falciparum* by γ-interferon-activated monocyte derived macrophages. *J. Immunol.* **133**, 1601–8.

Patarroyo, M.E., Romero, P., Torres, M.L. *et al.* (1987). Induction of protective immunity against experimental infection with malaria using synthetic peptides. *Nature (London)* **328**, 629–32.

Patarroyo, M.E., Amador, R., Clavijo, P. *et al.* (1988). A synthetic vaccine protects humans against challenge with asexual blood stages of *Plasmodium falciparum* malaria. *Nature (London)* **332**, 158–61.

Pearson, C.D., McLean, S.A., Tetley, K. and Phillips, R.S. (1983). Induction of secondary antibody responses to *Plasmodium chabaudi in vitro*. *Clin. Exp. Immunol.* **52**, 121–8.

Peiris, J.S.M., Premawansa, S., Ranawaka, M.B.R. *et al.* (1988). Monoclonal and polyclonal antibodies both block and enhance transmission of human *Plasmodium vivax* malaria. *Am. J. Trop. Med. Hyg.* **39**, 26–32.

Perkins, M.E. and Rocco, L.J. (1988). Sialic acid-dependent binding of *Plasmodium falciparum* merozoite surface antigen, Pf200, to human erythrocytes. *J. Immunol.* **141**, 3190–6.

Perlmann, H.K., Berzins, K., Wahlgren, M. *et al.* (1984). Antibodies in malarial sera to parasite antigens in the membrane of erythrocytes infected with early stages of *Plasmodium falciparum*. *J. Exp. Med.* **159**, 1686–704.

Perlmann, H.K., Berzins, K., Wåhlin, B. *et al.* (1987). Absence of antigenic diversity in Pf155, a major parasite antigen in membranes of erythrocytes infected with *Plasmodium falciparum*. *J. Clin. Microbiol.* **25**, 2347–54.

Perlmann, H.K., Perlmann, P., Berzins, K. *et al.* (1989). Dissection of the human antibody response to the malaria antigen Pf155/RESA into epitope specific components. *Immunol. Rev.* **112**, 115–32.

Perlmann, P., Berzins, K., Carlsson, J. *et al.* (1986). Specificity and inhibitory activity of antibodies to a *Plasmodium falciparum* antigen (Pf155) and its major repeat sequence. In *Vaccines 86*, ed. R.A. Lerner, R.M. Chanock and F. Brown., pp. 149–55, Cold Spring Harbor Laboratories, New York.

Perrin, L.H., Ramirez, E., Lambert, P.H. and Miescher, P.A. (1981). Inhibition of *P. falciparum* growth in human erythrocytes by monoclonal antibodies. *Nature (London)* **289**, 301–3.

Perrin, L.H., Loche, M., Dedet, J.-P., Roussilhon, C. and Fandeur, T. (1984). Immunization against *Plasmodium falciparum* asexual blood stages using soluble antigens. *Clin. Exp. Immunol.* **56**, 67–72.

Perrin, L.H., Simitsek, P. and Srivastawa, I. (1988). Development of malaria vaccines. *Trop. Geog. Med.* **40**, S6–S21.

Petersen, E., Högh, B., Perlmann, H. *et al.* (1989). An epidemiological study of humoral and cell-mediated immune response to the *Plasmodium falciparum* antigen Pf155/RESA in adult Liberians. *Am. J. Trop. Med. Hyg.* **41**, 386–94.

Petersen, E., Högh, B., Marbiah, N.T. *et al.* (1990). A longitudinal study of antibodies to the *Plasmodium falciparum* antigen Pf155/RESA and immunity to malaria infection in adult Liberians. *Trans. Roy. Soc. Trop. Med. Hyg.* **84**, 339–45.

Peterson, M.G., Crewther, P.E., Thompson, J.K. *et al.* (1988). A second heat shock protein of *Plasmodium falciparum. DNA* **7**, 71–8.

Phillips, R.E. and Warrell, D.A. (1986). The pathophysiology of severe falciparum malaria. *Parasitol. Today* **2**, 271–82.

Pied, S., Nussler, A., Pontet, M. *et al.* (1989). C-reactive protein protects against preerythrocytic stages of malaria. *Infect. Immunity* **57**, 278–82.

Piessens, W.F., Hoffman, S.L., Wadee, A.A. *et al.* (1985). Antibody-mediated killing of suppressor T lymphocytes as a possible cause of macroglobulinemia in the tropical splenomegaly syndrome. *J. Clin. Invest.* **75**, 1821–7.

Ponnudurai, T., van Gemert, G.J., Bensink, T., Lensen, A.H.W. and Meuwissen, J.H.E.T. (1987). Transmission blockade of *Plasmodium falciparum*: its variability with gametocyte numbers and concentration of antibody. *Trans. Roy, Soc. Trop. Med. Hyg.* **81**, 491–3.

Pye, D., Edwards, S.J., Anders, R.F. *et al.* (1991). Failure of recombinant vaccinia viruses expressing *Plasmodium falciparum* antigens to protect *Saimiri* monkeys against malaria. *Infect. Immun.* **59**, 2403–11.

Quakyi, I.A., Matsumoto, Y., Carter, R. *et al.* (1989). Movement of a falciparum malarial protein through the erythrocyte cytoplasm to the erythrocyte membrane is associated with lysis of the erythrocyte and release of gametes. *Infect. Immunity* **57**, 833–9.

Richards, R.L., Hayre, M.D., Hockmeyer, W.T. and Alving, C.R. (1988). Liposomes, lipid A and aluminium hydroxide enhance the immune response to a synthetic malaria sporozoite antigen. *Infect. Immunity* **56**, 682–6.

Richards, R.L., Swartz, G.M., Schultz, C. *et al.* (1989). Immunogenicity of liposomal malaria sporozoites in monkeys: adjuvant effects of aluminium hydroxide on non-pyrogenic liposomal lipid A. *Vaccine* **7**, 506–11.

Rickman, L.S., Long, G.W., Oberst, R. *et al.* (1989). Rapid diagnosis of malaria by acridine orange staining of centrifuged parasites. *Lancet* **i**, 68–71.

Rieckmann, K.H., Carson, P.E., Beaudoin, R.L., Cassells, J. and Sell, K.W. (1974). Sporozoite induced immunity in man against an Ethiopian strain of *Plasmodium falciparum. Trans. Roy. Soc. Trop. Med. Hyg.* **68**, 258–9.

Riley, E.M., Jepsen, S., Andersson, G., Otoo, L.N. and Greenwood, B.M. (1988a). Cell-mediated immune responses to *Plasmodium falciparum* antigens in adult Gambians. *Clin. Exp. Immunol.* **71**, 377–82.

Riley, E.M., Andersson, G., Otoo, L.N., Jepsen, S. and Greenwood, B.M. (1988b). Cellular immune responses to *Plasmodium falciparum* antigens in Gambian children during and after an acute attack of falciparum malaria. *Clin. Exp. Immunol.* **73**, 17–22.

Robson, K.J.H., Hall, J.R.S., Jennings, M.W. *et al.* (1988). A highly conserved amino-acid sequence in thrombospondin, properdin and in proteins from sporozoites and blood stages of a human malaria parasite. *Nature (London)* **335**, 79–82.

Rockett, K.A., Targett, G.A.T. and Playfair, J.H.L. (1988). Killing of blood stage *Plasmodium falciparum* by lipid peroxidase from tumor necrosis serum. *Infect. Immunity* **56**, 3180–3.

Rodriguez, M.H. and Jungery, M. (1986). A protein on *Plasmodium falciparum* infected erythrocytes functions as a transferrin receptor. *Nature (London)* **324**, 388–91.

Romero, P., Maryanski, J.L., Corradin, G., Nussenzweig, R.S., Nussenzweig, V. and Zavala, F. (1989). Cloned cytotoxic T cells recognize an epitope in the circumsporozoite protein and protect against malaria. *Nature (London)* **341**, 323–6.

Rosenberg, E.B., Strickland, G.T., Yang, S.-L. and Whalen, G.E. (1973). IgM antibodies to red cells and autoimmune anemia in patients with malaria. *Am. J. Trop. Med. Hyg.* **22**, 146–52.

Rosenberg, Y.J. (1978). Autoimmune and polyclonal B cell responses during murine malaria. *Nature (London)* **274**, 170–2.

Ruangjirachuporn, W., Wåhlin, B., Perlmann, H.K. *et al.* (1988). Monoclonal antibodies to a synthetic peptide corresponding to a repeated sequence in the *Plasmodium falciparum* antigen Pf155. *Mol. Biochem. Parasitol.* **29**, 19–28.

Russo, D.M. and Weidanz, W.P. (1988). Activation of antigen-specific suppressor T cells by the intravenous injection of soluble blood-stage malarial antigen. *Cell. Immunol.* **115**, 437–46.

Rzepczyk, C.M., Saul, A.J. and Ferrante, A. (1984). Polyamine oxidase-mediated intraerythrocytic killing of *Plasmodium falciparum*: evidence against the role of reactive oxygen metabolites. *Infect. Immunity* **43**, 238–44.

Rzepczyk, C.M., Ramasamy, R., Ho, P.C.-L. *et al.* (1988). Identification of T epitopes within a potential *Plasmodium falciparum* vaccine antigen: a study of human lymphocyte responses to repeat and nonrepeat regions of Pf155/RESA. *J. Immunol.* **141**, 3197–202.

Sadoff, J.C., Ballou, W.R., Baron, L.S. *et al.* (1988). Oral *Salmonella typhimurium* vaccine expressing circumsporozoite protein protects against malaria. *Science* **240**, 336–8.

Sam-Yellowe, T.Y., Shio, H. and Perkins, M.E. (1988). Secretion of *Plasmodium falciparum* rhoptry protein into the plasma membrane of host erythrocytes. *J. Cell Biol.* **106**, 1507–13.

Santoro, F., Cochrane, A.H., Nussenzweig, V. *et al.* (1983). Structural similarities among the protective antigens of sporozoites from different species of malaria parasites. *J. Biol. Chem.* **258**, 3341–5.

Scherf, A., Hilbich, C., Sieg, K., Mattei, D., Mercereau-Puijalon, O. and Müller-Hill, B. (1988). The 11-1 gene of *Plasmodium falciparum* codes for distinct fast evolving repeats. *EMBO J.* **7**, 1129–37.

Schmidt-Ullrich, R., Brown, J., Whittle, H. and Lin, P.-S. (1986). Human–human hybridomas secreting monoclonal antibodies to the M_r 195 000 *Plasmodium falciparum* blood stage antigen. *J. Exp. Med.* **163**, 179–88.

Schofield, L., Villaquiran, J., Ferreira, A., Schellekens, H., Nussenzweig, R. and Nussenzweig, V. (1987). γ-Interferon, $CD8^+$ T cells and antibodies required for immunity to malaria sporozoites. *Nature (London)* **330**, 664–6.

Scuderi, P., Lam, K.S., Ryan, K.J. *et al.* (1986). Raised serum levels of tumour necrosis factor in parasite infections. *Lancet* **ii**, 1364–5.

Seed, T.M. and Kreier, J.P. (1980). Erythrocyte destruction mechanisms in malaria. In *Malaria*, ed. J.P. Kreier, vol. II, pp. 1–46, Academic Press, New York.

Shear, H.L., Srinivasan, R., Nolan, T. and Ng, C. (1989). Role of IFN-γ in lethal and non-lethal malaria in susceptible and resistant murine hosts. *J. Immunol.* **143**, 2038–44.

Siddiqui, W.A., Tam, L.Q., Kramer, K.J. *et al.* (1987). Merozoite surface coat precursor protein completely protects *Aotus* monkeys against *Plasmodium falciparum* malaria. *Proc. Nat. Acad. Sci. (USA)* **84**, 3014–18.

Sinigaglia, F. and Pink J.R.L. (1985) Human T lymphocyte clones specific for malaria (*Plasmodium falciparum*) antigens. *EMBO J.* **4**, 3819–22.

Sinigaglia, F. and Pink, J.R.L. (1990). A way round the 'real difficulties' of malaria sporozoite vaccine development? *Parasitol. Today* **6**, 17–19.

Sinigaglia, F., Guttinger, M., Gillessen, D. *et al.* (1988a). Epitopes recognized by human T lymphocytes on malaria circumsporozoite protein. *Eur. J. Immunol.* **18**, 633–6.

Sinigaglia, F., Guttinger, M., Kilgus, J. *et al.* (1988b). A malaria T-cell epitope recognized in association with most mouse and human MHC class II molecules. *Nature (London)* **336**, 778–80.

Sinigaglia, F., Takacs, B., Jacot, H. *et al.* (1988c). Nonpolymorphic regions of p190, a protein of the *Plasmodium falciparum* erythrocytic stage, contain both T and B cell epitopes. *J. Immunol.* **140**, 3568–72.

Smythe, J.A., Coppel, R.L., Brown, G.V., Ramasamy, R., Kemp, D.J. and Anders, R.F. (1988). Identification of two integral membrane proteins of *Plasmodium falciparum*. *Proc. Nat. Acad. Sci. (USA)* **85**, 5195–9.

Smythe, J.A., Peterson, M.G., Coppel, R.L., Saul, A.J., Kemp, D.J. and Anders, R.F. (1990). Structural diversity in the 45-kilodalton merozoite surface antigen of *Plasmodium falciparum*. *Mol. Biochem. Parasitol.* **39**, 227–34.

Srivastava, I.K., Takacs, B., Caspers, P. *et al.* (1989). Recombinant polypeptides for serology of malaria. *Trans. Roy. Soc. Trop. Med. Hyg.* **83**, 317–21.

Stahl, H.D., Kemp, D.J., Crewther, P.E. *et al.* (1985). Sequence of a cDNA encoding a small polymorphic histidine- and alanine-rich protein from *Plasmodium falciparum*. *Nucleic Acids Res.* **13**, 7837–46.

Stahl, H.D., Bianco, A.E., Crewther, P.E. *et al.* (1986). An asparagine-rich protein from blood stages of *Plasmodium falciparum* shares determinants with sporozoites. *Nucleic Acid Res.* **14**, 3089–3102.

Stevenson, M.M. and Ghadirian, E. (1989). Human recombinant tumor necrosis factor alpha protects susceptible A/J mice against lethal *Plasmodium chabaudi* AS infection. *Infect. Immunity* **57**, 3936–9.

Stevenson, M.M., Tam, M.F., Belosevic, M., van der Meide, P.H. and Podoba, J.E. (1990). Role of endogenous gamma interferon in host response to infection with blood-stage *Plasmodium chabaudi* AS. *Infect. Immunity* **58**, 3225–32.

Süss, G., Eichmann, K., Kury, E., Linke, A. and Langhorne, J. (1988). Roles of CD4- and CD8-bearing T lymphocytes in the immune response to the erythrocytic stages of *Plasmodium chabaudi*. *Infect. Immunity* **56**, 3081–8.

Szarfman, A., Lyon, J.A., Walliker, D. *et al.* (1988). Mature liver stages of cloned *Plasmodium falciparum* share epitopes with proteins from sporozoites and asexual blood stages. *Parasite Immunol.* **10**, 339–51.

Tam, J.P. (1988). Synthetic peptide vaccine design: synthesis and properties of a high-density multiple antigenic peptide system. *Proc. Nat. Acad. Sci. (USA)* **85**, 5409–13.

Tam, J.P., Clavijo, P., Lu, Y., Nussenzweig, V., Nussenzweig, R. and Zavala, F. (1990). Incorporation of T and B epitopes of the circumsporozoite protein in a chemically defined synthetic vaccine against malaria. *J. Exp. Med.* **171**, 299–306.

Tanabe, K., Mackay, M., Goman, M. and Scaife, J.G. (1987). Allelic dimorphism in a surface antigen gene of the malaria parasite *Plasmodium falciparum*. *J. Mol. Biol.* **195**, 273–87.

Tapchaisri, P., Chomcharn, Y., Poonthong, C. *et al.* (1983). Anti-sporozoite antibodies induced by natural infection. *Am. J. Trop. Med. Hyg.* **32**, 1203–8.

Targett, G.A.T. (1988). *Plasmodium falciparum*: natural and experimental transmission-blocking immunity. *Immunol. Lett.* **19**, 235–40.

Taverne, J., Tavernier, J., Fiers, W. and Playfair, J.H.L. (1987). Recombinant tumour necrosis factor inhibits malaria parasites *in vivo* but not *in vitro*. *Clin. Exp. Immunol.* **67**, 1–4.

Taylor, D.W., Parra, M., Chapman, G.B. *et al.* (1987). Localization of *Plasmodium falciparum* histidine-rich protein 1 in the erythrocyte skeleton under knobs. *Mol. Biochem. Parasitol.* **25**, 165–74.

Togna, A.R., Del Giudice, G., Verdini, A.S. *et al.* (1986). Synthetic *Plasmodium falciparum* circumsporozoite peptides elicit heterogenous L3T4$^+$ T-cell proliferative responses in H-2^b mice. *J. Immunol.* **137**, 2956–60.

Torii, M., Adams, J.H., Miller, L.H. and Aikawa, M. (1989). Release of merozoite dense granules during erythrocyte invasion by *Plasmodium knowlesi*. *Infect. Immunity* **57**, 3230–3.

Trager, W. and Jensen, J.B. (1976). Human malaria parasites in continuous culture. *Science* **193**, 673–5.

Trager, W., Rudzinska, M.A. and Bradbury, P.C. (1966). The fine structure of *Plasmodium falciparum* and its host erythrocyte in natural malarial infections in man. *Bull. WHO* **35**, 883–5.

Triglia, T., Stahl, H.-D., Crewther, P.E., Silva, A., Anders, R.F. and Kemp, D.J. (1988). Structure of a *Plasmodium falciparum* gene that encodes a glutamic acid-rich protein (GARP). *Mol. Biochem. Parasitol.* **31**, 199–202.

Troye-Blomberg, M. and Perlmann, P. (1988). T cell functions in *Plasmodium falciparum* and other malarias. *Prog. Allergy* **41**, 253–87.

Troye-Blomberg, M., Romero, P., Patarroyo, M.-E., Björkman, A. and Perlmann, P. (1984). Regulation of the immune response in *Plasmodium falciparum* malaria. III. Proliferative response to antigen *in vitro* and subset composition of T cells from patients with acute infection or from immune donors. *Clin. Exp. Immunol.* **58**, 380–7.

Troye-Blomberg, M., Kabilan, L., Andersson, G., Patarroyo, M.E. and Perlmann, P. (1987). Cellular regulation of the immune response in *Plasmodium falciparum* malaria *in vitro*. In *Immune Regulation by Characterized Polypeptides*, ed. G. Goldstein, J.-F. Bach and H. Wigzell, pp. 699–709, Alan R. Liss, New York.

Troye-Blomberg, M., Kabilan, L., Riley, E.M. *et al.* (1988). T cell reactivity of defined peptides from a major *Plasmodium falciparum* vaccine candidate: the Pf155/RESA antigen. *Immunol. Lett.* **19**, 229–34.

Troye-Blomberg, M., Riley, E.M., Perlmann, H. *et al.* (1989). T and B cell responses of *Plasmodium falciparum* malaria immune individuals to sequences in different regions of the *P. falciparum* antigen Pf155/RESA. *J. Immunol.* **143**, 3043–8.

Troye-Blomberg, M., Riley, E.M., Kabilan, L. *et al.* (1990). Production by activated human T cells of interleukin 4 but not interferon-γ is associated with elevated levels of serum antibodies to activating malaria antigens. *Proc. Nat. Acad. Sci. (USA)* **87**, 5484–8.

Udeinya, I.J., Leech, J., Aikawa, M. and Miller, L.H. (1985). An *in vitro* assay for sequestration: binding of *Plasmodium falciparum*-infected erythrocytes to formalin-fixed endothelial cells and amelanotic melanoma cells. *J. Protozool.* **32**, 88–90.

Udomsangpetch, R., Aikawa, M., Berzins, K., Wahlgren, M. and Perlmann, P. (1989a). Cytoadherence of knobless *Plasmodium falciparum* infected erythrocytes and its inhibition by a human monoclonal antibody. *Nature (London)* **338**, 763–5.

Udomsangpetch, R., Carlsson, J., Wåhlin, B. *et al.* (1989b). Reactivity of the human monoclonal antibody 33G2 with repeated sequences of three distinct *Plasmodium falciparum* antigens. *J. Immunol.* **142**, 3620–6.

Udomsangpetch, R., Wåhlin, B., Carlson, J. *et al.* (1989c). *Plasmodium falciparum*-infected erythrocytes from spontaneous erythrocyte rosettes. *J. Exp. Med.* **169**, 1835–40.

Uni, S., Masuda, A., Stewart, M.J., Igarashi, I., Nussenzweig, R. and Aikawa, M. (1987). Ultrastructural localization of the 150/130 kd antigens in sexual and asexual blood stages of *Plasmodium falciparum*-infected human erythrocytes. *Am. J. Trop. Med. Hyg.* **36**, 481–8.

Vergara, U., Ferreira, A., Schellekens, H. and Nussenzweig, V. (1987). Mechanism of escape of exoerythrocytic forms (EEF) of malaria parasites from the inhibitory effects of interferon-γ. *J. Immunol.* **138**, 4447–9.

von Brunn, A., Früh, K., Stunnenberg, B. and Bujard, H. (1988). 22 nm-like particles of the hepatitis B surface antigen containing epitopes of p190 of *P. falciparum*. In *Technological Advances in Vaccine Development*, ed. L. Lasky, pp. 167–73, Alan R. Liss, New York.

Wahlgren, M. (1986). Antigens and antibodies involved in humoral immunity to *Plasmodium falciparum*. Thesis, Karolinska Institute, Stockholm, ISBN 91-7900-026-6.

Wahlgren, M., Berzins, K., Perlmann, P. and Björkman, A. (1983). Characterization of the humoral immune response in *Plasmodium falciparum* malaria. I. Estimation of antibodies to *P. falciparum* or human erythrocytes by means of microELISA. *Clin. Exp. Immunol.* **53**, 127–34.

Wahlgren, M., Åslund, L., Franzén, L. *et al.* (1986a). A *Plasmodium falciparum* antigen containing clusters of asparagine residues. *Proc. Natl. Acad. Sci. (USA)* **83**, 2677–81.

Wahlgren, M., Björkman, A., Perlmann, H.K., Berzins, K. and Perlmann, P. (1986b). Anti-*Plasmodium falciparum* antibodies acquired by residents in a holoendemic area of Liberia during development of clinical immunity. *Am. J. Trop. Med. Hyg.* **35**, 22–9.

Wahlgren, M., Perlmann, H.K., Berzins, K. *et al.* (1986c). Characterization of the humoral immune response in *Plasmodium falciparum* malaria. III. Factors influencing the coexpression of antibody isotypes (IgM and IgG-1 to 4). *Clin. Exp. Immunol.* **63**, 343–53.

Wahlgren, M., Carlson, J., Udomsangpetch, R. and Perlmann, P. (1989). Why do *Plasmodium falciparum*-infected erythrocytes form spontaneous erythrocyte rosettes? *Parasitol. Today* **5**, 183–5.

Weber, J.L., Lyon, J.A, Wolff, R.H., Hall, T., Lowell, G.H. and Chulay, J.D. (1988). Primary structure of a *Plasmodium falciparum* malaria antigen located at the merozoite surface and within the parasitophorous vacuole. *J. Biol. Chem.* **263**, 11421–5.

Weidanz, W.P. and Long, C.A. (1988). The role of T cells in immunity to malaria. *Prog. Allergy* **41**, 215–52.

Weiss, W.R., Sedegah, M., Beaudoin, R.L., Miller, L.H. and Good, M.F. (1988). $CD8^+$ T cells (cytotoxic/suppressors) are required for protection in mice immunized with malaria sporozoites. *Proc. Nat. Acad. Sci. (USA)* **85**, 573–6.

Weiss, W.R., Mellouk, S., Houghten, R.A. *et al.* (1990) Cytotoxic T cells recognize a peptide from the circumsporozoite protein on malaria-infected hepatocytes. *J. Exp. Med.* **171**, 763–73.

Wernsdorfer, W.H. (1980). The importance of malaria in the world. In *Malaria*, ed. J.P. Kreier, vol. I, pp. 1–93, Academic Press, New York.

Whittle, H.C., Brown, J., Marsh, K. *et al.* (1984). T-cell control of Epstein–Barr virus-infected B cells is lost during *P. falciparum* malaria. *Nature (London)* **312**, 449–50.

Wilson, R.J.M. (1980). Serotyping *Plasmodium falciparum* malaria with S-antigens. *Nature (London)* **284**, 451–2.

Wilson, R.J.M., McGregor, I.A., Hall, P., Williams, K. and Bartholomew, R. (1969). Antigens associated with *Plasmodium falciparum* infections in man. *Lancet* **ii**, 201–5.

Winograd, E. and Sherman, I.W. (1989). Characterization of a modified red cell membrane protein expressed on erythrocytes infected with the human malaria parasite *Plasmodium falciparum*: possible role as a cytoadherent mediating protein. *J. Cell Biol.* **108**, 23–30.

World Health Organization (1986). Severe and complicated malaria. *Trans. Roy. Soc. Trop. Med. Hyg.* **80**, 1–50.

World Health Organization (1987). In *Tropical Disease Research: A Global Partnership*, ed. J. Maurice and A.M. Pearce, p. 20, World Health Organization, Geneva.

World Health Organization (1988). Malaria diagnosis: memorandum from a WHO meeting. *Bull. WHO* **66**, 575–94.

World Health Organization (1991) In *Weekly Epidemiol. Rec.* **66**, 156–64.

Yoshida, N., Nussenzweig, R.S., Potocnjak, P., Nussenzweig, V. and Aikawa, M. (1980). Hybridoma produces protective antibodies directed against the sporozoite stage of malaria parasite. *Science* **207**, 71–3.

Zavala, F., Gwadz, R.W., Collins, F.H., Nussenzweig, R.S. and Nussenzweig, V. (1982). Monoclonal antibodies to circumsporozoite protein identify the species of malaria parasite in infected mosquitoes. *Nature* **299**, 737–8.

Zavala, F., Tam, J.P., Cochrane, A.H., Quakyi, I., Nussenzweig, R.S. and Nussenzweig, V. (1985). Rationale for development of a synthetic vaccine against *Plasmodium falciparum* malaria. *Science* **228**, 1436–40.

Zevering, Y., Houghten, R.A., Frazer, I.H. and Good, M.F. (1990). Major population differences in T cell response to a malaria sporozoite vaccine candidate. *Int. Immunol.* **2**, 945–55.

Zouali, M., Druilhe, P., Gentilini, M. and Eyquem, A. (1982). High titres of anti-T antibodies and other haemagglutinins in human malaria. *Clin. Exp. Immunol.* **50**, 83–91.

Zouali, M., Druilhe, P. and Eyquem, A. (1986). IgG-subclass expression of anti-DNA and anti-ribonucleoprotein autoantibodies in human malaria. *Clin. Exp. Immunol.* **66**, 273–8.

80: Immunology of Leishmaniasis

J.M. Blackwell

Introduction

The application of advanced molecular and cellular technology to the study of parasite immunology has given new insight into the interactions between parasite and host which regulate the outcome of infection and thus provide potential targets for disease control. Leishmaniasis, in particular, provides a model system in which to observe the impact of advanced technology in sorting out what appeared 5 years ago to be largely phenomenology. The means by which leishmanial parasites could, for example, activate the complement cascade and yet remain infective for the host was not well understood, while ill-defined concepts of 'suppression' of cell-mediated immunity led to the 'proliferation' of operationally defined T cell subsets now more rationally defined in functional terms by their cytokine profiles. To provide a logical sequence to our examination of the latest developments in *Leishmania* immunology this review will follow the fate of the parasite as it enters the host and its interactions with the immune system (see Fig. 80.1). In so doing we will examine: (i) what constitutes an infective leishmanial parasite; (ii) how this parasite evades the lytic consequences of activating the complement cascade, using it instead to advantage in gaining access to its preferred host cell; (iii) the intracellular fate of the parasite in naïve and activated macrophage populations; (iv) the induction, maintenance and characterization of antigen-specific T cell responses; and (v) immunotherapy, immunoprophylaxis and the design of a vaccine suitable for use in genetically diverse human populations. Before transmitting our parasite by way of its sandfly vector into the host, a brief update on current *Leishmania* taxonomy in relation to clinical patterns and immunological features of human disease will be given.

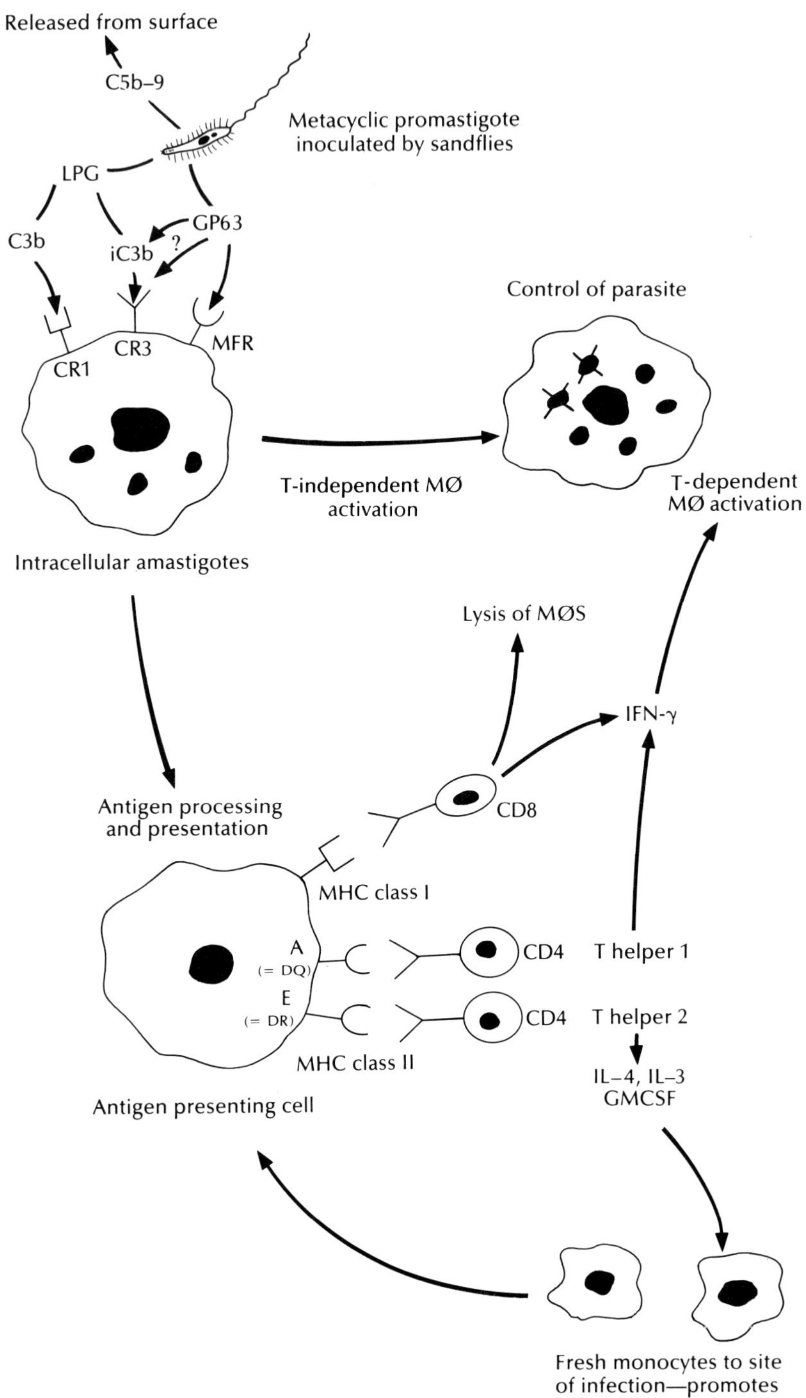

Fig. 80.1. Model of molecular interactions between leishmanial parasites (and their products) and the vertebrate immune system which influence the course of infection.

Leishmania taxonomy and clinical patterns of disease

Early separation of *Leishmania* species was based on clinical patterns of disease and later included other distinguishing characteristics such as geographical distribution, reservoir host species, vectors, and behaviour in hamsters and in culture *in vitro* (Lainson and Shaw 1972, 1979). Most of the early species and subspecies classified in this way have since been confirmed using isoenzyme (Gardener *et al*. 1974; Chance *et al*. 1977; Gardener 1977; Miles *et al*. 1981; Chance 1982; Miles 1985), monoclonal antibody (McMahon Pratt and David

1981; McMahon Pratt *et al.* 1982, 1985; Jaffe and McMahon Pratt 1983, 1984) or DNA probe (Arnot and Barker 1981; Barker and Butcher 1983; Barker *et al.* 1986) techniques. Based on these criteria, many (though not all) taxonomists now favour raising the major sub-species to full species status (Lainson and Shaw 1987). This paper will follow this updated classification as outlined in Table 80.1. Clinical patterns and broad immunological features (e.g. skin test response to specific antigen *in vivo*; proliferative response of peripheral blood T cells to specific antigen *in vitro*) of disease associated with these species are as follows.

Visceral leishmaniasis

Visceral infection is classically associated with *L. donovani* and *L. infantum* in the Old World and *L. chagasi* in the New World. Immunoepidemiological studies carried out in different areas indicate that only a small proportion (probably less than one in five) of infections with these species lead to severe visceral disease, many people in endemic regions developing positive skin test responses to leishmanial antigen (Ho *et al.* 1982; Badaro *et al.* 1986a, b; Sacks *et al.* 1987), proliferative responses to specific antigen in T cell assays *in vitro* (Sacks *et al.* 1987), or hepatic granulomata (Pampiglione *et al.* 1974), without ever having presented with clinical disease. Clinical disease is characterized by profound non-responsiveness to leishmanial antigen both in skin tests (Rezai *et al.* 1978; Ho *et al.* 1983) and T cell assays (Carvalho *et al.* 1981; Haldar *et al.* 1983; Ho *et al.* 1983; Sacks *et al.* 1987). Primary cutaneous lesions preceding *L. donovani* are rarely reported from endemic regions, although self-healing lesions have been observed in laboratory infections with an Ethiopian strain of *L. donovani* (pers. obs.), again associated with development of skin test and T cell reactivity to leishmanial antigen (Melby *et al.* 1989). Rioux *et al.* (1980) and Belazzoug *et al.* (1985) have also reported cases of solitary self-healing lesions, caused by natural infection with *L. infantum* in France and Algeria, with no visceral disease. Secondary cutaneous lesions, post-kala-azar dermal leishmaniasis or PKDL, are observed following successful drug cure of visceral disease in 20% of Indian and 5% of East African cases of *L. donovani* (Bryceson 1986). Patients with PKDL vary in skin test positivity (Sen Gupta and Mukherjee 1962; Munro *et al.* 1972) and responsiveness to leishmanial antigen in T cell assays *in vitro* (Haldar *et al.* 1983).

Table 80.1. Species of *Leishmania* belonging to four major species complexes. Disease profiles observed in man are shown along with the broad geographical distribution for each species. Data compiled from Zuckerman and Lainson (1977), Lainson (1983) and Lainson and Shaw (1987).

Species complex	Species	Disease in man	Geographical distribution
L. tropica	*L. tropica*	LCL; LR	Asia, Africa, Europe
	L. major	LCL	Asia, Africa
	L. aethiopica	LCL; DCL; MCL	Ethiopia, Kenya
L. donovani	*L. donovani*	VL; PKDL	India, Nepal, China, Kenya, Sudan
	L. infantum	VL	Mediterranean, China, Africa, Asia
	L. chagasi	VL	South America
L. mexicana	*L. mexicana*	LCL; DCL	Central America
	L. amazonensis	LCL; DCL	Brazil, Amazon basin
	L. pifanoi	LCL; DCL	Venezuela
L. braziliensis	*L. braziliensis*	LCL; MCL	Brazil, Venezuela
	L. panamensis	LCL	Panama, Costa Rica
	L. guyanensis	LCL	Brazil, Guyana, Surinam
	L. peruviana	LCL	Peru, Argentina

LCL = localized cutaneous lesion; LR = leishmaniasis recidivans; DCL = diffuse cutaneous leishmaniasis; MCL = mucocutaneous leishmaniasis; VL = visceral leishmaniasis; PKDL = post-kala-azar dermal leishmaniasis.

Old World cutaneous leishmaniasis

Three different species of *Leishmania*, *L. major*, *L. tropica* and *L. aethiopica*, are associated with cutaneous leishmaniasis in the Old World. Infection with *L. major*, classically recognized as rural or zoonotic cutaneous leishmaniasis, leads to rapid lesion development typically resulting in necrosis, ulceration, exudation and crust formation with surrounding inflammation (Bryceson 1986). Lesions self-heal in 3–6 months, infection being accompanied by development of skin test and T cell reactivity (Witzum *et al.* 1978; Wyler *et al.* 1979). Lesions caused by urban, anthroponotic *L. tropica* infection generally take longer (5–14 months) to heal. In some cases the primary lesion fails to heal, new nodules arising at the edge of the scar which may ulcerate and cause destructive sores (Bryceson 1986). This condition, known as recidivans, is associated with tuberculoid histology, lesions containing histiocytic granulomas with or without giant cells, with pronounced lymphocyte infiltration and very few parasites (Zuckerman and Lainson 1977). Patients develop strong skin test responses to leishmanial antigen (Ardehali *et al.* 1980). The third Old World cutaneous species, *L. aethiopica*, produces small nodules with little local inflammation which take 1–3 years to heal (Bryceson 1986). Patients with localized lesions generally develop skin test (Bryceson 1970) and T cell (Schurr *et al.* 1986) reactivity to leishmanial antigen. Local spreading of nodules to produce larger tumour-like lesions is frequent. In rare cases, metastases occur elsewhere in the skin and diffuse cutaneous leishmaniasis (DCL), characterized by lack of responsiveness to specific antigen in skin test (Bryceson 1970) and T cell (Schurr *et al.* 1986) assays, develops. Diffuse cutaneous leishmaniasis occurs only with *L. aethiopica*. Neither recidivans nor DCL are seen with *L. major* infection. Lesions may occur on the mucocutaneous border of the nose with any of the Old World cutaneous species (e.g. Al-Ginden *et al.* 1983) but destruction of nasal cartilage is usually only observed with *L. aethiopica* (Bryceson 1986) and is never as severe as the mucocutaneous leishmaniasis (MCL) seen with New World species.

New World cutaneous leishmaniasis

The taxonomy of Central and South American species of *Leishmania* causing cutaneous disease is complex, although the broad division (see Table 85.1) into *L. braziliensis* and *L. mexicana* species complexes is supported by sequence homology analysis using kinetoplast deoxyribonucleic acid (DNA) (Barker and Butcher 1983; Barker *et al.* 1986). All species produce localized lesions which self-heal at varying rates in the majority of patients and are associated with skin test (Lynch *et al.* 1982) and T cell (Castes *et al.* 1983, 1984) responsiveness to leishmanial antigen. *Leishmania mexicana* produces small nodular lesions which crust and heal in 3–5 months (Bryceson 1986). Lesions on the ear occur in up to 40% of cases (Zuckerman and Lainson 1977) and result in invasion of the cartilage and slow destruction of the pinna over many years. Diffuse cutaneous leishmaniasis has been reported in a few cases of *L. mexicana* in Mexico (Ramos Aguire 1970) but is more generally associated with *L. amazonensis* in the Amazon region of Brazil (Lainson 1983) and with the related parasite *L. pifanoi* in Venezuela (Convit *et al.* 1972). Histologically, DCL lesions are composed almost entirely of highly vacuolated macrophages containing numerous parasites and with very few lymphocytes present (Convit *et al.* 1972). Patients with DCL fail to respond to leishmanial antigen in skin tests *in vivo* (Petersen *et al.* 1982, 1984; Castes *et al.* 1983) or T cell proliferation assays *in vitro* (Petersen *et al.* 1982; Castes *et al.* 1983, 1984). *Leishmania amazonensis* has also recently been isolated from bone marrow aspirated from a typical visceral leishmaniasis patient in Brazil (Barral *et al.* 1986).

Leishmania braziliensis causes large, deep and destructive lesions of 12 or more months' duration (Bryceson 1986), and can be followed by severe and disfiguring MCL, which may appear as the primary lesion is healing or at any time from months to many years later (Walton *et al.* 1973; Zuckerman and Lainson 1977; Marsden 1986). Mucocutaneous leishmaniasis is characterized by strong skin test (Shaw and Lainson 1975; Moriearty *et al.* 1978) and T cell reactivity (Castes *et al.* 1983, 1984; Carvalho *et al.* 1985a). Recent reports also suggest that DCL-like conditions may occur with *L. braziliensis* infection (Goto *et al.* 1989) but immunological studies have not been performed. Other members of this complex, *L. guyanensis* and *L. panamensis*, also cause cutaneous leishmaniasis with one or more lesions but have not been reported from MCL cases. *Leishmania peruviana* causes solitary lesions on the face, which self-heal in less than 1 year, and has not been associated with MCL or DCL (Bryceson 1986).

Metacyclogenesis

Parasites entering the host from the sandfly vector meet with first-line non-specific immune mechanisms: complement and phagocytes. Although earlier investigation (Killick-Kendrick 1979) had pointed to the possibility that flagellated promastigotes underwent a morphological transformation from non-infective to infective 'metacyclic' forms during development in the sandfly gut, this has only more recently been defined in terms of functionally important, developmentally regulated changes at the molecular level, which can be mimicked in culture form promastigotes (Sacks and Perkins 1984; Sacks *et al.* 1985; da Silva and Sacks 1987; Sacks and da Silva 1987). The most dramatic developmentally regulated change which has been observed during metacyclogenesis involves additional glycosylation (Sacks and da Silva 1987; Sacks *et al.* 1989) of a major surface lipophosphoglycan (LPG) molecule which, for *L. major*, alters the width of the glycocalyx on the cell surface from 7 to 17 nm (Pimenta *et al.* 1989). For *L. major* (Sacks *et al.* 1985; da Silva and Sacks 1987) and *L. donovani* (Howard *et al.* 1987; Cooper *et al.* 1988), glycosylation of the LPG molecule alters the ability of the promastigote to bind the lectin peanut agglutinin (PNA). This provides a convenient means of characterizing (Cooper *et al.* 1988) or separating (Sacks *et al.* 1985; da Silva and Sacks 1987) populations of PNA +ve logarithmic-phase promastigotes and PNA −ve metacyclics. Although comparative studies of the two populations now serve to demonstrate preadaptation of metacyclics to the host environment, it should be recognized that most studies predating 1985 (and many since) were carried out using logarithmic or, at best, mixed promastigote populations and should therefore be scrutinized rather carefully. Unfortunately, South American cutaneous species do not share the same lectin-binding characteristics so it is not possible to separate populations by the same criteria. It should, nevertheless, be possible to develop monoclonal antibodies which will recognize metacyclic LPG in these species.

The LPG molecule of *L. donovani* has been characterized biochemically (Turco *et al.* 1984, 1987; Turco 1988) as a heterogeneous glycoconjugate of around 9 kD with an average of 16 repeating phosphorylated disaccharide units ($PO_4 \rightarrow 6$ Gal (β1,4) Man α1) linked in a linear array by α-glycosidic linkages. The antigenically distinct *L. major* LPG has multiple phosphorylated tri- and tetrasaccharide units containing galactose, mannose, glucose and arabinose (McConville *et al.* 1987), the tetrasaccharides being modified in metacyclic LPG (Sacks *et al.* 1989). The repeating phosphorylated disaccharide units of *L. donovani* LPG are attached to a unique heptasaccharide carbohydrate core containing three galactose, two mannose, one glucose and one glucosamine residues (Turco *et al.* 1987). The molecule is anchored in the membrane via a novel lyso-1-*O*-alkyl-phosphatidylinositol (PI) lipid (Turco *et al.* 1987), the first PI lipid anchor reported for a polysaccharide. As a major component (at least 1.25×10^6 copies per promastigote; Orlandi and Turco 1987) of the promastigote, and especially the metacyclic (Pimenta *et al.* 1989), surface the LPG molecule provides an important interface between parasite and host. The molecule, known from the earlier literature as excreted factor, is also said to be found on amastigotes (Schnur *et al.* 1972) and on the surface of infected macrophages (Berman and Dwyer 1981) but these observations have not been confirmed with specific monoclonal reagents.

Another major surface component which changes in expression during development of *Leishmania* promastigotes in culture (Kweider *et al.* 1987) and in the sandfly gut (Davies *et al.* 1990) is the glycoprotein known as GP63 (or GP65) (Bouvier *et al.* 1985). Glycoprotein 63 is a protease (Etges *et al.* 1986a; Bordier 1987) which is also anchored to the membrane by a PI lipid anchor (Etges *et al.* 1986b), probably via a more conventional diacylated PI as found for many other eukaryote membrane proteins (Cross 1987; Ferguson and Williams 1988), including trypanosome variable surface glycoproteins (Ferguson *et al.* 1985) and mammalian Thy-1 (Low and Kincade 1985). For GP63 there are an estimated 500 000 copies at the surface of each promastigote, representing 0.5–1% of the total cellular protein (Bouvier *et al.* 1985). The molecule is highly conserved across species of *Leishmania* (Colomer-Gould *et al.* 1985; Etges *et al.* 1986a; Bouvier *et al.* 1987). Glycoprotein 63 has been cloned and sequenced for *L. major* (Button and McMaster 1988; McMaster 1990), *L. chagasi* (Miller *et al.* 1989) and *L. donovani* (W.R. McMaster, pers. comm.), with 87% sequence conservation observed between *L. major* and *L. donovani* at the DNA level and 84% at the protein level. Monoclonal antibody studies originally suggested that GP63 was not expressed on amastigotes (Fong and Chang 1982; Chang *et al.* 1986) but more recent data using Western blot analysis with monoclonals raised against fusion protein, as well as studies at the ribonucleic acid (RNA) level, confirm that GP63 is synthesized and expressed in amastigotes (W.R. McMaster and D.G. Russell, pers. comm.). Using the anti-GP63 monoclonal antibody 3.8, Davies and co-workers (1990) did not observe GP63 on promastigotes transforming in sandflies fed on murine blood containing *L. major* amastigotes until 4 days after the blood feed. This may parallel the observation that GP63 increases in expression as *L. braziliensis* (but not *L. chagasi*) promastigotes proceed from logarithmic to stationary phase in culture (Kweider *et al.* 1987) but this has not been correlated precisely with metacyclogenesis as defined by changes in the LPG molecule. Since this is a quantitative rather than a qualitative difference, it cannot be used to distinguish metacyclic parasites. Nevertheless, as we shall see, both LPG and GP63 feature strongly in studies examining the interaction between the parasite and the host's immune system.

Interaction with complement

The complement system provides two important ways in which the non-immune host can attack invading micro-organisms: (i) by formation of the membrane attack complex and direct lysis of the organism; or (ii) to opsonize the invader for uptake by phagocytes such as polymorphonuclear leucocytes (PMN) and macrophages. Entry of leishmanial promastigotes (Chang 1981; Pearson and Steigbigel 1981) or amastigotes (Chang 1978) into PMN generally results in destruction of the parasite, but successful entry into macrophages is crucial since *Leishmania* spp. are obligate intracellular pathogens of the mononuclear phagocyte system. Hence, opsonization and binding to complement receptors might provide the parasite with an easy means of entry into the preferred host cell. It would therefore be advantageous for metacyclic parasites to activate the alternative or classical complement pathways, but how do they avoid formation of, or lysis by, the terminal membrane attack complex?

Complement activation and resistance to lysis

Franke and co-workers (1985) demonstrated that stationary-phase promastigotes of various species of *Leishmania* are relatively resistant to fresh non-immune human serum compared with the exquisite serum sensitivity of log-phase organisms. Using promastigotes of *L. major* separated into log and metacyclic populations according to PNA-binding characteristics, Puentes *et al.* (1988) found that, although both forms activate complement and deposit C3 (predominantly in the form C3b rather than iC3b) on their surface, different mechanisms are involved. Log-phase organisms activate the alternative pathway and bind C3 covalently via O-ester linkages. Metacyclics activate the classical pathway (independently of antibody) and bind C3 non-covalently. Immunoprecipitation experiments demonstrated that the LPG molecule is the major C3 acceptor on both log and metacyclic parasites. Hence, failure to activate complement and bind C3 could not account for serum resistance in metacyclic forms. In pursuing the mechanisms of serum resistance, Puentes and co-workers (1989) have gone on to demonstrate that, while deposition of C5b-7 is stable in metacyclics, the majority of C5b-9 is spontaneously released. This suggests that the developmental modification of the LPG molecule (Sacks and da Silva 1987) and the increase in width of the glycocalyx (Pimenta *et al.* 1989) block insertion of lytic C5b-9 into the promastigote membrane in a manner analogous to that previously reported for smooth, serum-resistant isolates of *Salmonella* (Joiner *et al.* 1982). As for rough, serum-sensitive *Salmonella*, C5b-9 inserts stably into the membranes of log promastigotes and results in lysis.

Detailed studies of this kind using well-characterized log and metacyclic promastigote populations of other species of *Leishmania* have not been performed, previous reports on complement activation by unfractionated populations of promastigotes oscillating between the demonstration of antibody-dependent classical pathway activation, even with non-immune serum (Pearson and Steigbigel 1980), and alternative pathway activation (Mosser and Edelson 1984; Blackwell *et al.* 1985a; Franke *et al.* 1985; Mosser *et al.* 1986). Clearly more refined studies are required.

Leishmanial parasites may be exposed to complement products again when amastigotes transfer from one macrophage to another. In this case interesting species differences are observed, amastigotes of *L. major* being sensitive to lysis by fresh human serum whereas those of *L. donovani* are resistant (Hoover *et al.* 1984; Mosser *et al.* 1985). Using the Riches and Stanworth (1980) method for measuring alternative pathway activation, we found amastigotes of *L. donovani* LV9 to be very poor activators (Blackwell *et al.* 1985a). In similar, assays using *L. donovani* 1-S, Mosser and co-workers (1985) reported equivalent complement consumption to that observed with *L. major* and *L. mexicana*, although the number of ^{125}I-labelled C3 molecules bound per amastigote was only about half (3.7×10^4) that measured for *L. major* ($6.6. \times 10^4$) or *L. mexicana* (5.9×10^4). Since amastigotes of the strain of *L. mexicana* used are also resistant to lysis by human serum (Mosser *et al.* 1985), the simple conclusion that cutaneous species bind C3 more efficiently and are therefore serum-sensitive while visceral species bind C3 inefficiently and are serum-resistant cannot be drawn. Nor can the observation that some strains of *L. mexicana* or *L. major* visceralize in mice be used to distinguish visceralizing from cutaneous human strains since the same strain (NIH173) of *L. major* amastigotes may be resistant to lysis in murine serum (pers. obs.) but sensitive in human serum (Hoover *et al.* 1984). It is clear nevertheless that, as with log and metacyclic promastigotes, the fate of bound C3 may be different for amastigotes from different leishmanial strains and might therefore help to determine their fate *in vivo*.

Entry into macrophages

Studies from our laboratory (Blackwell *et al.* 1985a) were amongst the first to demonstrate a role for complement receptors in binding promastigotes to macrophages. These studies were of particular interest at the time because inhibition of binding of *L. donovani* promastigotes to the murine macrophage type 3 complement (iC3b) receptor (CR3) using the anti-CR3 monoclonal antibody M1/70 (Beller *et al.* 1982) could be demonstrated in the absence of an exogenous (serum) complement source. Mosser and Edelson (1985) made a similar observation for *L. major* promastigotes. Additional data on the ability to block *L. donovani* promastigote binding in the presence either of an anti-C3 antibody or of the nucleophile sodium salicyl hydroxamate (Saha), which inhibits covalent binding of C3 to an activator surface (Sim *et al.* 1981), suggested that binding of promastigotes to murine CR3 was mediated by local opsonization with macrophage-derived complement components (Blackwell *et al.* 1985a). This, in turn, could be demonstrated using the anti-C3 antibody, protein A–gold labelling and transmission electron microscopy (Wozencraft *et al.* 1986). Addition of an exogenous (serum) source of complement greatly enhanced C3 deposition on promastigotes, mediating a 5–10-fold increase in their M1/70-inhibitable binding to macrophages (Blackwell *et al.* 1985a). These early results required clarification following (i) the demonstration that CR3 has multiple epitopes or binding sites, one of which mediates the binding of iC3b via an arginine–glycine–aspartic acid (RGD)-containing sequence (Wright *et al.* 1987) while another or others are involved in direct interactions with molecules other than C3 (e.g. yeast zymosan (Ross *et al.* 1985); β-glucan (Ross *et al.* 1987); bacterial lipopolysaccharides (LPS) (Wright and Jong 1986)); (ii) the molecular characterization of log-form and metacyclic promastigotes (Sacks and da Silva 1987); and (iii) the demonstration that GP63 contains an RGD sequence (Button and McMaster 1988).

In further studies (Cooper *et al.* 1988) carried out using murine macrophages and populations of *L. donovani* and *L. major* promastigotes characterized according to their ability to bind the lectin PNA, we obtained differential inhibition for the serum-independent binding of log forms versus metacyclics using different anti-CR3 antibodies, M1/70 and 5C6 (Rosen and Gordon 1987), and Saha. The Saha inhibition data suggested that 5C6- and M1/70-inhibitable binding of PNA +ve log forms was mediated by covalently bound C3 (iC3b) while the M1/70-inhibitable binding of metacyclics was not. In parallel studies examining the serum-independent binding and ingestion of stationary-phase *L. donovani* promastigotes to human monocyte-derived macrophages, Wilson and Pearson (1988) also found differential inhibition using monoclonal antibodies which bind to different epitopes on CR3. OKM10, which blocks EiC3b-rosetting (Wright *et al.* 1983a), failed to inhibit while OKM1, which is believed to block the lectin-binding site, was a potent inhibitor. One possibility for the direct binding of metacyclics to CR3 lay in the observation that GP63, identified by earlier studies (Russell and Wilhelm 1986) as a possible parasite ligand for macrophage attachment, has the capacity to bind directly* to the iC3b-binding site of human CR3 via its RGD-containing sequence (Russell and Wright 1988). Whether this holds true for murine CR3 or is differentially inhibitable by the two antibodies, M1/70 and 5C6, is not known. This hypothesis would, in any case, be inconsistent with the human study (Wilson and Pearson 1988) since antibodies (e.g. OKM10) which block the iC3b-binding site would also be expected to block direct binding of the GP63 RGD sequence to CR3. An alternative hypothesis for direct binding to CR3 is that LPG, also identified as a parasite ligand for macrophages (Handman and Goding 1985), may bind directly to the LPS-binding site of CR3, a possibility consistent with the parallel macrophage-activating capacities of LPS (Hamilton and Adams 1987), M1/70 (Ding *et al*. 1987) and PNA −ve promastigotes (Blackwell *et al*. 1988; (see below)). Considering the density of LPG expressed on the metacyclic surface and the increase in width of the glycocalyx mediated by the additional glycosylation of the LPG molecule (Sacks and da Silva 1987; Pimenta *et al*. 1989), it is difficult to imagine that molecules other than LPG (or C3 bound to it) would be exposed to interact with the macrophage.

Reduced efficiency of serum-independent binding of *L. major* metacyclic promastigotes to human monocyte-derived macrophages, together with the observation (Puentes *et al*. 1988) that only a small proportion of non-covalently bound C3 is in the form iC3b, led da Silva and co-workers (1989) to examine the role of CR1, the macrophage receptor for C3b, in uptake of metacyclic promastigotes. The most efficient (50−80%) inhibition of serum-dependent binding of *L. major* metacyclics was obtained using the anti-CR1 monoclonal antibody 1B4. The entry of log forms was mediated by both CR1 and CR3 in the presence of serum, and by CR3 in the absence of serum. In this case, differential inhibition using OKM10 versus OKM1 suggested that serum-independent binding of log forms was via the lectin-binding site of CR3. Parallel studies on serum-dependent binding of *L. donovani* log and metacyclic parasites to human macrophages have not been reported but the observation (Puentes *et al*. 1988) that 75% of C3 bound to *L. donovani* metacyclics is in the form iC3b suggests that CR3 rather than CR1 might be important.

The interpretation of monoclonal inhibition data raises problems since the antibody may block by steric hindrance rather than by direct binding to the epitope of interest. Hence, the mapping of parasite binding to precise epitopes on receptors will require a level of precision above that currently applied. The more refined studies of Russell and Wright (1988) using purified parasite molecules coupled to beads in conjunction with peptide inhibitors are a step in the right direction, but it will be some time before all the individual components of parasite binding have been examined so that the 'whole parasite' picture can be reconstructed. Such studies are important since binding to different epitopes of the same receptor may stimulate different physiological responses. In previous studies with CR3, for example, it has been suggested that binding to the lectin-binding site leads to stimulation of the respiratory burst by PMN and monocytes (Ross *et al*. 1985, 1987), whereas binding to the iC3b-binding site mediates the release neither of respiratory burst products (Wright and Silverstein 1983; Yamamoto and Johnston 1984) nor of arachidonic acid metabolites (Aderem *et al*. 1985). Respiratory burst products (superoxide anion and hydrogen peroxide) are important antimicrobial agents. Along with arachidonic acid metabolites (prostaglandins and leucotrienes), they are also important mediators of an inflammatory response. Binding of C3b to CR1 also fails to signal a respiratory burst response (Wright and Silverstein 1983). Hence, opsonin (C3b or iC3b)-dependent binding of metacyclics to either CR1 or CR3 could provide an advantageous route of entry into the macrophage for the parasite. However, studies by Wright and colleagues (Wright and Silverstein 1982; Wright *et al*. 1983b) indicate that, although CR1 and CR3 show avid binding of C3b- or iC3b-coated particles, their phagocytosis-promoting capacity is low. Both re-

* The work of Russell and Wright (1988) reporting on the direct binding of GP63 to CR3 via an RGD sequence requires reinterpretation (Russell 1990) in the light of more recent data (McMaster 1990) showing that the original sequence data for GP63 were incorrect. The molecule does not contain an RGD sequence.

ceptors can be activated for opsonin-dependent phagocytic activity by spreading of macrophages on to surfaces coated with the extracellular matrix proteins fibronectin or laminin (Pommier *et al.* 1983; Wright *et al.* 1984), the interaction of surface-bound fibronectin with fibronectin receptors on the underside of the macrophage affecting a change in the phagocytosis-promoting capacity of CR3 or CR1 on the apical portion of the membrane. A change in state of the receptors might therefore be dependent upon the site of the macrophage *in vivo* and its ability to interact with local extracellular matrix proteins. Cross-linking of receptors may also be important in determining whether the parasite transmits the correct signal for endocytosis. Russell and Wright (1988) found, for example, that beads coated with GP63 alone bound avidly to CR3 but were not endocytosed. Coupling of an additional ligand, LPG, to the beads mediated endocytosis, but it was not clear to which receptor the LPG was binding or whether this resulted in stimulation of a respiratory burst response. Studies from a number of laboratories indicate that receptors other than CR1 and CR3, e.g. the mannose/fucose receptor (MFR; Channon *et al.* 1984; Blackwell *et al.* 1985a; Wilson and Pearson 1986; Wilson and Hardin 1988), the fibronectin receptor (Wyler *et al.* 1985), the receptor for advanced glycosylation end-products (Mosser *et al.* 1987), may also play a role in binding promastigotes of different species of *Leishmania* to macrophages. In the case of the MFR, studies by Olafson and colleagues (R. Olafson, pers. comm.) have demonstrated appropriate ligands on the glycosylated portion of the GP63 molecule, but this interaction may prove detrimental to the parasite since this receptor is associated with signal transduction for respiratory burst activity (Berton and Gordon 1983; Channon *et al.* 1984). In counter-defence, McNeely and Turco (1987) have demonstrated that isolated LPG can inhibit protein kinase C activity and may thus inhibit the respiratory burst response. This could account for the observation of Handman *et al.* (1986) that passive transfer of LPG into macrophages along with an LPG-deficient avirulent strain conferred survival. If LPG inhibits protein kinase C during uptake, endocytosis would have to rely on alternative transmembrane signalling pathways. Whilst studies on non-complement receptor-mediated endocytosis have, in most cases, yet to be repeated on defined metacyclic promastigote populations, it is possible that mechanisms involving dual recognition by more than one receptor (Blackwell *et al.* 1985a) and/or synergism between receptors (Pommier *et al.* 1983; Wright *et al.* 1984) might apply. In cross-linking particular combinations of receptors different parasites might elicit distinct transmembrane signalling events which differ in their capacity to stimulate endocytic, respiratory burst or macrophage priming/activation (cf. below) pathways. This may help to determine not only the fate of the infecting organism but that of the expanding parasite population as well.

In attempting to draw together current data on whole parasite binding to macrophages it should be emphasized that, while a range of macrophage receptors may be available to the parasite, it can only make use of them according to their relative expression on a particular macrophage population and its own composition of available ligands (including opsonins). The fact, for example, that metacyclic promastigotes of *L. major* make heavy use of CR3 in entering murine macrophages (Cooper *et al.* 1988; Davies *et al.* 1989) but use CR1 to enter human monocyte-derived macrophages (da Silva *et al.* 1989) may simply reflect the relative expression of the two receptors on the different macrophage populations. With more iC3b than C3b on its surface, *L. donovani*, on the other, may preferentially use CR3 even in entering human monocyte-derived macrophages. The use of human monocyte-derived macrophages may be closer to reality in terms of human infection, although it is not clear at present how representative this might be of the macrophage subpopulations available at the site of infection in the skin. Locksley and co-workers (1988) compared the interaction of *L. major* promastigotes with dermal macrophages and epidermal Langerhans cells from primates. Only the dermal macrophage population, which was oxidatively deficient and expressed CR3, could be successfully infected. The importance of this resident skin population, as opposed to a fresh influx of monocytes arriving at the site of the sandfly bite, in initiating infection is unknown.

Expansion of the parasite population in the host may also be dependent upon an inflammatory response (Wilson *et al.* 1987; Davies *et al.* 1988) and upon the receptor interactions between macrophages and amastigote forms of the parasite. Few studies had successfully addressed the question of receptors involved in amastigote binding, our own earlier studies having failed to demonstrate a conclusive role for CR3 or the MFR in serum-independent binding of *L. donovani* amastigotes to murine macrophages which was consistent (i) with their inability to activate the alternative complement pathway; (ii) with their lack of surface expression of GP63 (Fong and Chang 1982; Chang *et al.* 1986) which might mediate direct binding to CR3 or MFR; and (iii) with our inability to demonstrate any serum-enhanced binding to macrophages. We therefore decided to raise antimurine macrophage antibodies in rats and screen in functional assays for their ability to inhibit amastigote binding (A.M. Cooper and J.M. Blackwell, unpublished). One monoclonal antibody, HE4, raised in this manner inhibits the binding of *L. donovani* amastigotes in the presence or absence of normal mouse serum but has no effect on *L. major* amastigote binding. The affinity-purified antibody recognizes a macrophage protein of 83 000 daltons on Western blots which we are currently attempting to characterize. Binding of *L. donovani* but not *L. major* amastigotes to murine macrophages is also inhibited by 1 mg/ml of: (i) a 17-mer RGD-containing synthetic peptide based on the *L. major* GP63 sequence (Button and McMaster 1988); (ii) the RGDS fibronectin receptor-binding peptide; and (iii) the fibronectin analogue GRGDSPL. We have yet to establish whether the peptide inhibition is additive with HE4 or whether the HE4 antigen is a member of the larger family of RGD-recognizing integrins (Hynes 1987). These differences observed in inhibition of binding of amastigotes of *L. donovani* versus *L. major* may, nevertheless, help to explain the different tissue tropisms of these two species of the parasite.

Macrophage response to infection

Studies outlined above demonstrate that molecular interactions between leishmanial parasites and host macrophages may be critical in determining the fate of the infecting organism and subsequent expansion of the parasite population. One aspect of these interactions which has not been considered is that both parasite and host may be polymorphic for genes which regulate these interactions. Epidemiological studies in man certainly provide evidence that not all members of an endemic population are uniformly susceptible to infection (see above), but the extent to which this is genetically determined has hitherto been difficult to demonstrate. Data available from murine studies now provide powerful evidence that genes regulating the primary macrophage response to infection may be important determinants of host susceptibility to leishmanial infections.

Genetically regulated primary macrophage responses

The best studied gene regulating the host response to leishmanial infections is the gene *Lsh* (*Ity*/*Bcg*), known also for its role in regulating the early response to infection with *Salmonella typhimurium* (Plant *et al.* 1982), *Mycobacterium bovis* (Skamene *et al.* 1982), *M. lepraemurium* (Brown *et al.* 1982; Skamene *et al.* 1984), and *M. intracellulare* (Goto *et al.* 1984). Early studies indicated that resistance encoded by this gene was not dependent upon a functional T cell population (O'Brien and Metcalf 1982; Gros *et al.* 1983; Bonventre and Nickol 1984), and was expressed most efficiently against *L. donovani* in resident tissue macrophages (e.g. Kupffer cells (Crocker *et al.* 1984, 1987)). A 1–3-day delay in expression of resistance *in vivo* (Crocker *et al.* 1984) and *in vitro* (Crocker *et al.* 1987) was also observed. Resistance could be enhanced by pretreating mice with bacterial LPS (Crocker *et al.* 1984), suggesting that macrophage priming/activation may form the basis to the resistance mechanism. In carrying out the receptor studies described above (see above) we were struck by the parallel observations: (i) that leishmanial parasites share in common with bacterial LPS (Wright and Jong 1986) and *Mycobacterium* (M. Horowitz, pers. comm.) the capacity to bind to one or more members (CR3, lymphocyte function-associated antigen (LFA)-1, p150,95) of the adhesion/activation-promoting integrin family of receptors; and (ii) that the anti-CR3 monoclonal antibody M1/70 had the capacity to activate macrophages (Ding *et al.* 1987) in a manner analogous to that observed with the T cell product interferon-γ (see above). In preliminary studies (Blackwell *et al.* 1988), in which macrophage activation was measured in terms of phorbol myristate acetate (PMA)-elicited superoxide anion release or anti-leishmanial activity, differential responsiveness to 48-hour activation with M1/70 or low doses of metacyclic promastigotes or amastigotes of *L. donovani* was observed for macrophages from B10(*Lsh*^{s}) versus congenic B10.L-*Lsh*^{r} mice. Subsequent two-dimensional gel analysis (Blackwell *et al.* 1989) of proteins phosphorylated in response to the activating signals (metacyclic promastigotes or amastigotes) show low-molecular-weight (10–12 kD and 14 kD; PI 5.9–6.1) proteins phosphorylated in B10(*Lsh*^{s}) but not B10.L-*Lsh*^{r} macrophages. PMA fails to elicit this specific protein phosphorylation, suggesting that a signal transduction pathway independent of protein kinase C, perhaps involving cyclic adenosine monophosphate (AMP)-dependent protein kinase A, operates to inhibit macrophage activation in susceptible macrophages. These studies provide a promising breakthrough in the search for a protein product for the *Lsh* gene which would facilitate molecular characterization of the gene at the DNA level. In the mean time, mapping of the gene on to a region of mouse chromosome 1 with known homology to human 2q (reviewed Blackwell 1988a, b) provides numerous linked marker loci which can be used in family linkage analysis to obtain evidence for a homologous gene in man.*

The secondary effect of *Lsh* gene-mediated T cell-independent macrophage activation is the upregulation of Class II major histocompatibility complex (MHC) molecules, which leads to the earlier establishment of a specific T cell response in resistant mice (Kaye *et al.* 1988). Hence, although the gene can operate independently of T cells, an enhanced ability to respond to leishmanial antigens in skin test or T cell assays (e.g. Ho *et al.* 1982; Badaro *et al.* 1986a, b; Sacks *et al.* 1987) without clinical symptoms of disease may provide a marker to identify individuals with primary macrophage resistance to infection. For *L. mexicana* infection *Lsh* fails to influence growth of the primary lesion but prevents visceralization of the infection (Roberts *et al.* 1989). Other genes, *Scl-1* and *Scl-2*, which may also act at the level of the primary macrophage response to regulate (*Scl-1*) or prevent (*Scl-2*) lesion growth following infection with *L. major* and *L. mexicana* (reviewed in Blackwell 1988b), have also been identified and mapped to regions of known homology with human chromosomes.

* The current status of research on *Lsh* is reviewed in Blackwell *et al.* (1991).

T-cell-dependent macrophage activation

The role of lymphokines released by antigen-specific T cells in activating macrophages for enhanced antileishmanial activity is now well established, early studies employing crude T cell supernatants to activate macrophages *in vitro* (Behin *et al.* 1979; Chang and Chiao 1981; Nacy *et al.* 1981; Murray *et al.* 1983) now being substantiated by the use of recombinant cytokines, principally interferon-γ *in vitro* (Titus *et al.* 1984; Murray *et al.* 1985; Nacy *et al.* 1985) and *in vivo* (Murray *et al.* 1987). Administration of anti-interferon-γ antibodies during infection in mice demonstrates the importance of this cytokine as a mediator of macrophage activation and clearance of parasites *in vivo* (Gutierrez *et al.* 1984; Squires *et al.* 1986). Both oxygen-dependent (Buchmuller and Mauel 1981; Murray 1981a, b, 1982) and oxygen-independent (Scott *et al.* 1986) leishmanicidal mechanisms are important, the ability of interferon-γ to activate macrophages also being temperature-dependent (Scott 1985). The latter may be particularly important in cutaneous leishmaniasis, where the temperature at the site of the lesion ranges from 27°C to 32°C. A role for other cytokines (e.g. granulocyte–macrophage colony-stimulating factor (GM-CSF) and interleukin 4 (IL-4)) in mediating macrophage activation has also been suggested, Handman and Burgess (1979) and Weishui *et al.* (1987) having observed enhanced leishmanicidal activity following activation of macrophages with GM-CSF and other workers (Crawford *et al.* 1987) having shown upregulation of Class II MHC molecules and enhanced tumoricidal activity in macrophages treated with IL-4. Paradoxically, the presence of antigen-specific CD4 T cells releasing these cytokines is negatively correlated with resolution of infection *in vivo* (see below) and mice treated with recombinant GM-CSF *in vivo* show enhanced lesion growth (Solbach *et al.* 1987). The complexity of interactions between the cytokines of different T cell subsets, which may be secreted in different amounts at the site of infected macrophages in the viscera or the skin, has yet to be fully explored, although there are preliminary reports (Liew 1989; P. Scott, pers. comm.) that the products (IL-4, IL-3, GM-CSF) of T helper 2 cells may inhibit the ability of interferon-γ the principal product of T helper 1 cells, to activate macrophages for leishmanicidal activity *in vitro*. In our hands (A. Kiderlen, P.M. Kaye and J.M. Blackwell unpubl. obs.) IL-4 promotes the intracellular growth of *L. donovani* in non-activated macrophages but does not inhibit interferon-γ-mediated macrophage activation for killing of amastigotes. Similarly, Louis and co-workers (1987) report that IL-3 and GM-CSF promote intracellular growth of *L. major* amastigotes in macrophages *in vitro*. Interestingly, subcutaneous injection of recombinant IL-4 in a 'slow-release' gel preparation under the site of *L. major* lesions results in healing (Carter *et al.* 1989). The mechanism for this action is unknown but the authors suggest a role for IL-4 in localized activation of macrophages and/or up-regulation of Class II MHC expression and enhanced antigen-presenting cell function by macrophages and B cells. The mice are resistant to rechallenge and protection can be transferred to naïve mice with splenic T cells from IL-4-treated mice.

Activation of specific T cell responses

The immunobiology of leishmaniasis was the subject of a recent forum in *Annales de l'Institut Pasteur, Immunologie* (Louis and Milon 1987). This heralded the first real evidence for a functional split in CD4 T cell subsets according to cytokine profiles (Locksley *et al.* 1987), which begins to make some sense of the earlier (Howard *et al.* 1980, 1981; Liew *et al.* 1982; Blackwell and Ulczak 1984) demonstration of CD4 +ve 'suppressor' cells in leishmanial infections. The importance of CD8 cells in resolution of leishmanial infection has also begun to receive fresh attention. The evidence for different roles for these T cell subsets will be examined before determining how their differential expansion might be regulated at the level of antigen-presenting cell function *in vivo*.

CD4 T cell subsets

Locksley and co-workers (1987) showed dramatically different levels of cytokines in the draining lymph nodes of non-healing BALB/c (high IL-4, no interferon-γ) mice infected with *L. major* compared with healing CBA/Ca (high interferon-γ, no IL-4) mice. This was in broad agreement with the split in CD4 subsets published earlier by Mosman and co-workers (1986), T helper 1 cells producing interferon-γ and IL-2 while T helper 2 cells produce predominantly IL-4 and little IL-2. According to the Mosman *et al.* (1986) data, both CD4 subsets produce IL-3 and GM-CSF. Subsequent studies on T cell lines generated from BALB/c mice vaccinated with different soluble fractions of leishmanial antigens (Scott *et al.* 1988) show a clear split between those of the T helper 1 phenotype which produce interferon-γ and IL-2 and transfer protection, and T helper 2 cells which produce IL-4 and IL-5 and exacerbate disease. The T helper 2 line also produced significantly more colony-stimulating factor (GM-CSF and/or IL-3). One of the explanations for the disease-promoting capacity of T helper 2 cells in non-healing/non-curing mice is their ability to call in a fresh influx of monocytes to the site of infection which, in the absence of interferon-γ, provide safe targets within which the parasite population can expand (Modabber 1987). *Leishmania major* amastigotes, in particular, appear to target preferentially into young monocytes, in which they survive and grow (Davies *et al.* 1988). The concept of safe targets is supported by the observations of Mirkovitch and co-workers (1986) demonstrating enhanced myelopoiesis in the spleen and bone marrow of susceptible BALB/c mice following *L. major* infection, and by the work of Lelchuck and co-workers (1987) showing a clear difference in conconavalin A- or specific antigen-induced IL-3 production by T cells from spleens of non-healing BALB/c versus healing CBA/Ca mice. Both IL-3 (Kindler *et al.* 1986) and GM-CSF (Metcalf 1986) are known to enhance myelopoiesis *in vivo*. Hence, the so-called 'suppression' mediated by CD4 T cells in leishmaniasis (Howard *et al.* 1980; Blackwell and Ulczak 1984) may simply reflect over-stimulation of the T helper 2 subset. Different routes of vaccination also presumably preferentially stimulate T helper 1 versus T helper 2 CD4 subsets, the work of Liew and co-workers (reviewed in Liew 1987) having shown quite clearly that an irradiated promastigote vaccine given intravenously or intraperitoneally protects susceptible BALB/c mice against challenge infection with *L. major* whereas subcutaneous inoculation of the vaccine results in exacerbation of the disease.

Studies in man do not show the same clear-cut separation of CD4 T cells into T helper 1 and T helper 2 phenotypes (Powrie and Mason 1988). However, as with the BALB/c mouse studies, Carvalho and co-workers (1985b) have demonstrated the absence of interferon-γ and IL-2 production during active visceral leishmaniasis in man. Similarly, T cells from patients with DCL fail to express IL-2 receptors and do not produce interferon-γ in response to leishmanial antigen *in vitro* (Rada *et al.* 1987; Castes *et al.* 1988). Conversely, CD4 T cells associated with localized cutaneous lesions or MCL (Rada *et al.* 1987; Castes *et al.* 1988) or with resolution of Old World cutaneous or visceral leishmaniasis (Melby *et al.* 1989) do produce interferon-γ in response to specific antigen stimulation *in vitro*. Using two-dimensional gel T cell blotting Melby *et al.* (1989) have demonstrated that 50–70 distinct leishmanial antigens stimulate interferon-γ production and/or proliferative responses in T cells from patients who have either self-cured or been drug-cured following leishmanial infection (Fig. 80.2). Further characterization of these antigens and the MHC restriction of T cells responding to them should provide a battery of candidate protective antigens for vaccine development (see below).

CD8 T cell subsets

Several laboratories have demonstrated that antigen-specific CD8 +ve T cells are also important in resolution of cutaneous and visceral leishmanial infections. Depletion of CD8 cells *in vivo* by administration of anti-CD8 monoclonal antibodies before and during infection with *L. major* causes exacerbation of lesion growth in both susceptible and resistant mice (Titus *et al.* 1987). Limiting dilution analyses of T cells capable of transferring antigen-specific delayed hypersensitivity to naïve mice have shown a high frequency of CD8 cells in the draining lymph nodes of resistant mice just prior to onset of resolution of *L. major* lesions (Milon *et al.* 1986) and, in the livers of self-curing mice infected with *L. donovani*, only CD8 +ve antigen-specific T cells were observed during the period of maximum resolution of parasite load (Roberts *et al.* 1988). The latter is consistent with immunocytochemical studies also demonstrating exclusively CD8 +ve T cells in liver sections from curing mice (McElrath *et al.* 1988). The role played by these CD8 cells in disease resolution is not clear. Stern *et al.* (1988) have demonstrated their ability to secrete interferon-γ in response to mitogen or antigen stimulation but they are not as potent producers as CD4 cells purified from the same infected mice. These workers have also shown that athymic nude (congenitally T cell-deficient) mice reconstituted with either CD4- or CD8-enriched immune spleen cells alone fail to control visceral parasite replication despite the fact that, with CD4 cells in particular, the capacity to secrete interferon-γ is restored. The problem appears to lie in their inability to develop effective tissue granulomas. Treatment of normal euthymic mice with anti-CD4 or anti-CD8 monoclonal antibodies also prevents self-cure and impairs the tissue granulomatous response. Genetically non-curing mice also fail to develop an effective granulomatous response (Bradley and Kirkley 1977), fusion of infected Kupffer cells in the livers of chronically infected mice resulting in heavily parasitized giant cells (Bradley and Kirkley 1977; Murray *et al.* 1987). Another possible role for CD8 cells might be to lyse this oxidatively inert resident macrophage population to release parasites for uptake by younger macrophages still capable of responding to activating signals. The concept of cytotoxic T cell lysis of infected macrophages is not new (Bryceson *et al.* 1970) but it should now be possible to define this role more precisely in terms of antigen specificity, MHC restriction and molecular interactions between the infected macrophage and the effector T cell population.

Antigen presentation

One of the more remarkable observations which the use of genetically defined mouse strains has permitted is that mice bearing different *H-2* haplotypes on a common (B10 or BALB) genetic background show dramatically different disease profiles following infection with *L. donovani* (Blackwell *et al.* 1980). It is now known that the MHC (*H-2* in mice, HLA in man) encodes the Class I and Class II MHC molecules to which foreign antigens bind for presentation to CD8 and CD4 T cells respectively. Immunogenetic studies (Blackwell 1983) suggested that the major influence of *H-2* on disease phenotype mapped to the I region, to the A (= HLA-DQ) and E (= HLA-DR) Class II MHC molecules which present antigen to CD4 T cells. Treatment of non-curing ($H\text{-}2^d$) mice with monoclonal antibodies directed against these two molecules led to another striking observation (Blackwell and Roberts 1987). Administration of anti-I-E^d promoted resolution of liver and spleen

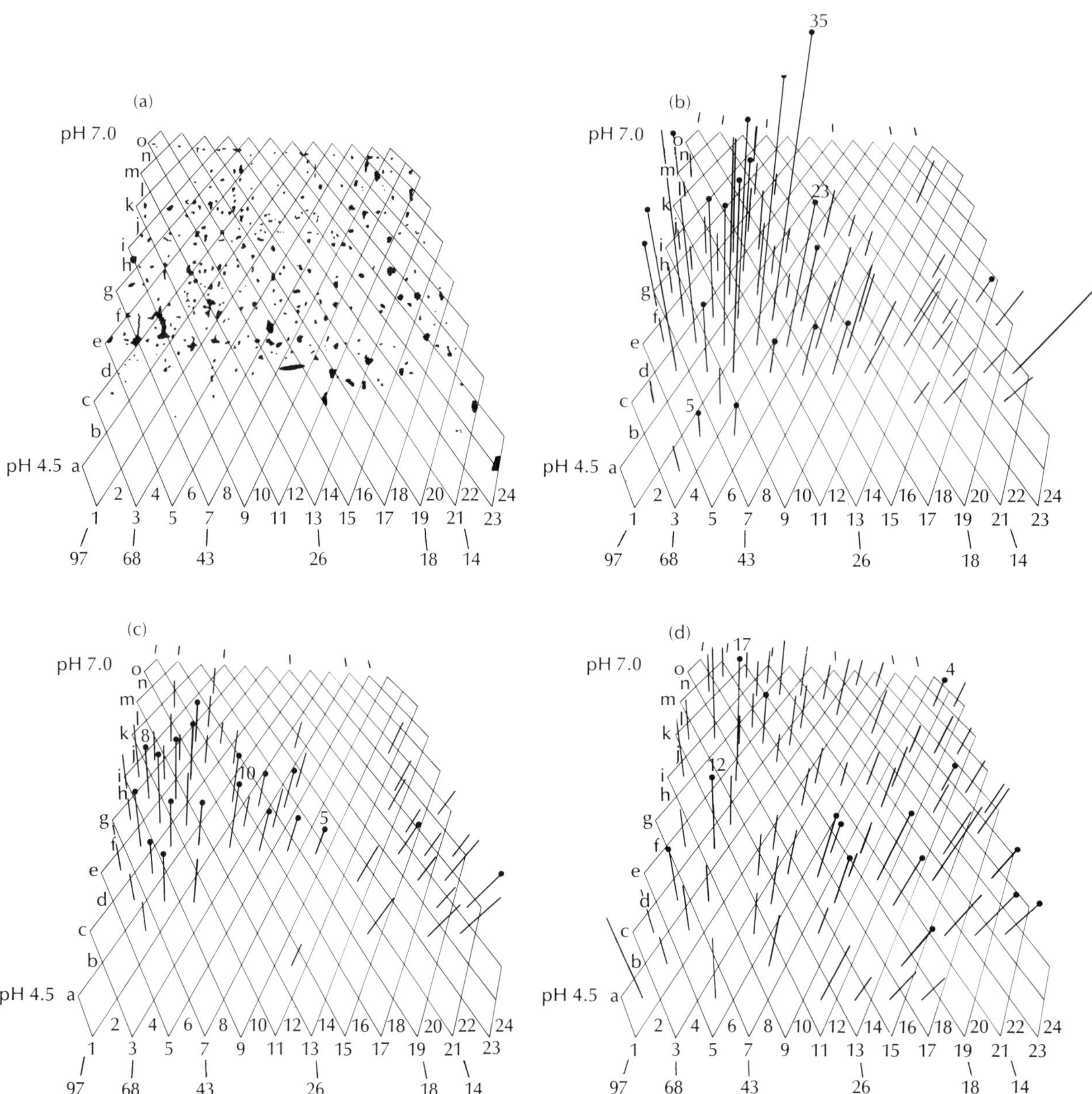

Fig. 80.2. Profile of antigen-specific proliferative and interferon-γ responses in peripheral blood lymphocytes from healed MCL and LCL patients. Bars represent stimulation indices for proliferative responses. Dotted bars indicate wells in which significant levels of interferon-γ were secreted. A schematic representation of individual silver-stained antigens from the two-dimensional immunoblot which were punched into the wells of two 96-well plates is shown in (a). Results from a cured MCL patient are shown in (b); from a localized *L. donovani* infection in (c); and from an *L. major* LCL patient in (d). Diagram kindly supplied by Peter Melby and David Sacks of the National Institutes of Health, Bethesda, Maryland, USA.

parasite loads, whereas anti-I-A^d resulted in exacerbation of disease. The reason why these observations are rather surprising is that, in the context of an antigenically complex whole parasite infection, one might hardly have expected to observe such dramatic MHC restriction, the more so since one-dimensional T cell blotting shows that T cells from curing strains (*H-2*^{b}, *H-2*^{r}) respond to a wide range of parasite antigens of different molecular weights (Kaye *et al.* 1987; A.J. Curry and P.M. Kaye, unpubl. obs.). Considering the array of antigens which promote interferon-γ-producing T cells during cure (Melby *et al.* 1989), it might be expected that, if a particular antigen failed to bind to the

Class II MHC molecules of a given haplotype, many others could substitute in triggering appropriate CD4 T cell responses. How then does a change in *H-2* haplotype or the blocking of I-E exert such a dramatic effect?

One possibility is that one or a few dominant antigens presented in the context of *H-2*^{d} and, more specifically I-E^{d}, preferentially stimulates T helper 2 cells early in infection. Our preliminary observation (A.J. Curry and P.M. Kaye, unpubl. obs.) is that T cells from *H-2*^{d} mice proliferate in response to a broad array of antigens early (8 days) in infection but become markedly restricted in their response as infection progresses. A more detailed analysis of cytokine profiles and Class II MHC (I-A versus I-E) restriction of these T cells should reveal whether one or a few 'suppressor' antigens dominate in terms of CD4 T cell responses. Another possibility is that any antigen presented in the context of I-E^{d} preferentially stimulates a T helper 2 response. This might, in turn, reflect a restricted repertoire of T cells available for recognition of antigen in this strain. Bill and co-workers (1988) have shown, for example, that congenic mice bearing different *H-2* haplotypes on a B10 genetic background show significant differences in the relative contributions of one Vα gene family (Vα3) and several Vβ gene segments (Vβ5.1, -5.2, -11 and -12) to their T cell repertoires, while work on well-defined antigen plus Class II MHC molecule combinations (e.g. pigeon cytochrome C peptide 88–104 plus I-E; ovalbumin peptide 323–330 plus I-A^{d}) shows that T cell receptor recognition involves restricted use of particular members of the Vβ and Vα gene families (Marrack and Kappler 1988). Further work on the molecular interaction between Class II MHC molecules and T cell receptor complexes of antigen-specific CD4 subsets will be crucial to understanding how a curative and/or protective T cell response can be generated and why some combinations lead to non-curing/non-healing responses. Important too are studies examining the roles of different accessory cell populations in processing and presenting antigen to different T cell subsets (CD4 versus CD8; T helper 1 versus T helper 2). Whilst receptor-mediated endocytosis of parasites might readily lead to processing of antigen in acid endosomes, binding to Class II MHC and presentation to CD4 T cells, endocytosed antigen cannot be presented by Class I MHC molecules (reviewed by Long and Jacobson 1989). Hence, although it is clear that antigen-specific CD8 T cells are generated during leishmanial infection and are important in the curing response (see below) the intracellular pathway to processing of parasite antigen and binding to Class I MHC molecules for presentation to CD8 T cells remains unclear. This may be crucial to vaccination, especially against *L. donovani* where vaccination schedules (e.g. intravenous killed promastigotes) effective against *L. major* (Liew 1987, 1989) fail to protect BALB/c mice against *L. donovani* (Blackwell *et al*. 1985b).

Immunotherapy and vaccination

The demonstration by Melby *et al*. (1989) that interferon-γ-producing T cells generated during cure from leishmanial infections recognize a broad range of leishmanial antigens suggests that the search for a single major protective antigen for vaccination against disease may be inappropriate. In any case, polymorphism at the loci encoding Class I and Class II MHC molecules in genetically diverse human populations makes single-antigen vaccines less attractive since the MHC molecules of some members of the population may fail to bind the antigen for presentation to T cells. A recombinant vaccine combining T cell epitopes from an array of protein antigens might therefore be more attractive. The most worrying concern in designing such a vaccine is that the same protein antigen bound to the MHC molecules of one individual might stimulate a protective T cell response whereas, in the context of alternative MHC alleles, a disease-promoting T cell response might predominate. In attempting to resolve these problems, valuable information can be gained by application of more sophisticated immunological techniques in the context of ongoing immunotherapy and immunoprophylaxis trials using crude antigen preparations.

Immunotherapy

A randomized trial carried out in Venezuela (Convit *et al*. 1987) has demonstrated that intradermal inoculation of live bacillus Calmette–Guérin (BCG) together with heat-killed *Leishmania* promastigotes provides effective immunotherapy against localized cutaneous leishmaniasis. Three vaccinations over 32 weeks gave a similar cure rate (94%) to three 20-day courses of meglumine antimonate. The great advantage of the immunotherapy is that side-effects are few, the cost of production and administration is a fraction of that of chemotherapy, and the vaccine can be administered by primary health services. Studies in progress will examine in detail the changing T cell response in patients undergoing immunotherapy and chemotherapy. Analysis of antigen recognition and cytokine profiles of T cells in conjunction with HLA typing for DR and DQ should assist in the search for a battery of candidate protective protein antigens suitable for prophylactic vaccination.

Immunoprophylaxis

The basic observation that healing of the primary lesion in cutaneous leishmaniasis provides lasting immunity against reinfection led to the traditional practice of 'leishmanization' to protect against prominent disfiguring scars. This involved either exposure of certain areas of skin to sandfly bites or scratching the skin area with material from active lesions. The technique was standardized when methods for culturing promastigotes became available but variability in the size and duration of lesions resulting from the inoculation of virulent strains has caused the practice to be discontinued in Israel and the Soviet Union (Greenblatt 1988). The spread of immunosuppressive infections such as human immunodeficiency virus (HIV) and the use of immunosuppressive drugs in transplantation surgery mean that future prospects for a live (albeit apparently avirulent in an immunocompetent host) vaccine might also be inappropriate. It is to be hoped that modern technology can ultimately provide a safe antigenically defined molecular vaccine, but what has been/can be learned from the use of crude killed promastigote vaccines?

Mayrink and co-workers (1985) have reported on the use of a cocktail of five strains of methiolate-treated *L. braziliensis* promastigotes given as two or three weekly injections intramuscularly as a prophylactic vaccine against cutaneous leishmaniasis in Brazil. Protection in the first year ranged from 67 to 85% in vaccinees who showed skin test conversion, but skin test positivity waned with time (78.4–54% after 2 years; 31% at 3 years) after vaccination. Detailed T cell studies have not been carried out in the context of these Brazilian trials. Success with the immunotherapy regimen of live BCG plus heat-killed promastigotes has led Convit and colleagues to proceed with a prophylactic vaccination trial in Venezuela. Again, more detailed genetic and T cell studies, incorporating the two-dimensional T cell Western blotting techniques of Melby and co-workers (1989), are being used (M. Castes, J.M. Blackwell and co-workers, collaborative studies in progress) to assess the potential efficacy of the vaccine in genetically diverse individuals of the study population, results of which should be known before epidemiological follow-up can determine the impact of the vaccine on natural incidence rates in the region. In the context of this trial, which includes groups vaccinated with and without BCG, it will be especially interesting to determine the role of BCG in promoting CD8 versus CD4 subsets as well as the split within the CD4 T cell compartment.

Future vaccine strategies

Studies of human and experimental leishmaniasis presented above provide some encouragement for the development of a defined molecular vaccine against leishmaniasis. Indeed, some degree of success with purified protein (e.g. GP63; Russell and Alexander 1987) and protein fractions (Scott *et al*. 1987), as well as with purified LPG (Handman and Mitchell 1985), has been reported in experimental cutaneous leishmaniasis. In summary, the indications are that a successful vaccine against leishmaniasis should: (i) contain a battery of protein epitopes which can be presented to T cells in the context of genetically diverse Class I and Class II MHC molecules; and (ii) be administered with an appropriate adjuvant or in a vector which can promote activation of both CD4 and CD8 T cell subsets, the latter being perhaps more difficult to achieve in the light of current knowledge of differential intracellular trafficking pathways for endogenous and exogenous protein antigens.

If the golden dreams come true, a defined molecular vaccine against leishmaniasis could provide parasitologists with their first real success in promoting disease control through the administration of an antiparasite vaccine.

Acknowledgements

The author gratefully acknowledges the generosity of friends and colleagues in making available prepublication manuscripts during the preparation of this review.

References

Aderem, A.A., Wright, S.D., Silverstein, S.C. and Cohn, Z.A. (1985). Ligated complement receptors do not activate the arachidonic acid cascade in resident peritoneal macrophages. *J. Exp. Med.* **161**, 617–22.

Al-Ginden, Y., Omer, A.H.S., Al-Humaidan, Y., Peters, W. and Evans, D.A. (1983). A case of mucocutaneous leishmaniasis in Saudi Arabia caused by *Leishmania major* and its response to treatment. *Clin. Exp. Dermatol.* **8**, 185–8.

Ardehali, S., Sodeiphy, M., Haghighi, P., Rezai, H. and Vollum, D. (1980). Studies on chronic (lupoid) leishmaniasis. *Ann. Trop. Med. Parasitol.* **74**, 439–45.

Arnot, D.E. and Barker, D.C. (1981). Biochemical identification of *Leishmania* by analysis of kinetoplast DNA. II. Sequence homologies in *Leishmania* kDNA. *Mol. Biochem. Parasitol.* **3**, 47–56.

Badaro, R., Jones, T.C., Lorenco, B.J.C. *et al.* (1986a). A prospective study of visceral leishmaniasis in an endemic area of Brazil. *J. Infect. Dis.* **154**, 639–49.

Badaro, R., Jones, T.C., Carvalho, E.M. *et al.* (1986b). New perspectives on a subclinical form of visceral leishmaniasis. *J. Infect. Dis.* **154**, 1003–11.

Barker, D.C. and Butcher, J. (1983). The use of DNA probes in the identification of leishmanias: discrimination between isolates of the mexicana and braziliensis complex. *Trans. Roy. Soc. Trop. Med. Hyg.* **77**, 285–98.

Barker, D.C., Gibson, L.J., Kennedy, W.P.K., Nasser, A.A.A.A. and Williams, R.H. (1986). The potential of using recombinant DNA species-specific probes for the identification of tropical *Leishmania*. *Parasitology* **91**, s139–74.

Barral, A., Badaro, R., Barral-Netto, M., Grimaldi, G., Momem, H. and Carvalho, E.M. (1986). Isolation of *Leishmania mexicana amazonensis* from the bone marrow in a case of American visceral leishmaniasis. *Am. J. Trop. Med. Hyg.* **35**, 732–4.

Behin, R., Mauel, J. and Sordat, B. (1979). *Leishmania tropica*: pathogenicity and *in vitro* macrophage function in strains of inbred mice. *Exp. Parasitol.* **48**, 81–91.

Belazzoug, S., Lanotte, G., Maazoun, R., Pratlong, F. and Rioux, J.A. (1985). Un nouveau variant enzymatique de *Leishmania infantum*, Nicolle, 1908, agent de la leishmaniose cutanée du Nord de l'Algerie. *Ann. Parasitol. Hum. Comp.* **60**, 1–3.

Beller, D.I., Springer, T.A. and Schreiber, R.D. (1982). Anti-Mac-1 selectively inhibits the mouse and human type three complement receptor. *J. Exp. Med.* **156**, 1000–9.

Berman, J.D. and Dwyer, D.M. (1981). Expression of *Leishmania* antigen on the surface membrane of infected human macrophages *in vitro*. *Clin. Exp. Immunol.* **44**, 342–8.

Berton, G. and Gordon, S. (1983). Modulation of macrophage mannose-specific receptors by cultivation on immobilised zymosan: effects on phagocytosis and superoxide anion release. *Immunology* **49**, 705–15.

Bill, J., Appel, V.B. and Palmer, E. (1988). An analysis of T-cell receptor variable region gene expression in major histocompatibility complex disparate mice. *Proc. Nat. Acad. Sci. (USA)* **85**, 9184–8.

Blackwell, J.M. (1983). *Leishmania donovani* infection in heterozygous and recombinant *H-2* haplotype mice. *Immunogenetics* **18**, 101–9.

Blackwell, J.M. (1988a). Bacterial infections. In *Genetics of Resistance to Bacterial and Parasitic Infection*, ed. D. Wakelin and J.M. Blackwell, pp. 63–101, Taylor & Francis, London, Philadelphia and New York.

Blackwell, J.M. (1988b). Protozoan infections. In *Genetics of Resistance to Bacterial and Parasitic Infection*, ed. D. Wakelin and J.M. Blackwell, pp. 103–51, Taylor & Francis, London, Philadelphia and New York.

Blackwell, J.M. and Roberts, M.B. (1987). Immunomodulation of murine visceral leishmaniasis by administration of anti-Ia antibodies: differential effects of anti-IA versus anti-IE antibodies. *Eur. J. Immunol.* **17**, 1669–72.

Blackwell, J.M. and Ulczak, O.M. (1984). Immunoregulation of genetically controlled acquired responses to *Leishmania donovani* infection in mice: demonstration and characterization of suppressor T cells in noncure mice. *Infect. Immunity* **44**, 97–102.

Blackwell, J.M., Freeman, J. and Bradley, D. (1980). Influence of *H-2* complex on acquired resistance to *Leishmania donovani* infection mice. *Nature* **283**, 72–4.

Blackwell, J.M., Ezekowitz, R.A.B., Roberts, M.B., Channon, J.Y., Sim, R.B. and Gordon, S. (1985a). Macrophage complement and lectin-like receptors bind *Leishmania* in the absence of serum. *J. Exp. Med.* **162**, 324–31.

Blackwell, J.M., Roberts, M. and Alexander, J. (1985b). Response of BALB/c mice to leishmanial infection. *Curr. Topics Microbiol. Immunol.* **122**, 97–106.

Blackwell, J.M., Roaeh, T.I.A., Kiderlein, A. and Kaye, P.M. (1989). Role of *LsL* in regulating macrophage priming activation. *Res. Immunol.* **140**, 798–805.

Blackwell, J.M., Roaeh, T.I.A., Atkinson, S.E., Ajioka, J.W., Barton, C.H. and Shaw, M.-A. (1991). Genetic regulation of macrophage primary activation. *Res. Immunol.* **140**, 798–805.

Blackwell, J.M., Toole, S., King, M., Dawda, P., Roach, T.I.A. and Cooper, A. (1988). Analysis of *Lsh* gene expression in congenic B10.L-*Lsh*^{r} mice. *Curr. Topics Microbiol. Immunol.* **137**, 301–9.

Bonventre, P.F. and Nickol, A.D. (1984). *Leishmania donovani* infection in athymic mice derived from parental strains of the susceptible (*Lsh*^{s}) or resistant (*Lsh*^{r}) phenotype. *J. Leukocyte Biol.* **36**, 651–8.

Bordier, C. (1987). The promastigote surface protease of *Leishmania*. *Parasitol. Today* **3**, 151–3.

Bouvier, J., Etges, R. and Bordier, C. (1985). Identification and purification of membrane and soluble forms of the major surface protein of *Leishmania* promastigotes. *J. Biol. Chem.* **260**, 15504–9.

Bouvier, J., Etges, R. and Bordier, C. (1987). Identification of the promastigote surface protease in seven species of *Leishmania*. *Mol. Biochem. Parasitol.* **24**, 73–9.

Bradley, D.J. and Kirkley, J. (1977). Regulation of *Leishmania* populations within the host. I. The variable course of *Leishmania donovani* infections in mice. *Clin. Exp. Immunol.* **30**, 119–29.

Brown, I.N., Glynn, A.A. and Plant, J. (1982). Inbred mouse strain resistance to *Mycobacterium lepraemurium* follows the *Ity/Lsh* pattern. *Immunology* **47**, 149–56.

Bryceson, A.D.M. (1970). Diffuse cutaneous leishmaniasis in Ethiopia. III. Immunological studies. *Trans. Roy. Soc. Trop. Med. Hyg.* **64**, 380–7.

Bryceson, A.D.M. (1986). Clinical variations associated with various taxa of *Leishmania*. In *Leishmania. Taxonomie et phylogenes. Applications eco-epidemiologiques*, ed. J. Rioux, pp. 221–8, Colloquiem Internationale CNRS/INSERM, 1984, IMEEE Publishers, Montpellier.

Bryceson, A.D.M., Bray, R.S., Wolstencroft, R.A. and Dumonde, D.C. (1970). Immunity in cutaneous leishmaniasis of the guinea-pig. *Clin. Exp. Immunol.* **7**, 301–41.

Buchmuller, Y. and Mauel, J. (1981). Studies on the mechanisms of macrophage activation: possible involvement of oxygen metabolites in killing of *Leishmania enrietti* by activated mouse macrophages. *J. Reticulendothelial Soc.* **29**, 181–93.

Button, L.L. and McMaster, W.R. (1988). Molecular cloning of the major surface antigen of *Leishmania*. *J. Exp. Med.* **167**, 724–9.

Carter, K.C., Gallagher, G., Baillie, A.J. and Alexander, J. (1989). The induction of protective immunity to *Leishmania major* in the BALB/c mouse by interleukin-4 treatment. *Eur. J. Immunol.* **19**, 779–82.

Carvalho, E.M., Teixeira, R.S. and Johnson, W.D. (1981). Cell-mediated immunity in American visceral leishmaniasis: reversible immunosuppression during acute infection. *Infect. Immunity* **33**, 498–502.

Carvalho, E.M., Johnson, W.D., Barreto, E. *et al.* (1985a). Cell mediated immunity in American cutaneous and mucosal leishmaniasis. *J. Immunol.* **135**, 4144–8.

Carvalho, E.M., Badaro, R., Reed, S.G., Jones, T.C. and Johnson, W.D. (1985b). Absence of gamma interferon and interleukin-2 production during active visceral leishmaniasis. *J. Clin. Invest.* **76**, 2066–9.

Castes, M., Agnelli, A., Verde, O. and Rondon, A.J. (1983). Characterization of the cellular immune response in American cutaneous leishmaniasis. *Clin. Immunol. Immunopathol.* **27**, 176–86.

Castes, M., Agnelli, A. and Rondon, A.J. (1984). Mechanisms associated with immunoregulation in human American cutaneous leishmaniasis. *Clin. Exp. Immunol.* **57**, 279–86.

Castes, M., Cabrera, M., Trujillo, D. and Convit, J. (1988). T cell subpopulations, expression of interleukin-2 receptor, and production of interleukin-2 and gamma interferon in human American cutaneous leishmaniasis. *J. Clin. Microbiol.* **26**, 1207–13.

Chance, M.L. (1982). Nomenclature of enzyme variants with regard to functional taxonomic classification of *Leishmania*. In *Proceedings of a Workshop held at the Pan American Health Organization, Washington, DC (9–11 December 1980)*, pp. 115–21, UNDP/World Bank/WHO Special Programme for Research and Training in Tropical Diseases, Geneva, Switzerland.

Chance, M.L., Gardener, P.J. and Peters, W. (1977). Biochemical taxonomy of *Leishmania* as an ecological tool. In *Ecologie des leishmanioses*, Colloquiem Internationale CNRS no. 239, Montpellier, 18–24 August 1974, pp. 53–61.

Chang, C.-S., Inserra, T.J., Kink, J.A., Fong, D. and Chang, K.-P. (1986). Expression and size heterogeneity of a 63 kilodalton membrane glycoprotein during growth and transformation of *Leishmania mexicana amazonensis*. *Mol. Biochem. Parasitol.* **18**, 197–210.

Chang, K.-P. (1978). Phagocytosis and intracellular digestion of leishmanial amastigotes by human polymorphonuclear phagocytes. *J. Protozool.* **25**, 20a.

Chang, K.-P. (1981). Leishmanicidal mechanisms of human polymorphonuclear, phagocytes. *Am. J. Trop. Med. Hyg.* **30**, 322–33.

Chang, K.-P. and Chiao, J.W. (1981). Cellular immunity of mice to *Leishmania donovani in vitro*: lymphokine-mediated killing of intracellular parasites in macrophages. *Proc. Nat. Acad. Sci. (USA)* **78**, 7083–7.

Channon, J.Y., Roberts, M.B. and Blackwell, J.M. (1984). A study of the differential respiratory burst elicited by promastigotes and amastigotes of *Leishmania donovani* in murine resident peritoneal macrophages. *Immunology* **53**, 345–55.

Colomer-Gould, V., Galvao Quintao, L., Keithly, J. and Nogueira, N. (1985). A common major surface antigen on amastigotes and promastigotes of *Leishmania* species. *J. Exp. Med.* **162**, 902–16.

Convit, J., Pinardi, M.E. and Rondon, A. (1972). Diffuse cutaneous leishmaniasis. A disease due to an immunological defect. *Trans. Roy. Soc. Trop. Med. Hyg.* **66**, 603–10.

Convit, J., Castellanos, P.L., Rondon, A. *et al.* (1987). Immunotherapy versus chemotherapy in localised cutaneous leishmaniasis. *Lancet*, **i**, 401–5.

Cooper, A.M., Rosen, H. and Blackwell, J.M. (1988). Monoclonal antibodies which recognise distinct epitopes of macrophage type three complement receptor differ in their ability to inhibit binding of *Leishmania* promastigotes harvested at different phases of their growth cycle. *Immunology* **65**, 511–14.

Crawford, R.M., Finbloom, D.S., Ohara, J., Paul, W.E. and Meltzer, M.S. (1987). B cell stimulatory factor-1 (interleukin 4) activates macrophages for increased tumoricidal activity and expression of Ia antigens. *J. Immunol.* **139**, 135–41.

Crocker, P.R., Blackwell, J.M. and Bradley, D.J. (1984). Expression of the natural resistance gene *Lsh* in resident liver macrophages. *Infect. Immunity* **43**, 1033–40.

Crocker, P.R., Davies, E.V. and Blackwell, J.M. (1987). Variable expression of the natural resistance gene *Lsh* in different macrophge populations infected *in vitro* with *Leishmania donovani*. *Parasite Immunol.* **9**, 705–19.

Cross, G.A.M. (1987). Eukaryote protein modification and membrane attachment via, phosphatidylinositol. *Cell* **48**, 179–81.

da Silva, R.P. and Sacks, D.L. (1987). Metacyclogenesis is a major determinant of *Leishmania* promastigote virulence and attenuation. *Infect. Immunity* **55**, 2802–6.

da Silva, R.P., Hall, B.F., Joiner, K.A. and Sacks, D.L. (1989). CR1, the C3b receptor, mediates binding of infective *Leishmania major* metacyclic promastigotes to human macrophages. *J. Immunol.* **143**, 617–22.

Davies, C.R., Cooper, A.M., Peacock, C., Blackwell, J.M. and Lane, R.P. (1990). Expression of LPG and GP63 by different developmental stages of *Leishmania* major in the sandfly *Phlebotomus papatasi Parasitology* **101**, 337–46.

Davies, E.V., Singleton, A.M.T. and Blackwell, J.M. (1988).

Differences in *Lsh* gene control over systemic *Leishmania major* and *Leishmania donovani* or *Leishmania mexicana mexicana* infections are caused by differential targeting to infiltrating and resident liver macrophage populations. *Infect. Immunity* **56**, 1128–34.

Ding, A., Wright, S.D. and Nathan, C.F. (1987). Activation of mouse peritoneal macrophages by monoclonal antibodies to Mac-1 (complement receptor type 3). *J. Exp. Med.* **165**, 733–49.

Etges, R., Bouvier, J. and Bordier, C. (1986a). The major surface protein of *Leishmania* promastigotes is a protease. *J. Biol. Chem.* **261**, 9098–101.

Etges, R., Bouvier, J. and Bordier, C. (1986b). The major surface protein of *Leishmania* promastigotes is anchored in the membrane by a myristic acid-labeled phospholipid. *EMBO J.* **5**, 597–601.

Ferguson, M.J.A. and Williams, A.F. (1988). Cell-surface anchoring of proteins via glycosylphosphatidylinositol structures. *Ann. Rev. Biochem.* **57**, 285–320.

Ferguson, M.J.A., Low, M.G. and Cross, G.A.M. (1985). Glycosyl-*sn*-1,2-dimyristylphosphatidylinositol is covalently linked to *Trypanosoma brucei* variant surface glycoprotein. *J. Biol. Chem.* **260**, 14547–55.

Fong, D. and Chang, K.-P. (1982). Surface antigen change during differentiation of a parasitic protozoan, *Leishmania mexicana*: identification by monoclonal antibodies. *Proc. Nat. Acad. Sci. (USA)* **79**, 7366–70.

Franke, E.D., McGreevy, P.B., Katz, S.P. and Sacks, D.L. (1985). Growth cycle dependent generation of complement resistant *Leishmania* promastigotes. *J. Immunol.* **134**, 2713–18.

Gardener, P.J. (1977). Taxonomy of the genus *Leishmania*: a review of nomenclature and classification. *Trop. Dis. Bull.* **74**, 1069–88.

Gardener, P.J., Chance, M.L. and Peters, W. (1974). Biochemical taxonomy of *Leishmania*. II. Electrophoretic variation of malate dehydrogenase. *Ann. Trop. Med. Parasitol.* **68**, 317–25.

Goto, H., Sotto, M.N., Corbett, C.E.P. *et al.* A case of disseminated mucocutaneous leishmaniasis due to *Leishmania braziliensis braziliensis* infection. *J. Trop. Med. Hyg.* (in press).

Goto, Y., Nakamura, R.M., Takahashi, H. and Tokunaga, T. (1984). Genetic control of resistance to *Mycobacterium intracellulare* infection in mice. *Infect. Immunity* **46**, 135–40.

Greenblatt, C.L. (1988). Cutaneous leishmaniasis: the prospects for a killed vaccine. *Parasitol. Today* **4**, 53–4.

Gros, P., Skamene, E. and Forget, A.J. (1983). Cellular mechanisms of genetically controlled host resistance to *Mycobacterium bovis* (BCG) in mice. *J. Immunol.* **127**, 2417–21.

Gutierrez, Y., Maksem, J.A. and Reiner, N.E. (1984). Pathologic changes in murine leishmaniasis (*Leishmania donovani*) with special reference to the dynamics of granuloma formation in the liver. *Am. J. Pathol.* **114**, 222–30.

Haldar, J.P., Ghose, S., Saha, K.C. and Ghose, A.C. (1983). Cell-mediated immune response in Indian kala-azar and post-kala-azar dermal leishmaniasis. *Infect. Immunity* **42**, 702–7.

Hamilton, T.A. and Adams, D.O. (1987). Molecular mechanisms of signal transduction in macrophages. *Immunol. Today* **8**, 151–8.

Handman, E. and Burgess, A.W. (1979). Stimulation by granulocyte-macrophage colony-stimulating factor of *Leishmania tropica* killing by macrophages. *J. Immunol.* **122**, 1134–7.

Handman, E. and Goding, J.W. (1985). The *Leishmania* receptor for macrophages is a lipid containing glycoconjugate. *EMBO J.* **4**, 329–36.

Handman, E. and Mitchell, G.F. (1985). Immunization with *Leishmania* receptor for macrophages protects mice against cutaneous leishmaniasis. *Proc. Nat. Acad. Sci. (USA)* **82**, 5910–14.

Handman, E., Schnur, L.F., Spithill, T.W. and Mitchell, G.F. (1986). Passive transfer of *Leishmania* lipopolysaccharide confers parasite survival in macrophages. *J. Immunol.* **137**, 3608–13.

Ho, M., Siongok, T.K., Lyerly, W.H. and Smith, D.H. (1982). Prevalence and disease spectrum in a new focus of visceral leishmaniasis in Kenya. *Trans. Roy. Soc. Trop. Med. Hyg.* **76**, 741–6.

Ho, M., Koech, D.K., Iha, D.W. and Bryceson, A.D.M. (1983). Immunosuppression in Kenyan visceral leishmaniasis. *Clin. Exp. Immunol.* **51**, 207–14.

Hoover, D.L., Berger, M., Nacy, C.A., Hockmeyer, W.T. and Meltzer, M.S. (1984). Killing of *Leishmania tropica* amastigotes by factors in normal human serum. *J. Immunol.* **132**, 893–7.

Howard, J.G., Hale, C. and Liew, F.Y. (1980). Immunological regulation of experimental cutaneous leishmaniasis. III. Nature and significance of specific suppression of cell-mediated immunity in mice highly susceptible to *Leishmania tropica*. *J. Exp. Med.* **152**, 594–607.

Howard, J.G., Hale, C. and Liew, F.Y. (1981). Immunological regulation of experimental cutaneous leishmaniasis. IV. Prophylactic effect of sublethal irradiation as a result of abrogation of suppressor T cell generation in mice genetically susceptible to *Leishmania tropica*. *J. Exp. Med.* **153**, 557–68.

Howard, M.K., Sayers, G. and Miles, M.A. (1987). *Leishmania donovani* metacyclic promastigotes: transformation *in vitro*, lectin agglutination, complement resistance and infectivity. *Exp. Parasitol.* **64**, 147–56.

Hynes, R.O. (1987). Integrins: a family of cell surface receptors. *Cell* **48**, 549–54.

Jaffe, C.L. and McMahon Pratt, D. (1983). Monoclonal antibodies specific for *Leishmania tropica*. I. Characterization of antigens associated with stage and species specific determinants. *J. Immunol.* **131**, 1987–93.

Jaffe, C.L., Bennett, E., Grimaldi, G. and McMahon Pratt, D. (1984). Production of species specific monoclonal antibodies against *Leishmania donovani* for immunodiagnosis. *J. Immunol.* **133**, 440–7.

Joiner, K.A., Hammer, C.H., Brown, E.J. and Frank, M.M. (1982). Studies on the mechanism of bacterial resistance to complement-mediated killing. II. C8 and C9 release C5b67 from the surface of *Salmonella minnesota* S218 because the terminal complex does not insert into the bacterial outer membrane. *J. Exp. Med.* **155**, 809–19.

Kaye, P.M., Patel, N.K. and Blackwell, J.M. (1988). Acquisition of cell-mediated immunity to *Leishmania*. II. *Lsh* gene regulation of accessory cell function. *Immunology* **65**, 17–22.

Kaye, P.M., Roberts, M.B. and Blackwell, J.M. (1987). Analysing the immune response to *L. donovani* infection. *Ann. Inst. Pasteur Immunol.* **138**, 762–8.

Killick-Kendrick, R. (1979). The biology of *Leishmania* in Phlebotomine sandflies. In *Biology of the Kinetoplastida*, vol. II, ed. W.H.R. Lumsden and D.H. Evans, pp. 395–460,

Academic Press, London.

Kindler, V., Thorens, B. de Kossodo, S. *et al*. (1986). Stimulation of hematopoiesis *in vivo* by recombinant bacterial interleukin 3. *Proc. Nat. Acad. Sci. (USA)* **83**, 1001–5.

Kweider, M., Lemesre, J.-L., Carcy, F., Kusnierz, J.-P., Capron, A. and Santoro, F. (1987). Infectivity of *Leishmania braziliensis* promastigotes is dependent on the increasing expression of a 65 000 dalton surface antigen. *J. Immunol.* **138**, 299–305.

Lainson, R. (1983). The American leishmaniases: some observations on their ecology and epidemiology. *Trans. Roy. Soc. Trop. Med. Hyg.* **77**, 569–96.

Lainson, R. and Shaw, J.J. (1972). Leishmaniasis of the New World: taxonomic problems. *Br. Med. Bull.* **28**, 44–8.

Lainson, R. and Shaw, J.J. (1979). The role of animals in the epidemiology of South American leishmaniasis. In *Biology of the Kinetoplastida*, ed. W.H.R. Lumsden and D.A. Evans, vol. II, pp. 1–116, Academic Press, London, New York & San Francisco.

Lainson, R. and Shaw, J.J. (1987). Evolution, classification and geographical distribution. In *The Leishmaniases in Biology and Medicine*, ed. W. Peters and R. Killick-Kendrick, pp. 1–120, Academic Press, London, New York & San Francisco.

Lelchuck, R., Gravely, R. and Liew, F.Y. (1987). Susceptibility to murine cutaneous leishmaniasis correlates with the capacity to generate interleukin-3 in response to leishmania antigen *in vitro*. *Cell. Immunol.* **111**, 66–76.

Liew, F.Y. (1987). Analysis of host-protective and disease-promoting T cells. *Ann. Inst. Pasteur Immunol.* **138**, 749–55.

Liew, F.Y. (1989). Functional heterogeneity of $CD4^+$ T cells in leishmaniasis. *Immunol. Today* **10**, 40–5.

Liew, F.Y., Hale, C. and Howard, J.G. (1982). Immunological regulation of experimental cutaneous leishmaniasis. V. Characterization of effector and suppressor T cells. *J. Immunol.* **128**, 1917–22.

Locksley, R.M., Heinzel, F.P., Sadick, M.D., Holaday, B.J. and Gardner, K.D. (1987). Murine cutaneous leishmaniasis: susceptibility correlates with differential expansion of helper T-cell subsets. *Ann. Inst. Pasteur Immunol.* **138**, 744–9.

Locksley, R.M., Heinzel, F.R., Fankhauser, J.E., Nelson, C.S. and Sadick, M.D. (1988). Cutaneous host defense in leishmaniasis: interaction of isolated dermal macrophages and epidermal Langerhans cells with the insect-stage promastigote. *Infect. Immunity* **56**, 336–42.

Long, E.O. and Jacobson, S. (1989). Pathways of viral antigen processing and presentation to CTL. *Immunol. Today* **10**, 45–8.

Louis, J. and Milon, G. (Convenors) (1987). Twentieth Forum in Immunology: Immunobiology of Experimental Leishmaniasis. *Ann. Inst. Pasteur Immunol.* **138**, 737–95.

Louis, J.A., Pedrazzini, T., Titus, R.G. *et al*. (1987). Subsets of specific T cells and experimental cutaneous leishmaniasis. *Ann. Inst. Pasteur Immunol.* **138**, 755–8.

Low, M.G. and Kincade, P.W. (1985). Phosphatidylinositol is the membrane-anchoring domain of the Thy-1 glycoprotein. *Nature* **318**, 62–4.

Lynch, N.R., Yarzabal, L., Verde, O., Avila, J.L., Monzon, H. and Convit, J. (1982). Delayed-type hypersensitivity and immunoglobulin E in American cutaneous leishmaniasis. *Infect. Immunity* **38**, 877–81.

McConville, M.J., Bacic, A., Mitchell, G.F. and Handman, E. (1987). Lipophosphoglycan of *Leishmania major* that vaccinates against cutaneous leishmaniasis contains an alkylglycerophospho-inositol. *Proc. Nat. Acad. Sci. (USA)* **84**, 8941–5.

McElrath, M.J., Murray, H.W. and Cohn, Z.A. (1988). The dynamics of granuloma formation in experimental visceral leishmaniasis. *J. Exp. Med.* **167**, 1927–37.

McMahon Pratt, D. and David, J.R. (1981). Monoclonal antibodies that distinguish between New World species of *Leishmania*. *Nature* **291**, 581–3.

McMahon Pratt, D., Bennett, E. and David, J.R. (1982). Monoclonal antibodies that distinguish subspecies of *Leishmania braziliensis*. *J. Immunol.* **129**, 926–7.

McMahon Pratt, D., Bennett, E., Jaffe, C.L. and Grimalde, G. (1985). Subspecies and species-specific antigens of *Leishmania mexicana* characterized by monoclonal antibodies. *J. Immunol.* **134**, 1935–40.

McMaster, W.R. (1990). Correction. *J. Exp. Med.* **171**, 599.

McNeely, T.B. and Turco, S.J. (1987). Inhibition of protein kinase C activity by the *Leishmania donovani* lipophosphoglycan. *Biochem. Biophys. Res. Comm.* **148**, 653–7.

Marrack, P. and Kappler, J. (1988). The T-cell repertoire for antigen and MHC. *Immunol. Today* **9**, 308–14.

Marsden, P.D. (1986). Mucosal leishmaniasis. *Trans. Roy. Soc. Trop. Med. Hyg.* **80**, 859–76.

Mayrink, W., Williams, P., da Costa, C.A. *et al*. (1985). An experimental vaccine against American dermal leishmaniasis: experience in the State of Espirito Santo, Brazil. *Ann. Trop. Med. Parasitol.* **79**, 259–69.

Melby, P.C., Neva, F.A. and Sacks, D.L. (1989). Profile of human T cell response to leishmanial antigens: analysis by immunoblotting. *J. Clin. Invest.* **83**, 1868–72.

Metcalf, D. (1986). The molecular biology and functions of the granulocyte–macrophage colony-stimulating factors. *Blood* **67**, 257–67.

Miles, M.A. (1985). Biochemical identification of the leishmanias. *Bull. Pan Am. Health Org.* **19**, 343–53.

Miles, M.A., Lainson, R., Shaw, J.J., Povoa, M. and de Souza, A.A. (1981). Leishmaniasis in Brazil. XV. Biochemical distinction of *Leishmania mexicana amazonensis*, *L. braziliensis braziliensis*, and *L. braziliensis guyanensis*, aetiological agents of cutaneous leishmaniasis in the Amazon basin of Brazil. *Trans. Roy. Soc. Trop. Med. Hyg.* **75**, 524–9.

Miller, R.A., Parsons, M. and Reed, S.G. (1989). Cloning of the GP63 gene of *Leishmania donovani chagasi*. *J. Cell. Biochem.* **S13E**, 112.

Milon, G., Titus, R.G., Cerottini, J.-C., Marchal, G. and Louis, J.A. (1986). Higher frequency of *Leishmania major*-specific $L3T4^+$ T cells in susceptible BALB/c as compared with resistant CBA mice. *J. Immunol.* **136**, 1467–71.

Mirkovich, A.M., Gallelli, A., Allison, A.C. and Modabber, F.Z. (1986). Increased myelopoiesis during *Leishmania major* infection in mice: generation of 'safe targets', a possible way to evade the effector immune mechanism. *Clin. Exp. Immunol.* **64**, 1–7.

Modabber, F. (1987). A model for the mechanism of sensitivity of BALB/c mice to *L. major* and premunition in leishmaniases. *Ann. Inst. Pasteur Immunol.* **138**, 781–6.

Moriearty, P.L., Bittencourt, A.L., Pereira, C., Teixeira, R., Barreto, E. and Guimaraes, N.A. (1978). Borderline cutaneous leishmaniasis: clinical, immunological and histological differences from mucocutaneous leishmaniasis. *Rev. Inst. Med. Trop. São Paulo* **20**, 15–21.

Mosman, T.R., Cherwinski, H., Bond, M.W., Giedlin, M.W. and Coffman, R.L. (1986). Two types of murine helper T-cell clone. I. Definition according to profiles of lymphokine activities and secreted proteins. *J. Immunol.* **136**, 2348–57.

Mosser, D.M. and Edelson, P.J. (1984). Activation of the alternative complement pathway by *Leishmania* promastigotes: parasite lysis and attachment to macrophages. *J. Immunol.* **132**, 1501–5.

Mosser, D.M. and Edelson, P.J. (1985). The mouse macrophage receptor for C3bi (CR3) is a major mechanism in the phagocytosis of *Leishmania* promastigotes. *J. Immunol.* **135**, 2785–9.

Mosser, D.M., Wedgewood, J.F. and Edelson, P.J. (1985). *Leishmania* amastigotes: resistance to complement-mediated lysis is not due to a failure to fix C3. *J. Immunol.* **134**, 4128–31.

Mosser, D.M., Burke, S.K., Coutavas, E.E., Wedgewood, J.F. and Edelson, P.J. (1986). *Leishmania* species: mechanisms of complement activation by five strains of promastigotes. *Exp. Parasitol.* **62**, 394–404.

Mosser, D.M., Vlassara, H., Edelson, P.J. and Cerami, A. (1987). *Leishmania* promastigotes are recognized by the macrophage receptor for advanced glycosylation endproducts. *J. Exp. Med.* **165**, 140–5.

Munro, D.D., du Vivier, A. and Jopling, W.H. (1972). Post-kala azar dermal leishmaniasis. *Br. J. Dermatol.* **87**, 374–8.

Murray, H.W. (1981a). Susceptibility of *Leishmania* to oxygen intermediates and killing by normal macrophages. *J. Exp. Med.* **153**, 1302–15.

Murray, H.W. (1981b). Interaction of *Leishmania* with a macrophage cell line: correlation between intracellular killing and the generation if oxygen intermediates. *J. Exp. Med.* **153**, 1690–5.

Murray, H.W. (1982). Cell-mediated immune response in experimental visceral leishmaniasis. II. Oxygen-dependent killing of intracellular *Leishmania donovani* amastigotes. *J. Immunol.* **129**, 351–7.

Murray, H.W., Rubin, B.Y. and Rothermel, C.D. (1983). Killing of intracellular *Leishmania donovani* by lymphokine-stimulated human mononuclear phagocytes. Evidence that interferon-gamma is the activating lymphokine. *J. Clin. Invest.* **72**, 1506–10.

Murray, H.W., Spitalny, G.L. and Nathan, C.F. (1985). Activation of mouse peritoneal macrophages *in vitro* and *in vivo* by interferon-gamma. *J. Immunol.* **134**, 1619–22.

Murray, H.W., Stern, J.J., Welte, K., Rubin, B.Y., Carriero, S.M. and Nathan, C.F. (1987). Experimental visceral leishmaniasis: production of interleukin 2 and interferon-gamma, tissue immune reaction, and response to treatment with interleukin 2 and interferon-gamma. *J. Immunol.* **138**, 2290–7.

Nacy, C.A., Meltzer, M.S., Leonard, E.J. and Wyler, D.J. (1981). Intracellular replication and lymphokine-induced destruction of *Leishmania tropica* in C3H/HeN mouse macrophages. *J. Immunol.* **127**, 2381–6.

Nacy, C.A., Fortier, A.H., Meltzer, M.S., Buchmeier, N.A. and Schreiber, R.D. (1985). Macrophage activation to kill *L. major*: activation of macrophages for intracellular destruction of amastigotes can be induced by both recombinant interferon and non-interferon lymphokines. *J. Immunol.* **135**, 3505–11.

O'Brien, A.D. and Metcalf, E.S. (1982). Control of early *Salmonella typhimurium* growth in innately *Salmonella*-resistant mice does not require functional T lymphocytes. *J. Immunol.* **129**, 1349–51.

Orlandi, P.A. and Turco, S.J. (1987). Structure of the lipid moiety of the *Leishmania donovani* lipophosphoglycan. *J. Biol. Chem.* **262**, 10384–91.

Pampiglione, S., Manson-Bahr, P.E.C., Giungi, F., Giunti, G., Parenti, A. and Trotti, G.C. (1974). Studies on Mediterranean leishmaniasis. 2. Asymptomatic cases of visceral leishmaniasis. *Trans. Roy. Soc. Trop. Med. Hyg.* **68**, 447–53.

Pearson, R.D. and Steigbigel, R.T. (1980). Mechanism of lethal effect of human serum upon *Leishmania donovani*. *J. Immunol.* **125**, 2195–201.

Pearson, R.E. and Steigbigel, R.T. (1981). Phagocytosis and killing of the protozoan *Leishmania donovani* by human polymorphonuclear leucocytes. *J. Immunol.* **127**, 1438–43.

Petersen, E.A., Neva, F.A., Oster, C.N. and Bogaert-Diaz, H. (1982). Specific inhibition of lymphocyte-proliferation responses by adherent suppressor cells in diffuse cutaneous leishmaniasis. *N. Engl. J. Med.* **306**, 387–92.

Petersen, E.A., Neva, F.A., Barral, A. *et al.* (1984). Monocyte suppression of antigen-specific lymphocyte responses in diffuse cutaneous leishmaniasis patients from the Dominican Republic. *J. Immunol.* **132**, 2603–6.

Pimenta, P.F.P., da Silva, R.P., Sacks, D.L. and da Silva, P.P. (1989). Cell surface nanoanatomy of *Leishmania major* as revealed by fracture-flip: a surface meshwork of 44 nm fusiform filaments identifies infective developmental stage promastigotes. *Eur. J. Cell Biol.* **48**, 180–90.

Plant, J.E., Blackwell, J.M., O'Brien, A.D., Bradley, D.J. and Glynn, A.A. (1982). Are the *Lsh* and *Ity* disease resistance genes at one locus on mouse chromosome 1? *Nature* **297**, 510–11.

Pommier, C.G., Inada, S., Fries, L.F., Takahashi, T., Frank, M.M. and Brown, E.J. (1983). Plasma fibronectin enhances phagocytosis of opsonized particles by human peripheral blood monocytes. *J. Exp. Med.* **157**, 1844–54.

Powrie, F. and Mason, D. (1988). Phenotypic and functional heterogeneity of $CD4^+$ T cells. *Immunol. Today* **9**, 274–7.

Puentes, S.M., Sacks, D.L., da Silva, R.P. and Joiner, K.A. (1988). Complement binding by two developmental stages of *Leishmania major* promastigotes varying in expression of a surface lipophosphoglycan. *J. Exp. Med.* **167**, 887–902.

Puentes, S.M., da Silva, R.P., Sacks, D.L., Hammer, C.H. and Joiner, K.A. (1989). Serum resistance of metacyclic stage *Leishmania major* promastigotes is due to release of C5b-9. *J. Immunol.* **143**, 3743–9.

Rada, E., Trujillo, D., Castellanos, P.L. and Convit, J. (1987). Gamma interferon production induced by antigens in patients with leprosy and American cutaneous leishmaniasis. *Am. J. Trop. Med. Hyg.* **37**, 520–4.

Ramos Aguire, C. (1970). Leishmaniasis en la region carbonifera de Coahuila. Reporte de dos casos de la forma anergica difusa. *Dermatol. Mexico* **14**, 34–45.

Rezai, H.R., Ardehali, S.M., Amirhakimi, G. and Kharazmi, A. (1978). Immunological features of kala-azar. *Am. J. Trop. Med. Hyg.* **27**, 1079–83.

Riches, D.W.H. and Stanworth, D.R. (1980). A simple method of measuring the capacity to activate the alternative pathway.

Immunol. Lett. **1**, 363–6.

Rioux, J.A., Lanotte, G., Maazoun, R., Perello, R. and Pratlong, F. (1980). *Leishmania infantum* Nicolle, 1908, agent de bouton d'Orient autochtone. A propos de l'identification biochimique de deux souches isolées dans les Pyrenées-Orientales. *Comptes Rendus Hébdom. Séances Acad. Sci. D Sci. Nat. (Paris)* **291**, 701–3.

Roberts, M., Kaye, P.M., Milon, G. and Blackwell, J.M. (1988). Studies of immune mechanisms in *H-11*-linked genetic susceptibility to murine visceral leishmaniasis. In *Leishmaniasis: The Current Status and New Strategies for Control*, ed. D.T. Hart, pp. 259–66, Plenum Publishers.

Roberts, M., Alexander, J. and Blackwell, J.M. (1989). Influence of *Lsh*, *H-2* and an *H-11*-linked gene on visceralisation and metastasis associated with *Leishmania mexicana* infection in mice. *Infect. Immunity* **57**, 875–81.

Rosen, H. and Gordon, S. (1987). Monoclonal antibody to the murine type 3 complement receptor inhibits adhesion of myelomonocytic cells *in vitro* and inflammatory cell recruitment *in vivo*. *J. Exp. Med.* **166**, 1685–701.

Ross, G.D., Cain, J.A. and Lachmann, P.J. (1985). Membrane complement receptor type three (CR3) has lectin-like properties analogous to bovine conglutanin and functions as a receptor for zymosan and rabbit erythrocytes as well as a receptor for iC3b. *J. Immunol.* **134**, 3307–15.

Ross, G.D., Cain, J.A., Myones, B.L., Newman, S.L. and Lachman, P.J. (1987). Specificity of membrane complement receptor type three (CR3) for B-glucans. *Complement* **4**, 61–74.

Russell, D.G. (1990). *Leishmania* and the macrophage. *Immunol. Today* **11**, 74–5.

Russell, D.G. and Alexander, J. (1987). Effective immunization against cutaneous leishmaniasis with defined membrane antigens reconstituted into liposomes. *J. Immunol.* **140**, 1274–9.

Russell, D.G. and Wilhelm, H. (1986). The involvement of the major surface glycoprotein (gp63) of *Leishmania* promastigotes in attachment to macrophages. *J. Immunol.* **136**, 2613–20.

Russell, D.G. and Wright, S.D. (1988). Complement receptor type 3 (CR3) binds to an Arg–Gly–Asp-containing region of the major surface glycoprotein. gp63, of *Leishmania* promastigotes. *J. Exp. Med.* **168**, 279–92.

Sacks, D.L. and da Silva, R.P. (1987). The generation of infective *Leishmania major* promastigotes is associated with the cell-surface expression and release of a developmentally regulated glycolipid. *J. Immunol.* **139**, 3099–106.

Sacks, D.L. and Perkins, P.V. (1984). Identification of an infective stage of *Leishmania* promastigotes. *Science* **223**, 1417–19.

Sacks, D.L., Hieny, S. and Sher, A. (1985). Identification of cell surface carboyhydrate and antigenic changes between non-infective and infective developmental stages of *Leishmania major* promastigotes. *J. Immunol.* **135**, 564–9.

Sacks, D.L., Lal, S.L., Shrivastava, S.N., Blackwell, J.M. and Neva, F.A. (1987). An analysis of T cell responsiveness in Indian kala-azar. *J. Immunol.* **138**, 908–13.

Sacks, D.L. (1989). Metacyclogenesis in Leishmania promastigotes. *Exp. Parasit.* **69**, 100–3.

Schnur, L.F., Zuckerman, A. and Greenblatt, C.L. (1972). Leishmanial serotypes as distinguished by the gel diffusion of factors excreted *in vitro* and *in vivo*. *Israel J. Med. Sci.* **8**, 932–42.

Schurr, E., Kidane, K., Yemaneberhan, T. and Wunderlich, F. (1986). Cutaneous leishmaniasis in Ethiopia. I. Lymphocyte transformation and antibody titre. *Tropenmed. Parasitol.* **37**, 403–8.

Scott, P.E. (1985). Impaired macrophage leishmanicidal activity at cutaneous temperature. *Parasite Immunol.* **7**, 277–88.

Scott, P.E., James, S. and Sher, A. (1986). The respiratory burst is not required for killing of intracellular and extracellular parasites by lymphokine-activated macrophage cell line. *Eur. J. Immunol.* **15**, 553–8.

Scott, P.E., Natovitz, P., Coffman, R.L., Pearce, E. and Sher, A. (1988). Immunoregulation of cutaneous leishmaniasis: T cell lines which transfer protective immunity or exacerbation belong to different T helper subsets and respond to distinct parasite antigens. *J. Exp. Med.* **168**, 1675–84.

Scott, P.E., Pearce, E., Natovitz, P. and Sher, A. (1987). Vaccination against cutaneous leishmaniasis in a murine model. II. Immunologic properties of protective and non-protective subfractions of a soluble promastigote extract. *J. Immunol.* **139**, 3118–26.

Sen Gupta, P.C. and Mukherjee, A.M. (1962). Intradermal test with *Leishmania donovani* antigen in post-kala azar dermal leishmaniasis. *Ann. Biochem. Exp. Med.* **22**, 63–6.

Shaw, J.J. and Lainson, R. (1975). Leishmaniasis in Brazil. X. Some observations on intradermal reactions to different trypanosomatid antigens of patients suffering from cutaneous and mucocutaneous leishmaniasis. *Trans. Roy. Soc. Trop. Med. Hyg.* **69**, 323–35.

Sim, R.B., Twose, D.S., Peterson, D.S. and Sim, E. (1981). The covalent-binding reaction of complement component C3. *Biochem. J.* **193**, 115–27.

Skamene, E., Gros, P., Forget, A., Kongshavn, P.A.L., St Charles, C. and Taylor, B.A. (1982). Genetic regulation of resistance to intracellular pathogens. *Nature* **297**, 506–9.

Skamene, E., Gros, P., Forget, A., Patel, P.J. and Nesbitt, M.N. (1984). Regulation of resistance to leprosy by chromosome 1 locus in the mouse. *Immunogenetics* **19**, 117–24.

Solbach, W., Greil, J. and Rollinghoff, M. (1987). Anti-infectious responses in *Leishmania major*-infected BALB/c mice injected with recombinant granulocyte–macrophage colony-stimulating factor. *Ann. Inst. Pasteur Immunol.* **138**, 759–62.

Squires, K.E., Schreiber, R.D., McElrath, M.J. and Murray, H.W. (1986). Role of endogenous interferon-gamma in murine visceral leishmaniasis. *Clin. Res.* **35**, 492A.

Stern, J.J., Oca, M.J., Rubin, B.Y., Anderson, S.L. and Murray, H.W. (1988). Role of L3T4^{+} and Lyt-2^{+} cells in experimental visceral leishmaniasis. *J. Immunol.* **140**, 3971–7.

Titus, R.G., Kelso, A. and Louis, J.A. (1984). Intracellular destruction of *Leishmania tropica* by macrophages activated with macrophage activating factor/interferon gamma. *Clin. Exp. Immunol.* **55**, 157–65.

Titus, R.G., Milon, G., Marchal, G., Vassalli, P., Cerottini, J.C. and Louis, J.A. (1987). Involvement of specific Lyt-2^{+} T cells in the immunological control of experimentally induced murine cutaneous leishmaniasis. *Eur. J. Immunol.* **17**, 1429–33.

Turco, S.J. (1988). The lipophosphoglycan of *Leishmania*. *Parasitol. Today* **4**, 255–7.

Turco, S.J., Wilkerson, M.A. and Clawson, D.R. (1984). Expression of an unusual acidic glycoconjugate in *Leishmania*. *J. Biol. Chem.* **259**, 3883–9.

Turco, S.J., Hull, S.R., Orlandi, P.A., Shepherd, S.D. *et al.* (1987). Structure of the major carbohydrate fragment of the *Leishmania donovani* lipophosphoglycan. *Biochemistry* **26**, 6233–8.

Walton, B.C., Chinel, L.V. and Eguia, O.E. (1973). Onset of espundia after many years of occult infection with *Leishmania braziliensis*. *Am. J. Trop. Med. Hyg.* **22**, 696–8.

Weishui, W.Y., Van Niel, A., Clark, S.C., David, J.R. and Remold, H.G. (1987). Recombinant human granulocyte/macrophage colony-stimulating factor activates intracellular killing of *Leishmania donovani* by human monocyte-derived macrophages. *J. Exp. Med.* **166**, 1436–46.

Wilson, M.E. and Hardin, K.K. (1988). The major concanavalin A-binding surface glycoprotein of *Leishmania donovani chagasi* promastigotes is involved in attachment to human macrophages. *J. Immunol.* **141**, 265–72.

Wilson, M.E. and Pearson, R.D. (1986). Evidence that *Leishmania donovani* utilizes a mannose receptor on human mononuclear phagocyte to establish intracellular parasitism. *J. Immunol.* **136**, 4681–8.

Wilson, M.E. and Pearson, R.D. (1988). Roles of CR3 and mannose receptors in the attachment and ingestion of *Leishmania donovani* by human mononuclear phagocytes. *Infect. Immunity* **56**, 363–9.

Wilson, M.E., Innes, D.J., Sousa, A. de Q. and Pearson, R.D. (1987). Early histopathology of experimental infection with *Leishmania donovani* in hamsters. *J. Parasitol.* **73**, 55–63.

Witzum, E., Spira, D.T. and Zuckerman, A. (1978). Blast transformation in different stages of cutaneous leishmaniasis. *Israeli J. Med. Sci.* **14**, 244–7.

Wozencraft, A.O., Sayers, G. and Blackwell, J.M. (1986). Macrophage type 3 complement receptors mediate serum-independent binding of *Leishmania donovani*: detection of macrophage-derived complement on the parasite surface by immunoelectron microscopy. *J. Exp. Med.* **164**, 1332–7.

Wright, S.D. and Jong, M.T.C. (1986). Adhesion-promoting receptors on human macrophages recognize *E. coli* by binding to lipopolysaccharide. *J. Exp. Med.* **164**, 1876–88.

Wright, S.D. and Silverstein, S.C. (1982). Tumor-promoting phorbol esters stimulate C3b and C3b′ receptor-mediated phagocytosis in cultured human monocytes. *J. Exp. Med.* **156**, 1149–64.

Wright, S.D. and Silverstein, S.C. (1983). Receptors for C3b and C3bi promote phagocytosis but not the release of toxic oxygen from human phagocytes. *J. Exp. Med.* **158**, 2016–23.

Wright, S.D., Rao, P.E., Van Voorhis, W.C. *et al.* (1983a). Identification of the C3bi-receptor on human monocytes and macrophages by using monoclonal antibodies. *Proc. Nat. Acad. Sci. (USA)* **80**, 5699–703.

Wright, S.D., Criagmyle, L.S. and Silverstein, S.C. (1983b). Fibronectin and serum amyloid P component stimulates C3b- and C3bi-mediated phagocytosis in cultured human monocytes. *J. Exp. Med.* **158**, 1338–43.

Wright, S.D., Light, M.R., Craigmyle, L.S. and Silverstein, S.C. (1984). Communication between receptors for different ligands on a single cell: ligation of fibronectin receptors induces a reversible alteration in the function of C3 receptors in cultured human monocytes. *J. Cell Biol.* **99**, 336–9.

Wright, S.D., Reddy, P.A., Jong, M.T.C. and Erikson, B.W. (1987). C3bi-receptor (complement receptor type 3) recognizes a region of complement protein C3 containing the sequence Arg–Gly–Asp. *Proc. Nat. Acad. Sci. (USA)* **84**, 1965–8.

Wyler, D.J., Weinbaum, F.I. and Herrod, H.R. (1979). Characterization of *in vitro* proliferative responses of human lymphocytes to leishmanial antigens. *J. Infect. Dis.* **140**, 215–21.

Wyler, D.J., Sypek, J.P. and McDonald, J.A. (1985). *In vitro* parasite-monocyte interactions in human leishmaniasis: possible role of fibronectin in parasite attachment. *Infect. Immunity* **49**, 305–11.

Yamamoto, K. and Johnston, R.B. (1984). Dissociation of phagocytosis from stimulation of the oxidative metabolic burst in macrophages. *J. Exp. Med.* **159**, 405–16.

Zuckerman, A. and Lainson, R. (1977). Leishmania. In *Parasitic Protozoa. I. Taxonomy, Kinetoplastids and Flagellates of Fish*, ed. J.P. Kreier, pp. 57–133, Academic Press, New York, San Francisco, London.

81: The Immunology of African Trypanosomiasis

T.W. Pearson

African trypanosomiasis (African sleeping sickness in humans, nagana in cattle) is found in Africa and is caused by several different species and subspecies of related organisms, the African trypanosomes. The diseases in both humans and cattle are extremely serious and of profound medical and socio-economic importance (Kuzoe 1987).

African trypanosomes are notorious for their evasion of host immune responses and thus have been extensively utilized for studying antigenic variation. Because of several unique features, trypanosomes are increasingly being used as model organisms for research in biochemistry and molecular genetics but not, surprisingly, for immunology, despite the paramount role of the immune system in trypanosomiasis. This is probably due to the complexity of the immunological perturbations induced by infection with trypanosomes and our inability to envisage strategies for development of vaccines. Indeed, many knowledgeable researchers believe that vaccination against African trypanosomes will be impossible.

In this chapter I outline several features of African trypanosomes that are important for understanding host–parasite–vector interactions and discuss, where possible, their relationship to the host immune system. Information relevant to the immunology of trypanosomiasis is still too meagre to establish a solid base for pessimism regarding vaccine development.

Introduction

As protozoa, trypanosomes are unicellular eukaryotic organisms belonging to the genus *Trypanosoma*. Members of this genus are digenetic parasites which live alternately in the bloodstream and tissues of vertebrates and the gut of leeches or arthropods. The genus *Trypanosoma* is split into two divisions, Salivaria and Stercoraria. The African trypanosomes complete their development in the anterior parts of the tsetse fly (*Glossina* spp.) vector's digestive tract and are transmitted via vector saliva. They are thus called salivarian trypanosomes.

African trypanosomes cause disease in humans and their domestic animals in large areas of sub-Saharan Africa. More than 50 million people are at risk of African sleeping sickness and more than

200 million cattle at risk of nagana (from the Zulu, meaning poorly). Today, in Africa, the impact of cattle trypanosomiasis is much greater than that due to human trypanosomiasis since the number of human infections is relatively low. However, in the last decade the human disease has been increasing with more than 20 000 new cases reported each year. The true incidence is likely to be much higher. African trypanosomiasis is fatal unless treated and, as with all other human diseases caused by parasites, there is no vaccine.

Sleeping sickness was described as early as the fourteenth century by an Arab writer, al Qualquashaudi (Hoeppli 1959). The African trypanosomes themselves were discovered in the latter part of the nineteenth century. *Trypanosoma evansi*, which infects camels and horses, was discovered in 1880 and *T. brucei brucei*, which infects cattle, in 1894 (Hoare 1972). *T. brucei gambiense* and *T. brucei rhodesiense*, the causative organisms of African sleeping sickness in humans, were reported in 1902 and 1903, respectively (Hoare 1972). Although the disease and its causes have been known for a long time, there is still no prophylaxis available other than avoidance of the tsetse fly. This state of affairs is primarily due to the problem posed by antigenic variation.

Antigenic variation and the immune system

African trypanosomes are infamous for their ability to undergo antigenic variation, a process by which they are able as a population to avoid elimination from the mammalian host. At the beginning of this century it was noticed by several investigators that the parasitaemia levels in the bloodstream of infected humans fluctuated dramatically. Ross and Thompson (1910) measured and plotted parasitaemia levels in a trypanosome-infected patient and found successive peaks of parasitaemia, each followed by a decline in the number of bloodstream trypanosomes, often to undetectable levels. With remarkable insight they postulated that each new parasitaemic wave contained trypanosomes that somehow escaped the effects of host antibodies made against the parasites in the previous peak. In 1916, Ritz showed that infections initiated with a single trypanosome produced antigenically distinct variants, thus establishing that variation is a property of an individual trypanosome. The biochemical basis for antigenic variation was not understood until more than 50 years later. LePage (1968a, b) studied soluble antigens from trypanosomes isolated from a chronically infected rabbit and purified variant-specific antigens from cloned populations. He showed that each variant antigen had a unique tryptic fingerprint and thus different primary amino acid sequences. LePage concluded that the extent of such differences was unlikely to be caused by point mutations and that antigenic variation resulted from the expression of different genes. In a landmark study, Cross (1975) finally established the nature of the trypanosome surface coat and its relationship to antigenic variation. He showed that there was a major glycoprotein of M_r approximately 65 000 on the surface of bloodstream trypanosomes and that this glycoprotein differed in amino acid composition between antigenitically distinct clones. Since the publication of Cross's paper, the biochemistry of the variant surface glycoproteins (VSG) has been studied intensively (reviewed by Turner 1982). Surprisingly, though we know that the VSG molecule plays a central role in antigenic variation and survival of the trypanosome, its immunochemistry is not well understood. Nevertheless, it is now clear that African trypanosomes survive in their mammalian host in part by variation in their expression of VSG genes (see review by Donelson 1988) and subsequent avoidance of elimination by the immune system.

Although the trypanosome VSG is central to this parasite's *modus operandi* for success, many other aspects of trypanosome biology and biochemistry are important for understanding its interaction with the immune system and manifestations of the host–parasite interaction. Central to this understanding is a knowledge of the life cycle of the African trypanosome.

The life cycle

The prototypic African trypanosome follows a complex life cycle between the mammalian host and the tsetse fly vector and is thus said to be cyclically transmitted. A schematic representation of the life cycle of *T. brucei* is shown in Fig. 81.1. Several features of the life cycle are important for the following discussion. Firstly, the VSG coat is found only on the metacyclic stage in the tsetse fly and in all bloodstream stages in the infected mam-

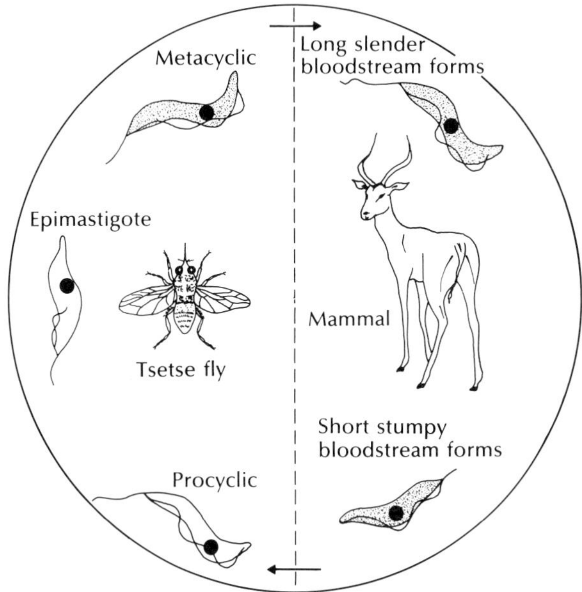

Fig. 81.1. A simplified representation of the life cycle of *Trypanosoma brucei* spp. The bloodstream forms in the mammalian host and the metacyclic form in the tsetse fly vector are covered with VSG (shaded grey). The procyclic and epimastigote forms in the tsetse fly are covered with the protein procyclin.

mal. Secondly, the forms of the parasite which lack VSG are covered with procyclin, an unusual molecule which may be important in parasite–vector interactions. Thirdly, the bloodstream parasites exist in several morphologically distinct forms, the rapidly dividing long-slender and intermediate forms and the non-dividing short-stumpy forms. For a review of the developmental biology of the African trypanosome see Vickerman (1985) and for a discussion of growth and use of the various life cycle stages in the laboratory see Shapiro and Pearson (1986).

Infection of the mammalian host is initiated by the injection into the skin of metacyclic forms from the tsetse fly vector's saliva. These rapidly differentiate into long-slender bloodstream forms, which are anaerobic and rely mainly on glycolysis for energy production. It is this form of the parasite that engages in antigenic variation. Short-stumpy bloodstream forms appear in the mammalian host presumably as a pre-adaptation to growth in the tsetse vector since they have a semideveloped mitochondrion and have ceased to divide (Shapiro *et al*. 1984). Both long-slender and short-stumpy life cycle stages are important for understanding the immunology of African trypanosomiasis, the former because of the phenomenon of antigenic variation and the latter because of its suspected involvement in limitation of parasitaemia levels and as a stage involved in transmission from the mammalian host to the tsetse fly vector. Both of these stages will be discussed in detail later.

The disease in humans, cattle and mice

Human trypanosomiasis (African sleeping sickness) has been responsible for hundreds of thousands of deaths in great epidemics (McKelvey 1973). Although such large epidemics have not occurred since the early part of this century, disruption of medical services and population movements caused by social instability have allowed recent smaller epidemics (Cattand 1988). The human disease exists in two forms although the criteria for distinguishing them are often subjective. Acute disease, attributed to *T. b. rhodesiense*, can lead to death in several weeks to a year and is found mainly in East and Southern Africa, whereas a more chronic disease, attributed to *T. gambiense*, may take several years to kill an untreated patient and is found primarily in West and Central Africa (Fig. 81.2). The two kinds of infection are distinguished on the basis of their locale and clinical course but, because the criteria used are somewhat subjective, definitive tests that discriminate between the two subspecies of parasites are still required.

The disease, in humans, progresses through three main stages: the first in which the trypanosomes are localized at the site of the tsetse fly bite; the second (systemic) stage in which the parasites are distributed in the bloodstream and tissues throughout the body; and the third in which the organisms invade the central nervous system. The first stage is sometimes characterized by a chancre at the bite site. The second stage is characterized by non-specific signs of infection, including intermittent fever, joint pains and general malaise, all of which are the result of the fluctuating parasitaemia and subsequent immunological and physiological responses to high parasite load and disruption of immunoregulation. The third stage is characterized by the consequences of meningoencephalitis resulting from invasion of the brain by the trypanosomes. The patient first appears irritated, may then appear psychotic and finally

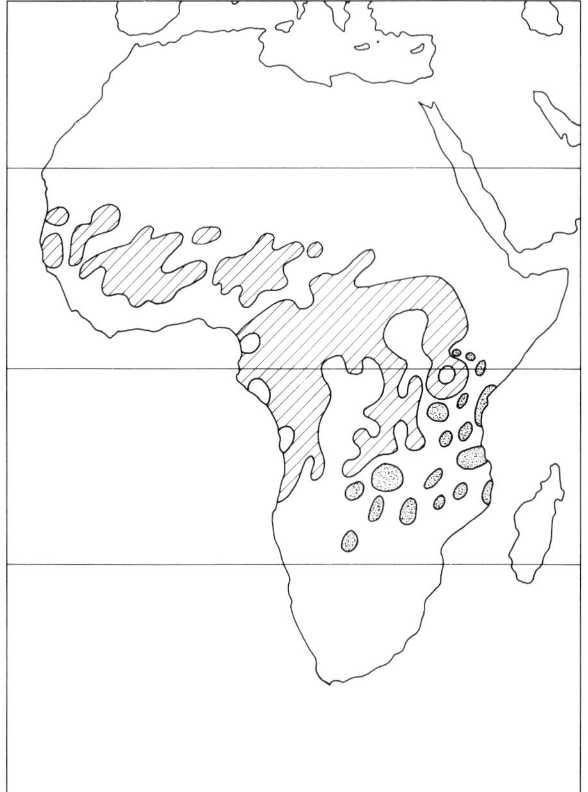

Fig. 81.2. The distribution of human African sleeping sickness on the African continent. Gambian sleeping sickness (hatched areas) caused by *T. b. gambiense* and Rhodesian sleeping sickness (shaded areas) caused by *T. b. rhodesiense* are shown in approximation. Redrawn from Peters and Gilles (1977).

loses consciousness: hence the name sleeping sickness. Once the parasite has invaded the central nervous system death is inevitable unless drug treatment ensues. Even with drug treatment the results are not always successful. Varying degrees of immunodepression occur during the middle and late stages of the disease and thus sometimes the patient will die of secondary infections.

In trypanosome infections of domestic animals the main livestock pathogens (*T. congolense*, *T. vivax*) rarely invade the central nervous system. The main causes of death are anaemia and cachexia (wasting) which cause severe weakness and inability to forage for food. Immunodepression can also occur in animal trypanosomiasis and some animals die from secondary infections (frequently pneumonia). However, animals do not necessarily die from trypanosomiasis; some species of wild animals are highly resistant to the disease (Mulla and Rickman 1988) and certain breeds of domestic animals show some resistance (Murray 1988).

A wide spectrum of disease susceptibility is seen with experimental trypanosome infections of inbred mice. In fact, most of our information on the immune response and the genetics of susceptibility and resistance to the parasite is based on the murine model. This will be discussed in detail later.

It is clearly evident that African trypanosomes cause a wide spectrum of disease phenotypes in both humans and animals and that both the host and parasite influence the course of the infection. Studies on the immunobiology of the host–trypanosome relationship illustrate this complexity. We do not understand the two essential features of the host–trypanosome interaction:

1 What determines the resistance or susceptibility of a host?

2 What determines the infectivity and/or pathogenicity of a trypanosome?

The immune system is central to understanding the above two questions but the mechanisms involved are poorly understood.

The immunology of trypanosomiasis

Both innate resistance and acquired immune responses are important in trypanosomiasis, the former being important in determination of parasite host range and the latter in parasite clearance and in the pathological consequences of infection.

Trypanocidal activity of sera

In 1902, the toxicity of normal human sera for *T. brucei* was first described (Laveran 1902). Several subsequent studies have shown that the morphologically indistinguishable subspecies of the *T. brucei* group showed different susceptibilities to this killing. Thus the human pathogens *T. b. rhodesiense* and *T. b. gambiense* are normally resistant to human sera whereas the cattle pathogen, *T. b. brucei*, is not. Serum resistance has thus been used to discriminate between *T. b. rhodesiense*, which is infective for humans, and *T. b. brucei*, which is not. This serum resistance in *T. b. rhodesiense* is not stable and both resistant and susceptible forms can switch after several generations (Van Meirvenne *et al.* 1976; Joshua 1985). It is probable that the designation of these two subspecies simply reflects the presence or absence of serum sensitivity since by all other criteria, including analysis by deoxyribonucleic acid (DNA) hybridization (Massamba and Williams 1984; Paindavoine *et al.* 1986), they are identical. The serum-resistant *T. b. gambiense* subspecies clearly differs from the *T. b. brucei* and *T. b. rhodesiense* organisms by DNA hybridization analysis. Serum sensitivity may not be absolute since there are clear examples of certain variable antigen types (within a series of antigenetically different clones derived from a single organism) that exhibit serum resistance whereas other antigenic types within the serodeme do not (Herbert *et al.* 1980). This is an important point since, in one instance, a research technician became accidentally infected with a particular variant antigen type of trypanosomes considered to be *T. b. brucei*. Clearly, in this case, the trypanosome stock had to be reclassified as *T. b. rhodesiense*. Since Jenni and Brun (1982) have shown that it is possible to grow a single serum-resistant trypanosome from a population of 10^5 serum-sensitive organisms, it is prudent to treat all *T. b. brucei* and *T. b. rhodesiense* stocks as potentially capable of infecting humans, that is, as if they are all *T. b. rhodesiense*.

Several investigators have attempted to identify the trypanocidal molecule(s) in human sera. Rifkin (1978a, b) showed that the active factor was associated with high-density lipoprotein (HDL). Rifkin did not claim that all of the HDL was trypanocidal and showed that only part of the HDL fraction was active. Indeed, Hajduk *et al.* (1989) have purified a subclass of HDL which is responsible for trypanolytic activity. The lytic factor is a very minor species of HDL, is unusually large and contains a number of unique proteins. A recent report describing a new method for purification of a trypanocidal factor from human serum (Barth 1989) showed that the active fraction was a protein complex of high molecular mass (>1000 kD) consisting of four proteins resolvable by sodium dodecyl sulphate polyacrylamide gel electrophoresis. No high-density lipoproteins were detectable in the active fraction, thus challenging the generally accepted view that HDL is responsible for the trypanolytic activity. Caution must be exercised in these types of studies, however, since it is possible that concentration of certain proteins or removal of inhibitory substances could result in the identification of trypanolytic molecules which are not functional in normal human sera. In addition, it is probable that multiple killing mechanisms exist. This possibility is suggested by the studies of Hawking (1978), who showed that some strains of *T. congolense* and *T. vivax* are highly resistant to human serum; yet these species do not infect humans. Also, a trypanocidal factor against *T. equiperdum* has been identified in human serum as naturally occurring immunoglobulin M (IgM) antibodies (Verducci *et al.* 1989). It has also been found that serum-resistant variants of *T. b. rhodesiense* express a messenger ribonucleic acid (mRNA) transcript that is not found in serum-sensitive variants (De Greef *et al.* 1989). The transcript was not found in *T. b. gambiense*, which is resistant to lysis by human sera, again suggesting that multiple killing mechanisms exist. Clearly both immunological and non-immunological trypanocidal components exist in sera. Such components, their mechanisms of action and their interaction with both susceptible and resistant parasites demand further study for possible exploitation against the trypanosome.

Immune responses during infection

Surprisingly, the biological relevance of host immune responses to trypanosome antigens is not well understood despite extensive literature on the subject. Part of the problem is that researchers have used a bewildering array of parasite species, stocks and clones in a variety of different mammalian hosts. Since trypanosomiasis is manifested by a wide spectrum of disease phenotypes, which is influenced by both parasite and host genetics, it is necessary, during the following discussion, to realize that the disease characteristics in one host–parasite combination may not be the same in another.

The immune system is radically affected in most animals infected with African trypanosomes and plays a central role in the attempted control of the parasite and in the pathogenesis of the disease. Trypanosome infections are initiated when metacyclic parasites are inoculated into a mammalian host by the bite of the tsetse fly (*Glossina* spp.). At the bite site, the organisms begin to replicate and mononuclear cells infiltrate and initiate the formation of a chancre. Trypanosomes are then disseminated throughout the host via the lymphatic vessels and blood and rapidly replicate extracellularly, giving rise to high parasitaemia levels which fluctuate throughout the infection. It is this rise and fall of parasite numbers which is associated with antigenic variation. Often, trypanosomes eventually invade the central nervous system (cerebrospinal fluid and the brain) and cause the death of the host.

The immune system is involved from the initiation of infection until the demise of the infected host. Immune reactions are responsible for events in the chancre and the immunoproliferative responses early in the infection are responsible for many of the characteristics of the disease: elevated immunoglobulin levels (especially IgM), splenomegaly and lymphadenopathy. Clearly specific antibody responses are responsible, in part, for clearance of parasites. Trypanosomal antigen–antibody complexes and autoantibodies induced by specific responses to parasite antigens and by non-specific B lymphocyte proliferation and differentiation to antibody-secreting plasma cells contribute to disease pathogenesis. Later in the infection, immune responses become depressed and the host is killed by the now uncontrollable trypanosomes or by secondary infections. The changes in the immune system will be discussed in terms of three different phases of parasite–immune system interaction.

THE CHANCRE

Five to ten days after the tsetse fly bite, a nodular lesion appears at the site. Bites from uninfected tsetse flies do not induce a chancre, indicating that the lesion is a specific response to the trypanosomes (Emery and Moloo 1981; Akol and Murray 1982), which along with an acute inflammatory response contribute to the formation of the lesion. Polymorphonuclear leucocytes and small lymphocytes initially infiltrate the lesion and, as the chancre develops, lymphoblasts appear, followed by macrophages and plasma cells as the lesion starts to subside. The chancre size is most probably related to the number of parasites at the site and the extent of the cellular infiltration. The exact role of the immune response in the chancre is not known although antibodies are probably made to the VSG of the predominant antigenic types. Animals that have been exposed previously to metacyclic trypanosomes of the same strain do not develop a chancre, probably because circulating anti-VSG antibodies limit the initial parasite proliferation at the site (Akol and Murray 1982). Events at the chancre possibly influence the selection of distinct parasite antigenic types that escape to the local draining lymph node and lymphatic system and then into the bloodstream, where the early systemic process of parasite replication initiates.

THE EARLY SYSTEMIC RESPONSE

Once in the bloodstream, the trypanosomes usually proliferate rapidly and become widely distributed throughout the animal. At this point, one or a few antigenic types give rise to a peak of parasitaemia in the blood and produce a concomitant immunoproliferative response in several lymphoid organs. The cellular changes are most profound in the mouse. There is a striking proliferation of splenic B and T lymphocytes, null cells which are mainly erythrocyte precursors and null lymphocytes (Corsini *et al.* 1977; Mayor-Withey *et al.* 1978) and phagocytic cells (Murray *et al.* 1974). The B lymphocyte proliferation results in a tremendous increase in levels of IgM antibodies (Luckins and Mehlitz 1976; Whittle *et al.* 1977). The B lymphocyte stimulation is polyclonal with the result that trypanosome-specific antibodies, autoantibodies and antibodies which do not bind to parasite or host molecules are produced (Hudson *et al.* 1976; Greenwood and Whittle 1980). The reason for the polyclonal proliferation of B lymphocytes is not known but has been hypothesized to be due to production or induction of a B lymphocyte mitogen by the bloodstream-form trypanosomes (Urquhart *et al.* 1973; Greenwood 1974). Indeed, activated macrophages from mice injected with lethally irradiated trypanosomes (Grosskinsky and Askonas 1981) or with trypanosome membranes (Sacks *et al.* 1982) have been shown to induce non-specific B lymphocyte proliferation. It is now generally believed that African trypanosomes induce host macrophages to stimulate both B and T lymphocyte proliferation and to influence several other aspects of the immune response, including immunodepression and immunosuppression (Askonas 1985; Mansfield 1990).

Trypanosome-specific (anti-VSG) antibodies are found in the serum 3–4 days after infection and, within hours of appearance, are usually extremely effective in eliminating most of the parasites. The antibody-aided decline in numbers of parasites and their subsequent reappearance is characteristically repeated and the host often develops a fluctuating chronic parasitaemia, the hallmark of African trypanosome infections and caused primarily by antigenic variation. Antibodies effective in the elimination of trypanosomes are primarily IgM and are directed to VSG epitopes that are exposed on the surface of living trypanosomes (Sendashonga and Black 1982). Evidence that VSG-specific antibodies are important in removal of trypanosomes is abundant (reviewed in Mansfield 1990). The specific anti-VSG antibody response is mainly T lymphocyte-independent and can occur in nude mice (Clayton *et al.* 1979). Variant surface glycoprotein-specific IgG antibodies are produced, however, but do not usually appear until after the parasites have been eliminated and are therefore probably not involved in parasite clearance. Variant surface glycoprotein-specific IgM antibodies are produced throughout most of an infection with African trypanosomes and there is evidence for a more effective IgM anti-VSG response in resistant strains of mice (Mitchell and Pearson 1983). In contrast, T lymphocyte-dependent IgG responses are soon down-regulated as the infection progresses. The trypanosomes are removed from the bloodstream by a combination of complement-mediated lysis (Murray and Urquhart 1977) and antibody-dependent phagocytosis (Greenblatt *et al.* 1983; Ngaira *et al.* 1983) which depends largely on Kupffer cells of the liver (Dempsey and Mansfield 1983). Even in mice, the liver appears to be where trypanosomes are cleared, despite the large number of macrophages in the greatly enlarged spleens of these animals.

That antibodies play an important role in trypanosome removal is clear. However, several observations have complicated our earlier somewhat simplistic views regarding the control of parasite levels during infection. Firstly, there is good evidence, in the murine system at least, that B lymphocyte responses are not linked genetically or functionally to the overall resistance to trypanosomiasis (see below under 'Genetics of resistance'). Secondly, non-immunological mechanisms appear to influence the transition of rapidly dividing trypanosomes to non-dividing forms, thus limiting parasite numbers (see below under 'Trypanosome differentiation'). Thus the role of the immune response in controlling trypanosome infections must be reassessed.

THE LATE SYSTEMIC RESPONSE

Most of the profound changes in the immune system of trypanosome-infected animals occur as a result of chronic parasitaemia. This is certainly true for the changes in cellular responses and for the immunosuppression observed in most species. However, many inbred mice become severely immunodepressed soon after experimental infection and exhibit drastic changes in their lymphocyte populations and lymphoid organ structure. These changes are most apparent in the murine spleen (Wellhausen and Mansfield 1980; Kar *et al.* 1981). Since most studies on the cellular immunology of trypanosomiasis have been performed using mice, it is important to remember that the situation in other animals may be quite different. Nevertheless, the murine models have been necessary for most of these studies and many of the phenomena observed in them have parallels, albeit not as profound, in other species.

The immunological changes that occur in mice result in a state of immunodepression in which both humoral and cell-mediated responses are affected (Corsini *et al.* 1977; Jayawardena and Waksman 1977; Pearson *et al.* 1978; Wellhausen and Mansfield 1980; Kar *et al.* 1981). The immunodepression is now thought to be caused primarily by a parasite-induced effect on macrophages, which actively suppress immune responses or fail to process or present antigen properly (Askonas 1985; Paulnock *et al.* 1988). Indeed, macrophages from infected mice expressed normal levels of Ia antigens, secreted stimulatory levels of interleukin 1, were able to process and present heterologous (non-trypanosome) antigen and yet were unable to respond normally to trypanosomes (Paulnock *et al.* 1988). The macrophages from trypanosome-infected animals thus possibly function to suppress responses in a parasite antigen-specific fashion. The mechanisms involved remain unknown.

The ultimate effect of the trypanosome-induced alterations in immunoregulation is that, throughout most of the infection, host T lymphocyte-dependent immune responses are depressed and T-independent B lymphocyte responses (to VSG surface antigens, for example) are left intact. Later in infection, even the T-independent antibody responses are inhibited, with the result that the trypanosomes are not effectively removed from the host animal (reviewed in Shapiro and Pearson

1986 and by Mansfield 1990). By suppressing T lymphocyte-dependent responses, the parasite may limit the immunopathology which occurs due to IgG autoantibodies and IgG immune complexes while still allowing parasite clearance and longer survival of the host. In this way, the trypanosome ensures its survival by increasing its chances of transmission to the tsetse vector and ultimately to a new host mammal.

Genetics of resistance

Humans, cattle and mice clearly show a wide spectrum of susceptibility to disease and of clinical symptoms of trypanosomiasis. Breeds of cattle which have been on the African continent for a long time show a degree of trypanotolerance (Murray *et al*. 1982) and some individual animals, although infected, show little pathology. Cattle introduced from Europe, however, rapidly succumb to the disease after experiencing severe disease and resultant cachexia. In humans, the disease ranges from mild to severe within a geographically defined population and there are anecdotal reports of spontaneous cure and even of people with persistent parasitaemia but no symptoms of disease.

The genetics of resistance has been studied in both cattle and mice although most of our information is from experimental infections of the latter with *T. brucei* spp. or with *T. congolense*. Indeed, strains of mice show varying degrees of susceptibility to disease, with some strains dying within a few days of infection and others surviving for several months. Therefore, relative resistance, based on time to death, is the usual parameter measured. Studies using major histocompatibility complex (MHC) congenic mice (strains with different *H-2* haplotypes on the same genetic background) have clearly shown for *T. b. congolense* and *T. b. rhodesiense* that resistance is not MHC-linked (Morrison and Murray 1979; Levine and Mansfield 1981) and that it is multigenic and complex (Morrison and Murray 1979; De Gee *et al*. 1988).

Evidence that antibody responses are not always linked to resistance has been obtained using both cattle and mice. No correlation between the magnitude of trypanosome-specific antibody responses and resistance was seen in cattle that demonstrated different degrees of resistance (Murray *et al*. 1982). In a murine model it was shown that F1 hybrids, derived from crosses between resistant and susceptible inbred mice, exhibited VSG-specific antibody responses and controlled the infecting trypanosome population (first peak of parasitaemia) but did not survive longer than the susceptible parental strain animals (Levine and Mansfield 1984). Thus antibody production and control of parasitaemia were inherited as a dominant trait whereas resistance to trypanosomiasis (as measured by relative survival time) was inherited as a recessive trait, the two segregating independently of one another. Further genetic analysis has clearly shown that anti-trypanosome antibodies and control of parasitaemia are controlled by genes different from those determining survival times (De Gee *et al*. 1988; Seed and Sechelski 1989a). Therefore, although VSG-specific antibody responses appear always to be linked to control of parasitaemia, they are not neccessarily linked to overall resistance to the trypanosome infection.

If the ability to make anti-VSG antibodies is not linked with overall survival, then what is the evidence that the immune response has anything to do with host survival and with our concept of antigenic variation as the mechanism by which the parasites evade the 'protective' host immune response? There is no doubt that immunosuppressed animals rapidly succumb to infection and that prior immunization with a parasite of a given antigenic type can protect against infection with homologous organisms. It is likely, then, that immune responses do play an important role in host resistance to trypanosomes but that other host factors play a major role. For example, strain differences in macrophage-mediated antigen processing, polyclonal B and T lymphocyte stimulation, or immunosuppression could easily alter long-term host survival by influencing immunoregulation and resultant immunopathology. It is clear that interleukin 1 and 2 production is markedly altered in trypanosome-infected mice (Mitchell *et al*. 1986) and, although there have been several subsequent publications on immunoregulatory factors involved in trypanosomiasis, this area of investigation remains relatively untouched. Under active investigation is the idea that there are non-immunological host factors which have an influence on parasite differentiation and which control parasitaemia levels in trypanosome-infected hosts (Black *et al*. 1985).

Trypanosome differentiation

During a parasitaemic wave in mice infected with trypanosomes, the long-slender bloodstream forms usually differentiate into short-stumpy non-dividing forms which accumulate prior to peak parasitaemia and wave remission (Robertson 1913; Balber 1972; Sendashonga and Black 1982). Trypanosomes able to undergo this transformation are said to be pleomorphic, in contrast to monomorphic parasites which are obtained by rapid syringe passage between host animals and which are rapidly dividing and remain as long-slender form parasites until they kill the host (Hoare 1970). Some imaginative work by Sam Black and his colleagues has shown that host immune responses are probably stimulated by VSG antigens from stumpy-form organisms and not from dividing long-slender forms (Black *et al*. 1982; Sendashonga and Black 1982). This suggests that the transition from long-slender to non-dividing short-stumpy forms influences the induction of VSG-specific antibody responses and thus control of the parasitaemia. The morphological transition to short-stumpy form parasites can occur in immunosuppressed animals (Balber 1972) and is thus not thought to be induced by specific immune responses (Black *et al*. 1985). Black and his colleagues have accumulated evidence that parasite numbers are regulated by the rate of transition of dividing long-slender bloodstream trypanosomes to non-dividing short-stumpy form organisms and that the parasite differentiation is controlled by host-derived molecules which inhibit parasite differentiation by promoting multiplication of the long-slender forms (Black *et al*. 1983a, b, 1985). Recently serum lipoproteins have been found to be necessary for multiplication of *T. brucei* (Black and Vanderweerd 1989) and an epidermal growth factor acceptor homologue has been found in trypanosomes (Hide *et al*. 1989), indicating that parasite growth might be controlled or at least influenced by host components. Evidence that differentiation to stumpy forms is due to a parasite-induced exogenous growth inhibitor has also been obtained (Seed and Sechelski 1989b). The significance of the slender-stumpy transition is not fully understood. Clearly it plays a major role in limiting parasitaemias and is intimately linked with the clearance of trypanosomes by the immune system.

Trypanosome virulence

No virulence factors (genes or gene products) have been identified in African trypanosomes. It has long been known, however, that different trypanosome species, subspecies and strains show a wide range of disease phenotypes, with some parasites being much more virulent or pathogenic than others (Mulligan 1970). This range in virulence has been shown to exist in antigenically different clones of trypanosomes isolated from a genetically homogeneous population (Inverso and Mansfield 1983). Nevertheless, virulence is not necessarily linked to VSG expression since both highly virulent and less virulent clones which express identical VSGs could be isolated (Inverso *et al*. 1988). These clones showed identical growth rates, induced similar antibody responses and were cleared from the host with similar kinetics. They did, however, induce different degrees of immunosuppression. For each clone, the virulence characteristics were observed to be stable in a given host and did not change during antigenic variation. The molecular basis for virulence differences in trypanosomes is not known but is clearly dependent on gene expression in the parasite since host animals do not determine whether or not a given clone is of high or low virulence.

The role of the surface coats

The plasma membrane of bloodstream forms of African trypanosomes is covered with a single species of glycoprotein, the VSG, which is central to antigenic variation. Surprisingly, the VSG molecules are highly immunogenic and cause the effective induction of host antibodies and subsequent removal of trypanosomes. The standard view, therefore, is that antibodies function to eliminate the parasites from the host and are thus host-protective. Why then would the trypanosome have evolved a highly antigenic coat? It has been suggested that anti-VSG antibodies decrease parasite numbers at the peak of parasitaemia when stumpy forms differentiate from long-slender forms (Black *et al*. 1985). This allows the host to re-establish conditions of homoeostasis which favour the growth of antigenically different long-slender forms (Seed and Sechelski 1987). The new parasite population forms the next parasitaemic wave and eventually establishes a population of intermediate forms thought to be important for transmission to the tsetse fly vector (Giffin *et al.* 1986; Giffin and McCann 1989). Removal of the stumpy forms would help maintain a vigorous population of dividing parasites and would ensure the availability of new intermediate forms during the periodic waves of parasitaemias. This results in the establishment of a chronic infection which increases the opportunity for transmission of trypanosomes to the tsetse fly vector. Thus specific antibodies are not only beneficial to the host, but also of benefit to the parasite, i.e. a successful host–parasite relationship is established.

It has long been thought that the insect stages of African trypanosomes are uncoated since they lose VSG upon differentiation from bloodstream forms (Barry and Vickerman 1979; Overath *et al.* 1983). The discovery of a stage-specific glycoprotein, procyclin (Richardson *et al.* 1988; Roditi *et al.* 1987) has changed this view, however, and it is now believed that at no point in the life cycle is the trypanosome uncoated (Roditi and Pearson 1990). Procyclin is a species-specific glycoprotein (Richardson *et al.* 1986, 1988) and both procyclin mRNA transcripts (Mowatt and Clayton 1987; Roditi *et al.* 1987) and encoded protein (Richardson *et al.* 1986, 1988) are expressed only in certain tsetse fly vector stages of the life cycle. In contrast to bloodstream forms, where the VSG is the only surface-exposed molecule, many different proteins can be labelled by surface iodination of procyclic culture forms (Gardiner *et al.* 1983). Among the procyclic surface proteins, however, procyclin is preponderant, since it is abundant (Clayton and Mowatt 1989) and immunodominant (Richardson *et al.* 1986). As differentiation proceeds, procyclin progressively replaces VSG on the trypanosome surface (Roditi *et al.* 1989), thus ensuring that the parasite is always coated. Despite its high immunogenicity it is not known if procyclin is naturally exposed to the immune system of the host, for example by parasites that begin to differentiate to procyclic forms in the bloodstream, if this occurs at all. Procyclin is not detected in short-stumpy trypanosomes (Colmerauer *et al.* 1989) but procyclin epitopes can be detected in the sera of trypanosome-infected mice (Liu and Pearson 1987). If the detected antigen is procyclin itself, it is possible that host antibodies may be produced and that these would immediately remove procyclic forms, ensuring that they would not be detected in the bloodstream. Also not known is whether antibodies to procyclin (or to other procyclic surface antigens) could effect trypanosome transmission rates in the field by influencing development of the parasite in the tsetse fly vector. Interference with trypanosome transmission has been seen after feeding tsetse flies on animals immunized with procyclic trypanosomes (Maudlin *et al.* 1984; Murray *et al.* 1985), suggesting that a transmission-blocking vaccine may be worth investigating.

Immunodiagnosis

Since there is no current vaccine or prophylaxis for trypanosomiasis and because the disease is usually lethal unless treated, diagnosis is essential in identifying infected individuals for immediate treatment. Two types of tests are currently in use, parasitological and serological. Both have serious drawbacks (Turner 1985). Parasitological diagnosis is based on detection of the parasite by light microscopy in blood films or biopsy material from lymph node punctures. The effectiveness of this technique is limited by low parasite levels, especially in *T. b. gambiense* infections, which are characterized by fluctuating parasitaemias (Doyle 1977).

Current serological methods for diagnosis of human sleeping sickness are based on the detection of anti-trypanosome antibodies in patient's sera (Van Meirvenne and Le Ray 1985). The card agglutination trypanosomiasis test (CATT) (Magnus *et al.* 1978), utilizing a fixed, stained bloodstream form of *T. b. gambiense* that expresses a ubiquitous VSG, is the most successfully applied screening technique for *T. b. gambiense* infection, found mainly in West and Central Africa (World Health Organization 1986). However, the CATT does not detect infections caused by *T. b. rhodesiense*, which occurs primarily in Southern and East Africa, because this subspecies does not express a ubiquitous VSG. In order to improve upon existing diagnostic tests for African sleeping sickness, the procyclic agglutination trypanosomiasis test (PATT) was developed (Pearson *et al.* 1986). This test uses living *T. b. rhodesiense* procyclic culture forms in an agglutination format and detects anti-procyclic antibodies in patient's sera. Antibodies to procyclic forms of *T. b. brucei*, *T. b. gambiense* and *T. b. rhodesiense* are detected in this test (Liu *et al*. 1989) and are presumably induced in the patient by cross-reacting antigens released by lysed bloodstream trypanosomes. The procyclic agglutination assay has proved to be effective in detecting anti-trypanosomal antibodies in the sera of *T. b. rhodesiense*-infected vervet monkeys (Pearson *et al*. 1986), in *T. b. gambiense*-infected humans (Liu *et al*. 1989) and in *T. b. rhodesiense*-infected humans (Liu *et al*. unpublished).

Serological tests based on the detection of anti-trypanosomal antibodies do not distinguish between past and currently active infections and thus are not ideal for revealing the infection status of patients. A diagnostic test for detection of circulating trypanosomal antigens may be more desirable. A double antibody sandwich enzyme-linked immunosorbent assay was therefore developed and has been found to detect antigen in the sera of trypanosome-infected mice (Liu and Pearson 1987), vervet monkeys (Liu *et al*. 1988) and humans from both West and East Africa (Liu *et al*. 1989, 1990a, b). The antigen capture assay gave results which were more indicative of infection status than the antibody detection assays (CATT and PATT) and in several cases predicted when patients were about to relapse after drug treatment (Liu *et al*. 1990b).

The CATT has been used extensively in the field and is inexpensive and elegantly simple although it takes some skill to obtain reliable results. It cannot be used for *T. b. rhodesiense* infections, however. In contrast, the PATT and the antigen capture assay are not restricted to detection of *T. b. gambiense* infections but they are currently only laboratory-based assays which require adaptation to simple formats for use in the field. This is a worthwhile technical and financial challenge, however, since early diagnosis of human trypanosomiasis is the first step in effective control of the disease, at least until other approaches become available.

Overview

Our understanding of the immunology of trypanosomiasis is incomplete and much of the scientific literature on the subject is complex and confusing. Although innate and adaptive host defence mechanisms are involved in determining the parasite host range and immunopathology of the disease, our earlier simplistic ideas about antibody control of the waves of parasitaemia during antigenic variation require reassessment in light of new information on parasite differentiation and the genetics of resistance. Unlike most other infectious micro-organisms, including many parasites, no trypanosome antigens with clear prospects for development of vaccines have been identified. It appears that control of trypanosomiasis will depend on information gained from basic research on the biochemistry, immunology and cell biology of the parasite. The use of the African trypanosome as a model organism in different disciplines is therefore of paramount importance.

Acknowledgements

I thank Drs Sam Black, Dick Seed and John Mansfield for sending me preprints of their work and Jennifer Duggan and Tanya Payne for typing the manuscript. Work in the author's laboratory received financial support from the Natural Sciences and Engineering Research Council of Canada and from the UNDP/World Bank/WHO Special Programme for Research and Training in Tropical Diseases.

References

Akol, G.W.O. and Murray, M. (1982). Early events following challenge of cattle with tsetse infected with *Trypanosoma congolense*: development of the local skin reaction. *Vet. Rec.* **110**, 295–302.

Askonas, B.A. (1985). Macrophages as mediators of immunosuppression in murine African trypanosomiasis. *Curr. Topics Microbiol. Immunol.* **117**, 119–27.

Balber, A.E. (1972). *Trypanosoma brucei*: fluxes of the morphological variants in intact and X-irradiated mice. *Exp. Parasitol.* **31**, 307–19.

Barry, J.D. and Vickerman, K. (1979). *Trypanosoma brucei*: loss of variable antigens during transformation from bloodstream to procyclic forms. *Exp. Parasitol.* **48**, 313–24.

Barth, P. (1989). A new method for the isolation of the trypanocidal factor from normal human serum. *Acta Trop.* **46**, 71–3.

Black, S.J. and Vandeweerd, V. (1989). Serum lipoproteins are required for multiplication of *Trypanosoma brucei brucei* under axenic culture conditions. *Mol. Biochem. Parasitol.* **37**, 65–72.

Black, S.J., Hewett, R.S. and Sendashonga, C.N. (1982). *Trypanosoma brucei* variable surface coat is released by degenerating parasites but not by actively dividing parasites. *Parasite Immunol.* **4**, 233–44.

Black, S.J., Jack, R.M. and Morrison, W.I. (1983a). Host : parasite interactions which influence the virulence of *Trypanosoma* (*Trypanozoon*) *brucei brucei* organisms. *Acta Trop.* **40**, 11–18.

Black, S.J., Sendashonga, C.N., Lalor, P.A. *et al*. (1983b). Regulation of the growth and differentiation of *Trypanosoma*

(*Trypanozoon*) *brucei brucei* in resistant (C57lB/6) and susceptible (C3H/He) mice. *Parasite Immunol.* **5**, 465–73.

Black, S.J., Sendashonga, C.N., O'Brien, C. *et al.* (1985). Regulation of parasitemia in mice infected with *Trypanosoma brucei*. *Curr. Topics Microbiol. Immunol.* **117**, 93–118.

Cattand, P. (1988). Sleeping sickness — re-awakes. *World Health* July, 24–5.

Clayton, C.R. and Mowatt, M.R. (1989). The procyclic acidic repetitive proteins of *Trypanosoma brucei*: purification and post-translational modification. *J. Biol. Chem.* **260**, 14547–55.

Clayton, C.E., Ogilvie, B.M. and Askonas, B.A. (1979). *Trypanosoma brucei* infection in nude mice: B lymphocyte function is suppressed in the absence of T lymphocytes. *Parasite Immunol.* **1**, 39–48.

Colmerauer, M.E.M., Davis, C.E. and Pearson, T.W. (1989). The trypanosome surface glycoprotein procyclin is expressed only on tsetse fly vector stages of the parasite. *Parasitol. Res.* **76**, 171–3.

Corsini, A.C., Clayton, C., Askonas, B.A. and Ogilvie, B.M. (1977). Suppressor cells and loss of B-cell potential in mice infected with *Trypanosoma brucei*. *Clin. Exp. Immunol.* **29**, 122–8.

Cross, G.A.M. (1975). Identification, purification and properties of clone-specific glycoprotein antigens constituting the surface coat of *Trypanosoma brucei*. *Parasitology* **71**, 393–417.

De Gee, A.L.W., Levine, R.F. and Mansfield, J.M. (1988). Genetics of resistance to the African trypanosomes. VI. Heredity of resistance and VSG specific immune responses. *J. Immunol.* **140**, 283–8.

DeGreef, C., Imberechts, H., Mathyssens, G. Van Meirvenne, N. and Hamers, R. (1989). A gene expressed only in serum-resistant variants of *Trypanosoma brucei rhodesiense*. *Mol. Biochem. Parasitol.* **36**, 169–76.

Dempsey, W.L. and Mansfield, J.M. (1983). Lymphocyte function in experimental African typanosomiasis. V. Role of antibody and the mononuclear phagocyte system in variant-specific immunity. *J. Immunol.* **130**, 405–11.

Donelson, J.E. (1988). Unsolved mysteries of trypanosome antigenic variation. In *The Biology of Parasitism*, ed. P.T. Englund and A. Sher, pp. 371–400, Alan R. Liss, New York.

Doyle, J.J. (1977). Antigenic variation in the salivarian trypanosomes. In *Immunity to Blood Parasites of Animals and Man*, ed. J. Pino, L. Miller and J.J. McKelvey Jr, pp. 31–63, Plenum Press, New York and London.

Emery, D.L. and Moloo, S.K. (1981). The dynamics of cellular reactions elicited in the skin of goats by *Glossina morsitans morsitans* infected with *Trypanosoma (Nannomanas) congolense* or *T. (Duttonella) vivax*. *Acta Trop.* **38**, 15–28.

Gardiner, P.L., Finerty, J.F. and Dwyer, D.M. (1983). Iodination and identification of surface membrane antigens in procyclic *Trypanosoma rhodesiense*. *J. Immunol.* **131**, 454–7.

Giffin, B.F. and McCann, P.P. (1989). Physiological activation of the mitochondrion and the transformation capacity of DFMO induced intermediate and short-stumpy bloodstream form trypanosomes. *Am. J. Trop. Med. Hyg.* **40**, 487–93.

Giffin, B.F., McCann, P.P., Bitonti, A.J. and Bacchi, C.J. (1986). Polyamine depletion following exposure to DL-alpha-difluoromethylornithine both *in vivo* and *in vitro* initiated morphological alterations and mitochondrial activation in a monomorphic strain of *Trypanosoma brucei brucei*. *J. Protozool.* **33**, 238–43.

Greenblatt, H.C., Diggs, C.L. and Aikawa, M. (1983). Antibody-dependent phagocytosis of *Trypanosoma rhodesiense* by murine macrophages. *Am. J. Trop. Med. Hyg.* **32**, 34–45.

Greenwood, B.M. (1974). Possible role of a B-cell mitogen in hypergamma-globulinemia in malaria and trypanosomiasis. *Lancet* **i**, 435–6.

Greenwood, B.M. and Whittle, H.C. (1980). The pathogenesis of sleeping sickness. *Trans. Roy. Soc. Trop. Med. Hyg.* **74**, 716–25.

Grosskinsky, C.M. and Askonas, B.A. (1981). Macrophages as primary target cells and mediators of immune dysfunction in African trypanosomiasis. *Infect. Immunity* **33**, 149–55.

Hajduk, S.L., Moore, D.R., Vasudevacharya, J. *et al.* (1989). Lysis of *Trypanosoma brucei* by a toxic subspecies of human high density lipoproteins. *J. Biol. Chem.* **264**, 5210–17.

Hawking, F. (1978). The resistance of *Trypanosoma congolense*, *T. vivax* and *T. evansi* to human plasma. *Trans. Roy. Soc. Trop. Med. Hyg.* **72**, 405–7.

Herbert, W.J., Parratt, D., Van Meirvenne, N. and Lennox, B. (1980). An accidental laboratory infection with trypanosomes of a defined stock. II. Studies on the serological response of the patient and the identity of the infecting organism. *J. Infect.* **2**, 113–24.

Hide, G., Gray, A., Harrison, C.M. and Tait, A. (1989). Identification of an epidermal growth factor receptor homologue in trypanosomes. *Mol. Biochem. Parasitol.* **36**, 51–60.

Hoare, C.A. (1970). Systematic description of the mammalian trypanosomes of Africa. In *The African Trypanosomiases*, ed. H.W. Mulligan, pp. 41–8, Allen and Unwin, Ministry of Overseas Development, London.

Hoare, C.A. (1972). *The Trypanosomes of Mammals*. Blackwell Scientific Publications, Oxford.

Hoeppli, I.R. (1959). *Parasites and Parasitic Infections in Early Medicine and Science*. University of Malaya Press, Singapore.

Hudson, K.M., Byner, C., Freeman, J. and Terry, R.J. (1976). Immunodepressing high IgM levels and evasion of the immune response in murine trypanosomiasis. *Nature* **264**, 256–8.

Inverso, J.A. and Mansfield, J.M. (1983). Genetics of resistance to the African trypanosomes. II. Differences in virulence associated with VSSA expression among clones of *Trypanosoma rhodesiense*. *J. Immunol.* **130**, 412–17.

Inverso, J.A., De Gee, A.L.W. and Mansfield, J.M. (1988). Genetics of resistance to the African trypanosomes. VII. Trypanosome virulence is not linked to variable surface glycoprotein expression. *J. Immunol.* **140**, 289–93.

Jayawardena, A.H. and Waksman, B.H. (1977). Suppressor cells in experimental trypanosomiasis. *Nature* **265**, 539–41.

Jenni, L. and Brun, R. (1982). A new *in vitro* test for human serum resistance of *Trypanosoma* (*T.*) *brucei*. *Acta Trop.* **39**, 281–4.

Joshua, R.A. (1985). Further studies on the acquisition of potential infectivity for man in closely related *Trypanosoma* (*Trypanozoon*) *brucei*. *Int. J. Zoonosis* **52**, 291–8.

Kar, S.K., Roelants, G.E., Mayor-Whitey, K.S. and Pearson, T.W. (1981). Immunodepression in trypanosome-infected mice. VI. Comparison of immune responses of different lymphoid organs. *Eur. J. Immunol.* **11**, 100–5.

Kuzoe, F.A.S. (1987). The African trypanosomiases. In *Tropical Disease Research: a Global Partnership*, ed. J. Maurice and A.M. Pearce, pp. 73–86, World Health Organization, Geneva.

Laveran, A. (1902). De l'action du sérum humain sur le trypanosome du nagana (*T. brucei*). *C. R. Acad. Sci. (Paris).* **134**, 735–9.

LePage, R.W.F. (1968a). Further studies on the variable antigen. of *T. brucei*. *Trans. Roy. Soc. Trop. Med. Hyg.* **62**, 131.

LePage, R.W.F. (1968b). Antigenic variation in *Trypanosoma brucei*. PhD thesis, University of Cambridge.

Levine, R.F. and Mansfield, J.M. (1981). Genetics of resistance to the African trypanosomes. I. Role of the H-2 locus in determining resistance of infection with *Trypanosoma rhodesiense*. *Infect. Immunity* **34**, 513–18.

Levine, R.F. and Mansfield, J.M. (1984). Genetics of resistance to the African trypanosomes. III. Variant-specific antibody responses of H-2 compatible resistant and susceptible mice. *J. Immunol.* **133**, 1564–9.

Liu, M.K. and Pearson, T.W. (1987). Detection of circulating trypanosomal antigens by double antibody ELISA using antibodies to procyclic trypanosomes. *Parasitology* **95**, 277–90.

Liu, M.K., Pearson, T.W., Sayer, P.D., Gould, S.S., Waitumbi, J.N. and Njogu, A.R. (1988). Serodiagnosis of African sleeping sickness in vervet monkeys by detection of parasite antigens. *Acta Trop.* **45**, 321–30.

Liu, M.K., Cattand, P., Gardiner, I.C. and Pearson, T.W. (1989). Immunodiagnosis of sleeping sickness due to *Trypanosoma brucei gambiense* by detection of anti-procyclic antibodies and trypanosome antigens in patient's sera. *Acta Trop.* **46**, 257–66.

Luckins, A.G. and Mehlitz, D. (1976). Observations on serum immunoglobulin levels in cattle infected with *Trypanosoma brucei, T. vivax* and *T. congolense*. *Ann. Trop. Med. Parasitol.* **70**, 479–80.

McKelvey, J.J. Jr, (1973). *Man Against Tsetse*. Cornwell University Press, Ithaca and London.

Magnus, E., Vervoort, T. and Van Meirvenne, N. (1978). A card agglutination test with stained trypanosomes (CATT) for the serological diagnosis of *T. b. gambiense* trypanosomiasis. *Ann. Soc. Belg. Med. Trop.* **58**, 169–76.

Mansfield, J.M. (1990). Immunology of African trypanosomiasis. In *Modern Parasite Biology. Cellular, Immunological, and Molecular Aspects*, ed. D.J. Wyler, pp. 222–46, W.H. Freeman, New York.

Massamba, N.N. and Williams, R.O. (1984). Distinction of African trypanosome species using nucleic acid hybridization. *Parasitology* **88**, 55–65.

Maudlin, J., Turner, M.J., Dukes, P. and Miller, N. (1984). Maintenance of *Glossina morsitans morsitans* on antiserum to procyclic trypanosomes reduces infection rates with homologous and heterologous *Trypanosoma congolense* stocks. *Acta Trop.* **41**, 253–7.

Mayor-Witney, D.S., Clayton, C.E., Roelants, G.E. and Askonas, B.A. (1978). Trypanosomiasis leads to extensive proliferation of B, T and null cells in spleen and bone marrow. *Clin. Exp. Immunol.* **34**, 359–63.

Mitchell, L.A. and Pearson, T.W. (1983). Antibody responses induced by immunization of inbred mice susceptible and resistant to African trypanosomes. *Infect. Immunity* **40**, 894–902.

Mitchell, L.A., Pearson, T.W. and Gauldie, J. (1986). Interleukin-1 and interleukin-2 production in resistant and susceptible inbred mice infected with *Trypanosoma congolense*. *Immunology* **57**, 291–6.

Morrison, W.I. and Murray, M. (1979). *Trypanosoma congolense*: inheritance of susceptibility to infection in inbred strains of mice. *Exp. Parasitol.* **48**, 364–74.

Mowatt, M.R. and Clayton, C.E. (1987). Developmental regulation of a novel repetitive protein of *Trypanosoma brucei*. *Mol. Cell Biol.* **7**, 2833–44.

Mulla, A.F. and Rickman, L.R. (1988). How do African game animals control trypanosome infections? *Parasitol. Today* **4**, 352–4.

Mulligan, H.W. (1970). *The African Trypanosomiases*. George Allen and Unwin, Ministry of Overseas Development, London.

Murray, M. (1988). Trypanotolerance, its criteria and genetic and environmental influences. In *Livestock Production in Tsetse Affected Areas of Africa*, pp. 133–51. ILCA/ILRAD, Nairobi.

Murray, M. and Urquhart, G.M. (1977). Immunoprophylaxis against African trypanosomiasis. In *Immunity to Blood Parasites of Animals and Man*, ed. L.H. Miller, J.A. Pino and J.J. McKelvey, Jr, pp. 209–41, Plenum Press, New York and London.

Murray, M., Morrison, W.J. and Whitelaw, D.D. (1982). Host susceptibility to African trypanosomiases: trypanotolerance. *Adv. Parasitol.* **21**, 1–68.

Murray, M., Hirumi, H. and Moloo, S.K. (1985). Suppression of *Trypanosoma congolense, T. vivax* and *T. brucei* infection rates in tsetse flies maintained in goats immunized with uncoated forms of trypanosomes grown *in vitro*. *Parasitology* **95**, 277–90.

Murray, P.K., Jennings, F.W., Murray, M. and Urquhart, G.M. (1974). The nature of immunosuppression in *Trypanosoma brucei* infections in mice. I. The role of the macrophage. *Immunology* **27**, 815–21.

Ngaira, J.M., Nantulya, V.M., Musoke, A.J. and Hirumi, K. (1983). Phagocytosis of antibody-sensitized *Trypanosoma brucei in vitro* by bovine peripheral blood macrophage. *Immunology* **49**, 393–400.

Overath, P., Czichos, J., Stock, U. and Nonnengasser, C. (1983). Repression of glycoprotein synthesis and release of surface coat during transformation of *Trypanosoma brucei*. *EMBO J.* **2**, 1721–8.

Paindavoine, P., Pays, E., Laurent, M. *et al.* (1986). The use of DNA hybridization and numerical taxonomy in determining relationships between *Trypanosoma brucei* stocks and subspecies. *Parasitology* **92**, 31–50.

Paulnock, D.M., Smith, C. and Mansfield, J.M. (1988). Antigen presenting cell function in African trypanosomiasis. In *Antigen Presenting Cells: Diversity, Differentiation and Regulation*, pp. 135–41, Alan R. Liss, New York.

Pearson, T.W., Roelants, G.E., Lundin, L.B. and Mayor-Witney, D.S. (1978). Immune depression in trypanosome-infected mice. I. Depressed T-lymphocyte responses. *Eur. J. Immunol.* **8**, 723–7.

Pearson, T.W., Liu, M.K., Gardiner, I.C. *et al.* (1986). Use of procyclic trypanosomes for detection of antibodies in sera from vervet monkeys infected with *Trypanosoma rhodesiense*: an immunodiagnosis test for African sleeping sickness. *Acta Trop.* **43**, 391–9.

Peters, W. and Gilles, H.M. (1977). *A Color Atlas of Tropical Medicine and Parasitology*, Wolfe, London.

Richardson, J.P., Jenni, L., Beecroft, R.P. and Pearson, T.W. (1986). Procyclic tsetse fly midgut forms and culture forms of African trypanosome share stage- and species-specific surface antigens identified by monoclonal antibodies. *J. Immunol.* **136**, 2259–64.

Richardson, J.P., Beecroft, R.P., Tolson, D.L., Liu, M.K. and Pearson, T.W. (1988). Procyclin: an unusual immunodominant glycoprotein surface antigen from the procyclic stage of African trypanosomes. *Mol. Biochem. Parasitol.* **31**, 203–16.

Rifkin, M.R. (1978a). *Trypanosoma brucei*: some properties of the cytotoxic reaction induced by normal human serum. *Exp. Parasitol.* **46**, 189–206.

Rifkin, M.R. (1978b). Identification of the trypanocidal factor in normal human serum: high density lipoprotein. *Proc. Nat. Acad. Sci. (USA)* **75**, 3450–4.

Ritz, H. (1916). Uber Rezidive bei experimenteller Trypanosomiasis. II. Mitteilung. *Arch. Schiffs Tropenhyg.* **20**, 397–420.

Robertson, M. (1913). Notes on the behavior of a polymorphic trypanosome in the bloodstream of the mammalian host. *Rep. Sleeping Sickness Com. Roy. Soc.* **13**, 111–19.

Roditi, I. and Pearson, T.W. (1990). The procyclin coat of African trypanosomes (or the not-so-naked trypanosome). *Parasitol. Today* **6**, 79–81.

Roditi, I., Carrington, M. and Turner, M.J. (1987). Expression of a polypeptide containing a dipeptide repeat is confined to the insect stage of *Trypanosoma brucei*. *Nature* **352**, 272–4.

Roditi, I., Schwarz, H., Pearson, T.W. *et al.* (1989). Procyclin gene expression and loss of the variant surface glycoprotein during differentiation of *Trypanosoma brucei*. *J. Cell Biol.* **108**, 737–46.

Ross, D. and Thomson, D. (1910). A case of sleeping sickness studied by precise enumerative methods: regular periodic increase in the parasites disclosed. *Proc. Roy. Soc. (London) Biol.* **82**, 411–15.

Sacks, D.L., Bancroft, G., Evans, W.H. and Askonas, B.A. (1982). Incubation of trypanosome-derived mitogenic and immunosuppressive products with peritoneal macrophages allows recovery of biological activity from soluble parasite fractions. *Infect. Immunity* **36**, 160–8.

Seed, J.R. and Sechelski, J.B. (1987). The role of antibody in African trypanosomiasis. *J. Parasitol.* **73**, 840–2.

Seed, J.R. and Sechelski, J.B. (1989a). African trypanosomes: inheritance of factors involved in resistance. *Exp. Parasitol.* **69**, 1–8.

Seed, J.R. and Sechelski, J.B. (1989b). Mechanism of long slender (LS) to short stumpy (SS) transformation in the African trypanosomes. *J. Protozool.* **36**, 572–7.

Sendashonga, C.N. and Black, S.J. (1982). Humoral immune responses against *Trypanosoma brucei* variable surface antigens are induced by degenerating parasites. *Parasite Immunol.* **4**, 245–57.

Shapiro, S. and Pearson, T.W. (1986). African trypanosomiasis: antigens and host–parasite interactions. In *Parasite Antigens: Toward New Strategies for Vaccines*, ed. T.W. Pearson, pp. 215–74, Marcel Dekker, New York and Basle.

Shapiro, S.Z., Naessens, J., Liessgang, B., Moloo, S.K. and Magondu, J. (1984). Analysis by flow cytometry of DNA synthesis during the life cycle of African trypanosomes. *Acta Trop.* **41**, 313–23.

Turner, M.J. (1982). Biochemistry of the variant surface glycoproteins of salivarian trypanosomes. *Adv. Parasitol.* **21**, 69–153.

Turner, M.J. (1985). Antigens of African trypanosomes. In *Parasite Antigens in Protection, Diagnosis and Escape*, ed. R.M.E. Parkhouse, pp. 141–58, Springer-Verlag, New York.

Urquhart, G.M., Murray, M., Murray, P.K., Jennings, F.W. and Bate, E. (1973). Immunosuppression in *Trypanosoma brucei* infections in rats and mice. *Trans. Roy. Soc. Trop. Med. Hyg.* **67**, 528–35.

Van Meirvenne, N. and Le Ray, D. (1985). Diagnosis of African and American trypanosomiasis. Technical Report Series 739, WHO, Geneva.

Van Meirvenne, N., Magnus, E. and Janssens, P.G. (1976). The effect of normal human serum on trypanosomes of distinct antigenic type isolated from a strain of *T. b. rhodesiense. Ann. Soc. Belg. Med. Trop.* **56**, 55–63.

Verducci, G., Perito, S., Rossi, R., Mannarino, E., Bistoni, F. and Marconi, P. (1989). Identification of a trypanocidal factor against *Trypanosoma equiperdum* in normal human sera. *Parasitology* **98**, 401–7.

Vickerman, K. (1985). Developmental cycles and biology of pathogenic trypanosomes. *Br. Med. Bull.* **41**, 105–14.

Wellhausen, S.R. and Mansfield, J.M. (1980). Lymphocyte function in experimental African trypanosomiasis. II. Splenic suppressor cell activity. *J. Immunol.* **122**, 818–24.

Whittle, H.C., Greenwood, B.M., Bidwell, D.E., Bartlett, A. and Voller, A. (1977). IgM and antibody measurement in the diagnosis and management of Gambian trypanosomiasis. *Am. J. Trop. Med. Hyg.* **26**, 1129–34.

World Health Organization (1986). Epidemiology and control of African trypanosomiasis. Technical Report Series 739, WHO, Geneva.

82: Immunology of Amoebiasis and Giardiasis

R.R. Kretschmer

Introduction

Amoebiasis — harbouring *Entamoeba histolytica* with or without disease — affects yearly about 500 million people worldwide. Ten per cent of these suffer from disease varying in severity from trivial to life-threatening. Amoebiasis causes the death of about 50 000 people a year, a toll second only to that of malaria among protozoal diseases and a remarkable feat for a parasite that could be kept at bay by apparently simple sanitary measures (Walsh 1986).

Amoebiasis is a non-epidemic, cosmopolitan parasitosis that strikes primarily at people living in the insanitary conditions and the malnutrition of poverty. These are found today more frequently in tropical and subtropical climates: hence the erroneous belief that this 'pathology of poverty' is just another tropical disease. The clinical spectrum of amoebiasis ranges from asymptomatic carriers of pathogenic and non-pathogenic strains of *E. histolytica*, all the way to invasive intestinal (dysentery, toxic fulminant colitis, amoeboma, appendicitis and the highly debatable chronic amoebic colitis) and extraintestinal (amoebic abscess of the liver (AAL), pulmonary, cutaneous and cerebral amoebiasis, etc.) amoebic disease (Guerrant 1986). Excellent reviews on many aspects of this disease have recently appeared and can be consulted by the interested reader (Martínez-Palomo 1986; Ravdin 1988). This chapter is devoted to the immunology of amoebiasis, a subject of relatively recent development, and to the somewhat related, but less advanced field of immunology of giardiasis. Immunology has contributed substantially to a better understanding of these parasitoses, even though a consistent picture of what is strictly cause, effect or epiphenomenon has yet to emerge in both cases.

Life cycle and general aspects of *Entamoeba histolytica*

Despite certain important immunological observations made in the past, amoebiasis entered the mainstream of modern immunology with Diamond's successful axenic cultivation of *E. histolytica* trophozoites (Diamond 1961). This in turn provided a reliable source of antigenic material from this parasite. Inasmuch as immune responses to *E. histolytica* are claimed to occur only following tissue invasion by the amoeba, a central issue for the understanding of this disease – and the immune phenomena it elicits – is the remarkable apparent 'switch' of the parasite from a harmless intestinal commensal (most of the cases) to an active and sometimes vicious invader. Some humoral antibodies against *E. histolytica* remain detectable for years and, on the other hand, intestinal invasion by amoebae can be subclinical and self-limited in some cases. Thus, there remains a certain imprecision in the terms 'luminal amoebiasis' and 'subclinical invasive intestinal amoebiasis' that is particularly disturbing for epidemiological and serological purposes. Pathogenic (with a broad range of virulence) and non-pathogenic strains of *E. histolytica* look totally alike under light and electron-microscopy, and do not appear to differ in antigenic repertoire. To be sure, some critical differences have been found, i.e. agglutination with low concentrations of concanavalin A (Con A), phagocytosis of erythrocytes and certain bacteria, lack of surface charge, *in vitro* cytopathic effects, resistance to complement-mediated lysis, proteolytic enzyme content, collagenase production, and GalNAc-inhibitable adhesin (Martínez Palomo 1982) and have been endorsed by the traditional virulence criteria, i.e. the presence of erythrophagocytizing *E. histolytica* in material obtained either directly from tissue lesions or from dysenteric stools, and the ability to induce caecal or hepatic lesions in experimental animals (rats and hamsters respectively and more recently gerbils, an experimental animal suited for both caecal and hepatic lesions) (Chadee and Meerovitch 1985b). Pursuing all these criteria can be quite cumbersome and they have not entered the clinical scenario of amoebiasis. The recently described zymodemes (isoenzymatic patterns) of *E. histolytica* appear to be more promising, as only certain (eight) zymodemes (II, XI, etc.) have been distinctly associated with invasive amoebiasis (Sargeaunt 1987). There is some debate as to the stability of such zymodemes, because changes in zymodemic patterns have been recorded, though, only under strict laboratory conditions (Mirelman *et al*. 1986). A new epidemiological dimension may be dawning for amoebiasis, as exemplified by recent studies of male homosexual carriers of non-pathogenic *E. histolytica*, who are only rarely invaded by the parasite (Allason-Jones *et al*. 1986), and by surveys of the pathogenic and non-pathogenic *E. histolytica* zymodeme ratios in communities where the disease is endemic (Gutiérrez and Muñoz 1989). Amoebiasis entered modern immunology relatively late, among other reasons, because *E. histolytica* and the effector cells of immunity (i.e. leucocytes), despite some important differences, are remarkably well matched foes in size and functions (locomotion, chemotaxis, adherence, membrane flow and capping of attached ligands, phagocytosis and cytolysis) and, when confronted, provide a complex picture of actions and evasions that is not easy to analyse (Kretschmer 1986).

Entamoeba histolytica, the only species of the genus *Entamoeba* known to be pathogenic for man and for subhuman primates in captivity (Amyx *et al*. 1978), is a small (average size 25 μm, ranging from 10 to 60 μm), essentially anaerobic, intestinal, extracellular protozoan with a simple life cycle that lacks sexual stages or intermediate hosts. The vegetative form, or trophozoite, feeds on the intestinal contents and reproduces by binary fission (Fig. 82.1). Under conditions that are not well understood encystment occurs, thus generating the only infective form of the parasite. From a few to up to 45×10^6 *E. histolytica* cysts (average size 8–20 μm) are passed daily with the stools by infected individuals and survive outside the host for weeks or months in a moist environment. If ingested (faecalism), the chitin-containing cyst wall provides protection against gastric acidity; excystation follows in the intestine, leading first to quadrinucleated metacysts and then to eight uninucleated trophozoites. Trophozoites are short-lived when eliminated in the stools and, if ingested, they would certainly not survive the acid journey in the upper gastrointestinal tract. Such faecal trophozoites, however, can cause perineal skin and mucosal lesions. Some trophozoites undergo encystment and close this simple, yet enormously successful, life cycle. The life cycle of the amoeba evidently does not require a tissue-invasive stage. In fact, in the vast majority of cases *E. histolytica* lives as a harmless (useful?) commensal in the colon (luminal or asymptomatic amoebiasis). In a few instances, however, trophozoites, aided in a complex way by otherwise harmless bacteria, adhere to the mucosal cells through a lectin-like ligand and tissue invasion is

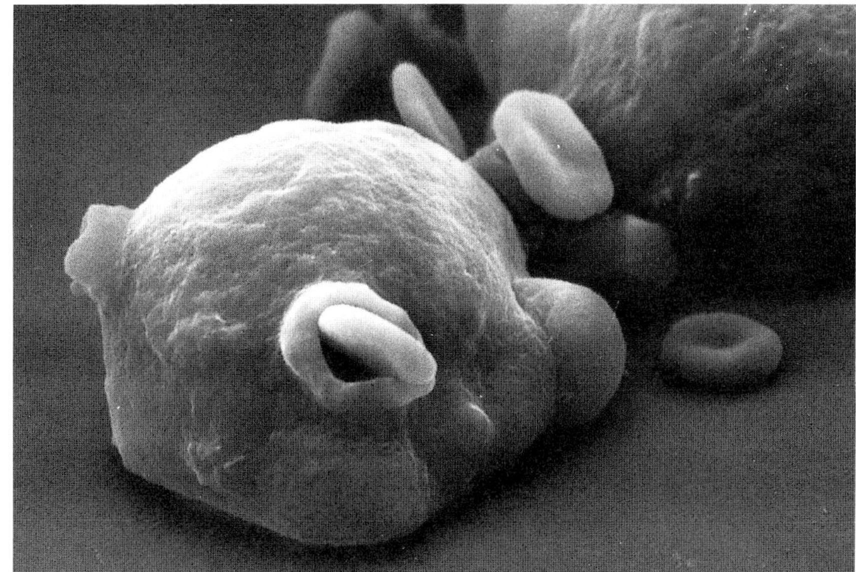

Fig. 82.1. Scanning electron micrograph of a trophozoite of *E. histolytica* ingesting erythrocytes. × 1860. Micrograph courtesy of A. Martínez-Palomo.

set in motion. Further in the evolution of some of these cases, trophozoites enter the bloodstream and reach their prime extraintestinal target, the liver, via the portal vein. From here they may erode their way directly into other organs (intestinal viscera, pericardium and lungs) or, by re-entering the bloodstream, they may even reach the brain, causing cerebral amoebiasis, the most dreaded and elusive of its complications.

A subtle balance between virulence and encystment may have been critical in the evolution of this host–parasite relationship, since cysts are not found in invaded tissues and only rarely in dysenteric stools (Kretschmer 1986). Thus, the more virulent forms of *E. histolytica*, by invading the tissues of a perhaps selected group of individuals are *de facto* lost for the purpose of transmission and preservation of the species, while the less virulent amoebae encyst, transmit and preserve the parasite. This is perhaps also the reason why *E. histolytica*, unlike *Giardia lamblia*, seldomly strikes in epidemic form in open populations. Incidentally, both properties, i.e. encystment and virulence, are lost more or less simultaneously in axenization of *E. histolytica*.

Characterization and topology of amoebic antigens

Antigens from axenically grown *E. histolytica* can be studied using whole cells, homogenates (with subcellular, particulated and soluble fractions thereof) and secreted products. The framework of our immunological knowledge in amoebiasis was built on one such antigen, histolyticin, a complex mixture of antigenic material not devoid of contaminants from the axenic medium that stick and remain attached to the amoebae even after thorough washing (Noya *et al.* 1980). Much progress has been made in the last 25 years, yet, despite some isolated and unconfirmed findings, a definite relationship between virulence and antigenic composition of *E. histolytica* has not been established.

Based on immunoelectrophoretic studies of aqueous extracts of virulent and non-virulent axenically grown amoebae, several authors concluded that the 'antigenic skeleton' of *E. histolytica* consists of 14–32 antigenic components, the range and variations being explained as periodic waves of emergence and hiding of antigens, a phenomenon that apparently does not correlate with virulence (Chang *et al.* 1979). It was hypothesized, however, that, by rendering previously acquired antibodies irrelevant, the shifting in the antigenic make-up could explain the tendency for reinfection and intestinal invasion in patients with high anti-*E. histolytica* antibody titres. Gel–sieve chromatography (Sephadex G-200) of whole amoebic extracts yields up to five fractions, only the larger three (fractions, I, II and III) immunoprecipitating, and only the largest (fraction I) haemagglutinating with reactive sera. When injected prior to inoculation with *E. histolytica*, all three glycoprotein fractions protected guinea-pigs against experimental amoebiasis. The best results (90–100% protection) were clearly obtained with fraction I (MW 650 kD), even though all three fractions shared antigens by immunoprecipitation (Krupp 1974). In an exhaustive analysis of a soluble extract of whole *E. histolytica* NIH-200, Aust-Kettis *et al.* (1983) found the same five fractions by gel–sieve chromatography (Sephadex G-200) with MW ranging from 9 to 150 kD by sodium dodecyl sulphate polyacrylamide gel electrophoresis (SDS-PAGE), twelve bands by autoradiography, seven polypeptides immunoabsorbing with human anti-amoeba immunoglobulin G (IgG) and eight bands by Western blot. For all its complexity, *E. histolytica* appeared antigenically quite uniform, and the wisdom of pursuing highly purified antigens for serological purposes in amoebiasis was thus questioned (Aust-Kettis *et al.* 1983) even though sera from invasive amoebiasis at different stages may tend to react with different antigens of the amoebic repertoire.

Surface antigens of *E. histolytica* are of special immunological interest. Parkhouse *et al.* (1978) radiolabelled the surface proteins of amoebae and isolated a major antigenic surface glycoprotein of 81 kD. By selective radiolabelling of external surface proteins, Aley *et al.* (1980) identified 12 glycoproteins ranging from 12 to 200 kD by autoradiography, thus revealing a membrane complexity more reminiscent of mammalian cells than of fellow amoebae (*Acanthamoeba*, *E. invadens*). Using protease inhibitors and SDS-PAGE, Joyce and Ravdin (1988) identified six surface proteins with MW ranging from 19.5 to 170 kD, the larger three being Con A-inhibitable glycoproteins. Two of these (37 kD and 90 kD) were more frequently recognized by sera from patients with amoebic abscess of the liver, coinciding neatly with two of the proteins isolated by Aust-Kettis *et al.* (1983). Recently the use of monoclonal antibodies has allowed the definition of a 96 kD surface antigenic glycoprotein determinant (Meza *et al.* 1987). Carbohydrate-free proteins and surface proteins involved in the *in vitro* adhesion of *E. histolytica* to various cells (including the Gal/GalNAc 170 kD inhibitable adherence lectin) (Petri *et al.* 1988) have been identified by different methods, with MW ranging from 112 to 220 kD. The precise antigenic properties of such material remains to be clarified but patients recovering from invasive amoebiasis regularly have antibodies against these lectins. The agglutination of *E. histolytica* with Con A and the activation of the alternative complement pathway by *E. histolytica* suggested the presence of carbohydrates on the surface of the parasite. A glycogen-free, polysaccharide surface antigen containing glucose, galactose, and xylose was purified from a lipopeptide phosphoglycan (LPPG) obtained from both virulent (HM1-IMSS) and non-virulent (HK-9) *E. histolytica*, and was found to react strongly with sera of patients with amoebic abscess of the liver. Moreover, the aminophospholipid residue of this LPPG constituted an epitope of its own, a rather unexpected feature for such a lipid. Preliminary data suggest the existence of structural differences between LPPG from virulent and non-virulent amoebae (Isibasi and Kumate 1989).

In vitro expression of surface antigens appears to be at its lowest in metabolically active *E. histolytica*. In fact, the relatively low immunogenicity of *E. histolytica* has been blamed on intracellular concealment of antigens, but the exceedingly rapid cytoplasmic/surface turnover and the periodic expression of surface antigens found *in vitro* should caution against such a conclusion. Nevertheless, lysosomal and ribosomal antigenic material obtained by differential ultracentrifugation of *E. histolytica* homogenates has attracted special attention. The lysosomal fraction, characterized by its acid phosphatase content and by electron microscopy, reveals several precipitation bands when exposed to serum of patients with amoebic abscess of the liver. This material is harmless, immunogenic (even in subhuman primates) and protective against experimental amoebiasis. On the other hand acid and basic proteins ranging from 14 to 112 kD have been found in ribosomes, but surprisingly not the 54 kD protein regularly found in all procaryotic and eucaryotic cells (Isibasi and Kumate 1989).

Axenically grown *E. histolytica* release complex protein toxins (exotoxins) that can be inhibited by immune but also by normal serum, suggesting some protease activity. Amoebic enterotoxins (23–25 kD enzymes), pore-forming proteins (amoebopore) and a trailing microexudate may also fall into this category of putative antigens. On the other hand there is strong passive, hydrophobic attachment of antigenic material, foremost bovine serum albumin, from the axenic medium on to the amoebae. Whether or not *E. histolytica* is capable of doing likewise with host antigens *in vivo* is not known, but other parasites, in particular *Schistosoma*, attach to themselves blood group substances and histocompatibility antigens of the host and may use this as an evasion mechanism (Cher 1978). The question of stage-specific antigens in *E. histolytica* warrants further studies that will come when the *in vitro* encystment of the parasite is fully achieved. Stage-specific (cyst) antigens cross-reacting with *E. histolytica* have been found in *E. invadens* (an amoeba of reptiles). The microscopical detection of *E. histolytica* in stools can be cumbersome and easily prone to interpretative errors. Deoxyribonucleic acid probes and enzyme-linked immunosorbent assay (ELISA) detection of amoebic antigens in stools using monoclonal antibodies appear to be sensitive, specific, rapid and precise diagnostic tools that still await the test of daily practice (Del Muro *et al*. 1987).

Humoral immune responses in amoebiasis

A prompt, alas transient, local secretory response followed by an equally prompt systemic antibody response ensues upon intestinal invasion by *E. histolytica*.

A mixture of IgA, IgG and IgM coproantibodies have been found by indirect haemagglutination (IHA) in about 80% of cases of amoebic dysentery, as opposed to 2% in healthy controls and 4% in non-amoebic parasitic infections (Table 82.1). Three weeks later this figure falls to 55%, just as serum antibodies make their appearance. A comparable local anti-amoebic antibody production has been experimentally induced in the rat gut. Secretory IgA anti-*E. histolytica* antibodies have also been found in human milk and colostrum and in the bile of intracaecally immunized rats (Acosta *et al*. 1983). A recent African survey found anti-*E. histolytica* antibodies in both milk and serum in only a few nursing females, most having either milk or serum antibodies but not both, thus revealing not only the transient character of the secretory anti-amoebic immune response, but also the effective traffic and 'homing' of gut-stimulated immune cells to other secretory areas (Grundy *et al*. 1983). Secretory IgE antibodies have not been investigated in amoebiasis although, as in the case of *Giardia lamblia*, a strictly local anaphylactic reaction in the gut could explain some of the clinical and early histopathological changes seen in amoebic dysentery.

Circulating antibodies to *E. histolytica* can be demonstrated as early as one week after the onset of symptoms in man and experimental animals. All immunoglobulin classes are involved, but most anti-amoebic antibodies belong to the IgG (IgG-2) class. Virtually all known serological methods have been employed in amoebiasis, starting with the pioneer work of Izar (1914), using complement fixation and precipitation tests, all the way to indirect immunofluorescence assay (IFA), IHA, RIA, CIE and ELISA, the latter being the most sensitive (0% false negatives in AAL), specific (3.6% false positives in controls), opportune (earliest detection, <1 week) and persistent (>3 years) in measuring such antibodies (reviewed by Kretschmer 1986). Much of the earlier work was done with IHA and CIE, which combined a high

Table 82.1. Positive reactions (%) to *Entamoeba histolytica* antigens[a]

Assay	Controls[b]	Asymptomatic cyst carriers	Symptomatic	
			Intestine	Liver
Serum antibody[c]	0–18	0–70	60–90	80–100
Coproantibodies[d]	0–2	NA[e]	35–80	NA
Immediate-type skin reaction	0–13	30–80	70–90	75–95
Delayed-type skin reaction	0–20	NA	30–50	6–100[f]

a Figures represent ranges based on references cited in the text (reviewed by Kretschmer 1986).
b Figures primarily dependent on endemicity.
c Indirect haemagglutination (IHA)/indirect immunofluorescence assay (IFA) enzyme-linked immunosorbent assay.
d Complement fixation (CF)/indirect haemoagglutination (IHA)/counter immunoelectrophoresis (CIE).
e Data not available.
f Stage-dependent.

degree of specificity (only 6.6 and 5.8% positivity respectively, in healthy controls living in endemic areas) and sensitivity (94.8 and 96.4% positivity respectively in proved cases of AAL), coinciding in over 90% of both negative and positive cases. The IFA test also deserves to be mentioned since it outdoes all other tests in simplicity, and when combined with IHA reaches a 100% positivity in cases of AAL. The Center for Disease Control in Atlanta, Georgia, has chosen IHA as its standard serological reference for amoebiasis with a 1:256 cut-off titre (Jones 1984). Counter immunoelectrophoresis on the other hand is particularly well suited for epidemiological surveys: 19442 non-selected individual serum samples revealed a 5.95% positivity in Mexico (range 2.53–9.95% depending on the geo-economic area). The same group found a comparable 6.6% positivity in *bona fide E. histolytica* cyst passers, a reassuring finding made in other surveys as well (Gutiérrez *et al.* 1976) (Table 82.1).

There is no doubt that antibody detection is a valuable tool in the diagnosis of amoebic abscess of the liver and amoeboma, where, in ascending order of sensitivity, IHA, CIE, ager gel diffusion (AGD), IFA, IHA-IFA and ELISA give virtually no false negatives even in very early sera (Table 82.1). Serology has a much less prominent role in the diagnosis of intestinal invasive amoebiasis, yielding only 60–90% positivity. Unfortunately standard serological tests cannot distinguish between present, recent or past (≥3 years) amoebic invasion and, furthermore, titres do not correlate with clinical severity in human amoebiasis (Petri and Ravdin 1989). The use of a suitable repertoire of antigens for amoebic serology may, however, improve its diagnostic selectivity. The broad range of positivity found in alleged cyst passers (0–70%) and the background problem of sub-clinical amoebic invasion cast further doubts on the usefulness of serology in intestinal amoebiasis, especially in communities where amoebiasis is endemic. Nevertheless, no patient suspected of inflammatory bowel disease should go without a diagnostic probe for amoebiasis (i.e. stool examinations and serology), lest a potentially fatal steroid treatment be started (Krogstad *et al.* 1978).

Immediate-hypersensitivity skin reactions to amoebic antigens are found in 70–95% of cases with amoebic dysentery or AAL (Table 82.1), and the presence of specific class IgE anti-*E. histolytica* antibodies in serum has been established in rodents and man (Usawattanakul *et al.* 1982; Kretschmer 1986).

Complement levels have been found both elevated and decreased in human and experimental invasive amoebiasis. This inconsistency contrasts with the observation that virulent and non-virulent strains of *E. histolytica* are equally capable of activating both pathways of the complement system, the classical pathway more vigorously and even in the absence of antibody. This activation is lethal for the non-virulent strains, while virulent strains resist lysis (Calderón and Tovar 1986). Moreover, cobra venom factor-decomplemented hamsters are more susceptible to experimental hepatic amoebiasis than controls (Capin *et al.* 1980). In contrast, patients with agammaglobulinaemia and B cell-immunosuppressed animals do not appear more susceptible to invasive amoebiasis than the normal population (Kretschmer 1986).

Finally, high rates of intestinal amoebic reinfection have been recorded in the presence of elevated titres of anti-amoebic antibodies (and of cell-mediated immunity for that matter (see next section)) (Krupp and Powell 1971). This and the apparent irrelevance of humoral antibodies — and complement — in *in vitro* lytic tests have led to the widespread consensus that circulating humoral anti-amoebic antibodies are not protective against intestinal (and perhaps extraintestinal) amoebiasis. If no protective value is granted to circulating anti-amoebic antibodies, neither do they appear to be harmful, as immune complex disease is not a feature in amoebiasis, even though such complexes have been found (Pillai and Mohinen 1982) and Indian authors believe a small group of patients with amoebiasis and arthritis may constitute the rare exception (Jalan 1984). The protective role of secretory IgA and IgE antibodies in amoebiasis remains to be clarified. *Entamoeba histolytica* trophozoites appear capable of degrading secretory IgA (Isibasi and Kumate 1989).

Cellular immune responses in amoebiasis

Information on the existence of a local cell-mediated immune response in amoebiasis is virtually non-existent, yet it would not come as a surprise to find one, since the basic ingredients are regularly present (i.e. the mucosal exudates contain mononuclear phagocytes and lymphoid cells, perhaps of the T suppressor/cytotoxic type, and there is close contact of amoebae and lymphoid cells in the ulcer rim), and a local version of cell-mediated immunity has been found for other micro-organisms (Arnaud-Battandier *et al.* 1978). Furthermore, local reactivity of submucosal lymphoid follicles and mesenteric lymph nodes consists of initial blastogenesis, T cell exhaustion–depletion and disorganization of the paracortical areas, followed by replenishment upon recovery, a sequence that fits into the peculiar chronobiology of cell-mediated immunity in amoebiasis (see below) (Chadee and Meerovitch 1985a).

On the other hand, systemic cell-mediated immunity, revealed by delayed-hypersensitivity skin reaction, *in vitro* lymphocyte transformation, lymphokine production and lymphocytotoxic assays, is regularly present and long-lasting (years) in virtually all patients upon recovery from AAL, albeit preceded by a transient anergy phase (Kretschmer 1986). This cellular anergy is apparently restricted to the amoebic antigens and to such antigens that are met for the first time during this period, since reactions to recall antigens (streptokinase-streptodornase (SSKD), purified protein derivative (PPD) and candidin) are positive from the onset. Confirmatory results of this peculiar chronobiology of cell-mediated immunity in amoebiasis have been obtained in experimental animals, and there is a decrease in the T4/T8 cell ratio in early human invasive amoebiasis (Salata *et al.* 1986).

Based on these observations it has been claimed that tissue invasion by *E. histolytica* must be preceded by, and associated with, some degree of T cell suppression, a condition that may be met by selection and/or induction (Harris and Bray 1976). The increased susceptibility of T cell-immunosuppressed experimental animals and man to invasive amoebiasis, the presence of malnutrition in over 90% of the autopsies of AAL, the increased susceptibility of children to amoebiasis in spite of transplacental maternal antibodies and the significant increase in human leucocyte antigens (HLA)-DR3 (Arellano *et al.* 1991) found in patients with AAL support the selective proposition, while the inductive proposal — not incompatible with the former — is supported by observations that free extracts of *E. histolytica* can exhaust, and thus suppress, the host's cellular immune response (Diamantstein *et al.* 1981). Patients with acquired immune deficiency syndrome (AIDS) are suprisingly not more susceptible to amoebic disease than homosexual men without AIDS. Conversely, it has been suggested that mitogenic stimulation of human immunodeficiency virus (HIV)-infected T cells by amoebic lectins could result in HIV expression and AIDS (Petri and Ravdin 1989). This indictment of cell-mediated immunity in amoebiasis does not necessarily disqualify it as a likely repository of the acquired protective immunity claimed to occur in this disease, especially with respect to AAL. Recurrences of AAL have been claimed to be rare in humans (0.04% recurrences vs. 0.2% first AAL cases per year calculated in Mexico City) (Kretschmer 1986) and experimental animals, allegedly due to a state of acquired protective cell-mediated immunity, although strictly speaking this isolated and still unconfirmed report could support a protective role of humoral antibodies as well. However, prospective selective immunization and immunosuppression of experimental animals, the few studies of passive transfer of immunity with cells and the straightforward outcome of the *in vitro* interaction of virulent *E. histolytica* with activated lymphocytes, eosinophils and mononuclear phagocytes, as opposed to polymorphonuclear leucocytes, humoral antibodies and complement (see next section), all favour the existence of cellular rather than humoral protective immunity against extraintestinal amoebiasis (Salata and Ravdin 1986). While humoral antibodies have a more diagnostic than protective value, the reverse is true for cellular immune phenomena, since delayed-hypersensitivity skin testing is of little diagnostic value, except perhaps in epidemiological surveys.

Important as cell-mediated immunity may be in amoebiasis, the actual defence strategy gravitates around the mononuclear phagocyte, an essential cell in natural immunity and the effector cell *par excellence* in cell-mediated immunity. Depressing the mononuclear phagocyte function with silica or antimacrophage serum or enhancing it with bacillus Calmette-Guérin (BCG) increases or decreases respectively the development of experimental amoebiasis in hamsters and mice (Ghadirian and Meerovitch 1982). In fact congenitally athymic Nu/nu mice (devoid of T lymphocytes) and genetically susceptible mice (C57BL/6 and C3H/HeJ) only developed AAL and intestinal amoebic disease respectively after mononuclear phagocyte blockade with silica (Stern *et al.* 1984). Furthermore, mononuclear phagocyte function is depressed in humans with amoebic dysentery and AAL, which may explain the increased susceptibility to opportunistic infections observed in patients with AAL (González-Mendoza and Aguirre-Garcia 1971).

In vitro interaction of *Entamoeba histolytica* with antibodies and inflammatory cells

Earlier studies of the *in vitro* interaction of *E. histolytica* with immune serum or γ-globulin revealed dramatic changes (i.e. inhibition of erythrophagocytosis and cytopathogenicity) and eventual killing of the parasite, an effect that was heat-stable and absorbable by preincubation of the serum with trophozoites or amoebic homogenates (Ortiz-Ortiz and Avella 1984). More recently, however, exceptions to these deleterious effects have been recorded. Both pathogenic and non-pathogenic amoebae redistribute membrane-attached antibodies (and lectins) into patches and caps at the uroid area, whence they are either internalized or released into the surrounding media as pieces of membrane-containing caps. The amoebae themselves emerge unharmed, 'trimmed' of antigens and therefore less vulnerable to further antibody attachment and damage. This may be a possible evasion mechanism of the amoebae, nicely matched by the capacity of virulent amoebae to avoid lysis by complement (Calderón *et al.* 1980).

When virulent amoebae interact with human or mammalian polymorphonuclear neutrophils (PMN) (and eosinophils (López-Osuna and Kretschmer 1989)), the leucocytes succumb after first showing positive chemotaxis towards the parasite and then firm pseudopodial attachment to it, using the amoebic GalNAc-inhibitable lectin (adhesin). The ensuing cytolytis requires Ca^{2+} ions and normal amoebic microfilament function, and is mediated by hydrolytic and proteolytic enzymes, cytotoxins, phospholipase A, protein kinase C and active lysosomal material. Some of the lysed leucocytes are eventually phagocytized by the amoebae. Not even 3000 neutrophils per virulent amoeba or the presence of antibodies or complement in the reaction prevents the virulent amoebae from destroying the leucocytes. Only when less virulent, emetine-treated or heat-attenuated amoebae are involved, and with PMN–amoeba ratios in excess of 200 : 1, are the leucocytes capable of destroying amoebae in a non-oxidative manner. It thus appears that PMN, the 'professional' phagocytic cell so effectively responsive to opsonins, is a remarkably incompetent effector cell against virulent *E. histolytica* (Ravdin and Guerrant 1982). Given this innate incompetence of neutrophils towards *E. histolytica*, it is small wonder that anti-amoebic humoral antibodies have not established much of a protective reputation in amoebiasis. Furthermore, *E. histolytica* resist and suppress the vigorous oxidative activity of the neutrophil. Recent evidence suggests that destroyed neutrophils, through the release of non-oxidative constituents (proteases, cathepsins, lysozyme), may play an important role in tissue damage in amoebiasis (Tsutsumi *et al.* 1984).

On the other hand, while non-stimulated lymphocytes also succumb to amoebic cytolytic activity, immune T8 lymphocytes or PHA-stimulated non-immune T lymphocytes kill virulent *E. histolytica* (Salata *et al.* 1986). Supernatant fluid of stimulated lymphocytes in turn inhibits amoebic protein synthesis. Antibody-dependent cell-mediated cytotoxity (ADCC), effective against other parasites (including perhaps *G. lamblia*), does not appear to operate against *E. histolytica*. Interaction of virulent *E. histolytica* and normal, non-activated human mononuclear phagocytes culminates in contact-dependent, serum-independent lysis of these cells without a concomitant decrease in amoebic viability. Again, the presence of anti-amoebic antibody and complement fails to reverse this effect. In contrast, lectin- or lymphokine-activated mononuclear phagocytes effectively kill virulent amoebae through an extracellular, immunologically non-specific, serum-independent, time- and contact-dependent oxidative as well as non-oxidative process. This occurs in mononuclear phagocyte : amoebae ratios as low as 10 : 1 and increases as the ratio reaches 100 : 1. Interestingly, it is followed by a concomitant decrease in mononuclear phagocyte viability, ostensibly due to toxic products released from the killed amoebae (Salata *et al.* 1985). These results suggest that the activated mononuclear phagocyte is a proficient effector cell against virulent *E. histolytica*, and studies with peritoneal and colostrum mononuclear phagocytes have supported this concept. The confrontation of amoebae and mononuclear phagocytes is none the less a reciprocated phenomenon, as many of the latter eventually succumb in the process as well, although, in the long run, the mononuclear phagocyte appears to emerge, by however small a margin, the overall victor, as opposed to the impressive *in vitro* superiority of virulent amoebae over PMN. The mononuclear phagocyte thus appears to be the leucocyte that under convenient conditions (i.e. activation) possesses a potential phagocytic/cytolytic superiority over *E. histolytica*, an asset that may be critical in controlling or preventing invasive amoebiasis (Kretschmer and López-Osuna 1990). A similar role may be played by the 'activated' eosinophils (Kretschmer and López-Osuna 1991).

Inflammation and tissue repair in amoebiasis

Since the classic description of Councilman and Lafleur (1891), invasive amoebiasis has been known for the paucity of its inflammatory reaction. Today, early endoscopic biopsies and of course the evidence gathered from experimental amoebiasis have, however, established the existence of an intense, albeit ephemeral, acute inflammatory reaction that soon fades and blends with the products of tissue necrosis (Pérez-Tamayo and Brandt 1971). The very early lesions of invasive intestinal and extraintestinal amoebiasis reveal an intense, acute inflammatory reaction followed by extensive necrosis due to ischaemic changes but, as it appears, also due to the non-oxidative cytolytic action of lysosomal enzymes released from host PMN that are so effectively destroyed by amoebae. Intraportal inoculation of axenically grown *E. histolytica* into hamsters have revealed that, in the very early stages, trophozoites lodged in the sinusoids of the liver are soon surrounded by 'cuffs' of densely packed neutrophils. These soon undergo lysis and, by releasing their non-oxidative cytolytic products help to destroy the surrounding liver parenchyma, without much evidence of a direct cytolytic effect by the amoebae (Tsutsumi *et al*. 1984). This destruction of leucocytes in turn fails to sustain the progress towards the later stages of the inflammatory reaction, and amoebae may also produce anti-inflammatory factors capable of delaying the arrival of mononuclear phagocytes to the scene (Kretschmer *et al*. 1985). The paucity of late inflammatory elements may be related to the equally remarkable lack of scarring and the consequent extensive parenchymal regeneration of the affected organs (colon, liver and skin) following recovery that is so typical of amoebiasis (Pérez-Tamayo 1986).

Biological significance of immunity in amoebiasis and prospects of immunoprotection

The case for the existence of acquired protective immunity in amoebiasis rests essentially on two basic observations: (i) the widely held belief that recurrent human AAL is exceedingly rare; and (ii) the refractoriness of most experimental animals to hepatic reinvasion with *E. histolytica* after spontaneous or therapeutic recovery, or after immunization with live trophozoites, with crude antigen plus adjuvant, with fractionated and chromatographed glycoproteins and lectins, or with ribosomal or lysosomal amoebic fractions (Sepúlveda 1978). Because of the artificiality of the animal models used, it may be that induced acquired immunity is just compensating for the breach of natural immunity in such animals. Furthermore, the increasing morbidity and mortality due to *E. histolytica* with age surely cast an uneasy doubt upon the concept of acquired protective immunity in amoebiasis (Ravdin and Guerrant 1982). Nevertheless, immunoprotection remains a reasonable proposition in human amoebiasis, especially since the public health control of the disease by other means would require radical socio-economic and political strategies that are more easily phrased than implemented. Several antigenic fractions of *E. histolytica* including the adhesion lectins have been studied as potential vaccines, but much remains to be learned before such a goal can be reached (Salata and Ravdin 1988).

Immunology of giardiasis

Giardia lamblia (*G. intestinalis* or *G. duodenalis*), presumably one of the first micro-organism seen by the human eye under the microscope 300 years ago, is together with *E. histolytica* the most important intestinal protozoan in man. Like the latter,

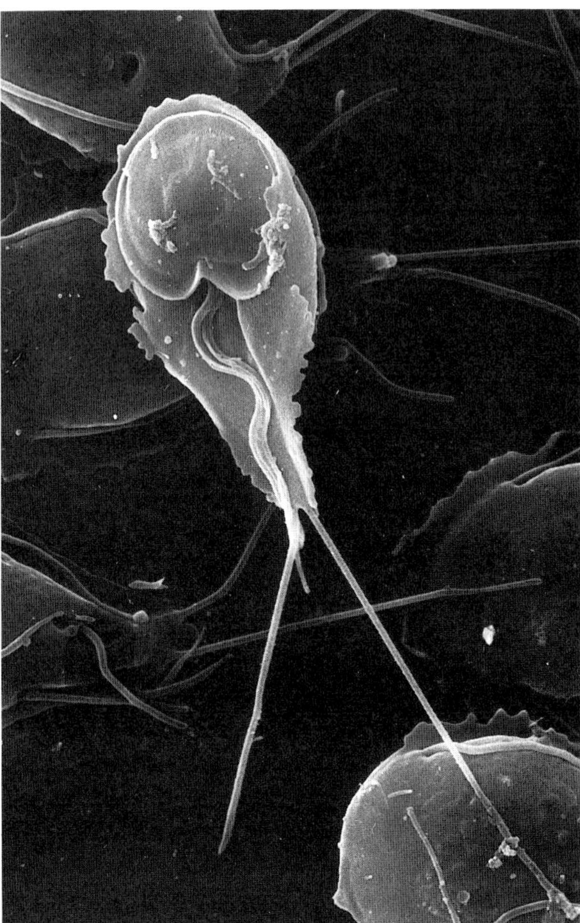

Fig. 82.2. Scanning electron micrograph of a trophozoite of *G. lamblia*. The ventral flagella and the adhesive disc are shown. × 1470. Micrograph courtesy of A. Martínez-Palomo.

this highly photogenic parasite has both a trophozoite (9–15 μm wide, 9–21 μm long and 2–4 μm thick pear-shaped body with four pairs of flagella) and a cyst (8–12 μm by 7–10 μm ovoid-shaped body) stage, the former causing clinical disease and the latter being responsible for the transmission of the parasite (Fig. 82.2). *Giardia lamblia* is the most common human intestinal parasite in the United States and Great Britain, affecting primarily the lower socio-economic class but not sparing the more affluent groups in suitable circumstances (e.g. skiing resorts, cruise ships, tourism in Leningrad, etc.) (Craft 1982).

Like amoebae, giardiae are cosmopolitan, endemic, extracellular parasites with widely spread infection rates (i.e. 3–13% in developed countries and up to 20–90% in day-care centres and Third World countries), low and age-dependent morbidity rates, person-to-person (faecal–oral) water and food transmission (faecalism) and a comparable response to drugs (metronidazole). Unlike *E. histolytica*, however, *Giardia* colonization is limited to the distal duodenum and proximal jejunum, epidemic outbreaks are common and mortality is virtually nil. Cross-species transmission occurs with dogs, cats, rodents and wild beavers and the parasite causes disease through direct, essentially non-invasive, mechanical microvillous injury and functional derangement of brush border enzymes. Limited penetration of the mucosa beyond the epithelial layer can, but need not occur and, when present, may increase the immune response to the parasite (Smith 1985). Tissue damage and symptoms have also been blamed on hypersensitivity to *Giardia* antigens as suggested by the increase in epithelial cell turnover and interepithelial lymphocyte counts, and by the local interactions between the parasite and itinerant leucocytes leading to mediator release (i.e. prostaglandin E_2) (Smith 1989). Formerly proposed mechanisms such as mechanical occlusion, bile salt deconjugation, bacterial overgrowth and enterotoxin secretion have not been confirmed.

As in amoebiasis, the vast majority of individuals infected with *G. lamblia* are asymptomatic. In fact, doubts over the pathogenicity of this parasite (first suggested by Lambl a century ago) were still aired as late as 1960. Why giardiae become pathogenic in certain individuals (causing diarrhoea, cramps, flatulence, nausea, vomiting and, when the infestation is chronic, malabsorption and protein–caloric malnutrition that can occasionally be life-threatening) is not known. Differences in virulence have been documented in animal and human volunteer models (Nash *et al*. 1987). Host risk factors claimed to be significant include hypochlorhydria, hypogammaglobulinaemia, blood group A, HLA antigens A1 and B12 and phenotypes A1/A2 and B12/B27, and cystic fibrosis, but the majority of patients with symptomatic giardiasis do not fit these categories (Smith 1989).

Modern immunology of giardiasis began with axenic cultivation of *G. lamblia* in 1976 (Meyer 1976). However, two early observations clearly pointed to immunological involvement in this parasitosis: (i) the remarkable susceptibility of patients with acquired adult common variable hypogammaglobulinaemia (particularly if IgA-deficient) to chronic, indolent and severe giardiasis

(Webster 1980); and (ii) the existence of acquired protective immunity, as suggested by a steady decrease in susceptibility with increasing age, by the results from experimental infections in prisoners and by the fact that residents of hyperendemic areas are much less affected than incidental travellers to such areas (Wright *et al.* 1977). As with *E. histolytica* we are far from understanding the exact adaptative role of the different immune phenomena observed in giardiasis.

Deoxyribonucleic acid (DNA) endonuclease restriction studies and surface antigen radiolabelling with ^{125}I have shown that DNA of most *Giardia* isolates differ and these differences are reflected in the surface antigens and excretory–secretory products of the parasite. *Giardia lamblia* isolates have both different and common antigens, the former mostly located on the surface, the latter appearing to be internal or somatic (Nash 1985; Ungar and Nash 1987). Antigenic variation has been described for a 170 kD cystine-rich antigen of *G. lamblia* (Adam *et al.* 1988), reflecting a possible evasion mechanism used by the parasite in chronic infection. More recently two additional surface antigens of 82 and 34 kD were described (Smith 1989).

The immune response in giardiasis most probably starts when trophozoites invading the mucosal cells are trapped by the extended pseudopodia of basal lamina mononuclear phagocytes, and these in turn interact with lymphoid cells. There is a weaker immune response to *Giardia* antigens when mucosal damage is severe. Nu/nu and T helper-depleted mice are particularly susceptible to severe *G. muris* infection and do not reveal either macrophage–lymphoblast interactions or the development of resistance upon recovery (Stevens *et al.* 1978). A secretory immune response with proliferation of IgM-, IgG- and finally IgA-bearing cells occurs regularly and is expressed even in milk (Miotti *et al.* 1985). The functional importance of secretory anti-*Giardia* antibodies, especially those of the surface IgA (sIgA) class, is not clear, although in a murine model they play a crucial role in parasite elimination (Andrews and Hewlett 1981). A systemic humoral immune response follows shortly thereafter. Healthy individuals have IgG anti-*Giardia* antibodies by IFA as frequently as patients with proved giardiasis, but in significantly lower titres. Cross-reaction with unrelated immunogens, or past overt or subclinical giardial disease, may explain this lack of specificity, which seriously limits the use of diagnostic serology in giardiasis, although a redeeming value may remain for sero-epidemiological surveys. Serological results have been quite discrepant, ranging from almost perfect distinction to complete overlap of titres in patients and controls. The conventional methods (CF, IFA, IgG-ELISA, using antigenic material from axenic trophozoites or cysts) fail to differentiate between individuals with and without giardiasis, and the persistence of antibodies can be variable as well (Smith 1989). Specific IgM antibody ELISA may eventually overcome these shortcomings as it combines excellent (96%) sensitivity and specificity and titres fade almost regularly 2–3 weeks after treatment (John-Goka *et al.* 1986). At any rate, serum antibodies as such do not appear to be of any value in the host's ability to eliminate the parasite, although they may be critical in preventing invasion beyond the intestinal mucosa.

The cellular immune response in giardiasis has been studied mainly in animal models (mice, rats, gerbils). Normal mice spontaneously resolve infections with *G. muris* and in due course acquire resistance to reinfection (Roberts-Thomson *et al.* 1976). Nu/nu mice, on the other hand, suffer protracted giardial infection and do not become resistant upon recovery, although when reconstituted with immune lymphocytes such protection is established (Roberts-Thomson and Mitchell 1978). The loss of protective immunity in the lactating female mice is due to migration of immunocompetent cells from the gut and eventual excretion in the milk (Craft 1982). Intraepithelial lymphocyte counts peak after 4 weeks, coinciding with the decline in trophozoite counts. It is thus fair to assume that a local cellular immune response contributes to the clearing of the infection. The role of a systemic cellular immune response in *Giardia* clearance remains unknown, although human patients with cellular immunodeficiences, including AIDS (Smith 1989), do not appear to be more susceptible to *Giardia*, and even Nu/nu mice eventually clear their giardial infection with time, without of course becoming resistant (Roberts-Thomson *et al.* 1976).

The possibility of a strictly local anaphylactic reaction contributing to either defence or disease in giardiasis remains an intriguing question, as isolated systemic allergic reactions have been claimed to exist in giardiasis (Halstead and Sadun 1965).

Giardia lamblia trophozoites are readily killed when exposed *in vitro* to fresh human serum lacking detectable antibody, apparently through activation of the classical complement pathway. Antibody (supposedly only of the IgM class) heightened this effect. The alternative complement pathway is not activated, but a unique pathway requiring Ca^{2+}, C1 and factor B, but not factors C2, C4 or C9, has been described (Deguchi *et al.* 1987). Studies of the interaction of *Giardia lamblia* with mononuclear phagocytes have yielded conflicting results. Some studies found that human, mouse and rabbit mononuclear phagocytes, aided or not by antibodies, have the capacity to ingest and kill intracellular giardiae through oxidative mechanisms (Hill and Peerson 1987), while other studies found the survival of giardiae in unfavourable culture conditions (i.e. 5% CO_2, 95% air) to be much better precisely when mononuclear phagocytes were present (Aggarwal and Nash 1986). Furthermore, neither cytotoxic T lymphocytes nor mononuclear phagocytes obtained from the intestinal lumen of *Giardia*-infected mice appear to be involved in the clearance of *G. muris* infection (Heyworth *et al.* 1985). Although lymphocytes and PMN are not spontaneously cytotoxic against *G. lamblia*, in the presence of immune serum they may kill the parasite, perhaps through an ADCC mechanism (Smith 1989). In summary, the present state of the art concerning the clearance of *G. lamblia* in humans would tentatively incriminate a combination of local humoral and cellular immune factors, but much remains to be learned on this subject (Owen 1980; Smith 1989).

The sensitivity of microscopic examinations of stools for the presence of *G. lamblia* cysts or — rarely — trophozoites is low and quite variable (≤50%) and examining duodenal fluid or performing a duodenal biopsy in search of giardiae, although reliable (sensitivity of 80–100%), is uncomfortable. Diagnostic serology is, as we have seen, apparently to no avail (Smith 1989). Clearly, there is room for more sensitive, non-invasive methods for diagnosing giardiasis. CIE or ELISA for *Giardia* antigen in the stools, perhaps employing monoclonal antibodies, appears at least as promising as its counterpart in the field of amoebiasis (Rosoff and Stibbs 1986).

Acknowledgements

The author wishes to express his gratitude to Dr Ruy Pérez-Tamayo for his critical review of the manuscript and to Dr Adolfo Martínez-Palomo for providing the scanning electron micrographs of *E. histolytica* and *G. lamblia*.

References

Acosta, G., Campus, R., Bayranco, C., Isibasi, A. and Kumate, J. (1983). Secretory IgA antibodies from bile of immunized rats reactive with trophozoites of *E. histolytica Ann. NY Acad. Sci.* **409**, 760–5.

Adam, R.D., Aggarwal, A., Lal, A.A., de la Cruz, V., McCutchan, T. and Nash, T.E. (1988). Antigenic variation of a cysteine-rich protein in *Giardia lamblia*. *J. Exp. Med.* **167**, 109–18.

Aggarwal, A. and Nash, T.E. (1986). Lack of cellular cytotoxicity by human mononuclear cells to Giardia. *J. Immunol.* **136**, 3486–8.

Aley, S.B., Scott, W.A. and Cohn, Z.A. (1980). Plasma membrane of *Entamoeba histolytica*. *J. Exp. Med.* **152**, 391–404.

Allason-Jones, E., Mindel, A., Sergeaunt, P. and Williams, P. (1986). *Entamoeba histolytica* as a commensal intestinal parasite in homosexual men. *N. Engl. J. Med.* **315**, 353–6.

Amyx, H.L., Asher, D.M. and Nash, T.E. (1978). Hepatic amebiasis in spider monkeys. *Am. J. Trop. Med. Hyg.* **27**, 888–91.

Andrews, J.S. and Hewlett, E.L. (1981). Protection against infection with *Giardia muris* by milk containing antibody to *Giardia*. *J. Infect. Dis.* **143**, 242–6.

Arellano, J., Granader, J., Pérez, E., Félix, C. and Kretschmer, R.R. (1991). Increased frequency of HLA-DR3 and completype SCO1 in Mexican mestizo patients with amoebic abscess of the liver. *Parasitic Immunol.* **13**, 23–9.

Arnaud-Battandier, F., Bundy, B.M., O'Neill, M., Bienenstock, J. and Nelson, D.L. (1978). Cytotoxic activities of gut mucosal lymphoid cells in guinea pigs. *J. Immunol.* **121**, 1059–65.

Aust-Kettis, D., Thorstensson, R. and Utter, G. (1983). Antigenicity of *Entamoeba histolytica* strain NIH-200: a survey of clinically relevant antigenic components. *Am. J. Trop. Med. Hyg.* **32**, 512–22.

Calderón, J. and Tovar, R. (1986). Loss of susceptibility to complement lysis in *Entamoeba histolytica* HM1 by treatment with human serum. *Immunology* **58**, 467–71.

Calderón, J., Muñoz, M.L. and Acosta, H.M. (1980). Surface redistribution and release of antibody-induced caps in *Entamoebae*. *J. Exp. Med.* **151**, 184–93.

Capin, R., Capin, N.R., Carmona, M. and Ortiz-Ortiz, L. (1980). Effect of complement depletion on the induction of amebic liver abscess in the hamster. *Arch. Invest. Méd. (Méx.)* **11** (1), 173–80.

Chadee, K. and Meerovitch, E. (1985a). *Entamoeba histolytica*: lymphoreticular changes in gerbils (*Meriones unguiculatus*) with experimentally induced caecal amoebiasis. *J. Parasitol.* **71**, 566–75.

Chadee, K. and Meerovitch, E. (1985b). The pathology of experimentally induced amebic liver abscess in the gerbil (*Meriones unguiculatus*). *Am. J. Pathol.* **119**, 485–94.

Chang, S.M., Lin, C.M., Dusanic, D.G. and Cross, J.H. (1979). Antigenic analysis of two axenized strains of *E. histolytica* by two-dimentional immunoelectrophoresis. *Am. J. Trop. Med. Hyg.* **28**, 845–53.

Cher, A. (1978). Acquisition of murine major histocompatibility complex gene products by schistosomula of *Schistosoma mansoni*. *J. Exp. Med.* **148**, 46–57.

Councilman, W.T. and Lafleur, H.A. (1891). Amebic dysentery. *Johns Hopkins Hosp. Rep.* **2**, 395–548.

Craft, J.C. (1982). Giardia and giardiasis in childhood. *Pediatr. Infect. Dis.* **1**, 196–211.

Deguchi, M., Gillin, F.D. and Gigli, I. (1987). Mechanism of killing of *Giardia lamblia* trophozoites by complement. *J. Clin. Invest.* **79**, 1296–302.

Del Muro, R., Oliva, A., Herion, P., Capin, R. and Ortiz-Ortiz, L. (1987). Diagnosis of *Entamoeba histolytica* in feces by ELISA. *J. Clin. Lab. Anal.* **1**, 322–5.

Diamantstein, T., Klos, M., Gold, D. and Hahn, H. (1981). Interaction between *Entamoeba histolytica* and the immune system. I. Mitogenicity of *Entamoeba histolytica* extracts for human peripheral T lymphocytes. *J. Immunol.* **126**, 2084–6.

Diamond, L.S. (1961). Axenic cultivation of *Entamoeba histolytica*. *Science* **134**, 336–7.

Ghadirian, E. and Meerovitch, E. (1982). Macrophages requirement for host defense against experimental hepatic amebiasis in the hamster. *Parasite Immunol.* **4**, 219–25.

González-Mendoza, A. and Aguirre-Garcia, J. (1971). Micosis oportunistas en amibiasis invasora. *Arch. Invest. Méd. (Méx.)* **2** (1), 321–6.

Grundy, M.S., Cartwright-Taylor, L., Lundin, L., Thors, C. and Huldt, G. (1983). Antibodies against *Entamoeba histolytica* in human milk and serum in Kenya. *J. Clin. Microbiol.* **17**, 753–8.

Guerrant, R.L. (1986). Amoebiasis: introduction, current status and research questions. *Rev. Infect. Dis.* **8**, 218–27.

Gutiérrez-Trujillo, G. and Muñoz, O. (1990). Epidemiology of amebiasis. In *Amebiasis*, ed. R.R. Kretschmer, pp. 173–89, CRC Press, Boca Raton.

Gutiérrez-Trujillo, G., Ludlow, A., Espinosa, G. *et al.* (1976). Encuesta serológica nacional. II. Investigación de anticuerpos contra *E. histolytica* en la República Mexicana. In *Proceedings of an International Conference on Amebiasis*, ed. B. Sepúlveda and L.S. Diamond, pp. 599–608, Instituto Mexicano del Seguro Social, Mexico, D.F.

Halstead, S.B. and Sadun, E.H. (1965). Alimentary hypersensitivity induced by *Giardia lamblia*. *Ann. Intern. Med.* **62**, 564–9.

Harris, W.G. and Bray, R.S. (1976). Cellular sensitivity in amoebiasis: preliminary results of lymphocytic transformation in response to specific antigen and mitogen in carrier and disease states. *Trans. Roy. Soc. Trop. Med. Hyg.* **70**, 340–3.

Heyworth, M.F., Owen, R.L. and Jones, A.L. (1985). Comparison of leukocytes obtained from the intestinal lumen of *Giardia*-infected immunocompetent mice and nude mice. *Gastroenterology* **89**, 1360–5.

Hill, D.R. and Pearson, R.D. (1987). Ingestion of *Giardia lamblia* trophozoites by human mononuclear phagocytes. *Infect. Immunity* **55**, 3155–61.

Isibasi, A. and Kumate, J. (1990). Antigens. In *Amebiasis*, ed. R.R. Kretschmer, pp. 61–76, CRC Press, Boca Raton.

Izar, G. (1914). Studien über das Vorkommen spezifischer Antikörper in Serum von Amoebennruhrkranken. *Arch. Schiffs. Tropenhyg.* **18** (suppl.), 45–79.

Jalan, N.K. (1984). Clinical amebiasis and pathology. In *Proceedings of the Eleventh International Congress in Tropical Medicine and Hygiene*, vol. I, p. 68, Calgary.

John-Goka, A.K., Mathan, V.I., Rolston, D.D.K. and Farthing, M.J.G. (1986). Diagnosis of giardiasis by specific IgM antibody enzyme-linked immunosorbent assay. *Lancet* **ii**, 184–6.

Jones, J.F. (1984). Serodiagnosis in parasitic infections. *Clin. Immunol. Newslett.* **5**, 103–5.

Joyce, M.P. and Ravdin, J.I. (1988). Antigens of *Entamoeba histolytica* recognized by immune sera from liver abscess patients. *Am. J. Trop. Med. Hyg.* **38**, 74–80.

Kretschmer, R.R. (1986). Immunology of amebiasis. In *Amebiasis*, ed. A. Martínez-Palomo, pp. 96–167, Elsevier, Amsterdam.

Kretschmer, R.R. and López-Osuna, M. (1990). Effector mechanisms and immunity to amebas. In *Amebiasis*, ed. R.R. Kretschmer, pp. 105–22, CRC Press, Boca Raton.

Kretschmer, R.R. and López-Osuna, M. (1991). Destruction of virulent *E. histolytica* by f-MLP activated human eosinophils. *FLSEB J.* **5**, A640.

Kretschmer, R.R., Collado, M.L., Pacheco, M.G. *et al.* (1985). Inhibition of human monocyte locomotion by products of axenically grown *E. histolytica*. *Parasite Immunol.* **7**. 527–43.

Krogstad, D.J., Spencer, H.C. and Healy, G.R. (1978). Current concepts in parasitology: amebiasis. *N. Engl. J. Med.* **298**, 262–5.

Krupp, I.M. (1974). Protective immunity to amebic infection demonstrated in guinea pigs. *Am. J. Trop. Med. Hyg.* **23**, 355–60.

Krupp, I.M. and Powell, S.J. (1971). Comparative study of the antibody response in amebiasis: persistence after successful treatment. *Am. J. Trop. Med. Hyg.* **20**, 421–4.

López-Osuna, M. and Kretschmer, R.R. (1989). Destruction of normal human eosinophils by *Entamoeba histolytica*. *Parasite Immunol.* **11**, 403–11.

Martínez-Palomo, A. (1982). *The Biology of Entamoeba Histolytica*. Research Studies Press/Wiley, Chichester.

Martínez-Palomo, A. (1986). *Amebiasis*, Elsevier, Amsterdam.

Meyer, E.A. (1976). *Giardia lamblia*: isolation and axenic cultivation. *Exp. Parasitol.* **39**, 101–5.

Meza, I., Cazarez, F., Rosales, J.L., Talamas, P. and Rojkind, H. (1987). Use of antibodies to characterize a 220-kilodalton surface protein from *E. histolytica*. *J. Infect. Dis.* **156**, 798–805.

Miotti, P.G., Gilman, R.H., Pickering, L.K., Ruiz-Palacior, G., Park, H.S. and Yolken, R.H. (1985). Prevalence of serum and milk antibodies to *Giardia lamblia* in different populations of lactating women. *J. Infect. Dis.* **152**, 1025–31.

Mirelman, D., Bracha, R., Wexler, A. and Chayen, A. (1986). Alteration of isoenzyme patterns of a cloned culture of non pathogenic *Entamoeba histolytica* upon changes in growth conditions. *Arch. Invest. Méd. (Méx.)* **17** (1), 187–93.

Nash, T. (1985). Comparison of different isolates of *Giardia*. *Microbiol. Ther.* **15**, 121–32.

Nash, T.E., Herrington, D.A., Losonsky, G.A. and Levine, M.M. (1987). Experimental human infections with *Giardia lamblia*. *J. Infect. Dis.* **156**, 974–84.

Noya, O., Warren, L.G. and Goha, R. (1980). Serum proteins in the plasma membrane in *Entamoeba histolytica*. *Arch. Invest. Méd. (Méx.)* **11** (1), 109–11.

Ortiz-Ortiz, L. and Avella, M.L. (1984). Respuesta inmune en infecciones por *E. histolytica*. *Immunología* **3**, 5–11.

Owen, R.L. (1980). The immune response in clinical and experimental giardiasis. *Trans. Roy. Soc. Trop. Med. Hyg.* **74**, 443–5.

Parkhouse, M., Cid, M.E. and Calderón, J. (1978). Identificación de antígenos de membrana de *Entamoebas* y su caracterización en inmunoquimica. *Arch. Invest. Méd. (Méx.)* **9** (1), 211–18.

Pérez-Tamayo, R. (1986). Pathology of amebiasis. In *Amebiasis*, ed. A. Martínez-Palomo, pp. 45–94, Elsevier, Amsterdam.

Pérez-Tamayo, R. and Brandt, H. (1971). Amebiasis. In *Pathology of Protozoan and Helminthic Diseases*, ed. M.A. Marcial-Rojas, pp. 145–88, Williams & Wilkins, Baltimore.

Petri, W.A. and Ravdin, J.I. (1989). *Entamoeba. histolytica*. In *Parasitic Infections in the Compromised Host*, ed. P.D. Walzer and R.M. Genta, pp. 385–437. Marcel Dekker, New York/Basle.

Petri, W.A., Smith, R.D., Schlesinger, P.H., Murphy, C.F. and Ravdin, J.I. (1988). Isolation of the galactose-binding lectin that mediates the *in vitro* adherence of *Entamoeba histolytica*. *J. Clin. Invest.* **80**, 1238–44.

Pillai, S. and Mohimen, A. (1982). A solid-phase sandwich radioimmunoassay for *E. histolytica* proteins and the detection of circulating antigens in amoebiasis. *Gastroenterology* **83**, 1210–16.

Ravdin, J.I. (1988). *Amebiasis: Human Infection by Entamoeba histolytica*. John Wiley, New York.

Ravdin, J.I. and Guerrant, R.L. (1982). A review of the parasite cellular mechanisms involved in the pathogenesis of amebiasis. *Rev. Infect. Dis.* **4**, 1184–207.

Roberts-Thomson, I.C. and Mitchell, G.F. (1978). Giardiasis in mice. I. Prolonged infections in certain mouse strains and hypothymic (nude) mice. *Gastroenterology* **75**, 42–6.

Roberts-Thomson, I.C. *et al.* (1976). Giardiasis in the mouse: an animal model. *Gastroenterology* **71**, 57–61.

Rosoff, J.D. and Stibbs, H.H. (1986). Isolation and identification of a *Giardia lamblia* species stool antigen (GSA65) useful in coprodiagnosis of giardiasis. *J. Clin. Microbiol.* **23**, 905–10.

Salata, R.A. and Ravdin, J.I. (1986). Review of the human immune mechanism directed against *Entamoeba histolytica*. *Rev. Infect. Dis.* **8**, 261–72.

Salata, R.A. and Ravdin, J.I. (1988). Immunoprophylaxis. In *Amebiasis: Human Infection by Entamoeba histolytica*, ed. J.I. Ravdin, pp. 784–92, John Wiley, New York.

Salata, R.A., Cox, J. and Ravdin, J.I. (1985). Interaction of human leucocytes and *Entamoeba histolytica*: killing of virulent amebas by the activated macrophage. *J. Clin. Invest.* **76**, 491–9.

Salata, R.A., Pearson, R.D. and Ravdin, J.I. (1986). Patients treated for amebic liver abscess develop cell-mediated immune responses effective *in vitro* against *Entamoeba histolytica*: killing of virulent amoeba by lectin dependent lymphocytes. *Parasite Immunol.* **9**, 249–61.

Sargeaunt, P.G. (1987). The reliability of *Entamoeba histolytica* zymodemes in clinical diagnosis. *Parasitol. Today* **3**, 40–3.

Sepúlveda, B. (1978). Induccion de inmunidad protectora antiamibiana con 'nuevos' antígenos en el hamster lactante. A. Introducción. *Arch. Invest. Méd. (Méx.)* **9** (1), 309–10.

Smith, P.D. (1985). Pathophysiology and immunology of giardiasis. *Ann. Rev. Med.* **36**, 295–307.

Smith, P.D. (1989). *Giardia lamblia*. In *Parasitic Infections in the Compromised Host*, ed. P.D. Walzer and R.M. Genta, pp. 343–84, Marcel Dekker, New York/Basle.

Stern, J.J., Graybill, J.A. and Drutz, D.J. (1984). Murine amebiasis: the role of the macrophage in host defense. *Am. J. Trop. Med. Hyg.* **33**, 372–80.

Stevens, D.P. *et al.* (1978). Thymus dependency of host resistance to *Giardia muris* infection: studies in nude mice. *J. Immunol.* **120**, 680–2.

Tsutsumi, V., Mena-Lopez, R., Anaya-Velazquez and Martinez-Palomo, A. (1984). Cellular bases of experimental liver abscess formation. *Am. J. Pathol.* **117**, 81–91.

Ungar, B.L.P. and Nash, T.E. (1987). Cross-reactivity among different *Giardia lamblia* isolates using immunofluorescent antibody and enzyme immunoassay techniques. *Am. J. Trop. Med. Hyg.* **37**, 283–9.

Usawattanakul, W., Tapchaisri, P., Thammapalerd, N., Tharavanyij, S. and Kojima, S. (1982). Mouse IgE response to an allergen from *E. histolytica*. *J. Parasitol.* **68**, 398–401.

Walsh, J.A. (1986). Problems in recognition and diagnosis of amebiasis: estimation of the global magnitude of morbidity and mortality. *Rev. Infect. Dis.* **8**, 228–38.

Webster, A.D.B. (1980). Giardiasis and immunodeficiency diseases. *Trans. Roy. Soc. Trop. Med. Hyg.* **74**, 440–3.

Wright, R.A., Spencer, H.C., Brodsky, R.E. and Vernon, T.M. (1977). Giardiasis in Colorado: an epidemiologic study. *Am. J. Epidemiol.* **105**, 330–6.

83: The Immunology of Helminth Infections

A.E. Butterworth

Introduction

The immune response to helminth parasites does not differ in any fundamental way from that to any other infectious agent. However, several special aspects of the host–parasite relationship in helminth infections result in the consequences of the response showing some unusual features. These features are broadly outlined below, and are then discussed in detail by reference to a few selected examples drawn from parasites of human or veterinary importance.

Helminths as macroparasites

Anderson and May (1979) have drawn a sharp distinction between microparasites, such as viruses, bacteria and protozoa, and macroparasites, such as helminths. Microparasites, apart from their small size, are characterized by rapid direct reproduction leading to an infection that is frequently (although not invariably) of short duration, culminating in death of the host or in recovery with immunity to reinfection. In contrast, macroparasites — especially adult helminths within their definitive hosts — do not replicate: the organisms are long-lived in relation to the lifespan of the host and any immunity that is engendered is, at best, incomplete. In such a situation, the unit of measurement of infection is the individual parasite, rather than the infected host: it is both possible and necessary to record intensities of infection, rather than simply its presence or absence.

The distribution of the intensity of helminth infection in a naturally exposed community is usually over-dispersed: a small number of individuals harbour most of the worms (Anderson and May 1985). The reason for this over-dispersal or aggregation is usually not known, but may include a predisposition of certain individuals to heavy infections attributable to either environmental or genetic factors (e.g. Bensted-Smith *et al.* 1987; Haswell-Elkins *et al.* 1988): and genetically determined variations in host responses are of crucial importance in many experimental helminth infections (Wakelin 1988). In addition, and in contrast to microparasitic infections, the manifestation of clinical disease is frequently dependent on intensity of infection.

These differences between micro- and macroparasites have several implications. First, the continued survival of the adult worm for long periods in the infected host suggests that the worm has evolved mechanisms for evading the effects of the host's immune response. Secondly, although an immune response that protects a host against superinfection or against reinfection after treatment or spontaneous cure may be only partially effective, it may be of great value in preventing disease, by reducing the proportion of individuals who acquire high-intensity infections. An implication of this is that, in order to be useful as a control measure, a vaccine need not be completely effective in any individual: a partial reduction in the mean number of worms acquired by the host may lead to a considerable reduction in morbidity (Butterworth and Hagan 1987).

Evasion of the host's immune response

The mechanisms whereby the adult worms of a primary infection may evade the host's immune response have been reviewed in detail elsewhere (Ogilvie and Wilson 1977; Parkhouse 1984; Behnke 1987a; Lightowlers and Rickard 1988), and include:

1 Sequestration of the parasite in a site that is anatomically protected from host effector mechanisms (e.g. *Trichinella spiralis* larvae within host muscle cells).

2 Possession of a tegument that is resistant to immune attack (e.g. many adult nematodes, which possess a tough, rigid cuticle).

3 Uptake of host-derived macromolecules that mask the expression of the parasite's own surface antigens (e.g. *Schistosoma mansoni* (Smithers *et al.* 1969; Goldring *et al.* 1977)).

4 Loss of expression of parasite antigens from the tegumental surface, such that the worm presents to the host an immunologically inert surface (e.g. *Schistosoma mansoni* (Pearce *et al.* 1986a)).

5 Rapid shedding of surface material in the face of immune attack (e.g. *Fasciola hepatica* (Duffus and Franks 1980), *Toxocara canis* (Badley *et al.* 1987)).

6 Production and release of moieties that inhibit the induction or expression of the host response. These moieties may include, for example; anti-complementary factors in *Taenia taeniaeformis* infections (Hammerberg and Williams 1978; Letonja and Hammerberg 1983); proteases that cleave immunoglobulins in *Schistosoma mansoni* (Auriault *et al.* 1981) and *Fasciola hepatica* (Chapman and Mitchell 1982) infections; and factors that modify lymphocyte, macrophage, granulocyte or mast cell functions in infections with *Schistosoma mansoni* (Mazingue *et al.* 1980; Vieira *et al.* 1986), *Taenia taeniaeformis* (Leid *et al.* 1986) and *Trichinella spiralis* (Rhoads 1983).

These and other evasion mechanisms reflect adaptations on the part of the parasite rather than unusual features of the host response, and are not discussed in further detail. The important point is that the adult worm may continue to survive for long periods, even in the face of a protective immune response that allows the host to resist reinfection with a secondary challenge of fresh infective larvae.

Evidence for protective immunity against helminth infections in man

The continued survival of adult worms from early infections and the incomplete nature of immunity to reinfection render difficult the study of the mechanisms of such immunity. Three approaches have been adopted, each of which has disadvantages. First, the study of helminth parasites of rodents in their natural hosts, such as *Nippostrongylus brasiliensis* in the rat or *Nematospiroides dubius* (*Heligmosoides polygyrus*) in the mouse, allows the analysis of a 'natural' host–parasite relationship; but results from such studies cannot necessarily be extrapolated to comparable parasites of man or his domestic animals. Secondly, the use of 'unnatural' rodent models to study human parasites (e.g. *Schistosoma mansoni* in the mouse or rat (Dean 1983; Capron and Capron 1986)) allows the identification of immune effector mechanisms that may be involved in human immunity, but again yields no direct proof that such mechanisms are indeed involved. Instead, therefore, more recent attempts have been made to demonstrate the presence and understand the mechanisms of immunity to human helminths in their natural host, man. Apart from the problem that evidence for the role of any particular immune effector mechanism must be correlative rather than experimental in nature, there is an additional difficulty in distinguishing between immunity and reduced exposure as possible reasons for a lack of superinfection or of reinfection after treatment. However, epidemiological studies now strongly support the hypothesis that an acquired immunity to reinfection develops slowly with age against at least some helminth parasites of man.

In schistosomiasis, for example, there is a characteristic decline with age in the prevalence and intensity of infection among individuals living in endemic areas. Until recently, it was argued that this decline might be attributable to a slow, spontaneous death of adult worms from early infections, together with a reduced contact with contaminated water in the older age groups (Warren 1973: Dalton and Pole 1978). However, direct observations of the patterns of water contact among individuals treated for primary infections with either *Schistosoma haematobium* (Wilkins *et al.* 1987) or *Schistosoma mansoni* (Butterworth *et al.* 1985, 1988; Dessein *et al.* 1988) have allowed the demonstration that, although water contact levels do indeed decline with age, there is in addition the slow development of an acquired resistance to reinfection. Similarly, studies of the epidemiology of infection with the hookworms *Ancylostoma duodenale* and *Necator americanus* suggest that, at least in some individuals, there is some evidence both for a rapid expulsion of adult worms and for a resistance to reinfection with fresh infective larvae (Behnke 1987b). In contrast, other nematode parasites, such as *Ascaris lumbricoides*, show no evidence of eliciting an effective protective response: adult worm numbers can continue to increase throughout the life of the host and, following treatment, there is a very rapid return of worm burdens to pretreatment levels (Elkins *et al.* 1988).

Evidence from human infections suggests that protective immunity against helminth infections, when it is demonstrable, is relatively weak; the development of effective vaccines (discussed below) must therefore depend not only on the identification and production of appropriate antigens, but also on their delivery at a time and in a manner that elicits an appropriate response. In contrast, several helminth parasites of veterinary importance clearly elicit high levels of immunity in their natural hosts; a commercial vaccine based on live irradiated larvae has been in use for many years for the cattle lungworm, *Dictyocaulus viviparus*, and the development of new vaccines may depend solely on the identification and production through recombinant deoxyribonucleic acid (DNA) techniques of sufficient amounts of the appropriate antigen.

Pathological consequences of the immune response to helminth infections

In some helminth infections, the extent of disease is determined solely by the intensity of infection, and the parasite exerts a dose-dependent pathophysiological effect on the host, an example being the extensive blood loss and anaemia in heavy hookworm infestations. More frequently, however, the extent of disease is determined not only by the intensity of infection (which may still be crucial), but also by the nature and extent of the host response. In the lymphatic filariases attributable to *Wuchereria bancrofti* or *Brugia malayi*, for example, acute or chronic lymphangitis or lymphatic obstruction is associated with high levels of cell-mediated responses to adult worm and microfilarial antigens, and with low numbers of circulating microfilariae; individuals with weak or absent immune responses and a high microfilarial load may show little in the way of clinical features. Similarly, in *Onchocerca volvulus* infections, the severe skin and eye lesions are associated with an immunologically mediated damage to the microfilariae, a situation that may be enhanced, in the Mazzotti reaction, by treatment with microfilaricidal drugs (Mackenzie *et al.* 1985). In *Schistosoma mansoni* infections, the severity of disease is determined by the extent of granuloma formation around eggs deposited in the tissues; such a reaction may be simultaneously beneficial, in protecting the host against the toxic effects of released egg products, and deleterious, in leading to subsequent fibrosis and obstruction of hepatic portal blood vessels.

An important aspect of helminth infections, therefore, is the study of not only antigens and mechanisms that may be involved in protective immunity, but also those that may be involved in immunopathology. In this context, it should be recalled that, in comparison with other parasites, the helminth presents to its host a complex array of different life cycle stages, each of which may express different, stage-specific antigens that may elicit different categories of response, which may be either protective or deleterious to the host. It is difficult to make broad generalizations about the nature and effects of such responses: each parasite and each stage should be considered separately. In the following sections, some examples are given that illustrate these points in more detail.

Effector mechanisms of immunity

Helminth parasites present to their hosts a wide variety of target structures, ranging from the double plasma membrane of the bloodstream trematode to the thick, collagen-containing cuticle of the adult nematode, the only common feature of such organisms being that they are all large, multicellular and non-phagocytosable particles. It is therefore not surprising that a diverse range of immune effector mechanisms can operate against these targets, each one being more or less effective in different circumstances.

Potential immune effector mechanisms can be identified *in vitro* by the use of assays that permit the demonstration of damage to any particular helminth by appropriate combinations of purified effector cells, antibodies and other effector molecules. Such assays have the advantage that they allow a detailed analysis of each effector mechanism; they also offer the only realistic approach, by appropriate analysis of correlations, towards determining which effector mechanisms may be operative in man. However, it is not possible to affirm, solely from experiments *in vitro*, that any given effector mechanism is active, or is the most important, in the intact host. Studies *in vitro* must therefore be supported by experimental observations *in vivo*, but in this case care must be taken not to extrapolate excessively from the experimental laboratory host under study to the natural host.

Studies on immune effector mechanisms *in vitro*

A wide range of effector mechanisms active against helminths *in vitro* has now been demonstrated (reviewed by Butterworth 1984). Some that are highly effective against other infectious agents are relatively inefficient in killing helminths, while others are particularly active and may have evolved selectively to deal with these large, non-phagocytosable organisms.

Cell-independent effects, including neutralization by antibody and killing or lysis by antibody and complement, are generally poorly active against most helminths. Although some killing of schistosomula of *Schistosoma mansoni* is observed in the presence of immunoglobulin G (IgG) antibodies and complement, large amounts of complement are required and the effect is both weak and slow (Clegg and Smithers 1972); the same is true of most other helminths that have been studied. Exceptions to this general rule are the marked susceptibility of immature metacestodes of some taeniid worms, in particular *Taenia taeniaeformis*, to damage by antibody and complement (Rickard and Williams 1982), and the action of antibody alone, possibly reacting with excretory/secretory products, in neutralizing some intestinal nematodes and permitting their expulsion from the gut (reviewed by Lloyd and Soulsby 1988).

Similarly, lymphocyte-mediated damage by either cytolytic T lymphocytes (CTL) or K cells acting in the presence of appropriate antibodies is either slight or indetectable. In the case of CTL, the most likely explanation is that the parasite does not bear on its surface the appropriate major histocompatibility complex (MHC) products for cell recognition; but even when adherence is induced, either through passively acquired MHC products or by the use of a non-specific ligand, little damage is observed with murine CTLs (Butterworth *et al.* 1979b: Vadas *et al.* 1979a). However, one group has reported that human peripheral blood lymphocytes can kill schistosomula of *Schistosoma mansoni* after stimulation with phytohaemagglutinin or concanavalin A, the cell involved being of the CD8 phenotype (Ellner *et al.* 1982). This interesting observation deserves further exploration.

In contrast, antibody-dependent cell-mediated cytotoxic (ADCC) reactions mediated by granulocytes or macrophages, with or without enhancement of the effect by complement, are highly active against many helminths. Two aspects of such reactions deserve particular comment.

First, although neutrophils have been reported to be active against a range of helminths, including both schistosome larvae (Dean *et al.* 1974, 1975; Anwar *et al.* 1979; Kazura *et al.* 1981; Moser and Sher 1981) and more particularly a variety of nematode larvae (Bass and Sjezda 1979; Kazura 1981; Mehta *et al.* 1981, 1982; El-Sadr *et al.* 1983), eosinophils exert a particularly marked effect (Butterworth *et al.* 1977; Capron *et al.* 1978a, b; McLaren and Ramalho-Pinto 1979; Vadas *et al.* 1979b). The antibody-dependent effect of eosinophils, which is enhanced both by complement (Anwar *et al.* 1979) and by mast cell mediators (Capron *et al.* 1978a, b; Anwar *et al.* 1980), is associated with an initial tight attachment of the cell, followed by the release on to the parasite surface of a series of highly toxic, cationic proteins (Butterworth *et al.* 1979a; McLaren *et al.* 1981). These include the eosinophil major basic protein (MBP) (Gleich *et al.* 1974) and the eosinophil cationic protein (ECP) (Olsson *et al.* 1977). Both are toxic in isolation for schistosomula: and, although ECP, which has recently been characterized as a member of the perforin family (Young *et al.* 1986), is the more potent on a molar basis (Ackerman *et al.* 1985), the higher concentrations of MBP in the granule probably account for most of the toxicity of the intact cell.

The marked capacity of the eosinophil to damage helminths may be associated with its propensity to degranulate upon contact with large, non-phagocytosable surfaces (Butterworth 1984); but other mechanisms may also be involved, including the generation of active oxygen metabolites (Kazura *et al.* 1981). In addition, eosinophils recovered from the blood of individuals with enhanced eosinophil levels, attributable either to helminth infections or to allergic disorders, show an enhanced killing capacity (David *et al.* 1980), which may be attributable to the release from monocytes of one or more eosinophil-activating moieties (Veith and Butterworth 1983; Dessein *et al.* 1983; Thorne *et al.* 1986). An extreme form of eosinophil activation is seen in the hypereosinophilic syndrome, in which the low-density eosinophils that are recovered are able to mediate damage in the presence of IgE antibodies (Capron *et al.* 1984 and below).

A second striking feature of ADCC reactions to helminths is the involvement of IgE antibodies. These may not only amplify the effects of a reaction, through an antigen/IgE-induced release of mast cell mediators which may enhance effector cell function, but also serve directly as ligands in the ADCC reaction itself. Capron *et al.* (1975, 1977) first demonstrated that IgE antibodies, in the form of immune complexes with antigen, were both sufficient and necessary to mediate macrophage-dependent killing of schistosomula in the rat, a finding that has since been extended to other host species (Joseph *et al.* 1978) and other parasites (Haque *et al.* 1980; Mehta *et al.* 1980). Subsequently, IgE has also been shown to mediate damage in the presence of rat and human platelets (Joseph *et al.* 1984; Capron *et al.* 1987b) and eosinophils (Capron *et al.* 1981b). As with the macrophage (Dessaint *et al.* 1979; Melewicz and Spiegelberg 1980; Pestel *et al.* 1988), both rat and human eosinophils have been found to bear low-affinity receptors for IgE (Capron *et al.* 1981a, 1984); the expression of such receptors is increased in conditions of eosinophil activation, and in particular the hypereosinophilic syndrome (Capron *et al.* 1986; Jouault *et al.* 1988).

Increased circulating eosinophil numbers and high levels of both total and parasite-specific IgE are hallmarks of helminth infections, which have frequently been used as models for studying the regulation of IgE responses. It may be speculated that the presence of tissue-stage helminths selectively elicits a highly specialized host protective response, involving:

1 An increase in both the numbers and functional activity of circulating eosinophils.

2 A local IgE-dependent immediate-hypersensitivity reaction, with the release of mast cell mediators that both localize eosinophils and further enhance their functional properties.

3 Destruction of the invading helminth by eosinophils, mediated not only by IgG but also by IgE antibodies.

The pathological consequences of immediate-hypersensitivity reactions can be regarded as secondary to this basic protective role.

A completely separate effector mechanism that is highly active against many helminths is the antibody-independent effect of macrophages activated by T cell products. The potential importance of this reaction, from the point of view of vaccine development (below), is that parasite surface antigens need not be involved; released products may be equally effective, in both inducing the initial T cell response and eliciting a subsequent local macrophage activation at the site of invasion. Killing of both *Schistosoma mansoni* and *Trichinella spiralis* larvae has been described following activation of murine macrophages through T cell responses to irrelevant antigens (bacillus Calmette–Guérin (BCG) or *Corynebacterium parvum*) (Mahmoud *et al.* 1979): the mechanism is uncertain, although release of arginase (Olds *et al.* 1980) and of active oxygen species (Peck *et al.* 1983) have both been implicated. More recently, macrophage activation leading to killing of schistosomula has been described following either infection with *Schistosoma mansoni* or immunization under conditions that lead to the development of protective immunity to challenge (James *et al.* 1982, 1983; James 1986a, b, 1987). In man, macrophages appropriately cultured and activated by T cell products or by recombinant interferon-γ have been shown to damage schistosomula in some experiments (Olds *et al.* 1981; Cottrell *et al.* 1989), although others have not confirmed this effect (Remold *et al.* 1988).

Studies on immunity in experimental animal models

Immunity to helminth infections in experimental animal models has been studied by the conventional techniques of histological examination of the site of immune damage to the invading parasite, cell or antibody transfer or depletion studies, the use of inbred animals deficient in particular components of the immune system, and the use of immunization protocols designed selectively to elicit a particular category of response. Although broad generalizations can be drawn concerning the nature of the effector mechanisms that are operative *in vitro*, this is not possible for experiments *in vivo*: results vary not only with the parasite species under investigation, but also with the host strain or species and the mode of immunization.

In schistosomiasis, for example, there are marked differences between the rat and the mouse as experimental models. The rat is a non-permissive host, in the sense that adult worms of a primary infection mature but fail to lay eggs; instead, the worms are killed (not necessarily by immunological mechanisms) and the animal is markedly resistant to reinfection (Capron and Capron 1986). Resistance can be consistently transferred to naïve animals with infection serum (Ford *et al.* 1987) or with monoclonal antibodies with specificity for schistosomulum surface antigens (Grzych *et al.* 1982; Verwaerde *et al.* 1987). The antibodies (monoclonal or otherwise) that transfer protection are of the IgE and IgG2a isotypes; IgG2c blocks the transfer of immunity (Grzych *et al.* 1984). In addition, eosinophils recovered from rats at appropriate times after infection can also transfer immunity: such cells can be demonstrated to bear on their surface cytophilic anti-schistosomulum IgG2a antibodies. In this model, therefore, immunity appears to depend on ADCC reactions that involve anaphylactic antibodies and various cell types, including eosinophils and possibly also macrophages and platelets. Immune effector mechanisms are thus directed against the surface of the young schistosomulum, either soon after penetration of the skin or during or immediately after its migration through the lungs (Ford *et al.* 1987).

The mouse, in contrast, is a permissive host of *Schistosoma mansoni*, in that the adult worms of a primary infection mature, lay eggs and can persist for the lifespan of the host. The resistance to reinfection that is observed following a chronic primary infection is now considered to be attributable largely to non-specific effects, including structural changes in the lungs and liver, which follow egg-induced pathology (McHugh *et al.* 1987); studies on specific immunity have therefore more recently involved the use of animals immunized with irradiated cercariae or with crude or purified antigen preparations (Dean 1983). In these models, although both sera from immunized animals and some monoclonal antibodies against schistosomulum surface antigens have been shown to transfer protection (Zodda and Phillips 1982; Harn *et al.* 1984; Mangold and Dean 1986), the effect is weaker and less consistent than in the rat, and only in some systems is there evidence for ADCC reactions acting on skin-stage parasites (Ward and McLaren 1988). Instead, experiments by James and colleagues and by others (reviewed by James 1986b) have indicated a major role for T cell-mediated responses with macrophage activation in animals immunized either with irradiated larvae or by the intradermal inoculation of crude or purified worm antigens in the presence of BCG. In this case, killing occurs at a stage after the migrating schistosomulum leaves the skin, and may be associated with the expulsion of the parasite into the alveoli of the lung.

These findings for schistosomiasis have been described in some detail, simply to exemplify the complexity of the host responses involved in protective immunity, and the very major differences that may be observed between different experimental models. Similar problems are encountered in most helminth infections, but these can only be summarized. Intestinal nematodes, for example, elicit a range of protective responses that may mediate the rapid expulsion of adult worms from the intestine, reduce the fecundity of the adult worms, or mediate protection against reinfection by fresh larvae. Each of these effects may be mediated by different mechanisms, which may include the direct interaction of IgG or IgA antibodies, changes in mucus composition and formation, and IgE-mediated effects with the release of mucosal mast cell mediators (Miller 1987). Antibody-dependent cell-mediated cytotoxic reactions may be involved in protection against tissue-invasive nematodes; such reactions may also mediate clearance of microfilariae from the skin or blood, although this effect may be associated with the manifestations of pathology (below). In cestode infections, immunity to reinfection against the invading oncosphere may involve both prevention of invasion by antibody and killing of the oncosphere by antibody, complement and various effector cells (Lightowlers and Rickard 1988).

Correlative studies in man

The wide discrepancies in results from different experimental hosts imply that, although such results can provide useful pointers towards the immune effector mechanisms that should be sought in man, they cannot be taken as evidence that such mechanisms do occur. Investigations on the nature of human immunity must therefore depend on a direct analysis of human materials and, since an experimental approach is almost invariably impossible, they must be correlative in nature; that is, attempts must be made to relate a given immune response or set of responses to the presence or absence of immunity. Apart from the intrinsic danger in the interpretation of observed correlations, such investigations are extremely difficult for many reasons, including the partial nature of immunity, the difficulty in estimating exposure, and the long time period over which infection or reinfection slowly and cumulatively occurs. At present, the most extensive studies have been undertaken in the field of schistosomiasis; separate studies on lymphatic filariasis relate more to the mechanisms of immunopathology, and are described below.

Following the demonstration of an age-dependent acquired resistance to schistosome infection in man, distinguishable from age-dependent changes in exposure through water contact (Butterworth *et al.* 1985; Wilkins *et al.* 1987), various groups have attempted to relate such resistance to a range of immune responses. In *Schistosoma haematobium* infections in The Gambia, Hagan *et al.* (1985, 1987) have shown that resistance to reinfection after treatment of children is associated with an increase in circulating eosinophil counts — suggesting a role for eosinophil-mediated ADCC reactions — and with the development with age of antibodies with specificity for adult worm and schistosomulum membrane antigens. The finding that these antibodies can include IgE (Hagan *et al.* 1991) represents the first demonstration of a potential protective role for IgE in man. In studies on *Schistosoma mansoni* in Kenya, the association of resistance with eosinophil levels has not proved consistent (Sturrock *et al.* 1983; Butterworth *et al.* 1985), and all children show a range of potentially protective responses, including high levels of antibodies mediating eosinophil-dependent killing of schistosomula *in vitro*. Instead, the continued susceptibility of younger children to reinfection after treatment may be attributable to the presence of 'blocking' antibodies of an inappropriate isotype (IgM, IgG2 and IgG4), that may cross-react with egg carbohydrate antigens and that prevent the binding and functional activity of effector antibodies with specificity for schistosomulum surface antigens (Butterworth *et al.* 1987, 1988; Dunne *et al.* 1988). In separate studies in Brazil, Dessein *et al.* (1988) have reported a marked heterogeneity in individual resistance to reinfection in older children, and have ascribed such resistance to the presence of antibodies recognizing a 37 kD schistosomulum surface antigen. All of these observations are consistent with a major role in man for ADCC reactions against the young schistosomulum. However, a role for T cell responses with macrophage activation has not yet been excluded, and Colley *et al.* (1986a), in studies in Egypt, have reported a relationship between resistance to reinfection and lymphocyte proliferative responses to cercarial antigens.

Identification and molecular cloning of protective antigens

In spite of much effort, only two vaccines against helminth infections, for *Dictyocaulus viviparus* in cattle and *Ancylostoma caninum* in dogs, have been developed to the stage of commercial exploitation; both of these vaccines consist of irradiation-attenuated infectious larvae (Miller 1971; reviewed by Heidrich 1988). The main reasons for this relative lack of progress have been the incomplete nature of the immunity that is engendered, either by natural infection or by a potential vaccine preparation, and the difficulty in producing sufficient amounts of parasite material for large-scale preparation of antigens. During recent years, however, two advances have rekindled interest in vaccine development: first, the realization that a vaccine need not be completely effective in order to be of value in preventing morbidity; and, secondly, the application of recombinant DNA techniques to the potential large-scale production of parasite antigens in *Escherichia coli* or other hosts. Most work has been undertaken in the field of schistosomiasis, but significant advances have also been made in *Taenia ovis* infections of sheep and in various nematode infections.

Two broad groups of peptides have been identified as candidate vaccine antigens in schistosomiasis: those that are expressed at the surface of the young schistosomulum, and may therefore serve as targets for ADCC reactions, and those that are released from the migrating schistosomulum or adult worm, and that may either elicit delayed-type hypersensitivity (DTH) reactions with macrophage activation or play some major functional role in the parasite's physiology. The most promising candidate, the p28 of *Schistosoma mansoni*, falls into both of these categories. It is produced by parenchymal cells, but is transiently expressed at the surface of the schistosomulum, and monospecific antisera against the molecule mediate eosinophil-dependent killing of schistosomula (Balloul *et al*. 1987b): in addition, it is a glutathione S-transferase. Identification of a complementary DNA (cDNA) encoding p28 has allowed the expression of the corresponding peptide in *E. coli* and in yeast, and the expressed peptides elicit high levels of protection in rats, mice and hamsters (Balloul *et al*. 1987a). Pilot trials have also been carried out in baboons (Capron *et al*. 1987a), but the results have not yet been published in detail. Another glutathione S-transferase, the Sj26 of *Schistosoma japonicum*, has been characterized as uniquely recognized by resistant strains of mice (Mitchell *et al*. 1985; Smith *et al*. 1987; Tiu *et al*. 1988) and is also available as a recombinant peptide for vaccination studies (Smith and Johnson 1988; Smith *et al*. 1988). A major schistosomulum surface antigen (gp38) has been identified by monoclonal antibodies that transfer immunity in rats (Grzych *et al*. 1982) and mice (Harn *et al*. 1984): these monoclonal antibodies recognize carbohydrate epitopes that are also expressed on egg antigens, and anti-idiotypic monoclonal 'second' antibodies elicit both protective immunity and anti-schistosomulum surface antibodies in both rats and mice (Grzych *et al*. 1985; Percy and Harn 1988). Other cloned surface peptides include particularly an 18 kD molecule (Dalton and Strand 1987; Dalton *et al*. 1987). In contrast, another major candidate as a vaccine antigen, Sm97 (Pearce *et al*. 1986b), is not expressed at the surface: it has been identified as schistosome paramyosin (Lanar *et al*. 1986), and, following immunization of mice with either the native molecule or the recombinant peptide, protective immunity is associated with delayed hypersensitivity and macrophage activation for killing of schistosomula (Pearce *et al*. 1988).

Other candidate vaccine antigens have also been identified, but are in a less advanced stage of development. These include surface peptides of 22, 28 and 37 kD (Harn *et al*. 1985; Dessein *et al*. 1988; Oligino *et al*. 1988) and molecules of 68 and 50 kD (King *et al*. 1987; Havercroft *et al*. 1988). Since no antigen so far identified elicits absolute protection, considerable work remains to be done on identifying the optimal antigen or combination of antigens, and the optimal mode of administration with suitable adjuvants, in both rodent and primate models. However, there are now realistic prospects for the development of a vaccine suitable for use in man within the foreseeable future.

In cestode infections, the most promising candidates for vaccine antigens are those excreted or released from the early larval oncosphere stage (Lightowlers and Rickard 1988). Early work with *Taenia ovis* showed that sheep could be fully protected against a challenge infection by immunization with native antigens from this stage (Rickard and Bell 1971; Rickard and Williams 1982). One such antigen, of M_r 45 000, has recently been cloned and expressed in *E. coli* as a fusion peptide with Sj26, and the fusion peptide shown to elicit high levels of protection in sheep (Johnson *et al.* 1989). This antigen has immediate potential as a commercial vaccine and, since oncosphere antigens of a range of taeniid cestodes can stimulate cross-species immunity, there are possibilities for the development of vaccines against a range of cestodes including those (such as *Echinococcus granulosus*) that are pathogenic in man. Substantial progress has been made in the identification, characterization and molecular cloning of potentially protective oncosphere antigens from a range of other cestodes, including *Taenia taeniaeformis* (Bowtell *et al.* 1983, 1984, 1986) and *Taenia saginata* (Harrison and Parkhouse 1986; Harrison *et al.* 1986).

A problem that is common to all helminth parasites, but that is particularly important in nematode infections, is that potentially protective responses against the invasive larvae may be associated with pathogenic responses to the same antigens expressed in other life cycle stages. Although some nematodes, such as *Trichinella spiralis*, do bear stage-specific surface antigens (Parkhouse *et al.* 1981), in others there is extensive cross-reactivity between the life cycle stages. Selkirk *et al.* (1986), for example, have identified a 75 kD antigen of *Brugia malayi* that is recognized selectively by sera from patients who are presumptively immune to superinfection, and Canlas *et al.* (1984) have generated monoclonal antibodies against a similar (possibly the same) antigen that mediate clearance of microfilariae *in vivo*. However, this antigen is also found in adult worms, and could be involved in the immunopathological reactions seen in chronically infected patients; vaccination with such an antigen might therefore be counter-productive. In spite of this, Kazura and colleagues (Kazura *et al.* 1986; Nilsen *et al.* 1988) have reported the identification and molecular cloning of a potentially protective antigen of *Brugia malayi*.

For any helminth infection of man, the cloning and expression of candidate vaccine antigens is only the first step on a long road towards its eventual clinical use. Subsequent problems include the demonstration of protection in appropriate experimental hosts, which in many cases may have to be primates; the exclusion of the possible induction or exacerbation of pathology; the design and execution of initial and large-scale trials in man; and the determination of the potential benefit of a vaccine in relation to the costs of manufacture and delivery, this problem being particular marked in those Third World countries in which such vaccines would be used. However, the first prerequisite, before such problems can be tackled, is the identification and molecular cloning of appropriate antigens, and progress in this area is now being made in many helminths of clinical importance.

Mechanisms of immunopathology

As with protective immunity, the immunopathological reactions that are observed in helminth infections do not differ in any fundamental way from those found in other infectious diseases. By virtue of their chronic nature, however, with a prolonged persistence of the adult worm, hypersensitivity reactions are particular common in helminth infections and may account for many of the clinical effects associated with infection; in conditions in which there is little or no immune response, as in infections with *Mansonella ozzardi*, few symptoms are observed, even though high parasite burdens may be present. It is again emphasized that clinical disease is dependent on intensity of infection; this is true whether the disease is attributable directly to the parasite or, as is more commonly the case, to the host response to the parasite.

The strong association between helminth infections and high IgE responses would suggest that immediate-hypersensitivity reactions with IgE-dependent mast cell degranulation should be particularly common, and this is the case. Acute systemic anaphylactic reactions are a common cause of death following rupture of a hydatid cyst attributable to *Echinococcus granulosus* infection (Rickard and Williams 1982), while more localized immediate-hypersensitivity reactions account for the early phase of the cercarial dermatitis, or 'swimmer's itch', that may follow penetration of the skin by cercariae of species that are both pathogenic and non-pathogenic for man. Sustained immediate-hypersensitivity reactions may account for the intense eosinophil infiltrate observed in tropical pulmonary eosinophilia attributable to cryptic filarial infections (Ottesen *et al.* 1979; Partono 1987). Helminth infections are also associated with a potentiation of IgE responses to unrelated antigens, and total as well as specific IgE levels are elevated, but this is not usually associated with an increase in prevalence of other allergic disorders.

Localized delayed hypersensitivity reactions, with T cell responses leading to macrophage activation, are also a common and important feature of helminth infections. A good example of this is the reaction to the schistosome egg: the granulomatous reaction, with its ensuing fibrosis, is responsible for almost all of the clinical manifestations of the disease. Early work by Warren and colleagues (reviewed by Warren 1982) demonstrated that the initial, cellular reaction around the egg was the result of a conventional T cell-mediated delayed-hypersensitivity reaction, and it was subsequently shown that the ensuing fibroblast proliferation and collagen synthesis was also the consequence of a T cell response (Wyler *et al.* 1987). However, two aspects of this reaction are of particular interest. First, T cell-depleted mice do not show a granulomatous reaction around eggs deposited during infection, nor do they develop the later manifestations of portal hypertension. Instead, however, they show an early mortality, associated with hepatic parenchymal cell damage, which has been attributed to a potent hepatotoxin released from the egg (Dunne *et al.* 1981). In this case, therefore, the granulomatous reaction represents a two-edged sword: it both damages the host, by causing subsequent fibrosis, and protects the host against the more serious consequences of an egg toxin. Secondly, the granulomatous reactions that are formed during late infection are smaller and lead to less tissue damage and fibrosis than those that are formed during early acute infection, a process that has been referred to as 'modulation' (Warren 1982). The mechanisms of this modulation have been extensively studied in man as well as mice, and adherent suppressor cells, soluble suppressor factors, CD8 +ve lymphocytes and antibody have all been implicated (Colley *et al.* 1977, 1978, 1986b; Gazzinelli *et al.* 1985). More recently, studies in man by Gazzinelli, Colley and colleagues (Lima *et al.* 1986; Parra *et al.* 1988; Gazzinelli *et al.* 1988; Colley *et al.* 1987) have raised an interesting alternative possibility. They have demonstrated the presence, in patients with chronic but well-compensated schistosomiasis mansoni, of T cells with an idiotypic specificity for anti-egg antibodies. Such cells are generally absent in patients with the severe, hepatosplenic form of disease. In addition, they have shown that some neonates born of infected mothers carry in their cord blood T cells with specificity for maternal anti-egg antibodies. The possible implications of these findings, in terms of regulation of the granulomatous reaction to egg antigens by an idiotypic network and the possible role of maternally transmitted antibody in modifying this network, have yet to be explored in detail.

By virtue of their chronic nature and high parasite burden, type III reactions attributable to circulating immune complexes are also common in helminth infections, including schistosomiasis and onchocerciasis. Manifestations may include a chronic glomerulonephritis, although the extent of pathology that is caused is still uncertain (Steward 1987).

In many infections the observed immunopathological reactions, although of major clinical importance, cannot be assigned to a single category. In the lymphatic filariases, for example, the chronic lymphadenopathy that develops in a minority of patients is associated with high levels of lymphocyte proliferation to adult worm antigens, high levels of anti-microfilarial antibodies, and low levels of microfilaraemia (Partono 1987; Piessens *et al.* 1987). Individuals with marked microfilaraemia, in contrast, show no antibodies or lymphocyte proliferative responses. In this case, therefore, the development of clinical disease is associated with responses to adult worms and microfilariae that prevent the release of microfilariae into the circulation, but the nature of the important responses, and of the unresponsiveness observed in many patients, remains to be determined. Similarly, in onchocerciasis, the severe clinical manifestations of blindness and pruritus are associated with the death of microfilariae in the eye and skin. Histological examination has shown that dying microfilariae are surrounded by degranulating eosinophils (Mackenzie *et al.* 1985), and there is evidence from studies *in vitro* of ADCC reactions mediated by eosinophils against microfilariae (Greene *et al.* 1981). These effects are exacerbated in the Mazzotti reactions that follow treatment with microfilaricidal drugs (Ottesen 1987).

These selected diseases serve to exemplify the range of immunopathological reactions that may be of clinical importance in helminth infections. The striking feature is that such reactions contribute significantly to the pathogenesis of disease: in their absence, there may be no clinical effects.

Conclusions

It is not possible, in a chapter of this nature, to cover comprehensively all aspects of the immunology of each medically important helminth parasite: major areas, including the role and methodology of immunodiagnosis, have inevitably been omitted. However, certain general features emerge.

1 Adult helminths are characteristically long-lived within their definitive hosts. They do not replicate, and disease is dependent on intensity of infection.

2 Adult worms have evolved a range of mechanisms for evading host immune responses that may be capable of damaging the young larvae of a fresh infection. Immunity to reinfection is usually incomplete, but the dose dependence of disease means that even an incomplete immunity may be of value in protecting the host against the severe effects of an overwhelming infection.

3 Immunity to reinfection is frequently mediated by ADCC reactions directed against the surface of the invading larva. However, other mechanisms, including an effect of activated macrophages, may also be important.

4 There are major differences in the mechanisms of immunity in experimental laboratory hosts of helminths that infect man. Such experimental models can provide useful pointers towards mechanisms that may be operative in man, but correlative studies in man are also necessary. Results of such studies are beginning to emerge.

5 One of the constraints on vaccine development is the availability of parasite material. This may be overcome by the application of recombinant DNA techniques, which have yielded several promising candidate vaccine antigens. However, much work remains to be done before such vaccines are ready for use in man.

6 Immune responses are also of major importance in the pathogenesis of disease in helminth infections, and may include immediate-hypersensitivity reactions, immune complex-mediated damage, and delayed-hypersensitivity reactions, alone or in combination.

References

Ackerman, S.J., Gleich, G.J., Loegering, D.A., Richardson, B.A. and Butterworth, A.E. (1985). Comparative toxicity of purified human eosinophil granule cationic proteins for schistosomula of *Schistosoma mansoni*. *Am. J. Trop. Med. Hyg.* **34**, 735–45.

Anderson, R.M. and May, R.M. (1979). Population biology of infections diseases: Part I. *Nature (London)* **280**, 361–7.

Anderson, R.M. and May, R.M. (1985). Helminth infections of humans: mathematical models, population dynamics and control. *Adv. Parasitol.* **24**, 1–101.

Anwar, A.R.E., Smithers, S.R. and Kay, A.B. (1979). Killing of schistosomula of *Schistosoma mansoni* coated with antibody and/or complement by human leukocytes *in vitro*: requirement for complement in preferential killing by eosinophils. *J. Immunol.* **122**, 628–37.

Anwar, A.R.E., McKean, J.R., Smithers, S.R. and Kay, A.B. (1980). Human eosinophil- and neutrophil-mediated killing of schistosomula of *Schistosoma mansoni in vitro*. I. Enhancement of complement-dependent damage by mast cell-derived mediators and formyl methionyl peptides. *J. Immunol.* **124**, 1122–9.

Auriault, C., Ouassi, M.A., Torpier, G., Eisen, H. and Capron, A. (1981). Proteolytic cleavage of IgG bound to the Fc receptor of *Schistosoma mansoni* schistosomula. *Parasite Immunol.* **3**, 33–44.

Badley, J.E., Grieve, R.B., Rockey, J.H. and Glickman, L.T. (1987). Immune-mediated adherence of eosinophils to *Toxocara canis* infective larvae: the role of excretory-secretory antigens. *Parasite Immunol.* **9**, 133–43.

Balloul, J.M., Sondermeyer, P., Dreyer, D. *et al.* (1987a). Molecular cloning of a protective antigen against schistosomiasis. *Nature (London)* **326**, 149–53.

Balloul, J.M., Grzych, J.M., Pierce, R.J. and Capron, A. (1987b). A purified 28 000 dalton protein from *Schistosoma mansoni* protects rats and mice against experimental schistosomiasis. *J. Immunol.* **138**, 3448–53.

Bass, D.A. and Sjezda, P. (1979). Eosinophils versus neutrophils in host defense: killing of newborn larvae of *Trichinella spiralis* by human granulocytes. *J. Clin. Invest.* **64**, 1415–22.

Behnke, J.M. (1987a). Evasion of immunity by nematode parasites causing chronic infections. *Adv. Parasitol.* **26**, 1–71.

Behnke, J.M. (1987b). Do hookworms elicit protective immunity in man? *Parasitol. Today* **3**, 200–6.

Bensted-Smith, R., Anderson, R.M., Butterworth, A.E. *et al.* (1987). Evidence for the predisposition of individual patients to reinfection with *Schistosoma mansoni* after treatment. *Trans. Roy. Soc. Trop. Med. Hyg.* **81**, 651–4.

Bowtell, D.D.L., Mitchell, G.F., Anders, R.F., Lightowlers, M.W. and Rickard, M.D. (1983) *Taenia taeniaeformis*: immunoprecipitation analysis of the protein antigens of oncospheres and larvae. *Exp. Parasitol.* **56**, 416–27.

Bowtell, D.D.L, Saint, R.B., Rickard, M.D. and Mitchell, G.F. (1984). Expression of *Taenia taeniaeformis* antigens in *Escherichia coli*. *Mol. Biochem. Parasitol.* **13**, 173–85.

Bowtell, D.D.L., Saint, R.B., Rickard, M.D. and Mitchell, G.F. (1986). Immunochemical analysis of *Taenia taeniaeformis* antigens expressed in *Escherichia coli*. *Parasitology* **93**, 599–610.

Butterworth, A.E. (1984). Cell-mediated damage to helminths. *Adv. Parasitol.* **23**, 143–235.

Butterworth, A.E. and Hagan, P. (1987). Immunity in human schistosomiasis. *Parasitol. Today* **3**, 11–16.

Butterworth, A.E., David, J.R., Franks, D. *et al.* (1977). Antibody-dependent eosinophil-mediated damage to 51Cr-labeled schistosomula of *Schistosoma mansoni*: damage by purified eosinophils. *J. Exp. Med.* **145**, 136–50.

Butterworth, A.E., Wassom, D.L., Gleich, G.J., Loegering, D.A. and David, J.R. (1979a). Damage to schistosomula of *Schistosoma mansoni* induced directly by eosinophil major basic protein. *J. Immunol.* **122**, 221–9.

Butterworth, A.E., Vadas, M.A., Martz, E. and Sher, A. (1979b). Cytolytic T lymphocytes recognize alloantigens on schistosomula of *Schistosoma mansoni*, but fail to induce damage. *J. Immunol.* **122**, 1314–21.

Butterworth, A.E., Capron, M., Cordingley, J.S. *et al.* (1985). Immunity after treatment of human schistosomiasis mansoni. II. Identification of resistant individuals, and analysis of their immune responses. *Trans. Roy. Soc. Trop. Med. Hyg.* **79**, 393–408.

Butterworth, A.E., Bensted-Smith, R., Capron, A. *et al.* (1987). Immunity in human schistosomiasis mansoni: prevention by blocking antibodies of the expression of immunity in young children. *Parasitology* **94**, 281–300.

Butterworth, A.E., Fulford, A.J.C., Dunne, D.W., Ouma, J.H. and Sturrock, R.F. (1988). Longitudinal studies on human schistosomiasis. *Phil. Trans. Roy. Soc. (London) B* **321**, 495–511.

Canlas, M., Wadee, A., Lamontagne, L. and Piessens, W.F. (1984). A monoclonal antibody to surface antigens on microfilariae of *Brugia malayi* reduces microfilaraemia in infected jirds. *Am. J. Trop. Med. Hyg.* **33**, 420–4.

Capron, A. and Capron, M. (1986). Rats, mice and men — models for immune effector mechanisms against schistosomiasis. *Parasitol. Today* **2**, 69–75.

Capron, A., Dessaint, J.P., Capron, M. and Bazin, H. (1975). Specific IgE antibodies in immune adherence of normal macrophages to *Schistosoma mansoni* schistosomules. *Nature (London)* **253**, 474–5.

Capron, A., Dessaint, J.P., Joseph, M., Capron, M. and Bazin, H. (1977). Interaction between IgE complexes and macrophages in the rat: a new mechanism of macrophage activation. *Eur. J. Immunol.* **7**, 315–22.

Capron, A., Dessaint, J.P., Capron, M., Ouma, J.H. and Butterworth, A.E. (1987a). Immunity to schistosomes: progress towards vaccine. *Science* **238**, 1065–72.

Capron, A., Joseph, M., Ameisen, J.C., Capron, M., Pancre, V. and Auriault, C. (1987b). Platelets as effectors in immune and hypersensitivity reactions. *Int. Arch. Allergy Appl. Immunol.* **82**, 307–12.

Capron, M., Capron, A., Torpier, G., Bazin, H., Bout, D. and Joseph, M. (1978a). Eosinophil-dependent cytotoxicity in rat schistosomiasis: involvement of IgG2a antibody and role of mast cells. *Eur. J. Immunol.* **8**, 127–33.

Capron, M., Rousseaux, J., Mazingue, C., Bazin, H., Bout, D. and Joseph, M. (1978b). Rat mast cell–eosinophil interaction in antibody-dependent eosinophil cytotoxicity to *Schistosoma mansoni* schistosomula. *J. Immunol.* **121**, 2518–25.

Capron, M., Bazin, H., Joseph, M. and Capron, A. (1981a). Evidence for IgE-dependent cytotoxicity by rat eosinophils. *J. Immunol.* **126**, 1764–8.

Capron, M., Capron, A., Dessaint, J.P., Torpier, G., Johansson, S.G.O. and Prin, L. (1981b). Fc receptors for IgE on human and rat eosinophils. *J. Immunol.* **126**, 2087–92.

Capron, M., Spiegelberg, H.L., Prin, L. *et al.* (1984). Role of IgE receptors in effector function of human eosinophils. *J. Immunol.* **132**, 462–8.

Capron, M., Jouault, T., Prin, L. *et al.* (1986). Functional study of a monoclonal antibody to IgE Fc receptor (FceR2) of eosinophils, platelets and macrophages *J. Exp. Med.* **164**, 72–89.

Chapman, C.B. and Mitchell, G.F. (1982). Proteolytic cleavage of immunoglobulins by enzymes released from *Fasciola hepatica*. *Vet. Parasitol.* **11**, 165–78.

Clegg, J.A. and Smithers, S.R. (1972). The effects of immune rhesus monkey serum on schistosomula of *Schistosoma mansoni* during cultivation *in vitro*. *Int. J. Parasitol.* **2**, 79–98.

Colley, D.G., Hieny, S.E., Bartholomew, R.K. and Cook, J.A. (1977). Immune responses during human schistosomiasis mansoni. III. Regulatory effect of patients' sera on human lymphocyte blastogenic responses to schistosomal antigen preparations. *Am. J. Trop. Med. Hyg.* **26**, 917–25.

Colley, D.G., Lewis, F.A. and Goodgame, R.W. (1978). Immune responses during human schistosomiasis mansoni. IV. Induction of suppressor cell activity by schistosome antigen preparations and concanavalin A. *J. Immunol.* **120**, 1225–32.

Colley, D.G., Barsoum, I.S., Dahawi, H.S., Gamil, F., Habib, M. and el Alamy, M.A. (1986a). Immune responses and immunoregulation in relation to human schistosomiasis in Egypt. III. Immunity and longitudinal studies of *in vitro* responsiveness after treatment. *Trans. Roy. Soc. Trop. Med. Hyg.* **80**, 952–7.

Colley, D.G., Garcia, A.A., Lambertucci, J.R. *et al.* (1986b). Immune responses during human schistosomiasis. XII. Differential responsiveness in patients with hepatosplenic disease. *Am. J. Trop. Med. Hyg.* **35**, 793–802.

Colley, D.G., Parra, J.C., Montesano, M.A. *et al.* (1987). Immunoregulation in human schistosomiasis by idiotypic interactions and lymphokine-mediated mechanisms. *Mem. Inst. Oswaldo Cruz*, **82** (Suppl. 4), 105–9.

Cottrell, B., Pye, C. and Butterworth, A.E. (1989). Cytotoxic effects *in vitro* of human monocytes and macrophages on schistosomula of *Schistosoma mansoni*. *Parasite Immunol.* **11**, 91–104.

Dalton, J.P. and Strand, M. (1987). *Schistosoma mansoni* polypeptides immunogenic in mice vaccinated with radiation-attenuated cercariae. *J. Immunol.* **139**, 2474–81.

Dalton, J.P., Tom, T.D. and Strand, M. (1987). Cloning of a cDNA encoding a surface antigen of *Schistosoma mansoni* schistosomula recognized by sera of vaccinated mice. *Proc. Nat. Acad. Sci. (USA)* **84**, 4268–72.

Dalton, P.R. and Pole, D. (1978). Water-contact patterns in relation to *Schistosoma haematobium* infection. *Bull. World Health Org.* **56**, 417–26.

David, J.R., Vadas, M.A., Butterworth, A.E. *et al.* (1980). Enhanced helminthotoxic capacity of eosinophils from patients with eosinophils. *N. Engl. J. Med.* **303**, 1147–52.

Dean, D.A. (1983). A review. *Schistosoma* and related genera: acquired resistance in mice. *Exp. Parasitol.* **55**, 1–104.

Dean, D.A., Wistar, R. and Murrell, K.D. (1974). Combined

in vitro effects of rat antibody and neutrophilic leukocytes on schistosomula of *Schistosoma mansoni*. *Am. J. Trop. Med. Hyg.* **23**, 420–8.

Dean, D.A., Wistar, R. and Chen, P. (1975). Immune responses of guinea pigs to *Schistosoma mansoni*. I. *In vitro* effects of antibody and neutrophils, eosinophils and macrophages on schistosomula. *Am. J. Trop. Med. Hyg.* **24**, 74–82.

Dessaint, J.P., Torpier, G., Capron, M., Bazin, H. and Capron, A. (1979). Cytophilic binding of IgE to the macrophage. I. Binding characteristics of IgE on the surface of macrophages in the rat. *Cell. Immunol.* **46**, 12–23.

Dessein, A.J., Lenzi, H.L., Vadas, M.A. and David, J.R. (1983). A new class of eosinophil activators that enhance eosinophil helminthotoxicity. In *Immunobiology of the Eosinophil*, ed. T. Yoshida and M. Torisu, pp. 369–82, Elsevier Biomedical, New York.

Dessein, A.J., Begley, M., Demeure, C. *et al.* (1988). Human resistance to *Schistosoma mansoni* is associated with IgG reactivity to a 37-kDa larval surface antigen. *J. Immunol.* **140**, 2727–36.

Duffus, W.P.H. and Franks, D. (1980). *In vitro* effect of immune serum and bovine granulocytes on juvenile *Fasciola hepatica*. *Clin. Exp. Immunol.* **41**, 430–40.

Dunne, D.W., Lucas, S., Bickle, Q. *et al.* (1981). Identification and partial purification of an antigen (w1) from *Schistosoma mansoni* eggs which is putatively hepatotoxic in T-cell deprived mice. *Trans. Roy. Soc. Trop. Med. Hyg.* **75**, 54–71.

Dunne, D.W., Grabowska, A.M., Fulford, A.J.C. *et al.* (1988). Human antibody responses to *Schistosoma mansoni*: the influence of epitopes shared between different life cycle stages on the response to the schistosomulum. *Eur. J. Immunol.* **18**, 123–31.

Elkins, D.B., Haswell-Elkins, M. and Anderson, R.M. (1988). The importance of host age and sex to patterns of reinfection with *Ascaris lumbricoides* following mass anthelminthic treatment in a South Indian fishing community. *Parasitology* **96**, 171–84.

Ellner, J.J., Olds, G.R., Lee, C.W., Kleinhenz, M.E. and Edwards, K.L. (1982). Destruction of the multicellular parasite *Schistosoma mansoni* by T lymphocytes. *J. Clin. Invest.* **70**, 369–78.

El-Sadr, W.M., Aikawa, M. and Greene, B.M. (1983). *In vitro* immune mechanisms associated with clearance of microfilariae of *Dirofilaria immitis*. *J. Immunol.* **130**, 428–34.

Ford, M.J., Dissous, C., Pierce, R.J., Taylor, M.J., Bickle, Q.D. and Capron, A. (1987). The isotypes of antibody responsible for the 'late' passive transfer of immunity in rats vaccinated with highly irradiated cercariae. *Parasitology* **94**, 509–22.

Gazzinelli, G., Lambertucci, J.R., Katz, N., Rocha, R.S., Lima, M.S. and Colley, D.G. (1985). Immune responses during human schistosomiasis mansoni. XI. Immunologic status of patients with acute infections and after treatment. *J. Immunol.* **135**, 2121–7.

Gazzinelli, R.T., Parra, J.F.C., Correa-Oliveira, R. *et al.* (1988). Idiotypic/anti-idiotypic interactions in schistosomiasis and Chagas' disease. *Am. J. Trop. Med. Hyg.* **39**, 288–94.

Gleich, G.J., Loegering, D.A., Kueppers, F., Bajaj, S.P. and Mann, K.G. (1974). Comparative properties of the Charcot–Leyden crystal protein and the major basic protein from human eosinophils. *J. Clin. Invest.* **57**, 633–40.

Goldring, O.L., Sher, A., Smithers, S.R. and McLaren, D.J. (1977). Host antigens and parasite antigens of murine *Schistosoma mansoni*. *Trans. Roy. Soc. Trop. Med. Hyg.* **71**, 144–8.

Greene, B.M., Taylor, H.R. and Aikawa, M. (1981). Cellular killing of microfilariae of *Onchocerca volvulus*: eosinophil and neutrophil mediated immune serum dependent destruction. *J. Immunol.* **127**, 1611–18.

Grzych, J.M., Capron, M., Bazin, H. and Capron, A. (1982). *In vitro* and *in vivo* effector function of rat IgG2a monoclonal anti-*Schistosoma mansoni* antibodies. *J. Immunol.* **129**, 2739–43.

Grzych, J.M., Capron, M., Dissous, C. and Capron, A. (1984). Blocking activity of rat monoclonal antibodies in experimental schistosomiasis. *J. Immunol.* **133**, 998–1004.

Grzych, J.M., Capron, M., Lambert, P.H., Dissous, C., Torres, S. and Capron, A. (1985). An anti-idiotype vaccine against experimental schistosomiasis. *Nature (London)* **316**, 74–6.

Hagan, P., Wilkins, H.A., Blumenthal, U.J., Hayes, R.J. and Greenwood, B.M. (1985). Eosinophilia and resistance to *Schistosoma haematobium* in man. *Parasite Immunol.* **7**, 625–32.

Hagan, P., Blumenthal, U.J., Chaudri, M. *et al.* (1987). Resistance to reinfection with *Schistosoma haematobium* in Gambian children: analysis of their immune responses. *Trans. Roy. Soc. Trop. Med. Hyg.* **81**, 938–46.

Hagan, P., Blumenthal, U.J., Dunn, D. and Wilkins, H.A. (1991). Human IgE, IgG4 and resistance to reinfection with *Schistosoma haematobium*. *Nature* **349**, 243–5.

Hammerberg, B. and Williams, J.F. (1978). Interaction between *Taenia taeniaeformis* and the complement system. *J. Immunol.* **120**, 1033–8.

Haque, A., Joseph, M., Ouaissi, M.A., Capron, M. and Capron, A. (1980). IgE antibody-mediated cytotoxicity of rat macrophages against microfilariae of *Dipetalonema viteae in vitro*. *Clin. Exp. Immunol.* **40**, 487–95.

Harn, D.A., Mitsuyama, M. and David, J.R. (1984). *Schistosoma mansoni*: anti-egg monoclonal antibodies protect against cercarial challenge *in vivo*. *J. Exp. Med.* **159**, 1371–87.

Harn, D.A., Mitsuyama, M., Huguenel, E.D., Oligino, L. and David, J.R. (1985). Identification by monoclonal antibody of a major (28 kDa) surface membrane antigen of *Schistosoma mansoni*. *Mol. Biochem. Parasitol.* **16**, 345–54.

Harrison, L.J.S. and Parkhouse, R.M.E. (1986). Passive protection against *Taenia saginata* infection in cattle by a mouse monoclonal antibody reactive with the surface of the invasive oncosphere. *Parasite Immunology* **8**, 319–32.

Harrison, L.J.S., Joshua, G.W.P. and Parkhouse, R.M.E. (1986). Identification of protective antigens in *Taenia saginata* cysticercosis. In *Proceedings of the Sixth International Congress for Parasitology*, p. 146.

Haswell-Elkins, M., Elkins, D.B., Manjula, K., Michael, E. and Anderson, R.M. (1988). An investigation of hookworm infection and reinfection following mass anthelminthic treatment in the South Indian fishing community of Vairankuppam. *Parasitology* **96**, 565–77.

Havercroft, J.C., Huggins, M.C., Nene, V. *et al.* (1988). Cloning of the gene encoding a 50 kilodalton potential surface antigen of *Schistosoma mansoni*. *Mol. Biochem. Parasitol.* **30**, 83–8.

Heidrich, H.G. (1988). Parasites and vaccination. In *Parasitology in Focus: Facts and Trends*, ed. H. Mehlhorn, pp. 719–38,

Springer-Verlag, Berlin.

James, S.L. (1986a). Induction of protective immunity against *Schistosoma mansoni* by a nonliving vaccine. III. Correlation of resistance with induction of activated larvacidal macrophages. *J. Immunol.* **136**, 3872–7.

James, S.L. (1986b). Activated macrophages as effector cells of protective immunity to schistosomiasis. *Immunol. Res.* **5**, 139–48.

James, S.L. (1987). Induction of protective immunity against *Schistosoma mansoni* by a non-living vaccine. V. Effects of varying the immunization schedule and site. *Parasite Immunol.* **9**, 531–41.

James, S.L., Sher, A., Lazdins, J.K. and Meltzer, M.S. (1982). Macrophages as effector cells of protective immunity in murine schistosomiasis. II. Killing of newly transformed schistosomula *in vitro* by macrophages activated as a consequence of *Schistosoma mansoni* infection. *J. Immunol.* **128**, 1535–40.

James, S.L., Lazdins, J.K., Heiny, S. and Natovitz, P. (1983). Macrophages as effector cells of protective immunity in murine schistosomiasis. V. T cell-dependent, lymphokine-mediated activation of macrophages in response to *Schistosoma mansoni* antigens. *J. Immunol.* **131**, 1481–6.

Johnson, K.J., Harrison, G.B.L., Lightowlers, M.W. *et al.* (1989). Vaccination against ovine cysticercosis using a defined recombinant antigen. *Nature*, **338**, 585–7.

Joseph, M., Capron, A., Butterworth, A.E., Sturrock, R.F. and Houba, V. (1978). Cytotoxicity of human and baboon mononuclear phagocytes against schistosomula *in vitro*: induction by immune complexes containing IgE and *Schistosoma mansoni* antigens. *Clin. Exp. Immunol.* **33**, 48–56.

Joseph, M., Ameisen, J.C., Kusnierz, J.P., Pancre, V., Capron, M. and Capron, A. (1984). Participation du récepteur pour l'IgE à la toxicité des plaquettes sanguinés contre les schistosomes. *C. R. Acad. Sci. Ser. III Sci. Vie* **298**, 55–62.

Jouault, T., Capron, M., Balloul, J.M., Ameisen, J.C. and Capron, A. (1988). Quantitative and qualitative analysis of the Fc receptor for IgE Fc epsilon RII on human eosinophils. *Eur. J. Immunol.* **18**, 237–41.

Kazura, J.W. (1981). Host defense mechanisms against nematode parasites: destruction of newborn *Trichinella spiralis* larvae by human antibodies and granulocytes. *J. Infect. Dis.* **143**, 712–18.

Kazura, J.W., Fanning, M.M., Blumer, J.L. and Mahmoud, A.A.F. (1981). Role of cell-generated hydrogen peroxide in granulocyte-mediated killing of schistosomula of *Schistosoma mansoni in vitro* . *J. Clin. Invest.* **67**, 93–102.

Kazura, J.W., Cicirello, H. and McCall, J.W. (1986). Induction of protection against *Brugia malayi* infection in jirds by microfilarial antigens. *J. Immunol.* **136**, 1422–6.

King, C.H., Lett, R.R., Nanduri, J. *et al.* (1987). Isolation and characterization of a protective antigen for adjuvant-free immunization against *Schistosoma mansoni*. *J. Immunol.* **139**, 4218–24.

Lanar, D., Pearce, E.J., James, S.L. and Sher, A. (1986). Identification of paramyosin as the schistosome antigen recognised by intradermally vaccinated mice. *Science* **234**, 593–6.

Leid, R.W., Suquet, C.M., Bouwer, H.G. and Henrich, D.J. (1986). Interleukin inhibition by a parasite proteinase inhibitor, taeniaestatin. *J. Immunol.* **137**, 2700–2.

Letonja, T. and Hammerberg, B. (1983). Third component of complement, immunoglobulin deposition, and leucocyte attachment related to surface sulphate on larval *Taenia taeniaeformis*. *J. Parasitol.* **69**, 637–44.

Lightowlers, M.W. and Rickard, M.D. (1988). Excretory–secretory products of helminth parasites: effects on host immune responses. *Parasitology* **96**, S123–S166.

Lima, M.S., Gazzinelli, G., Nascimento, E., Carvalho Parra, J., Montesano, M.A. and Colley, D.G. (1986). Immune responses during human schistosomiasis mansoni: evidence for anti-idiotypic T cell responsiveness. *J. Clin. Invest.* **78**, 983–8.

Lloyd, S. and Soulsby, E.J.L. (1988). Immunological responses of the host. In *Parasitology in Focus: Facts and Trends*, ed. H. Mehlhorn, pp. 619–50, Springer-Verlag, Berlin.

McHugh, S.M., Coulson, P.S. and Wilson, R.A. (1987). The relationship between pathology and resistance to reinfection with *Schistosoma mansoni* in mice: a causal mechanism of resistance in chronic infections. *Parasitology* **94**, 69–80.

Mackenzie, C.D., Williams, J.F., Sisley, B.M., Steward, M.W. and O'Day, J. (1985). Variations in host responses and the pathogenesis of onchocerciasis. *Rev. Infect. Dis.* **7**, 802–8.

McLaren, D.J. and Ramalho-Pinto, F.J. (1979). Eosinophil-mediated killing of schistosomula of *Schistosoma mansoni in vitro*: synergistic effect of antibody and complement. *J. Immunol.* **123**, 1431–8.

McLaren, D.J., McKean, J.R., Olsson, I., Venge, P. and Kay, A.B. (1981). Morphological studies on the killing of schistosomula of *Schistosoma mansoni* by human eosinophil and neutrophil cationic proteins *in vitro*. *Parasite Immunol.* **3**, 359–73.

Mahmoud, A.A.F., Peters, P.A., Civil, R.H. and Remington, J.S. (1979). *In vitro* killing of schistosomula of *Schistosoma mansoni* by BCG and *Corynebacterium parvum*-activated macrophages. *J. Immunol.* **122**, 1655–7.

Mangold, B.L. and Dean, D.A. (1986). Passive transfer with serum and IgG antibodies of irradiated cercaria-induced resistance against *Schistosoma mansoni* in mice. *J. Immunol.* **136**, 2644–8.

Mazingue, C., Camus, D., Dessaint, J.P., Capron, M. and Capron, A. (1980). *In vitro* and *in vivo* inhibition of mast cell degranulation by a factor from *Schistosoma mansoni*. *Int. Arch. Allergy Appl. Immunol.* **63**, 178–89.

Mehta, K., Sindhu, R.K., Subramanyam, D. and Nelson, D.S. (1980). IgE-dependent adherence and cytotoxicity of rat spleen and peritoneal cells to *Litomosoides carinii* microfilariae. *Clin. Exp. Immunol.* **41**, 107–14.

Mehta, K., Sindhu, R.K., Subramanyam, D., Hopper, K., Nelson, D.S. and Rao, C.K. (1981). Antibody-dependent cell-mediated effects in bancroftian filariasis. *Immunology* **43**, 117–23.

Mehta, K., Sindhu, R.K., Subramanyam, D., Hopper, K. and Nelson, D.S. (1982). IgE-dependent cellular adhesion and cytotoxicity to *Litomosoides carinii* microfilariae — nature of effector cells. *Clin. Exp. Immunol.* **48**, 477–84.

Melewicz, F.M. and Spiegelberg, H.L. (1980). Fc receptors for IgE on a subpopulation of human peripheral blood monocytes. *J. Immunol.* **125**, 1026–31.

Miller, H.R.P. (1987). Gastrointestinal mucus, a medium for survival and for elimination of parasitic nematodes and protozoa. *Parasitology* **94**, S77–S100.

Miller, T.A. (1971). Vaccination against the canine hookworm diseases. *Adv. Parasitol.* **9**, 153–83.

Mitchell, G.F., Beall, J.A., Cruise, K.M., Tui, W.V. and Garcia, E.G. (1985). Antibody responses to the antigen Sj26 of *Schistosoma japonicum* worms that is recognized by genetically resistant 129/J mice. *Parasite Immunol.* **7**, 165–78.

Moser, G. and Sher, A. (1981). Studies of the antibody-dependent killing of schistosomula of *Schistosoma mansoni* employing haptenated target antigens. II. *In vitro* killing of TNP-schistosomula by human eosinophils and neutrophils. *J. Immunol.* **126**, 1025–9.

Nilsen, T.W., Maroney, P.A., Goodwin, R.G. *et al.* (1988). Cloning and characterization of a potentially protective antigen in lymphatic filariases. *Proc. Nat. Acad. Sci. (USA)* **85**, 3604–7.

Ogilvie, B.M. and Wilson, R.J.M. (1977). Evasion of the immune response by parasites. *Br. Med. Bull.* **32**, 177–81.

Olds, G.R., Ellner, J.J., Kearse, L.A., Kazura, J.W. and Mahmoud, A.A.F. (1980). Role of arginase in killing of schistosomula of *Schistosoma mansoni*. *J. Exp. Med.* **151**, 1557–62.

Olds, G.R., Ellner, J.J., el-Kholy, A. and Mahmoud, A.A.F. (1981). Monocyte-mediated killing of schistosomula of *Schistosoma mansoni*: alterations in human schistosomiasis mansoni and tuberculosis. *J. Immunol.* **127**, 1538–42.

Oligino, L.D., Percy, A.J. and Harn, D.A. (1988). Purification and immunochemical characterization of a 22 kilodalton surface antigen from *Schistosoma mansoni*. *Mol. Biochem. Parasitol.* **28**, 95–104.

Olsson, I., Venge, P., Spitznagel, J.K. and Lehrer, R.I. (1977). Arginine-rich cationic proteins of human eosinophil granules: comparison of the constituents of eosinophilic and neutrophilic leukocytes. *Lab. Invest.* **36**, 493–500.

Ottesen, E.A. (1987). Description, mechanisms and control of reactions to treatment in the human filariases. In *Filariasis* (CIBA Foundation Symposium 127), ed. D. Evered and S. Clark, pp. 265–83, Wiley, Chichester.

Ottesen, E.A., Neva, F.A., Paranjape, R.S., Tripathy, S.P., Thriuvengadam, K.V. and Beaven, M.A. (1979). Specific allergic sensitization to filarial antigens in the tropical eosinophilia syndrome. *Lancet* **i**, 1158–62.

Parkhouse, R.M.E. (1984). Editor: Parasite evasion of the immune response (Symposia of the British Society for Parasitology, 21), *Parasitology* **88**, 571–682.

Parkhouse, R.M.E., Philipp, M. and Ogilvie, B.M. (1981). Characterisation of surface antigens of *Trichinella spiralis*. *Parasite Immunol.* **3**, 339–52.

Parra, J.C., Lima, M.S., Gazzinelli, G. and Colley, D.G. (1988). Immune responses during human schistosomiasis mansoni. XV. Anti-idiotypic T cells can recognize and respond to anti-SEA idiotypes directly. *J. Immunol.* **140**, 2401–5.

Partono, F. (1987). The spectrum of disease in filariasis. In *Filariasis* (CIBA Foundation Symposium 127), ed. D. Evered and S. Clark, pp. 15–31, Wiley, Chichester.

Pearce, E.J., Basch, P.F. and Sher, A. (1986a). Evidence that the reduced antigenicity of developing *Schistosoma mansoni* schistosomula is due to antigen shedding rather than host molecule acquisition. *Parasite Immunol.* **3**, 339–52.

Pearce, E.J., James, S.L., Dalton, J.P. *et al.* (1986b). Immunochemical characterization and purification of Sm97, a *Schistosoma mansoni* antigen monospecifically recognized by antibodies from mice protectively immunized with a non-living vaccine. *J. Immunol.* **137**, 3593–600.

Pearce, E.J., James, S.L., Hieny, S., Lanar, D.E. and Sher, A. (1988). Induction of protective immunity against *Schistosoma mansoni* by vaccination with schistosome paramyosin (Sm97), a nonsurface parasite antigen. *Proc. Nat. Acad. Sci. (USA)* **85**, 5678–82.

Peck, C.A., Carpenter, M.D. and Mahmoud, A.A.F. (1983). Species-related innate resistance to *Schistosoma mansoni*: role of mononuclear phagocytes in schistosomula killing *in vitro*. *J. Clin. Invest.* **71**, 66–72.

Percy, A. and Harn, D.A. (1988). Monoclonal anti-idiotypic and anti-anti-idiotypic antibodies from mice immunized with a protective monoclonal antibody against *Schistosoma mansoni*. *J. Immunol.* **140**, 2760–2.

Pestel, J., Joseph, M., Dessaint, J.P. and Capron, A. (1988). Variation in the expression of macrophage Fc epsilon receptors in relation to experimental rat schistosome infection. *Int. Arch. Allergy Appl. Immunol.* **85**, 55–62.

Piessens, W.F., Wadee, A.A. and Kurniawan, L. (1987). Regulation of immune responses in lymphatic filariasis. In *Filariasis* (CIBA Foundation Symposium 127), ed. D. Evered and S. Clark, pp. 164–87, Wiley, Chichester.

Remold, H.G., Mednis, A., Hein, A. and Caulfield, J.P. (1988). Human monocyte-derived macrophages are lysed by schistosomula of *Schistosoma mansoni* and fail to kill the parasite after activation with interferon gamma. *Am. J. Pathol.* **131**, 146–55.

Rhoads, M.L. (1983). *Trichinella spiralis*: identification and purification of superoxide dismutase. *Exp. Parasitol.* **56**, 41–54.

Rickard, M.D. and Bell, K.J. (1971). Successful vaccination of lambs against infection with *Taenia ovis* using antigens produced during *in vitro* cultivation of the larval stages. *Res. Vet. Sci.* **12**, 401–2.

Rickard, M.D. and Williams, J.F. (1982). Hydatidosis/cysticercosis: immune mechanisms and immunization against infection. *Adv. Parasitol.* **21**, 229–96.

Selkirk, M.E., Denham, D.A., Partono, F., Sutanto, I. and Maizels, R.M. (1986). Molecular characterization of antigens of lymphatic filarial parasites. *Parasitology* **91**, S15–S38.

Smith, D.B. and Johnson, K.S. (1988). Single-step purification of polypeptides expressed in *Escherichia coli* as fusions with glutathione S-transferase. *Gene* **67**, 31–40.

Smith, D.B., Davern, K.M., Board, P.G., Tiu, W.V., Garcia, E.G. and Mitchell, G.F. (1987). The Mr 26 000 antigen of *Schistosoma japonicum* recognized by resistant WEHI 129/J mice is a parasite glutathione-S-transferase. *Proc. Nat. Acad. Sci. (USA)* **83**, 8703–7.

Smith, D.B., Rubira, M.R., Simpson, R.J. *et al.* (1988). Expression of an enzymatically-active parasite molecule in *Escherichia coli*: *Schistosoma japonicum* glutathione S-transferase. *Mol. Biochem. Parasitol.* **27**, 249–56.

Smithers, S.R., Terry, R.J. and Hockley, D.J. (1969). Host antigens in schistosomiasis. *Proc. Roy. Soc. (London) B.* **171**, 483–94.

Steward, M.W. (1987). Immunopathological mechanisms in the induction of parasitic diseases with particular reference to type III hypersensitivity reactions. *Parasitology* **94**, S139–S158.

Sturrock, R.F., Kimani, R., Cottrell, B. *et al.* (1983). Observations on possible immunity to reinfection among Kenyan schoolchildren after treatment for *Schistosoma mansoni*. *Trans. Roy. Soc. Trop. Med. Hyg.* **77**, 363–71.

Thorne, K.J.I., Richardson, B.A., Taverne, J., Williamson, D.J., Vadas, M.A. and Butterworth, A.E. (1986). A comparison of eosinophil activating factor (EAF) with other monokines and lymphokines. *Eur. J. Immunol.* **16**, 1143–9.

Tiu, W.U., Davern, K.M., Wright, M.D., Board, P.G. and Mitchell, G.F. (1988). Molecular and serological characteristics of the glutathione S-transferases of *Schistosoma japonicum* and *Schistosoma mansoni*. *Parasite Immunol.* **10**, 693–706.

Vadas, M.A., Butterworth, A.E., Burakoff, S. and Sher, A. (1979a). Major histocompatibility complex products restrict the adherence of cytolytic T lymphocytes to minor histocompatibility antigens or to trinitrophenyl determinants on schistosomula of *Schistosoma mansoni*. *Proc. Nat. Acad. Sci. (USA)* **76**, 1982–5.

Vadas, M.A., David, J.R., Butterworth, A.E., Pisani, N.T. and Siongok, T.A. (1979b). A new method for the purification of human eosinophils and neutrophils, and a comparison of the ability of these cells to damage schistosomula of *Schistosoma mansoni*. *J. Immunol.* **122**, 1228–36.

Veith, M.C. and Butterworth, A.E. (1983). Enhancement of human eosinophil-mediated killing of *Schistosoma mansoni* larvae by mononuclear cell products *in vitro*. *J. Exp. Med.* **157**, 1828–43.

Verwaerde, C., Joseph, M., Capron, M. *et al.* (1987). Functional properties of a rat monoclonal IgE antibody specific for *Schistosoma mansoni*. *J. Immunol.* **138**, 4441–6.

Vieira, L.Q., Gazzinelli, G., Kusel, J.R., de Souza, C.P.S. and Colley, D.G. (1986). Inhibition of human peripheral blood mononuclear cell proliferative responses by released materials from *Schistosoma mansoni*. *Parasite Immunol.* **8**, 333–43.

Wakelin, D. (1988). Genetic control of immunity to helminth infections. In *Parasitology in Focus: Facts and Trends*, ed. H. Mehlhorn, pp. 651–70, Springer-Verlag, Berlin.

Ward, R.E. and McLaren, D.J. (1988). *Schistosoma mansoni*: evidence that eosinophils and/or macrophages contribute to skin-phase challenge attrition in vaccinated CBA/Ca mice. *Parasitology* **96**, 63–84.

Warren, K.S. (1973). Regulation of the prevalence and intensity of schistosomiasis in man: immunology or ecology? *J. Infect. Dis.* **127**, 595–699.

Warren, K.S. (1982). The secret of the immunopathogenesis of schistosomiasis: *in vivo* models. *Immunol. Rev.* **61**, 189–213.

Wilkins, H.A., Blumenthal, U.J., Hagan, P., Hayes, R.J. and Tulloch, S. (1987). Resistance to reinfection after treatment of urinary schistosomiasis. *Trans. Roy. Soc. Trop. Med. Hyg.* **81**, 29–35.

Wyler, D.J., Ehrlich, H.P., Postlethwaite, A.E., Raghow, R. and Murphy, M.M. (1987). Fibroblast stimulation in schistosomiasis. VII. Egg granulomas secrete factors that stimulate collagen and fibronectin synthesis. *J. Immunol.* **138**, 1581–6.

Young, J.D., Peterson, C.G., Venge, P. and Cohn, Z.A. (1986). Mechanisms of membrane damage mediated by human eosinophil cationic protein. *Nature (London)* **321**, 613–16.

Zodda, D.M. and Phillips, S.M. (1982). Monoclonal antibody-mediated protection against *Schistosoma mansoni* infection in mice. *J. Immunol.* **129**, 2326–8.

84: Immunity to Fungi

P.F. Lehmann

The fungi that cause disease form a diverse group. Few species are frank pathogens in the healthy immunocompetent host; however, a large number of different species have been found as the aetiological agents of disease in severely immunocompromised patients. Such patients include those who receive cytotoxic and immunosuppressive drugs, those with acquired immune deficiency syndrome (AIDS), severely burnt patients and a number of other patient groups who will be described in the appropriate sections.

Although these agents are under-studied, there has been an increased interest in the nature of fungal antigens and immunity to fungi during the last decade and the interested reader is referred to recent books that cover the topic to a greater extent than is possible herein (Reiss 1986; Cox 1989a). In addition, the immunology of fungal diseases in animals has been reviewed (Lehmann 1985; Smith 1989).

In discussing immunity to fungi and any associated immunopathological responses, the diseases will be grouped (Table 84.1). Such grouping is not always satisfactory as there may be a spectrum of disease types produced by any single organism. For example, *Candida albicans* commonly produces mucosal and cutaneous disease but is also a common cause of invasive fungal disease in the severely neutropenic patient. The mechanisms of resistance differ for the two situations and, for this reason, there is extensive discussion of the organism in two sections of the text. Also, the reader should recognize that the true fungal pathogens are able to cause disease in both immunocompetent and immunocompromised

Table 84.1. Major groups of fungal diseases[a]

Allergies
Fungi cause asthma, allergic rhinitis, allergic alveolitis, hypersensitivity pneumonitis, skin sensitization. The fungi do not grow within the host. Numerous species involved, e.g. *Alternaria* spp., *Aspergillus* spp.
Cutaneous and mucosal infections
1 *Superficial infections*
Fungi growing on hair or the surface of the skin and eliciting almost no inflammatory response; e.g. *Malassezia furfur* (tinea versicolor) and the agents of tinea nigra, black piedra and white piedra
2 *Dermatophyte infections*
Trichophyton spp., *Microsporum* spp. and *Epidermophyton floccosum* grow in keratinized sites (skin, hair, nails). Cause ringworm disease; e.g. tinea capitis, tinea cruris, tinea imbricata, favus and tinea pedis
3 *Mucosal and cutaneous candidiasis*
Candida albicans and other *Candida* spp. causing oral thrush, chronic mucocutaneous candidiasis, vaginitis
Subcutaneous infections
A heterogeneous group of fungi which grow subcutaneously and produce an inflammatory lesion at the site of inoculation. Infection usually results from implantation of fungus after trauma, e.g. skin puncture by a contaminated thorn; e.g. *Sporothrix schenckii* (sporotrichosis); *Fonsecaea pedrosoi* and other spp. (chromoblastomycosis); *Loboa loboi* (Lobo's disease); *Rhinosporidium seeberi* (rhinosporidiosis); numerous species (mycetoma and phaeohyphomycosis)
Systemic infections
1 *Pathogens*
Fungi, which usually infect via the lung, may produce disease in a normal host after exposure to large doses of inoculum. The fungi show a different morphology in tissues from that in culture at room temperature; e.g. *Histoplasma capsulatum* (histoplasmosis); *Blastomyces dermatitidis* (blastomycosis); *Coccidioides immitis* (coccidioidomycosis); *Paracoccidioides brasiliensis* (paracoccidioidomycosis)
2 *Opportunists*
Fungi with low virulence for systemic disease. Infections almost always occur in immunosuppressed or immunodeficient patients. Numerous species involved:
(a) Opportunists associated with T cell deficiencies and AIDS *Cryptococcus neoformans* (cryptococcosis); *Pneumocystis carinii* (pneumocystosis)
(b) Opportunists associated with neutropenia and PMN dysfunction; e.g. *Aspergillus fumigatus* and other *Aspergillus* spp. (invasive aspergillosis); *Candida albicans* and some other *Candida* spp. (invasive candidiasis); *Rhizopus oryzae* (invasive mucormycosis)

a Several fungi form a spectrum of clinical types but in this table they have been grouped together, largely on the basis of their most common clinical features. *Candida albicans* is placed in two major groups.

people; however, the interplay of the organism with the components of the immune system will be very different in each setting and virulence factors required for successful infection of the former may not be required for production of disease in the latter.

Finally, when considering the role of the immune response in most fungal diseases that are seen in immunocompetent hosts, the reader should realize that little is known about the relative importance of variations in strain virulence, inoculum size and host susceptibility in determining the outcome of the infection.

Allergies

Many fungi have an ability to induce allergies. While *Alternaria alternata* seems the most common cause of respiratory system allergy, it should be remembered that relatively few fungi have been studied closely and several species of *Penicillium*, *Aspergillus*, mushrooms and other fungi may also be common causes of asthma, rhinitis or hives. Food allergies are reported also. In these studies, it is notable that the various stages of fungal differentiation can be distinct antigenically, e.g. the dominant antigenic components on spores can differ from those found on vegetative mycelium. Also, many different fungi can share antigenic determinants; this can cause problems in determining the aetiology of a hypersensitivity disease (O'Neil *et al.* 1987). For example, the pathogen *Cryptococcus neoformans* was originally implicated as the cause of an early summer hypersensitivity pneumonitis in Japan; however, later studies have shown *Trichosporon cutaneum*, a common mould that is rarely pathogenic, to be the most likely cause (Yoshida *et al.* 1988). Spores are the major problem in that these structures have often been designed for aerial spread and can be present in vast numbers in certain settings. Unlike foods, they may be difficult to avoid. Because most fungal spores are smaller than pollen grains, single spores are capable of penetrating far into the airways; indeed the smaller spores may reach the alveoli. However, for many fungi, the spores exist in the atmosphere primarily in clusters which sediment in the upper airways so the number reaching the alveoli may be small.

Prolonged exposure to high concentrations of fungal spores can give rise to chronic lung disease;

Table 84.2. Occupational allergies and hypersensitivity diseases associated with fungi or mouldy materials[a]

Mushroom workers' lung[b]
Paprika cutters' lung
Bakers' lung
Malt workers' lung
Chiropodists' (podiatrists') lung[c]
Farmers' lung
Maple bark disease
Woodworkers' lung
Cheese washers' lung
Sauna takers' lung
Lycoperdonosis

a From Al-Doory and Domson (1984) and Fink (1984).
b Commercial mushroom growers try to breed varieties that release only small numbers of spores, but moulds in composts may also be problematical.
c Sensitization to dermatophyte antigens has been noted in persons who generate dusts from treating hardened skin on the feet (Davies *et al.* 1983).

some of these are occupation-related (Table 84.2). Such disease may be complicated further when the fungus is capable of growing within the airways as is found in allergic bronchopulmonary aspergillosis and allergic bronchopulmonary alternariosis. The former is briefly discussed in the section 'Other diseases'. As the thrust of this chapter concerns infectious fungi, the reader is referred to other sources for more thorough discussions of the allergenic fungi and the associated hypersensitivity diseases (Al-Doory and Domson 1984; Fink 1984; Burge 1985; Lopez and Salvaggio 1985, 1987; Bush and Yuninger 1987; Butcher *et al.* 1987).

Cutaneous and mucosal infections

Tinea versicolor

Tinea versicolor, also known as pityriasis versicolor, is caused by the lipid-requiring yeast *Malassezia furfur (Pityrosporum orbiculare).* Disease, which is associated with patches of discoloration on the skin, appears to be associated with overgrowth of *M. furfur*, as the fungus may be found on healthy skin. Little is known of the role of an immune response in resistance to tinea versicolor. Usually, no observable inflammatory process is seen, though this may be found in patients who develop folliculitis (Bäck *et al.* 1985; Yohn *et al.* 1985; Faergemann *et al.* 1986). The finding that some persons develop multiple recurrences of tinea versicolor would be consistent with a defect in an effective immune response, as would the increased incidence of the disease in people receiving corticosteroids (Roberts 1969); however, other factors, such as the composition of the skin, could explain the susceptibility.

Antibody, which is routinely present in all adults, has been studied by several researchers but conflicting results have been found as to whether the titres are significantly different in patients and in healthy controls (DaMert *et al.* 1980; Faergemann 1983; Bergbrant and Faergemann 1989). It has been suggested that *M. furfur* is less antigenic than other fungi (Sohnle and Collins-Lech 1980). Antibodies might play some role in initiating inflammatory responses, which are seen most prominently in folliculitis and seborrhoeic dermatitis, but *M. furfur* is capable of activating complement via the alternative pathway (Belew *et al.* 1980; Sohnle and Collins-Lech 1983) and so could initiate such inflammation in the absence of antibodies.

Any possible role of T lymphocyte-mediated immunity in resistance to tinea versicolor must be clarified further. Sohnle and Collins-Lech (1978, 1982) reported that chronic infection was associated with lower than normal production of LMIF (leucocyte migration inhibition factor) when *Candida albicans* or *M. furfur* was used as antigen. The LMIF deficiency was linked to the presence of a serum blocking factor in some, but not all, of the patients. In addition, patients appeared to have less antigen-reactive cells than did normal persons. The defective production of LMIF was not seen when streptokinase/streptodornase was used as antigen, nor did the researchers find any defects in the lymphocyte transformation response to mitogens or other fungal antigens. However, as the T lymphocytes found in the skin below tinea versicolor lesions are dominated by CD4 +ve cells (Scheynius *et al.* 1984) and as increased colonization by *M. furfur* is not found in AIDS (Håkansson *et al.* 1988), it appears that simple reduction in T lymphocyte activity is unlikely to explain chronic susceptibility to the superficial form of this disease. However, T cell deficiencies may very well be important in predisposing the seborrhoeic dermatitis folliculitis seen in AIDS (Groisser *et al.* 1989).

Malassezia furfur has been reported as a rare

cause of invasive infection in premature infants fed a high lipid diet; but, the importance of an immune response in resolution of these infections remains unknown.

Cutaneous and mucosal candidiasis

Many species of yeasts can cause mucosal and cutaneous infections. The most common species, *Candida albicans*, is a constituent of the normal oral flora of most healthy people, though the apparent carriage rate varies substantially in association with the methods used to detect it. It is clear that the organism is more common, or present in higher numbers, in a number of patient groups, such as the immunosuppressed, the diabetic or the hospitalized (Odds 1988). Almost all research on the nature of immunity to cutaneous and mucosal candidiasis has concentrated on *C. albicans*; however, the reader should be aware that the current state of fungal taxonomy is such that the other Candida species may be very different genetically; the genus contains a highly heterogeneous group of organisms. Furthermore, while *C. albicans* shows some intraspecific variability similar to many fungi, some species, such as *C. parapsilosis*, are clearly composed of a mixture of genetically different organisms (P.F. Lehmann, L.C. Wu and M.G. Rinaldi unpublished). Therefore, it may be unwise to assume that all the findings for *C. albicans* may be directly applicable to the other *Candida* species.

The basic method by which T cell responses lead to control of *Candida* on surfaces is an area of limited understanding. Indeed, control of infection at the skin surface can also involve other cell types. Two major forms of cellular response to cutaneous infections have been seen in rodents (Sohnle *et al.* 1976b). These are illustrated in Fig. 84.1. One form of resistance involves a rapid polymorphonuclear leucocyte (PMN) response to *Candida* when this has been applied under an occlusive dressing which maintains a hot, moist environment favouring fungal growth. The response leads to the formation of a dry crust and sloughing of the skin. It appears that the main reason for the PMN infiltrate is the activation of complement, which can be brought about via activation of both the alternative and the classical pathways; however, fungal chemotactic factors may also play some role (Ray and Wuepper 1976, 1978; Sohnle *et al.* 1976a, b).

The second form of response is seen in infections of dry skin, where an occlusive dressing has not been used (Sohnle *et al.* 1976b; Sohnle and Kirkpatrick 1978). Here there is the production of a mononuclear cell infiltrate in the dermis. This infiltrate develops rapidly in immune animals, and in non-immunized animals it is greatly delayed. It appears to be induced by T cell-mediated responses to the *Candida* antigens. The keratinized epidermis then undergoes profuse scaling in response to stimulated growth of the epidermal cells. The nature of the epidermal cell stimulant is not known but it may be composed of a number of different cytokines including interleukin 3 (IL-3) and granulocyte/monocyte colony-stimulating factor (Hancock *et al.* 1988). Other reactions, such as those involving cutaneous basophil hypersensitivity, may play some role (Sohnle and Kirkpatrick 1977). The report that keratinocytes are capable of killing *C. albicans* must await verification as the cell populations were not completely devoid of other cell types; however, these may provide yet another defence against invasion of the lower layers of the epidermis (Csato *et al.* 1987).

In humans, it is clear that the T cell-mediated immune response is important for the restriction of *C. albicans* on the skin and mucosae. Oral candidiasis is associated with T cell deficiencies, and this is particularly obvious in AIDS, where oral and oesophageal candidiasis are among the first symptoms of the disease. In contrast, high concentrations of antibody are found in adults with mucosal candidiasis and extremely high levels occur in patients with chronic mucocutaneous candidiasis (CMCC), a particularly serious form of the disease which can involve extensive areas of the nails, skin and mucosal surfaces. Therefore, circulating antibodies are not protective at the body surfaces.

The role of secreted antibodies in mucosal defence has been the subject of much argument. High levels of immunoglobulin G (IgG), IgA and IgE in mucosal secretions have been detected but there is no definitive evidence that these play an important role in prevention or induction of disease. The studies have been reviewed (Domer and Carrow 1989). It is likely that the specificity of the antibodies may be important; those that target the ligands involved in attachment may be more effective at preventing disease than those that merely attach to sites on the fungal surface. The possibility that IgE-mediated mast cell degranulation compromises the mucosal surface is further discussed in the section 'Immunotherapy and vaccination'.

The immunodeficiency in CMCC has been the subject of much study. As is also the case in AIDS, systemic candidiasis is rarely encountered. After the first descriptions of the immunodeficiency (Chilgren *et al*. 1967, 1969), it became clear that the T cell response was abnormally poor with respect to *Candida* antigens; both lymphocyte transformation *in vitro* and skin tests showed a diminished response. In contrast, in most patients, there was no observable inhibition of T cell-mediated responses to a panel of unrelated antigens (Kirkpatrick *et al*. 1971; Stiehm 1978). There have been multiple other abnormalities reported in CMCC, including disorders of monocytes (Yamazaki *et al*. 1984), and it should be remembered that many of the patients have coexistent endocrinopathies which may seriously affect the normal function of the immune system. However, failure of T cell function seems not the only factor responsible for preventing the overgrowth of Candida as CMCC patients with normal T-cell mediated immunity are found (Higgs and Wells 1972; Valdimarsson *et al*. 1973; Stiehm 1978). Reference to original papers on many of the abnormalities seen is available in reviews (Edwards *et al*. 1978; Domer and Carrow 1989).

There has been increasing interest in the cause

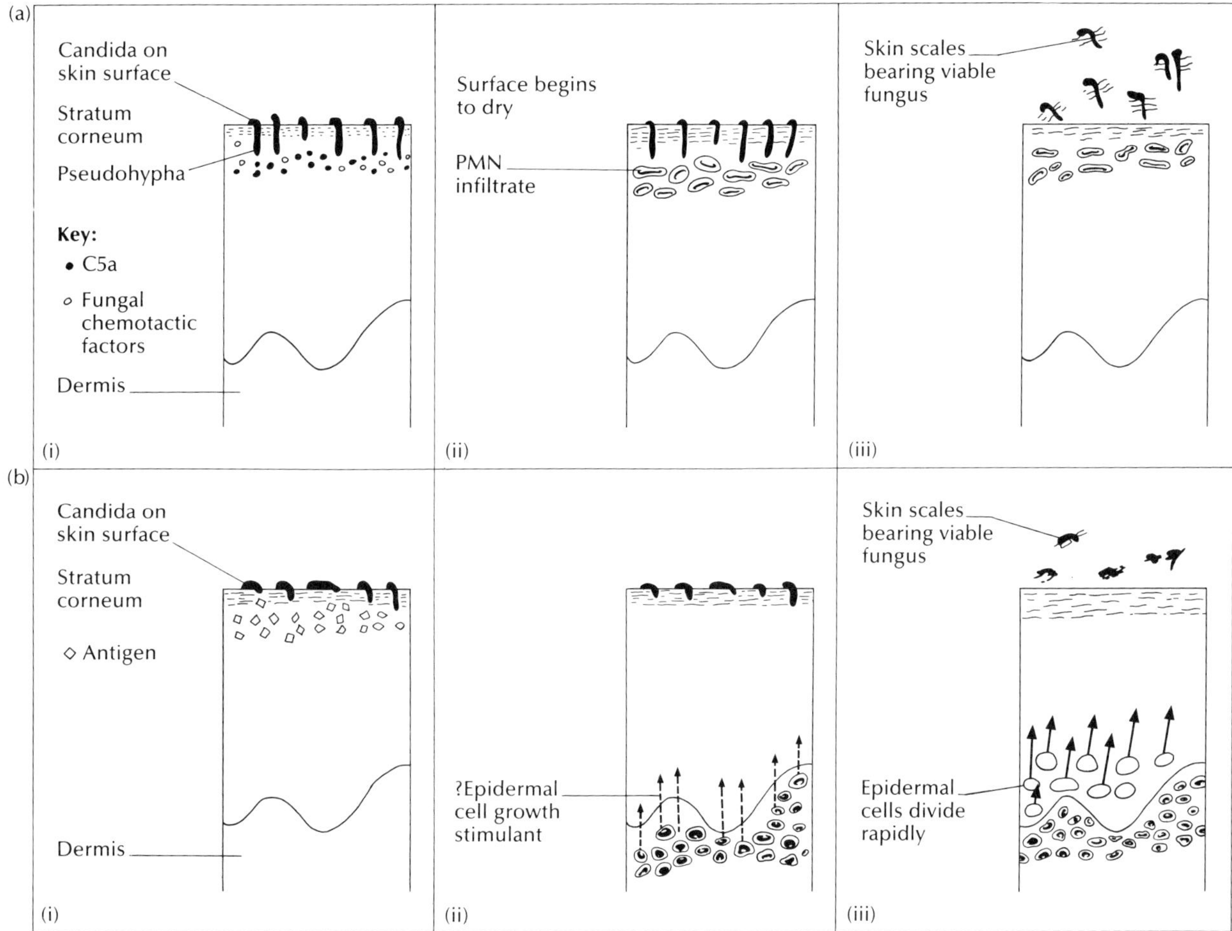

Fig. 84.1. Mechanisms for elimination of *Candida albicans* from the skin surface. (a) Infiltration of PMNs into epidermis in response to chemotactic factors released by the pseudohyphae or by complement fixation involving the alternative pathway. The infected surface dries out and is sloughed off. (i) Penetration and production of chemotactic factors; (ii) infiltration of PMNs; (iii) sloughing of infected surface. (b) Infiltration of mononuclear cells into dermis in response to the presence of antigens. Epidermal cells are stimulated to divide rapidly, resulting in an increased turnover of the epidermis and sloughing of infected scales. (i) Antigen release into epidermis; (ii) antigen processing by antigen-presenting cells and T cells giving rise to a mononuclear cell infiltrate; (iii) sloughing of infected skin.

of the immunodeficiency in CMCC and in the chronic mucosal infections such as vaginitis. Suppressor cells may be present, including monocytes and macrophages with inhibitory properties (Witkin *et al.* 1986). The demonstration of circulating inhibitors, which appeared to be mannan (Fischer *et al.* 1978, 1982), has been of interest. Inhibitor levels can vary in persons undergoing plasmaphaeresis or receiving antifungals (Paterson *et al.* 1971; Twomey *et al.* 1975). Studies with mannan that had been extracted from *C. albicans* with cetyltrimethylammonium bromide, a gentle extraction procedure, showed that such mannan was strongly antigenic, but that small mannose oligosaccharides, which could be released from the larger molecules, were strong inhibitors of the anti-*Candida* lymphocyte transformation response *in vitro* (Podzorski *et al.* 1990). These small oligomers induced a significant inhibition of the response to tetanus toxoid and herpes simplex virus (HSV)-1, apparently unrelated antigens; in contrast, they did not inhibit lymphocyte transformation brought about by the lectin from *Phaseolus limensis*. Such fragments, which would be expected to behave as haptens, could participate in the reduction of T cell-mediated responses that are associated with CMCC.

Dermatophytosis

The immune response to the dermatophytes has been the subject of several reviews (Lepper 1969; Grappel *et al.* 1974; Calderon 1989; Sohnle 1989). These cover much of the early literature and provide more extensive coverage than is possible here. The three genera of dermatophytes, *Trichosporon*, *Epidermophyton* and *Microsporum*, are closely related and share antigenic determinants. This allows trichophytin, the skin test antigen preparation, to be used as a general recall antigen. There are numerous different species of dermatophytes, but all are characterized by being able to utilize keratin present in the hair, skin and nails. Various theories are given for the inability of the organisms to form deep-seated infections except in very unusual patients. These include the killing of the fungi by neutrophils (they show an acute sensitivity to the products of the oxidative burst (Calderon and Hay 1987; Calderon and Shennan 1987)), and the inability of dermatophytes to obtain iron when unsaturated transferrin is present (King *et al.* 1975). In addition, many of the fungi grow poorly at a temperature of 37 °C or higher.

Infection by these fungi gives rise to a variety of responses; inflamed lesions may result in some people while, in others, inflammation is negligible. Increased resistance to infection is observed in persons who have been treated for, or who have recovered naturally from, the most inflammatory infections. These include favus, which is caused by *T. schoenleinii*, and the tinea capitis caused by *M. canis* (Friedman and Derbes 1960). In both these cases, reinfections are resolved rapidly.

Host methods for removing dermatophytes are complex and not well understood. Resistance to infection of the skin is associated with keratinization, with increased epidermal cell division rates allowing a significant reduction in the transit time from basal cell layer to skin surface. This seems to be a major component of defence against several skin-infecting fungi including *Candida* (above) and has been reviewed (Lehmann 1985; Calderon 1989; Sohnle 1989). Associated with this response is the normal finding of T cell-mediated immunity with strong delayed-type hypersensitivity (DTH) reactions characterizing clearance. The tissue reaction may also mimic a contact sensitivity response (Green *et al.* 1980). As discussed below, immediate hypersensitivity is more characteristic of chronic infections (reviewed by Calderon 1989). Circulating antibodies are routine but levels do not reflect disease status; however, cross-reactivity with other fungi and the host (Hopfer *et al.* 1975; Young and Roth 1979) may be responsible for some of the variations found in the inflammatory response.

Most animal models of dermatophyte infection have failed to produce the chronic infections that are the most troublesome form for humans. However, studies with guinea-pigs and rats have shown that clearance of infection is associated with the production of T cell-mediated responses (Kerbs *et al.* 1977; Hunjan and Cronholm 1979; Green *et al.* 1983). Resistance to infection was transferable with immune cells, but not serum, and was dependent on T cells (Green *et al.* 1987). That some form of immunomodulation was present was reported by Green and Balish (1979) but has been most thoroughly explored in a mouse model of dermatophytosis by Hay, Calderon and their colleagues (Hay *et al.* 1983a). Their findings, which are covered briefly below, have been fully reviewed (Calderon 1989).

After inoculation with *T. quinckeanum*, most of the mice were able to clear the infection by 2–3 weeks via crusting and shedding infected skin; however, a few mice developed a chronic infection which was associated with a suppression in cell-mediated immune responses. Transfer of resistance from infected to uninfected mice was T helper-dependent; interestingly, mice having chronic infections were capable of transferring immunity, suggesting that the T helper cell activity was blocked in infections. Blocking factors, which have been observed in human leucocyte cultures, did not appear to be antibody but rather fungal products. Circulating antigen, found using an antibody reactive with phosphorylcholine determinants, has since been detected in chronic dermatophyte infections (Calderon *et al.* 1987).

Suppression by antigen is known in humans. Repeated injections of trichophytin resulted in the replacement of a delayed-type with an immediate-type hypersensitivity response (Jillson and Huppert 1949). Whether this would lead to an increased susceptibility to infections is not clear; but, both in experimental infection studies in humans and in routine studies on patients, immediate-type skin reactions are far more common with chronic infections than in persons who are not carriers of dermatophytes (Wood and Cruickshank 1962; Jones *et al.* 1973, 1974; Hanifin *et al.* 1974; Hay and Brostoff 1977; Jones 1980).

Tinea imbricata, a chronic body ringworm that may cover most of the body, is found in the Malay archipelago, Papua New Guinea, Oceania and parts of South and Central America. Susceptibility to the disease, which is caused by *T. concentricum*, seems to be associated with an autosomal recessive gene in some populations, but the gene product is unknown (Serjeantson and Lawrence 1977; Ravine *et al.* 1980). There is no general agreement on the presence of such a gene (Hay 1988); and it seems likely that non-genetic factors, including nutrition, play a major role in immunity (Schofield *et al.* 1963). The immune response to antigens of *T. concentricum* has been studied by Hay and his colleagues. Most infected persons had elevated levels of specific IgE and had typical immediate-type skin tests when challenged intradermally; 9% of the group showed a DTH response in spite of chronic infection (Hay *et al.* 1983b). *In vitro* assays using LMIF demonstrated that there was no significant increase in T cell response to the *T. concentricum* antigen in patients, though antibodies were present. An elevated specific IgE response in patients with tinea imbricata was also suggested by MacLennan (1972); here the antigen used was derived from a different *Trichophyton* species but the result can be explained by the presence of cross-reactivity between species of dermatophytes.

It is very unusual to get such extensive disease as is found in tinea imbricata in other forms of tinea corporis (body ringworm). In temperate regions, chronic tinea corporis is caused by *T. rubrum* or *E. floccosum* while other species seem less likely to cause chronic infections unless underlying diseases are present (Hay 1982). These disorders include diabetes, atopy, collagen vascular diseases and AIDS.

Subcutaneous diseases

Sporotrichosis

There have been few studies on immunity to the agents of subcutaneous mycoses. For *Sporothrix schenckii*, the temperature sensitivity of the fungus may be important in determining its ability to spread along the lymphatics from the initial site of trauma (Kwon-Chung 1979); however, others have questioned the importance of temperature sensitivity (de Albornoz *et al.* 1986). Delayed-type hypersensitivity is found in the lymphocutaneous disease, but it can be absent, or at least suppressed, in patients with systemic infection (Plouffe *et al.* 1979); this may merely reflect the immunosuppressed state of the latter group of patients (Lynch *et al.* 1970). Neutrophils are capable of killing yeast-phase cells *in vitro* and the killing may involve the myeloperoxidase–H_2O_2–iodide system as this was found to be toxic *in vitro* (Cunningham *et al.* 1979). As iodide is used as a therapy for lymphocutaneous sporotrichosis, it is noteworthy that these investigators found that the replacement of iodide with chloride led to loss of killing of *S. schenckii*, though *C. albicans* yeasts remained susceptible.

The evolution of the inflammatory reaction in tissues of infected mice has been followed over a 6-month period by light and electron microscopy (Hiruma *et al.* 1988). Both PMNs and macrophages were present at an early stage and were capable of phagocytosing the yeasts; however, later on the only yeasts remaining were restricted within macrophages, where they appeared to be capable of proliferating. Possibly, the macrophages provide a niche where PMNs are unable to attack the fungus. The PMNs in the inflammatory response may be attracted, at least in part, by C5a released during the activation of complement by the yeasts (Torinuki and Tagami 1985; Scott *et al*. 1986). The importance of T cells in resistance to sporotrichosis is still unclear. Nude mice show an increased susceptibility to infection; however, the difference between these and their T cell-competent littermates was only seen when they were challenged with large inoculum doses (Shiraishi *et al*. 1979; Dickerson *et al*. 1983). Immunization of nude mice with dead yeasts, after they had been reconstituted with thymus cells, led to an increase in resistance; in contrast, the unreconstituted nude mice showed an increased susceptibility to challenge after the immunization (Dickerson *et al*. 1983). The cause of this suppressive effect is unclear.

Chromoblastomycosis

Little is known in detail about the role of the immune system in restricting the growth of agents of other subcutaneous mycoses. *Fonsecaea pedrosoi* is a fairly typical agent of chromoblastomycosis, a disease where the fungus is seen in tissues as a round pigmented structure. The species has been shown to be capable of activating complement (Torinuki *et al*. 1984); and it is likely that this is a general property for these fungi for the tissue reactions routinely show an inflammatory infiltrate in which neutrophils and mononuclear cells are mixed (Uribe-J. *et al*. 1989). The fungi, which normally enter the tissue via some site of trauma, can be eliminated from superficial layers of the body by transepithelial passage of microabscesses; however, granuloma formation followed by fibrosis is found in deeper tissues. In such sites, the fungi can persist for many years.

The role of T cell-mediated immunity has been studied by use of nude mice (Nishimura and Miyagi 1981). Nude mice were more susceptible to large doses of *F. pedrosoi* than were the controls. However, no differences were found when the mice were challenged with smaller doses. Therefore, T cells may play only a partial role in defence against *F. pedrosoi*. Using another species, *Exophiala dermatitidis*, the same authors reported nude mice to have an increased susceptibility to infection and that they needed a longer time to clear infected organs of viable fungus (Nishimura and Miyagi 1983). Both these studies utilized animal models in which the mice were infected by intravenous injection and this is very different from the situation with human disease, where infection normally follows trauma and implantation of the fungus subcutaneously.

A recent report from Brazil has indicated that persons of European origin, who carry human leucocyte antigen (HLA)-A29, have a 10-fold increased risk of developing chromoblastomycosis: this is an area of the world where *F. pedrosoi* is the most common aetiological agent (Tsuneto *et al*. 1989).

Systemic diseases

The true systemic fungal pathogens are agents that cause pulmonary infection and may spread from the lungs to other sites. There are a number of results to an infection. Recovery is the most common. Little is known about the behaviour of *Blastomyces dermatitidis*, but the other fungi may survive in the calcified lesions for a number of years and reactivation is known in persons who become immunodeficient. Cavitary disease can develop, but is a less common finding. Reactivation is much rarer for mycoses than for tuberculosis; it seems that the fungi die after some years.

Histoplasmosis

Of the varieties of *Histoplasma capsulatum*, the variety *capsulatum* is the most common cause of disease. The varieties *duboisii*, which is found in parts of Africa, and *farcimosum*, which infects horses, will not be discussed.

Histoplasmosis occurs in a number of forms, including a rare fulminant disease of childhood where it is likely that there is a defect in the macrophage killing functions, a cavitary disease and the disease following reactivation of latent infection (Goodwin and Des Prez 1978). Most research has concentrated on primary pulmonary infections. The disease is acquired from inhalation of the microconidia (spores). These are produced by the fungus, which grows in soils that have been heavily manured with bird and bat excrement. The microconidia reach the alveoli, where they are ingested by the alveolar macrophages. The fungus grows intracellularly as a yeast and may spread to other parts of the body, typically the spleen, bone marrow and liver, where the yeasts are found within the phagocytic cells. Some time after infection of the normal individual, an intense granulomatous response is mounted. This results in either the inhibition or the death of the fungus and the subsequent production of necrotic lesions, which eventually calcify.

Most of our knowledge of pulmonary histoplasmosis has been derived from studies of epidemics. It is clear that many people are exposed to the fungus at low doses, and they may have a benign infection where no symptoms are observed. Such people develop a delayed-type skin test reaction for histoplasmin, a fairly specific reagent. The acute form of the disease occurs after exposure to higher numbers of spores.

The incubation time for acute pulmonary disease differs in naïve and immune individuals. Primary infections typically produce symptoms between 2 and 3 weeks after exposure while, in secondary infections, symptoms develop more rapidly and are seen at about 10 days following a heavy exposure (Goodwin and Des Prez 1978). The symptoms, which can range from a mild chest cold to a severe influenza-like illness, appear to be determined by the intensity of the hypersensitivity response occurring in the lung, which is in turn related to the actual dose of microconidia inhaled. Presumably, host factors play a role in addition, but there is little known concerning these for the normal individual. Very serious disease is in fact rare; of the estimated 500 000 persons infected each year, 200 000 may develop symptoms, but only about 4000 require to be hospitalized (Ajello 1977). Occasionally, erythema nodosum and erythema multiforme are associated with pulmonary histoplasmosis. Almost all these cases are found in women (Sellers *et al.* 1965). These painful swellings are probably caused by immune reactions to fungal antigens and immune complexes.

Surveys of skin test reactivity to histoplasmin have been made in the USA. In areas where the disease is common, the majority of the population show a positive delayed-type reaction, while in other areas of the country, and in other parts of the world, there are lower levels both of exposure and the concomitant development of an immune state (Edwards *et al.* 1969; Ajello 1971). The skin test has limitations in a lack of total specificity, there being cross-reactions with other fungi; in addition, it may provoke the production of complement-fixing antibodies, which are used diagnostically (Kaufman *et al.* 1967). Serodiagnostic techniques have improved over the years and both antibodies and antigens are detectable during active disease (Wheat 1989).

The interaction of *H. capsulatum* with the immune system starts with infection. Both the microconidia and the yeasts are able to bind to the surfaces of alveolar macrophages and other macrophage types. The binding involves attachment to the CD18 (complement receptor 3 (CR3), lymphocyte function-associated antigen (LFA)-1 and p150, 95) glycopeptides (Bullock and Wright 1987; Newman *et al.* 1990). This obviates any requirement for opsonization for there to be successful phagocytosis. Following phagocytosis, phagolysosome fusion occurs (Dumont and Robert 1970); however, the oxidative burst fails to develop to full capacity (Eissenberg and Goldman 1987; Wolf *et al.* 1987) and the yeasts are capable of multiplying freely. This multiplication can be greatly restricted by the activation of the macrophages by immune T cells or some of their products, such as interferon gamma (IFN-γ) (Howard 1975; Howard and Otto 1977; Wu-Hsieh and Howard 1987, 1989a).

Other factors may be important in restricting growth of the fungus. These include iron deprivation (Sutcliffe *et al.* 1980; Caldwell and Sprouse 1982) and intracellular killing by PMNs (Howard 1973), though the importance of the latter has been questioned. Natural killer (NK) cells seem unlikely to be important (Suchyta *et al.* 1988), in spite of an increased susceptibility of beige (*bg*/*bg*) mice (Patiño *et al.* 1987), as treatment of *bg*/+ mice with anti-asialo GM1, which should inactivate NK cells, did not increase their susceptibility to histoplasmosis.

Evidence for the central role of T cells in inducing immunity to histoplasmosis comes from their ability to mediate the adoptive transfer of immunity in animal models (Tewari *et al.* 1978) and includes their transfer of immunity to athymic mice, which are very susceptible to histoplasmosis (Williams *et al.* 1981). Further evidence comes from the finding of increased susceptibility in T cell deficiencies, such as AIDS, where PMNs seem unaffected (Wheat *et al.* 1985). As is found for patients with other systemic mycoses, modulation of immune responses clearly occurs during the development of histoplasmosis. Acute, self-limited infections resolve with the development of a T cell-mediated inflammatory response and a DTH skin test, while progressive disseminated infections show the development of anergy and suppression of specific responses to *Histoplasma* and, on occasion, suppression of responses to mitogens and other antigens (Newberry *et al.* 1968; Reddy *et al.* 1970; Smith and Utz 1972; Cox 1979). Mouse models of infection show the development of immunosuppression and suppressor cells during disseminated disease and injection of antibodies to the T helper cell population significantly reduces resistance to the disease (Gomez *et al.* 1988). The animal studies have been thoroughly reviewed (Wu-Hsieh and Howard 1989b).

The development of suppressor cells in human histoplasmosis has been observed (Stobo *et al.* 1976), and flow cytometric analysis of T lymphocyte subpopulations shows that the proportion of CD8 +ve (suppressor/cytotoxic) T cells can increase in disseminated disease (Lehmann *et al.* 1983; Payan *et al.* 1984). Immune complexes may also be of some importance in the induction of suppression. Another form of immunosuppression may result from a lowered total T cell count, and from the production of unusual subpopulations of T cells (CD2 −ve, CD3 +ve, CD4 −ve, CD8 −ve and Tγδ +ve) which have been reported in one instance (Lehmann *et al.* 1989). Overall, the studies with animals and humans support the idea that the progression of disease depends, in large part, upon the suppression of T cell responses and that this suppression can be induced as part of the immune response to infection. The development of disseminated disease, though most common in persons with T cell deficiencies, can occur in apparently normal persons. These people may have unknown abnormalities in their ability to process *Histoplasma* antigens or, as seems more likely to this author, may have had the misfortune to have been exposed to large amounts of inoculum. Then, much as is found in animals which have been injected with large numbers of organisms, the resulting infection overwhelms the normal cell-mediated immune response and induces immunosuppression.

Coccidioidomycosis

The causal agent, *Coccidioides immitis*, is found in restricted areas of the Americas. As with histoplasmosis and paracoccidioidomycosis, a spectrum of disease types is seen and the majority of exposed persons show no, or minor, symptoms (Smith *et al.* 1946). Indeed, skin test reactivity to coccidioidin (CDN) indicates that the infection is asymptomatic in most people. Infection follows the inhalation of arthrospores which, under the influence of the lung environment and increased $P\text{CO}_2$ (Klotz *et al.* 1984), swell to form large (10–80 μm diameter) spherical structures named spherules. Mature spherules contain hundreds of endospores (2–5 μm diameter) which are released on rupture of the wall and can be spread throughout the body (Sun and Huppert 1976). Female sex hormones, at levels found during pregnancy, stimulate the growth rate of *C. immitis* and may explain the profound susceptibility of non-immune, pregnant women to coccidioidomycocis (Drutz and Huppert 1983).

The different forms of the fungus vary in their resistance to killing. Arthrospores have an antiphagocytic outer coat that inhibits neutrophil phagocytosis (Drutz and Huppert 1983) and both the endospores and spherules resist phagocytosis and are coated with an antiphagocytic material (Frey and Drutz 1986; Galgiani 1986). Killing of the endospores and arthroconidia by PMNs is not very extensive; however, specific antibody and complement may increase the ability of these phagocytes to ingest the organism.

Normal macrophages are unable to kill ingested arthrospores or endospores; this seems to be related to an inhibition of phagolysosome fusion. In contrast, once activated via T cell-mediated immune responses, the macrophages are capable of killing the fungus (Beaman *et al.* 1983). Mere increases in macrophage activity, as are found in nude mice, are not enough (Clemons *et al.* 1985), for effective activation seems to require the action of lymphokines from T helper cells. In this regard it is notable that IFN-γ will convert murine alveolar macrophages into efficient killers of arthrospores and endospores (Beaman 1987).

The central role of the T cell-mediated immune

response in the induction of immunity has been reviewed (Cox 1989b). Though PMNs and possibly NK cells (Petkus and Baum 1987) may have some ability to reduce the amount of initial inoculum, the need for adequate T cell responses is clear. As evidence, Cox cites the susceptibility of athymic (*nu/nu*) and thymectomized mice, the ability to transfer immunity between mice using T cells, and the lack of an effect of B cell depletion on such transfers. *In vitro* studies point to the Lyt-1 +ve Lyt-2 −ve (T helper) lymphocytes as being responsible for the activation of the effector macrophages; the lymphocytes alone were not fungitoxic (Beaman *et al.* 1981; Beaman 1987). Supporting the central role for T cell-mediated immunity is the finding of a very severe form of coccidioidomycosis in AIDS patients; here, it is often unclear whether the disease results from the activation of endogenous organisms, from a new infection or from a mixture of both (Bronnimann *et al.* 1987).

Modulation of the immune responses occurs in human disease; in many ways the findings are similar to those for other infections that show both acute self-limited and chronic disseminating forms of disease. In self-limited disease, the fungus may be largely restricted to the lung and symptoms, if observed, correlate with the inflammatory response. A number of patients develop erythema nodosum and erythema multiforme (Smith 1940), and eosinophilia may be encountered (Goldstein and Louie 1943). Resolution of disease is accompanied by a DTH skin test response to CDN. Typically, in progressive disease, T cell-mediated responses are markedly suppressed and anergy to CDN is common both *in vivo* and *in vitro* (Smith *et al.* 1948). Occasionally, the anergy may extend to unrelated antigens (Cox 1989b). There is also evidence for some polyclonal activation of the humoral response; for elevations in most immunoglobulin isotypes and in specific antibodies are normal. Complement-fixing antibodies (IgG isotype) and IgE (Cox *et al.* 1982) are routinely elevated, with the former forming the basis of a serological test having some prognostic value (Smith *et al.* 1956). These responses have been reviewed (Drutz and Catanzaro 1978; Cox 1989b).

Reductions in the specific lymphocyte response to CDN *in vitro* are found in disseminated coccidioidomycosis. Suppression is associated with blocking serum factors, which may include immune complexes (Opelz and Scheer 1975; Yoshinoya *et al.* 1980; Cox *et al.* 1983; Cox and Pope 1987), and with the generation of suppressor cells that can be detected functionally and in tissues (Catanzaro 1981; Modlin *et al.* 1985). When skin tests show the presence of profound anergy involving multiple antigens, it is generally found that the lymphocyte transformation responses are likewise reduced (Cox 1989b).

Blastomycosis

Blastomyces dermatitidis, the causative agent of blastomycosis, produces a focus of pulmonary infection which disseminates to a number of other sites. Males are more susceptible than females, a feature that is also seen in canine blastomycosis, and this might be brought about by the immunosuppressive action of male hormones (Furcolow *et al.* 1970; Legendre *et al.* 1981). Several factors determine whether severe disease will occur and many of these are not obviously linked to the functioning of the immune system. Differences in strain virulence can be great; Cox *et al.* (1974) demonstrated that cell wall fractions of a virulent strain induced granulomata while those of an avirulent strain, which had been taken from a human lesion, failed to induce a granulomatous response. The age of the host and the strain of mouse are important; certain strains are more susceptible than others and this susceptibility depends on the route of inoculation. While C3H/HeJ mice are more resistant than DBA/1J mice when challenged intranasally with yeasts, the reverse applies when intraperitoneal injection is used (Morozumi *et al.* 1981a, b).

The infectious forms of *B. dermatitidis* are assumed to be the conidia (conidiospores). These convert within the lung to the yeast form. Resistance to the two morphological forms is not identical. Human PMNs are capable of phagocytosing the conidia *in vitro*, though killing is not very efficient; both phagocytosis and killing are enhanced by complement (Drutz and Frey 1985; Schaffner *et al.* 1986). In addition, monocyte-derived macrophages and murine bronchoalveolar macrophages have been shown to be capable of ingesting and killing the conidia (Drutz and Frey 1985; Deepe 1989).

Compared with the conidia, the yeasts are more resistant to killing. They produce a factor which is chemotactic for PMNs and monocytes (Sixbey *et al.* 1979), but the PMNs seem relatively unable to kill the yeasts (Thurmond and Mitchell 1984; Drutz and Frey 1985; Schaffner *et al.* 1986). Indeed, PMNs may actually enhance yeast growth both *in vitro* and *in vivo* (Brummer and Stevens 1982, 1983). However, yeasts can be killed by the H_2O_2–myeloperoxidase–iodide and the iron–hydrogen peroxide systems (Sugar *et al.* 1983, 1984). The *in vitro* administration of IFN-γ has been claimed to result in the production of PMNs that can kill the yeast form *in vitro* (Morrison *et al.* 1989); furthermore, IFN-γ will activate alveolar macrophages to enhance their killing of *Blastomyces* yeasts (Brummer *et al.* 1988). Resistance to infection is associated with the development of T cell-mediated immunity (Cozad and Chang 1980) and T cells are the effector cells in adoptive transfer of immunity (Brummer *et al.* 1982). Compared with cells from uninfected controls, monocyte-derived macrophages from infected and recovered patients are better able to phagocytose yeasts and to prevent intracellular replication of the yeast form (Bradsher *et al.* 1987). The addition of lymphokines to the phagocyte cultures can increase their anti-*Blastomyces* activity substantially (Brummer *et al.* 1985; Brummer and Stevens 1987).

In human infections, there appears to be a modulation of the immune response which involves finding enhanced levels of CD8 +ve (suppressor) T cells in the lungs during treatment of pulmonary blastomycosis (Jacobs *et al.* 1985). However, there have been relatively few studies on lymphocyte populations in blastomycosis so the general nature of this phenomenon and its possible association with treatment need to be confirmed. Generalized anergy, including lymphopaenia, is often found in serious disseminated disease in both dogs and humans and is associated with a poor prognosis (Legendre and Becker 1982; Bradsher 1984). After treatment, this suppression of immune responses may be very rapidly resolved. In mice, infection can give rise to a generalized suppression of immune response but this appears late in infection (Deepe *et al.* 1985). Antibody responses are present in infected persons and are useful in establishing a diagnosis (Klein *et al.* 1987). They may have some value as opsonins but, based on studies on the adoptive transfer of immunity, they play at best a minor role in resistance to infection (Brummer *et al.* 1982).

Paracoccidioidomycosis

The natural reservoir for *Paracoccidioides brasiliensis* is unknown. Epidemiological studies using the skin test reagent paracoccidioidin (PCN) show that the disease is endemic to South and Central America and that the majority of infected persons do not develop disease (Conti-Díaz 1972). In persons past the age of puberty, males develop disease far more commonly than females. This may be related to the action of the female sex hormone 17β-oestradiol, which directly inhibits the formation of the yeast phase of *P. brasiliensis*, the form that is seen in tissues (Loose *et al.* 1983).

The virulence of the fungus seems to be directly related to the wall content of α-glucan, a carbohydrate that is not degraded by macrophages. The fungus is capable of activating complement via the alternative pathway (Calich *et al.* 1979) but this is not essential to disease resistance or for inducing inflammation as chemotactic factors are produced by *P. brasiliensis* (Silva and Fazioli 1985).

The immune responses in paracoccidioidomycosis have been reviewed recently (Restrepo-M. 1988; Jimenez-Finkel and Restrepo-Moreno 1989). As with blastomycosis, the disease develops from a pulmonary focus (Restrepo *et al.* 1970). There are different forms of the disease: a fulminant form found in juveniles and a chronic, slowly progressing form seen in adults. The adult disease has been most thoroughly studied. It is associated with a spectrum of immune responses similar to what is found in histoplasmosis, coccidioidomycosis and mycobacterioses. In the self-limited infections, strong T cell-mediated immune responses are the rule, while chronic progressive infections are associated with numerous abnormalities in T cell-mediated immune responses. These include anergy to PCN and unrelated antigens, reduced mitogen-induced lymphocyte transformation, reduced or absent contact sensitivity responses to dichloronitrobenzene and reduced numbers of circulating T lymphocytes (Mendes and Raphael 1971; Mendes *et al.* 1971; Musatti *et al.* 1976; Mok and Greer 1977). Changes in T cell subpopulations have been found with elevations in the population of CD8 +ve (suppressor) T cells in chronic infections (Jimenez-Finkel and Restrepo-Moreno 1989). Humoral factors are also modified. Newly diagnosed infections appear to be associated with some degree of polyclonal activation of the humoral immune system. Elevations in IgE antibodies have been found in chronic infections (Musatti *et al.* 1976; Yarzábal *et al.* 1980). The specific IgG level tended to be higher in acute progressing disease than in long-lasting chronic infections (Biagnoni *et al.* 1984). In addition, immune complexes are present in the blood of chronically infected persons (Arango *et al.* 1982). These, or possibly some other factors in plasma, seem responsible for the inhibition of lymphocyte transformation *in vitro* which is seen when serum from patients is added to normal lymphocytes (Musatti *et al.* 1976; Arango *et al.* 1982).

Antibodies may play an accessory role in immunity to paracoccidioidomycosis but T cell-mediated immunity seems vital for resolution of infections. Nude (*nu*/*nu*) mice were susceptible to infection but littermates (+/+ or *nu*/+), or nude mice that had received a thymus transplant, were resistant (Robledo *et al.* 1982; Miyaji and Nishimura 1983). Activated macrophages seem to be the effector cells for successful resistance (Brummer *et al.* 1989).

Other cell types and opsonins may be important in reducing the effective size of the original inoculum. Peripheral blood PMNs have been shown to be capable of killing yeasts, although PMNs from patients with chronic infections were not so effective (Goihman-Yahr *et al.* 1980). Incubation of the cultures with immune serum led to better phagocytosis and killing by PMNs, and, as the H_2O_2−myeloperoxidase−halide system is known to generate effective killing capacity (McEwen *et al.* 1984), phagocytosis by PMNs may be one form of natural resistance. Natural killer cells may also be important in restricting the initial development of *P. brasiliensis* (Jimenez and Murphy 1984).

Opportunistic infections

The widespread use of chemotherapy and immunosuppressive drugs in the treatment of cancer, transplant recipients and autoimmune diseases, as well as the development of the AIDS epidemic, have brought into being a large population of patients who show increased susceptibility to fungal diseases. Not only do these people develop very severe infections when a true pathogen colonizes them, but they become susceptible to a multitude of novel organisms that are rarely, if ever, found in the normal healthy person. Though many treatments affect both the PMN−humoral immune system and the T cell-mediated immune system, in certain settings only one system is severely impaired. It has been found that different fungi predominate in each situation. Some of the more common opportunistic diseases are discussed in the following sections.

Infections in T cell deficiencies

Cryptococcosis

The aetiological agent *Cryptococcus neoformans* is an encapsulated yeast. Two varieties exist; the variety *neoformans* is found in pigeon guano and has a world-wide distribution, while the *gattii* variety is found in warmer areas associated with red gum trees (Kwon-Chung and Bennett 1984; Ellis and Pfeiffer 1990). The varieties are separated readily using a selective medium or serotype-specific antibodies that bind to the capsule. The variety *gattii* is serotype B or C while the variety *neoformans* is either serotype A or D. Almost all the research on the interaction of *Cryptococcus neoformans* with the immune system has involved the *neoformans* variety. This is the main variety that causes AIDS-related infection, even in areas of the world where the *gattii* variety is also present (Swinne *et al.* 1986; Bottone *et al.* 1987). Disease follows pulmonary infection and the fungus can then disseminate to other areas of the body, most notably the brain, where it causes a meningitis. The pulmonary disease may be unapparent, so the first noticeable symptoms are often associated with the disseminated forms of cryptococcosis. These are characterized by the presence of soluble polysaccharide, derived from the yeast capsule, which is detectable in body fluids and is useful in aiding in diagnosis, and for monitoring treatment and for prognosis (Diamond and Bennett 1974).

The capsule is composed of an acidic polysaccharide, which differs in chemical structure depending on the serotype (Cherniak 1988). Mutants that lack the capsule are avirulent (Kozel and Cazin 1971). It has been suggested that the capsular surface is 'invisible' to host phagocytes which do not have receptors capable of binding the polysaccharides (Kozel 1983). Phagocytosis, therefore, requires that the yeasts are opsonized. This can be achieved via binding of IgG antibody and iC3b (Tacker *et al.* 1972; Diamond *et al.* 1974), the latter being deposited on the surface of the capsule after activation of the complement alternative pathway (Kozel *et al.* 1989). By itself, iC3b appears to be less effective as an opsonin than whole serum, which usually contains antibody as well as other possible opsonins (Kozel and McGaw 1979; Kozel *et al.* 1989).

The role of the capsule in inhibition of phagocytosis has been shown in two ways. Yeasts bearing thin capsules are more easily phagocytosed by macrophages and PMNs than are yeasts that have thick capsules (Bulmer and Sans 1968; Diamond *et al.* 1972; Kozel and Mastroianni 1976; Davies *et al.* 1982; Granger *et al.* 1985). Secondly, exogenous application of soluble polysaccharide to unencapsulated cells leads to their becoming coated with capsular polysaccharide and resistant to phagocytosis (Kozel and Mastroianni 1976). In addition, solutions of the polysaccharide inhibit phagocytosis and have been reported to interfere with PMN chemotaxis (Drouhet and Segretain 1951). The presence of the capsular polysaccharide in serum may be the reason for the suppressed level of leucocyte phagocytosis that is found when testing cells in the presence of autologous serum taken from patients (Mohr *et al.* 1974). In addition, complement may become depleted in some patients with severe cryptococcaemia; this would result in a loss of opsonins from the serum (Macher *et al.* 1978).

The role of PMNs in resistance to disease is somewhat confusing. They are capable of killing phagocytosed yeasts, but these require to be opsonized. Polymorphonuclear leucocytes are seen in lesions, presumably arriving as a response to the generation of C5a during activation of complement (Laxalt and Kozel 1979; Diamond and Erickson 1982). The importance of C5a generation is underscored by the finding that C5-deficient mice are extremely susceptible to disease (Rhodes *et al.* 1980). Once phagocytosed, the yeasts are killed primarily by oxidative mechanisms. These appear to involve H_2O_2–myeloperoxidase, for cells from chronic granulomatous disease patients have a reduced efficiency at killing cryptococci (Diamond *et al.* 1972). In addition, non-oxidative killing is somewhat effective and may include the action of cytotoxic peptides or 'defensins' (Ganz *et al.* 1985). Finally, PMNs may encircle yeasts and attack them by an extracellular mechanism (Kalina *et al.* 1974). In spite of the effectiveness of PMNs *in vitro*, it should be pointed out that PMN dysfunction is not associated with human cryptococcosis and that many cryptococcosis patients have what appear to be fully functional PMNs. These cells may, therefore, provide only a portion of the defence against infection and may act by reducing the level of effective inoculum (Murphy 1989).

Studies on monocytes and macrophages have generally concluded that they are not efficient killers of *C. neoformans* (Murphy 1989). Few studies have involved the alveolar macrophage, which would be the first macrophage type to encounter the organism. Guinea-pig alveolar macrophages were unable to kill the yeasts, even if taken from animals where they had become activated after injection of killed bacteria (Bulmer and Tacker 1975). In contrast, human alveolar macrophages were found to be fungistatic when incubated with cryptococci in the absence of human serum; in its presence, yeasts became phagocytosed and a limited number were killed (Weinberg *et al.* 1987). Fungistasis was also observed when incubating yeasts with murine peritoneal macrophages; these had been activated *in vivo* using killed bacteria (Granger *et al.* 1986). Earlier reports that monocytes were efficient killers (Diamond *et al.* 1972) have been questioned as the mononuclear cell preparations were likely to have contained NK cells.

Since their report showing the action of NK cells on *C. neoformans* (Murphy and McDaniel 1982), the role of NK cells in cryptococcosis has been studied extensively, most prominently by Murphy and her collaborators (Murphy 1989). Binding of NK cells to yeasts was observed to be independent of capsule size. The levels of NK cells in mice, including mice treated with cyclophosphamide and the nude and beige strains, correlated very closely with the early clearance of *C. neoformans* from host organs following infection. Furthermore, NK cells injected as components of cell preparations appeared capable of reconstituting cyclophosphamide-treated mice; the same cell preparations, when pretreated with anti-asialo GM1, which reacts with NK cells, did not confer any resistance to the recipient (Hidore and Murphy 1986). However, in spite of their apparent effectiveness, NK cells do not seem to provide a complete defence, for the mice eventually die. T cell-mediated immunity is vital for complete clearance of an infection.

The evidence for a central role of T cell-mediated immunity comes from a number of different areas. Clinically, T cell deficiencies and AIDS predispose to cryptococcosis (Zuger *et al.* 1986) and cryptococcosis patients rarely have defective antibody production or defects in complement or phagocyte function (Murphy 1989). Athymic nude mice show an increased susceptibility to infection (Graybill and Drutz 1978; Cauley and Murphy 1979) and do not clear the organism from the liver (Nishimura and Miyagi 1979). T cell-enriched preparations from sensitized mice are able to transfer immunity (Lim and Murphy 1980), and depletion of the CD4 +ve population, using a monoclonal antibody, impairs resistance to cryptococcosis in mice (Mody *et al.* 1990). T cells may act by stimulating macrophages; in contrast to most findings with macrophages and monocytes that were not activated immunologically, murine peritoneal macrophages that had been activated with IFN-γ were capable of killing yeasts intracellularly (Levitz and DiBenedetto 1988). Also, in cultures of bone marrow-derived macrophages, IFN-γ was found to induce killing of *C. neoformans* via an extracellular mechanism (Flesch *et al.* 1989).

In addition to the activation of macrophages, T cells can help in production of antibody; this action could be important in defence against cryptococcosis. The B cell-defective CBA/N mouse was found to be more susceptible to intravenous challenge with *C. neoformans* than were other mouse strains; however, this susceptibility was not correlated with an increase in numbers of yeasts colonizing the brain (Marquis *et al.* 1985). Thus, effective defence mechanisms appeared to differ depending on the host organ. Most studies have shown that antibodies do not provide complete protection (Murphy 1989). The amount of antibody to capsular polysaccharide that is produced in an immune response seems ineffective (Goren 1967), but passive transfer of enough monoclonal antibody reactive with the capsule was found to protect mice from a quick death following intravenous challenge. The protection was not complete as the mice died later of cryptococcosis (Dromer *et al.* 1987).

There have always been some persons who develop cryptococcosis without having obvious predisposing conditions. Even after cure, these people show a variety of deficiences in a number of parameters associated with T cell-mediated immune responses but the pattern of defects can vary substantially. Poor lymphocyte transformation to cryptococcal antigens *in vitro* as well as to unrelated antigens, poor delayed-type skin test reactivity to killed *C. neoformans*, and a failure of leucocytes to respond to leucocyte migration inhibitory factor are among some of the defects seen. This indicates that several different cell types can be abnormal (Schimpff and Bennett 1975). The abnormal responses may also be brought about by the expansion of the CD8 +ve subset and by changes in the kinetics of lymphocyte responses (Miller and Puck 1984). In mice, during infection, suppression of immune responses has been seen and this can be induced by the intravenous administration of serum from infected animals. The same effect can be found in mice receiving solely the serum antigen after its purification using antibody to *C. neoformans* in affinity chromatography (Murphy and Cox 1988; Murphy 1989). A network of suppressor cells producing soluble suppressor factors has been implicated in being responsible for the immunosuppression.

In summary, T cell-mediated immune responses are essential to defence against *C. neoformans*; however, the early colonization phases following infection may be controlled to a substantial extent by the interactions of NK cells, antibodies and PMNs.

Pneumocystosis

Pneumocystis carinii, like *C. neoformans*, has gone from being an uncommon cause of pneumonia to being widely encountered as an AIDS-associated infection. The organism, which has recently been considered to have affinities to fungi, can only be passaged for a short time *in vitro* and animals require to be immunosuppressed to allow their infection. Its close link to AIDS suggests that T cell-mediated immunity is central to defence against *P. carinii*.

Infections in neutropenic hosts

Invasive aspergillosis, invasive candidiasis, invasive mucormycosis and a variety of other mycoses are considered to be opportunistic diseases of the neutropenic host. The hyphae, and in the case of *Candida* species the pseudohyphae, are far too large for simple intracellular destruction by phagocytes. In contrast, spores and individual yeasts can be phagocytosed. Extracellular methods of attacking the large filamentous structures of the causative fungi have been described and recently reviewed (Waldorf and Diamond 1989). Neutrophils, monocytes and macrophages can be involved. While great similarities exist for resistance to many of the pathogens in the setting of invasive disease, significant differences can be found with different fungal species and in different clinical settings.

Invasive aspergillosis

Pulmonary infection which can lead to systemic disease is the most common form of invasive aspergillosis in the neutropenic host. The most common agent is *Aspergillus fumigatus*, though other species of *Aspergillus* can be found. Infection follows inhalation of conidia (spores), which swell and germinate to form invasive branching hyphae. Though there is a strong association with neutropenia, PMNs do not kill the conidia (Lehrer and Jan 1970); however, the PMNs are capable of damaging and killing the filamentous hyphae (Diamond *et al*. 1978a; Schaffner *et al*. 1982; Waldorf and Diamond 1985). Activation of complement appears to act as a chemotactic stimulus for the PMNs (Waldorf and Diamond 1985).

Though monocytes can damage hyphae (Diamond *et al*. 1983), the PMNs seem the dominant defence against this form of the fungus. This is clear from studies in nitrogen mustard-treated mice which exhibit neutropenia, yet in which the monocytes and macrophages remain functional. Such mice are very susceptible to infection with pre-germinated conidia, yet remain resistant to ungerminated conidia which are killed by macrophages (Schaffner *et al*. 1982). Others have shown that normal murine alveolar macrophages are capable of killing the conidia of aspergilli (Merkow *et al*. 1971; Waldorf *et al*. 1984); however, macrophages taken from cortisone-treated mice lose their ability to prevent fungal growth. A different situation is seen for the effect of cortisone in infected mice. These mice develop resistance to reinfection when the macrophages would be likely to be fully activated (Smith 1972; Sandhu *et al*. 1976). In such mice, treatment with cortisone no longer induces susceptibility to infection by spores; furthermore, there is no apparent reduction in defences against mycelial invasion (Lehmann and White 1976). Here, it seems likely that activated, cortisone-resistant macrophages are sufficient for defence against invasive infection.

The methods by which phagocytes kill *Aspergillus* spores and hyphae have been reviewed (Waldorf and Diamond 1989). The myeloperoxidase$-H_2O_2-$halide system is likely to play an important role in killing by neutrophils and monocytes; but macrophages, which lack myeloperoxidase, appear to kill spores by a different mechanism. It has been suggested that the active components are derived from a mixture of Fe^{2+}, H_2O_2 and I^-

A comparison of the methods of killing *Aspergillus* hyphae and the hyphae of *Rhizopus* (an agent of mucormycosis, see next section) shows that some features differ. Invasive aspergillosis is not uncommon in X-linked chronic granulomatous disease (CGD), and the monocytes from CGD patients produce only small amounts of H_2O_2. While these monocytes fail to damage *Rhizopus* hyphae, they are capable of damaging *Aspergillus* hyphae (Diamond *et al*. 1982). The effectiveness of the damage appears to be limited, for PMNs have been shown to inhibit the action of CGD monocytes (Diamond *et al*. 1983). In myeloperoxidase deficiency, the reverse situation is found; monocytes are capable of damaging *Rhizopus* hyphae but not those of *Aspergillus*. In addition, differences in the ability of alveolar macrophages to kill *Rhizopus* and *Aspergillus* spores are reported. Though the macrophages from normal mice were effective inhibitors of both fungi, those taken from streptozotocin-treated diabetic mice were incapable of resisting the spores of *Rhizopus* though they were capable of resisting those of *Aspergillus* (Waldorf *et al*. 1984). Studies such as these demonstrate that multiple killing mechanisms are involved in resistance to opportunistic fungi and that the methods for resisting the different morphological forms of the fungus may vary.

No clear evidence for a role of antibodies in resistance to invasive aspergillosis has been shown. Antibodies may be opsonic and play some role in situations where spores enter the bloodstream such as might be found during the intravenous administration of contaminated materials.

Mucormycosis

Several fungi in the order Mucorales have been found to cause mucormycosis, a rarely encountered disease. There are different disease patterns, including rhinocerebral mucormycosis, which is associated with diabetic ketoacidosis, and invasive mucormycosis, which is an invasive disease in the profoundly immunocompromised patient. As in aspergillosis, the PMNs act as a major line of defence against the hyphae (Diamond *et al.* 1978a) and the alveolar macrophages resist the spores. However, in contrast to *Aspergillus fumigatus* spores, which are killed in the alveolar macrophages, spores of *Rhizopus oryzae* are not destroyed. Instead, the macrophages prevent their successful germination (Waldorf *et al.* 1984). The activation of complement and the direct production of chemotactic factors for PMNs are found when spores are assayed for these activities; but swollen spores and hyphae are more effective than fresh spores, a situation also seen with the conidia of *A. fumigatus* (Waldorf and Diamond 1985). More details on the basis of resistance to agents of mucormycosis can be found in a recent review (Waldorf and Diamond 1989).

Invasive candidiasis

In contrast to severe mucosal candidiasis, where the T cell-mediated immune response is often compromised, typically, severe invasive candidiasis is not seen in the absence of frank neutrophil dysfunction or neutropenia. In addition, foci of infection may develop following haematogenous spread of fungi from infected indwelling catheters. Thus, invasive candidiasis in not an AIDS-related infection. *Candida albicans* is the most common agent, though other species are not uncommon. The fungus can activate complement via the alternative pathway (Ray and Wuepper 1976; Solomkin *et al.* 1978) and C5-deficient mice have an increased susceptibility to infection (Morelli and Rosenberg 1971). Not only dose *C. albicans* activate complement, but it also has receptors for iC3b and C3d (Heidenreich and Deirich 1985; Hostetter *et al.* 1990; Ollert *et al.* 1990). These are more abundant on the filamentous form than on the yeast form. The iC3b receptor is antigenically cross-reactive with human CR_3 (Edwards *et al.* 1986; Eigentler *et al.* 1989). The receptors have not been detected on a number of other species of Candida, including *C. tropicalis*, which produces similar forms of disease. Their role is far from clear; they may be involved in inhibition of phagocytosis and, like human CR_3 (Wright *et al.* 1988), they may be multifunctional and bind other compounds. In this regard, binding by *C. albicans* of several other proteins, including fibrinogen, albumin, transferrin and plasmin, has been reported (Bouali *et al.* 1987; Page and Odds 1988; Hsiao *et al.* 1990).

Candida albicans grows in both a filamentous form and a yeast form. The filaments, also known as hyphae and pseudohyphae, are too large to be phagocytosed. Diamond and his colleagues have shown that PMNs will attach to these *in vitro*. Once attached, a process aided by opsonins, the PMNs are able to damage the cells. Polymorphonuclear leucocytes from persons with chronic granulomatous disease do not produce this damage, suggesting that oxidative mechanisms may be involved in the killing (Diamond and Krzesicki 1978; Diamond *et al.* 1978b, 1980). The interaction of the filamentous forms and PMNs can occur even under conditions where there is no PMN-mediated response to the yeast form. There are also significant differences in the detailed nature of the metabolic changes found in PMNs as they respond to opsonized and unopsonized filaments (Levitz *et al.* 1987; Kolotila and Diamond 1988; Wysong *et al.* 1989).

Under certain conditions, bystander cells involved in inflammation and T cell-mediated responses may contribute to resistance via the production of cytokines which enhance the antifungal activity of PMNs, macrophages and monocytes. The active cytokines include tumour necrosis factor, IFN-γ, IL-3, granulocyte–macrophage colony-stimulating factor (CSF) and macrophage CSF. In addition some uncharacterized compounds are described (Djeu *et al.* 1986; Djeu and Blanchard 1987; Karbassi *et al.* 1987; Perfect *et al.* 1987; Wang *et al.* 1989).

The recent demonstration of high rates of phenotypic switching of morphology in several isolates of *C. albicans* (Slutsky *et al.* 1985, 1987) raises the question as to whether the different morphological forms differ in their resistance to antifungal defences. Using the white–opaque switching system, Kolotila and Diamond (1990) reported that, compared with yeasts of the white form, the yeasts of the opaque form were more readily killed by PMNs and were more potent as stimuli of superoxide production by PMNs.

General features of immunity

The T cell-mediated immune response is important for the restriction of several fungal infections. A number of features found in common in these are shown in Table 84.3. There is a spectrum of responses found in patients. In many cases the only evidence for a past infection is the demonstration of the presence of T cell-mediated immunity in a person. However, when chronic and disseminated disease are found, the antigen-specific T cell-mediated responses become suppressed. This suppression can develop during the course of an infection. Enhanced levels of IgE antibody, DTH skin test anergy, antigen-specific suppressor cells and soluble suppressor factors, including immune complexes, are found routinely. Immune responses appear to progress towards one or other end of the spectrum shown in Table 84.3.

For invasive candidiasis, invasive aspergillosis and invasive mucormycosis, the infections are associated with neutropenia.

Other diseases

In addition to invasive disease, *Aspergillus fumigatus* and other aspergilli cause a number of pulmonary diseases including aspergilloma, where the fungus grows as a mass in a pulmonary cavity, and syndromes that result from hypersensitivity. The latter include allergic bronchopulmonary aspergillosis, a disease in which the fungus remains within the lumen of the bronchioles and bronchi. It does not invade deeper tissues; presumably, this is on account of the effective population of PMNs. Inflammation results as a reaction to fungal materials that escape into the lung. Immune complex-mediated and IgE-mediated reactions, as well as the direct activation of complement and delayed-type responses, can be found. The spectrum of the diseases caused by aspergilli has been reviewed (Bardana 1980a, b).

There are other mycoses, many of which are quite unusual. Certain of these have been reviewed previously as regards their immunological features (Lehmann 1985; Smith 1989). Included are adiaspiromycosis, conidiobolomycosis, phaeohyphomycosis, pythiosis, basidiobolomycosis, rhinosporidiomycosis, and a variety of opportunistic diseases.

Immunotherapy and vaccination

There have been successes in the application of vaccines to mycoses of veterinary animals and these have been reviewed previously (Lehmann 1985). Vaccination of cattle, using an intramuscular injection of a live attenuated strain of *Trichophyton*

Table 84.3. Poles of the spectrum of T cell-mediated responses in fungal infections[a]

	Features	
	'Helper pole'	'Suppressor pole'
Coccidioidomycosis[b]		
Histoplasmosis[b]	Mild or absent disease	Chronic or progressive disease
Paracoccidioidomycosis[b]	DTH$^+$	DTH$^-$ or ↓
Cryptococcosis	LT$^+$	LT$^-$ or ↓
Pneumocystosis		Suppressor factors[c]
Dermatophytosis		Suppressor cells ↑
Mucosal and cutaneous candidiasis		IgE antibody ↑
Malassezia folliculitis		

a Not all the markers have been reported in all the diseases and other changes are seen as described in the appropriate sections of the text.
b Complement-fixing antibody is elevated in disseminated disease.
c Soluble factors, including fungal products and immune complexes, in serum.
$^+$ = positive; $^-$ = negative; ↑ = elevated; ↓ = suppressed; DTH = delayed-type hypersensitivity skin test; LT = antigen-specific lymphocyte transformation.

verrucosum, has been very effective at preventing disease and appears to speed the recovery of animals once they are infected. The vaccine is not totally innocuous, for some calves have died after receiving it (Aamodt *et al.* 1982). Subcutaneous pythiosis in horses has been treated by immunotherapy. Extremely large, chronic suppurative lesions were found to heal, but again the crude 'vaccine' was not without severe side-effects in a number of animals (Miller 1981; Miller *et al.* 1983). In another instance, vaccination with killed fungus was used to limit an epidemic of venereal disease in geese. The causative agent was *Candida albicans* (Kuttin *et al.* 1980).

In each of the above cases, the 'vaccines' were administered intramuscularly or intradermally. With the antigen administered in a bolus at an unusual site, it seems that it is possible to induce a response in a different population of immune cells from those in which a response was induced by antigens released during natural infections. Maybe such as effect can explain the successes reported for similar 'vaccines' in the immunotherapy of human disease. Bazyka reported treatment of tinea pedis (cited in Lepper 1969), and other remarkable responses have been seen from time to time (e.g. Beemer *et al.* 1977). Possibly, desensitization may be occurring in some patients; indeed desensitization injections have been claimed to be effective for vaginal candidiasis (Kudelko 1971). There are indications that mast cell degranulation may sometimes predispose candidiasis (Simon *et al.* 1979) and, certainly, IgE antibodies are prominent in vaginal secretions of some women with recurrent vaginal candidiasis (Mathur *et al.* 1977). However, the value of immunotherapy or desensitization for treatment of candidiasis or any other human mycosis remains to be proved and will require the use of properly controlled trials. Many features of vaccines, primarily based on studies in animal models, are discussed by Segal (1987).

Secondary manifestations of the immune response

Many allergic reactions to fungi can develop during infections. They include the 'id' reaction in ringworm infections, erythema nodosum and erythema multiforme, both of which can develop during prolonged infection of immunocompetent hosts. The basis for these skin reactions is not well understood. They are likely to be inflammatory reactions to fungal materials that have entered the circulation and been deposited at distant sites, but several other causes can be suggested.

Kerion celsi is a boggy swelling which can appear on the face of persons with tinea capitis or tinea barbae. Fungal antigens have been detected within the tumour, but living fungal cells are not present (Zaslow and Derbes 1969; Imamura *et al.* 1975).

Immunodiagnosis

Immunological methods of diagnosis have been summarized by Kaufman and Reiss (1986). They are valuable in helping establish the diagnosis of cryptococcosis, where capsular antigen in body fluids is detectable using a simple latex agglutination test. Antibody detection may help in alerting the physician to the possibility of a systemic mycosis (histoplasmosis, coccidioidomycosis, blastomycosis or paracoccidioidomycosis) and in establishing a diagnosis of allergic bronchopulmonary aspergillosis and aspergilloma. Because of antigenic cross-reactivity between fungi, very few antigenic preparations are specific for a single aetiological agent.

Skin test responses and antibody levels can be useful in monitoring patients; in general, a fall in antibody levels and a strong delayed-type skin test are good prognostic signs. Skin tests alone are not diagnostic, as they merely show the presence of previous sensitization; however, skin tests have been useful in establishing the boundaries of endemic areas for *Coccidioides immitis*, *Paracoccidioides brasiliensis* and *Histoplasma capsulatum*. The use of antigen and antibody detection for diagnosis of most opportunistic infections, except cryptococcosis, must still be considered experimental, though a number of tests seen extremely promising. Several specific antibody reagents are available at reference laboratories for the direct identification of fungi in culture or in tissue sections using immunofluorescence. A recently described technique (Kaufman and Standard 1987), the exoantigen test, is useful in identifying fungal cultures several days before they produce spores; here, soluble extracts of mycelium are analysed with reference reagents using Öuchterlony immunodiffusion in agar.

References

Aamodt, O., Naess, B. and Sandvik, O. (1982). Vaccination of Norwegian cattle against ringworm. *Zentralbl. Veterinärmed. B* **29**, 451–6.

Ajello, L. (1971). Distribution of *Histoplasma capsulatum* in the United States. In *Histoplasmosis. Proceedings of the Second National Conference*, ed. L. Ajello, E.W. Chick and M.L. Furcolow, pp. 103–22, C.C. Thomas, Springfield, Illinois.

Ajello, L. (1977). Systemic mycoses in modern medicine. *Contrib. Microbiol. Immunol.* **3**, 2–6.

Al-Doory, Y. and Domson, J.F. (1984). *Mould Allergy*. Lea & Febiger, Philadelphia.

Arango, M., Oropeza, F., Anderson, O., Contreras, C., Bianco, N. and Yarzábal, L.A. (1982). Circulating immune complexes and *in vitro* cell-reactivity in paracoccidioidomycosis. *Mycopathologia* **79**, 153–8.

Bäck, O., Faergemann, J. and Hörnqvist, R. (1985). *Pityrosporum* folliculitis: a common disease of the young and middle-aged. *J. Am. Acad. Dermatol.* **12**, 56–61.

Bardana, E.J. (1980a). The clinical spectrum of aspergillosis — Part 1: Epidemiology, pathogenicity, infection in animals and immunology of *Aspergillus*. *CRC Crit. Rev. Clin. Lab. Sci.* **13**, 21–83.

Bardana, E.J. (1980b). The clinical spectrum of aspergillosis — Part 2: Classification and description of saprophytic, allergic, and invasive variants of human disease. *CRC Crit. Rev. Clin. Lab. Sci.* **13**, 85–159.

Beaman, L. (1987). Fungicidal activation of murine macrophages by recombinant gamma interferon. *Infect. Immunity* **55**, 2951–5.

Beaman, L., Benjamini, E. and Pappagianis, D. (1981). Role of lymphocytes in macrophage-induced killing of *Coccidioides immitis in vitro*. *Infect. Immunity* **34**, 347–53.

Beaman, L., Benjamini, E. and Pappagianis, D. (1983). Activation of macrophages by lymphokines: enhancement of phagosome–lysosome fusion and killing of *Coccidioides immitis*. *Infect. Immunity* **39**, 1201–7.

Beemer, A.M., Kuttin, E.S. and Pinto, M. (1977). Treatment with antifungal vaccines. *Contrib. Microbiol. Immunol.* **4**, 136–46.

Belew, P.W., Rosenberg, E.W. and Jennings, B.R. (1980). Activation of the alternate pathway of complement by *Malassezia ovalis (Pityrosporum ovale)*. *Mycopathologia* **70**, 187–91.

Bergbrant, I.-M. and Faergemann, J. (1989). Seborrhoeic dermatitis and *Pityrosporum ovale*: a cultural and immunological study. *Acta Dermatol. Venereol. (Stockholm)* **69**, 332–5.

Biagnoni, L., Souza, M.J., Chamma, L.G. *et al.* (1984). Serology of paracoccidioidomycosis. II. Correlation between class-specific antibodies and clinical forms of the disease. *Trans. Roy. Soc. Med. Hyg.* **78**, 617–21.

Bottone, E.J., Salkin, I.F., Hurd, N.J. and Wormser, G.P. (1987). Serogroup distribution of *Cryptococcus neoformans* in patients with AIDS. *J. Infect. Dis.* **156**, 242.

Bouali, A., Robert, R., Tronchin, G. and Senet, J.-M. (1987). Characterization of binding of human fibrinogen to the surface of germ-tubes and mycelium of *Candida albicans*. *J. Gen. Microbiol.* **133**, 545–51.

Bradsher, R.W. (1984). Live *Blastomyces dermatitidis* yeast-induced responses of immune and nonimmune human mononuclear cells. *Mycopathologia* **87**, 159–66.

Bradsher, R.W., Balk, R.A. and Jacobs, R.F. (1987). Growth inhibition of *Blastomyces dermatitidis* in alveolar and peripheral macrophages from patients with blastomycosis. *Am. Rev. Respir. Dis.* **135**, 412–17.

Bronnimann, D.A., Adam, R.D., Galgiani, J.N. *et al.* (1987). Coccidioidomycosis in the acquired immunodeficiency syndrome. *Ann. Intern. Med.* **106**, 372–9.

Brummer, E. and Stevens, D.A. (1982). Opposite effects of human monocytes, macrophages, and polymorphonuclear neutrophils on replication of *Blastomyces dermatitidis in vitro*. *Infect. Immunity* **36**, 297–303.

Brummer, E. and Stevens, D.A. (1983). Enhancing effect of murine polymorphonuclear neutrophils (PMN) on the multiplication of *Blastomyces dermatitidis in vitro* and *in vivo*. *Clin. Exp. Immunol.* **54**, 587–94.

Brummer, E. and Stevens, D.A. (1987). Activation of pulmonary macrophages for fungicidal activity by gamma-interferon or lymphokines. *Clin. Exp. Immunol.* **70**, 520–8.

Brummer, E., Morozumi, P.A., Vo, P.T. and Stevens, D.A. (1982). Protection against pulmonary blastomycosis: adoptive transfer with T lymphocytes, but not serum, from resistant mice. *Cell. Immunol.* **74**, 349–59.

Brummer, E., Morrison, C.J. and Stevens, D.A. (1985). Recombinant and natural gamma-interferon activation of macrophages *in vitro*: different dose requirements for induction of killing activity against phagocytizable and nonphagocytizable fungi. *Infect. Immunity* **49**, 724–30.

Brummer, E., Hanson, L.H., Restrepo, A. and Stevens, D.A. (1988). *In vivo* and *in vitro* activation of pulmonary macrophages by IFN-γ for enhanced killing of *Paracoccidioides brasiliensis* or *Blastomyces dermatitidis*. *J. Immunol.* **140**, 2786–9.

Brummer, E., Hanson, L.H., Restrepo, A. and Stevens, D.A. (1989). Intracellular multiplication of *Paracoccidioides brasiliensis* in macrophages: killing and restriction of multiplication by activated macrophages. *Infect. Immunity* **57**, 2289–94.

Bullock, W.E. and Wright, S.D. (1987). Role of the adherence-promoting receptors, CR3, LFA-1, and p150,95, in binding of *Histoplasma capsulatum* by human macrophages. *J. Exp. Med.* **165**, 195–210.

Bulmer, G.S. and Sans, M.D. (1968). *Cryptococcus neoformans*. III Inhibition of phagocytosis. *J. Bacteriol.* **95**, 5–8.

Bulmer, G.S. and Tacker, J.R. (1975). Phagocytosis of *Cryptococcus neoformans* by alveolar macrophages. *Infect. Immunity* **11**, 73–9.

Burge, H.A. (1985). Fungus allergens. *Clin. Rev. Allergy* **3**, 319–29.

Bush, R.K. and Yunginger, J.W. (1987). Standardization of fungal allergens. *Clin. Rev. Allergy* **5**, 3–21.

Butcher, B.T., O'Neil, C.E., Reed, M.A., Altman, L.C., Lopez, M. and Lehrer, S.B. (1987). Basidiomycete allergy: measurement of spore-specific IgE antibodies. *J. Allergy Clin. Immunol.* **80**, 803–9.

Calderon, R.A. (1989). Immunoregulation of dermatophytosis. *CRC Crit. Rev. Microbiol.* **16**, 339–68.

Calderon, R.A. and Hay, R.J. (1987). Fungicidal activity of human neutrophils and monocytes on dermatophyte fungi, *Trichophyton quinckeanum* and *Trichophyton rubrum*. *Immunology* **61**, 289–95.

Calderon, R.A. and Shennan, G.I. (1987). Susceptibility of

Trichophyton quinckeanum and *Trichophyton rubrum* to products of oxidative metabolism. *Immunology* **61**, 283–8.

Calderon, R.A., Hay, R.J. and Shennan, G.I. (1987). Circulating antigens and antibodies in human and mouse dermatophytosis: use of monoclonal antibodies reactive to phosphorylcholine-like epitopes. *J. Gen. Microbiol.* **133**, 2699–705.

Caldwell, C.W. and Sprouse, R.F. (1982). Iron and host resistance in histoplasmosis. *Am. Rev. Respir. Dis.* **125**, 674–7.

Calich, V.L.G., Kipnis, T.L., Mariano, M., Fava Neto, C. and da Silva, W.D. (1979). The activation of the complement system by *Paracoccidioides brasiliensis in vitro*: its opsonic effect and possible significance for an *in vivo* model of infection. *Clin. Immunol. Immunopathol.* **12**, 20–30.

Catanzaro, A. (1981). Suppressor cells in coccidioidomycosis. *Cell. Immunol.* **64**, 235–45.

Cauley, L.K. and Murphy, J.W. (1979). Response of congenitally athymic (nude) and phenotypically normal mice to *Cryptococcus neoformans* infection. *Infect. Immunity* **23**, 644–51.

Cherniak, R. (1988). Soluble polysaccharides of *Cryptococcus neoformans*. *Curr. Topics Med. Mycol.* **2**, 40–54.

Chilgren, R.A., Meuwissen, H.J., Quie, P.G. and Hong, R. (1967). Chronic mucocutaneous candidiasis, deficiency of delayed hypersensitivity, and selective local antibody defect. *Lancet* **ii**, 688–93.

Chilgren, R.A., Quie, P.G., Meuwissen, H.J., Good, R.A. and Hong, R. (1969). The cellular immune defect in chronic mucocutaneous candidiasis. *Lancet* **i**, 1286–8.

Clemons, K.V., Leathers, C.R. and Lee, K.W. (1985). Systemic *Coccidioides immitis* infection in nude and beige mice. *Infect. Immunity* **47**, 814–21.

Conti-Díaz, I.A. (1972). Skin tests with paracoccidioidin and their importance. *Sci. Publ. Pan Am. Health Org.* **254**, 197–202.

Cox, R.A. (1979). Immunologic studies of patients with histoplasmosis. *Am. Rev. Respir. Dis.* **120**, 143–9.

Cox, R.A. (ed.) (1989a). *Immunology of the Fungal Diseases*. CRC Press, Boca Raton, Florida.

Cox, R.A. (1989b). Coccidioidomycosis. In *Immunology of the Fungal Diseases*, ed. R.A. Cox, pp. 165–97, CRC Press, Boca Raton, Florida.

Cox, R.A. and Pope, R.M. (1987). Serum-mediated suppression of lymphocyte transformation responses in coccidioidomycosis. *Infect. Immunity* **55**, 1058–62.

Cox, R.A., Mills, L.R., Best, G.K. and Denton, J.F. (1974). Histologic reactions to cell walls of an avirulent and a virulent strain of *Blastomyces dermatitidis*. *J. Infect. Dis.* **129**, 179–86.

Cox, R.A., Baker, B.S. and Stevens, D.A. (1982). Specificity of immunoglobulin E in coccidioidomycosis and correlation with disease involvement. *Infect. Immunity* **37**, 609–16.

Cox, R.A., Pope, R.M. and Stevens, D.A. (1983). Immune complexes in coccidioidomycosis: correlation with disease involvement. *Am. Rev. Respir. Dis.* **126**, 439–43.

Cozad, G.C. and Chang, C.-T. (1980). Cell-mediated immunoprotection in blastomycosis. *Infect. Immunity* **28**, 398–403.

Csato, M., Kenderessy, A.S. and Dobozy, A. (1987). Enhancement of *Candida albicans* killing activity of separated human epidermal cells by ultraviolet radiation. *Br. J. Dermatol.* **116**, 469–75.

Cunningham, K.M., Bulmer, G.S. and Rhoades, E.R. (1979). Phagocytosis and intracellular fate of *Sporothrix schenckii*. *J. Infect. Dis.* **140**, 815–17.

DaMert, G.J., Kirkpatrick, C.H. and Sohnle, P.G. (1980). Comparison of antibody responses in chronic mucocutaneous candidiasis and tinea versicolor. *Int. Arch. Allergy Appl. Immunol.* **63**, 97–104.

Davies, R.R., Ganderton, M.A. and Savage, M.A. (1983). Human nail dust and precipitating antibodies to *Trichophyton rubrum* in chiropodists. *Clin. Allergy* **13**, 309–15.

Davies, S.F., Clifford, D.P., Hoidal, J.R. and Repine, J.E. (1982). Opsonic requirements for the uptake of *Cryptococcus neoformans* by human polymorphonuclear leukocytes and monocytes. *J. Infect. Dis.* **145**, 870–4.

de Albornoz, M.B., Mendoza, M. and de Torres, E.D. (1986). Growth temperatures of isolates of *Sporothrix schenckii* from disseminated and fixed cutaneous lesions of sporotrichosis. *Mycopathologia* **95**, 81–3.

Deepe, G.S. (1989). Blastomycosis. In *Immunology of the Fungal Diseases*, ed. R.A. Cox, pp. 139–63, CRC Press, Boca Raton, Florida.

Deepe, G.S., Taylor, C.L. and Bullock, W.E. (1985). Evolution of inflammatory response and cellular immune responses in a murine model of disseminated blastomycosis. *Infect. Immunity* **50**, 183–9.

Diamond, R.D. and Bennett, J.E. (1974). Prognostic factors in cryptococcal meningitis: a study in 111 cases. *Ann. Intern. Med.* **80**, 176–81.

Diamond, R.D. and Erickson, N.F. (1982). Chemotaxis of human neutrophils and monocytes induced by *Cryptococcus neoformans*. *Infect. Immunity* **38**, 380–2.

Diamond, R.D. and Krzesicki, R. (1978). Mechanisms of attachment of neutrophils to *Candida albicans* psuedohyphae in the absence of serum, and of subsequent damage to pseudohyphae by microbicidal processes *in vitro*. *J. Clin. Invest.* **61**, 360–9.

Diamond, R.D., Root, R.K. and Bennett, J.E. (1972). Factors influencing killing of *Cryptococcus neoformans* by human leukocytes *in vitro*. *J. Infect. Dis.* **125**, 367–76.

Diamond, R.D., May, J.E., Kane, M.A., Frank, M.M. and Bennett, J.E. (1974). The role of the classical and alternate complement pathways in host defenses against *Cryptococcus neoformans* infection. *J. Immunol.* **112**, 2260–70.

Diamond, R.D., Krzesicki, R., Epstein, B. and Jao, W. (1978a). Damage to hyphal forms of fungi by human leukocytes *in vitro*: a possible host defense mechanism in aspergillosis and mucormycosis. *Am. J. Pathol.* **91**, 313–28.

Diamond, R.D., Krzesicki, R. and Jao, W. (1978b). Damage to pseudohyphal forms of *Candida albicans* by neutrophils in the absence of serum *in vitro*. *J. Clin. Invest.* **61**, 349–59.

Diamond, R.D., Clark, R.A. and Haudenschild, C.C. (1980). Damage to *Candida albicans* hyphae and pseudohyphae by the myeloperoxidase system and oxidative products of neutrophil metabolism *in vitro*. *J. Clin. Invest.* **66**, 908–17.

Diamond, R.D., Haudenschild, C.C. and Erickson, N.F. (1982). Monocyte-mediated damage to *Rhizopus oryzae in vitro*. *Infect. Immunity* **38**, 292–7.

Diamond, R.D., Huber, E. and Haudenschild, C.C. (1983). Mechanisms of destruction of *Aspergillus fumigatus* hyphae mediated by human monocytes. *J. Infect. Dis.* **147**, 474–83.

Dickerson, C.L., Taylor, R.L. and Drutz, D.J. (1983). Susceptibility of congenitally athymic (nude) mice to sporotrichosis. *Infect. Immunity* **40**, 417–20.

Djeu, J.Y. and Blanchard, D.K. (1987). Regulation of human

polymorphonuclear neutrophil (PMN) activity against *Candida albicans* by large granular lymphocytes via release of a PMN-activating factor. *J. Immunol.* **139**, 2761–7.

Djeu, J.Y., Blanchard, D.K., Halkias, D. and Friedman, H. (1986). Growth inhibition of *Candida albicans* by human polymorphonuclear neutrophils: activation by interferon-γ and tumor necrosis factor. *J. Immunol.* **137**, 2980–4.

Domer, J.E. and Carrow, E.W. (1989). Candidiasis. In *Immunology of the Fungal Diseases*, ed. R.A. Cox, pp. 57–92, CRC Press, Boca Raton, Florida.

Dromer, F., Charreire, J., Contrepois, A., Carbon, C. and Yeni, P. (1987). Protection of mice against experimental cryptococcosis by anti-*Cryptococcus neoformans* monoclonal antibody. *Infect. Immunity* **55**, 749–52.

Drouhet, E. and Segretain, G. (1951). Inhibition de la migration leucocytaire *in vitro* par un polyoside capsulaire de *Torulopsis (Cryptococcus) neoformans*. *Ann. Inst. Pasteur* **81**, 674–6.

Drutz, D.J. and Catanzaro, A. (1978). Coccidioidomycosis. *Am. Rev. Respir. Dis.* **117**, 559–85, 727–71.

Drutz, D.J. and Frey, C.L. (1985). Intracellular and extracellular defenses of human phagocytes against *Blastomyces dermatitidis* conidia and yeasts. *J. Lab. Clin. Med.* **105**, 737–50.

Drutz, D.J. and Huppert, M. (1983). Coccidioidomycosis: factors affecting the host–parasite interaction. *J. Infect. Dis.* **147**, 372–90.

Dumont, A. and Robert, A. (1970). Electron microscopic study of phagocytosis of *Histoplasma capsulatum* by hamster peritoneal macrophages. *Lab. Invest.* **23**, 278–86.

Edwards, J.E., Lehrer, R.I., Stiehm, E.R., Fischer, T.J. and Young, L.S. (1978). Severe candidal infections: clinical perspective, immune defense mechanisms, and current concepts of therapy. *Ann. Intern. Med.* **89**, 91–106.

Edwards, J.E., Gaither, T.A., O'Shea, J.J. *et al.* (1986). Expression of specific binding sites on *Candida* with functional and antigenic characteristics of human complement receptors. *J. Immunol.* **137**, 3577–83.

Edwards, L.B., Acquaviva, F.A., Livesay, V.T., Cross, F.W. and Palmer, C.E. (1969). An atlas of sensitivity to tuberculin, PPD-B, and histoplasmin in the United States. *Am. Rev. Respir. Dis.* **99** (suppl.), 1–132.

Eigentler, A., Schulz, T.F., Larcher, C. *et al.* (1989). C3bi-binding protein on *Candida albicans*: temperature-dependent expression and relationship to human complement receptor type 3. *Infect. Immunity* **57**, 616–22.

Eissenberg, L.G. and Goldman, W.E. (1987). *Histoplasma capsulatum* fails to trigger release of superoxide from macrophages. *Infect. Immunity* **55**, 29–34.

Ellis, D.H. and Pfeiffer, T.J. (1990). Natural habitat of *Cryptococcus neoformans* var. *gattii*. *J. Clin. Microbiol.* **28**, 1642–4.

Faergemann, J. (1983). Antibodies to *Pityrosporum orbiculare* in patients with tinea versicolor and controls of various ages. *J. Invest. Dermatol.* **80**, 133–5.

Faergemann, J., Johansson, S., Bäck, O. and Scheynius, A. (1986). An immunologic and cultural study of *Pityrosporum* folliculitis. *J. Am. Acad. Dermatol.* **14**, 429–33.

Fink, J.N. (1984). Hypersensitivity pneumonitis. *J. Allergy Clin. Immunol.* **74**, 1–9.

Fischer, A., Ballet, J.-J. and Griscelli, C. (1978). Specific inhibition of *in vitro Candida*-induced lymphocyte proliferation by polysaccharidic antigens present in the serum of patients with chronic mucocutaneous candidiasis. *J. Clin. Invest.* **62**, 1005–13.

Fischer, A., Pichat, L., Audinot, M. and Griscelli, C. (1982). Defective handling of mannan by monocytes in patients with chronic mucocutaneous candidiasis resulting in a specific cellular unresponsiveness. *Clin. Exp. Immunol.* **47**, 653–60.

Flesch, I.E.A., Schwamberger, G. and Kaufmann, S.H.E. (1989). Fungicidal activity of IFN-γ-activated macrophages: extracellular killing of *Cryptococcus neoformans*. *J. Immunol.* **142**, 3219–24.

Frey, C.L. and Drutz, D.J. (1986). Influence of fungal surface components on the interaction of *Coccidioides immitis* with polymorphonuclear neutrophils. *J. Infect. Dis.* **153**, 933–43.

Friedman, L. and Derbes, V.J. (1960). The question of immunity in ringworm infections. *Ann. NY Acad. Sci.* **89**, 178–83.

Furcolow, M.L., Chick, E.W., Busey, J.D. and Menges, R.W. (1970). Prevalence and incidence studies of human and canine blastomycosis. I. Cases in the United States, 1885–1968. *Am. Rev. Respir. Dis.* **102**, 60–7.

Galgiani, J.N. (1986). Inhibition of different phases of *Coccidioides immitis* by human neutrophils or hydrogen peroxide. *J. Infect. Dis.* **153**, 217–22.

Ganz, T., Selsted, M.E., Szklarek, D. *et al.* (1985). Defensins: natural peptide antibiotics of human neutrophils. *J. Clin. Invest.* **76**, 1427–35.

Goihman-Yahr, M., Essenfeld-Yahr, E., de Albornoz, M.C. *et al.* (1980). Defect of *in vitro* digestive ability of polymorphonuclear leukocytes in paracoccidioidomycosis. *Infect. Immunity* **28**, 557–66.

Goldstein, D.M. and Louie, S. (1943). Primary pulmonary coccidioidomycosis: report of an epidemic of seventy-five cases. *War Med. (Chicago).* **4**, 299–317.

Gomez, A.M., Bullock, W.E., Taylor, C.L. and Deepe, G.S. (1988). Role of L3T4$^+$ T cells in host defense against *Histoplasma capsulatum*. *Infect. Immunity* **56**, 1685–91.

Goodwin, R.A. and Des Prez, R.M. (1978). Histoplasmosis. *Am. Rev. Respir. Dis.* **117**, 929–56.

Goren, M.B. (1967). Experimental murine cryptococcosis: effect of hyperimmunization to capsular polysaccharide. *J. Immunol.* **98**, 914–22.

Granger, D.L., Perfect, J.R. and Durack, D.T. (1985). Virulence of *Cryptococcus neoformans*: regulation of capsule synthesis by carbon dioxide. *J. Clin. Invest.* **76**, 508–16.

Granger, D.L., Perfect, J.R. and Durack, D.T. (1986). Macrophage-mediated fungistasis: requirement for a macromolecular component in serum. *J. Immunol.* **137**, 693–701.

Grappel, S.F., Bishop, C.T. and Blank, F. (1974). Immunology of dermatophytes and dermatophytosis. *Bacteriol. Rev.* **38**, 222–50.

Graybill, J.R. and Drutz, D.J. (1978). Host defenses in cryptococcosis. II. Cryptococcosis in the nude mouse. *Cell. Immunol.* **40**, 263–74.

Green, F. and Balish, E. (1979). Suppression of *in vitro* lymphocyte transformation during an experimental dermatophyte infection. *Infect. Immunity* **26**, 554–62.

Green, F., Anderson, J.W. and Balish, E. (1980). Cutaneous basophil hypersensitivity and contact sensitivity after cutaneous *Trichophyton mentagrophytes* infection. *Infect. Immunity* **29**, 758–67.

Green, F., Weber, J.K. and Balish, E. (1983). The thymus dependency of acquired resistance to *Trichophyton mentagrophytes* dermatophytosis in rats. *J. Invest. Dermatol.* **81**, 31–8.

Green, F., Weber, J.K. and Balish, E. (1987). Acquired immunity to *Trichophyton mentagrophytes* in thymus-grafted or peritoneal exudate cell-injected nude rats. *J. Invest. Dermatol.* **88**, 345–9.

Groisser, D., Bottone, E.J. and Lebwohl, M. (1989). Association of *Pityrosporum orbiculare (Malassezia furfur)* with seborrheic dermatitis in patients with acquired immunodeficiency syndrome (AIDS). *J. Am. Acad. Dermatol.* **20**, 770–3.

Håkansson, C., Faergemann, J. and Löwhagen, G.-B. (1988). Studies on the lipophilic yeast *Pityrosporum ovale* in HIV-seropositive and HIV-seronegative homosexual men. *Acta Dermatol. Venereol. (Stockholm)* **68**, 422–6.

Hancock, G.E., Kaplan, G. and Cohn, Z.A. (1988). Keratinocyte growth regulation by the products of immune cells. *J. Exp. Med.* **168**, 1395–402.

Hanifin, J.M., Ray, L.F. and Lobitz, W C. (1974). Immunological reactivity in dermatophytosis *Br. J. Dermatol.* **90**, 1–8.

Hay, R.J. (1982). Chronic dermatophyte infections. I. Clinical and mycological features. *Br. J. Dermatol.* **106**, 1–7.

Hay, R.J. (1988). Tinea imbricata. *Curr. Topics Med. Mycol.* **2**, 55–72.

Hay, R.J. and Brostoff, J. (1977). Immune responses in patients with chronic *Trichophyton rubrum* infections. *Clin. Exp. Dermatol.* **2**. 373–80.

Hay, R.J., Calderon, R.A. and Collins, M.J. (1983a). Experimental dermatophytosis: the clinical and histopathologic features of a mouse model using *Trichophyton quinckeanum* (mouse favus). *J. Invest. Dermatol.* **81**, 270–4.

Hay, R.J., Reid, S., Talwat, E. and Macnamara, K. (1983b). Immune responses of patients with tinea imbricata. *Br. J. Dermatol.* **108**, 581–6.

Heidenreich, F. and Dierich, M.P. (1985). *Candida albicans* and *Candida stellatoidea*, in contrast to other *Candida* species, bind iC3b and C3d but not C3b. *Infect. Immunity* **50**, 598–600.

Hidore, M.R. and Murphy, J.W. (1986). Correlation of natural killer activity and clearance of *Cryptococcus neoformans* from mice after adoptive transfer of splenic nylon wool-non-adherent cells. *Infect. Immunity* **51**, 547–55.

Higgs, J.M. and Wells, R.S. (1972). Chronic mucocutaneous candidiasis: associated abnormalities of iron metabolism. *Br. J. Dermatol.* **86**, (suppl. 8), 88–102.

Hiruma, M., Yamaji, K., Shimizu, T., Ohata, H. and Kukita, A. (1988). Ultrastructural study of tissue reaction of mice against *Sporothrix schenckii* infection. *Arch. Dermatol. Res.* **280**, S94–S100.

Hopfer, R.L., Grappel, S.F. and Blank, F. (1975). Antibodies with affinity for epithelial tissue in chronic dermatophytosis. *Dermatologica* **151**, 135–43.

Hostetter, M.K., Lorenz, J.S., Preus, L. and Kendrick, K.E. (1990). The iC3b receptor on *Candida albicans*: subcellular location and modulation of receptor expression by glucose. *J, Infect. Dis.* **161**, 761–8.

Howard, D.H. (1973). Fate of *Histoplasma capsulatum* in guinea pig polymorphonuclear leukocytes. *Infect. Immunity* **8**, 412–19.

Howard, D.H. (1975). The role of phagocytic mechanisms in defense against *Histoplasma capsulatum*. *Sci. Publ. Pan Am. Health Org.* **304**, 50–7.

Howard, D.H. and Otto, V. (1977). Experiments on lymphocyte-mediated cellular immunity in murine histoplasmosis. *Infect. Immunity* **16**, 226–31.

Hsiao, C.B., Lehmann, P.F. and Boyle, M.D.P. (1990). Plasmin-binding by *Candida albicans*. In *Second Conference on Candida and Candidiasis: Biology, Pathogenesis and Management, Philadelphia*. Abstract B3, American Society for Microbiology, Washington.

Hunjan, B.S. and Cronholm, L.S. (1979). An animal model for cell-mediated immune responses to dermatophytes. *J. Allergy Clin. Immunol.* **63**, 361–9.

Imamura, S., Tanaka, M. and Watanabe, S. (1975). Use of immunofluorescence staining in kerion. *Arch. Dermatol.* **111**, 906–9.

Jacobs, R.F., Marmer, D.J., Balk, R.A. and Bradsher, R.W. (1985). Lymphocyte subpopulations of blood and alveolar lavage in blastomycosis. *Chest* **88**, 579–85.

Jillson, O.F. and Huppert, M. (1949). The immediate wheal and the 24–48 hour tuberculin type edematous reactions to trichophytin. *J. Invest. Dermatol.* **12**, 179–85.

Jimenez, B.E. and Murphy, J.W. (1984). *In vitro* effects of natural killer cells against *Paracoccidioides brasiliensis* yeast phase. *Infect. Immunity* **46**, 552–8.

Jimenez-Finkel, B. and Restrepo-Moreno, A. (1989). Paracoccidioidomycosis. In *Immunology of the Fungal Diseases*, ed. R.A. Cox, pp. 227–47, CRC Press, Boca Raton, Florida.

Jones, H.E. (1980). The atopic-chronic-dermatophytosis syndrome. *Acta Dermatol. Venereol. (Stockholm)* **92** (suppl.), 81–5.

Jones, H.E., Reinhardt, J.H. and Rinaldi, M.G. (1973). A clinical, mycological, and immunological survey for dermatophytosis. *Arch. Dermatol.* **108**, 61–5.

Jones, H.E., Reinhardt, J.H. and Rinaldi, M.G. (1974). Immunologic susceptibility to chronic dermatophytosis. *Arch. Dermatol.* **110**, 213–20.

Kalina, M., Kletter, Y. and Aronson, M. (1974). The interaction of phagocytes and the large-sized parasite *Cryptococcus neoformans*: cytochemical and ultrastructural study. *Cell Tissue Res.* **152**, 165–74.

Karbassi, A., Becker, J.M., Foster, J.S. and Moore, R.N. (1987). Enhanced killing of *Candida albicans* by murine macrophages treated with macrophage colony-stimulating factor: evidence for augmented expression of mannose receptors. *J. Immunol.* **139**, 417–21.

Kaufman, L. and Reiss, E. (1986). Serodiagnosis of fungal diseases. In *Manual of Clinical Laboratory Immunology*, 3rd edn, ed. N.R. Rose, H. Friedman and J.L. Fahey, pp. 446–66, American Society for Microbiology, Washington, D.C.

Kaufman, L. and Standard, P.G. (1987). Specific and rapid identification of medically important fungi by exoantigen detection. *Ann. Rev. Microbiol.* **41**, 209–25.

Kaufman, L., Terry, R.T., Schubert, J.H. and McLaughlin, D. (1967). Effects of a single histoplasmin skin test on the serological diagnosis of histoplasmosis. *J. Bacteriol.* **94**, 798–803.

Kerbs, S., Greenberg, J. and Jesrani, K. (1977). Temporal correlation of lymphocyte blastogenesis, skin test responses and erythema during dermatophyte infections. *Clin. Exp. Immunol.* **27**, 526–30.

King, R.D., Khan, H.A., Foye, J.C., Greenberg, J.H. and Jones, H.E. (1975). Transferrin, iron, and dermatophytes. I. Serum dermatophyte inhibitory component definitively identified as unsaturated transferrin. *J. Lab. Clin. Med.* **86**, 204–12.

Kirkpatrick, C.H., Rich, R.R. and Bennett, J.E. (1971). Chronic mucocutaneous candidiasis: model-building in cellular immunity. *Ann. Intern. Med.* **74**, 955–78.

Klein, B.S., Vergeront, J.M., Kaufman, L. *et al.* (1987). Serological tests for blastomycosis: assessments during a large point-source outbreak in Wisconsin. *J. Infect. Dis.* **155**, 262–8.

Klotz, S.A., Drutz, D.J., Huppert, M., Sun, S.H. and DeMarsh, P.L. (1984). The critical role of CO_2 in the morphogenesis of *Coccidioides immitis* in cell-free subcutaneous chambers. *J. Infect. Dis.* **150**, 127–34.

Kolotila, M.P. and Diamond, R.D. (1988). Stimulation of neutrophil actin polymerization and degranulation by opsonized and unopsonized *Candida albicans* hyphae and zymosan. *Infect. Immunity* **56**, 2016–22.

Kolotila, M.P. and Diamond, R.D. (1990). Effects of neutrophils and *in vitro* oxidants on survival and phenotypic switching of *Candida albicans* WO-1. *Infect. Immunity* **58**, 1174–9.

Kozel, T.R. (1983). Dissociation of a hydrophobic surface from phagocytosis of encapsulated and non-encapsulated *Cryptococcus neoformans*. *Infect. Immunity* **39**, 1214–19.

Kozel, T.R. and Cazin, J. (1971). Nonencapsulated variant of *Cryptococcus neoformans*. I. Virulence studies and characterization of soluble polysaccharide. *Infect. Immunity* **3**, 287–94.

Kozel, T.R. and McGaw, T.G. (1979). Opsonization of *Cryptococcus neoformans* by human immunoglobulin G: role of immunoglobulin G in phagocytosis by macrophages. *Infect. Immunity* **25**, 255–61.

Kozel, T.R. and Mastroianni, R.P. (1976). Inhibition of phagocytosis by cryptococcal polysaccharide: dissociation of the attachment and ingestion phases of phagocytosis. *Infect. Immunity* **14**, 62–7.

Kozel, T.R., Wilson, M.A., Pfrommer, G.S.T. and Schlageter, A.M. (1989). Activation and binding of opsonic fragments of C3 on encapsulated *Cryptococcus neoformans* by using an alternative complement pathway reconstituted from six isolated proteins. *Infect. Immunity* **57**, 1922–7.

Kudelko, N.M. (1971). Allergy in chronic monilial vaginitis. *Ann. Allergy* **29**, 266–7.

Kuttin, E.S., Beemer, A.M. and Pinto, M. (1980). Vaccination of geese suffering from candidosis. In *Human and Animal Mycology, Proceedings of the Seventh Congress of ISHAM, Jerusalem, Israel, March 11–16, 1979*, ed. E.S. Kuttin and G.L. Baum, pp. 64–7, Excerpta Medica, Amsterdam.

Kwon-Chung, K.J. (1979). Comparison of isolates of *Sporothrix schenckii* obtained from fixed cutaneous lesions with isolates from other types of lesions. *J. Infect. Dis.* **139**, 424–31.

Kwon-Chung, K.J. and Bennett, J.E. (1984). Epidemiologic differences between the two varieties of *Cryptococcus neoformans*. *Am. J. Epidemiol.* **120**, 123–30.

Laxalt, K.A. and Kozel, T.R. (1979). Chemotaxigenesis and activation of the alternative complement pathway by encapsulated and non-encapsulated *Cryptococcus neoformans*. *Infect. Immunity* **26**, 435–40.

Legendre, A.M. and Becker, P.U. (1982). Immunologic changes in acute canine blastomycosis. *Am. J. Vet. Res.* **43**, 2050–3.

Legendre, A.M., Walker, M., Buyukmihci, N. and Stevens, R. (1981). Canine blastomycosis: a review of 47 clinical cases. *J. Am. Vet. Med. Assoc.* **178**, 1163–8.

Lehmann, P.F. (1985). Immunology of fungal infections in animals. *Vet. Immunol. Immunopathol.* **10**, 33–69.

Lehmann, P.F. and White, L.O. (1976). Acquired immunity to *Aspergillus fumigatus*. *Infect. Immunity* **13**, 1296–8.

Lehmann, P.F., Gibbons, J., Senitzer, D., Ribner, B.S. and Freimer, E.H. (1983). T lymphocyte abnormalities in disseminated histoplasmosis. *Am. J. Med.* **75**, 790–4.

Lehmann, P.F., Sawyer, T. and Donabedian, H. (1989). Novel abnormality in subpopulations of circulating lymphocytes: $T\gamma\delta$ and $CD2^-$, 3^+, 4^-, 8^- lymphocytes in histoplasmosis-associated immunodeficiency. *Int. Arch. Allergy Appl. Immunol.* **90**, 213–18.

Lehrer, R.I. and Jan, R.G. (1970). Interaction of *Aspergillus fumigatus* spores with human leukocytes and serum. *Infect. Immunity* **1**, 345–50.

Lepper, A.W.D. (1969). Immunological aspects of dermatomycoses in animals and man. *Rev. Med. Vet. Mycol.* **6**, 435–46.

Levitz, S.M. and DiBenedetto, D.J. (1988). Differential stimulation of murine resident peritoneal cells by selectively opsonized encapsulated and acapsular *Cryptococcus neoformans*. *Infect. Immunity* **56**, 2544–51.

Levitz, S.M., Lyman, C.A., Murata, T., Sullivan, J.A., Mandell, G.L. and Diamond, R.D. (1987). Cytosolic calcium changes in individual neutrophils stimulated by opsonized and unopsonized *Candida albicans* hyphae. *Infect. Immunity* **55**, 2783–8.

Lim, T.S. and Murphy, J.W. (1980). Transfer of immunity to cryptococcosis by T-enriched splenic lymphocytes from *Cryptococcus neoformans*-sensitized mice. *Infect. Immunity* **30**, 5–11.

Loose, D.S., Stover, E.P., Restrepo, A., Stevens, D.A. and Feldman, D. (1983). Estradiol binds to a receptor-like cytosol binding protein and initiates a biological response in *Paracoccidioides brasiliensis*. *Proc. Nat. Acad. Sci. (USA)* **80**, 7659–63.

Lopez, M. and Salvaggio, J.E. (1985). Mold-sensitive asthma. *Clin. Rev. Allergy* **3**, 183–96.

Lopez, M. and Salvaggio, J.E. (1987). Epidemiology of hypersensitivity pneumonitis/allergic alveolitis. *Monog. Allergy* **21**, 70–86.

Lynch, P.J., Voorhees, J.J. and Harrell, E.R. (1970). Systemic sporotrichosis. *Ann. Intern. Med.* **73**, 23–30.

McEwen, J.G., Sugar, A.M., Brummer, E., Restrepo, A. and Stevens, D.A. (1984). Toxic effects of products of oxidative metabolism on the yeast form of *Paracoccidioides brasiliensis*. *J. Med. Microbiol.* **18**, 423–8.

Macher, A.M., Bennett, J.E., Gadek, J.E. and Frank, M.M. (1978). Complement depletion in cryptococcal sepsis. *J. Immunol.* **120**, 1686–90.

MacLennan, R. (1972). The trichophytin test in chronic tinea imbricata. *Papua New Guinea Med. J.* **15**, 201–2.

Marquis, G., Montplaisir, S., Pelletier, M., Mousseau, S. and Auger, P. (1985). Genetic resistance to murine cryptococcosis: increased susceptibility in the CBA/N XID mutant strain of mice. *Infect. Immunity* **47**, 282–7.

Mathur, S., Goust, J.-M., Horger, E.O. and Fudenberg, H.H. (1977). Immunoglobulin E anti-*Candida* antibodies and candidiasis. *Infect. Immunity* **18**, 257–9.

Mendes, E. and Raphael, A. (1971). Impaired delayed hypersensitivity in patients with South American blastomycosis. *J. Allergy* **47**, 17–22.

Mendes, N.F., Musatti, C.C., Leão, R.C., Mendes, E. and Naspitz, C.K. (1971). Lymphocyte cultures and skin allograft survival in patients with South American blastomycosis. *J. Allergy Clin. Immunol.* **48**, 40–5.

Merkow, L.P., Epstein, S.M., Sidransky, H., Verney, E. and Pardo, M. (1971). The pathogenesis of experimental pulmonary aspergillosis: an ultrastructural study of alveolar macrophages after phagocytosis of *A. flavus* spores *in vivo*. *Am. J. Pathol.* **62**, 57–74.

Miller, G.P.G. and Puck, J. (1984). *In vitro* human lymphocyte responses to *Cryptococcus neoformans*: evidence for primary and secondary responses in normals and infected subjects. *J. Immunol.* **133**, 166–72.

Miller, R.I. (1981). Treatment of equine phycomycosis by immunotherapy and surgery. *Aust. Vet. J.* **57**, 377–82.

Miller, R.I., Wold, D., Lindsay, W.A. *et al.* (1983). Complications associated with immunotherapy of equine phycomycosis. *J. Am. Vet. Med. Assoc.* **182**, 1227–9.

Miyaji, M. and Nishimura, K. (1983). Granuloma formation and killing functions of granuloma in congenitally athymic nude mice infected with *Blastomyces dermatitidis* and *Paracoccidioides brasiliensis*. *Mycopathologia* **82**, 129–41.

Modlin, R.L., Segal, G.P., Hofman, F.M. *et al.* (1985). *In situ* localization of T lymphocytes in disseminated coccidioidomycosis. *J. Infect. Dis.* **151**, 314–19.

Mody, C.H., Lipscomb, M.F., Street, N.E. and Toews, G.B. (1990). Depletion of CD4$^+$ (L3T4$^+$) lymphocytes *in vivo* impairs murine host defense to *Cryptococcus neoformans*. *J. Immunol.* **144**, 1472–7.

Mohr, J.A., Muchmore, H.G. and Tacker, R. (1974). Stimulation of phagocytosis of *Cryptococcus neoformans* in human cryptococcal meningitis. *J. Reticuloendothelial Soc.* **15**, 149–54.

Mok, P.W.Y. and Greer, D.L. (1977). Cell-mediated immune responses in patients with paracoccidioidomycosis. *Clin. Exp. Immunol.* **28**, 89–98.

Morelli, R. and Rosenberg, L.T. (1971). Role of complement during experimental *Candida* infection in mice. *Infect. Immunity* **3**, 521–3.

Morozumi, P.A., Halpern, J.W. and Stevens, D.A. (1981a). Susceptibility differences of inbred strains of mice to blastomycosis. *Infect. Immunity* **32**, 160–8.

Morozumi, P.A., Brummer, E. and Stevens, D.A. (1981b). Strain differences in resistance to infection reversed by route of challenge: studies in blastomycosis. *Infect. Immunity* **34**, 623–5.

Morrison, C.J., Brummer, E. and Stevens, D.A. (1989). *In vivo* activation of peripheral blood polymorphonuclear neutrophils by gamma interferon results in enhanced fungal killing. *Infect. Immunity* **57**, 2953–8.

Murphy, J.W. (1989). Cryptococcosis. In *Immunology of the Fungal Diseases*, ed. R.A. Cox, pp. 93–138, CRC Press, Boca Raton, Florida.

Murphy, J.W. and Cox, R.A. (1988). Induction of antigen-specific suppression by circulating *Cryptococcus neoformans* antigen. *Clin. Exp. Immunol.* **73**, 174–80.

Murphy, J.W. and McDaniel, D.O. (1982). *In vitro* reactivity of natural killer (NK) cells against *Cryptococcus neoformans*. *J. Immunol.* **128**, 1577–83.

Musatti, C.C., Rezkallah, M.T., Mendes, E. and Mendes, N.F. (1976). *In vivo* and *in vitro* evaluation of cell-mediated immunity in patients with paracoccidioidomycosis. *Cell. Immunol.* **24**, 365–78.

Newberry, W.M., Chandler, J.W., Chin, T.D.Y. and Kirkpatrick, C.H. (1968). Immunology of the mycoses. I. Depressed lymphocyte transformation in chronic histoplasmosis. *J. Immunol.* **100**, 436–43.

Newman, S.L., Bucher, C., Rhodes, J. and Bullock, W.E. (1990). Phagocytosis of *Histoplasma capsulatum* yeasts and microconidia by human cultured macrophages and alveolar macrophages: cellular cytoskeleton requirement for attachment and ingestion. *J. Clin. Invest.* **85**, 223–30.

Nishimura, K. and Miyagi, M. (1979). Histopathological studies on experimental cryptococcosis in nude mice. *Mycopathologia* **68**, 145–53.

Nishimura, K. and Miyagi, M. (1981). Defense mechanisms of mice against *Fonsecaea pedrosoi* infection. *Mycopathologia* **76**, 155–66.

Nishimura, K. and Miyagi, M. (1983). Defense mechanisms of mice against *Exophiala dermatitidis* infection. *Mycopathologia* **81**, 9–21.

Odds, F.C. (1988). *Candida and Candidosis*, 2nd edn, Baillière Tindall, London.

Ollert, M.W., Wadsworth, E. and Calderone, R.A. (1990). Reduced expression of the functionally active complement receptor for iC3b but not for C3d on an avirulent mutant of *Candida albicans*. *Infect. Immunity* **58**, 909–13.

O'Neil, C.E., Reed, M.A., Hughes, J.M., Butcher, B.T. and Lehrer, S.B. (1987). *Fusarium solani*: evidence for common antigenic/allergenic determinants with other Fungi Imperfecti. *Clin. Allergy* **17**, 127–33.

Opelz, G. and Scheer, M.I. (1975). Cutaneous sensitivity and *in vitro* responsiveness of lymphocytes in patients with disseminated coccidioidomycosis. *J. Infect. Dis.* **132**, 250–5.

Page, S. and Odds, F.C. (1988). Binding of plasma proteins to *Candida* species *in vitro*. *J. Gen. Microbiol.* **134**, 2693–702.

Paterson, P.Y., Semo, R., Blumenschein, G. and Swelstad, J. (1971). Mucocutaneous candidiasis, anergy and a plasma inhibitor of cellular immunity: reversal after amphotericin B therapy. *Clin. Exp. Immunol.* **9**, 595–602.

Patiño, M.M., Williams, D., Ahrens, J. and Graybill, J.R. (1987). Experimental histoplasmosis in the beige mouse. *J. Leukocyte Biol.* **41**, 228–35.

Payan, D.G., Wheat, L.J., Brahmi, Z. *et al.* (1984). Changes in immunoregulatory lymphocyte populations in patients with histoplasmosis. *J. Clin. Immunol.* **4**, 98–107.

Perfect, J.R., Granger, D.L. and Durack, D.T. (1987). Effects of antifungal agents and γ interferon on macrophage cytotoxicity for fungi and tumor cells. *J. Infect. Dis.* **156**, 316–23.

Petkus, A.F. and Baum, L.L. (1987). Natural killer cell inhibition of young spherules and endospores of *Coccidioides immitis*. *J. Immunol.* **139**, 3107–11.

Plouffe, J.F., Silva, J., Fekety, R., Reinhalter, E. and Browne, R. (1979). Cell-mediated immune responses in sporotrichosis. *J. Infect. Dis.* **139**, 152–8.

Podzorski, R.P., Gray, G.R. and Nelson, R.D. (1990). Different effects of native *Candida albicans* mannan and mannan-derived oligosaccharides on antigen-stimulated lymphoproliferation *in vitro*. *J. Immunol.* **144**, 707–16.

Ravine, D., Turner, K.J. and Alpers, M.P. (1980). Genetic inheritance of susceptibility to tinea imbricata. *J. Med. Genet.* **17**, 342–8.

Ray, T.L. and Wuepper, K.D. (1976). Activation of the alternative (properdin) pathway of complement by *Candida albicans* and related species. *J. Invest. Dermatol.* **67**, 700–3.

Ray, T.L. and Wuepper, K.D. (1978). Experimental cutaneous candidiasis in rodents. II. Role of the stratum corneum barrier and serum complement as a mediator of a protective inflammatory response. *Arch. Dermatol.* **114**, 539–43.

Reddy, P., Gorelick, D.F., Brasher, C.A. and Larsh, H. (1970). Progressive disseminated histoplasmosis as seen in adults. *Am. J. Med.* **48**, 629–36.

Reiss, E. (1986). *Molecular Immunology of Mycotic and Actinomycotic Infections*. Elsevier Science, New York.

Restrepo, A., Robledo, M., Gutiérrez, F., Sanclemente, M., Castañeda, E. and Calle, G. (1970). Paracoccidioidomycosis (South American blastomycosis): a study of 39 cases observed in Medellín, Colombia. *Am. J. Trop. Med. Hyg.* **19**, 68–76.

Restrepo-M., A. (1988). Immune response to *Paracoccidioides brasiliensis* in human and animal hosts. *Curr. Topics Med. Mycol.* **2**, 239–77.

Rhodes, J.C., Wicker, L.S. and Urba, W.J. (1980). Genetic control of susceptibility to *Cryptococcus neoformans* in mice. *Infect. Immunity* **29**, 494–9.

Roberts, S.O.B. (1969). Pityriasis versicolor: a clinical and mycological investigation. *Br. J. Dermatol.* **81**, 315–26.

Robledo, M.A., Graybill, J.R., Ahrens, J., Restrepo, A., Drutz, D.J. and Robledo, M. (1982). Host defense against experimental paracoccidioidomycosis. *Am. Rev. Respir. Dis.* **125**, 563–7.

Sandhu, D.K., Sandhu, R.S., Khan, Z.U. and Damodaran, V.N. (1976). Conditional virulence of a *p*-aminobenzoic acid-requiring mutant of *Aspergillus fumigatus*. *Infect. Immunity* **13**, 527–32.

Schaffner, A., Douglas, H. and Braude, A.I. (1982). Selective protection against conidia by mononuclear and against mycelia by polymorphonuclear phagocytes in resistance to *Aspergillus*: observations on these two lines of defence *in vivo* and *in vitro* with human and mouse phagocytes. *J. Clin. Invest.* **69**, 617–31.

Schaffner, A., Davis, C.E., Schaffner, T., Markert, M., Douglas, H. and Braude, A.I. (1986). *In vitro* susceptibility of fungi to killing by neutrophil granulocytes discriminates between primary pathogenicity and opportunism. *J. Clin. Invest.* **78**, 511–24.

Scheynius, A., Faergemann, J., Forsum, U. and Sjöberg, O. (1984). Phenotypic characterization *in situ* of inflammatory cells in pityriasis (tinea) versicolor. *Acta Dermatol. Venereol. (Stockholm)* **64**, 473–9.

Schimpff, S.C. and Bennett, J.E. (1975). Abnormalities in cell-mediated immunity in patients with *Cryptococcus neoformans* infection. *J. Allergy Clin. Immunol.* **55**, 430–41.

Schofield, F.D., Parkinson, A.D. and Jeffrey, D. (1963). Observations on the epidemiology, effects and treatment of tinea imbricata. *Trans. Roy. Soc. Trop. Med. Hyg.* **57**, 214–27.

Scott, E.N., Muchmore, H.G. and Fine, D.P. (1986). Activation of the alternative complement pathway by *Sporothrix schenckii*. *Infect. Immunity* **51**, 6–9.

Segal, E. (1987). Vaccines against fungal infections. *CRC Crit. Rev. Microbiol.* **14**, 229–71.

Sellers, T.F., Price, W.N. and Newberry, W.M. (1965). An epidemic of erythema multiforme and erythema nodosum caused by histoplasmosis. *Ann. Intern. Med.* **62**, 1244–62.

Serjeantson, S. and Lawrence, G. (1977). Autosomal recessive inheritance of susceptibility to tinea imbricata. *Lancet* **i**, 13–15.

Shiraishi, A., Nakagaki, K. and Arai, T. (1979). Experimental sporotrichosis in congenitally athymic (nude) mice. *J. Reticuloendothelial Soc.* **26**, 333–6.

Silva, C.L. and Fazioli, R.A. (1985). A *Paracoccidioides brasiliensis* polysaccharide having granuloma-inducing, toxic and macrophage stimulating activity. *J. Gen. Microbiol.* **131**, 1497–501.

Simon, M.R., Tubergen, D., Cassidy, J., Silva, J. and Magilavy, D. (1979). Chronic mucocutaneous candidiasis clinically exacerbated by type I hypersensitivity. *Clin. Immunol. Immunopathol.* **14**, 56–63.

Sixbey, J.W., Fields, B.T., Sun, C.N., Clark, R.A. and Nolan, C.M. (1979). Interactions between human granulocytes and *Blastomyces dermatitidis*. *Infect. Immunity* **23**, 41–4.

Slutsky, B., Buffo, J. and Soll, D.R. (1985). High-frequency switching of colony morphology in *Candida albicans*. *Science* **230**, 666–9.

Slutsky, B., Staebell, M., Anderson, J., Risen, L., Pfaller, M. and Soll, D.R. (1987). 'White–opaque transition': a second high-frequency switching system in *Candida albicans*. *J. Bacteriol.* **169**, 189–97.

Smith, C.E. (1940). The epidemiology of acute coccidioidomycosis with erythema nodosum ('San Joaquin' or 'valley fever'). *Am. J. Public Health* **30**, 600–11.

Smith, C.E., Beard, R.R., Whiting, E.G. and Rosenberger, H.G. (1946). Varieties of coccidioidal infection in relation to the epidemiology and control of the diseases. *Am. J. Public Health* **36**, 1394–402.

Smith, C.E., Whiting, E.G., Baker, E.E., Rosenberger, H.G., Beard, R.R. and Saito, M.T. (1948). The use of coccidioidin. *Am. Rev. Tuberculosis* **57**, 330–60.

Smith, C.E., Saito, M.T. and Simons, S.A. (1956). Pattern of 39 500 serologic tests in coccidioidomycosis. *JAMA* **160**, 546–52.

Smith, G.R. (1972). Experimental aspergillosis in mice: aspects of resistance. *J. Hyg. (Cambridge)* **70**, 741–54.

Smith, J.M.B. (1989). *Opportunistic Mycoses of Man and Other Animals*. CAB International, Wallingford.

Smith, J.W. and Utz, J.P. (1972). Progressive disseminated histoplasmosis: a prospective study of 26 patients. *Ann. Intern. Med.* **76**, 557–65.

Sohnle, P.G. (1989). Dermatophytosis. In *Immunology of the Fungal Diseases*, ed. R.A. Cox, pp. 1–27, CRC Press, Boca Raton, Florida.

Sohnle, P.G. and Collins-Lech, C. (1978). Cell-mediated immunity to *Pityrosporum orbiculare* in tinea versicolor. *J. Clin. Invest.* **62**, 45–55.

Sohnle, P.G. and Collins-Lech, C. (1980). Relative antigenicity of *P. orbiculare* and *C. albicans*. *J. Invest. Dermatol.* **75**, 279–83.

Sohnle, P.G. and Collins-Lech, C. (1982). Analysis of the lymphocyte transformation response to *Pityrosporum orbiculare* in patients with tinea versicolor. *Clin. Exp. Immunol.* **49**, 559–64.

Sohnle, P.G. and Collins-Lech, C. (1983). Activation of complement by *Pityrosporum orbiculare*. *J. Invest. Dermatol.* **80**, 93–7.

Sohnle, P.G. and Kirkpatrick, C.H. (1977). Study of possible mechanisms of basophil accumulation in experimental cutaneous candidiasis in guinea pigs. *J. Allergy Clin. Immunol.* **59**, 171–7.

Sohnle, P.G. and Kirkpatrick, C.H. (1978). Epidermal proliferation in the defense against experimental cutaneous candidiasis. *J. Invest. Dermatol.* **70**, 130–3.

Sohnle, P.G., Frank, M.M. and Kirkpatrick, C.H. (1976a). Deposition of complement components in the cutaneous lesions of chronic mucocutaneous candidiasis. *Clin. Immunol. Immunopathol.* **5**, 340–50.

Sohnle, P.G., Frank, M.M. and Kirkpatrick, C.H. (1976b). Mechanisms involved in elimination of organisms from experimental cutaneous *Candida albicans* infections in guinea pigs. *J. Immunol.* **117**, 523–30.

Solomkin, J.S., Mills, E.L., Giebink, G.S., Nelson, R.D., Simmons, R.L. and Quie, P.G. (1978). Phagocytosis of *Candida albicans* by human leukocytes: opsonic requirement. *J. Infect. Dis.* **137**, 30–7.

Stiehm, E.R. (1978). Chronic mucocutaneous candidiasis: clinical aspects, pp. 96–9 in J.E. Edwards (moderator). Severe candidal infections: clinical perspective, immune defense mechanisms, and current concepts of therapy. *Ann. Intern. Med.* **89**, 91–106.

Stobo, J.D., Paul, S., Van Scoy, R.E. and Hermans, P.E. (1976). Suppressor thymus-derived lymphocytes in fungal infection. *J. Clin. Invest.* **57**, 319–28.

Suchyta, M.R., Smith, J.G. and Graybill, J.R. (1988). The role of natural killer cells in histoplasmosis. *Am. Rev. Respir. Dis.* **138**, 578–82.

Sugar, A.M., Chahal, R.S., Brummer, E. and Stevens, D.A. (1983). Susceptibility of *Blastomyces dermatitidis* strains to products of oxidative metabolism. *Infect. Immunity* **41**, 908–12.

Sugar, A.M., Chahal, R.S., Brummer, E. and Stevens, D.A. (1984). The iron–hydrogen peroxide–iodide system is fungicidal: activity against the yeast phase of *Blastomyces dermatitidis*. *J. Leukocyte Biol.* **36**, 545–8.

Sun, S.H. and Huppert, M. (1976). A cytological study of morphogenesis in *Coccidioides immitis*. *Sabouraudia* **14**, 185–98.

Sutcliffe, M.C., Savage, A.M. and Alford, R.H. (1980). Transferrin-dependent growth inhibition of yeast-phase *Histoplasma capsulatum* by human serum and lymph. *J. Infect. Dis.* **142**, 209–19.

Swinne, D., Nkurikiyinfura, J.B. and Muyembe, T.L. (1986). Clinical isolates of *Cryptococcus neoformans* from Zaire. *Eur. J. Clin. Microbiol.* **5**, 50–1.

Tacker, J.R., Farhi, F. and Bulmer, G.S. (1972). Intracellular fate of *Cryptococcus neoformans*. *Infect. Immunity* **6**, 162–7.

Tewari, R.P., Sharma, D.K. and Mathur, A. (1978). Significance of thymus-derived lymphocytes in immunity elicited by immunization with ribosomes or live yeast cells of *Histoplasma capsulatum*. *J. Infect. Dis.* **138**, 605–13.

Thurmond, L.M. and Mitchell, T.G. (1984). *Blastomyces dermatitidis* chemotactic factor: kinetics of production and biological characterization evaluated by a modified neutrophil chemotaxis assay. *Infect. Immunity* **46**, 87–93.

Torinuki, W. and Tagami, H. (1985). Complement activation by *Sporothrix schenckii*. *Arch. Dermatol. Res.* **277**, 332–3.

Torinuki, W., Okohchi, H., Takematsu, H. and Tagami, H. (1984). Activation of the alternative complement pathway by *Fonsecaea pedrosoi*. *J. Invest. Dermatol.* **83**, 308–10.

Tsuneto, L.T., Arce-Gomez, B., Petzl-Erler, M.L. and Queiroz-Telles, F. (1989). HLA-A29 and genetic susceptibility to chromoblastomycosis. *J. Med. Vet. Mycol.* **27**, 181–5.

Twomey, J.J., Waddel, C.C., Krantz, S., O'Reilly, R., L'Esperance, P. and Good, R.A. (1975). Chronic mucocutaneous candidiasis with macrophage dysfunction, a plasma inhibitor, and coexistent aplastic anemia. *J. Lab. Clin. Med.* **85**, 968–77.

Uribe-J., F., Zuluaga, A.I., Leon, W. and Restrepo, A. (1989). Histopathology of chromoblastomycosis. *Mycopathologia* **105**, 1–6.

Valdimarsson, H., Higgs, J.M., Wells, R.S., Yamamura, M., Hobbs, J.R. and Holt, P.J.L. (1973). Immune abnormalities associated with chronic mucocutaneous candidiasis. *Cell. Immunol.* **6**, 348–61.

Waldorf, A.R. and Diamond, R.D. (1985). Neutrophil chemotactic responses induced by fresh and swollen *Rhizopus oryzae* spores and *Aspergillus fumigatus* conidia. *Infect. Immunity* **48**, 458–63.

Waldorf, A.R. and Diamond, R.D. (1989). Aspergillosis and mucormycosis. In *Immunology of the Fungal Diseases*, ed. R.A. Cox, pp. 29–55, CRC Press, Boca Raton, Florida.

Waldorf, A.R., Levitz, S.M. and Diamond, R.D. (1984). *In vivo* bronchoalveolar macrophage defense against *Rhizopus oryzae* and *Aspergillus fumigatus*. *J. Infect. Dis.* **150**, 752–60.

Wang, M., Friedman, H. and Djeu, J.Y. (1989). Enhancement of human monocyte function against *Candida albicans* by the colony-stimulating factors (CSF): IL-3 granulocyte–macrophage-CSF, and macrophage-CSF. *J. Immunol.* **143**, 671–7.

Weinberg, P.B., Becker, S., Granger, D.L. and Koren, H.S. (1987). Growth inhibition of *Cryptococcus neoformans* by human alveolar macrophages. *Am. Rev. Respir. Dis.* **136**, 1242–7.

Wheat, L.J. (1989). Diagnosis and management of histoplasmosis. *Eur. J. Clin. Microbiol. Infect. Dis.* **8**, 480–90.

Wheat, L.J., Slama, T.G. and Zeckel, M.L. (1985). Histoplasmosis in the acquired immune deficiency syndrome. *Am. J. Med.* **78**, 203–10.

Williams, D.M., Graybill, J.R. and Drutz, D.J. (1981). Adoptive transfer of immunity to *Histoplasma capsulatum* in athymic nude mice. *Sabouraudia* **19**, 39–48.

Witkin, S.S., Hirsch, J. and Ledger, W.J. (1986). A macrophage defect in women with recurrent *Candida* vaginitis and its reversal *in vitro* by prostaglandin inhibitors. *Am. J. Obstet. Gynecol.* **155**, 790–5.

Wolf, J.E., Kerchberger, V., Kobayashi, G.S. and Little, J.R. (1987). Modulation of the macrophage oxidative burst by *Histoplasma capsulatum*. *J. Immunol.* **138**, 582–6.

Wood, S.R. and Cruickshank, C.N.D. (1962). The relation between trichophytin sensitivity and fungal infection. *Br. J. Dermatol.* **74**, 329–36.

Wright, S.D., Weitz, J.I., Huang, A.J., Levin, S.M., Silverstein, S.C. and Loike, J.D. (1988). Complement receptor type three (CD11b, CD18) of human polymorphonuclear leukocytes recognizes fibrinogen. *Proc. Nat. Acad. Sci. (USA)* **85**, 7734–8.

Wu-Hsieh, B.A. and Howard, D.H. (1987). Inhibition of the intracellular growth of *Histoplasma capsulatum* by recombinant murine gamma interferon. *Infect. Immunity* **55**, 1014–16.

Wu-Hsieh, B. and Howard, D.H. (1989a). Macrophage cell lines $P388D_1$ and IC-21 stimulated with gamma interferon fail to inhibit the intracellular growth of *Histoplasma capsulatum. Infect. Immunity* **57**, 2903–5.

Wu-Hsieh, B. and Howard, D.H. (1989b). Histoplasmosis. In *Immunology of the Fungal Diseases*, ed. R.A. Cox, pp. 200–25, CRC Press, Boca Raton, Florida.

Wysong, D.R., Lyman, C.A. and Diamond, R.D. (1989). Independence of neutrophil respiratory burst oxidant generation from the early cytosolic calcium response after stimulation with unopsonized *Candida albicans* hyphae. *Infect. Immunity* **57**, 1499–505.

Yamazaki, M., Yasui, K., Kawai, H., Miyagawa, Y., Komiyama, A. and Akabane, T. (1984). A monocyte disorder in siblings with chronic candidiasis. *Am. J. Dis. Child.* **138**, 192–6.

Yarzábal, L., Dessaint, J.P., Arango, M., de Albornoz, M.C.B. and Campins, H. (1980). Demonstration and quantification of IgE antibodies against *Paracoccidioides brasiliensis* in paracoccidioidomycosis. *Int. Arch. Allergy Appl. Immunol.* **62**, 346–51.

Yohn, J.J., Lucas, J. and Camisa, C. (1985). *Malassezia* folliculitis in immunocompromised patients. *Cutis* **35**, 536–8.

Yoshida, K., Ando, M., Sakata, T. and Araki, S. (1988). Environmental mycological studies on the causative agent of summer-type hypersensitivity pneumonitis. *J. Allergy Clin. Immunol.* **81**, 475–83.

Yoshinoya, S., Cox, R.A. and Pope, R.M. (1980). Circulating immune complexes in coccidioidomycosis: detection and characterization. *J. Clin. Invest.* **66**, 655–63.

Young, E. and Roth, F.J. (1979). Immunological cross-reactivity between a glycoprotein isolated from *Trichophyton mentagrophytes* and human isoantigen A. *J. Invest. Dermatol.* **72**, 46–51.

Zaslow, L. and Derbes, V.J. (1969). The immunologic nature of kerion celsi formation. *Dermatol. Int.* **8**, 1–4.

Zuger, A., Louie, E., Holzman, R.S., Simberkoff, M.S. and Rahal, J.J. (1986). Cryptococcal disease in patients with the acquired immune deficiency syndrome: diagnostic features and outcome of treatment. *Ann. Intern. Med.* **104**, 234–40.

85: Autoimmunity and Infection

R.C. Williams, Jr

When the subject of autoimmunity and autoimmune diseases is broached, there is usually a real and theoretical gap between the concept of autoimmune disease and its occurrence within the human host. One of the most attractive explanations for autoimmune phenomena has always centred on various infections as possible natural events capable of initiating the process. Although there are several autoimmune disease models clearly related to well-defined initiating infections, most autoimmune diseases are still looking for a bench-mark infection to provide a plausible explanation for their pathogenesis. Nevertheless there now exists a considerable body of evidence to support infection as one triggering event for autoimmune disorders. This chapter aims to review those well-established models of autoimmune disease that have an infectious aetiology and to consider other, less well-defined disorders and their possible relation to initial or concurrent infection.

The *Streptococcus* and post-streptococcal sequelae

Acute post-streptococcal glomerulonephritis

Much early thinking on the role of infection in giving rise to autoimmune disease is based on clinical findings and epidemiological studies on acute and, possibly, later subacute/chronic glomerulonephritis following group A streptococcal infection (Rammelkamp 1957; Rammelkamp *et al.* 1952; Andres *et al.* 1966; Michael *et al.* 1966; Treser *et al.* 1969). Epidemiological studies clearly implicated group A β-haemolytic streptococcal infection in subsequent acute glomerulonephritis. Moreover, as the clinical and epidemiological studies were extended, it became obvious that group A streptococcal skin infection frequently preceded subclinical or obvious clinical evidence of acute nephritis (Dillon 1967; Potter *et al.* 1968; Anthony *et al.* 1969). Certain streptococcal serotypes, M-type 12, 14 or 49, were often associated with acute glomerulonephritis and this gave rise to the concept of nephritogenic streptococcal strains. Following the initial recognition that group A streptococcal infection can result in acute nephritis, immunochemical studies both of streptococcal antigens and of the immune complex deposits within involved glomeruli have attempted to explain the preferential renal localization of immune complex components and the exact steps in disease pathogenesis. The demonstration of elevated levels of circulating immune complexes (van de Rijn *et al.* 1978) during the course of post-streptococcal nephritis and the characterization of various streptococcal products which may be important in producing immune complex-mediated lesions in glomeruli during the course of the disease have extended knowledge in these areas (Treser *et al.* 1970; Villarreal *et al.* 1979). Moreover, immune complexes isolated from sera of patients with post-streptococcal glomerulonephritis have been shown to contain streptococcal antigens using crossed immunoelectrophoresis and hetero-antisera made against defined streptococcal antigens (Friedman *et al.* 1984).

Whether or not a more direct relationship exists between certain strains of the group A *Streptococcus* and important or accessible antigens within the kidney is, however, still not completely resolved. Fillit *et al.* (1985) reported that sera from patients with post-streptococcal glomerulonephritis contained antibodies reacting with glomerular heparan sulphate proteoglycan. It was not clear whether these antibodies were formed to the initial streptococcal infection inducing the glomerulonephritis or whether they were a response to autologous glomerular tissue components altered by the disease. In similar fashion, antibodies reacting with basement membrane collagen and laminin have also been found in sera from patients with post-streptococcal glomerulonephritis (Kefalides *et al.* 1986). It was suggested that true autoantibodies to such self-components as basement membrane collagen might result from ongoing tissue damage and release of antigenic glomerular components into the circulation. Taken together the reports of antibodies both against glomerular heparan sulphate proteoglycan and against basement membrane collagen in sera from patients with post-streptococcal nephritis indicate that after the initial immune complex injury a secondary chain of tissue injury and anti-tissue antibody production may occur. Whether such a process should be regarded as autoimmune cannot be resolved in the current state of our knowledge.

Work continues to define the particular components of certain strains of group A streptococci which define the initial nephrogenicity of such antigens. Although it has been established that acute post-streptococcal glomerulonephritis results from infection with a limited number of serological types of group A streptococci (Rammelkamp 1954; Stollerman 1971) it has been noted that, even within a known nephritogenic type, not all strains cause nephritis. Such findings suggest that only certain strains within a given putative nephritogenic subgroup may produce an antigen or streptococcal product responsible for actual induction of nephritis. Immunohistochemical data obtained largely from studies of glomerular biopsy material (Seegal *et al.* 1965; Lange *et al.* 1983) have demonstrated the presence of streptococcal antigens in glomeruli. A 46 000 dalton extracellular protein described by Villareal *et al.* (1979) appeared to be related to nephritic strains; later purification and partial sequence analysis by Johnston and Zabriskie (1986) have indicated that it was a streptokinase. However, how such nephritic streptococcal components are related to disease pathogenesis is still not clear.

ULTIMATE OUTCOME — CAN ACUTE POST-STREPTOCOCCAL GLOMERULONEPHRITIS BE CONSIDERED AN AUTOIMMUNE DISORDER?

Opinion is still divided as to the long-term consequences of acute post-streptococcal glomerulonephritis. Some studies employing careful clinical and laboratory parameters, including 7–12 years of follow-up, have shown an extremely low (<1.0%) incidence of chronic renal disease (Perlman *et al.* 1965; Nissenson *et al.* 1979). However, other observations on the long-term outcome in such post-streptococcal glomerulonephritis patients indicate a much higher proportion with features of irreversible renal damage or eventual progression to uraemia (Baldwin *et al.* 1974; Schacht *et al.* 1976). This unresolved problem makes it difficult to evaluate the role of the initial active infection as a precipitating event in the induction of chronic tissue damage to various target organs.

Acute rheumatic fever

Acute rheumatic fever probably provides the most convincing clinical example of an initial bacterial infection inducing subsequent widespread tissue damage and inflammation through a variety of autoimmune mechanisms. Until recently the disease was thought to be relatively common only in Third World regions such as India, Pakistan, Egypt and south-east Asia, but during the last few years small but convincing epidemics of acute rheumatic fever have once again made their appearance in a number of widely distributed regions of the United States (Hosier *et al.* 1987; Veasy *et al.* 1987; Wald *et al.* 1987). It appears that rheumatic fever may have returned to North America after a relative hiatus of three or four decades.

CLINICAL EVENTS AND PRESENTATION

Acute rheumatic fever most often occurs in children between the ages of 3 and 12, and, where epidemiological data are most reliable, the peak incidence of the first attack appears to be between the ages of 5 and 8. Initial episodes may be seen within the first 2 years of life, particularly in areas such as India where the clinical picture of juvenile mitral stenosis with far-advanced valvular changes at ages 5 or 6 has been recognized for some time (Vaishnava *et al.* 1960; Roy *et al.* 1963). However, in geographical areas outside the Third World, well-documented episodes of acute rheumatic fever may occur also in the second, third or even fourth decades of life.

In most patients, clinical, bacteriological or serological evidence suggests that streptococcal infection precedes the first clinical manifestations of acute rheumatic fever by 2–3 weeks. Epidemiological data accumulated during World War II epidemics (Rammelkamp *et al.* 1952) showed that, in relatively closely housed military recruits, clinical pharyngitis due to group A streptococci was followed by a rheumatic fever attack rate of approximately 3%. Unlike the well-established nephritogenic streptococcal M-types 12, 14 or 49, no clear-cut M- or T-type association for rheumatogenic streptococci has thus far been established.

Many studies have emphasized the necessity for the initial group A streptococcal infection to occur in the pharynx. In many instances where streptococcal isolates have been studied from both the skin and the pharynx in the same patients, it has been established that the strains, responsible for rheumatic fever must be present in the oropharynx. By contrast, particularly in tropical areas, epidemic post-streptococcal nephritis can usually be related to streptococcal pyoderma (Poon-King *et al.* 1967; Bisno *et al.* 1970).

Acute rheumatic fever begins 2–3 weeks after initial streptococcal pharyngeal infection — typically with a broad constellation of signs and symptoms which include acutely swollen and painful joints in a true migratory arthritis and crops of multiple small subcutaneous nodules usually located at sites of minor daily trauma or pressure such as the extensor surfaces of the elbows, knuckles, Achilles tendons or ischial areas. In several clinical correlative studies, the presence of multiple subcutaneous nodules has been directly linked to the severity of the associated carditis. Occasional patients with acute rheumatic fever show a strange serpiginous bordered skin eruption over the thorax, buttocks or upper arms (erythema marginatum).

The most ominous aspect of acute rheumatic fever is the cardiac involvement, where an intense inflammatory process generally involves the myocardium, endocardium, valvular structures and pericardium. The clinical presentation may be that of rapid onset of acute biventricular heart failure along with high fever and persistent tachycardia. A typical appearance of massive cardiac enlargement in an 11-year-old child is shown in Fig. 85.1. Systolic and diastolic mitral and aortic murmurs, in association with physical signs of pericardial fluid accumulation or with a pericardial friction rub, may be a prominent feature of the clinical picture.

In some patients (10–15%) the only clinical manifestation of acute rheumatic fever may be that of Sydenham's chorea. In these patients the interval between the initial group A streptococcal throat infection and chorea may be as long as 6–9 weeks (Taranta and Stollerman 1956). A long-term follow-up study conducted two decades after the initial chorea episodes (Bland and Jones 1951; Bland 1961) showed that 25–30% of chorea patients eventually showed detectable rheumatic valvular involvement.

MOLECULAR MIMICRY AND RHEUMATIC FEVER

The mechanisms whereby pharyngeal infection with β-haemolytic group A streptococci induce acute rheumatic fever 3 weeks later are still not completely defined. However, a strong case can be made for what can be called 'molecular mimicry'. A number of examples have now been identified of antigenic cross-reactions between group A streptococcal components and human tissues

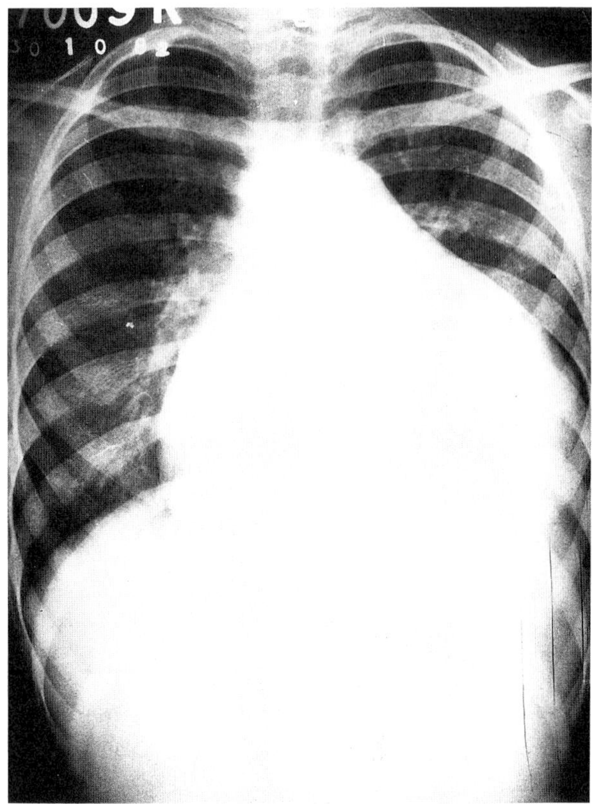

Fig. 85.1. Chest film showing massive cardiomegaly in an 11-year-old child with recent onset of acute rheumatic fever and pancarditis.

involved in the course of rheumatic fever. The first indications that molecular mimicry might be present between the *Streptococcus* and key human tissue epitopes came from studies by Kaplan and co-workers (Kaplan and Meyeserian 1962; Kaplan 1963). These studies showed that group A streptococcal cell walls contained heart cross-reactive antigens and that the antigenic cross-reactivity was restricted particularly to M-types 5 and 19 frequently isolated from patients with rheumatic fever. Several years later similar cross-reactions were demonstrated by Lyampert *et al.* (1966) using antisera produced in rabbits against M-types 1 and 5. Cross-reacting streptococcal and human heart antigens were also reported by Zabriskie and Freimer (1966), who found that the cross-reactive epitopes were particularly concentrated within group A protoplast membranes or sarcolemmal membrane preparations isolated from human heart tissue. Later, relative purification of heart-reactive antibody from serum of rheumatic fever patients by van de Rijn *et al.* (1977), using affinity isolation and elution from streptococcal or sarcolemmal membranes, showed that a broad variety of cross-reacting antigens could be identified. An example of heart-reactive antibody staining normal cardiac myofibres is shown in Fig. 85.2. These immunochemical studies were amplified by correlative clinical work which showed that levels of heart-reactive antibody were directly related to clinical rheumatic fever activity (Zabriskie *et al.* 1970) when patients were studied serially over the course of their illness. Similar findings of circulating heart-reactive antibody during the course of acute rheumatic carditis (Kaplan and Svec 1964; Kaplan *et al.* 1964) were extended by the demonstration that large amounts

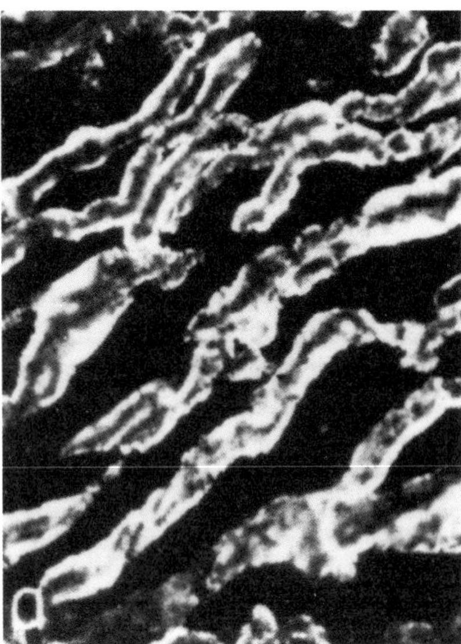

Fig. 85.2. Immunofluorescence demonstration of heart-reactive antibody from a patient with acute rheumatic fever showing staining of heart muscle, particularly around sarcolemmal membrane regions (a), the photograph on the right shows same field after absorption of the patient's serum with isolated group A streptococcal membranes. From van de Rijn *et al.* (1977).

of immunoglobulin and complement are deposited within the myocardium during acute carditis (Kaplan *et al.* 1964).

Additional studies of other cardiac muscle and streptococcal relationships have now uncovered an impressive degree of cross-reactivity between components of streptococcal M protein itself and human cardiac antigens located both in sarcolemmal membrane and in cardiac myosin (Dale and Beachey 1982, 1985, 1986). These extensive cross-reactions between components of M proteins and intrinsic human cardiac epitopes have provided a major theoretical problem in using M proteins as components of any protective streptococcal vaccine. Further evidence for molecular mimicry involving antigens shared by group A streptococci and human heart was presented by Cunningham and Russell (1983) and Krisher and Cunningham (1985), using murine monoclonal antibodies against group A streptococci which reacted with skeletal muscle and cardiac myosin. All of these studies emphasize the multiple cross-reactive antigenic epitopes which occur in human cardiac muscle and streptococci.

Other potentially important cross-reactions between heart valve glycoproteins and those of group A streptococci were originally described by Goldstein *et al.* (1967, 1968). Shortly thereafter Dudding and Ayoub (1968) reported that elevated levels of antibody to streptococcal group A carbohydrate appeared to persist for very long periods of time in patients with rheumatic valvular heart disease. This occurred despite the absence of overt clinical recurrences of acute rheumatic fever, and, when affected valves were surgically removed, a decrease in anti-streptococcal group A carbohydrate antibody was recorded in this group of patients (Ayoub *et al.* 1974). Persistence of markedly elevated antibodies to group A carbohydrate antigens among subjects with rheumatic valvular heart disease (when compared with normal controls or other patients with valvular dysfunction such as mitral valve prolapse (Appleton *et al.* 1985)) suggests that heart valves damaged by the initial rheumatic episode may subsequently serve as the source of antigens capable of perpetuating the original anti-carbohydrate immune response. Gowrishankar and Agarwal (1980), using migration inhibition assays with glycoprotein fractions from cardiac valves, have reported significant levels of cell-mediated immunity in many patients with established rheumatic heart disease.

The peculiar clinical manifestation of acute Sydenham's chorea has also been implicated as a possible manifestation of molecular mimicry. Cross-reactions between antigens of group A streptococci and the human nervous system were described by Kingston and Glynn (1976) with antisera produced against streptococcal components. More convincingly, Husby *et al.* (1976) found immunoglobulin G (IgG) antibody reacting with cytoplasmic antigens of neurons within subthalamic and caudate nuclei in the sera of patients with active chorea, which was completely removed by absorption with purified membranes of group A streptococci. An example of anti-neuronal antibody present in serum from a patient with active Sydenham's chorea is shown in Fig. 85.3. Whether such cross-reacting anti-streptococcal antibody actually causes the chorea episodes and central nervous system manifestations of acute rheumatic fever has never been clarified but the striking localization of anti-neuronal antibody binding to the very sites in the central nervous system known to be involved in the peculiar Sydenham's movement disorder is intriguing.

Mechanisms which might operate by molecular mimicry in rheumatic fever

Molecular mimicry mechanisms may be involved in the genesis of acute rheumatic fever and subsequent rheumatic heart disease by initially generating an immune response to components of the *Streptococcus* such as group A membrane, carbohydrate or M protein. However, because these components share antigenic determinants with a wide variety of key human tissues, including cardiac muscle sarcolemmal membranes, cardiac myosin, valvular glycoproteins, or antigens also present within caudate nucleus neurons, the initial anti-streptococcal immune response eventually becomes self-directed and is capable of initiating a true inflammatory autoimmune process. While there are many attractive features to such a hypothesis, several problems must be considered. One is why only a small fraction of individuals exposed to a particular strain of group A *Streptococcus* develop rheumatic fever. It seems likely that individual susceptibility may be analogous to major histocompatibility complex (MHC) restriction. A

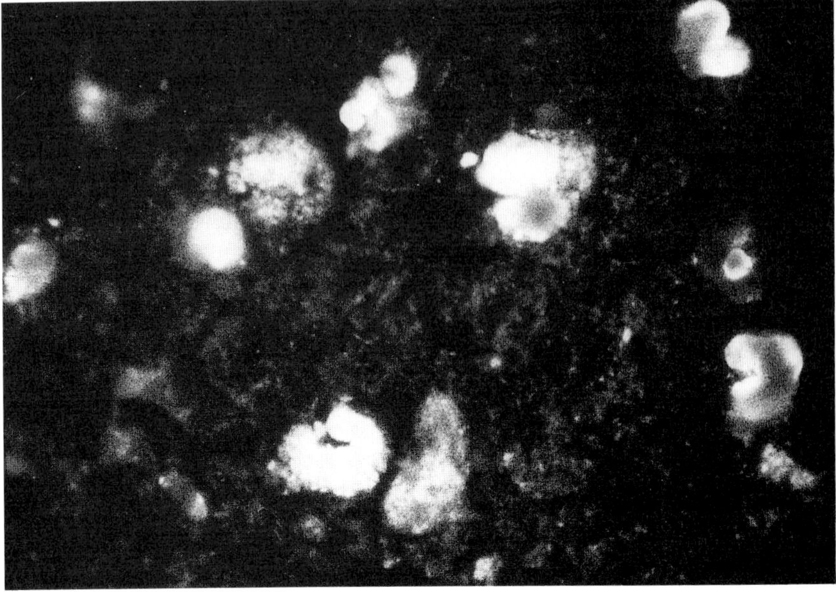

(a)

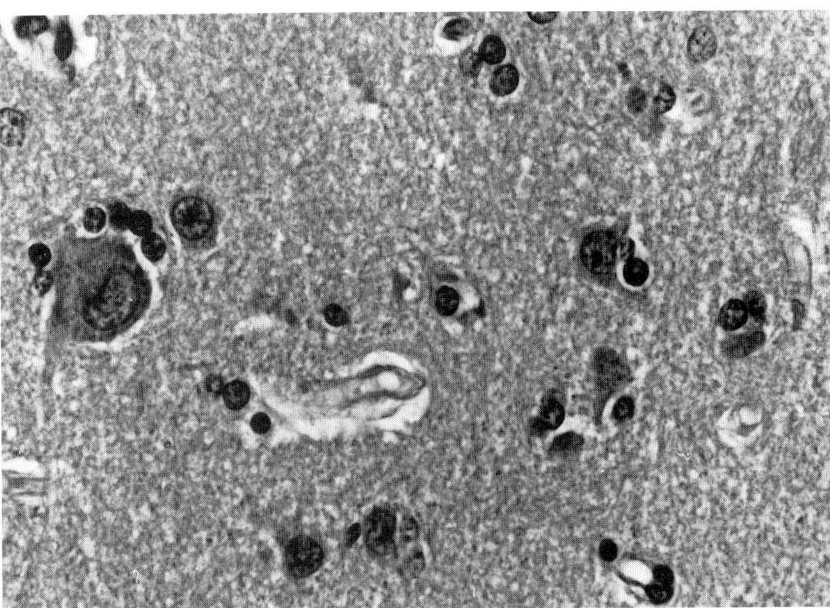

(b)

Fig. 85.3. (a) Immunofluorescence demonstration of anti-neuronal antibody in serum from a child with acute Sydenham's chorea. The serum was overlaid on a 4 μm frozen section of normal human caudate nucleus and counter-stained with fluorescein-conjugated $F(ab')_2$ fragment of goat antibody to human IgG. Positive fluorescence staining involving the cytoplasmic antigens of large- and intermediate-sized neurons is shown (× 270). (b) Haematoxylin- and eosin-stained section similar to field shown in (a), indicating medium- and large-sized neurons present within this particular tissue.

number of earlier studies had attempted to link variations within the human leucocyte antigen (HLA)-DR system to rheumatic fever susceptibility (Falk *et al*. 1973; Murray *et al*. 1978), but no consistent association was found until studies by Ayoub *et al*. (1986) defined a relationship with HLA-DR2 and DR4 phenotypes in Black and Caucasian rheumatic subjects respectively. In addition to these findings, studies of a B cell alloantigen linked to rheumatic fever susceptibility (Patarroyo *et al*. 1979) suggested that other genetic factors might be involved in initiation of the disease. Subsequent work using several monoclonal antibodies with similar B cell alloantigen specificity have extended insight into this area (Zabriskie *et al*. 1985; Khanna *et al*. 1988). It appears that not only is initial group A pharyngeal streptococcal infection essential, but also individual patient susceptibility may be controlled by genetically determined B cell antigens which are present in 15–17% of the normal population but which can be identified in most patients with rheumatic fever.

Reactive arthritis and ankylosing spondylitis

Since the recognition that ankylosing spondylitis (AS) and later a number of other spondyloarthropathies were associated with HLA-B27 (Brewerton *et al.* 1973; Schlosstein *et al.* 1973), interest in the so-called seronegative spondyloarthropathies has increased. Moreover, a number of parallel and intriguing findings have raised the question of some sort of enteric infection possibly initiating the disease. In the case of AS, Reiter's syndrome, psoriatic arthritis, colitis arthritis and reactive arthritis — in addition to the frequent positive relationship with HLA-B27 — molecular mimicry, or interaction, of bacteria or bacterial factors with HLA Class I MHC antigens has frequently been suggested as a pathogenic mechanism. Since only a limited number of enteric or other pathogens may cause Reiter's syndrome or reactive arthritis (Keat 1983; Leirisalo *et al.* 1982; Martin *et al.* 1984), it has been suggested that various Enterobacteriaceae capable of initiating disease may share a common arthritis-inducing factor (Toivanen *et al.* 1985; Yu *et al.* 1985). Some evidence for such shared factors has been provided. *Yersinia enterocolitica*, serotype 3, which is recognized as a major aetiological agent of Reiter's disease in European countries shares an outer membrane component with arthritogenic strains of *Shigella flexneri*. T cells from American patients with Reiter's syndrome divide *in vitro* when stimulated with a European *Yersinia* isolate (Brenner *et al.* 1984).

No definite organism has yet been linked with AS but several reports suggest *Klebsiella pneumoniae* as a candidate since increased numbers of this organism have been recorded in faecal samples from patients with AS (Ebringer *et al.* 1985) and active inflammatory disease appears to be associated with the presence of *Klebsiella* in the faeces (Ebringer *et al.* 1978).

Several lines of evidence have linked AS to various bacterial organisms as possible inciting factors. One possibility is that B27 molecules (or other components genetically associated with B27) may function as specific cell surface receptors for products released by bacteria (Seager *et al.* 1979; Geczy *et al.* 1983). After such surface receptors have been modified by bacterial components, they may become vulnerable as targets for antibodies against these or similar bacteria and this in turn could lead to an inflammatory reaction and be the initial basis for starting the disease. This postulated scheme of pathogenesis is somewhat different from that usually put forward as being centrally involved in autoimmune mechanisms; however, a substantial body of evidence has now been marshalled, largely by one group, to support such a mechanism. Human leucocyte antigen B27 +ve lymphocytes from normal individuals incubated with some strains of *Klebsiella* organisms, or certain other Gram-negative bacteria, appear to express new antigens (Edmonds *et al.* 1981; Cameron *et al.* 1983) which can also be found on lymphocytes from B27 +ve patients with AS or Reiter's syndrome without prior incubation of bacterial supernatants. Moreover, experiments were reported which indicated that these same determinants/receptors could be transferred from supernatants of cultured lymphocytes (from patients with spondylitis) to normal subjects' B27 +ve cells. Cell-mediated lymphocytotoxicity may be involved in the pathogenesis since cytotoxic T lymphocytes produced by stimulating peripheral blood mononuclear cells of an HLA-B27 +ve normal individual with peripheral blood cells from an HLA-identical sibling with AS (B27 +ve) could be shown to kill B27 +ve AS +ve lymphocytes but not cells from HLA-B27 +ve subjects without AS or from B27 −ve AS or from normal controls (Geczy *et al.* 1986). Moreover, similar cytotoxic specificities could be demonstrated after *in vitro* stimulation of B27 +ve AS −ve cells with autologous cells modified by cross-reactive bacterial antigens (Geczy *et al.* 1986). Antiserum produced against a factor produced by peripheral blood cells of an HLA-B27 +ve patient with AS was shown to specifically lyse B27 +ve but not B27 −ve cells of AS patients or those of B27 +ve or B27 −ve normal controls (Sullivan and Geczy 1987). The interpretation of these interesting findings is open to question since there have been difficulties reproducing the same pattern of results in other laboratories. However, the possibility that components derived from *Klebsiella* or other Gram-negative bacteria might be capable of altering cell-localized HLA-B27 epitopes and somehow inducing self-directed immune reactions represents a fascinating new area for further investigation.

Molecular mimicry between human leucocyte antigen B27 and bacterial products

Antigenic similarity between HLA-B27 and various bacterial components has been identified using rabbit antisera (Welsh *et al.* 1980) and human tissue-typing sera (Avakian *et al.* 1980) and with monoclonal antibodies (van Bohemen *et al.* 1984; Kono *et al.* 1985; Chen *et al.* 1987; Raybourne *et al.* 1988). The idea that this molecular mimicry may be involved in the pathogenesis of ankylosing spondylitis was given additional momentum when Schwimmbeck *et al.* (1987) demonstrated that the HLA-B27 molecule shares a sequence of six amino acids (QTDRED) at residues 69–78 with an exactly similar sequence at positions 185–194 in the *Klebsiella pneumoniae* nitrogenase protein. Moreover, when these sequences were prepared as parts of small synthetic peptides showing appropriate amino acids at either end based on known HLA-B27 or nitrogenase sequences, a substantial proportion of sera from patients with AS or Reiter's syndrome showed antibodies reacting with these peptides. Hydrophobicity plots indicated that the respective homologous HLA-B27 and *Klebsiella* peptides were both hydrophilic and therefore more likely to be exposed on the surface of their individual molecules. These findings have recently been extended by our group (Tsuchiya *et al.* 1989) confirming the presence of antibodies to the HLA-B27 peptide in sera from AS patients. However, no significant elevation in antibodies reacting with the QTDRED-containing *Klebsiella* peptide was recorded. Moreover, a substantial difference in the proportion of AS patients with anti-B27 peptide antibody was noted between AS patients from Tromso, Norway, and those from New Mexico, USA. These findings may indicate that various previously defined HLA-B27 subtypes with single amino acid substitutes within the 69–78 sequence may significantly influence the mechanisms of molecular mimicry. There is great interest in this general area and, clearly, more investigative work is now necessary.

If various enteric organisms (and other bacteria) share important antigens with self determinants, such as HLA-B27, then this might explain the tissue distribution of lesions in diseases such as ankylosing spondylitis or Reiter's syndrome. Thus rat hetero-antisera to HLA-B27 and to *Klebsiella* peptides were used to stain articular tissues from AS patients in an attempt to localize the distribution of any possible cross-reacting epitopes (Husby *et al.* 1988). Extensive expression of structures reacting both with rat anti-B27 and with anti-*Klebsiella* peptide antibodies was found, particularly within synovial lining cells and endothelial cells of blood vessels in inflamed AS tissues. An example of such cross-reactivity expressed in articular tissue is shown in Fig. 85.4. Unfortunately, these studies do not help to explain the strange 'enthesopathy' or frequent localization of inflammatory foci at regions of ligament or tendon insertions in AS or other spondyloarthropathies.

Reactive arthritis and molecular mimicry

The organisms which have most commonly been associated with reactive arthritis in the past have been *Shigella*, *Salmonella*, *Yersinia* and, in some instances, *Campylobacter* species. Several observations concerning possible alternative mechanisms for molecular mimicry have recently appeared. A small plasmid shared by several strains of *Shigella flexneri* isolated from different patients with reactive arthritis was studied by Stieglitz and Lipsky (1988), who found that the proteins expressed by the plasmid shared part of the sequence of the original QTDRED reported by Schwimmbeck *et al.* (1987). These findings were of great interest since they indicated that a common cross-reacting determinant might be shared among a number of bacterial strains (or alternatively by their plasmids) which might be associated with arthritogenic potential. However, subsequently no homology was shown between deoxyribonucleic acid (DNA) from arthritogenic *Yersinia* strains and HLA-B27 DNA using *in vitro* hybridization and Southern blotting techniques (Viitanen *et al.* 1988). Clearly, now that the area of molecular mimicry has been raised by these and similar studies, considerably more work is needed in this general area using molecular biological techniques.

Molecular mimicry and human leucocyte antigen DR subtypes in rheumatoid arthritis

(see also Chapter 60)

Another aspect of infections and autoimmune disorders relates to virus infection. It has repeatedly been demonstrated that susceptibility to rheumatoid arthritis is associated with the Class II MHC

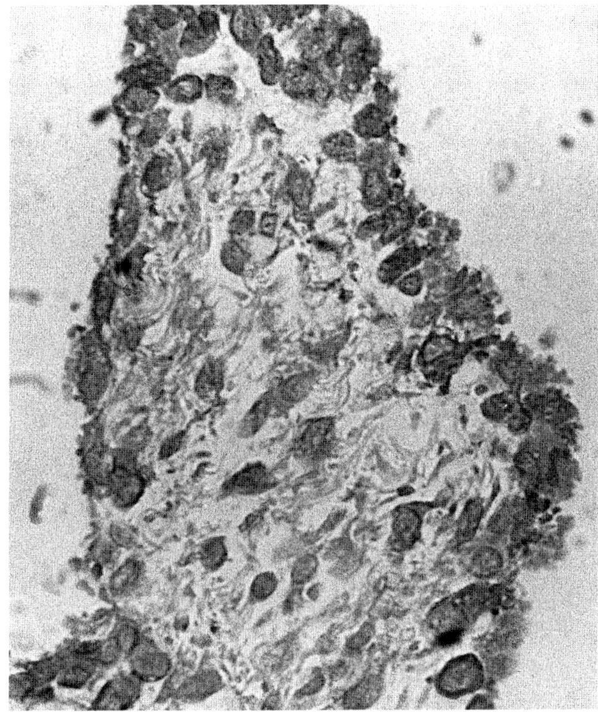

(a)

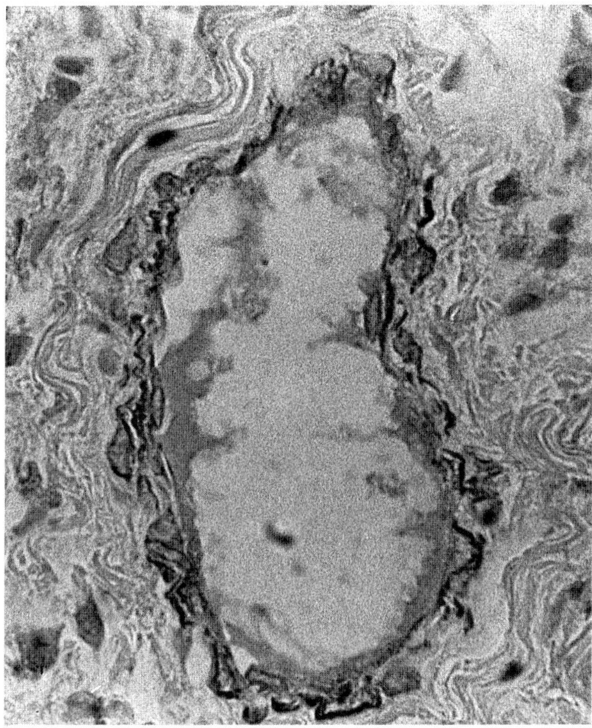

(b)

Fig. 85.4. Synovial tissue from patient with ankylosing spondylitis stained with rat antiserum against HLA-B27 peptide containing QTDRED hexamer showing homology with a sequence within *Klebsiella* nitrogenase. Strong staining of synovial lining cells (a) and endothelial structures (b) is seen with immunoperoxidase technique (× 200).

antigens HLA-DR4 and HLA-DR1 (Stastny 1978; Woodrow *et al.* 1981). The reasons for this apparent MHC restriction in genetic predisposition are not yet known. However, the major role of Class II MHC antigens is believed to be to present processed antigen to T lymphocytes (Schwartz 1987). Roudier *et al.* (1988) suggest that molecular mimicry between antigens of Epstein–Barr virus glycoprotein gp110 and regions within Class II MHC molecules might be involved in antigen presentation to T cell receptors. Within DR β chains, subtypes can be identified which include HLA-DR4, Dw4, Dw14 and Dw15 — all of which are associated with rheumatoid arthritis, whereas HLA-DR4 subtypes Dw10 and Dw13 are not (Ohta *et al.* 1982; Nepom *et al*, 1986; Zoschke and Segall 1986). The sequences which distinguish the rheumatoid arthritis Dw subtypes from non-rheumatoid have now been identified with amino acids 70–74 of the third hypervariable region of the DR β1 chain. These comparisons are illustrated in Table 85.1. When considered together, HLA-DR4 and DR1 include ~93% of cases of rheumatoid arthritis. With this background, the sequence QKRAA/QRRAA is present on the third hypervariable region of the DR β1 chain in most rheumatoid arthritis patients. Present evidence suggests that Class II MHC molecule β chains include an antigen-binding site and a site for interaction with the T cell receptor (Ronchese *et al.* 1987). The third hypervariable region within the DR β chain represents a portion of the site for direct interaction between the T cell receptor and the Class II MHC molecule. Moreover, this particular region is involved in the HLA-DR1 and HLA-Dw4 subtypes and the region QKRAA/QRRAA may very probably represent a portion of the actual interaction

Table 85.1. Comparative sequences of the third hypervariable region of the DR β1 chain of Dw subtypes. From Roudier *et al.* (1988).

65	70 74	80	
HLA DR1 KDLLE	QRRAA	VDTYCR	RA-associated haplotypes
HLA Dw4 DDLLE	QKRAA	VDTYCR	
HLA Dw14 KDLLE	QRRAA	VDTYCR	
HLA Dw15 KDLLE	QRRAA	VDTYCR	
HLA Dw13 KDLLE	QRRAE	VDTYCR	Not associated with RA
HLA Dw10 KDLLE	DERAA	VDTYCR	

RA = rheumatoid arthritis.

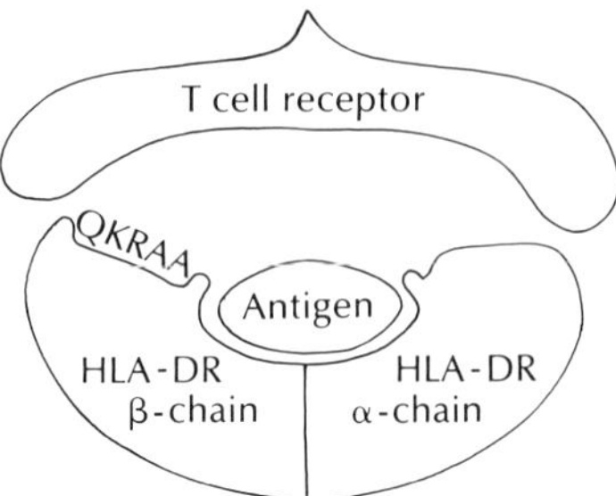

Fig. 85.5. Relationship between the possible rheumatoid arthritis susceptibility determinant QKRAA within the third hypervariable region of the DR β1 chain of HLA-Dw4 and the recognition site for T cells. The putative antigen is shown within the cleft known to be made up of the interacting DR β and α chains. Adapted with permission from Roudier *et al.* (1988).

site for T cells on the HLA-DR β1 chain. This is diagrammed in Fig. 85.5. Roudier *et al.* (1988) have found that sequences 807–816 of the Epstein–Barr virus glycoprotein GP110 contains a six-amino acid sequence EQKRAA which matches HLA-Dw4 and that is followed by a similar second copy (QRAA) of the susceptibility determinant for rheumatoid arthritis.

The GP110 glycoprotein represents a nucleocapsid glycoprotein which is found in the nucleus and cytoplasm of Epstein–Barr virus-infected cells. The hypothesis proposed by Roudier *et al.* (1988) suggests that autoreactive T cells recognizing HLA-Dw4/Dw14/Dw15/DR1 might conceivably trigger rheumatoid arthritis and that such T cells could be expanded by additional stimulation by GP110. T cells reacting with autologous HLA molecules have been found in large numbers within synovial fluid from rheumatoid arthritis patients (Klareskog *et al.* 1982; Duke *et al.* 1987). This remarkable theory represents yet another example of how infection — in this case ubiquitous residence of Epstein–Barr virus — might help trigger an autoimmune disease such as rheumatoid arthritis.

Molecular mimicry and myasthenia (see also Chapter 106)

A further extension of the concept of molecular mimicry between infectious agents and host tissues has recently been defined by Schwimmbeck *et al.* (1989) in studies of myasthenia gravis. These investigators showed that sequences defined by residues 160–167 within the alpha subunit of the human acetylcholine receptor showed direct immunological cross-reactivity with a shared homologous domain on herpes simplex virus glycoprotein D, residues 286–293. The immunological cross-reactivity in this instance was demonstrated both by direct binding and by inhibition studies. Immunological cross-reactivity of this self determinant (represented by the defined peptide within the alpha subunit of the human acetylcholine receptor) and an exactly homologous epitope on the herpes simplex virus could conceivably function in a way to provide a rational explanation for genesis of the disease in some patients. This concept is particularly appealing since herpes viruses are known to be widely distributed among the general population, often in asymptomatic carriers.

There are many other mechanisms not covered in detail here which could be used to link infection of one kind or another to various autoimmune disorders. The representative examples discussed here provide only a suggestion as to how the two processes may in some instances be intertwined. Clearly a great deal more work will be necessary before many of the hypotheses or concepts already presented can be either extended or shown to be incorrect.

References

Andres, G.A., Accinni, L., Hsu, K.C., Zabriskie, J.B. and Seegal, B.C. (1966). Electron microscopic studies of human glomerulonephritis with ferritinconjugated antibody. *J. Exp. Med.* **123**, 399–412.

Anthony, B.F., Kaplan, E.L., Wannamaker, L.W., Briese, F.W. and Chapman, S.S. (1969). Attack rates of acute nephritis after type 49 streptococcal infection of the skin and of the respiratory tract. *J. Clin. Invest.* **48**, 1697–704.

Appleton, R.S., Victoria, B.E., Tamer, D. and Ayoub, E.M. (1985). Specificity of persistence of antibody to the streptococcal group A carbohydrate in rheumatic valvular heart disease. *J. Lab. Clin. Med.* **105**, 114–19.

Avakian, H., Welsh, J., Ebringer, A. and Entwistle, C.C. (1980). Ankylosing spondylitis, HLA-B27 and *Klebsiella*. II, Cross-reactivity studies with human tissue typing sera. *Br. J. Exp. Pathol.* **61**, 92–7.

Ayoub, E.M., Taranta, A. and Bartley, J.D. (1974). Effect of valvular surgery on antibody to the group A streptococcal carbohydrate. *Circulation* **50**, 144–50.

Ayoub, E.M., Barrett, D.J., MacLaren, N.K. and Krischer, J.P. (1986). Association of class II human histocompatibility leukocyte antigens with rheumatic fever. *J. Clin. Invest.* **77**, 2019–26.

Baldwin, D.S., Gluck, M.C., Schacht, R.G. and Gallo, G. (1974). The long-term course of poststreptococcal glomerulonephritis. *Ann. Intern. Med.* **80**, 342–58.

Bisno, A.L., Pearce, I.A., Wall, H.P., Moody, M.D. and Stollerman, G.H. (1970). Contrasting epidemiology of acute rheumatic fever and acute glomerulonephritis: nature of the antecedent streptococcal infection. *N. Engl. J. Med.* **283**, 561–5.

Bland, E.F. (1961). Chorea as a manifestation of rheumatic fever, a long term perspective. *Trans. Am. Clin. Climatol. Assoc.* **73**, 209–13.

Bland, E.F. and Jones, T.D. (1951). Rheumatic fever and rheumatic heart disease — a 20 year report on 1000 patients followed since childhood. *Circulation* **4**, 836–43.

Brenner, M.B., Kobayaski, S., Wiesenhutter, C.W., Huberman, A.K., Bales, P. and Yu, D.T.Y. (1984). *In vitro* T lymphocyte proliferative response to *Yersinia enterocolitica* in Reiter's syndrome. *Arthritis Rheum.* **27**, 250–7.

Brewerton, D.A., Hart, F.D., Nicholls, A., Caffrey, M., James, D.C.O. and Sturrock, R.D. (1973). Ankylosing spondylitis and HL-A27. *Lancet* **i**, 904–7.

Cameron, F.H., Russell, P.J., Sullivan, J. and Geczy, A.F. (1983). Is a *Klebsiella* plasmid involved in the aetiology of ankylosing spondylitis in HLA-B27-positive individuals? *Mol. Immunol.* **20**, 563–6.

Chen, J.-H., Kono, D., Yong, Z., Park, M.S., Oldstone, M.B.A. and Yu, D.T.Y. (1987). A *Yersinia pseudotuberculosis* protein which cross reacts with HLA-B27. *J. Immunol.* **139**, 3003–11.

Cunningham, M.W. and Russell, S.M. (1983). Study of heart-reactive antibody in antisera and hybridoma culture fluids against group A streptococci. *Infect. Immunity* **42**, 531–7.

Dale, J.B. and Beachey, E.H. (1982). Protective antigenic determinant of streptococcal M protein shared with sarcolemmal membrane protein of human heart. *J. Exp. Med.* **156**, 1165–76.

Dale, J.B. and Beachey, E.H. (1985). Multiple heart-cross-reactive epitopes of streptococcal M proteins. *J. Exp. Med.* **161**, 113–22.

Dale, J.B. and Beachey, E.H. (1986). Sequence of myosin cross-reactive epitopes of streptococcal M protein. *J. Exp. Med.* **164**, 1785–90.

Dillon, H.C., Jr (1967). Pyoderma and nephritis. *Ann. Rev. Med.* **18**, 207–18.

Dudding, B.A. and Ayoub, E.M. (1968). Persistence of streptococcal group A antibody in patients with rheumatic valvular disease. *J. Exp. Med.* **128**, 1081–98.

Duke, O., Gordon, Y. and Panayi, G.S. (1987). Synovial fluid mononuclear cells exhibit a spontaneous HLA DR driven proliferative response. *Clin. Exp. Immunol.* **70**, 10–17.

Ebringer, A., Baines, M. and Plaszynska, T. (1985). Spondylitis, uveitis, HLA-B27 and *Klebsiella*. *Immunol. Rev.* **86**, 101–6.

Ebringer, R.W., Cawdell, D.R., Cowling, P. and Ebringer, A. (1978). Sequential studies in ankylosing spondylitis: association of *Klebsiella pneumoniae* with active disease. *Ann. Rheum, Dis.* **37**, 146–51.

Edmonds, J., McCauley, D., Tyndall, A. *et al.* (1981). Lymphocytotoxicity of anti-*Klebsiella* antisera in ankylosing spondylitis and related arthropathies. *Arthritis Rheum.* **24**, 1–7.

Falk, J.A., Fleischman, J.L., Zabriskie, J.B. and Falk, R.E. (1973). A study of HLA antigen phenotype in rheumatic fever and rheumatic heart disease patients. *Tissue Antigens* **3**, 173–8.

Fillit, H., Damle, S.P., Gregory, J.D., Volin, C., Poon-King, T. and Zabriskie, J. (1985). Sera from patients with post-streptococcal glomerulonephritis contain antibodies to glomerular heparan sulfate proteoglycan. *J. Exp. Med.* **161**, 277–89.

Friedman, J., van de Rijn, I., Ohkuni, H., Fischetti, V.A. and Zabriskie, J.B. (1984). Immunological studies of post-streptococcal sequelae evidence for presence of streptococcal antigens in circulating immune complexes. *J. Clin. Invest.* **74**, 1027–34.

Geczy, A.F., Alexander, K., Bashir, H.V., Edmonds, J.P., Upfold, L. and Sullivan, J. (1983). HLA-B27, *Klebsiella*, and ankylosing spondylitis: biological and chemical studies. *Immunol. Rev.* **70**, 23–50.

Geczy, A.F., McGuigan, L.E., Sullivan, J.S. and Edmonds, J.P. (1986). Cytotoxic T lymphocytes against disease-associated determinant(s) in ankylosing spondylitis. *J. Exp. Med.* **164**, 932–7.

Goldstein, I., Halpern, B. and Robert, L. (1967). Immunological relationship between *Streptococcus* A polysaccharide and the structural glycoproteins of heart valve. *Nature* **213**, 44–7.

Goldstein, I., Reybeyotte, P., Parlebas, J. and Halpern, B. (1968). Isolation from heart valves of glycopeptides which share immunological properties with *Streptococcus haemolyticus* group A polysaccharides. *Nature* **219**, 866–8.

Gowrishankar, R. and Agarwal, S.C. (1980). Leukocyte migration inhibition with human heart valve glycoproteins and group A streptococcal ribonucleic acid proteins in rheumatic heart disease and post-streptococcal glomerulonephritis. *Clin. Exp. Immunol.* **39**, 519–25.

Hosier, D.M., Craenen, J.M., Teske, D.W. and Wheller, J.J. (1987). Resurgence of acute rheumatic fever. *Am. J. Dis. Child.* **141**, 730–3.

Husby, G., van de Rijn, I., Zabriskie, J.B., Abdin, Z.H. and Williams, R.C., Jr (1976). Antibodies reacting with cytoplasm of subthalamic and caudate nuclei neurons in chorea and acute rheumatic fever. *J. Exp. Med.* **144**, 1094–110.

Husby, G., Tsuchiya, N., Schwimmbeck, P.L. *et al.* (1988). *Klebsiella pneumoniae* nitrogenase cross-reactive epitope in articular tissues of HLA-B27(+) patients with ankylosing spondylitis. *Clin. Res.* **36**, 879A.

Johnston, K.H. and Zabriskie, J.B. (1986). Purification and partial characterization of the nephritis strain-associated protein from *Streptococcus pyogenes* group A. *J. Exp. Med.* **163**, 697–712.

Kaplan, M.H. (1963). Immunologic relation of streptococcal and tissue antigens. I. Properties of an antigen in certain strains of group A streptococci exhibiting an immunologic cross-reaction with human heart tissue. *J. Immunol.* **90**, 595–606.

Kaplan, M.H. and Meyeserian, H. (1962). An immunologic cross-reaction between group A streptococcal cells and human heart. *Lancet* **ii**, 706–10.

Kaplan, M.H. and Svec, K.H. (1964). Immunologic relations of streptococcal and tissue antigens. III. Presence in human sera of streptococcal antibody cross-reactive with heart tissue: association with streptococcal infection, rheumatic fever, and glomerulonephritis. *J. Exp. Med.* **119**, 651–66.

Kaplan, M.H., Bolande, R., Rakita, L. and Blair, J. (1964). Presence of bound immunoglobulins and complement in the myocardium in acute rheumatic fever. *N. Engl. J. Med.* **271**, 637–45.

Keat, A. (1983). Reiter's syndrome and reactive arthritis in perspective. *N. Engl. J. Med.* **309**, 1606–15.

Kefalides, N.A., Pegg, M.T., Ohno, N., Poon-King, T., Zabriskie, J. and Fillit, H. (1986). Antibodies to basement membrane collagen and to laminin are present in sera from patients with post-streptococcal glomerulonephritis. *J. Exp. Med.* **163**, 588–602.

Khanna, A., Gibofsky, A., Buskirk, D.R. *et al.* (1989). The presence of a non HLA B-cell antigen in rheumatic fever patients and their families as defined by a monoclonal antibody. *J. Clin. Invest.* **83**, 1710–16.

Kingston, D. and Glynn, L.E. (1976). Antistreptococcal antibodies reacting with brain tissue. I. Immunofluorescent studies. *Br. J. Exp. Pathol.* **57**, 114–28.

Klareskog, L., Forsum, U., Scheynius, A., Kabelitz, D. and Wigzell, H. (1982). Evidence in support of a self-perpetuating HLA-DR dependent delayed type cell reaction in rheumatoid arthritis. *Proc. Nat. Acad. Sci. (USA)* **79**, 3632–6.

Kono, D.H., Ogasawara, M., Effros, R.B., Park, M.S., Valdord, R.L. and Yu, D.T.Y. (1985). Ye-1, a monoclonal antibody that cross-reacts with HLA-B27 lymphoblastoid cell lines and an arthritis causing bacteria. *Clin. Exp. Immunol.* **61**, 503–8.

Krisher, K. and Cunningham, M.W. (1985). Myosin: a link between streptococci and heart, *Science* **227**, 413–15.

Lange, K., Seligson, G. and Cronin, W. (1983). Evidence for the *in situ* origin of poststreptococcal glomerulonephritis: glomerular localization of endostreptosin and the clinical significance of the subsequent antibody response. *Clin. Nephrol.* **19**, 3–10.

Leirisalo, M., Skylv, G., Kousa, M. *et al.* (1982). Follow-up study on patients with Reiter's disease and reactive arthritis with special reference to HLA-B27. *Arthritis Rheum.* **25**, 249–59.

Lyampert, I.M., Vedenskaya, O.L., and Danilova, T.A. (1966). Study on *Streptococcus* group A antigens common with heart tissue elements. *Immunology* **11**, 313–20.

Martin, D.H., Pollock, S., Kuo, C.C., Wang, S.P., Brunham, R.C. and Holmes, K.K. (1984). Chlamydia trachomatis infections in men with Reiter's syndrome. *Ann. Int. Med.* **100**, 207–13.

Michael, A.F., Drummond, K.N., Good, R.A. and Vernier, R.L. (1966). Acute post-streptococcal glomerulonephritis: immune deposit disease. *J. Clin. Invest.* **45**, 237–47.

Murray, G.C., Montiel, M.M. and Persellin, R.H. (1978). A study of antigens in adults with acute rheumatic fever. *Arthritis Rheum.* **21**, 652–6.

Nepom, G., Seyfried, C.E., Holbekc, S.L., Wilske, F.R. and Nepom, B.S. (1986). Identification of HLA Dw14 genes in DR4+ rheumatoid arthritis. *Lancet* **i**, 1002–5.

Nissenson, A.R., Mayon-White, R., Potter, E.V. *et al.* (1979). Continued absence of clinical renal disease seven to 12 years after poststreptococcal acute glomerulonephritis in Trinidad. *Am. J. Med.* **67**, 255–62.

Ohta, N., Nishimura, Y.K., Tanimoto, K. *et al.* (1982). Association between HLA and Japanese patients with rheumatoid arthritis. *Hum. Immunol.* **5**, 123–32.

Patarroyo, M.E., Winchester, R.J., Vejerano, A. *et al.* (1979). Association of a B-cell alloantigen with susceptibility to rheumatic fever. *Nature* **278**, 173–4.

Perlman, L.V., Herdman, R.C., Kleinman, H. and Vernier, R.L. (1965). Poststreptococcal glomerulonephritis: a ten-year follow-up of an epidemic. *JAMA* **194**, 63–70.

Poon-King, T., Mohammed, I., Cox, R. *et al.* (1967). Recurrent epidemic nephritis in South Trinidad. *N. Engl. J. Med.* **277**, 728–33.

Potter, E.V., Moran, A.F., Poon-King, T. and Earle, D.P. (1968). Characteristics of beta hemolytic streptococci associated with acute glomerulonephritis in Trinidad, West Indies. *J. Lab. Clin. Med.* **71**, 126–37.

Rammelkamp, C.H., Jr (1954). Acute hemorrhage glomerulonephritis. In *Streptococcal Infections*, ed. M. McCarty, pp. 197–207, Columbia University Press, New York.

Rammelkamp, C.H., Jr (1957). Microbiologic aspects of glomerulonephritis. *J. Chron. Dis.* **5**, 28–33.

Rammelkamp, C.H., Jr, Weaver, R.S. and Dingle, J.H. (1952). Significance of the epidemiological differences between acute nephritis and rheumatic fever. *Trans. Assoc. Am. Physicians* **65**, 168–79.

Raybourne, R.B., Bunning, V.K. and Williams, K.M. (1988). Reaction of anti-HLA-B monoclonal antibodies with envelope proteins of *Shigella* species: evidence for molecular mimicry in the spondyloarthropathies. *J. Immunol.* **140**, 3489–95.

Ronchese, F., Schwartz, R.H. and Germain, R.N. (1987). Functionally distinct subsites on a class II major histocompatibility complex molecule. *Nature* **329**, 254–6.

Roudier, J., Rhodes, G., Petersen, J., Vaughan, J.H. and Carson, D.A. (1988). The Epstein–Barr virus glycoprotein gp110, a molecular link between HLA DR4, HLA DR1 and rheumatoid arthritis. *Scand. J. Immunol.* **27**, 367–71.

Roy, S.B., Bhatia, M.L., Lazaro, E.J. and Ramalingaswami, V. (1963). Juvenile mitral stenosis in India. *Lancet* **ii**, 1193–5.

Schacht, R.G., Gluck, M.C., Gallo, G.R. and Baldwin, D.S. (1976). Progression to uremia after remission of acute post-streptococcal glomerulonephritis. *N. Engl. J. Med.* **295**, 977–81.

Schlosstein, L., Terasaki, P.I., Bluestone, R. and Pearson, C.M. (1973). High association of an HLA-A antigen, W27, with ankylosing spondylitis. *N. Engl. J. Med.* **288**, 704–6.

Schwartz, R. (1987). Fugue in T-lymphocyte recognition. *Nature* **326**, 738–9.

Schwimmbeck, P.L., Yu, D.T.Y. and Oldstone, M.B.A. (1987). Autoantibodies to HLA B27 in the sera of HLA B27 patients with ankylosing spondylitis and Reiter's syndrome molecular mimicry with *Klebsiella pneumoniae* as potential mechanism of autoimmune disease. *J. Exp. Med.* **166**, 173–81.

Schwimmbeck, P.L., Dyrberg, T., Drachman, D.B. and Oldstone, M.D. (1989). Molecular mimicry and myasthenia gravis. An autoantigenic site of the acetylcholine receptor alpha-subunit that has biologic activity and reacts immunocytochemically with herpes simplex virus. *J. Clin. Invest.* **84**, 1174–80.

Seager, K., Bashir, H.V., Geczy, A.F., Edmonds, J. and De Vere-Tyndall, A. (1979). Evidence for a specific B27-associated cell surface marker on lymphocytes of patients with ankylosing spondylitis. *Nature* **277**, 68–70.

Seegal, B.C., Andres, G.A., Hsu, K.C. and Zabriskie, J.B. (1965). Studies on the pathogenesis of acute and progressive glomerulonephritis in man by immunofluorescence and immunoferritin techniques. *Fed. Proc.* **24**, 100–8.

Stastny, P. (1978). Association of the B-cell alloantigen DRw4 with rheumatoid arthritis. *N. Engl. J. Med.* **298**, 869–71.

Stieglitz, H. and Lipsky, P.E. (1988). Identification of a plasmid shared by *Shigella flexneri* strains associated with reactive arthritis. *Arthritis Rheum.* **31**, S-14.

Stollerman, G.H. (1971). Rheumatogenic and nephritogenic streptococci. *Circulation* **43**, 915–21.

Sullivan, J.S. and Geczy, A.F. (1987). An antiserum to a disease-associated factor from the cells of an HLA-B27 positive patient with ankylosing spondylitis specifically recognizes an HLA-B27 associated determinant. *Arthritis Rheum.* **30**, 439–42.

Taranta, A. and Stollerman, G.H. (1956). The relationship between Sydenham's chorea to infection with Group A streptococci. *Am. J. Med.* **20**, 170–5.

Toivanen, A., Granfors, K., Lahesmaa-Rantala, R., Leino, R., Stahlberg, T. and Vuento, R. (1985). Pathogenesis of *Yersinia*-triggered reactive arthritis: immunological, microbiological and clinical aspects. *Immunol. Rev.* **86**, 47–70.

Treser, G., Semar, M., McVicar, M., Franklin, M.A., Ty, A., Sagel, I. and Lange, K. (1969). Antigenic streptococcal components in acute glomerulonephritis. *Science* **163**, 676–7.

Treser, G., Semar, M., Ty, A., Sagel, I., Franklin, M.A. and Lange, K. (1970). Partial characterization of antigenic streptococcal plasma membrane components in acute glomerulonephritis. *J. Clin. Invest.* **49**, 762–8.

Tsuchiya, N., Husby, G. and Williams, R.C., Jr (1989). Studies of humoral and cell-mediated immunity to peptides shared by HLA-B27.1 and *Klebsiella pneumoniae* nitrogenase in ankylosing spondylitis. *Clin. Exp. Immunol.* **76**, 354–60.

Vaishnava, S., Webb, J.K.G. and Cherian, J. (1960). Juvenile rheumatism in S. India: a clinical study of 166 cases. *Indian J. Child Health* **9**, 290–9.

van Bohemen, C.G., Brumet, F.C. and Zanen, H.C. (1984). Identification of HLA-B27M1 and -M2 cross-reactive antigens in *Klebsiella*, *Shigella* and *Yersinia*. *Immunology* **52**, 607–10.

van de Rijn, I., Zabriskie, J.B. and McCarty, M. (1977). Group A streptococcal antigens cross-reactive with myocardium: purification of heart-reactive antibody and isolation and characterization of the streptococcal antigen. *J. Exp. Med.* **146**, 579–99.

van de Rijn. I., Fillit, H., Brandeis, W.E. *et al.* (1978). Serial studies on circulating immune complexes in post-streptococcal sequelae. *Clin. Exp. Immunol.* **34**, 318–25.

Veasy, L.G., Wiedmeier, S.E., Orsmond, G.S. *et al.* (1987). Resurgence of acute rheumatic fever in the intermountain area of the United States. *N. Engl. J. Med.* **316**, 421–7.

Viitanen, A.M., Lahesmaa-Rantala, R., Weiss, E. and Toivanen, A. (1988). Lack of hybridization between *Yersinia enterocolitica* and HLA-B27 DNA. *J. Rheumatol.* **15**, 1123–5.

Villarreal, H., Jr, Fischetti, V.A., van de Rijn, I. and Zabriskie, J.B. (1979). The occurrence of a protein in the extracellular products of streptococci isolated from patients with acute glomerulonephritis. *J. Exp. Med.* **149**, 459–72.

Wald, E.R., Dashefsky, B., Feidt, C., Chiponis, D. and Byers, C. (1987). Acute rheumatic fever in Western Pennsylvania and the tri-state area. *Pediatrics* **80**, 371–4.

Welsh, J., Avakian, H., Cowling, P. *et al.* (1980). Ankylosing spondylitis, HLA-B27, and *Klebsiella*. I. Cross-reactivity studies with rabbit antisera. *Br. J. Exp. Pathol.* **61**, 85–91.

Woodrow, J.C., Nichol, F.E. and Zaphiropoulos, G. (1981). DR antigens and rheumatoid arthritis: a study of two populations. *Br. Med. J.* **283**, 1287–8.

Yu, DTY, Ogasawara, M., Hill, J.L. and Kono, D.H. (1985). Study of Reiter's syndrome with special emphasis on *Yersinia enterocolitica*. *Immunol. Rev.* **86**, 27–45.

Zabriskie, J.B. and Freimer, E.H. (1966). An immunological relationship between the group A *Streptococcus* and mamalian muscle. *J. Exp. Med.* **124**, 661–78.

Zabriskie, J.B., Hsu, K.C. and Seegal, B.C. (1970). Heart-reactive antibody associated with rheumatic fever: characterization and diagnostic significance. *Clin. Exp. Immunol.* **7**, 147–59.

Zabriskie, J.B., Lavency, D., Williams, R.C., Jr *et al.* (1985). Rheumatic fever associated B-cell alloantigen as identified by monoclonal antibodies. *Arthritis Rheum.* **28**, 1047–51.

Zoschke, D. and Segall, M. (1986). Dw subtypes of DR4 in rheumatoid arthritis: evidence for a preferential association with Dw4. *Hum. Immunol.* **15**, 118–24.

Section 10
Transplantation

86: The Allograft Response

R.I. Lechler and K.J. Wood

The clinical transplantation of organs and tissues is now practised in most major medical centres around the world. The techniques of transplantation have spread rapidly since the first successful human renal transplants were carried out by Hume, Merrill and Miller in 1952. Success rates vary according to the transplanted tissue; however, for kidney grafts that are exchanged between unrelated individuals 12-month survival rates of 80% are generally achieved. Transplantation immunology as a research area has a special place in the history of cellular immunology because of the insights that it has contributed. Most notably the strength of immune responses against transplanted allogeneic tissues led to the detection of the major histocompatibility complex (MHC) products, which were first known as transplantation antigens and now are known to play a central role in T cell recognition.

Given our current understanding of immune recognition, it is remarkable that tissues from any source other than an identical twin can be successfully transplanted. In this chapter we examine the immune response to incompatible tissues, how they are recognized and the effector mechanisms that can lead to their destruction. This is followed by a review of the forms of immunoregulation that can be induced or administered. Extensive reference will be made to experimental models of transplantation, from which much knowledge has been gained, and clinical applications will be discussed.

Overview of the allograft response

The events involved in allograft rejection are complex and knowledge of the underlying cellular and molecular interactions is still developing. The rejection process can be divided into two stages:

1 The afferent stage: this involves the activation of the recipient's immune system as a result of recognition of the donor alloantigens. Activation can occur in lymphoid tissue following the release of donor cells or antigen from the graft, or within the graft itself.

2 The efferent stage: this results from triggering of

the humoral and cellular effector mechanisms that are responsible for destroying and eliminating the transplanted tissue from the body.

An outline of these events is shown in Fig. 86.1. In brief, the donor alloantigens are presented by immunostimulatory antigen-presenting cells (APC) to the recipient's T cells, which are essential for allograft rejection (Rolstad and Ford 1974; Rygaard 1974; Hall *et al.* 1978). As shown in Fig. 86.1, both donor and recipient APC are thought to be responsible for the activation of allospecific helper T cells (T_h) (Lechler and Batchelor 1982a; Austyn and Steinman 1988). The T_h population in turn influences qualitative and quantitative aspects of alloimmune responses (Loveland *et al.* 1981; Dallman *et al.* 1982). In general the T_h have the CD4 +ve phenotype; however, recent evidence suggests that T cells expressing the CD8 antigen can also act as helper cells during allograft rejection (Rosenberg *et al.* 1986, 1987; Sprent *et al.* 1986). Helper T cells recognize the donor antigen(s) via the T cell receptor (TCR)/CD3 complex and as a result become activated, producing a number of soluble mediators collectively called lymphokines, including interleukin 2 (IL-2), IL-4 and interferon gamma (IFN-γ). Through direct cellular as well as lymphokine-mediated interactions T_h trigger the effector arm of the rejection response. The cellular events supported by activated T_h include: (i) triggering the maturation of T cell cytotoxic precursors (T_{cp}) into mature effector cytotoxic cells (T_c) that can kill cells of the transplanted organ; (ii) the growth and differentiation of B cells which produce antibody reactive against the graft; (iii) the activation of macrophages which develop cytocidal activity; (iv) an increase in the lytic activity of natural killer (NK) cells; (v) the attraction of other leucocytes to the site of the immune response, resulting in amplification of the response; and (vi) the increased expression of MHC antigens on tissues in the vicinity of the activated helper cells by the release of IFN-γ which may amplify the

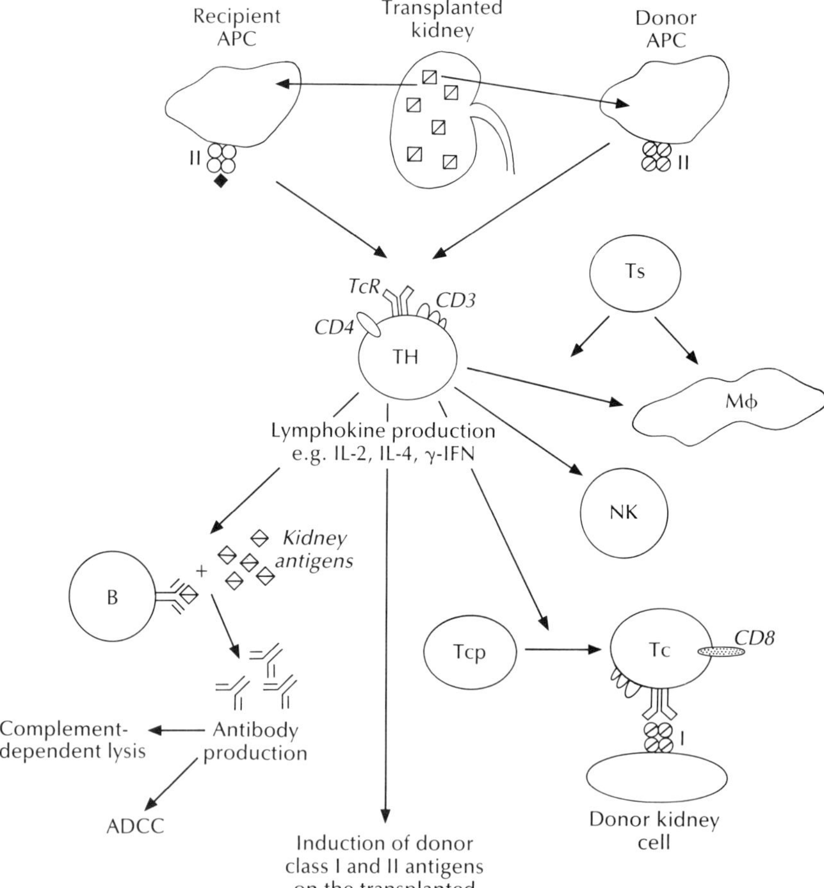

Fig. 86.1. Overview of the immune response to a kidney allograft. The cellular interactions involved in the immune response to a renal allograft and the effector mechanisms that may contribute to graft rejection are shown. Each of the cellular events displayed schematically in the figure are discussed in detail in the text. APC, antigen-presenting cell; T_h, helper T lymphocyte; NK, natural killer cell; B, B lymphocyte; ADCC, antibody-dependent cellular cytotoxicity.

rejection response. The relative contribution of each of these effector mechanisms to graft destruction is still a matter for debate and the contribution of each mechanism may be dependent on the organ transplanted.

Allorecognition

Fundamental to unravelling how the immune system is triggered by foreign tissues is understanding the molecular mechanisms by which transplanted donor alloantigens are recognized by T lymphocytes.

Transplantation antigens, so called because of their discovery as the stimulus to allograft rejection, can be divided into major and minor systems. The major antigens are the products of the MHC genes, which are described in detail elsewhere, and will be discussed extensively below. Minor transplantation or minor histocompatibility (mH) antigen are less well defined. The evidence for their existence is provided by the proliferative and cytotoxic responses of T lymphocytes to MHC-compatible allogeneic cells *in vitro* and by allograft rejection *in vivo*. The identity of minor antigens has yet to be elucidated; the current hypotheses about their nature are outlined below.

Recognition of allogeneic major histocompatibility complex antigens

It has long been known that MHC-incompatible cells induce uniquely strong primary immune responses *in vitro*, giving rise to the mixed lymphocyte reaction (MLR), and, *in vivo*, induce rapid graft rejection and/or graft-versus-host disease (GVHD). These reactions can largely be accounted for by the unusually high precursor frequency of T cells that are capable of recognizing and responding to foreign MHC molecules (Fischer-Lindahl and Wilson 1977). However, the ultimate cause of the high frequency of potentially alloreactive cells remains unclear (see below).

Any model proposed to explain allorecognition needs to take account of the three-dimensional structure of the human Class I MHC molecule, human leucocyte antigen (HLA)-A2 (Bjorkman *et al.* 1987), and the hypothetical model of Class II MHC structure that arises from it (Brown *et al.* 1988). The probable structure of a Class II MHC molecule is shown in Fig. 86.2 in schematic form.

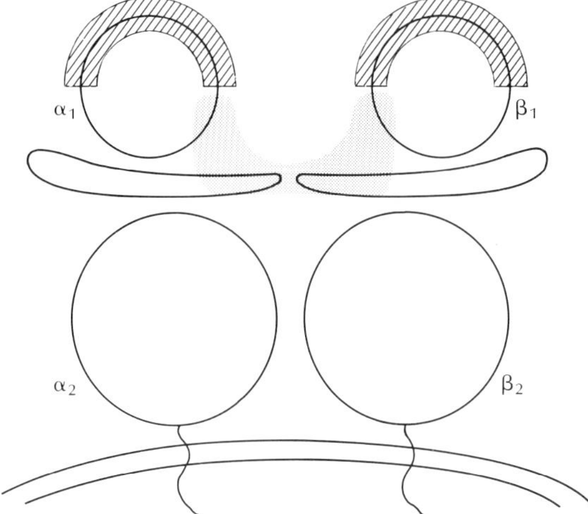

Fig. 86.2. Schematic diagram of the three-dimensional structure of a Class II MHC molecule. A cross-section through a Class II MHC molecule is represented schematically. Class II molecules are heterodimers composed of two transmembrane glycoproteins with molecular weights of approximately 33 kD and 28 kD. The hypothetical model of Class II MHC three-dimensional structure shown here is based on the published structure of the HLA-A2 molecule (Bjorkman *et al.* 1987; Brown *et al.* 1988). The membrane-proximal, α_2 and β_2, domains are predicted to resemble closely the structure of an immunoglobulin domain. The membrane-distal, α_1 and β_1, domains are predicted to have a unique structure comprising a platform of anti-parallel strands, overlain by a stretch of α-helical sequence, shown in cross-section here. This arrangement creates an antigen-binding groove bounded on either side of the inner aspects of the α-helices and beneath by the anti-parallel strands. The two regions of the molecule thought to be directly involved in controlling antigen recognition by T cells are highlighted. The surface predicted to make physical contact with bound antigens, the 'desetopic' surface, is stippled and the 'histotopic', T cell receptor-contacting, surface is cross-hatched in the figure.

The two structural components of the amino-terminal domains, namely the platform of anti-parallel strands overlain by stretches of α-helical sequence, can be clearly seen. As a result of this arrangement a groove is formed, flanked on either side by the α-helices, and beneath by the floor of antiparallel strands. This groove appears to be the site of antigen binding, and several lines of evidence suggest that many, if not all, such sites are occupied most of the time by endogenous peptides derived from self proteins.

Two major hypotheses have been proposed to account for the high precursor frequency of alloreactive cells. The first envisages that the specific ligand for most alloreactive T cells is the native foreign MHC molecule alone, and therefore predicts that an allogeneic, MHC-incompatible cell will display a high determinant density for T cell recognition (Bevan 1984). This model assumes either that a substantial fraction of the MHC molecules on the stimulator cell surface are 'vacant' (that is, unoccupied by peptide fragments) at any one time, or that alloreactive T cells pay no attention to endogenous peptides that may be bound to the foreign MHC molecules. In contrast the surface density of binary complexes of autologous MHC and nominal antigen recognized by antigen-specific T cells is predicted to be much lower, since only a small fraction of the MHC molecules on an APC surface are likely to be occupied with the relevant peptide for a particular T cell. If this were the case, the high determinant density of allo ligands would mean that cells of medium and of low affinity for allogeneic MHC could contribute to the alloreactive repertoire, thereby raising the precursor frequency relative to the number of nominal antigen-specific cells, which need to be of higher affinity.

The second hypothesis envisages that a single MHC molecule can give rise to multiple different antigenic specificities by forming binary complexes with an array of endogenous peptides that are continuously being generated by the endocytosis and processing of plasma and cellular proteins. Each of these binary complexes will be recognized by one or more clones of alloreactive T cells. In this case the 'determinant density' may be no higher than for a nominal antigen response. However, a single foreign MHC molecule should be capable of giving rise to multiple foreign MHC–peptide complexes and thus stimulate a large number of alloreactive cells, each with different fine specificities (Lombardi *et al.* 1989a). When this hypothesis was first proposed it was envisaged that cell surface molecules could interact directly with MHC products and give rise to multiple neo-antigenic determinants (Matzinger and Bevan 1977). This predated knowledge of the general requirement for antigen to be processed prior to its association with MHC.

Although these hypotheses help to explain why a single incompatible Class I or Class II MHC molecule may be capable of stimulating a large number of alloreactive T cells, they do not explain why T cells which usually recognize nominal antigens in conjunction with host MHC molecules should be capable of recognizing foreign MHC products. One of the early suggestions was that alloreactive T cells were a distinct population of cells, separate from the self-MHC-restricted, antigen-specific repertoire. However, the frequent detection of T cell clones with two defined specificities, one for self MHC and nominal antigen, the other for an allogeneic MHC molecule, suggests that alloreactive and antigen-specific T cell repertoires are overlapping (Bevan and Fink 1978; Finberg *et al.* 1978; Hunig and Bevan 1982). Definition of the T cell $\alpha\beta$ antigen-specific receptor (Ti) at the protein and genetic level has further established that alloreactive and self-restricted T cells are of the same lineage. A fundamental issue in determining whether or not the cross-reactive T cells described above are the exception or the rule is how the mature T cell repertoire is selected. The confluence of several lines of evidence strongly suggests that, in the thymus, differentiating T cells are positively selected for their ability to recognize antigen with host MHC molecules. This conclusion is derived from: (i) a large series of murine chimera and thymus graft experiments which demonstrate that T cells are restricted by the MHC type of the thymus in which they differentiated (Zingernagel *et al.* 1978; Lo and Sprent 1986); (ii) *In vivo* treatment of neonatal F_1 mice with monoclonal antibodies directed against one or other parental Class II MHC type resulted in T cell responses which were strongly biased towards restriction through the untreated MHC type (Marrack *et al.* 1988); and (iii) T cell receptor transgenic experiments in which the transgene-expressing T cells emerging from the thymus have the CD4 or CD8 phenotype appropriate to the MHC class specificity of the transgene-encoded receptor (Teh *et al.* 1988). Based on such evidence for selection of a self-MHC-restricted T cell repertoire, it has generally been assumed that allorecognition reflects some kind of molecular mimicry by foreign MHC molecules, with or without bound endogenous peptides, of the complex of self-MHC + '*x*' for which the T cell has a primary specificity. The difficulty in accounting for allorecognition by a cross-reactive hypothesis is that, at face value, this would appear to violate the well-established rules of T cell specificity. Most clonal populations of T cells have specificity for both the fragment of antigen and the MHC restriction element with which the antigen is associated.

The structural basis of this cross-reactivity can be more clearly understood in the light of current models of MHC three-dimensional structure as described above. It appears that two functionally distinct sites on MHC molecules are responsible for restricted recognition of antigen. The first, referred to as the 'desetope', is responsible for the binding of antigen and comprises amino acid residues that point into the antigen-binding groove. The surface of the Class II MHC molecule contributing to the desetope is stippled in Fig. 86.2. The second site is termed the 'histotope', and is predicted to interact directly with the Ti molecule, comprising residues that are predicted to point up towards Ti, and to determine MHC restriction specificity (Heber-Katz *et al.* 1983; Ronchese *et al.* 1987). This region is cross-hatched in Fig. 86.2. When all the different human Class II MHC HLA-DR types are compared it emerges that there is extensive similarity of histotopic, or MHC restriction-determining, regions between groups of variants. Examples of this are displayed in Fig. 86.3. The variable histotopic residues are highlighted. In contrast, the desetopic, or antigen-binding, portions of these groups of molecules contain multiple differences in most cases. This is likely to mean that they will each bind and display a different, although overlapping, array of endogenous peptides derived from the processing of self proteins. These observations suggest that, in many donor–recipient DR-incompatible combinations, allorecognition may mimic self-restricted recognition (because of histotopic similarity) of novel endogenous peptides bound by donor but not by responder MHC (because of desetopic differences) (Lombardi *et al.* 1989b). In these combinations allorecognition may follow the conventional rules of nominal antigen-specific, self-restricted, T cell responses. In combinations where extensive histotopic differences exist and self-MHC restriction cannot be mimicked, an alternative mechanism may be operative. It is possible, for example, that, although thymocytes appear to be selected for self-restricted recognition, a small minority may, by chance, interact with higher affinity with a histotopically distinct MHC molecule. These structural differences in allorecognition between particular donor–recipient combinations may have importance in determining individual precursor frequencies of alloreactive T cells, and as a consequence may influence the strength of T cell responses generated against allografts.

Thus far the role of donor cells acting directly as APC in the stimulation of alloimmune reactions has been discussed. An alternative mechanism exists for the generation of Class II MHC-restricted T cell help for alloresponses against Class I or II MHC-incompatible tissues. This involves the presentation of shed allogeneic molecules, including MHC products, by recipient APC. This is portrayed in Fig. 86.1. The self-restricted presentation of processed foreign MHC may be of particular importance in the absence of donor cells

				60				70						80		90	
DR cons	RP	—	AE	—	WNSQKD	–	LE	–	–	R	– –	VD	–	YCRHNYGV	—	ESFTVQRR	Source
1w1		D		Y		L		Q	R		AA		T		G		Tonelle *et al.* (1985)
4w4		D		Y		L		Q	K		AA		T		G		Spies *et al.* (1985)
4w14		D		Y		L		Q	R		AA		T		V		Gregerson *et al.* (1986)
4w15		S		Y		L		Q	R		AA		T		G		Gregerson *et al.* (1986)
w14w16		D		Y		L		Q	R		AA		T		G		Gorski (1989)
w15w2		D		Y		F		D	R		AA		T		G		
w15w12		D		Y		F		D	R		AA		T		G		Lee *et al.* (1987)
w16w21 (βIII)		D		Y		F		D	R		AA		T		G		Wu *et al.* (1986)
w11w5		DE		Y		F		D	R		AA		T		G		Tieber *et al.* (1986)
w8w8.1		S		Y		F		D	R		AL		T		G		Bell *et al.* (1987)
4w10		D		Y		I		D	E		AA		T		V		Gregerson *et al.* (1986)
w11wNew		DE		Y		I		D	E		AA		T		V		Bell *et al.* (1987)
w13w18		D		Y		I		D	E		AA		T		V		Gorski and Mach (1986)
w13w19		D		Y		I		D	E		AA		T		G		Tiercy *et al.* (1989)
w17w3		D		Y		L		Q	K		GR		N		V		Gorski and Mach (1986)
w52a		V		S		L		Q	K		GR		N		G		Gorski and Mach (1986)

Fig. 86.3. Sharing of β_1 domain polymorphic histotopic residues between groups of HLA-DR molecules. Amino acid sequences of the carboxy-terminal half of multiple DRβ_1 domains are presented. Only those residues that differ from the DRβ consensus sequences are shown. Residues at the five allelically polymorphic positions that are predicted to contribute to the histotopic surface of the domain are boxed. The sequences are presented in groups that share conserved residues at these five positions.

with the ability to induce strong primary responses, as discussed below in the section on immunogenicity. This was first proposed by Lechler and Batchelor (1982a), and has been extensively explored by Golding and Singer (1984) and by Sherwood *et al.* (1986). In view of the observation that Class I MHC-restricted antigen presentation appears to be predominantly concerned with intracellular proteins, rather than internalized extracellular material (Germain 1986; Morrison *et al.* 1986), this alternative route of allosensitization is likely to be confined to the stimulation of self Class II MHC-restricted T cells.

Recognition of minor histocompatibility antigens

In man, the transplantation of tissues between HLA-identical individuals, other than identical twins, leads to graft rejection unless immunosuppression is employed. Similarly in bone marrow transplantation, T cells present in the (untreated) donor bone marrow can mount severe GVHD. The same applies to experimental animals. Rejection of murine allografts, particularly of skin, transplanted from a H-2-identical donor of a different strain, led to the discovery of mH antigens (reviewed in Loveland and Simpson 1986). Incompatibility at mH loci leads to a slower tempo of graft rejection than for MHC mismatched combinations. This ranges from 15–30 to >70 days for mouse skin and heart grafts according to the degree of minor incompatibility. The important features of mH responses are that they are invariably MHC-restricted, and that they are under immune response (Ir) gene control by both MHC and non-MHC genes (Peugh *et al.* 1986).

Although many murine mH loci have been genetically mapped, including the male H-Y antigen, no mH product has yet been delineated. The facts that these antigens are seen by T cells but that no convincing anti-minor antibodies have been reported may be taken to imply that many mH antigens are allelically polymorphic intracellular molecules which are seen by T cells as processed peptides, complexed to cell surface MHC molecules. The intracellular location of the parent molecules may explain the absence of serological recognition. In man, mH antigen-specific T cells have been described, and five mH antigenic determinants defined (Goulmy 1988). Attempts to identify the molecules responsible are in progress.

Immunogenicity of transplanted tissues

A number of factors influence the immunogenicity of transplanted allogeneic tissues. In addition to the important differences between major and minor histoincompatibilities, there is variation between different strain combinations in experimental animal models. This is most clearly seen in rats; for example, rejection of (DA × Lewis) kidneys by Lewis recipients is very difficult to suppress, but the response of DA recipients to kidneys from the same F_1 strain is weak and easily suppressed. There is also a gene dosage effect in that the response to fully MHC-incompatible allografts is usually much stronger than that to semi-allogeneic tissues (Lechler and Batchelor 1982b). This is reflected in clinical human transplantation where kidney graft survival correlates with the number of matched HLA loci (Opelz 1987). The type of tissue allografted is another variable in this context, such that a rough rank order of vulnerability of different tissues to graft rejection is (from most to least vulnerable) bone marrow, skin, pancreatic islets, gut, lung, heart, kidney and liver (Calne 1983). The strong immunogenicity of allografted lung and gut tissues can be accounted for by the large number of lymphoid cells that reside at these sites.

A set of *in vitro* studies with obvious relevance to the kind of response made against an allograft has demonstrated that the specific recognition of antigen–MHC by T cells does not necessarily lead to activation. Under certain conditions antigen recognition can induce a state of specific non-responsiveness (tolerance). This seems to be determined by the nature of the APC. Thus, presentation of peptides of antigen by purified human T cells (Lamb *et al.* 1983), by artificial planar membranes impregnated with Class II MHC molecules (Quill and Schwartz 1987) or by chemically modified splenic APC (Jenkins and Schwartz, 1987) can lead to a specific state of tolerance in T cell clones. It is also clear that different lineages of Class II MHC-expressing cells have differing abilities in inducing a primary *in vitro* MLR response. For example, MHC-incompatible resting mouse B cells fail to stimulate proliferation in the MLR (Steinman and Inaba 1986), while activated B cells are capable of primary *in vitro* allostimulation. This cannot be accounted for by differing levels of MHC expression. The cell type with the greatest potency as an MLR stimulator appears to be the bone marrow-derived dendritic cell, which has been extensively studied by Steinman and Inaba (1986).

These *in vitro* observations have *in vivo* parallels in experimental models of organ transplantation. Depletion of bone marrow-derived cells from rodent kidney (Batchelor *et al.* 1979) and thyroid (Lafferty *et al.* 1975; Lafferty and Woolnough 1977) allografts by passage through an intermediate recipient or by low-temperature *in vitro* culture caused a marked reduction of immunogenicity. This led to indefinite survival without immunosuppression in some strain combinations, and significantly prolonged survival in others. Further, the immunogenicity of the retransplanted kidney was fully restored if chimerism was induced in the intermediate recipient with donor strain bone marrow (Lechler and Batchelor 1982b). The effect of bone marrow chimerism was to reconstitute the transplanted kidney with donor-strain passenger cells prior to retransplantation. In keeping with the *in vitro* data the allogeneic dendritic cell was the most potent passenger cell in restoring the immunogenicity of depleted kidneys, in that small numbers of donor-strain dendritic cells injected into the recipient at the time of retransplantation led to brisk graft rejection. A hundredfold more donor strain macrophages were required to have the same effect (Lechler and Batchelor 1982a). The design of these experiments is shown in Fig. 86.4. The possible relevance and application of these results to clinical transplantation will be discussed below in the section entitled 'Specific immunoregulation'.

Another factor that influences the immunogenicity of transplanted allogeneic tissue is the

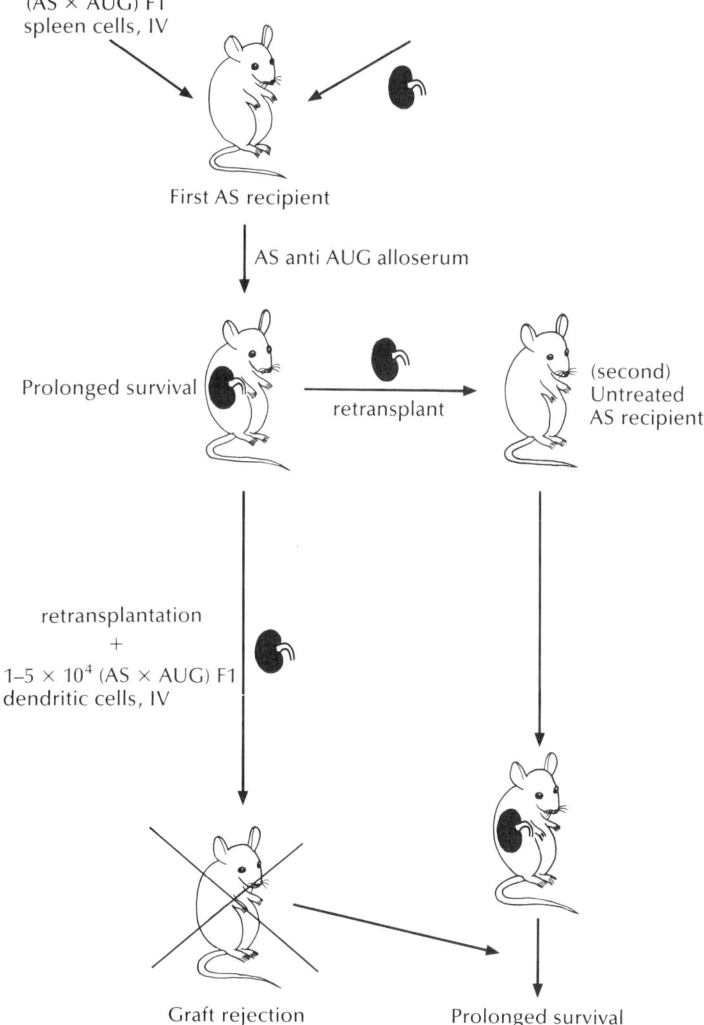

Fig. 86.4. Restoration of immunogenicity to passenger cell-depleted rat kidney allografts by the addition of donor-strain dendritic cells. AS × AUG kidneys transplanted into AS rats pretreated with AS × AUG spleen cells (active enhancement) and/or injected with AS anti-AUG alloantiserum perioperatively (passive enhancement) survive indefinitely (reviewed in Lechler and Batchelor 1982c). If the AS × AUG kidney is then retransplanted 4 weeks or more later into an untreated AS recipient, the allograft is not rejected and enjoys indefinite survival. This is due to the elimination of donor-strain, bone marrow-derived passenger cells. In contrast, if the second recipient is injected with as few as 10^4 donor-strain dendritic cells at the time of transplantation, the retransplanted graft is rejected at the same tempo as a primary transplant.

effect of Ir genes. This is clearly seen in the wide variation in survival times of rat kidney allografts transplanted between different strain combinations as described above, and has been extensively studied for rat liver allografts. For example, DA ($RT1^a$) livers transplanted into PVG ($RT1^c$) recipients enjoy indefinite survival, whereas LEW ($RT1^l$) livers placed in PVG recipients are rejected in approximately 30 days (reviewed in Kamada 1988). Immune response gene control of the antibody response to allogeneic red blood cells has been carefully studied by Butcher *et al.* 1982). Using a series of congenic rat strains that only differed in the MHC, they detected clear differences between MHC-disparate strains in response to the same alloantigen. The mechanism underlying these Ir gene effects is not clear, and any of the three major mechanisms — determinant selection (i.e. differential peptide binding, determined by MHC sequence variation), holes in the repertoire, or suppression — that have been proposed to account for Ir gene control of nominal antigen responses could apply in this context.

Effector mechanisms in allograft rejection

Activated T_h support the generation of several different immune effector mechanisms, all or any of which may contribute to or mediate graft de-

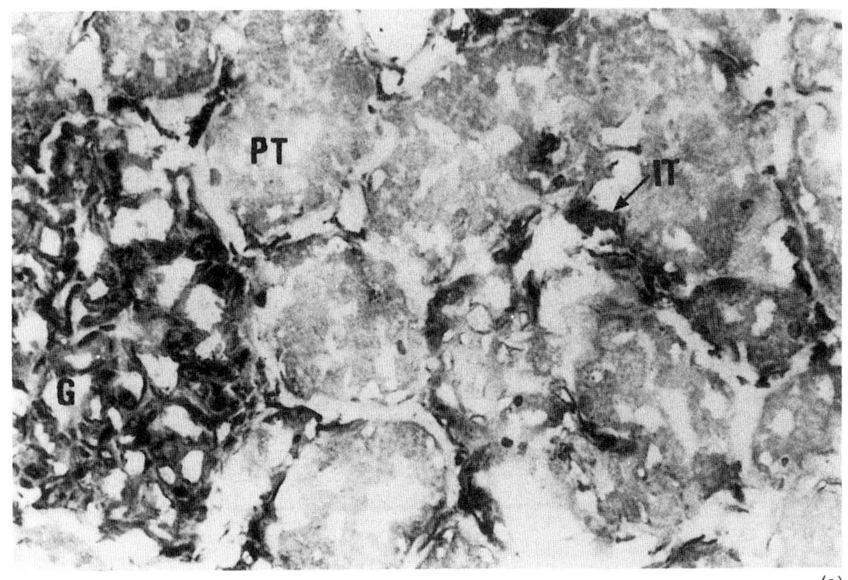

(a)

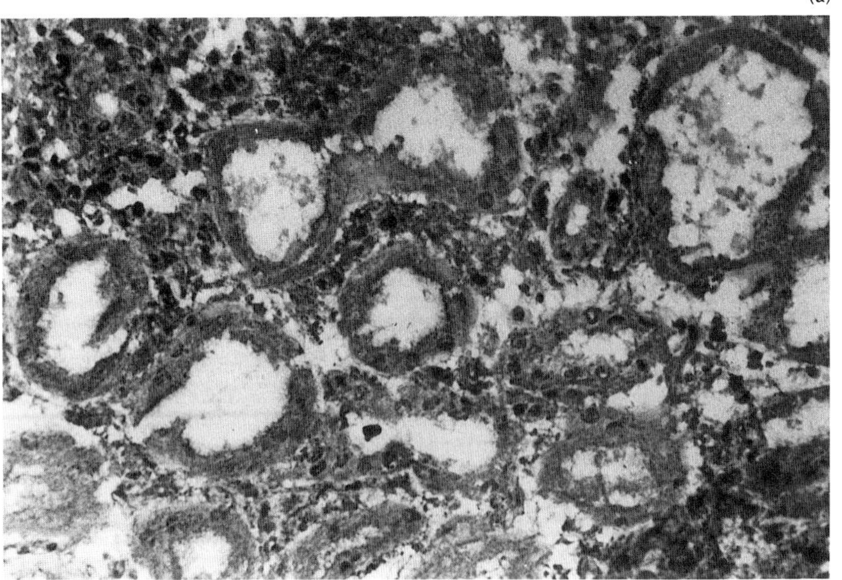
(b)

Fig. 86.5. Needle core biopsies from normal kidney before transplantation and from a graft during an acute rejection episode. (a) Cryostat section prepared from a pregraft biopsy, stained using a monoclonal antibody specific for HLA-DR, Class II MHC antigens and the indirect immunoperoxidase technique. Class II molecules are expressed weakly on some structures in normal kidney. G = glomerulus, PT = proximal tubule, IT = intertubular structures. (b) Cryostat section prepared from a biopsy taken during an episode of acute cellular rejection, stained in the same way. During graft rejection there is massive induction of HLA-DR antigens on all structures in the kidney.

struction (Fig. 86.1). These include cellular effector mechanisms: cell lysis mediated by antigen-specific cytotoxic T cells, activated macrophages as effectors of delayed-type hypersensitivity (DTH) reactions, and NK cells; and humoral mechanisms: the production of antibodies by B cells leading to antibody-dependent cell-mediated cytotoxicity (ADCC) and complement-dependent antibody-mediated cytotoxicity. The contribution of each of these mechanisms to the ultimate destruction of a graft is still a matter for debate and may depend on many different factors, including the immune status of the recipient and the tissue transplanted. One of the characteristic features of acutely rejecting allografts, namely the induction of Class II MHC antigen expression by tubular epithelial cells and the appearance of a mononuclear cell infiltrate are illustrated in Fig. 86.5. The 'activated' phenotype of the infiltrating cells is shown in a fine-needle aspirate from a rejecting kidney graft in Fig. 86.6. Each of the major candidate mechanisms of graft rejection is discussed below.

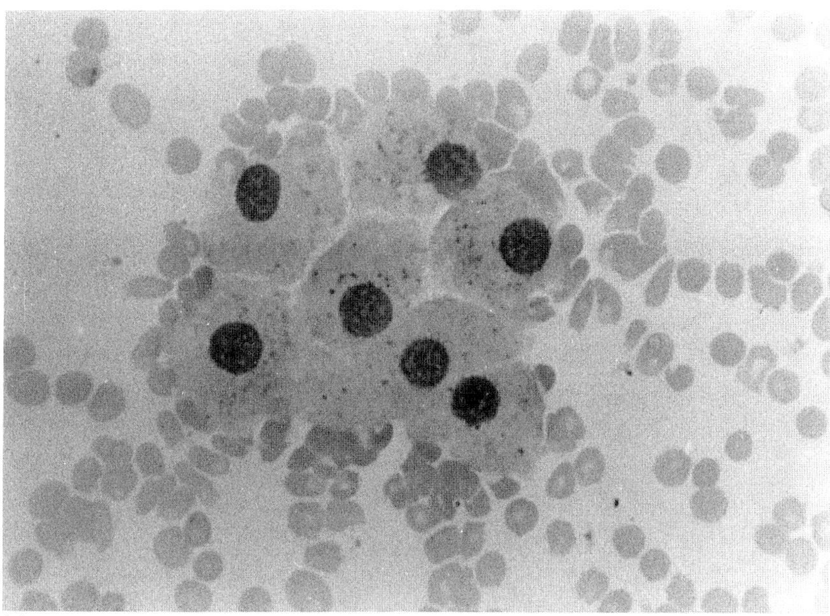

(a)

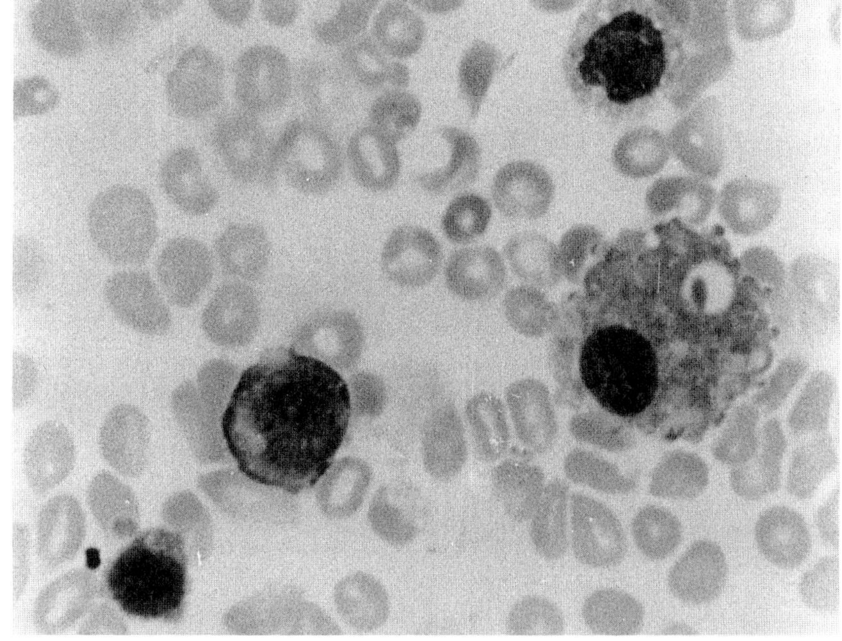

(b)

Fig. 86.6. Cells infiltrating rejected and non-rejected renal grafts. Fine-needle aspirates taken from (a) a renal graft showing good function and (b) a renal graft during a rejection episode. Fine-needle aspiration cytology allows the course of a graft to be monitored on a daily basis after transplantation, and thus offers advantages over needle core biopsies (Fig. 91.5). Infiltrating leucocytes and renal cells aspirated from a transplanted kidney are analysed morphologically and using monoclonal antibodies to define cell surface antigens. (a) The biopsy shows a collection of normal tubular cells and red blood cells. No infiltrating leucocytes are present. This example is typical of a fine-needle aspirate biopsy taken from a graft showing normal function and no signs of rejection. (b) This biopsy contained a large number of infiltrating leucocytes and damaged renal cells. The field selected shows a damaged tubular cell and three leucocytes in various stages of activation.

Cytotoxic T cells

Evidence is available for and against the role of the T_c as the main effector of allograft rejection. Although the idea that T_c are involved is attractive, there remains a shortage of clear evidence implicating this cell type as the major effector of cell-mediated rejection. The evidence for and against the role of T_c in the rejection process is outlined below.

SPECIFICITY

The specificity of the rejection process for cells expressing donor alloantigens has been interpreted as evidence supporting the role of T_c in graft destruction. In a series of experiments using tetraparental mice, bred by fusing embryos of two different genetic origins, Mintz and Silvers (1967, 1970) demonstrated the exquisite antigen specificity of the rejection process. The tissues of tetraparental mice are a mosaic made up of patches of cells from each parental type. When skin from the tetraparental offspring was transplanted to either parent, the cells of the other parental type were rejected leaving only cells of the recipient parental type intact in the skin graft. If the effector mechanisms mediating graft destruction were non-specific, such as those involved in DTH lesions (see later), bystander lysis of cells of both parental types in the skin graft would have been expected. In more recent studies Rosenberg *et al.* (1989) and Sutton *et al.* (1989) have also demonstrated exquisite specificity in the effector mechanisms mediating graft rejection.

THE EFFECTS OF CLONED CYTOTOXIC T CELLS

The clearest demonstration that T_c can mediate tissue damage comes from experiments in which cloned populations of donor-specific T_c have been used to reject tumour grafts in mice (Engers *et al.* 1982). These cells have been shown to cause local tissue necrosis when injected intradermally into mice expressing the skin-specific mH antigen, Epa-1, against which the T_c were directed (Tyler *et al.* 1984). Snider and co-workers (1986) have shown that cytotoxic cells specific for the Epa-1 antigen, isolated from lymph nodes draining rejected grafts and then cloned *in vitro*, will also induce tissue necrosis when injected intradermally. Although the results obtained using these cloned T_c are clear, these data have to be interpreted in the light of the fact that these cells were maintained *in vitro* for long periods after either *in vitro* or *in vivo* activation and as a result their functional activity may be different from cytotoxic cells activated and maintained *in vivo*.

DETECTION OF CYTOTOXIC T CELLS IN GRAFTS

Cells with specific cytotoxic effector activity can be recovered from rejected grafts (Tilney *et al.* 1974; Mason and Morris 1984; Bradley *et al.* 1985; Dallman *et al.* 1987). Furthermore, in some rat studies, where cyclosporin A was used to prevent graft rejection in certain rat strain combinations, specific T_c could not be recovered from non-rejected grafts (Mason and Morris 1984; Bradley *et al.* 1985). Together these data support the view that T_c play a vital role in graft rejection. However, recent experiments of Dallman and co-workers have demonstrated that donor-specific T_c can be recovered from non-rejected rat renal allografts in cyclosporin A-treated recipients, in some donor–recipient rat strain combinations (M.J. Dallman *et al.*, unpublished observation). Furthermore the presence of T_c in non-rejected grafts has also been demonstrated in recipients where preoperative donor-specific blood transfusion was used to prolong the survival of renal allografts indefinitely (Armstrong *et al.* 1987; Dallman *et al.* 1987). Indeed, in these grafts cytotoxic activity could still be detected 100 days after transplantation (K.J. Wood and M.J. Dallman, unpublished results). Thus the mere presence of a donor-specific T_c within a graft is not sufficient to result in its destruction. These findings do not necessarily imply that T_c are not involved in graft rejection. It is possible that the activity of the T_c is blocked within the graft, either by antibody or by suppressor cells, although as yet there is no firm evidence in support of this. Furthermore, when considering all of these data, it must be remembered that the cytotoxic activity of these graft-infiltrating cells is assayed *in vitro*, using the standard chromium release assay that has traditionally been used as a measure of cytoxicity. It may be that this assay system, and in particular the target cells used to determine the functional cytotoxic activity of graft-infiltrating cells, correlates poorly with the situation within the allograft itself *in vivo*. At present we do not know which cells are the main targets for the rejection response within the graft. The vascular endothelium has been suggested as the primary target (Paul *et al.* 1979), but until this issue is resolved or it is possible to develop a more relevant target to assay the activity of these cells *in vitro*, all of these data, including the detection of T_c in non-rejected grafts, are difficult to interpret.

Evidence derived in a different experimental system suggests, at least, that graft rejection can occur in the apparent absence of a specific T_c response. Male skin transplanted on to females of the same strain will normally be rejected, as a result of expression of the H-Y mH antigen by male tissue. Although female mice can reject male skin, they do not always generate H-Y-specific T_c (Hurme *et al.* 1978a, b). Thus in this case there is no correlation between the ability to reject a skin graft and the presence of T_c, implying that T_c are not required for the rejection of skin grafts resulting from mH antigen differences between donor and recipient.

RESTORATION OF GRAFT REJECTION BY CYTOTOXIC T CELLS

Experiments designed to determine the nature of the cells that are required to restore graft rejection have been performed in many laboratories. Skin allograft rejection can be restored in T-cell-depleted animals by reconstitution with CD4 +ve cells alone (Loveland *et al.* 1981; Dallman *et al.* 1982), suggesting at first sight that T_c are not important for the rejection process. However, as Dallman and her colleagues have pointed out, these data do not exclude a role for T_c in graft destruction for two reasons. First, these T-cell-depleted animals do contain T_{cp} that can be induced to mature into cytotoxic effector cells when T cells of the CD4 phenotype are provided (Mason *et al.* 1984). Second, it has been clearly demonstrated that T cell phenotype does not always correlate with the functional activity of the cell. Thus, although the majority of T_c are CD8 +ve and recognize antigen in association with Class I MHC antigens, a proportion of CD4 +ve T cells can also be cytotoxic for targets expressing antigen in association with Class II MHC molecules (Swain *et al.* 1981; Krensky *et al.* 1982). As a result of these findings interpretation of data from experiments based on the phenotype of the cells alone is difficult.

MONOCLONAL ANTIBODY INHIBITION

Monoclonal antibodies directed to the predominantly helper/inducer (CD4) and cytotoxic (CD8) T cell subsets have been used to study the requirements for graft rejection. Treatment of naïve recipients with antibodies to the CD4 subset only was sufficient to prolong the survival of murine skin allografts (Cobbold and Waldmann 1986) and cardiac allografts in mice (Madsen *et al.* 1987) and rats (Herbert and Roser 1988). Cobbold and colleagues (Cobbold *et al.* 1984; Cobbold and Waldmann 1986) also showed that treatment with antibodies specific for the CD8 +ve as well as the CD4 +ve subset resulted in greater prolongation of graft survival, again implicating a role for CD8 +ve T_c in graft rejection. Further, in recipients sensitized to donor alloantigens before transplantation, anti-CD8 monoclonal antibodies have been shown to prolong the survival of heart grafts (Madsen *et al.* 1989), suggesting that the relative roles of the two subsets of T cells in graft rejection may depend on the immune status of the recipient being treated. A similar conclusion can be drawn from reconstitution experiments reported by Hall and his colleagues (1978). These workers showed that reconstitution of rat kidney allograft rejection in irradiated recipients required both CD4 +ve and CD8 +ve cells if naïve cells were used. In contrast, if the reconstituting cells were from a sensitized animal, only CD8 +ve cells were required.

Taking into account all the available evidence from experimental models of organ transplantation, it appears that allospecific T_c of both CD4 +ve and CD8 +ve phenotypes do provide an important mechanism of allograft destruction. The results discussed in this section suggest that additional mechanisms, acting in concert with T_c, may be necessary to effect rejection. It also appears that other factors, such as the transplanted tissue and the immune status of the recipient, may determine the contribution of T_c.

Delayed-type hypersensitivity reactions

The original suggestion that DTH reactions were involved in graft rejection was made by Brent and colleagues (1962), who observed that the histological picture of cellular infiltrates in rejected skin grafts was similar to that observed in DTH reactions. Delayed-type hypersensitivity reactions are antigen-specific during the induction phase, but the effector phase is non-specific. The cells that generate DTH reactions are known to be helper/inducer cells of the CD4 +ve phenotype. Thus the observation that CD4 +ve T cells could reconstitute the rejection response in T-cell-deficient recipients (Loveland *et al*. 1981; Dallman *et al*. 1982) was initially taken as evidence for DTH being the major mechanism of graft rejection. However, as mentioned above, these recipients do possess cytotoxic precursors that can be induced to differentiate into cytotoxic cells both *in vitro* and *in vivo*, when 'help' is provided. In addition it is clear that a proportion of CD4 +ve T cells can also be cytotoxic.

Evidence in support of DTH in graft rejection comes from the studies of rejection of H-Y-disparate skin grafts where no correlation is found between graft rejection and the presence of T_c, but where a correlation is found with the development of DTH reactions (Liew and Simpson 1980). Bystander destruction of tissue has also been observed as a result of an antigen-specific immune response, implicating a non-specific effector mechanism such as DTH (Rubin and Tolkoff-Rubin 1984). Interestingly, when T cell clones specific for mH antigens, including H-Y and Epa-1, are injected intradermally into syngeneic recipients, ulcerating skin lesions can develop. The cells present in these skin lesions were found to be sensitive to irradiation of the recipient mouse prior to injection of the clone. This implies that much of the tissue damage was caused by host-derived, non-specific effector cells, such as activated macrophages which can mediate DTH (Snider and Steinmuller 1987).

Natural killer cells

Natural killer cells represent another cytotoxic cell lineage, but do not apparently show any antigen specificity or MHC restriction when they lyse target cells. These cells have been implicated as being important in the elimination of certain types of tumour cells from the body (Pross 1986), but their significance in graft rejection remains to be established. High levels of NK activity are found in rejected grafts (Mason and Morris 1984); however, similar levels of NK activity are also found in the non-rejected grafts of cyclosporin-treated (Bradley *et al*. 1985) or blood-transfused recipients (M.J. Dallman, K.J. Wood and P.J. Morris, unpublished observations). Furthermore, depletion of NK cells from recipients by treatment with anti-asialo GM1 antibodies did not alter the course of the rejection response to cardiac allografts (Heidecke *et al*. 1985).

Antibodies and graft rejection

Hyperacute rejection of transplanted organs in humans is the most clearly defined example of the role of antibodies in graft rejection. In this situation the recipient has been sensitized to one or more of the donor alloantigens before transplantation, either by a previous organ graft, pregnancy or blood transfusion, and as a result has circulating antibodies that can mediate graft rejection within hours of transplantation (Kissmeyer-Nielsen *et al*. 1966; Patel and Terasaki 1969; Morris and Ting 1982). Hyperacute rejection is accompanied not only by the deposition of antibody and complement components on the transplanted tissue, but also by the infiltration of polymorphonuclear leucocytes into the graft (Kissmeyer-Nielsen *et al*. 1966; Williams *et al*. 1968; Patel and Terasaki 1969). These observations resulted in the introduction of the cross-match test into clinical transplantation, whereby serum from the recipient is tested for reactivity with donor cells before transplantation. The presence of donor-reactive HLA antibodies in the recipient's serum immediately prior to transplantation is a contraindication to the use of that donor–recipient combination. For a review of this area, see Ting (1988). For reasons that are not clear, hyperacute rejection of liver allografts is not seen even in the face of a positive cross-match, so that the rules for liver transplantation are more relaxed.

Antibody is also thought to contribute to acute or accelerated graft rejection where the rejection is resistant to treatment with steroids or anti-thymocyte globulin, although the evidence is somewhat tenuous.

In summary, the major effector mechanisms

of graft rejection appear to be T_c, DTH and alloantibodies directed against graft antigens. It may well be the case that more than one of these mechanisms, acting in concert, may be required for vigorous graft rejection.

Regulation of the allograft response

The multicellular, multimolecular nature of alloimmune responses creates scope for many different approaches to manipulation of the allograft response. In this section the possible strategies are discussed under two major headings, non-specific and specific. The non-specific strategies include immunosuppressive drugs and the use of antibodies which interfere with immunity against any antigen. The approaches with specificity for the immune response against the transplanted tissue include mechanisms of reducing allograft immunogenicity and of inducing regulatory cells that hold the rejection in check. These strategies have been extensively studied in experimental models. Although success in applying some of these insights to clinical transplantation has been elusive, the induction of immunological non-responsiveness specific for the transplanted alloantigens remains the chief goal of transplantation immunology. It should be noted that the diminishing requirement for immunosuppressive drugs, as the time interval following transplantation increases, is evidence for naturally occurring regulatory mechanisms. Such 'native' immunoregulation may well be necessary for long-term graft survival, and should be augmented by any successful immunosuppressive regimen.

Non-specific immunosuppressive therapy

Drugs

AZATHIOPRINE AND CORTICOSTEROIDS

Azathioprine with prednisolone, or prednisone, have been used as maintenance immunosuppressive therapy in clinical transplantation for many years. Azathioprine is one of a group of drugs known as the thiopurines and is only active following metabolism in the liver. The major effect of this agent is antiproliferative, although the biochemical effects of azathioprine are complex and have not been completely characterized. It is important to note that the effects of azathioprine therapy are not restricted to the cells of the immune system: its metabolites can inhibit both deoxyribonucleic acid (DNA) and ribonucleic acid (RNA) synthesis and can, for example, interfere with coenzyme formation and function in any cell (for review see Bach 1975). Studies have shown that azathioprine also blocks the production of IL-2 by lymphocytes (Mussche *et al*. 1976). As lymphokines play a critical role in amplifying the rejection response (Fig. 86.1), blocking IL-2 production may be an important feature of azathioprine as an immunosuppressive drug.

Corticosteroids, such as prednisolone, have multiple effects on the immune system. In addition to reducing circulating numbers of T and B lymphocytes, prednisolone inhibits the trafficking of monocytes. The activation of T cells is also particularly inhibited. However, as with azathioprine, the action of steroids is not limited to the immune system, and the side-effects of these drugs on skin, eyes, bones and other tissues continue to present problems in clinical transplantation. Although azathioprine and prednisolone can be used successfully to control graft rejection, both of these agents act non-specifically on the immune system. Thus all immune responses are suppressed in recipients receiving these drugs, not only the immune response against the organ graft.

CYCLOSPORIN A

An immunosuppressive drug with the advantage of relative selectivity for T lymphocytes is cyclosporin A (CYA). While attempting to identify new antifungal agents in 1970, workers at Sandoz in Switzerland discovered the cyclosporins. The extracts of two strains of fungi imperfecti had weak antifungal activity but very low toxicity, and subsequent *in vitro* and *in vivo* testing by Borel and colleagues revealed interesting selective immunosuppressive effects. By 1980 CYA, a neutral, hydrophobic, cyclic peptide composed of 11 amino acids, was being synthesized and applied to clinical practice (Borel, 1981). During the past decade the use of CYA has had a major impact on clinical transplantation, increasing 12-month kidney graft survival rates by approximately 10% and significantly reducing the incidence of severe GVHD following bone marrow transplantation (Calne 1979).

In vitro CYA exerts non-cytotoxic, reversible inhibitory effects on mitogen-, nominal antigen- and alloantigen-induced activation of resting T lymphocytes. This can be detected as inhibition of proliferation or of T_c generation. An extensive literature attests to the effort which has been applied to determining the mechanism by which CYA interrupts lymphocyte activation. Although the story is incomplete, some progress has been made, as reviewed by Schreiber and Crabtree (1992), and outlined below.

After some early conflicting results, it is now clear that the major effect on CYA on T cells results from inhibition of IL-2 secretion (Bunjes *et al.* 1981). The addition of exogenous IL-2 to CYA-treated cultures usually leads to restoration of proliferation and T_c generation. Evidence has also been reported for an inhibitory effect of CYA on IL-1 secretion (Bunjes *et al.* 1981). The results of studies of IL-2 monoclonal antibodies and by IL-2 binding assays remain confusing (Dos Reis and Shevach 1982; Palacios 1982; Miyawaki *et al.* 1983; Orosz *et al.* 1983; Lillehoj *et al.* 1984). Some of the confusion may be resolved by monitoring the high-affinity form of the IL-2 receptor (IL-2R).

Examination of the effects of CYA on the biochemical parameters of cellular activation that can currently be measured has shown that hydrolysis of inositol phospholipids and calcium mobilization proceed normally (Metcalfe 1984). However, CYA seems to selectively inhibit the activation of lymphocytes by agents which mobilize Ca^{2+} (e.g. receptor cross-linking or ionophores) (Kay *et al.* 1983; Simons *et al.* 1986). In contrast, responses to polyclonal activators which directly activate protein kinase C (e.g. phorbol esters) are CYA-resistant (Sugawara and Ishizaka 1983). These data suggest that the site of action of CYA is 'downstream' of second-messenger generation. The observation that CYA binds to the Ca^{2+}-binding protein calmodulin (Simons *et al.* 1986) is consistent with this conclusion; however, it is difficult to reconcile this with the target specificity of CYA, given the ubiquitous distribution of calmodulin in eukaryotic cells.

In addition to these important effects on T cell activation, CYA also influences B cell responses to certain stimuli. Activation of resting B cells by anti-immunoglobulin (Ig) is inhibited, but lipopolysaccharide-induced activation is not (Dongworth and Klaus 1982). There appear to be parallels with the effects of CYA on T cells, in that early activation events are blocked in B cells, but the later phases of B cell growth and maturation, which are regulated by T-cell-derived factors, are unaffected (Klaus and Hawrylowicz 1984).

One lymphocyte population that appears refractory to the effect of CYA is suppressor T cells (T_c). It was noted several years ago in rat allograft models that a 14-day course of CYA resulted in prolonged alloantigen-specific non-responsiveness (Nagao *et al.* 1982). The evidence suggested that this was mediated by T_s (Wang *et al.* 1982; Hall *et al.* 1984; Yoshimura and Kahan 1985) and was paralleled by *in vitro* studies of T_s generation in mixed lymphocyte reactions in the presence or absence of CYA (Hess *et al.* 1980; Mohagheghpour *et al.* 1983). It is clear that important interspecies differences exist in this area, but relative sparing of suppressor cells may contribute to the immunosuppression induced by CYA in clinical transplantation.

A final consideration is whether the *in vitro* effects of CYA on T cells are mirrored *in vivo*. Studies in experimental animals demonstrated that T cell priming occurred *in vivo* in the presence of levels of CYA that were fully immunosuppressive *in vitro*. Thus, while the drug suppressed the development of experimental allergic encephalomyelitis in monkeys, following immunization with myelin basic protein (MBP), if challenged with MBP after withdrawal of CYA the animals succumbed to demyelination of the same severity and at the same tempo as animals that had been primed in the absence of CYA (Borel 1981). Similar observations made in other species and with other antigens illustrate the same point, that, although CYA suppresses the function of T_h it does not prevent their priming.

During the last 10 years CYA has emerged as a very effective immunosuppressive agent in clinical transplantation. More precise understanding of its mechanism of action requires a more detailed grasp of the biochemical pathways of lymphocyte activation. Paradoxically the inclusion of CYA in *in vitro* studies of cellular activation may assist in their unravelling.

FK-506

A new fungal fermentation product with immunosuppressive properties has been isolated and investigated in the last 5 years (Ochiai *et al.* 1987). This agent appears to be very similar to CYA in its effects on the immune system, but has the advantage of minimal nephrotoxicity. In several rodent models of organ transplantation FK-506 proved to be a more potent immunosuppressive drug than CYA (Morris *et al.* 1989). However, CYA remains the most effective agent in canine allotransplantation (Sato *et al.* 1989; Yokota *et al.* 1989) and in xenotransplantation (Gudas *et al.* 1989). *In vitro* FK-506, like CYA, prevents the generation of T_c and inhibits the induction of IL-2R and T cell proliferation in response to allostimulation. One difference from CYA is that FK-506 appears not to spare suppressor cells (Yoshimura *et al.* 1989).

15-DEOXYSPERGUALIN

During the same period that FK-506 has been under study, a new drug, 15-deoxyspergualin (DSG), has emerged as a potent immunosuppressive agent (Nemoto *et al.* 1987). 15-Deoxyspergualin was derived from the anti-tumour antibiotic spergualin, which was originally isolated from *Bacillus laterosporus*. This drug has also proved to have powerful immunosuppressive effects in rodent allotransplantation (Schubert *et al.* 1987; Suzuki *et al.* 1987; Walter *et al.* 1987; Engermann *et al.* 1988). Its role in larger animals remains uncertain (Collier *et al.* 1988), and its use as a maintenance immunosuppressive agent is hampered by the fact that it cannot be administered orally. The mechanism of action of DSG has yet to be established, but it is clearly different from that of CYA and FK-506 (Okubo *et al.* 1989). 15-Deoxyspergualin has no inhibitory effect on IL-2 production, but may rather exert its action on alloantigen-presenting macrophages and B cells.

Antibodies

Once it was established that the T lymphocyte played an essential role in graft rejection (Rolstad and Ford 1974; Rygaard 1974), it followed that agents which acted selectively on this arm of the immune response might result in more specific immunosuppressive therapy. The drugs discussed in the preceding sections do exert some of their effects on T cells — this is particularly true of CYA; however, they are not truly specific. Lymphocytes, T cells and B cells express cell surface molecules that allow them to be distinguished from other cell types. Polyclonal and monoclonal antibodies can be made that react with cell surface molecules expressed by all lymphocytes, by T cells but not B cells, by some T cells, for example CD4 +ve or CD8 +ve subsets, or by activated but not resting T cells, for example the IL-2R (CD25). These reagents have all been shown to be effective in experimental systems, and are at various stages of clinical application.

The molecules against which therapeutic antibodies may be directed are illustrated, schematically, in Fig. 86.7. It should be noted that anti-MHC antibodies, although effective immunosuppressive agents in experimental animals, are not readily applicable in man. This reflects differences in the distribution of Class II MHC molecules, which are constitutively expressed on vascular endothelium in man but not in rodents, and variation in the efficiency of complement fixation and its consequences.

ANTILYMPHOCYTE AND ANTITHYMOCYTE GLOBULIN

The properties of antilymphocyte sera were studied as long as 60 years ago, although it is only

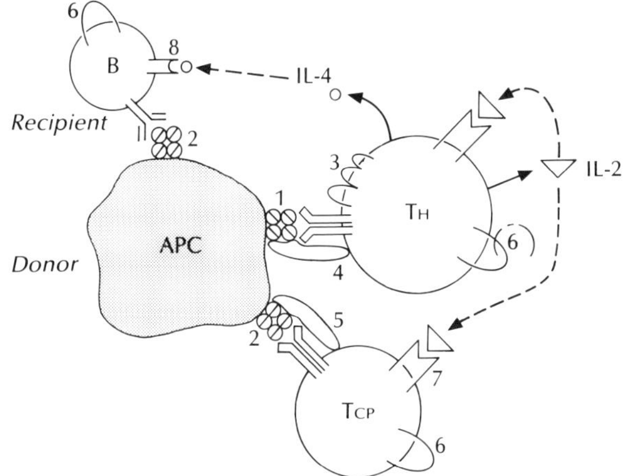

Fig. 86.7. Target molecules for immunotherapy. Some of the cell surface and secreted molecules that are involved in the generation of specific immune responses are shown. Antibodies have been produced against all these molecules, and several such reagents (directed against sites 3–7 in the figure) have been used in the clinical context. These are discussed in detail in the text. 1 = MHC Class II, 2 = MHC Class I, 3 = CD3, 4 = CD4, 5 = CD8, 6 = pan lymphocyte surface molecules (e.g. CD45), 7 = IL-2R, 8 = IL-4R.

more recently that their effects on graft rejection have been carefully investigated. Since the early 1980s antilymphocyte globulin (ALG) and antithymocyte globulin (ATG) have been used by many transplant centres for the treatment of rejection episodes in patients receiving azathioprine and steroids and/or CYA therapy (Matas *et al.* 1982). The polyclonal antisera are composed of multiple antibodies specific for lymphocyte cell surface molecules, including the pan-lymphocyte molecules shown in Fig. 86.7.

Both ALG and ATG are prepared by immunizing an animal (rabbit, horse or goat) with human lymphoid cells, either lymphoblasts for ALG or thymocytes for ATG. The thymus is greatly enriched in T cells; however, lymphoblasts include not only T and B cells but also other types of leucocyte, so that ALG preparations are usually less specific reagents than ATG. One of the problems associated with the production and use of ATG or ALG is variation between different preparations of antisera. Unfortunately there is no standardized *in vitro* test to determine the potency of ALG or ATG preparations, and this can only be assessed reliably *in vitro*, by examining their ability to prolong graft survival in non-human primates. Another complication of using these agents is the development of side-effects, mainly fever, in some patients. This probably results from the release of pyrogens due to rapid lympholysis. The mechanism of action of ALG and ATG is a matter of considerable debate. Treatment with ATG or ALG does result in a depletion of the lymphocyte count; however, it is not necessary to completely deplete the recipient of lymphocytes to achieve immunosuppression using these agents. In addition, ATG or ALG therapy decreases the proliferative capacity of lymphocytes in response to activation signals. Interestingly this remains impaired for some time after treatment with the antiserum has stopped, even though the numbers of lymphocytes in the circulation gradually return to normal (for review see Cosimi 1988). It has been suggested that these continued effects result from the generation of non-specific suppressor cells during ALG or ATG therapy, which continue to suppress the immune response after the antibody treatment has been completed. Such cells have been identified in both mouse (Maki *et al.* 1981) and monkey (Thomas *et al.* 1982) models.

MONOCLONAL ANTIBODIES (see also Chapter 47)

Monoclonal antibodies offer several advantages over conventional polyclonal antisera, partly because of their monospecificity, and partly because once a stable, antibody-secreting hybridoma has been cloned the antibody it secretes can be produced in large quantities and purified to homogeneity. This means that the dose of antibody administered can be determined accurately and precisely targeted immunotherapy can be achieved. It should be noted that many factors can influence the therapeutic potency of a particular monoclonal antibody. Not all monoclonal antibodies specific for the same molecule may have the same effects *in vivo*. For example, different antibodies may react with different antigenic epitopes on a molecule and as a result deliver a different signal to the cell, and antibodies with specificity for an identical epitope, but having different Fc regions, e.g. IgM vs. IgG, may have different properties. All of these parameters have to be considered when a monoclonal antibody is selected for use *in vivo*.

Anti-CD3

It was initially envisaged that monoclonal antibodies with similar specificities to the polyclonal antibody preparations might overcome some of the problems of batch variability and cross-reactivity associated with ALG and ATG preparations. A number of cell surface molecules, for example CD3 and CD2, are expressed by all T cells irrespective of their antigen specificity. Monoclonal antibodies specific for these molecules may mimic the action of ATG and be powerful immunosuppressive agents, specifically targeting the T lymphocytes.

The mouse monoclonal antibody OKT3, which recognizes the human CD3 antigen, has been used to treat recipients of renal allografts in clinical transplantation (Cosimi *et al.* 1981). Intravenous administration of OKT3 clears T cells from the circulation very efficiently, presumably by opsonization. Within minutes of the first infusion of the antibody, T cells are essentially undetectable as shown by the fall in the number of peripheral blood lymphocytes and loss of reactivity with monoclonal antibodies that detect other molecules present in the T cell membrane. Interestingly, as therapy with OKT3 continues, the number of lymphocytes present in the circulation that are not reactive with the monoclonal antibody OKT3 but are reactive with antibodies detecting T cell markers increases and, after a period of culture *in vitro*, the CD3 molecule is re-expressed by these T cells. These data suggest that, although elimination of T cells may occur initially on treatment with OKT3, modulation of the CD3 molecule from the surface of the T cells or repopulation of the peripheral blood by immature CD3 −ve T cells may occur subsequently.

The monoclonal antibody OKT3 was first evaluated as an immunosuppressive agent in 1981, when it was used in a pilot trial to treat acute graft rejection (Cosimi *et al.* 1981). It was found to be a very effective treatment for reversing acute rejection in all the cases tested. A multicentre controlled trial was then undertaken (Ortho Multi-Centre Transplant Study Group 1985) and OKT3 is now widely used to treat steroid-resistant rejection episodes by many transplant centres in the United States (for review see Waldmann 1989).

The major disadvantages of anti-CD3 monoclonal antibody treatment are its side-effects, which may be more severe than for polyclonal antisera, and the development of anti-mouse Ig antibodies in approximately 75% of patients (Jaffers *et al.* 1986). These antibodies effectively neutralize the therapeutic effects of the monoclonal antibody. As a result, OKT3 therapy can only effectively be used once to treat a rejection episode after transplantation. To try and reduce the recipient's immune response to the xenogeneic antibody, cyclosphosphamide may be included in the immunosuppressive protocol during and after OKT3 therapy.

This problem may be overcome in the future by using 'reshaped' human monoclonal antibody, where the hypervariable regions that contact the antigen have been transplanted from the mouse or rat Ig genes into human Ig genes. The hybrid heavy and light chain genes can be expressed and large quantities of the reshaped antibody isolated for use therapeutically (Reichmann *et al.* 1988).

Anti-CD4 and anti-CD8

Monoclonal antibodies specific for the two major subsets of T cells are also available. T cells expressing the CD4 molecule are specific for Class II MHC molecules and generally function as T_h, although CD4 +ve cell-mediated lysis has often been documented *in vitro* (Swain *et al.* 1981). In contrast, T cells expressing the CD8 molecule are specific for Class I MHC molecules, and in general function as T_c. Monoclonal antibodies specific for these molecules in many species, including man, have been made, and their role as immunosuppressive agents has been explored. In the mouse, anti-CD4 monoclonal antibodies have been shown to be potent immunosuppressive agents in naïve recipients (Cobbold *et al.* 1984; Cobbold and Waldmann 1986; Madsen *et al.* 1987; Shizuru *et al.* 1987). In some instances if monoclonal antibodies specific for CD4 and CD8 antigens are combined, more potent immunosuppression can be achieved (Cobbold and Waldmann 1986). Madsen *et al.* (1989) have shown that therapy with anti-CD8 monoclonal antibody may be more effective in recipients sensitized to the organ donor before transplantation, presumably because alloantigen-specific CD8 +ve T_c have previously been primed and clonally expanded. The immunosuppressive properties of monoclonal antibodies specific for the human CD4 molecule, OKT4 and OKT4A, have been tested in a primate model (Jonker *et al.* 1986); however, the results obtained were not very encouraging. Clinical trials of anti-CD4 monoclonal antibody therapy, are currently in progress.

Monoclonal antibodies specific for activation antigens

When T cells respond to antigen and become activated, they express new molecules at the cell surface that are not present on resting T cells. One such antigen is the IL-2R (CD25). Targeting activated lymphocytes using monoclonal antibody reagents may allow more selective immunosuppressive therapy, as only those T cells that are activated and expressing the appropriate activation molecule at the time the antibody is administered will be affected. The IL-2R is composed of two polypeptide chains, p55, which has low affinity for IL-2R, and p75, which has intermediate affinity for IL-2R. When these two chains are associated at the cell surface, a receptor with high affinity for IL-2 is produced (Dukovich *et al.* 1987). Monoclonal antibodies specific for the IL-2R have been developed. In each case, the antibodies produced react with the low-affinity polypeptide, p55.

These reagents have achieved effective immunosuppression in experimental transplant models (Kirkman *et al.* 1985; Kupiec-Weglinski *et al.* 1985; Tellides *et al.* 1989) and an anti-human IL-2R monoclonal antibody is currently being evaluated in clinical trials (Soullilou *et al.* 1987).

Targeted toxins

In order to circumvent the problems of inefficient complement fixation, and the formation of anti-mouse Ig antibodies, following conventional monoclonal antibody therapy, Williams *et al.* (1987) developed a chimeric IL-2–toxin fusion protein. A recombinant gene was constructed in which the sequence encoding the receptor-binding domain of diphtheria toxin was replaced with the IL-2 gene. This fusion protein was cytotoxic for cells bearing the high-affinity form of the IL-2R *in vitro* (Bacha *et al.* 1988) and has recently been shown to cause prolonged or indefinite survival of cardiac allografts in mice (Barrett *et al.* 1989). The preliminary success of this approach will encourage the future development of new agents, in which other immunological ligands are coupled to toxins. This may provide new options for manipulation of the alloimmune response.

Total lymphoid irradiation

In the late 1970s investigators at Stanford found that a state of temporary non-responsiveness was induced following fractionated total lymphoid irradiation (TLI). This led to the permanent acceptance of skin and solid organ allografts in various experimental rodent models (Slavin *et al.* 1978; Strober *et al.* 1980). The administration of TLI was usually accompanied by the infusion of bone marrow and establishing a state of stable chimerism. During the past decade this technique has been applied in larger animals such as dogs (Strober 1984) and baboons (Myburgh *et al.* 1983). It has been suggested that the immunosuppressed state that results from TLI is due, in part, to the effects of natural suppressor cells (Bennett *et al.* 1978). Natural suppressor cells have certain features in common with NK cells in that they have a null phenotype, they do not need to be primed and they are not genetically restricted. These cells are not lytic, however, and seem to exert their effect by inhibiting the proliferation of other cell types (for review see Claman *et al.* 1986). The place of TLI in clinical transplantation has yet to be determined. It may prove to be useful, in conjunction with other measures, in the preoperative preparation of highly sensitized patients. This has been explored in a canine model of allotransplantation into hyperimmunized recipients (Rapaport *et al.* 1987).

Specific immunoregulation

One of the long-term aims in transplantation is the development of an immunosuppressive therapy that would selectively suppress or abolish the recipient's ability to respond to and reject the transplanted organ, but that would not affect the capacity of the immune system to respond to other antigenic stimuli encountered after transplantation. Although some of the approaches discussed above target certain immune cell populations, none of them are truly antigen-specific.

In experimental systems specific, donor-directed, regulation of alloimmunity can be induced in a number of ways. These approaches can be divided into those that inhibit alloimmunization and those that inhibit alloimmune effector functions. Although many of these interventions cannot readily be applied in clinical transplantation, the quest for detailed understanding of experimental immunosuppressive mechanisms is motivated by the possibility of developing approaches that can be transferred to human organ transplantation.

Inhibition of alloimmunization

ELIMINATION OR INACTIVATION OF PASSENGER LEUCOCYTES

The contribution of donor, bone marrow-derived, 'passenger cells', most notably dendritic cells, to graft immunogenicity has been discussed in the section on immunogenicity. The experimental approaches to passenger cell depletion/inactivation, by passage of an allograft (kidney) through an intermediate recipient or by *in vitro* low-temperature organ culture (thyroid) prior to transplantation, have been referred to above. Attempts to reduce the immunogenicity of human allografts by treatment of the donor with cytotoxic drugs and X-irradiation or by perfusion of the isolated kidney with anti-Class II MHC or with anti-leucocyte antibodies have had mixed results. Given the expression of Class II MHC antigens on vascular endothelium in man, perfusion with anti-MHC antibody would be a hazardous approach. A recent trial of graft perfusion with a monoclonal antibody specific for the leucocyte common antigen showed some benefit in reducing the incidence of early acute rejection (Brewer *et al.* 1989). However, tissue penetration by perfused antibody, in order to bind to interstitial white cells, may be incomplete during the available perfusion time. Furthermore, it is possible that the indirect route of alloimmunization, due to presentation of alloantigens by recipient APC (see Fig. 86.1), is sufficient to induce strong *in vivo* alloimmunization in man.

An extensive literature exists describing the immunosuppressive effects, in experimental animals, of injecting the recipient with anti-donor MHC antibody at the time of transplantation. This technique, known as 'passive enhancement', can achieve indefinite survival in some rat strain combinations (reviewed in Lechler and Batchelor 1982c). The mechanism may, again, be that of eliminating passenger cells or of masking alloantigen display on these cells. Certainly, potent immunosuppression is achieved by amounts of antibody that are far from sufficient to mask the majority of graft MHC antigens. In addition, removal of the Fc portion of the injected antibody practically abolishes its immunosuppressive effect (Winearls *et al.* 1979), implying that opsonization or complement-mediated lysis of cells with bound antibody may be an important mechanism in passive enhancement.

ELIMINATION OR INACTIVATION OF ANTIGEN-REACTIVE CELLS

One of the mechanisms proposed to account for the immunosuppressive effects of anti-donor MHC, 'enhancing' antibody is the clearance of antigen-reactive cells via the reticuloendothelial system. This hypothesis has been referred to as antigen-reactive cell opsonization, or ARCO. It is envisaged that a large immune complex is formed with an allogeneic cell acting as a bridge, bound simultaneously by an alloreactive T cell and by anti-donor antibody. The whole complex could then be cleared by Fc receptor (FcR)-mediated binding, leading to the selective removal of antigen-reactive recipient T cells. Such a phenomenon has been observed in rats bearing long-term surviving kidney allografts (Hutchinson 1980) and in mice carrying tumour or skin allografts (Hutchinson and Brent 1981). The clearance of antigen-reactive cells by this mechanism long after any passively administered antibody has disappeared from the circulation depends on the continual production of anti-donor antibody by the recipient. This has not been formally demonstrated.

Inhibition of immune effector mechanisms

A vast literature on T_s has accumulated over the past two decades, mostly describing *in vitro* systems. Much of this is regarded with some suspicion because of the failure to produce well-characterized, purified, cellular or soluble reagents. However, by far the most convincing experiments demonstrating antigen-specific T_s have been performed in animal transplant systems. There have been multiple reports of the suppressive effects of splenic T cells from an animal carrying a long-surviving allograft, when adoptively transferred to a syngeneic recipient of a fresh allograft from the same donor strain (Brent and Opara 1979; Marquet and Heystek 1981; Batchelor *et al.* 1984; Barber *et al.* 1985). The phenotype of the cells that are capable of transferring suppression appears to be that of CD8+ve T lymphocytes. The specificity and mechanism of action of these T_s remain unclear, although it has been suggested that recognition of, and immunity against, processed fragments of the receptors expressed by alloreactive cells may be an important mechanism (Lancaster *et al.* 1985; Batchelor *et al.* 1989). Evidence has also been described which implicates T_s in the specific non-responsiveness induced by pretreatment of the recipient with donor antigen, known as 'active enhancement'. This has a possible parallel in the beneficial effect of third-party blood transfusion in clinical renal transplantation.

The presence of anti-idiotypic (anti-antigen receptor) antibodies with immunosuppressive effects in rats carrying long-surviving allografts has been described (Binz and Wigzell 1979). These observations have been difficult to reproduce in experimental systems; however, there have been reports of anti-idiotypic antibodies in blood-transfused human recipients which have inhibitory effects in the mixed lymphocyte reaction (Singal and Joseph 1982; Burlingham *et al.* 1985). Such antibodies could exert their effects by blocking or modulating alloantigen-specific receptors, by leading to the removal of idiotype-bearing cells or by delivering a negative signal to idiotype-expressing cells.

References

Armstrong, H.E., Bolton, E.M., McMillan, I., Spencer, S.C. and Bradley, J.A. (1987). Prolonged survival of actively enhanced rat renal allografts despite accelerated cellular infiltration and rapid induction of both class I and II MHC antigents. *J. Exp. Med.* **165**, 891–907.

Austyn, J.M. and Steinman, R.M. (1988). The passenger leukocyte: a fresh look. *Transplant. Rev.* **2**, 139–76.

Bach, J.F. (1975). *The Mode of Action of Immunosuppressive Agents*. North-Holland, Amsterdam, The Netherlands.

Bacha, P., Williams, D.P., Watos, C., Williams, J.M., Murphy, J.R. and Strom, T.B. (1988). Interleukin 2 receptor-targeted cytotoxicity. *J. Exp. Med.* **167**, 612–22.

Barber, W.H., Hutchinson, I.V. and Morris, P.J. (1985). Mechanisms of kidney allograft maintenance in rats treated with cyclosporin. *Transplant. Proc.* **17**, 1391–3.

Barrett, L.V., Murphy, J.R., Strom, T.B. and Kirkman, R.L. (1989). Treatment with a diphtheria toxin-related interleukin 2 fusion protein prolongs cardiac allograft survival in mice. *Transplant. Proc.* **21**, 1130–1.

Batchelor, J.R., Welsh, K.I., Maynard, A. and Burgos, H. (1979). Failure of long-surviving, passively enhanced kidney allografts to provoke T-dependent alloimmunity. *J. Exp. Med.* **150**, 455–64.

Batchelor, J.R., Phillips, B.E. and Grennan, D. (1984). Suppressor cells and their role in the survival of immunologically enhanced rat kidney allografts. *Transplantation* **37**, 43–6.

Batchelor, J.R., Lombardi G. and Lechler, R.I. (1989). Speculations on the specificity of suppression. *Immunol. Today* **10**, 37–40.

Bennett, J.A., Rao, V.S. and Mitchell, M.S. (1978). Systemic bacillus Calmette–Guérin (BCG) activates natural suppressor cells. *Proc. Nat. Acad. Sci. (USA)* **75**, 5142–4.

Bevan, M.J. (1984). High determinant density may explain the phenomenon of alloreactivity. *Immunol. Today* **5**, 128–30.

Bevan, M.J. and Fink, P.J. (1978). The influence of thymus H-2 antigens on the specificity of maturing killer and helper cells. *Immunol. Rev.* **42**, 3–19.

Binz, H. and Wigzell, H. (1979). Induction of specific transplantation tolerance in adult animals. *Transplant. Proc.* **11**, 914–18.

Bjorkman, P.J., Saper, M.A., Samraoui, B., Bennett, W.S., Strominger, J.L. and Wiley, D.C. (1987). Structure of the human class I histocompatibility antigen, HLA-A2. *Nature* **329**, 506–12.

Borel, J.F. (1981). In *Transplantation and Clinical Immunology*, Vol. XIII, ed. J.L. Jouraine, J. Traeger and H. Betuel, p. 3, Excerpta Medica, Amsterdam.

Bradley, J.A., Mason, D.W. and Morris, P.J. (1985). Evidence that rat renal allografts are rejected by cytotoxic T cells and not by nonspecific effectors. *Transplantation* **39**, 169–75.

Brent, L. and Opara, S.C. (1979). Specific unresponsiveness to skin allografts in mice. V. Synergy between donor tissue extract, procarbazine hydrochloride and antilymphocyte serum in creating a long lasting unresponsiveness mediated by suppressor T cells. *Transplantation* **27**, 120–6.

Brent, L., Brown, J.B. and Medawar, P.B. (1962). Quantitative studies on tissue transplantation immunity. IV. Hypersensitivity reactions associated with the rejection of homografts. *Proc. Roy. Soc. B* **156**, 187–209.

Brewer, Y., Bewick, M., Palmer, A., Servern, A., Welsh, K.I. and Taube, D. (1989). Prevention of renal allograft rejection by perfusion with antileucocyte common (LC) monoclonal antibodies (MCABs) is dependent on good uptake of antibody by interstitial dendritic cells. *Transplant. Proc.* **21**, 1772–3.

Brown, J.H., Jardetsky, T., Saper, M.A., Samraoui, B., Bjorkman, P.J. and Wiley, D.C. (1988). A hypothetical model of the foreign antigen binding site of class II histocompatibility molecules. *Nature* **332**, 845–50.

Bunjes, D., Hardt, C., Rollinghoff, M. and Wagner, H. (1981). Cyclosporin A mediates immunosuppression of primary cytotoxic T-cell responses by impairing the release of interleukin 1 and interleukin 2. *Eur. J. Immunol.* **11**, 657–61.

Burlingham, W.J., Sparks, E.M., Sandel, P.M., Glass, N.R., Belzer, F.O. and Sollinger, H.W. (1985). Improved renal allograft survival following donor specific transfusions. I. Antibodies that inhibit a primary antidonor mixed lymphocyte culture response. *Transplantation* **39**, 12–17.

Butcher, G.W., Corvalan, J.R., Licence, D.R. and Howard, J.C. (1982). Immune response genes controlling responsiveness to major transplantation antigens: specific major histocompatibility complex-linked defect for antibody responses to class I alloantigens. *J. Exp. Med.* **155**, 303–20.

Calne, R.Y. (1979). Immunosuppression for organ grafting — observations on cyclosporine A. *Immunol. Rev.* **46**, 113–24.

Calne, R.Y. (1983). Allografting in the pig. In *Immunological Aspects of Transplantation Surgery*, ed. R.Y. Calne, MTP, Lancaster, UK.

Claman, H.N., Holda, J.H. and Maier, T. (1986). Natural suppressor cell systems. In *Progress in Immunology VI*, ed. B. Cinader and R.G. Miller, pp. 1035–9. Academic Press.

Cobbold, S.P. and Waldmann, H. (1986). Skin allograft rejection by L3T4 and Lyt2 cell subsets. *Transplantation* **41**, 634–9.

Cobbold, S.P., Jayasuriya, A., Nash, A., Prospero, T.D., Waldmann, H. (1984). Therapy with monoclonal antibodies by elimination of T cell subsets *in vivo*. *Nature* **312**, 548–51.

Collier, D.St. J., Calne, R., Thiru, S., Kohno, H. and Levickis, J. (1988). 15-Deoxyspergualin in experimental dog renal allografts. *Transplant. Proc.* **20** (suppl. 1), 240–1.

Cosimi, A.B. (1988). Antilymphocyte globulin and monoclonal antibodies. In *Kidney Transplantation — Principles and Practice*, ed. P.J. Morris, pp. 343–69.

Cosimi, A.B., Burton, R.C., Colvin, R.B. *et al.* (1981). Treatment of acute renal allograft rejection with OKT3 monoclonal antibody. *Transplantation* **32**, 535–9

Dallman, M.J., Mason, D.W. and Webb, M. (1982). The roles of host and donor cells in the rejection of skin allografts by T cell deprived rats injected with syngeneic T cells. *Eur. J. Immunol.* **12**, 511–18.

Dallman, M.J., Wood, K.J. and Morris, P.J. (1987). Specific

cytotoxic cells are found in the non-rejected kidneys of blood transfused rats. *J. Exp. Med.* **165**, 566–71.

Dongworth, D.W. and Klaus, G.G.B (1982). Effect of cyclosporin A on the immune system of the mouse. I. Evidence for a direct selective effect of cyclosporin A on B cells responding to anti-immunoglobulin antibodies. *Eur. J. Immunol.* **12**, 1018–22.

Dos Reis, G.A. and Shevach, E. (1982). Effect of cyclosporin A on T cell function *in vitro*: the mechanism of suppression of T-cell proliferation depends on the nature of the T cell stimulus as well as the differentiation state of the responding T cells. *J. Immunol.* **129**, 2360–7.

Dukovich, M., Wano, Y., Bich Thuy, L-T. *et al.* (1987). A second human interleukin-2 binding protein that may be a component of high-affinity interleukin-2 receptors. *Nature* 327, 518–22.

Engermann, R., Gassel, H.J., Lafrenz, E., Stoffregen, C., Thiede, A. and Hamelmann, H. (1988). The use of 15-deoxyspergualin in orthotopic rat liver transplantation: induction of transplantation tolerance and treatment of acute rejection. *Transplant. Proc.* **20**(suppl. 1), 237–9.

Engers, H.D., Glasebrook, A.L. and Sorenson, G.D. (1982). Allogeneic tumour rejection induced by the intravenous injection of Lyt-2 positive cytotoxic T lymphocyte clones. *J. Exp. Med.* **156**, 1280–5.

Finberg, R., Burakoff, S.J., Cantor, H. and Benacerraf, B. (1978). Biological significance of alloreactivity: T cells stimulated by Sendai virus-coated syngeneic cells specifically lyse allogeneic target cells. *Proc. Nat. Acad. Sci. (USA)* **75**, 5145–9.

Fischer-Lindahl K. and Wilson, D.B. (1977). Histocompatibility antigen-activated cytotoxic T lymphocytes. *J. Exp. Med.* **145**, 500–7.

Germain, R.N. (1986). The ins and outs of antigen processing and presentation. *Nature* **322**, 687–9.

Golding, H. and Singer, A. (1984). Role of accessory cell processing and presentation of shed H-2 alloantigens in allospecific cytotoxic T cell responses. *J. Immunol.* **133**, 597–605.

Gorski, J. (1989). First domain sequence of the HLA-DRB1 chain from two HLA-DRw14 homozygous typing cell lines: TEM (Dw9) and AMALA (Dw16). *Hum. Immunol.* **24**, 145–9.

Gorski, J. and Mach, B. (1986). Polymorphism of human Ia antigens: gene conversion between two DRβ loci results in a new HLA-D/DR specificity. *Nature* **322**, 67–70.

Goulmy, E. (1988). Minor histocompatibility antigens in man and their role in transplantation. *Transplant. Rev.* **2**, 29–53.

Gregersen, P.K., Shen, M., Song, Q. *et al.* (1986). Molecular diversity of HLA-DR4 haplotypes. *Proc. Nat. Acad. Sci. (USA)* **83**, 2642–6.

Gudas, V.M., Carmichael, P.G. and Morris, R.R. (1989). Comparison of the immunosuppressive and toxic effects of FK506 and cyclosporine in xenograft recipients. *Transplant. Proc.* **21**, 1072–3.

Hall, B.M., Dorsch, S.E. and Roser, B. (1978). The cellular basis of allograft rejection in vivo. I. The cellular requirements for first-set rejection of heart grafts. *J. Exp. Med.* **148**, 878–89.

Hall, B.M., Jelbart, M.E. and Dorsch, S.E. (1984). Suppressor T cells in rats with prolonged cardiac allograft survival after treatment with cyclosporin. *Transplantation* **37**, 595–600.

Heber-Katz, E., Hansburg, D. and Schwartz, R.H. (1983). The Ia molecule of the antigen-presenting cell plays a critical role in immune response gene regulation of T cell activation. *J. Mol. Cell. Immunol.* **1**, 3–18.

Heidecke, C.D., Araujo, J.L., Kupiec-Weglinski, J.W., Abbudfilho, M. and Araneda, D. (1985). Lack of evidence for an active role for NK cells in acute rejection of organ allografts. *Transplantation* **40**, 441–4.

Herbert, J. and Roser, B. (1988). Strategies of monoclonal antibody therapy that induce permanent tolerance of organ transplants. *Transplantation* **46**, 1285–345.

Hess, A.D. and Tutschka, P.J. (1980). Effects of cyclosporine A on human lymphocyte responses *in vitro*. I CSA allows for the expression of alloantigen-activated suppressor cells while preferentially inhibiting the induction of cytolytic effector lymphocytes in MLR. *J. Immunol.* **124**, 2601–8.

Hume, D.M., Merrill, J.P., Miller, B.F. and Thorn, G.W. (1952). Experiences with renal homotransplantation in the human: report of nine cases. *J. Clin. Invest.* **34**, 327–82.

Hunig, T. and Bevan, M.J. (1982). Antigen recognition by cloned cytotoxic T lymphocytes follows rules predicted by the altered self hypothesis. *J. Exp. Med.* **155**, 111–25.

Hurme, M., Hetherington, C.M., Chandler, P.R. and Simpson, E. (1978a). Cytotoxic T-cell responses to H-Y: mapping of the Ir genes. *J. Exp. Med.* **147**, 758–67.

Hurme, M., Chandler, P.R., Hetherington, C.M. and Simpson, E. (1978b). Cytotoxic T-cell responses to H-Y: correlation with rejection of syngeneic male skin grafts. *J. Exp. Med.* **147**, 768–75.

Hutchinson, I.V. (1980). Antigen reactive cell opsonization (ARCO) and its role in antibody mediated immune suppression. *Immunol. Rev.* **49**, 167–90.

Hutchinson, I.V. and Brent, L. (1981). Immunological enhancement of tumour allografts following treatment of mice with TNP-conjugated alloantigen and anti-TNP antibody. *Nature* **292**, 353–5.

Jaffers, G.J., Fuller, T.C., Cosimi, A.B., Russell, P.S., Winn, H.J. and Colvin, R.B. (1986). Monoclonal antibody therapy: anti-idiotypic and non-anti-idiotypic antibodies to OKT3 arising despite intense immunosuppression. *Transplantation* **41**, 572–8.

Jenkins, M.K. and Schwartz, R.H. (1987). Antigen-presentation by chemically-modified splenocytes induces antigen-specific T cell unresponsiveness *in vitro* and *in vivo*. *J. Exp. Med.* **165**, 302–19.

Jonker, M., Neuhaus, P., Fucello, A. and Goldstein, G. (1986). OKT4 and OKT4a antibody treatment as immunosuppression for transplantation in rhesus monkeys. *Transplantation* **39**, 247–53.

Kamada, N. (1988). Genetics of liver graft rejection in the rat. In *Experimental Liver Transplantation*. CRC Press, Boca Raton.

Kay, J.E., Benzie, C.R. and Borghetti, A.F. (1983). Effect of cyclosporin A on lymphocyte activation by the calcium ionophore A23187. *Immunology* **50**, 441–6.

Kirkman, R.L., Barrett, L.V., Gaulton, G.N., Kelley, V.E., Ythier, A. and Strom, T.B. (1985). Administration of an anti-interleukin 2 receptor monoclonal antibody prolongs cardiac allograft survival in mice. *J. Exp. Med.* **162**, 358–62.

Kissmeyer-Nielsen, F., Olsen, S., Petersen, V.P. and Fjeldborg, O. (1966). Hyperacute rejection of kidney allografts, associated with pre-existing humoral antibodies against donor cells. *Lancet* **ii**, 662–5.

Klaus, G.G.B. and Hawrylowicz, C.M. (1984). Activation and proliferation signals in mouse B cells. II. Evidence for activation (G0 to G1) signals differing in sensitivity to cyclosporin. *Eur. J Immunol.* **14**, 250–4.

Krensky, A.M., Reiss, C.S., Mier, J.W., Strominger, J.L. and Burakoff, S.J. (1982). Long-term human cytolytic T-cell lines allospecific for HLA-DR6 antigen are OKT4+. *Proc. Nat. Acad. Sci. (USA)* **79**, 2365–9.

Kupiec-Weglinksi, J.W., Diamantstein, T., Tilney, N.L. and Strom, T.B. (1985). Therapy with monoclonal antibody to interleukin 2 receptor spares suppressor T cells and prevents or reverses acute allograft rejection in rats. *Proc. Nat. Acad. Sci. (USA)* **83**, 2624–7.

Lafferty, K.J. and Woolnough, J. (1977). The origin and mechanism of the allograft reaction. *Immunol. Rev.* **35**, 231–62.

Lafferty, K.J., Cooley, M.A., Woolnough, J. and Walker, K.Z. (1975). Thyroid allograft immunogenicity is reduced after a period in organ culture. *Science* **188**, 259–61.

Lamb, J.R., Skidmore, B.J., Green, N., Chiller, J.M. and Feldmann, M. (1983). Induction of tolerance in influenza virus-immune T lymphocyte clones with synthetic peptides of influenza haemagglutinin. *J. Exp. Med.* **157**, 1434–47.

Lancaster, F., Chui, Y.L. and Batchelor, J.R. (1985). Anti-idiotypic T cells suppress rejection of renal allografts in rats. *Nature* **315**, 336–7.

Lechler, R.I. and Batchelor, J.R. (1982a). Restoration of immunogenicity to passenger cell-depleted kidney allografts by the addition of donor strain dendritic cells. *J. Exp. Med.* **155**, 31–41.

Lechler, R.I. and Batchelor, J.R. (1982b). Immunogenicity of retransplanted rat kidney allografts: effect of inducing chimaerism in the first recipient and quantitative studies on immunosuppression of the second recipient. *J. Exp. Med.* **156**, 1835–41.

Lechler, R.I. and Batchelor, J.R. (1982c). Organ allograft enhancement: a review. *Heart Transplant.* **1**, 217–20.

Lee, B.S.M., Rust, N.A., McMichael, A.J. and McDevitt, H.O. (1987). HLA-DR2 subtypes form an additional supertypic family of DRβ alleles. *Proc. Nat. Acad. Sci. (USA)* **84**, 4591–5.

Liew, F.Y. and Simpson, E. (1980). Delayed-type hypersensitivity responses to H-Y: characterisation and mapping of Ir genes. *Immunogenetics* **11**, 255–66.

Lillehoj, H.S., Malek, T.R. and Shevach, E.M. (1984). Differential effect of cyclosporin A on the expression of T and B lymphocyte activation antigens. *J. Immunol.* **133**, 244–50.

Lo, D. and Sprent, J. (1986). Identity of cells that imprint H-2-restricted T-cell specificity in the thymus. *Nature* **319**, 672–5.

Lombardi, G., Sidhu, S., Lamb, J.R., Batchelor, J.R. and Lechler, R.I. (1989a). Co-recognition of endogenous antigens with HLA-DR1 by alloreactive human T cell clones. *J. Immunol.* **142**, 753–9.

Lombardi, G., Sidhu, S., Batchelor, J.R. and Lechler, R.I. (1989b). Allorecognition of DR1 by T cells from a DR4/6 responder may mimic self-restricted recognition of novel endogenous peptides. *Proc. Nat. Acad. Sci. (USA)* **86**, 4190–4.

Loveland, B.E. and Simpson, E. (1986). The non-MHC transplantation antigens: neither weak nor minor. *Immunol. Today* **7**, 223–9.

Loveland, B.E., Hogarth, P.M., Ceredig, R. and McKenzie, I.F.C. (1981). Cells mediating graft rejection in the mouse. I. Lyt-1 cells mediate skin graft rejection. *J. Exp. Med.* **153**, 1044–57.

Madsen, J.C., Pugh, W.N., Wood, K.J. and Morris, P.J. (1987). The effect of anti L3T4 monoclonal antibody on first set rejection of murine cardiac allografts. *Transplantation* **44**, 849–51.

Madsen, J.C., Wood, K.J. and Morris, P.J. (1989). Effects of anti-L3/T4 and anti-Lyt2 monoclonal antibody therapy on cardiac allograft survival in presensitised recipients. *Transplant. Proc.* **21**, 1022.

Maki, T., Gottschalk, R., Wood, M.L. and Monaco, A.P. (1981). Specific unresponsiveness to skin allografts in antilymphocyte serum treated, marrow injected mice: participation of donor marrow derived suppressor T cells. *J. Immunol.* **127**, 1433–8.

Marquet, R.L. and Heystek, G.A. (1981). Induction of suppressor cells by donor-specific blood transfusions and heart transplantation in rats. *Transplantation* **31**, 271–4.

Marrack, P., Kushnir, E., Born, W., McDuffie, M. and Kappler, J. (1988). The development of helper T cell precursors in mouse thymus. *J. Immunol.* **140**, 2508–14.

Mason, D.W. and Morris, P.J. (1984). Inhibition of the accumulation, in rat kidney allografts, of specific but not nonspecific cytotoxic cells by cyclosporin. *Transplantation* **37**, 46–51.

Mason, D.W., Dallman, M.J., Arthur, R.P. and Morris, P.J. (1984). Mechanisms of allograft rejection: the roles of cytotoxic T cells and delayed type hypersensitivity. *Immunol. Rev.* **77**, 167–84.

Matas, A.J., Tellis, V.A., Quinn, T. *et al.* (1982). ALG treatment of steroid resistant rejection in patients receiving cyclosporin. *Transplantation* **41**, 579–83.

Matzinger, P. and Bevan, M.J. (1977). Why do so many lymphocytes respond to the major histocompatibility antigens? *Cell. Immunol.* **29**, 1–5.

Metcalfe, S. (1984). Cyclosporin does not prevent cytoplasmic calcium changes associated with lymphocyte activation. *Transplantation* **38**, 161–4.

Mintz, B. and Silver, W.B. (1967). Intrinsic immunological tolerance in allophenic mice. *Science* **158**, 1484–6.

Mintz, B. and Silver, W.B. (1970). Histocompatibility antigens on melanoblasts and hair follicles: cell-localized homograft rejection in allophenic skin grafts. *Transplantation* **9**, 497–505.

Miyawaki, T., Yachie, A., Ohzeki, S., Nagaoki, T. and Taniguchi, N. (1983). Cyclosporin A does not prevent expression of the Tac antigen, a probable TCGF receptor molecule, on mitogen-stimulated human T cells. *J. Immunol.* **130**, 2737–42.

Mohagheghpour, N., Denicke, C.J., Karsas, G., Bieber, C. and Englerian, E.G. (1983). Activation of antigen-specific suppressor T cell in the presence of cyclosporin requires interactions between T cells of inducer and suppressor lineage. *J. Clin. Invest.* **72**, 2092–100.

Morris, P.J. and Ting, A. (1982). Studies of HLA-DR with relevance to renal transplantation. *Immunol. Rev.* **66**, 104–31.

Morris, R.E., Hoyt, E.G., Murphy, M.P. and Shorthouse, R. (1989). Immunopharmacology of FK 506. *Transplant. Proc.* **21**, 1042–4.

Morrison, L.A., Lukacher, A.E., Braciale, V.L., Fan, D.P. and Braciale, T.J. (1986). Differences in antigen presentation to MHC class I and class II restricted influenza virus-specific cytolytic T lymphocyte clones. *J. Exp. Med.* **163**, 903–21.

Mussche, M.M., Ringoir, S.M. and Lameire, N.N. (1976). High intravenous doses of methylprednisolone for acute cadaveric renal allograft rejection. *Obstet. Gynecol.* **16**, 287–91.

Myburgh, J.A., Smit, J.A., Browde, S. and Stark, J.H. (1983). Current status of total lymphoid irradiation. *Transplant. Proc.* **15**, 659–67.

Nagao, T., White, D.J. and Calne, R.Y. (1982). Kinetics of unresponsiveness induced by a short course of cyclosporin A. *Transplantation* **33**, 31–5.

Nemoto, K., Ito, J., Hayashi, M. *et al.* (1987). Effects of spergualin and 15-deoxyspergualin on the development of graft-versus-host disease in mice. *Transplant. Proc.* **19**, 3520–1.

Ochiai, T., Nakajima, K., Nagata, M. *et al.* (1987). Effect of a new immunosuppressive agent FK 506 on heterotopic cardiac allotransplantation in the rat. *Transplant. Proc.* **19**, 1284–6.

Okubo, M., Masaki, Y., Kamata, K., Sato, N., Inoue, K. and Umetani, N. (1989). Immunosuppressive mode of action of deoxyspergualin in mice, as compared with cyclosporin A and mizoribine. *Transplant. Proc.* **21**, 1085–7.

Opelz, G. (1987). Effect of HLA matching in 10 000 cyclosporin-treated cadaver kidney transplants. *Transplant. Proc.* **19**, 641–9.

Orosz, C.G., Roopenian, D.C., Widmer, M.B. and Bach, F.H. (1983). Analysis of cloned T cell function. II. Differential blockade of various cloned T cell functions by cyclosporin. *Transplantation* **36**, 706–11.

Ortho Multi-Centre Transplant Study Group (1985). A randomised trial of OCT3 monoclonal antibody for acute rejection of cadaveric renal transplantation. *N. Eng. J. Med.* **313**, 337–42.

Palacios, R. (1982). Concanavalin A triggers T lymphocytes by directly interacting with their receptors for activation. *J. Immunol.* **128**, 337–42.

Patel, R. and Terasaki, P.I. (1969). Significance of the positive crossmatch test in kidney transplantation. *N. Engl. J. Med.* **280**, 735–9.

Paul, L.C., van Es, L.A., van Rood, J.J., van Leeuwen, A., Brutel de la Riviere, G. and de Graeff, J. (1979). Antibodies directed against antigens on the endothelium of peritubular capillaries in patients with rejecting renal allografts. *Transplantation* **27**, 175–9.

Pross, H.F. (1986). The involvement of natural killer cells in human malignant disease. In *Immunobiology of Natural Killer Cells*, vol. II, ed. E. Lotzova and R.B. Herberman, pp. 11–27 CRC Press, Boca Raton, Florida.

Pugh, W.M., Superina, R.A., Wood, K.J. and Morris, P.J. (1986). The role of H-2 and non-H-2 antigens and genes in the rejection of murine cardiac allografts. *Immunogenetics* **23**, 30–7.

Quill, H. and Schwartz, R.H. (1987). T cell nonresponsiveness induced by antigen and purified Ia molecules. *J. Immunol.* **138**, 3704–12.

Rapaport, F.T., Meek, A.G., Arnold, A.N., Miura, S., Hayashi, R. and Strober, S. (1987). Preoperative preparation of high risk specifically hyperimmunized canine renal allograft recipients with total-lymphoid irradiation and cyclosporin. *Transplantation* **44**, 185–95.

Reichmann, L., Clark, M.R., Waldmann, H. and Winter, G. (1988). Reshaping human antibodies for therapy. *Nature* **332**, 323–7.

Rolstad, B. and Ford, W.L. (1974). Immune responses of rats deficient in thymus-derived lymphocytes to strong transplantation antigens (Ag-B): graft-versus-host activity, allograft rejection, and the factor of immunisation. *Transplantation* **17**, 405–15.

Ronchese, F., Schwartz, R.H. and Germain, R.N. (1987). Functionally distinct subsites on a class II major histocompatibility complex molecule. *Nature* **329**, 254–6.

Rosenberg, A.S., Mizuochi, T. and Singer, A. (1986). Analysis of T-cell subsets in rejection of Kb mutant skin allografts differing at class I MHC. *Nature* **322**, 829–31.

Rosenberg, A.S., Toshiaki, M., Sharrow, S.O. and Singer, A. (1987). Phenotype, specificity and function of T cell subsets and T cell interactions involved in skin allograft rejection. *J. Exp. Med.* **165**, 1296–315.

Rosenberg, A.S., Rose, P., Weatherly, B. and Singer, A. (1989). Antigen-specific effector mechanisms in skin allograft rejection. *Transplant. Proc.* **21**, 131–2.

Rubin, R.H. and Tolkoff-Rubin, N.E. (1984). The problems of cytomegalovirus infection in transplantation. In *Progress in Transplantation*, vol. I, ed. P.J. Morris and N.L. Tilney, Churchill Livingstone, Edinburgh.

Rygaard, J. (1974). Skin grafts in nude mice. *Ann. Intern. Med.* **82**, 93–104.

Sato, K., Yamagishi, K., Nakayama, Y. *et al.* (1989). Pancreatico-duodenal allotransplantation with cyclosporin and FK506. *Transplant. Proc.* **21**, 1074–5.

Schreiber, S.L. and Crabtree, G.R. (1992). The mechanism of action of cyclosporin A and FK506. *Immunol. Today* **13**, 136–42.

Schubert, G., Stoffregen, C., Timmerman, W., Schang, T. and Thiede, A. (1987). Comparison of the new immunosuppressive agent 15-deoxyspergualin and cyclosporin A after highly allogeneic pancreas transplantation. *Transplant. Proc.* **19**, 3978–9.

Sherwood, R.A., Brent, L. and Rayfield, L.S. (1986). Presentation of alloantigens by host cells. *Eur. J. Immunol.* **16**, 569–74.

Shizuru, J.A., Gregory, A.K., Tien-Bao Chao, C. and Fathman, C.G. (1987). Islet allograft survival after a single course of treatment with antibody to L3/T4. *Science* **237**, 278–80.

Simons, J.W., Noga, S.J., Colombani, P.M., Beschorner, N.E., Foffney, D.S. and Hess, A.D. (1986). Cyclosporin A, an *in vitro* calmodulin antagonist involves nuclear lobulations in human T lymphocytes and monocytes. *J. Cell Biol.* **102**, 145–50.

Singal, D.P. and Joseph, S. (1982). Role of blood transfusion on the induction of antibodies against recognition sites on T lymphocytes in renal transplant patients. *Hum. Immunol.* **4** 93–108.

Slavin, S., Reitz, B., Bieber, C.P., Kaplan, H.S. and Strober, S. (1978). Transplantation tolerance in adult rats using total lymphoid irradiation: permanent survival of skin, heart and marrow allografts. *J. Exp. Med.* **147**, 700–7.

Snider, M.E. and Steinmuller, D. (1987). Non-specific tissue destruction as a consequence of cytotoxic T lymphocyte interactions with antigen-specific target cells. *Transplant. Proc.* **19**, 421–3.

Snider, M.E., Armstrong, L., Hudson, J.L. and Steinmuller, D. (1986). *In vivo* and *in vitro* cytotoxicity of T cells cloned from rejecting allografts. *Transplantation* **42**, 171–7.

Soullilou, J.P., Peyronnet, P., Le Mauff, B. *et al.* (1987). Prevention of rejection of kidney transplants by monoclonal antibody directed against interleukin-2 receptor. *Lancet* **i**, 1339–42.

Spies, T., Sorrentino, R., Boss, J.M., Okada, K. and Strominger, J. (1985). Structural organization of the DR subregion of the major histocompatibility complex. *Proc. Nat. Acad. Sci. (USA)* **82**, 5165–9.

Sprent, J., Schaeffer, M., Lo, D. and Korngold, R. (1986). Properties of purified T cell subsets. *J. Exp. Med.* **163**, 998–1011.

Steinman, R.M. and Inaba, K. (1986). Stimulation of the primary mixed lymphocyte reaction. *CRC Crit. Rev. Immunol.* **5**, 331–3.

Strober, S. (1984). Natural suppressor (NS) cells, neonatal tolerance and total lymphoid irradiation. *Ann. Rev. Immunol.* **2**, 219–37.

Strober, S., Gottlieb, M.S., King, D.P. *et al.* (1980). Acceptance of bone marrow and organ allografts after total lymphoid irradiation (TLI). *Fed. Proc.* **39**, 1202.

Sugawara, I. and Ishizaka, S. (1983). The degree of monocyte participation in human B- and T-cell activation by phorbol myristate acetate. *Clin. Immunol. Immunopathol.* **26**, 299–308.

Sutton, R., Gray, D.W.R., Peters, M., McShane, P., Dallman, M. and Morris, P.J. (1989). Specificity of pancreatic islet allograft rejection in mixed strain rat islet transplants. *J. Exp. Med.* **170**, 751–62.

Suzuki, S., Kanashiro, M. and Amemiya, H. (1987). Effect of a new immunosuppressant, 15-deoxyspergualin, on heterotopic rat heart Transplantation in comparison with cyclosporin. *Transplantation* **44**, 483–7.

Swain, S.L., Dennert, G., Wormsley, S. and Dutton, R.W. (1981). The Lyt phenotype of a long-term allospecific T-cell line: both helper and killer activities to IA are mediated by Ly-1 cells. *Eur. J. Immunol.* **11**, 175–80.

Teh, H.S., Kisielow, P., Scott, B. *et al.* (1988). Thymic major histocompatibility complex antigens and the T-cell receptor determine the CD4/CD8 phenotype of T cells. *Nature* **335**, 229–33.

Tellides, G., Dallman, M.J. and Morris, P.J. (1989). Mechanism of action of interleukin-2 receptor (IL-2R) monoclonal antibody therapy: target cell depletion or inhibition of function. *Transplant. Proc.* **21**, 997–8.

Thomas, J.M., Carver, F.M., Haisch, C.E., Fahrenbruck, G., Deepe, R.M. and Thomas, F.T. (1982). Suppressor cells in rhesus monkeys treated with antithymocyte globulin. *Transplantation* **34**, 83–9.

Tieber, V.L., Abruzzini, L.F., Didier, D.K., Schwartz, B.D. and Rotwein, P. (1986). Complete characterization and sequence of an HLA class II DR chain cDNA from the DR5 haplotype. *J. Biol. Chem.* **261**, 2738–42.

Tiercy, J.M., Gorski, J., Betuel, H., Friedel, A.C., Jeannet, M. and Mach, B. (1989). DNA typing DRw6 subtypes: correlation with DRB1 and DRB3 allelic sequences by hybridization with oligonucleotide probes. *Hum. Immunol.* **24**, 1–14.

Tilney, N.L., Strom, T.B. and Macpherson, S.S. (1974). Populations of infiltrating cells removed from rejecting rat cardiac allografts. *Surg. Forum* **25**, 289–92.

Ting, A. (1988). HLA matching and crossmatching in renal transplantation. In *Kidney Transplantation — Principles and Practice*, ed. P.J. Morris, W.B. Saunders, Philadelphia.

Todd, J.A., Bell, J.I. and McDevitt, H.O. (1987). HLA-DQ gene contributes to susceptibility and resistance to insulin-dependent diabetes mellitus. *Nature* **329**, 599–604.

Tonnelle, C., De Mars, R. and Long, E.O. (1985). DOβ: a new β chain gene in HLA-D with a distinct regulation of expression. *EMBO J.* **4**, 2839–47.

Tyler, J.D., Galli, S.J., Snider, M.E., Dvorak, A.M. and Steinmuller, D. (1984). Cloned Lyt-2+ cytolytic T lymphocytes destroy allogeneic tissue *in vivo*. *J. Exp. Med.* **159**, 234–43.

Waldmann, H. (1989). Manipulation of T cell responses with monoclonal antibodies. *Ann. Rev. Immunol.* **7**, 407–44.

Walter, P., Dickneile, G., Feifel, G. and Thies, J. (1987). Deoxyspergualin induces tolerance in allogeneic kidney transplantation. *Transplant. Proc.* **19**, 3980–1.

Wang, B.S., Heacock, E.H., Chang-Xue, Z., Tilney, N.L., Strom, T.B. and Mannick, J.A. (1982). Evidence for the presence of suppressor T lymphocytes in animals treated with cyclosporin A. *J. Immunol.* **128**, 1382–5.

Williams, D.P., Parker, K., Bacha, P. *et al.* (1987). Diphtherial toxin receptor binding domain substitution with interleukin-2 genetic construction and properties of a diphtheria toxin-related interleukin-2 fusion protein. *Protein Engineering* **1**, 493–504.

Williams, G.M., Humer, D.M., Hudson, R.P., Morris, P.J., Kano, K. and Milgrom, F. (1968). Hyperacute renal homograft rejection in man. *N. Engl. J. Med.* **279**, 611–18.

Winearls, C.G., Fabre, J.W., Millard, P.R. and Morris, P.J. (1979). A quantitative comparison of whole antibody and F(ab')2 in kidney allograft enhancement. *Transplantation* **28**, 36–9.

Wu, S., Saunders, T.L. and Bach, F.H. (1986). Polymorphism of human Ia antigens generated by reciprocal intergenic exchange between two DR loci. *Nature* **324**, 676–9.

Yokota, K., Takishima, T., Sato, K. *et al.* (1989). Comparative studies of FK506 and cyclosporin in canine orthotopic hepatic allograft survival. *Transplant. Proc.* **21**, 1066–8.

Yoshimura, N. and Kahan, B.D. (1985). Suppressor cell activity of cells infiltrating rat renal allografts prolonged by perioperative administration of extracted histocompatibility antigen and cyclosporin. *Transplantation* **40**, 708–13.

Yoshimura, N., Matsui, S., Hamashima, T., Lee, C.J. and Oka, T. (1989). A new immunosuppressive agent, FK506, inhibits the expression of alloantigen-activated suppressor cells as well as the induction of alloreactivity. *Transplant. Proc.* **21**, 1045–7.

Zingernagel, R.M., Callahan, G.N., Klein, J. and Dennert, G. (1978). Cytotoxic T cells learn specificity for self H-2 during differentiation in the thymus. *Nature* **271**, 251–3.

87: Bone Marrow Transplantation

R.P. Witherspoon and R. Storb

Introduction

In the past 20 years bone marrow transplantation has become the standard treatment for congenital immunodeficiency diseases, selected haematological malignancies and aplastic anaemia for those patients who have a syngeneic (identical twin) or allogeneic human leucocyte antigen (HLA)-identical sibling. Until recently, many patients without identical siblings could not receive the potentially curative benefit of marrow grafting and died of their underlying disease. In the last decade, inroads have been made to identify prognostic factors for outcomes of HLA-non-identical grafts from family members, autologous marrow and, most recently, unrelated phenotypically HLA-identical marrow. The clinical experience now gained in allogeneic marrow grafting indicates that the degree of disparity at the major histocompatibility region of the sixth chromosome correlates with graft rejection and graft-versus-host disease (GVHD). The future challenge is to modify treatment to alter rejection and GVHD in high-risk patients. The use of chemoradiotherapy conditioning regimens targeted more specifically to the malignant disease rather than other host tissues, and a better understanding of whether lymphocytes can be separated into distinct cells with graft-versus-host or graft-versus-malignancy function, may lead to better results for a greater number of patients.

Histocompatibility and donor selection

The major histocompatibility complex (MHC) is located on the sixth chromosome in human beings, and consists of the Class I MHC A and B loci and the Class II MHC D locus. There are two alleles for each locus. Each allele is located on a separate haplotype. One haplotype is inherited from each parent. Therefore, four haplotypes are available for inheritance, and each child has a one-in-four chance of sharing the same haplotypes with a sibling. These siblings are genotypically HLA-identical, and they serve as the most common source of marrow. Due to differences in other areas of the chromosomes, recipients of these allogeneic HLA-identical marrow grafts are at risk of developing graft rejection or GVHD. Therefore, treatment of the recipient before grafting with immunosuppressive chemoradiotherapy is required to permit engraftment. The recipient must also receive post-grafting treatment to prevent GVHD. Patients with identical twins have an ideal source of marrow, eliminating the risk of rejection or GVHD. Transplantation of marrow from HLA-non-identical family members may be carried out if two individuals share one haplotype and are HLA-identical for one or more antigens on the other haplotype. Transplantation from these HLA-non-identical family members carries a higher risk of graft rejection or GVHD than transplantation from HLA-identical siblings. Transplantation from unrelated donors who happen to be identical with the recipient for the MHC loci is possible by identifying donors through national and international bone marrow registries. The risk and benefit of transplantation from these donors are currently being defined. Finally, for patients without donors, cryopreservation and storage of normal bone marrow taken during remission of haematological malignancy provide a source of marrow to rescue a patient from high doses of chemoradiotherapy which would otherwise be fatal to the bone marrow.

Bone marrow harvest and infusion

Between 10 and 15 ml of bone marrow per kg of recipient weight is harvested from the iliac crests and/or sternum of the donor who is under general or spinal anaesthesia. This marrow is filtered through screens to remove bone fragments and tissue particles, and shortly thereafter it is infused into the recipient through a peripheral vein (Buckner *et al.* 1984). When autologous marrow is harvested, it may be cryopreserved for infusion later, after the patient has received high-dose chemoradiotherapy. Prior to cryopreservation, the marrow may be treated with antibodies to remove the cell line which is malignant. Currently, however, depletion of malignant cells from marrow is controversial because no clear benefit of depletion has been demonstrated in the relapse rate after autologous bone marrow transplantation (Marmont *et al.* 1986). Alternatively, positive selection of bone marrow stem cells, using columns coated with antibodies which identify antigens on haemopoietic stem cells, may offer a means of utilizing marrow transplantation for patients with solid tumours metastatic to bone marrow (Berenson *et al.* 1988). Haemopoietic stem cells may also be collected from peripheral blood and have been used successfully to reconstitute haemopoietic function after total body irradiation (TBI) for people with tumour metastatic to the marrow, or for individuals who have previously had radiation to the pelvis and sternum. The procedure involves many hours of leucaphaeresis to collect a sufficient number of cells to ensure engraftment (Kessinger *et al.* 1988).

Conditioning the recipient

In order for the donor marrow to be accepted by the host, chemotherapy and/or radiotherapy must be used to suppress the immunological process of rejection and to create space in the bone marrow for engraftment to occur. In patients with malignancy, the conditioning regimen also has a major antitumour effect. Patients with malignant diseases are usually conditioned with cyclophosphamide and between 10 and 15.75 Gy TBI, delivered in daily fractions for 6–7 days (Storb 1989). However, for advanced stages of disease, the relapse rate after these conditioning regimens is high. Newer approaches are exploring chemotherapy with etoposide or cyclophosphamide and delivery of irradiation fractions two or three times daily to achieve 12–16 Gy in 3–4 days, a process termed hyperfractionated radiation (Blume 1987b). For acute lymphocytic leukaemia (ALL), initial reports suggest a reduction of relapse from more than 50% to less than 20% (Brochstein *et al.* 1987). Follow-up of studies for sufficient time to observe relapse should provide data about the effect of hyperfractionated TBI on the relapse rate for haematological malignancies.

A variety of chemotherapy programmes have been used for patients with non-malignant diseases, aplastic anaemia (Storb *et al.* 1988) and thalassaemia (Thomas *et al.* 1982). Experience with these chemotherapy regimens is also being explored for patients with malignant lymphomas who cannot receive TBI to the 12–16 Gy level because of previous treatment with irradiation to the limit of tolerable dose. Conditioning regimens of busulphan and cyclophosphamide, commonly used in conditioning for acute non-lymphocytic leukaemia (ANL) (Santos *et al.* 1983), as well as carmustine, etoposide and cyclophosphamide, are being utilized for such patients.

Results of bone marrow transplantation in specific diseases

Acute non-lymphocytic leukaemia

ALLOGENEIC MARROW

Patients with ANL who achieve a first complete remission by conventional chemotherapy have a likelihood of being cured of their disease. In contrast, around 45–60% of patients given marrow transplants in first remission from HLA-identical siblings are cured (Fig. 87.1) (Appelbaum *et al.* 1988; McGlave *et al.* 1988). If patients are transplanted in second remission, 30% may expect long-term disease-free survival. Patients given transplants in their first relapse have survival similar to that of patients transplanted in second remission (Clift *et al.* 1987). Even though results of marrow transplantation from HLA-identical siblings in first remission are superior to chemotherapy beyond first remission, patients who are older or have organ dysfunction (such as liver disease) are at higher risk for fatal hepatic veno-occlusive disease and cardiac or renal failure during the first few weeks to months after transplantation. For these patients it is often recommended to delay transplantation until it is certain that they are not cured by conventional chemotherapy. These patients may receive bone marrow transplantation early in their first relapse or second remission.

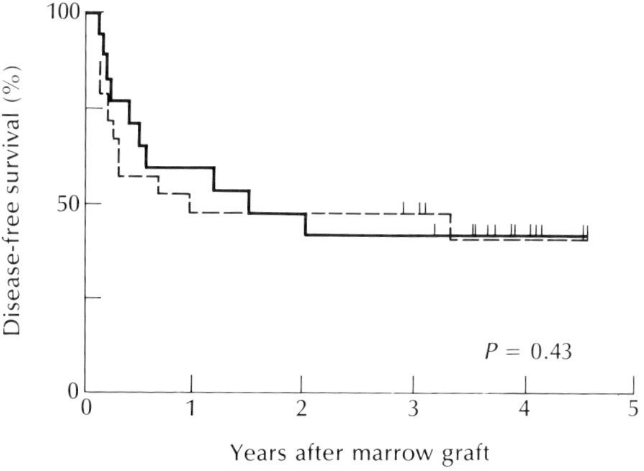

Fig. 87.1. Survival free from relapse is shown for patients transplanted in the last 5 years from HLA-identical siblings for ANL in first remission with either methotrexate and cyclosporin (solid line) or cyclosporin alone (dashed line) as post-grafting prophylaxis of acute GVHD. Vertical marks indicate patients censored by length of follow-up.

Some patients with ANL become refractory to chemotherapy. These patients carry a low but definite long-term survival rate of 10–12%. When marrow transplantation was first undertaken in Seattle in the early 1970s, most patients were refractory to chemotherapy, and 12% of those who survived transplantation and did not relapse continue alive today. They have not received any chemotherapy maintenance treatment since leaving Seattle. These patients illustrate the curative potential of bone marrow transplantation for a small but definite group of patients with refractory leukaemia (Thomas *et al.* 1977).

AUTOLOGOUS MARROW

For patients without HLA-identical siblings, autologous marrow transplantation may be considered. With marrow stored in first remission, transplants may be performed in first or second remission or early first relapse. In a small experience reported from Seattle, three of 13 patients given autologous marrow in first remission are alive free of leukaemia between 1 and 5 years from transplant (Stewart *et al.* 1985). Substantially larger numbers of patients have been reported from combined European centres with 48% of 102 patients grafted in first remission being alive and disease-free at 4 years. Disease-free survival for 36 patients grafted in second remission was 35% at 1 year (Marmont *et al.* 1986).

While the follow-up time is not as long as the nearly 20-year experience with allogeneic marrow transplantation, the survivors at 4 years suggest a potential for a long-term disease-free interval for some patients. However, if marrow was stored during or after the third remission, all patients have relapsed. Depletion of myeloid cells from autologous bone marrow utilizing 4-hydroxyperoxycyclophosphamide offers a method for potentially ensuring that leukaemia could be removed from marrow used for transplantation (Yeager *et al.* 1986). However, a comparison of studies from centres using depleted and non-depleted marrow does not show differences in the relapse rates (Marmont *et al.* 1986). Therefore, the effectiveness of depletion of leukaemia cells from the bone marrow remains to be defined.

Acute lymphocytic leukaemia

ALLOGENEIC MARROW

Nearly 50% of children with typical childhood ALL, positive for common ALL antigen, may be cured by conventional therapy. However, when ALL relapses the first time, there is no prospect for cure using conventional chemotherapy. Patients are usually reinduced during first relapse to attempt a second remission. Patients given marrow transplantation in their second remission have a 30–45% likelihood of long-term disease-free survival, depending upon their age, with children under 12 having the best results (Sanders *et al.* 1987). In contrast, chemotherapy alone after second remission results in shorter and shorter remissions, leading to resistant disease and death from leukaemia (Johnson *et al.* 1981). For patients whose leukaemia has become refractory to chemotherapy, marrow transplantation offers less than 10–15% chance for long-term disease-free survival. While the relapse rate may be as high as 60–70% for these patients after transplantation, marrow transplantation still offers the only means of curing end-stage leukaemic patients of their disease (Thomas *et al.* 1977). Conditioning regimens delivering TBI with hyperfractionated programmes suggest that the relapse rate may be reduced by this technique (Brochstein *et al.* 1987). In most cases, radiation doses approaching 18 Gy have been tried. Patients receiving more than 15.75–16 Gy TBI have experienced organ toxicity to the liver, gastrointestinal (GI) tract and perhaps lung, which limits the therapeutic benefit. These early results require confirmation before they can be considered standard therapy in conditioning regimens.

There are exceptions to the rule of waiting for the first relapse for patients with ALL. Those individuals whose disease is at high risk of early relapse, such as patients with T cell disease, who often present with mediastinal masses and central nervous system disease, or with Burkitt's leukaemia and adults with ALL with white counts in excess of 100 000, should be considered for transplantation when they achieve a remission and their tumour burden is low (Blume *et al.* 1987a; Doney *et al.* 1987).

AUTOLOGOUS MARROW

The patient without an HLA-identical family member should be considered for bone marrow storage during first remission of ALL. Autologous marrow transplantation should be considered at first relapse or second remission (Sanders *et al.* 1989). Often, however, bone marrow storage is delayed for non-medical reasons until the second remission. The combined European centres report 48% 2-year disease-free survival for autologous bone marrow transplantation accomplished in second remission (Marmont *et al.* 1986). This follow-up is short and more time is needed to establish a true relapse rate for autologous bone marrow transplantation for ALL. Like data for ANL, no benefit of depleting autologous marrow of leukaemia cells using monoclonal antibodies has been demonstrated for ALL.

Chronic myelogenous leukaemia

Patients with chronic myelogenous leukaemia (CML) who develop blast crisis have no opportunity for long-term disease-free survival by conventional chemotherapy. Marrow transplantation was first utilized in patients with blast crisis and 15% became long-term survivors cured of their leukaemia. The longest follow-up is now over 10 years from treatment. This result led to trials of marrow transplantation earlier in the chronic phase of the disease. Initially patients with identical twin donors were used and six of the first 10 patients did well and survived long-term (Fefer *et al.* 1982). Transplantation from HLA-identical siblings during the chronic phase resulted in between 65% and 75% long-term disease-free survival for more than 198 patients transplanted in the first 10–12 years (Fig. 87.2) (Thomas *et al.*

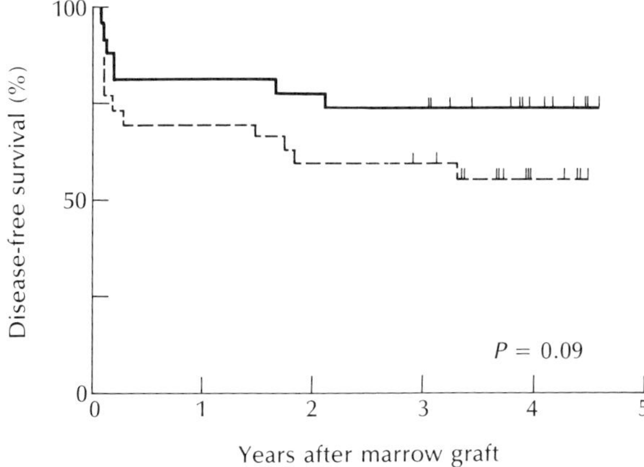

Fig. 87.2. Survival free from relapse is shown for patients transplanted from HLA-identical siblings in the last 5 years for CML in chronic phase with either methotrexate and cyclosporin (solid line) or cyclosporin alone (dashed line) as post-grafting prophylaxis of acute GVHD. Vertical marks indicate patients censored by length of follow-up.

1986; Goldman *et al.* 1988). Disease-free survival is better for patients transplanted in the first year from diagnosis than if transplantation is done in the second or third year from diagnosis (Thomas *et al.* 1986). Transplantation in the accelerated phase of CML results in long-term disease-free survival of about 30%. This poor result is due in part to higher relapse rates after transplantation, but also to other transplant-related complications such as hepatic veno-occlusive disease, or infection, presumably related to the more aggressive conditioning regimens commonly given to these patients. A minority of CML patients may develop lymphoid blast crisis and express the TdT surface marker. These patients may be easily returned to a second chronic phase by vincristine and prednisone treatment. This 'remission' of blast crisis is normally short-lived. Curiously, however, transplantation during this second chronic phase results in survival quite similar to that of patients transplanted in their first chronic phase (Thomas *et al.* 1986).

Patients with CML who do not have an HLA-identical family member donor face a more difficult decision about treatment. Since the morbidity and mortality of transplantation from a two-antigen-mismatched donor is high, transplantation should be delayed until the clinical condition worsens to warrant a riskier procedure. Patients whose only available donors are two- or three-antigen-mismatched would be considered for transplantation during the accelerated phase or blast crisis.

Lymphomas

Marrow transplantation has been used as an alternative to chemotherapy as salvage treatment for patients whose initial remission has failed. Results in 100 patients were reported by Appelbaum *et al.* (1987c). Patients were given syngeneic, allogeneic or autologous grafts following cyclophosphamide and 12 Gy TBI. Between 20% and 30% became long-term survivors. Many patients had extensive disease and did poorly, with early relapse. Patients with minimal disease at transplant did better and tended to be among the survivors. There was no difference in survival by source of marrow and no difference by histology of the lymphoma. These data suggest that marrow transplantation offers effective salvage treatment for patients with advanced lymphoma, but indicate that the cyclophosphamide–12 Gy TBI conditioning regimen is not sufficient to eradicate tumour in a majority of patients with extensive disease. Hyperfractionated TBI and high-dose chemotherapy regimens are under study to reduce the relapse rate for patients with extensive disease. For patients with aggressive lymphomas, who are likely to relapse soon after initial remission induction, marrow transplantation is being explored in first remission to determine if a higher proportion of patients could be given long-term survival by bone marrow transplantation, similar to results seen for ANL patients in first remission. Because results from patients receiving autologous bone marrow transplantation or allogeneic bone marrow transplantation for lymphomas are similar, those patients who do not have marrow involvement may benefit from the lower morbidity and mortality of autotransplantation than of allogeneic transplantation. There is no advantage in selecting allogeneic HLA-identical donor marrow over autologous marrow free of tumour. While the long-term follow-up for allogeneic recipients transplanted for lymphoma is more than 10 years, the experience with autologous grafts is now approaching 5 years, with leading patients in the 7-year length of follow-up. The absence of relapse in these autologous recipients 7 years after transplant suggests that many of the patients may be cured. More follow-up of the cohort transplanted

2–4 years ago is required before drawing more definite conclusions about the potential of curative therapy for autologous transplantation for lymphoma.

Depletion of autologous marrow by monoclonal antibodies directed against specific cell lines is common for T cell lymphomas and follicular (nodular) lymphomas. The advantage of deletion of bone marrow without known disease is not clear at this time.

Other haematological malignancies

Multiple myeloma

Recently there has been renewed interest in marrow transplantation for multiple myeloma. Data from European centres suggest that remissions can be achieved by chemotherapy conditioning regimens in patients with extensive bone disease, and these remissions may last for a number of months or years (Tura *et al*. 1988). Data from other centres have also pointed to remissions, but, unfortunately, monoclonal proteins have reappeared in several patients (Barlogie *et al*. 1986). These different results show that some myeloma patients with extensive disease may be brought into remission by transplantation. Longer follow-up is needed to determine the relapse rate and the therapeutic benefit of transplantation.

Chronic lymphocytic leukaemia

Due to the nature of cell division for patients with chronic lymphocytic leukaemia (CLL), marrow ablative therapy with alkylating agents and high-dose TBI may not halt progressive tumour growth. Most patients with this disease are elderly and would tolerate conditioning for grafting poorly. Younger patients might be considered for transplantation on an experimental basis when blood counts are compromised by replacement of bone marrow by CLL cells (Michallet *et al*. 1988).

Preleukaemia

Patients with myelodysplastic syndrome have been transplanted from HLA-identical siblings (Appelbaum *et al*. 1987b). These patients all had clonal cytogenetic abnormalities and pancytopenia accompanied by marrow cellularity ranging from moderately hypocellular to hypercellular. Slightly less than half of the patients have survived and are free of their disease with the longest-surviving patients being 8–9 years from transplantation. The non-surviving patients died of expected complications of transplantation, GVHD or interstitial pneumonia. The first three patients treated for this disorder were conditioned with cyclophosphamide alone and relapsed later, prompting a change to the use of total body irradiation in preparing patients for grafting. The main factors determining prognosis are the extent to which the myelodysplasia is associated with fibrosis or with previous treatment of malignancy.

Solid tumours

Neuroblastomas and breast carcinomas, as well as a variety of other solid tumours (August *et al*. 1983; Phillips 1983), have been targets for treatment by autologous or allogeneic marrow transplantation. Collection of autologous marrow hematopoietic stem cells for reinfusion in patients with solid tumours which occasionally metastasize to bone offers a means to rescue patients from otherwise marrow-lethal chemoradiotherapy. Results of such studies are only now emerging so the effectiveness of positive selection of haemopoietic stem cells remains to be defined.

Non-malignant disorders

Aplastic anaemia

Patients with idiopathic aplastic anaemia typically have a hypocellular marrow, anaemia with a corrected reticulocyte count less than 1, absolute neutrophil count less than $500/mm^3$ and platelet count less than $20\,000/mm^3$. When such patients have HLA-identical siblings, marrow transplantation prior to transfusion is the preferred method of treatment. Eighty-five per cent of patients treated become long-term survivors. Transfusions given more than 48 hours prior to initiation of the conditioning regimen result in sensitization of the recipient and increase the incidence of graft rejection to around 13%. Seventy-two per cent of these patients become long-term survivors. Whenever possible, therefore, it is important to identify potential HLA-identical family member donors in newly diagnosed cases of aplastic anaemia and refer the patients to transplant centres before transfusions become necessary (Storb *et al.* 1988).

In the absence of an HLA-identical sibling or identical twin donor, patients should be considered for treatment with antithymocyte globulin (ATG). Twenty to forty-two per cent of patients will respond within 3 months of ATG treatment and become transfusion-independent (Champlin *et al.* 1983; Doney and Storb 1987). Cyclosporin A may be an alternative to ATG if early studies suggesting similarity of response are confirmed with longer follow-up time (Gluckman *et al.* 1988).

Homozygous beta thalassaemia

Children with homozygous beta thalassaemia begin developing iron overload in liver, heart and other tissues by 2–3 years of life. Most die by their early 20s of complications resulting from organ damage by iron. Treatment utilizes chelating agents and phlebotomy, with varying success. An alternative approach is to use bone marrow transplantation from an HLA-identical sibling who is normal or at least heterozygous for the disease (Thomas *et al.* 1982). The largest series of such patients is reported from Pessaro, Italy, where 70% have been put into continuous remission by transplantation (Lucarelli *et al.* 1987). The complications of GVHD and infection have occurred with frequencies similar to those of transplants for leukaemia or aplastic anaemia. A decision to elect transplantation as treatment requires weighing the long-term mortality risk of the disease against the risk of dying during marrow transplantation.

Other congenital diseases

Fifty-five per cent of patients with severe combined immunodeficiency disease transplanted from HLA-identical siblings have their deficiencies cured. The main cause of failure after transplant is infection related to the poor immunological status early after grafting (O'Reilly 1983). Patients with Wiskott–Aldrich syndrome do quite well if donors are HLA-identical siblings. Transplantation from identical siblings is also definitive treatment for children with Fanconi anaemia (Deeg *et al.* 1983). Some patients experience unusual toxicity associated with the conditioning regimen. Patients with Fanconi anaemia may benefit from a less aggressive conditioning regimen.

Marrow grafts have been effective in patients with ataxia telangiectasia, chronic granulomatous disease, osteopetrosis, Diamond–Blackfan anaemia, Chediak–Higashi syndrome, chronic mucocutaneous candidiasis, congenital erythrocyte aplasia, mucopolysaccharidosis, cartilage–hair hypoplasia and Gaucher's and other glycogen storage diseases. For some of the storage diseases, organ damage from the disease may not be reversed by transplantation of haemopoietic cells (Krivit and Paul 1986). Children with congenital agranulocytosis may benefit from marrow grafts, but exogenous replacement with granulocyte colony-stimulating factor (G-CSF) appears to result in maturation of granulocytes: normal granulocyte levels are achieved and infections are reduced. Longer follow-up is needed to determine if G-CSF will provide sustained therapeutic benefit (Bonilla *et al.* 1988). Patients who fail treatment could be considered for bone marrow transplantation. Patients with congenital diseases may be the first to receive trials of gene transfer by autologous marrow transplantation. At present, animal models of adenosine deaminase deficiency are being used to study retroviral infection of marrow cells with the gene for adenosine deaminase (Bordignon *et al.* 1988). Factors controlling the expression of these transfected genes must be understood before these techniques can be given trials in human beings.

Human leucocyte antigen non-identical and unrelated donor grafts

Non-identical family member donors

Transplantation from family members who are phenotypically but not genotypically HLA-identical, usually a parent, or siblings matched for all three antigens on the non-shared haplotype, has a clinical course similar to that of HLA-identical siblings. Those matched for two but mismatched for one locus on the non-shared haplotype also have a clinical course very similar to that of HLA-identical siblings (Beatty *et al.* 1985). However, graft rejection risk is 7–9%, whereas rejection is 2% for recipients of HLA-identical sibling marrow. For all haematological malignancies for which transplantation from HLA-identical siblings is recommended, transplantation from phenotypically identical family members or family members not matched at one HLA locus is also recommended. However, when the family member is not matched at two or three positions on the non-shared haplotype, the risk of rejection is elevated to 20% or higher. Eighty per cent of those who engraft have severe GVHD and mortality is high (Beatty *et al.* 1985). Less than 10% of patients become long-term survivors of transplantation from two- and three-antigen mismatched donors. Transplantation from such donors is not recommended for patients with ANL in first remission, ALL in second remission or CML in chronic phase. Only when the underlying disease relapses or enters accelerated or blast crisis phases does the risk from the more aggressive malignancy justify marrow transplantation in a higher-risk donor–recipient combination.

Unrelated donors

The creation of a national marrow donor registry has made identification of unrelated phenotypically HLA-identical donors possible for patients who do not have suitable family member donors. Several centres in the United States and Europe are gaining experience with transplantation using unrelated donors. Early reports suggest that the transplant-related complications of graft rejection and GVHD appear similar to those of HLA-matched or one-antigen mismatched family members (Hows *et al.* 1986). The odds of finding an unrelated phenotypically HLA-identical donor are about 1 in 5 for a registry of 50 000–100 000 donors (Beatty *et al.* 1988). Unrelated donors may become preferred over two- and three-antigen mismatched family member donors because of the lower incidence of GVHD. Further, the similarity of results to that of HLA-identical sibling recipients has led to exploration of transplantation from unrelated donors for patients with chronic-phase CML and patients with acute leukaemia in remission. Forty-five per cent of CML patients receiving marrow have become long-term survivors with follow-up now approaching 4–5 years (Fig. 87.3). (McGlave *et al.* 1987; Beatty *et al.* 1989). One limitation is the time it takes to identify a donor — usually 3–4 months. This limitation often restricts the utility of transplantation to those patients who are in remission. Relapsed patients who cannot be brought into remission often die before a donor can be found.

Because the experience is early, the long-term effects on relapse and chronic GVHD remain to be defined for recipients of unrelated donor marrow.

Problems after marrow grafting

The major complications of marrow transplantation are graft rejection, acute and chronic GVHD, opportunistic infection, immunodeficiency and recurrence of malignancy.

Graft rejection

Graft rejection is a serious complication because second graft attempts are rarely successful and death is the usual outcome. Fortunately, marrow

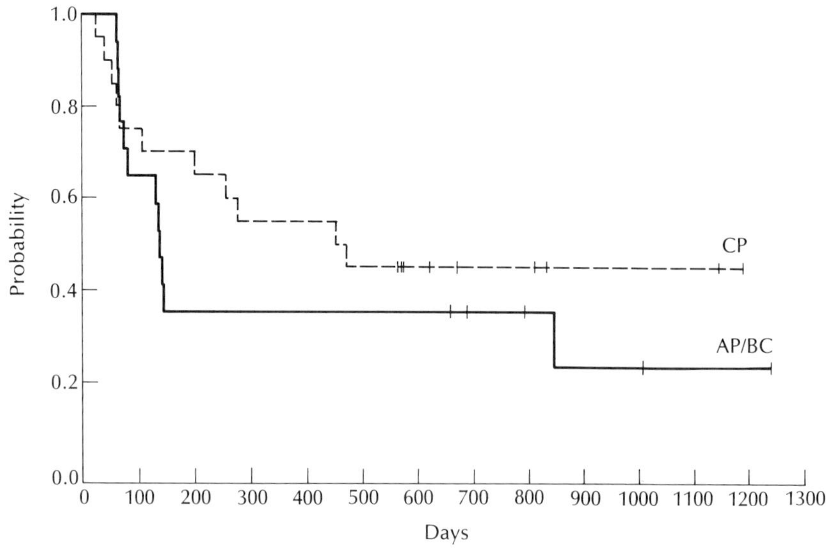

Fig. 87.3. Actuarial survival is shown for patients in chronic phase (CP), accelerated phase (AP) or blast crisis (BC) phase who received marrow from phenotypically HLA-identical unrelated donors. Vertical marks indicate patients censored by length of follow-up. Number of days after marrow grafting is indicated.

graft rejection is rare in HLA-identical sibling marrow recipients with haematological malignancy conditioned for grafting with chemotherapy and TBI. With disparity in HLA typing between donor and recipient, the risk of rejection rises. A study comparing rejection rates in 269 recipients of marrow from HLA-non-identical siblings and 930 recipients of HLA-identical marrow showed rejection rates to be 2% in HLA-genotypically identical siblings, 7% for phenotypically matched siblings, 9% for recipients matched at one locus and 20% for recipients of two-antigen mismatched marrow (Anasetti *et al.* 1989). Residual host lymphocytes could be detected in 11 of 14 informative patients with graft failure, suggesting that the underlying mechanism for rejection is a host-mediated immunological reaction. Research now under way is directed toward eliminating residual host immunity by higher-dose fractionated radiation and the addition of monoclonal antibodies directed against subsets of T lymphocytes.

Patients with aplastic anaemia who were extensively transfused before marrow grafting and conditioned with cyclophosphamide alone experienced graft rejection in 35% of cases. On the other hand, aplastic anaemia patients transplanted before any transfusions were given had 11% graft rejection. It has been possible to reduce the rejection rate for transfused aplastic anaemia patients by infusing haemopoietic stem cells, obtained from the peripheral blood buffy coat of the marrow donor, daily for 5 days post-transplant. The rejection rate was reduced to 13%. However, buffy coat cell infusion has resulted in an increase in *de novo* chronic GVHD (Storb *et al.* 1984). Some centres employ total lymphoid irradiation or thoraco-abdominal irradiation and report good results with engraftment in aplastic anaemia patients. However, for patients with non-malignant diseases, one would like to avoid irradiation in the conditioning regimen to reduce long-term irradiation complications such as cataracts, secondary malignancies and growth retardation.

Patients receiving marrow depleted of T lymphocytes carry rejection rates from 10% to as high as 30% reported in some series (Martin *et al.* 1985). It is believed that a subset of T lymphocytes which would otherwise suppress residual host immunity is removed from the transplanted marrow and permits host-mediated rejection to occur. Higher doses of irradiation have been employed to reduce graft rejection, with marginal success. Studies currently use monoclonal antibodies against T cell subsets delivered during the conditioning regimen with the aim of inactivating residual host immunity.

Graft-versus-host disease

Acute GVHD is a reaction of donor cells against histocompatibility differences with the host. The host must be immunosuppressed so as not to reject the donor graft, and the donor cells must persist in the host. Graft-versus-host disease is seen in 30–50% of patients with HLA-identical sibling donors, and in 80% or higher of recipients of two- and three-antigen mismatched marrow. Acute GVHD may be mild (grade I), moderately severe (grade II) or severe (grades III and IV). Patients with grades II–IV acute GVHD require treatment, and patients with grade IV GVHD generally die from acute GVHD or its complications, haemorrhage or infection (Glucksberg *et al.* 1974). Early studies with the canine littermate radiation chimera models pointed out the effectiveness of low doses of methotrexate given intermittently after grafting to reduce acute GVHD (Storb *et al.* 1970). Similar studies in human marrow transplant recipients illustrate that rates of acute GVHD are at high, unacceptable levels in patients not receiving prophylactic immunosuppression (Sullivan *et al.* 1986). Currently, the most effective treatment to prevent acute GVHD is a combination of methotrexate and cyclosporin, which results in reduction of the rate of acute GVHD in HLA-identical siblings to 25% (Storb *et al.* 1986). T depletion of marrow results in very low rates of GVHD but, unfortunately, is associated with graft rejection (Martin *et al.* 1985).

Treatment of established acute GVHD is with methylprednisolone, cyclosporin and/or ATG. Patients respond well to treatment if their disease involves skin alone, but less well when liver and GI tract are affected (Deeg *et al.* 1985). Monoclonal antibodies to T lymphocyte subsets or to interleukin (IL)-2 receptors on activated lymphocytes are being investigated to improve results of treatment.

Chronic GVHD may develop several months after acute GVHD has settled, or evolve from acute GVHD, or arise when no acute GVHD has preceded it. Chronic GVHD is a multisystem disease affecting the mouth, liver, GI tract, and skin and its appendages, eccrine and lacrimal glands, hair follicles and melanocytes. If left untreated, the disease will progress to dermal thickening, scarring, contractures and disability, chronic diarrhoea and nutritional deficiency, ocular sicca, immune suppression and susceptibility to infection (Sullivan *et al.* 1981). Fortunately, treatment early in the development of chronic GVHD usually controls the inflammation and leads to recovery in 9–18 months, when treatment may be discontinued (Sullivan *et al.* 1988a, b).

Graft-versus-host disease may have a subtle clinical benefit, however. Patients with relapsed ALL and AML who develop acute and chronic GVHD have lower relapse rates of leukaemia than do patients without GVHD. This graft-versus-leukaemia effect may be a result of incidental attack of donor cells on host HLA differences which the leukaemia shares, or it may be the result of attack on surface determinants specific to leukaemia cells (Sullivan *et al.* 1987). Murine models suggest the effect against leukaemia is distinct from the GVHD effect, but these differences have not been demonstrated in human beings.

Opportunistic infection

Early after grafting, patients are neutropenic and are at risk for bacterial and fungal infections. Viral infection is common and, in particular, cytomegalovirus (CMV) infection causes considerable morbidity, with viraemia, gastroenteritis and hepatitis. If CMV pneumonia develops, the outcome is usually fatal and does not respond to treatment with acyclovir. Patients who are seronegative for CMV and whose marrow donors are also seronegative may be protected from acquisition of CMV by using blood products from seronegative blood donors (Bowden *et al.* 1986). When patients become long-term survivors, those who are healthy and do not have chronic GVHD have very few infections. In contrast, patients with chronic GVHD are at high risk of developing fatal bacteraemia, pneumonia or meningitis from Gram-positive encapsulated organisms (Atkinson *et al.* 1979).

Immune deficiency

Granulocytes from the donor marrow achieve normal levels by 3–4 weeks after grafting. Patients become independent of platelet transfusions by 40–50 days after grafting and platelet counts are usually over 100 000/mm^3 by 3 months post-transplant. Independence of red cell transfusions occurs between 2 and 3 months after transplant. Time to granulocyte engraftment in recipients of autologous marrow has been accelerated by human recombinant growth factors (Nemunaitis *et al.* 1988). Lymphocyte counts are normal by the second post-transplant month, but usually more CD8 lymphocytes than CD4 lymphocytes are seen in the first 3–4 months after transplantation. Accompanying these low numbers of CD4 lymphocytes are low *in vitro* levels of IL-2 and diminished helper lymphocyte functions. Patients with chronic GVHD continue to have an imbalance of T lymphocyte subsets, whereas patients without chronic GVHD have a normal distribution of T lymphocyte subsets (reviewed in Witherspoon and Storb *et al.* 1989).

Early after grafting, all patients respond with poor antibody production to sensitization with the neo-antigens bacteriophage ϕX-174 and keyhole limpet haemocyanin and the recall pneumococcal antigens. When patients become long-term survivors, those without chronic GVHD respond appropriately to these antigens, but patients with chronic GVHD remain impaired, regardless of immunosuppressive treatment for chronic GVHD. Chronic GVHD patients have poor immunoglobulin G (IgG) antigen-specific antibody production in the secondary response to bacteriophage. *In vivo* delayed-type hypersensitivity skin testing shows that cellular immunity is impaired early after grafting and remains impaired in patients with chronic GVHD (Witherspoon *et al.* 1984).

Attempts to accelerate immunological reactivity to pathogens using thymic factors and thymic transplants have been unsuccessful (Witherspoon *et al.* 1988). Donor immunity may be transferred to the recipient as demonstrated by antigen-specific immunity to tetanus and diphtheria (Lum *et al.* 1988) and immediate hypersensitivity to common allergens (Agosti *et al.* 1988). At present, it has not been possible to utilize donor immunity to specific pathogenes, such as CMV, as a means of protecting the transplant recipient. Development of safe vaccines or anti-idiotype proteins to CMV may pave the way for safe trials of transfer of donor immunity to the recipient.

Relapse of malignancy

The high rate of relapse after transplantation for leukaemias is a major challenge in marrow transplantation. Modifications of the TBI conditioning regimen are being explored. However, the limit in the dose of TBI for acceptable non-life-threatening toxicity is about 14–15 Gy. Other means of targeting chemoradiotherapy to the tumour are under investigation. One approach is to employ radiolabelled monoclonal antibodies to the tumour cell line. These antibodies offer a means of delivering cytotoxic levels of irradiation directly to the tumour cell and sparing other organs, possibly reducing the toxicities of TBI (Appelbaum *et al.* 1987a). Additionally, bone-seeking isotopes are being developed which have the potential to destroy tumour in marrow and spare other organs, and in several days, when the radioactivity has passed out of the body, marrow from a sibling or autologous marrow previously stored in remission could be infused. Such studies are under way in animal models. Finally, retroviral infection of chemotherapy-resistant genes is an active area of investigation in animal models. If successful, it may be possible to render bone marrow safe from chemotherapy, permitting higher doses of the agent to be used in treatment of malignancy (Stead *et al.* 1988).

Conclusions and outlook

Marrow transplantation has progressed from its early beginnings when only patients with end-stage leukaemia were candidates. Now, when an identical twin or HLA-identical sibling donor is available, it is the therapy of choice for leukaemia which has relapsed once and for patients with chronic-phase CML and ANL in first remission. Marrow donors other than HLA-identical siblings may be used in certain high-risk stages of leukaemia and HLA-phenotypically identical unrelated donors may expand the application of marrow transplantation to more individuals who would not otherwise have a suitable donor.

Recurrence of malignancy after grafting is a major challenge for developing better conditioning regimens such as radiotherapy targeted to tumour by radiolabelled antibodies and bone-seeking isotopes. It is critical to lower the toxicity to other vital organs by these targeting methods. Also, a better understanding of which cells cause graft rejection and which cause GVHD could lead to more effective T lymphocyte depletion of marrow, wherein the cells causing graft acceptance could be enriched. A better understanding and delineation of distinct cells responsible for the graft-versus-leukaemia and GVHD effects could lead to selective infusion of marrow cells with anti-leukaemic effect and diminish recurrence of malignancy. Growth factor therapy has already enhanced the time to engraftment in recipients of autologous marrow, and additional factors may be discovered which boost immunological recovery and decrease infection. In the distant future, gene transfer of chemotherapy-resistance genes into autologous marrow recipients might provide a means of protecting marrow cells from otherwise lethal effects of chemotherapy, or alter the function of genes involved in the generation of disease.

Acknowledgements

This work is supported in part by grants CA 18029, CA 18221 and CA 15704 awarded by the National Cancer Institute, and by grant HL 36444 awarded by the National Heart, Lung and Blood Institute, NIH, DHHS.

References

Agosti, J.M., Sprenger, J.D. *et al.* (1988). Transfer of allergen-specific IgE-mediated hypersensitivity with allogeneic bone marrow transplantation. *N. Engl. J. Med.* **319**, 1623–8.

Anasetti, C., Amos, D. *et al.* (1989). Marrow graft failure after transplantation for malignancy: the role of donor compatibility for HLA. *N. Engl. J. Med.* **320**, 197–204.

Appelbaum, F.R., Badger, C. *et al.* (1987a). Use of iodine-131-labeled anti-immune response-associated monoclonal antibody as a preparative regimen prior to bone marrow transplantation: initial dosimetry. *Nat. Cancer Inst. Monog.* **3**, 67–71.

Appelbaum, F.R., Storb, R. *et al.* (1987b). Treatment of preleukemic syndromes with marrow transplantation. *Blood* **69**, 92–6.

Appelbaum, F.R., Sullivan, K.M. *et al.* (1987c). Treatment of malignant lymphoma in one hundred patients with chemotherapy, total body irradiation and marrow transplantation. *J. Clin. Oncol.* **5**, 1340–7.

Appelbaum, F.R., Fisher, L.D. *et al.* (1988). Chemotherapy versus marrow transplantation for adults with acute non-lymphocytic leukemia: a five-year follow-up. *Blood* **72**, 179–84.

Atkinson, K., Storb, R. *et al.* (1979). Analysis of late infections in 89 long-term survivors of bone marrow transplantation. *Blood* **53**, 720–31.

August, C.S., Serota, F.T. *et al.* (1983). Bone marrow transplantation for relapsed stage IV neuroblastoma. In *Recent Advances in Bone Marrow Transplantation*, ed. R.P. Gale, pp. 703–16, A.R. Liss, New York.

Barlogie, B., Alexanian, R. *et al.* (1986). High dose melphalan (HDM) + total body irradiation (TBI) and bone marrow transplantation (BMT) for refractory myeloma. *Blood* **68** (suppl. 1), 235a (abstract).

Beatty, P.G., Clift, R.A. *et al.* (1985). Marrow transplantation from related donors other than HLA-identical siblings. *N. Engl. J. Med.* **313**, 765–71.

Beatty, P.G., Dahlberg, S. *et al.* (1988). Probability of finding HLA-matched unrelated marrow donors. *Transplantation* **45**, 714–18.

Beatty, P.G., Ash, R. *et al.* (1989). The use of unrelated bone marrow donor in the treatment of patients with chronic myelogenous leukemia: experience of four marrow transplant centers. *Bone Marrow Transplant.* **4**, 287–90.

Berenson, R.J., Andrews, R.G. *et al.* (1988). Antigen $CD34^+$ marrow cells engraft lethally irradiated baboons. *J. Clin. Invest.* **81**, 951–5.

Blume, K.G., Forman, S.J. *et al.* (1987a). Allogeneic bone marrow transplantation for acute lymphoblastic leukemia during first complete remission. *Transplantation* **43**, 389–92.

Blume, K.G., Forman, S.J. *et al.* (1987b). Total body irradiation and high-dose etoposide: a new preparatory regimen for bone marrow transplantation in patients with advanced hematologic malignancies. *Blood* **69**, 1015–20.

Bonilla, M.A., Gillio, A.P. *et al.* (1988). Correction of neutropenia in patients with congenital agranulocytosis with recombinant human granulocyte colony stimulating factor *in vivo*. *Exp. Hematol.* **16**, 520 (abstract).

Bordignon, C., Hantzopoulos, P. *et al.* (1988). Retroviral vector mediated highly efficient expression of adenosine deaminase in hematopoietic long term cultures of ADA deficient marrow cells: lineage specific expression and reconstitution of proliferative capacity in lymphoid cells. *Blood* **72** (suppl. 1), 380a (abstract).

Bowden, R.A., Sayers, M. *et al.* (1986). Cytomegalovirus immune globulin and seronegative blood products to prevent primary cytomegalovirus infection after marrow transplant. *N. Engl. J. Med.* **314**, 1006–10.

Brochstein, J.A., Kernan, N.A. *et al.* (1987). Allogeneic bone marrow transplantation after hyperfractionated total body irradiation and cyclophosphamide in children with acute leukemia. *N. Engl. J. Med.* **317**, 1618–24.

Buckner, C.D., Clift, R.A. *et al.* (1984). Marrow harvesting from normal donors. *Blood* **64**, 630–4.

Champlin, R.E., Ho, W. *et al.* (1983). Antithymocyte globulin treatment in patients with aplastic anemia. *N. Engl. J. Med.* **308**, 113–18.

Clift, R.A., Buckner, C.D. *et al.* (1987). The treatment of acute nonlymphoblastic leukemia by allogeneic marrow transplantation. *Bone Marrow Transplant.* **2**, 243–58.

Deeg, H.J., Storb, R. *et al.* (1983). Fanconi's anemia treated by allogeneic marrow transplantation. *Blood* **61**, 954–9.

Deeg, H.J., Loughran, T.P. *et al.* (1985). Treatment of human acute graft-versus-host disease with antithymocyte globulin and cyclosporine with or without methylprednisolone. *Transplantation* **40**, 162–6.

Doney, K.C., Buckner, C.D. *et al.* (1987). Marrow transplantation for patients with acute lymphoblastic leukemia in first marrow remission. *Bone Marrow Transplant.* **2**, 355–63.

Doney, K.C., Storb, R. (1987). Treatment of aplastic anemia with anti-thymocyte globulin, high dose corticosteroids and androgens. *Exp. Hematol.* **15**, 239–42.

Fefer, A., Cheever, M.A. *et al.* (1982). Treatment of chronic granulocytic leukemia with chemoradiotherapy and transplantation of marrow from identical twins. *N. Engl. J. Med.* **306**, 63–8.

Gluckman, E., Esperou, H., Devergie, A. and the participating centers, Hospital Saint-Louis, Bone Marrow Transplant Unit, Paris, France (1988). Comparison of cyclosporine A (CyA) and horse antithymocyte globulin (H.ATG) for treatment of severe aplastic anemia (SAA): a multicenter prospective randomized study. *Blood* **72** (suppl. 1), 42a (abstract).

Glucksberg, H., Storb, R. *et al.* (1974). Clinical manifestations of graft-versus-host disease in human recipients of marrow from HLA-matched sibling donors. *Transplantation* **18**, 295–304.

Goldman, J.M., Gale, R.P. *et al.* (1988). Bone marrow transplantation for chronic myelogenous leukemia in chronic phase: increased risk for relapse associated with T-cell depletion. *Ann. Intern. Med.* **108**, 806–14.

Hows, J.M., Yin, J.L. *et al.* (1986). Histocompatible unrelated volunteer donors compared with HLA nonidentical family donors in marrow transplantation for aplastic anemia and leukemia. *Blood* **68**, 1322–8.

Johnson, F.L., Thomas, E.D. *et al.* (1981). A comparison of marrow transplantation with chemotherapy for children with acute lymphoblastic leukemia in second or subsequent remission. *N. Engl. J. Med.* **305**, 846–51.

Kessinger, A., Armitage, J.O. *et al.* (1988). Autologous peripheral hematopoietic stem cell transplantation restores hematopoietic function following marrow ablative therapy. *Blood* **71**, 723–7.

Krivit, W. and Paul, N.W. (eds.) (1986). *Bone Marrow Transplantation for Treatment of Lysosomal Storage Diseases*. A.R. Liss, New York.

Lucarelli, G., Galimberti, M. *et al.* (1987). Marrow transplantation in patients with advanced thalassemia. *N. Engl. J. Med.* **316**, 1050–6.

Lum, L.G., Noges, J.E. *et al.* (1988). Transfer of specific immunity in marrow recipients given HLA-mismatched, T cell-depleted, or HLA-identical marrow grafts. *Bone Marrow Transplant.* **3**, 399–406.

McGlave, P.B., Scott, E. *et al.* (1987). Unrelated donor bone marrow transplantation therapy for chronic myelogenous leukemia. *Blood* **70**, 877–81.

McGlave, P.B., Haake, R.J. *et al.* (1988). Allogeneic bone marrow transplantation for acute nonlymphocytic leukemia in first remission. *Blood* **72**, 1512–17.

Marmont, A.M., Bacigalupo, A. and Van Lint, M.T. (eds.) (1986). Proceedings of the XIIth annual meeting of the European Cooperative Group for Bone Marrow Transplantation. *Bone Marrow Transplant.* suppl. 1.

Martin, P.J., Hansen, J.A. *et al.* (1985). Effects of *in vivo* depletion of T cells in HLA-identical allogeneic marrow grafts. *Blood* **66**, 664–72.

Michallet, M., Corront, B. *et al.* (1988). Allogeneic bone marrow transplantation in chronic lymphocytic leukemia. *Blood* **72** (suppl. 1), 396a (abstract).

Nemunaitis, J., Singer, J. *et al.* (1988). Use of recombinant human granulocyte macrophage colony-stimulating factor in autologous marrow transplantation for lymphoid malignancies. *Blood* **72**, 834–6.

O'Reilly, R.J. (1983). Allogeneic bone marrow transplantation: current status and future directions. *Blood* **62**, 941–64.

Phillips, G.L. *et al.* (1983). Current clinical trials with intensive therapy and autologous bone marrow transplantation (ABMT) for lymphomas and solid tumors. In *Recent Advances in Bone Marrow Transplantation*, ed. R.P. Gale, pp. 567–97, A.R. Liss, New York.

Sanders, J.E., Thomas, E.D. *et al.* (1987). Marrow transplantation for children with acute lymphoblastic leukemia in second remission (concise report). *Blood* **70**, 324–6.

Sanders, J.E., Doney, K. *et al.* (1989). Autologous marrow transplant experience for acute lymphoblastic leukemia. In *Autologous Bone Marrow Transplantation: Proceedings of the Third International Symposium*, ed. K.A. Dicke, G. Spitzer, S. Jagannaths and M.J. Evinger-Hodges, pp. 155–60, Houston University of Texas, M.D. Anderson Hospital, Houston.

Santos, G.W., Tutschka, P.J. *et al.* (1983). Marrow transplantation for acute nonlymphocytic leukemia after treatment with busulfan and cyclophosphamide. *N. Engl. J. Med.* **309**, 1347–53.

Stead, R.B., Kwok, W.W. *et al.* (1988). Canine model for gene therapy: inefficient gene expression in dogs reconstituted with autologous marrow infected with retroviral vectors. *Blood* **71**, 742–7.

Stewart, P.S., Buckner, C.D. *et al.* (1985). Autologous marrow transplantation in patients with acute nonlymphocytic leukemia in first remission. *Exp. Hematol.* **13**, 267–72.

Storb, R. (1989). Bone marrow transplantation. In *Cancer: Principles and Practice of Oncology*, 3rd edn, ed. V.T. DeVita, S. Hellman and S.A. Rosenberg, pp. 2474–89, J.B. Lippincott, Philadelphia.

Storb, R., Epstein, R.B. *et al.* (1970). Methotrexate regimens for control of graft-versus-host disease in dogs with allogeneic marrow grafts. *Transplantation* **9**, 240–6.

Storb, R., Thomas, E.D. *et al.* (1984). Marrow transplantation for aplastic anemia. *Semin. Hematol.* **21**, 27–35.

Storb, R., Deeg, H.J. *et al.* (1986). Methotrexate and cyclosporine compared with cyclosporine alone for prophylaxis of acute graft versus host disease after marrow transplantation for leukaemia. *N. Engl. J. Med.* **314**, 729–35.

Storb, R., Doney, K.C. *et al.* (1988). Allogeneic and syngeneic marrow transplantation for aplastic anemia: overview of Seattle results. In *Recent Advances and Future Directions in Bone Marrow Transplantation (Experimental Hematology Today — 1987)*, ed. S.J. Baum, G.W. Santos and F. Takaku, pp. 119–24, Springer Verlag, New York.

Sullivan, K.M., Shulman, H.M. *et al.* (1981). Chronic graft-versus-host disease in 52 patients: adverse natural course and successful treatment with combination immunosuppression. *Blood* **57**, 267–76.

Sullivan, K.M., Deeg, H.J. *et al.* (1986). Hyperacute GVHD in patients not given immunosuppression after allogeneic marrow transplantation. *Blood* **67**, 1172–5.

Sullivan, K.M., Fefer, A. *et al.* (1987). Graft-versus-leukemia in man: relationship of acute and chronic graft-versus-host disease to relapse of acute leukemia following allogeneic bone marrow transplantation. In *Cellular Immunotherapy of Cancer*, ed. R.L. Truitt, R.P. Gale and M.M. Bortin, pp. 391–9, A.R. Liss, New York.

Sullivan, K.M., Witherspoon, R.P. *et al.* (1988a). Prednisone and azathioprine compared to prednisone and placebo for treatment of chronic graft-versus-host disease: prognostic influence of prolonged thrombocytopenia after allogeneic marrow transplantation. *Blood* **72**, 546–54.

Sullivan, K.M., Witherspoon, R.P. *et al.* (1988b). Alternating-day cyclosporine and prednisone for treatment of high-risk chronic graft-versus-host disease. *Blood* **72**, 555–61.

Thomas, E.D., Buckner, C.D. *et al.* (1977). One hundred patients with acute leukemia treated by chemotherapy, total body irradiation, and allogeneic marrow transplantation. *Blood* **49**, 511–33.

Thomas, E.D., Buckner, C.D. *et al.* (1982). Marrow transplantation for thalassemia. *Lancet* **ii**, 227–8.

Thomas, E.D., Clift, R.A. *et al.* (1986). Marrow transplantation for the treatment of chronic myelogenous leukemia. *Ann. Intern. Med.* **104**, 155–63.

Tura, S., Cavo, M. *et al.* (1988). Overview of bone marrow transplantation for multiple myeloma (abstract #K016). In UCLA Symposia on Molecular and Cellular Biology. *J. Cell. Biochem.* suppl. 12C, 69.

Witherspoon, R.P., Matthews, D. *et al.* (1984). Recovery of *in vivo* cellular immunity after human marrow grafting: influence of time postgrafting and acute graft-versus-host-disease. *Transplantation* **37**, 145–50.

Witherspoon, R.P., Sullivan, K.M. *et al.* (1988). Use of thymic grafts or thymic factors to augment immunologic recovery after bone marrow transplantation: brief report with 2.2–12.3 (median 6.7) years follow-up. *Bone Marrow Transplant.* **3**, 425–35.

Witherspoon, R.P., Storb, R. *et al.* (1989). Immunologic aspects of marrow transplantation. In *Immunology and Allergy Clinics of North America*, ed. P.F. Halloran, pp. 187–208, W.B. Saunders, Philadelphia.

Yeager, A.M., Kaizer, H. *et al.* (1986). Autologous bone marrow transplantation in patients with acute nonlymphocytic leukemia, using *ex vivo* marrow treatment with 4-hydroperoxy-cyclophosphamide. *N. Engl. J. Med.* **315**, 141–7.

88: Immunosuppression for Heart and Heart–Lung Transplantation

J. Wallwork and J.P. Scott

Introduction

It is now 25 years since the first human heart was transplanted (Barnard 1967). Following that operation there was a world-wide rush into cardiac transplantation with over 60 teams in 22 countries performing 150 transplants. The results, however, did not meet optimistic expectations, and it was left to a few centres to develop and refine the application of cardiac transplantation for patients with terminal heart disease.

In 1979 there were five active centres worldwide and by far the greatest experience had been gained by Shumway's group in Stanford (Baumgartner *et al.* 1979). Judicious adaptation of techniques and protocols developed in the experimental laboratory led to improvements in survival and quality of life. By 1980 more than half of the total 400 cardiac transplants performed had been undertaken at Stanford, where the proportion of patients surviving 1 year had risen from 22% in 1968 to 67% in 1979 (Pennock *et al.* 1982).

Encouraged by these improving results, interest by other centres has again been renewed, and currently there are some 250 active centres throughout the world and the number of transplants performed is continuing to rise (Heck *et al.* 1989).

Heart and heart–lung transplant recipients have tended to be more heavily immunosuppressed than other transplant patients, and consequently at greater risk of complications. The difficult balance between over-immunosuppression and under-immunosuppression is reflected by those early poor results and the small number of units prepared to apply the devotion necessary for success. There have been four advances in immunosuppression that stand out among the many. In 1972 antithymocytic globulin (ATG) was incorporated into the immunosuppressive regimen at Stanford (Bieber *et al.* 1976). Associated with this introduction, there was the ability to monitor its usage immunologically by daily T cell counts and assessing the pharmacokinetics of ATG (Bieber *et al.* 1977). After evaluation in the laboratory (Calne *et al.* 1978; Pennock *et al.* 1981; Reitz *et al.* 1981), cyclosporin A has been incorporated into the immunosuppressive regimen at Stanford since 1980 (Oyer *et al.* 1981) and in the United Kingdom since March 1982 (Wallwork *et al.* 1983). More controversial has been the use of Muvomonab —

CD3 monoclonal antibody (Orthoclone OKT3) — both as prophylaxis perioperatively instead of ATG (Laufer *et al*. 1989) and as a treatment for persistent rejection (Macris *et al*. 1989).

Heart transplantation

Human leucocyte antigen matching in cardiac transplantation

The importance of human leucocyte antigen (HLA) matching and cross-matching has been a matter of much debate. Previous single-centre studies have made various suggestions as to the importance of HLA-B and DR matching (Raffoux *et al*. 1987; Yacoub *et al*. 1987). These studies were limited by the small number of patients included. Papworth Hospital participated in a large collaborative heart transplant study on the importance of HLA matching in cardiac transplantation (Opelz 1989), which was started in 1985. Two thousand patients with HLA-typed heart transplants participated in the study. Despite the large numbers of patients included, the study was limited by the small number of well-matched grafts. Unlike renal transplantation, the possibility of donor/recipient heart transplants being completely matched is remote and occurs only by chance, as the tolerated ischaemic time is much shorter ($<4-6$ hours) (Kaye 1987). There were only nine patients with no HLA-B or DR mismatches in this study. However, it was noted that, in grafts with no mismatch, survival rates were better than in mismatched grafts. Larger numbers of patients are required to produce unequivocal results in this field.

A possible link between episodes of histologically detected rejection and HLA-DR mismatching has been noted in two small studies (Foerster *et al*. 1988; Pfeffer *et al*. 1988). The latter study (Pfeffer *et al*. 1988) included only 37 patients and was a univariate analysis, but it did show a statistically significant correlation with HLA-DR mismatch and an increased number of rejection episodes, plus an associated increase in rejection therapy administered to each patient. In a multivariate analysis (Pfeffer *et al*. 1988) in a larger study, the presence of two HLA-DR mismatches between donor and recipient was suggested as an independent risk factor for episodes of acute rejection. Confirmation of these findings in other centres is awaited. There is evidence in the rat model (Qian *et al*. 1988) of major histocompatibility complex (MHC) differences in Class I or in groups of MHC antigen producing mild and prolonged allograft rejection. Subsequent arterial changes 'identical' to graft arteriosclerosis were noted. Evidence of this in human cardiac transplantation is not available.

A comprehensive review of the possible role of cardiac allograft vascular endothelial cell antigen expression and the development of coronary occlusive disease (COD) has been performed by Libby *et al*. (1989).

Lymphocytotoxic antibody status and cross-match results

In our centre, lymphocytotoxic cross-match testing is not routinely performed except in patients in whom preformed HLA antibodies have been detected. McCloskey *et al*. (1988) have produced updated results on lymphocytotoxic antibody status and cross-match results in 301 cardiac transplant recipients. Lymphocytotoxic cross-match was performed in 277 patients; of these, lymphocytotoxic cross-match was positive in 36, using the modified National Institute of Health (NIH) technique. The 1- and 2-year graft survival was 56% compared with when the lymphocytotoxic cross-match was negative, when 1- and 2-year graft survival was 74% ($p<0.02$). However, lymphocytotoxic antibody status of the recipient had no effect on survival. Further work is required to establish these results.

Immunosuppressive therapy

Long-term survival of both graft and recipient depends on the prevention of acute and chronic immune injury to the transplanted heart. Immunosuppressive regimes to achieve this end can be divided into three phases: (i) early postoperative prophylactic suppression; (ii) maintenance immunosuppression; and (iii) enhanced immunosuppression for rejection episodes.

Until the introduction of cyclosporin A, immunosuppressive therapy for cardiac transplantation was universally based on a combination of corticosteroids, azathioprine and ATG. In contrast with other organ transplantation, ATG, following its introduction in 1972 (Bieber *et al*. 1976), has been widely accepted and incorporated into prophylactic regimens in the early postoperative period and for rejection episodes (Keith *et al.* 1988). However, no well-controlled trial has yet been performed; rather, ATG has become established by practice.

Conventional immunosuppressive therapy

The regimen developed by the Stanford group for prophylactic conventional immunosuppression is outlined in Table 88.1, and this has been the basis for subsequent groups' modifications according to the varied emphasis placed on the rejection/ infection axis. For example, in an attempt to reduce morbidity associated with high-dose steroids but to maintain good immunosuppression by reducing the T cell population for a 28-day period, the Papworth group adopted the protocol shown in Table 88.2. Essential differences are a lower initial steroid dose and a prolonged but less intense ATG course, with horse ATG rather than rabbit ATG, aiming to reduce the T cell count to, but not below, 5% of the total lymphocyte count.

The assessment of long-term survival on any regimen requires an assessment of the relative hazard or hazard ratio. This is the ratio of the instantaneous risk for a patient in group 1 divided by the instantaneous risk for a patient in group 2. The relative risk (RR) may apply to any measurable outcome, such as graft loss, graft rejection or infection. Theoretically, if the RR is equal to one, then the two groups have the same probability of graft loss. The 95% confidence intervals are always given and, if the 95% confidence interval contains the value one, we can say there is not strong evidence that the two groups have different survival profiles. Alternatively, if the value one lies above (below) the upper (lower) limit of the 95% confidence interval, the patients in group 1 can be said to have significantly lower (higher) risk of death than those in group 2.

Although we can assess factors individually to investigate their effect upon outcome, factors are not always independent of each other. As a result some factors may appear significant in a univariate context, but disappear when other factors are adjusted for. Cox regression permits investigation of multivariate models.

From such an analysis, it can be seen that triple therapy is the preferred therapy for overall graft survival and for a lower frequency of acute rejection, acute infection and COD (Tables 88.3–88.6).

Table 88.1. Conventional immunosuppression — Stanford

	Azathioprine	Prednisolone	ATG
Initial	4 mg/kg (IV) preop. 1.5–2.0 mg/kg per day orally[b]	500 mg IV 125 mg IV × 3 doses 1.5 mg/kg per day orally	Rabbit: alternating IV or IM for 14 days[a]
Maintenance	1.5–2.0 mg/kg per day orally[b]	1.5 mg/kg per day orally 1 mg/kg per day at 4 weeks 0.5–0.3 mg/kg per day at 6 months to 1 year	Additional course IM if T cell rise greater than 10% before 4 weeks
Rejection			
Early	No change	1 g IV × 3 doses ↑ 100 mg/day orally reduce to previous dose over 2 weeks	Additional course IM days 1, 2, 3, 5, 7 and 9
Late	No change	100 mg/day orally reduce to previous dose over 2 weeks	

a Daily dose adjusted to maintain T cell fraction of lymphocytes <1%.
b Dose adjusted to maintain white blood cells (WBC) >5000 cells/mm^3.

Table 88.2. Conventional immunosuppression — Papworth

	Azathioprine	Prednisolone	ATG
Initial	4 mg/kg (IV) preop. 1.5–2.0 mg/kg per day orally[b]	500 mg IV 125 mg IV × 3 doses 1 mg/kg per day orally	Horse: IV daily 28 days[a]
Maintenance	1.5–2.0 mg/kg per day orally[b]	1 mg/kg per day orally 0.5 mg/kg per day at 4 weeks 0.3–0.2 mg/kg per day at 3 months to 1 year	
Rejection			
Early	No change	1 g IV × 3 doses no change in oral dose	IV for initial course completed
Late	No change	Double oral dose and taper over 2 weeks	

a Daily dose adjusted to maintain T cell fraction of lymphocytes <5%.
b Dose adjusted to maintain WBC >5000 cells/mm^3.

Table 88.3. Overall graft survival by immunosuppression: relative risks adjusted for assay

Relationship	RR	95% CI
Pre-CyA/Triple	3.51	(1.97, 6.27)
Double/Triple	1.41	(0.82, 2.44)
Triple/Triple	1.00	

CI: confidence interval.
CyA: cyclosporin A.

Maintenance therapy

Whilst the major objective of long-term therapy is to reduce immunosuppression to the minimum required to prevent rejection, difficulties with adequate detection of rejection (Scott *et al.* 1991) make that less easy to define. With time, as the 'responsiveness' of the immune mechanism of the recipient is reduced, rejection episodes decrease in both frequency and intensity. This enables

Table 88.4. Acute rejection by immunosuppression group: unadjusted

Variable	Relationship	RR	95% CI
Immunotherapy	Pre-CyA/Triple	3.44	(1.25, 9.51)
	Double/Triple	2.24	(1.03, 4.85)
	Triple/Triple	1.00	

Table 88.5. Acute infection by immunosuppression group: unadjusted

Variable	Relationship	RR	95% CI
Immunotherapy	Pre-CyA/Triple	1.87	(0.37, 9.34)
	Double/Triple	3.15	(1.20, 8.24)
	Triple/Triple	1.00	

Table 88.6. Graft loss from coronary occlusive disease

		Univariate		Multivariate	
Variable	Relationship	RR	95% CI	RR	95% CI
Immuno-therapy	Pre-CyA/Triple	11.47	(1.16, 113.69)	17.52	(1.56, 196.87)
	Double/Triple	2.19	(0.22, 21.47)	3.18	(0.29, 34.81)
	Triple/Triple	1.00			

maintenance with low-dose steroids to be attained in the majority of cases, tapered to 0.2–0.3 mg/kg/day. Azathioprine is given daily in doses that allow the white blood count to be maintained above 5000 cells/mm^3. The risk to the patient of life-threatening complications of immunosuppressive therapy or of rejection are reduced but still remain, and long-term surveillance as an out-patient by both the patient's own physician and the transplant team is necessary.

Augmentation of immunosuppressive therapy for rejection

EARLY (0–3 MONTHS)

Suspected rejection episodes, confirmed by endomyocardial biopsy, are treated with an augmentation in immunosuppressive therapy. Intravenous methylprednisolone 1 g per day is given for 3 days, and an additional course of ATG therapy over several days according to the protocol adopted. The rejection episode is monitored by subsequent biopsies to assess the efficacy of the therapy given and to determine the amount and duration of anti-rejection therapy for a given rejection episode. During these episodes the patient is inevitably at greater risk of infection, and early detection and prompt treatment of rejection episodes is of prime importance in cardiac transplantation to minimize these risks. If early rejection persists, additional courses of methylprednisolone will be required, and occasionally episodes may be refractory to conventional therapy or may recur shortly after resolution. Under these circumstances ATG raised in a different species may be useful. If continuing high-dose methylprednisolone and further courses of ATG or OKT3 do not abort a rejection episode, other extraordinary intervention may be considered. Cardiac retransplantation, in the absence of active infection, was previously advocated (Copeland *et al.* 1977), but has in our experience been unrewarding and is a questionable use of scarce donor organs.

Immunosuppression with cyclosporin

The introduction of cyclosporin into heart transplant immunosuppression resulted in a re-evaluation of the techniques used for monitoring the patients. Whilst the addition of cyclosporin by itself does not decrease the number of rejection episodes, it does reduce their intensity and associated morbidity (Merian *et al.* 1983). As a result of its use, monitoring of E rosette numbers, previously helpful as a predictor of acute cardiac rejection (Bieber *et al.* 1977), is no longer helpful, T cell levels being normal in cyclosporin-immunosuppressed patients. Cyclosporin has also resulted in modifications in the interpretation of cardiac biopsy histology (Billingham 1981). Our cyclosporin regimen is given in Table 93.7.

As with all potent immunosuppressants, cyclosporin has numerous side-effects (Scott and Higenbottam 1988) (Table 93.8). Nephrotoxicity remains a major problem in the early and late post-transplant periods and is the main limitation on the dose of cyclosporin given to a patient. As a result doses of cyclosporin greater than 10 mg/kg/day are rarely achieved in our heart transplant recipients. Reliance on combination 'triple' immunosuppression with steroids and azathioprine supplementing cyclosporin remains our policy and that of Stanford, and, although such regimens may be associated with a greater incidence of lymphomas (White 1988), in our experience it is an uncommon occurrence, with only three possible lymphomas occurring in 300 patients over 5 years on 'tripple' therapy.

Studies of T cell subsets indicate that T cell numbers in the peripheral blood decrease with cyclosporin immunosuppression and with treatment of rejection and increase at the onset of rejection. However, the CD4/CD8 ratio has no predictive value (Pelletier *et al.* 1988). When discriminating rejection from infection or other inflammatory conditions, T cell subset studies have a sensitivity of only 43% and a specificity of 56% (Hanson *et al.* 1988).

The total concentration of cyclosporin in blood is a valuable indicator of possible toxicity, being linearly related to free drug concentration of cyclosporin up to 1000 μg/l or more (Awni and Sawchuck 1985).

The two methods in use of estimations of cyclosporin blood, plasma and serum concentrations are high-pressure liquid chromatography (HPLC) and a radio-immunoassay (RIA). The RIA test has usually come as a kit from Sandoz, the manufacturers, and is based on antibodies to cyclosporin originally raised in New Zealand white rabbits (Donatsch *et al.* 1981) and later in sheep (Rosano

Table 88.7. Immunosuppression for cardiac transplantation: Papworth Hospital protocol

	Cyclosporin A	Prednisolone	ATG
Initial	10 mg/kg per day	500 mg IV 125 mg IV × 3 doses 1 mg/kg per day	Rabbit: IV 2–4 days to T cells = 10–20%
Maintenance	Reduce gradually by 6 mg/kg per day[a]	1 mg/kg per day 0.3 mg/kg per day at 2 weeks	—
Rejection			
Early	No change	1 g IV × 2–3 doses	IV 3–5 days if moderate/ severe
Late	No change	1 mg/kg per day reduce to maintenance over 10 days or 1 g IV × 2–3 doses if rejection is recurrent	—

a Dose adjusted to drug level and nephrotoxicity.

Table 88.8. Cyclosporine side-effects

	Serum creatinine mmol/l mean (±15)			Systemic hypertension (% of all patients)
	1 year	3 years	5 years	
Conventional therapy	99	103	108	0
Double therapy using cyclosporin	175 (±6)	175 (±8)	157 (±5)	27
Triple therapy	171 (±5)	172 (±8)	—	31

et al. 1986a). In these two forms it was not sufficiently specific for clinical use as it reacted with cyclosporin metabolites. More recently a monoclonal antibody has been produced and this is the method we now use (Holt *et al.* 1986).

Comparisons of cyclosporin concentrations obtained with HPLC with those obtained with RIA have often been poor (Robinson *et al.* 1983; Abisch *et al.* 1986; Annesley *et al.* 1986). Comparisons between centres, sometimes very poor, have been best when HPLC and whole-blood samples have been used (Johnston *et al.* 1986).

Debate has arisen over whether serum, plasma or whole-blood cyclosporin concentrations are the best monitor for the pharmacological and toxic effects of the drug. Whole-blood samples are preferable from an analytical viewpoint, being unaffected by assay temperature or haematocrit (Rosano 1985; Van der Berg *et al.* 1985). Also, the ratio of the mildly toxic cyclosporin metabolite 17 to cyclosporin is similar in both whole blood and kidney, but differs greatly from that in serum (Rosano *et al.* 1986b).

However, if cyclosporin was added to samples of whole blood of varying haematocrit, various plasma cyclosporin concentrations were obtained, although whole-blood values were constant (Rosano 1985). This has led some to believe that whole blood does not reflect the pharmacologically effective concentration of the drug. We currently measure whole-blood levels by the specific monoclonal assay.

Careful attention must be given to the methods of collection and storage of blood preparation and analysis. Ethylenediamine tetra-acetic acid (EDTA) is probably a better anticoagulant than heparin, the blood pools prepared from the latter often having small clots (Van der Berg *et al.* 1985). Plasma samples must be allowed to equilibrate at a measured temperature — for 2 hours at room temperature or 30 minutes at body temperature (Rosano 1985).

When interpreting results and when considering adjustments in dosage, allowance must be made for time of dosage (Kahan *et al.* 1985), liver dysfunction (Grevel 1986) and general ill health, gastrointestinal disturbance (Agarwal *et al.* 1985), anaemia (Tufveson *et al.* 1986) and plasma lipoprotein levels (Task Force of Cyclosporine Monitoring 1987), to which the majority of plasma cyclosporin is bound.

Since the use of cyclosporin has made kinetic studies of ATG (Bieber *et al.* 1976) as well as T cell peripheral blood levels (Bieber *et al.* 1977) obsolete, dependence on endomyocardial biopsy for the early and sensitivity rejection has become greater than ever. The Papworth experience, like that of Stanford, has been to take three or at most four biopsies as a protocol of regular biopsy follow-up (Spiegelhalter and Stovin 1983). Recently, as a result of our experience with the increased sensitivity of increased numbers of adequate transbronchial biopsies, we have increased our cardiac biopsies to 8–12 biopsies at each session. This change has tripled the detection of acute cardiac rejection with evidence of myocyte necrosis, which we treat with intravenous and tapered oral steroids (Table 88.2). This increase in the detection of rejection has not been confined to the early postoperative period, but has also been a feature of long-term follow-up more than 6 years after transplantation. Most importantly, we have had no deaths from acute rejection or significant morbidity from rejection since starting our new policy.

The implication of our new policy is that previously endomyocardial biopsies had under-detected acute rejection. This raises serious doubts as to the validity of many earlier studies relating biopsy findings and treated rejection episodes to any other assessment of acute cardiac rejection. It may also enable us to assess more reliably any possible relationship between acute and chronic rejection in heart transplant recipients, which is so clearly present in heart–lung transplant recipients (Scott *et al.* 1990b).

The use of OKT3 remains more controversial. It may well be associated with a higher incidence of infection (Hegewald *et al.* 1989; Macris *et al.* 1989) than with alternative immunosuppressive regimens. Moreover, some groups have reported a higher incidence of rejection on OKT3 perioperative prophylaxis than on the ATG regimen described above (Kormos *et al.* 1988; Laufer *et al.* 1989). However, it is uncertain if valid comparisons can be made between these two immunosuppressants when the doses are often based on bodyweight rather than blood or tissue T cell levels or function.

Heart–lung transplantation

Human leucocyte antigens in heart–lung transplantation

Our own experience suggests that there is no statistically significant improvement in survival with HLA matching as yet. A trend of improved survival with HLA-DR match has been noted in a large collaborative study, although this trend did not reach statistical significance, probably as a result of small patient numbers (Opelz 1989).

There is controversy over the importance of Class II MHC antigen expression by bronchial epithelial cells as a marker of lung allograft rejection in humans. Taylor *et al.* (1989) found evidence of enhanced expression of Class II MHC antigens on endothelial and epithelial cells from lungs with end-stage obliterative bronchiolitis (OB). Its importance and relationship to the diagnosis of lung allograft rejection, however, have been disputed (Hruban *et al.* 1989). This is not surprising as infection and other stimuli can induce Class II MHC antigen expression (Barclay and Mason 1982).

Lymphocytotoxic antibody status and cross-match results

In a parallel study to one performed in cardiac transplant recipients, Festenstein *et al.* (1989) analysed data on 150 consecutive heart–lung transplant recipients. In contrast to the results in heart transplants, lymphocytotoxic cross-match results had minimal effect on graft survival. There was a trend towards improved survival with HLA Class I MHC matching but this did not reach statistical significance. Lymphocytotoxic antibody −ve patients survived longer than lymphocytotoxic antibody +ve patients. Again, small numbers of patients are involved.

Immunosuppression

The immunosuppressive regimen used clinically for heart–lung transplantation is outlined in Table 88.9. As with cyclosporin A protocols for cardiac transplant patients, the development clinically of suitable protocols for heart–lung transplantation is still in a state of flux. The important point is that oral steroids are not commenced until the first episode of acute rejection in order to minimize the effects on healing that steroids may have. Cyclosporin A immunosuppression is augmented during the period before steroids are commenced with azathioprine.

As with heart transplants, we continue to use ATG in the early postoperative period. The addition of steroid therapy to the double therapy of oral cyclosporin and azathioprine is tailored to the level of rejection found at transbronchial biopsy (Scott *et al.* 1990a).

We have not used endomyocardial biopsy for the detection of rejection in heart–lung transplant recipients since 1986, owing to the negligible yield of rejection when compared with transbronchial lung biopsies (Higenbottam *et al.* 1988). Again, we consider 18 biopsies — eight from the lower lobe, four from the lingula or middle lobe and six from the upper lobe — to be optimal for the diagnosis of lung rejection (Scott *et al.* 1991).

The first episode of lung rejection occurs 7–10 days after transplantation in most patients and is treated with intravenous steroids at 0.5–1 g daily for 3 days, followed by oral steroids at 1 mg/kg/day, reducing by 5 mg/day down to 0.25 mg/kg/day. Steroids are then kept at this level until the first biopsy, which is usually at 3 weeks before the intermediate discharge of the patient to a house near the hospital. If this shows only non-rejecting lung, the steroid therapy is tapered to zero over the next 3 weeks, and a further biopsy is performed at 3 months to confirm that there is no rejection off steroids.

If the first biopsy shows rejection at 3 weeks, intravenous and oral steroids are employed in the same way and the patient is rebiopsied at monthly intervals until all evidence of rejection has disappeared. We have reported the importance of the persistence, severity and frequency of rejection in identifying those patients who will develop chronic lung rejection, characterized by OB, vascu-

Table 88.9. Immunosuppression for heart–lung transplantation

	Cyclosporin A	Azathioprine	Prednisolone	ATG[a]
Initial	10 mg/kg per day	2 mg/kg IV preop	500 mg IV 125 mg IV × 3 doses	Rabbit: 2–4 doses (T cells 10–20%)
Maintenance	10 mg/kg per day[b]	1–2 mg/kg per day orally for 2 weeks	0.3 mg/kg per day orally, beginning 2 weeks and taper to 0.2 mg/kg per day	—
Rejection				
Early	No change	—	1 g IV × 3 doses	3–5 doses if persistent rejection
Late	No change	—	1 g IV × 3 doses	3–5 doses if persistent rejection

a Use under review.
b Dose adjusted according to drug level and nephrotoxicity.

lar sclerosis and interstitial fibrosis (Scott *et al.* 1989a, 1991). Severity of rejection is based on a simple grading system (Clelland *et al.* 1990) of the extent of perivascular acute mononuclear lung infiltrates. Of all these characteristics, persistent rejection is by far the most significant, reflecting the presence of rejection on subsequent biopsies following a previous biopsy-confirmed rejection episode. Persistent rejection reflects the likely persistence of the rejection process in the time between biopsies and the relative resistance of the process to the intravenous and tapering oral steroid immunosuppressive regimen (Scott *et al.* 1990c). It is becoming apparent that treatment in this way of moderate or severe rejection usually results in the presence of mild rejection at the next biopsy, suggesting that in such cases a further pulse of steroids or the addition of a further immunosuppressant such as ATG may be valuable. Since 1988, when we began employing this regimen consistently, we have had no further episodes of chronic rejection/OB. Moreover, at 1 year, the predicted average forced expiratory volume in 1 second (FEV_1)% is 15% higher in those transplanted, when compared with previous patients in whom close follow-up biopsies were not initially employed. This is not conclusive and it may be fortuitous, but it is encouraging.

We do not routinely use OKT3 in our heart–lung transplants, our very limited experience in three patients being consistent with the experience of others (C. Spratt 1989, pers. comm.) that its use is associated with a high incidence of infection.

The employment of more frequent, smaller doses of cyclosporin has been of use in our cystic fibrosis patients who have received heart–lung transplants (Scott *et al.* 1989b). The tailoring of dosage intervals to the reduced lipid absorption common in this group of patients has resulted in an average saving of £3000 a year on this expensive drug.

References

Abisch, E., Beveridge, T. Gratwohl, A., Niederberger, W. and Nussbaumer, K. (1986). Cyclosporine A: correlation between HPLC and RIA serum levels. *Pharmaceut. Weekbl. Sci. Ed.* **4**, 84–6.

Agarwal, R.P., McPherson, R.A. and Threatle, G.A. (1985). Assessment of cyclosporine A in whole blood and plasma in five patients with different haematocrit. *Ther. Drug Mon.* **7**, 61–5.

Annesley, T., Matz, K., Balogh, L., Clayton, L. and Glacerio, D. (1986). Liquid chromatographic analysis of cyclosporine using a microbore column and a reduced specimen requirement. *Clin. Chem.* **32**, 1407–9.

Awni, W.M. and Sawchuck, R.J. (1985). The pharmacokinetics of cyclosporine. II. Blood–plasma distribution and binding studies. *Drug Metab. Dispos.* **13**, 127–32.

Barclay, A.N. and Mason, D.W. (1982). Induction of Ia antigen in rat epidermal cells and gut epithelium by immunological stimuli. *J. Exp. Med.* **156**, 1665–7.

Barnard, C.N. (1967). A human cardiac transplant: interim report of a successful operation performed at Groote Schuur Hospital, Cape Town. *South Afr. Med. J.* **41**, 1271–4.

Baumgartner, W.A., Reitz, B.A., Oyer, P.E., Stinson, E.B. and Shumway, N.E. (1979). Cardiac homotransplantation. *Curr. Proc. Surg.* **16**, 1–61.

Bieber, C.P., Griepp, R.B., Oyer, P.E., Wary, J. and Stinson, E.B. (1976). Use of rabbit antithymocyte globulin in cardiac transplantation: relationship of serum clearance rates to clinical outcome. *Transplantation* **22**, 478–88.

Bieber, C.P., Griepp, R.B., Oyer, P.E., David, L.A. and Stinson, E.B. (1977). Relationship of rabbit ATB serum clearance rates to circulatory T-cell levels, rejection onset and survival in cardiac transplantation. *Transplant. Proc.* **9**, 1031–6.

Billingham, M.E. (1981). Diagnosis of cardiac rejection by endomyocardial biopsy. *J. Heart Transplant.* **1**, 25–30.

Calne, R.Y., White, D.J.C., Rolles, K., Smith, D.P. and Herbertson, B.M. (1978). Prolonged survival of pig orthotopic heart grafts treated with cyclosporin A. *Lancet* **i**, 1183–7.

Clelland, C.A., Higenbottam, T.W., Otulana, B.A. *et al.* (1990). Histological prognostic indicators for the lung allografts of heart–lung transplants. *J. Heart Transplant.* **9**, 177–86.

Copeland, J.G., Griepp, R.B., Bieber, C.P. *et al.* (1977). Successful re-transplantation of the human heart. *J. Thorac. Cardiovasc. Surg.* **73**, 242–7.

Donatsch, P., Abisch, E., Homberger, M., Traber, R. and Boges, R. (1981). A radioimmunoassay to measure cyclosporine A in plasma and serum samples. *J. Immunoassay* **2**, 19–32.

Festenstein, H., Banner, N., Smith, J. *et al.* (1989). The influence of HLA matching and lymphocytotoxic antibody status in heart–lung allograft recipients receiving cyclosporine and azathioprine. *Transplant. Proc.* **21**(1), 797–8.

Foerster, A., Abdelnoor, M., Froysaker, T. *et al.* (1988). Human heart transplantation. Rejection risk factors. *APMIS* **96** (suppl. 2), 160–73.

Grevel, J. (1986). Absorption of cyclosporine A after oral dosing. *Transplant. Proc.* **18** (suppl. 5), 9–15.

Hanson, C.A., Bolling, S.F., Stoolman, L.M. *et al.* (1988). Cytoimmunologic monitoring and heart transplantation. *J. Heart Transplant.* **7**, 424–9.

Heck, C.F., Shumway, S.J. and Kaye, M.P. (1989). The registry of the international society for heart transplantation: sixth official report. *J. Heart Transplant.* **8**, 271–6.

Hegewald, M.G., O'Connell, J.B., Renlurd, D.G. *et al.* (1989). OKT3 monoclonal antibody given for ten versus fourteen days as immunosuppressive prophylaxis in heart transplantation. *J. Heart Transplant.* **8**, 303–10.

Higenbottam, T.W., Stewart, S., Penketh, A. and Wallwork, J. (1988). Transbronchial lung biopsy for the diagnosis of rejection in heart–lung transplant patients. *Transplantation* **46**, 532–9.

Holt, D.W., Marsden, J.J. and Johnston, A. (1986). A measurement of cyclosporine: methodological problems. *Transplant. Proc.* **18** (suppl. 5), 101–10.

Hruban, R.H., Beschorner, W.E., Baumgartner, W.A. *et al.* (1989). Evidence that expression of Class II MHC antigens is not diagnostic of lung allograft rejection. *Transplant. Proc.* **48** (3), 529–30.

Johnston, A., Marsden, J.T. and Holt, D.W. (1986). The UK cyclosporine quality assessment scheme. *Ther. Drug Mon.* **8**, 200–4.

Kahan, B.D., Van Buren, C.T., Lorber, M.I. *et al.* (1985). Optimisation of cyclosporine immunosuppression for renal transplantation. *Transplant. Proc.* **17** (suppl. 2), 35–43.

Kaye, M.P. (1987). The registry of the International Society for Heart Transplantation: fourth official report — 1987. *J. Heart Transplant.* **6** (2), 63–7.

Keith, F.M., Mågilligan, D.J., Lakier, J.B., Drost, C.J. and Minesota, A.L.G. (1988). Safe and effective immunosuppression for cardiac transplantation. *Circulation* **78**, 11173–7.

Kormos, R., Herlon, D.B., Curran, M., Hardesty, R.L., Armitage, J. and Griffith, B.P. (1988). Monoclonal versus polyclonal antibody therapy for prophylaxis against rejection following cardiac transplantation. *J. Heart Transplant.* **7**, 80 (abstract).

Laufer, G., Laczkovic, S.A., Wollnek, G. *et al.* (1989). Impact of low-dose steroids and prophylactic monoclonal versus polyclonal antibodies on acute rejection in cyclosporin and azothioprine immunosuppressant cardiac allografts. *J. Heart Transplant.* **8**, 153–61.

Libby, P., Salomon, R.N., Payne, D.D., Schoen, F.J. and Pober, J.S. (1989). Functions of vascular wall cells related to development of transplantation-associated coronary arteriosclerosis. *Transplant. Proc.* **21**, 3677–84.

McCloskey, D., Festenstein, H., Banner, N. *et al.* (1988). The effect of HLA lymphocytotoxic antibody status in crossmatched results on cardiac transplant survival. *Transplant. Proc.* **21** (1), 804–6.

Macris, M.J., Frazier, O.H., Lammermeier, D., Radovoncevic, B. and Duncan, J.M. (1989). Clinical experience with Muromonal — CD3 monoclonal antibody (OKT3) in heart transplantation. *J. Heart Transplant.* **8**, 281–7.

Merian, R.M., White, D.J.G. and Calne, R.Y. (1983). Early renal rejection episodes are less aggressive with cyclosporine A immunosuppression. *Transplant. Proc.* **15**, 2172–3.

Opelz, G. (1989). Effects of HLA matching in heart transplantation. Collaborative heart transplant study. *Transplant. Proc.* **21** (1), 797–8.

Oyer, P.E., Stinson, E.B., Reitz, B.A. *et al.* (1981). Preliminary results with cyclosporin A in clinical cardiac transplantation. In *Cyclosporin A*, ed. D.J. White, pp. 461–71, Elsevier, Amsterdam.

Pelletier, L.C., Mont Plaisir, S., Pelletier, G. *et al.* (1988). Lymphocyte subpopulation monitoring in cyclosporine-treated patients following heart transplantation. *Ann. Thorac. Surg.* **45**, 11–15.

Pennock, J.L., Reitz, B.A., Bieber, C.P. *et al.* (1981). Cardiac allograft survival in cynomolgus monkeys treated with cyclosporin A in combination with conventional immunosuppression. *Transplant. Proc.* **13**, 390–2.

Pennock, J.L., Oyer, P.E., Reitz, B.A. *et al.* (1982). Cardiac transplantation in perspective for the future: survival complications, rehabilitation and cost. *J. Thorac. Cardiovasc. Surg.* **83**, 168–77.

Pfeffer, P., Foerster, A., Frosaker, T., Simonson, S. and Thorsby, E. (1988). HLA mismatch and histologically evaluated rejection episodes in cardiac transplants can be correlated. *Transplant. Proc.* **3**, 367–8.

Qian, S., Harnaha, J., Chapman, F.A., Estes, L.W., Starzl, T.E. and Makowka, L. (1988). Cardiac transplantation in the rat: the effect of histocompatibility differences on graft arteriosclerosis. *Transplantation* **47** (3), 414–19.

Raffaux, C., Mayor, V., Cabrol, C., Busson, M., Hors, J. and Colombani, J. (1987). The influence of HLA matching in cardiac allograft recipients in a single centre. *Transplant. Proc.* **19** (5), 3559–60.

Reitz, B.A., Bieber, C.P., Raney, A.A. *et al.* (1981). Orthotopic heart and combined heart and lung transplantation with cyclosporin A immunesuppression. *Transplant. Proc.* **13**, 393–6.

Robinson, W.T., Schran, H.F. and Barry, E.P. (1983). Methods to measure cyclosporine levels: high pressure liquid chromatography, radioimmunoassay and correlation. *Transplant. Proc.* **15** (suppl. 1), 2403–9.

Rosano, T.G. (1985). Effect of haematocrit on cyclosporine in whole blood and plasma of renal transplant patients. *Clin. Chem.* **31**, 410–12.

Rosano, T.G., Freed, B.M., Cerilli, J. and Lempert, N. (1986a). Immunosuppressive metabolites of cyclosporine in the blood of renal allograft recipients. *Transplantation* **42**, 262–6.

Rosano, T.G., Freed, B.M., Pell, M.A. and Lempert, N. (1986b). Cyclosporine metabolites in human blood and renal tissue. *Transplant. Proc.* **18** (suppl. 5), 35–40.

Scott, J.P. and Higenbottam, T.W. (1988). Adverse reactions and interactions of cyclosporine A. *Med. Toxicol. Adverse Drug Exp.* **3**, 212–27.

Scott, J.P., Higenbottam, T.W., Hutter, J.A., Stewart, S., Otulana, B.A. and Wallwork, J. (1989a). The natural history of obliterative bronchiolitis in heart–lung transplant recipients. *Transplant. Proc.* **21**, 2592–3.

Scott, J.P., Higgenbottam, T.W., Clelland, C.A. *et al.* (1989b). The value of three times a day cyclosporine dosing of cystic fibrosis patients. *Transplantation* **48**, 543–4 (letter).

Scott, J.P., Higenbottam, T.W., Clelland, C.A. *et al.* (1990a). Natural history of chronic rejection in heart–lung transplant recipients. *J. Heart Transplant.* **9**, 510–15.

Scott, J.P., Fradet, G., Smyth, R.L. *et al.* (1990b). Management following heart and lung transplantation: five years experience. *Eur. J. Cardiothorac. Surg.* **4**, 197–200.

Scott, J.P., Fradet, G., Smyth, R.L. *et al.* (1991). A prospective study of transbronchial biopsies in the management of heart–lung and single lung transplant patients. *J. Heart Transplant.* **10**, 626–37.

Spiegelhalter, D.J. and Stovin, P.G. (1983). An analysis of repeated biopsies following cardiac transplantation. *Stat. Med.* **2** (1), 33–40.

Task Force on Cyclosporine Monitoring (1987). Critical issues in cyclosporine monitoring. *Clin. Chem.* **33**, 1269–88.

Taylor, P.M., Rose, M.L. and Yacoub, M.H. (1989). Expression of MHC antigens in normal human lungs and transplant lungs with obliterative bronchiolitis. *Transplantation* **48** (3), 506–10.

Tufveson, G., Odlind, B., Sjoberg, A. *et al.* (1986). A longitudinal study of the pharmacokinetics of cyclosporine A and *in vitro* lymphocyte responses in renal transplant patients. *Transplant. Proc.* **xv** (4), 2559–66.

Van der Berg, J.W.O., Verhoef, M.L., de Boer, A.J.H. and Schalm, S.W. (1985). Cyclosporine A assay: conditions for sampling and processing of blood. *Clin. Chim. Acta* **147**, 291–7.

Wallwork, J., Cory-Pearce, R. and English, T.A.H. (1983). Cyclosporin A for cardiac transplantation — the UK trial. *Transplant. Proc.* **XV** (4), 2559–66.

White, D.J.G. (1988). Immunosuppression for cardiac transplantation. In *Heart and Heart–lung Transplantation,* ed. J. Wallwork, pp. 155–72, W.B. Saunders, London.

Yacoub, M., Festenstein, H., Doyle, P. *et al.* (1987). The influence of HLA matching in cardiac allograft recipients receiving cyclosporine and azathioprine. *Transplant. Proc.* **19** (1), 2487–9.

89: Kidney Transplantation

P.J. Morris

Introduction

Over the past 25 years kidney transplantation has moved from being an experimental procedure to the treatment of choice for most patients with end-stage renal failure. This is due to the dramatic improvement in graft survival over this time, both in the short and medium term, as a result of better and less toxic immunosuppression, tissue matching and better preparation of patients before transplantation, and to the ever-increasing experience of physicians and surgeons caring for transplant patients (Morris 1988a).

As the results have improved, this has allowed patients previously considered too high-risk for transplantation, such as the elderly and the diabetic, to be transplanted in increasing numbers. However, many problems remain to be resolved. Even with modern immunosuppression, 10–15% of kidneys are lost from rejection during the first year after transplantation, and chronic rejection is responsible for a steady attrition of grafts thereafter, while cardiovascular disease is now the commonest cause of death after renal transplantation. Nevertheless, advances in the understanding of the mechanisms of rejection are progressing rapidly, which will allow more specific immunosuppression to be designed, thus further improving graft survival and reducing the side-effects of current immunosuppression. Further attention needs to be given to long-term graft survival, for this still remains relatively poor, with predicted cadaveric graft survival at 10 years using current immunosuppression being around 50%.

Indications for transplantation

Glomerulonephritis, pyelonephritis, interstitial nephritis and diabetes mellitus represent the three major causes of end-stage renal failure leading to transplantation (Briggs 1988). There are no causes of end-stage renal failure for which renal transplantation has not been attempted, and indeed there are no conditions which represent an absolute contraindication to transplantation. However, oxalosis does represent a relative contraindication, although recently some success has been reported, at least in the short term, provided the transplanted kidney functions immediately (Scheinman *et al.* 1984). The results of transplantation in Fabry's disease remain uncertain because of a high mortality, but it does not appear that a successful renal transplant is able to replace the deficiency of the specific α-galactosidase enzyme (Maizel *et al.* 1981). Similarly, in amyloidosis there is a high mortality in these patients, although graft survival is acceptable after allowing for this increased mortality (Pasternack *et al.* 1986). Transplantation of children with the haemolytic uraemic syndrome would seem justified, although some, but not all, results have been poor in these patients.

Age is only a relative contraindication, although transplantation of infants under the age of 2 is possibly not justified as the results are not good, and it may be better to maintain these infants on dialysis until a little older before attempting transplantation. Patients up to the age of 70 are now being regularly transplanted with very good results, although, as would be expected, mortality in the years after transplantation is much greater, primarily due to cardiovascular disease. The supply of cadaver kidneys influences the number of elderly patients that can be transplanted, but, provided that an adequate supply of cadaver kidneys is available, then probably even for a significant number of patients over the age of 70 years a kidney transplant is preferable to dialysis.

Recurrent glomerulonephritis in the transplanted kidney is common. The nephritides which recur most commonly are membranous glomerulonephritis, mesangiocapillary type 1 and type 2 glomerulonephritis and immunoglobulin A (IgA) nephropathy (Cameron 1982). Although these conditions recur in 50–90% of transplanted kidneys, graft loss due to recurrent disease is relatively uncommon (around 10%). Thus transplantation is not contraindicated in those types of nephritis which have a high rate of recurrence.

Donor and donor nephrectomy

The donor of a kidney may be a living relative (in general, a first blood relative) or a cadaver. In certain situations a living unrelated donor may be used, provided that there is a special emotional relationship between the donor and recipient, e.g. transplantation between spouses (Council of the Transplantation Society 1985). Where a living related donor is used, then it is important to establish not only that renal function is normal in the donor but also that his/her general health is normal. Although in the relatively recent past it was felt that living related donors should be either human leucocyte antigen (HLA)-identical or at the most one-haplotype-disparate (e.g. parent to child), the better graft survival with current immunosuppressive protocols justifies transplants between two-haplotype-disparate siblings.

The donor nephrectomy in a living donor is a major operation and therefore carries the risks of such a procedure (Cosimi 1988a). It is performed either transperitoneally through an anterior incision or through a loin incision. The most important question concerning living related transplantation is whether the patient's renal function and general health in subsequent years is compromised by having donated one of two kidneys. Follow-up studies for between 15 and 20 years are now available for living related donors and there is no convincing evidence that up to that time any harm has arisen for the donor following donation of a kidney (Fehrman *et al.* 1986; Williams *et al.* 1986; Cosimi 1988a). Nevertheless, until it is possible to review a significant cohort of donors over a 30- to 40-year period, it is not possible to exclude any long-term detrimental affect on renal function as a result of donation.

The bulk of kidneys in Europe come from cadavers (approximately 70–85%). Nowadays cadaver kidneys are often removed as part of a multi-organ retrieval (Cosimi 1988a). This has occurred as the criteria for brain stem death have become widely accepted (Pallis 1988), and, although not essential for successful kidney transplantation, it is essential in the retrieval of hearts and livers for transplantation.

Preservation

Effective preservation is essential in all kidney transplant programmes, and there is no doubt that the use of donors for organs other than the kidney has led to improved clinical management of potential donors before removal of their organs. Preservation can be achieved either by continuous perfusion on a machine or by flushing with one of several appropriate flushing solutions and then storage in ice, which will allow preservation for at least 48 hours (Marshall *et al.* 1988). As a result, the latter approach has virtually displaced machine preservation of kidneys. However, it should be said that, if kidneys are to be kept for more than 48 hours, then ideally this should be done by machine preservation. The two flushing solutions used most commonly throughout the world are Collins solutions and citrate-based solutions. The major characteristics of these solutions are high concentrations of potassium, phosphate and mannitol, together with hypertonic or isotonic citrate in the citrate-based solutions. More recently, a new preservation solution developed at the University of Wisconsin (UW solution) has been described in an experimental pancreatic transplant model, which in clinical practice has dramatically lengthened the preservation time for livers, and early experience suggests that it may be a more effective flushing solution for kidneys (Wahlberg *et al.* 1987). It contains lactobionic acid and raffinose, together with a high potassium content.

Human leucocyte antigen matching and cross-matching

Human leucocyte antigen is the major histocompatibility system in man, as confirmed by the superior survival of transplants performed between siblings who are HLA-identical. Nevertheless, with current immunosuppression, the survival of kidneys between one-haplotype and two-haplotype family members has improved dramatically and is not much inferior to that in HLA-identical siblings. Nevertheless, as long-term follow-up of family transplants becomes available, the superior survival of HLA-identical sibling transplants is likely to become more pronounced, even with current cyclosporin protocols.

In cadaver transplantation, the enormous polymorphism of the HLA system has meant that it is virtually impossible to truly match two unrelated individuals. Nevertheless, the recognition by Ting and Morris in 1978 that matching for HLA-DR alone would significantly improve graft survival has enabled matching to be applied to unrelated cadaveric transplantation on a more limited basis, using HLA-DR or HLA-B and DR for matching (Ting 1988). The improved survival of patients receiving HLA-DR-compatible kidneys was striking in the azathioprine and prednisolone days (Fig. 89.1(a)). Although less striking in the cyclosporin era, matching for HLA-DR still shows a similar influence of compatibility for HLA-DR on first cadaver graft survival (Fig. 89.1(b)), but with a very striking influence on the outcome of cadaver regrafts (Fig. 89.1(c)).

An additional and very important part of typing potential donors and recipients is the cross-match between recipient sera and donor lymphocytes (Ting 1988). Since hyperacute rejection of a kidney allograft in the presence of pre-existing donor-specific cytotoxic antibodies was recognized in the late 1960s, a positive cross-match has been an absolute contraindication to transplantation. However, over the past 10 years, exceptions to this dogma have been recognized such that a number of situations can be found where transplantation can be safely carried out in the presence of a positive cross-match between donor and recipient. For example, the antibody causing a positive cross-match may be an autoantibody which can be directed against either donor B lymphocytes or donor B and T lymphocytes. The sera causing the positive cross-match may be from some remote time in the past while a current serum is negative (historically positive, current negative). In this situation, if the positive serum is due to an autoantibody, then this again is no contraindication to transplantation, but if it is directed against HLA it would appear that if the class of the positive antibody is IgM then it also is not a contraindication to transplantation, but if an IgG antibody then failure is likely. Thus it is only the presence of a positive cross-match due to antibodies against HLA Class I or Class II at the time of transplantation that represents an absolute contraindication to transplantation, whereas a historically positive but current negative cross-match where the positive cross-match is an HLA antibody of the IgM class represents a relative contraindication (Table 89.1).

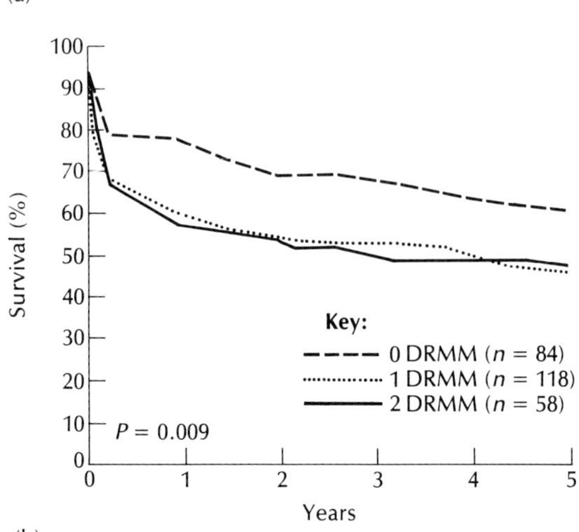

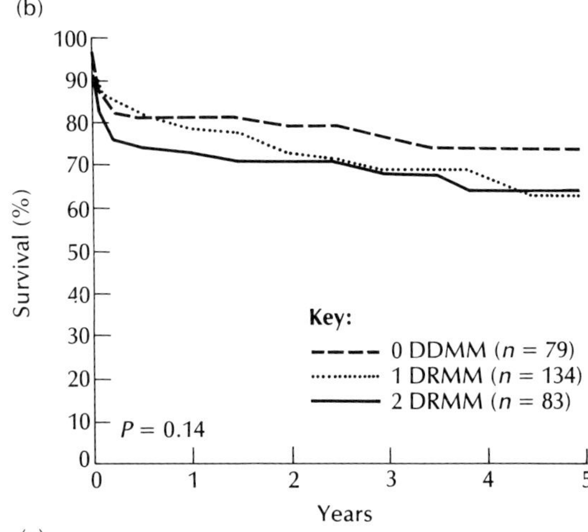

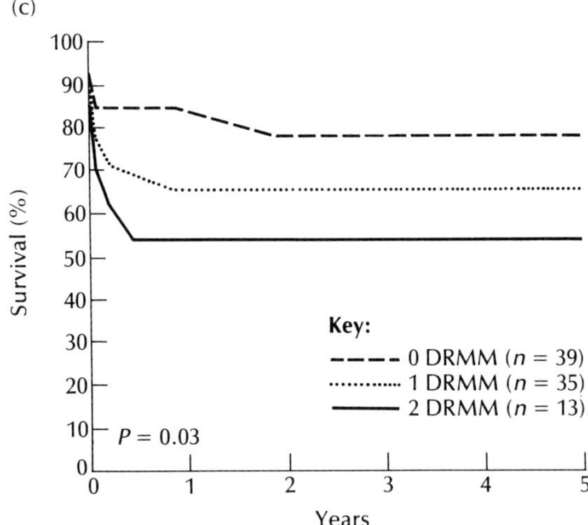

Fig. 89.1. The influence of matching for HLA-DR on the outcome of cadaver renal allografts in Oxford. (a) In patients with first cadaver grafts and treated with azathioprine and prednisolone. (b) In patients with first cadaver grafts and treated with cyclosporin. (c) In patients with cadaver regrafts and treated with cyclosporin. MM = mismatch; n = number of grafts.

Table 89.1. Renal transplants may be performed safely in the presence of positive cross-matches with donor lymphocytes (either B or B + T lymphocytes) (a, b) if the reactive antibody is non-HLA (usually IgM) or (c) if the current serum is negative and the previously positive serum was IgM but not IgG

Cross-match	Transplant	No.	Class	Graft survival at 6 months (%)
(a) B cell +ve	Living			
– non-HLA	related	7	IgM	100
	Cadaver	23	IgM	78
	Cadaver	2	IgG	100
(b) T + B cell +ve	Living			
– non-HLA	related	9	IgM	100
	Cadaver	35	IgM	89
(c) T + B cell +ve	Cadaver	16	IgM	69
– HLA Class I	Cadaver	13	IgG	8
– peak pos., current neg.				

Surgical techniques

The techniques of implantation of the kidney are very standard and certainly the technical complications in experienced units today are very low (Lee 1988). The kidney is placed extraperitoneally in one or other iliac fossa, the renal artery being joined either end-to-end to the internal iliac artery following its division or end-to-side to the external iliac artery using a cuff of the aorta with the renal artery. The vein is always anastomosed end-to-side to the external iliac vein. Multiple vessels on a kidney do not preclude its successful implantation and a number of techniques exist for dealing with the kidney that does have multiple vessels. Ideally, in the case of multiple arteries these vessels are implanted on a cuff of the aorta. In small children the kidney may have to be placed intraperitoneally with the vessels anastomosed to the vena cava and aorta. The ureter is usually implanted in the bladder, either directly into the dome of the bladder or inserted through a submocosal tunnel via an anterior cystotomy. The latter method is preferable, as it is a more satisfactory antireflux procedure.

Early course of the graft

In the case of living related transplantation all grafts would be expected to function immediately, whereas in the case of cadaver transplantation immediate function occurs in about 70% of patients. After cadaver transplantation, immediate function is determined by several factors, the most important of which is the time of preservation, but any untoward event causing hypotension in the donor before removal of the kidneys and the state of hydration of the recipient are also important.

The commonest cause of delayed function following transplantation is acute tubular necrosis due to ischaemia, but when function is delayed it is important to consider less common causes such as renal artery or renal vein thrombosis, ureteric obstruction and hyperacute rejection of the kidney. A renogram and an ultrasound of the kidney will exclude vascular thrombosis and ureteric obstruction respectively, while hyperacute rejection can be excluded by a trucut needle biopsy of the kidney (this would only be done in a highly sensitized patient who would be considered at risk of hyperacute rejection). Having excluded these other causes of delayed function, one can expect in most instances that the acute tubular necrosis will resolve and function of the kidney will be established, but this may take up to 4 weeks, particularly if cyclosporin is still being used as part of the immunosuppressive protocol.

When a kidney functions immediately, it is striking how quickly the patient's sense of well-being improves, and within a few days the plasma creatinine may be at normal levels. A massive osmotic diuresis may occur within the first few days, particularly in kidneys with little concentrating power initially, and this may require large amounts of fluid replacement, together with potassium.

Once function has been established, a deterioration in function during these first few weeks after transplantation is likely to be due to rejection or cyclosporin nephrotoxicity. Once again, an ultrasound will exclude ureteric obstruction and the diagnosis of rejection can be firmly estblished either by fine-needle aspiration cytology or a trucut core biopsy of the kidney. High cyclosporin blood levels will be found in the presence of cyclosporin nephrotoxicity.

A number of different types of rejection are recognized, based arbitrarily on their chronological time of occurrence after transplantation.

Hyperacute rejection

Hyperacute rejection occurs in the presence of donor-specific sensitization within the recipient and is an antibody-mediated destruction of the kidney. In the classical case, where a transplant is performed in the presence of HLA lymphocytotoxic antibodies in the recipient reacting with the donor, then within 20 minutes or so the kidney becomes blue and flabby and histology reveals a massive polymorphonuclear leucocyte infiltration (Williams *et al*. 1968; Fig. 89.2). However, with the recognition that positive cross-matches between recipient serum and donor lymphocytes are a contraindication to transplantation, this classical type of hyperacute rejection is rarely seen today

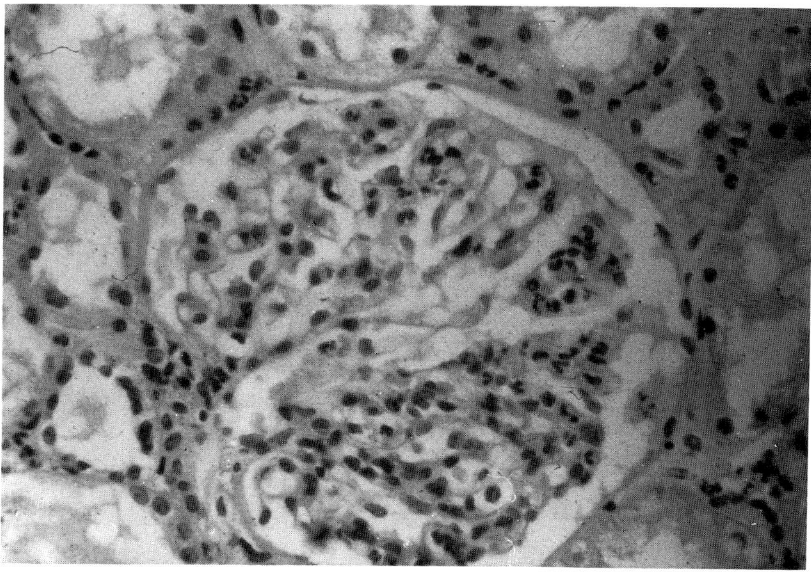

Fig. 89.2. A renal biopsy taken approximately 30 minutes after revascularization of a cadaver kidney that was to undergo hyperacute rejection, already showing a marked infiltration with polymorphonuclear leucocytes.

unless a transplant is carried out by error in the presence of a true HLA Class I positive cross-match or a major blood group incompatibility. Nevertheless, failure of grafts to function at all is far more common in regrafts, suggesting that there is an immunological reason for this non-function, which probably represents a less florid example of hyperacute rejection. A biopsy will confirm the diagnosis. It is also possible that this type of rejection can be mediated by cells, although there is no evidence for this in man. Hyperacute rejection is a very immediate reaction which is not treatable, and requires removal of the kidney once the diagnosis is established.

Accelerated rejection

Accelerated rejection is another manifestation of sensitization in the recipient. It occurs between 2 and 4 days after transplantation, is considered to be mediated by cells and represents the clinical homologue of a second-set type of rejection in the experimental model. In this case, the serum creatinine rises rapidly and the patient may exhibit fever and swelling and tenderness of the graft. The histology reveals oedema with an intense mononuclear cell infiltrate, and this may be associated with arteriolar fibrinoid necrosis and thrombosis. Early treatment of this type of rejection, if it is predominantly a cellular rejection histologically, may lead to salvage of the kidney and subsequent good long-term function.

Acute rejection

Acute rejection is the commonest type of rejection, occurring usually from 7 days to 3 weeks after transplantation. Deterioration in renal function and an associated fever and swelling and tenderness of the graft are classical signs that are usually less obvious with cyclosporin immunosuppression. Thus the clinical features associated with the deterioration of function may be very minimal or non-existent and hence confirmation of the diagnosis must be made by fine-needle aspiration cytology or a trucut needle biopsy of the graft. Histology again reveals oedema and cellular infiltration, with or without vascular changes (Fig. 89.3), the most severe of which are represented by fibrinoid necrosis of the arterial wall, thrombosis and interstitial haemorrhage (Dunnill 1988).

Both the accelerated and the acute types of rejection are treated in the first instance with high-dose methylprednisolone (e.g. 0.5 g intravenously each day for 3–5 days), but, if there is a failure to respond to steroids (steroid-resistant rejection), therapy with antithymocyte globulin (ATG) or a pan-T monoclonal antibody (OKT3) is commenced and some 75% of rejections will then respond (Richardson *et al.* 1989).

Chronic rejection

Chronic rejection is seen as an insidious deterioration of renal function occurring anywhere from

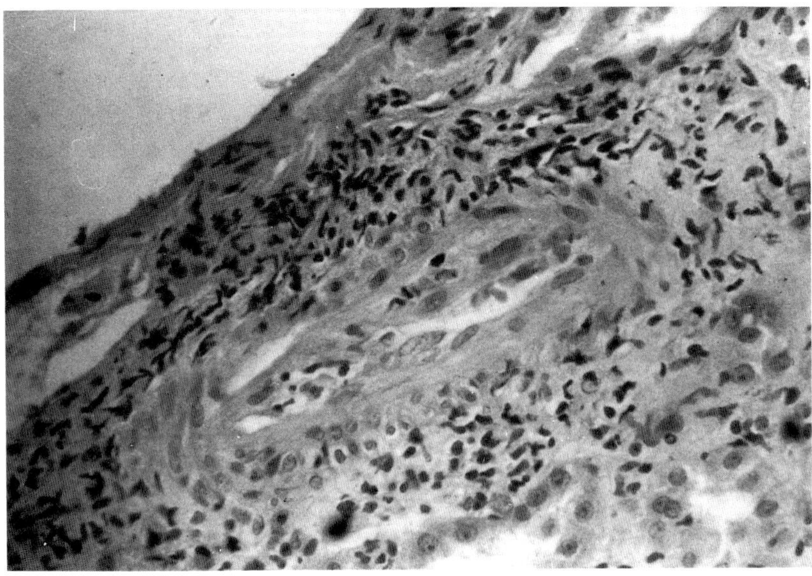

Fig. 89.3. A renal biopsy of a cadaver graft 21 days after transplantation, showing a perivascular cellular infiltrate and swelling of the endothelium lining a small artery, typical of a moderately severe acute rejection.

3 months to several years after transplantation. Renal biopsy shows interstitial fibrosis and intimal fibrosis of arteries and arterioles within the kidney (Dunnill 1988). This type of rejection is resistant to treatment with high doses of prednisolone unless there is an acute rejection superimposed on chronic rejection, which sometimes occurs, and in which case a response to treatment will be seen. Chronic rejection is of course the major reason for the steady attrition rate of kidneys after the first few months, and one can expect to lose 2–3% of kidneys from chronic rejection each year.

Immunosuppression

General comments

Since the early 1960s until relatively recently, azathioprine and prednisolone have been the basis of immunosuppression after renal transplantation (Walker and d'Apice 1988). To this basic protocol have been added antilymphocyte globulin (ALG), splenectomy, thymectomy, local graft irradiation and thoracic duct drainage, to name but a few of the additional therapies which have been used to any extent. The widespread availability of cyclosporin from the early 1980s led to a dramatic improvement in graft survival, ranging from 10 to 15% at 1 year, compared with that achieved with azathioprine and prednisolone. In the Western world all immunosuppressive protocols include cyclosporin. The first line of treatment for rejection remains high-dose methylprednisolone, with the use of either ALG or pan-T monoclonal antibodies for steroid-resistant rejection. Monoclonal antibodies to various leucocyte populations represent another advance in immunosuppression, which is just in its infancy. These antibodies will be used not only for the treatment of rejection but also prophylactically to produce better and hopefully more specific immunosuppression (see Chapters 46 and 47). The ultimate aim of research in transplantation biology would be to achieve specific immunosuppression, as all the immunosuppressive therapies currently available remain non-specific in their effect.

Azathioprine and prednisolone

Although no longer the conventional therapy in the Western world, azathioprine and prednisolone still have a role in patients who are intolerant to cyclosporin or who require conversion from cyclosporin for side-effects. Furthermore, in the developing world these two drugs must remain for some time yet the only available immunosuppressive therapy because of the cost of cyclosporin.

Azathioprine is one of the family of drugs known as thiopurines. Azathioprine is metabolized in the liver before it becomes active and one of its metabolic pathways is via conversion to 6-mercaptopurine and then to its active metabolite 6-thio-inosinic acid. Its biochemical effects are not completely understood but it can inhibit both deoxyribonucleic acid (DNA) and ribonucleic acid (RNA) synthesis and also blocks the production of interleukin 2 (IL-2).

It is relatively free from side-effects, the major complication being bone marrow aplasia, and regular monitoring of the white cell count is essential until a stable dose is established. In the presence of a leucopenia caused by intercurrent infection, especially cytomegalovirus, the dose of azathioprine may have to be significantly reduced, and this in turn can lead to rejection.

Steroids, which are used with azathioprine either as prednisone or prednisolone, are complex both in their pharmacology and in their effects on the immune system (Cupps and Fauci 1982). Although they do have an anti-inflammatory effect, steroids also particularly modify T lymphocytes, blocking their proliferation after interaction of the T cell receptor with antigen.

Until the late 1970s azathioprine was always used with high doses of steroids during the first 2 months after transplantation. This high dosage of steroids was undoubtedly the cause of the majority of infectious and non-infectious complications. The successful use of low-dose steroids by McGeown and colleagues (1977) and the confirmation of their efficacy in a prospective trial by the Oxford group in the late 1970s (Chan *et al.* 1980; Morris *et al.* 1982a) slowly led to the general adoption of low-dose steroids with azathioprine throughout the world. This in turn led to a dramatic reduction in steroid-related complications and a steady improvement in patient survival after transplantation as a result. However, if low-dose steroids are used, it is important to use an adequate dose of azathioprine (at least 2 mg/kg per day), for otherwise graft survival will be poor (d'Apice *et al.* 1984).

Cyclosporin

Cyclosporin is a powerful immunosuppressive drug and has proved to be a potent agent, both in a wide variety of experimental models of tissue transplantation and also in clinical organ transplantation (Morris 1981, 1988b). It was first isolated from two strains of fungi imperfecti by the Department of Microbiology at Sandoz in Basle as an antifungal agent of limited activity, but it was shown by Borel to have potent immunosuppressive activity in a variety of *in vitro* and *in vivo* experiments (Borel *et al*. 1976; Borel 1982). Following Borel's initial description of the immunosuppressive properties of this drug, it was then shown to suppress rejection of vascularized organ allografts in a variety of species (Morris 1981). Clinical trials of the drug in renal transplantation began in Cambridge in 1978 (Calne *et al*. 1979) and when cyclosporin became generally available in the early 1980s it rapidly became the major immunosuppressive drug used in all forms of organ transplantation.

Although the precise action of cyclosporin remains to be elucidated, it is clear that its major effect is directed at T lymphocytes at an early stage of the induction of the immune response to an antigen (Morris 1988b). Much of its immunosuppressive activity is related to the inhibition of the production of lymphokines such as IL-2 by the T helper cell, thus preventing the IL-2-produced proliferation of T helper cells and T cytotoxic cell precursors. Cyclosporin binds to a calcium-dependent intracellular protein, cyclophilin, thus blocking calcium-dependent activation of the normal induction signals initiating DNA synthesis of the various lymphokines such as IL-2.

Although it was quickly apparent that the use of cyclosporin led to fewer rejection episodes and certainly less irreversible rejection leading to loss of the kidney than was the case with azathioprine/prednisolone, it also became apparent that there were a number of significant side-effects associated with the use of this drug. The most serious side-effect is nephrotoxicity, but other side-effects include hypertrichosis, hypertension, hypercholesterolaemia, gingival hypertrophy and hepatotoxicity. Most of these side-effects are dose-related.

Three types of nephrotoxicity are observed with the use of cyclosporin (Morris 1988b). The first occurs immediately after transplantation, usually in a kidney already damaged by ischaemia. Thus, in patients with poorly functioning kidneys after transplantation due to ischaemia, cyclosporin dosages are reduced, or administration of the drug is delayed until renal function is well established. The second type of nephrotoxicity is seen any time after the first 2–3 weeks and is associated with deteriorating renal function, usually but not always associated with high-trough serum or blood levels of cyclosporin. This will respond to a reduction in dosage of cyclosporin but presents a diagnostic problem as it has to be distinguished from rejection. For rejection in patients on cyclosporin does not usually present with the florid signs previously seen with azathioprine and prednisolone therapy, as discussed earlier. Fine-needle aspiration cytology or a renal biopsy together with cyclosporin blood levels and the most satisfactory way to distinguish between the two. The third type of nephrotoxicity is a chronic condition associated with the histological appearance of severe interstitial fibrosis and which results in a steady deterioration in renal function. This does not usually respond very dramatically to a reduction in cyclosporin dosage and is thought to be related to cyclosporin-induced damage in an ischaemic kidney immediately after transplantation.

Because of the side-effects and especially the nephrotoxicity, various protocols have been devised to allow the use of lower doses of cyclosporin while maintaining the improved immunosuppression provided by the drug. Thus cyclosporin is now used at much lower doses, either alone or with steroids, than was the case at the time of its introduction, and starting doses ranged from 8 to 10 mg/kg daily. The need for steroids with cyclosporin remains controversial. Most units do use steroids and there is an increasing tendency for many units to use relatively high doses of steroids with cyclosporin in the early weeks after transplantation, even though several prospective randomized trials have not shown any beneficial effect from the use of steroids (Morris 1988b).

Possibly the commonest immunosuppressive protocol used at present is triple therapy, comprising low-dose cyclosporin, azathioprine and prednisolone (Simmons *et al*. 1986; Fries *et al*. 1987; Jones *et al*. 1988a). This protocol is particularly easy to use, is associated with few side-effects and has consistently good results (Fig. 89.4). Cyclosporin has also been used with azathioprine

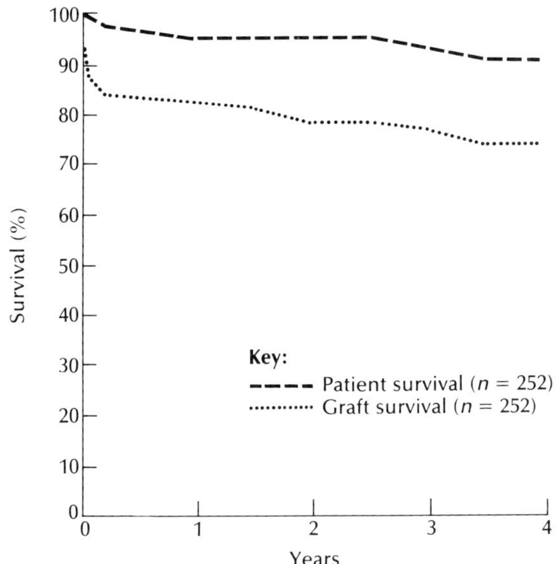

Fig. 89.4. Patient and cadaveric graft survival in 252 consecutive cadaver transplants immunosuppressed with triple therapy (low-dose cyclosporin, azathioprine and prednisolone) in Oxford.

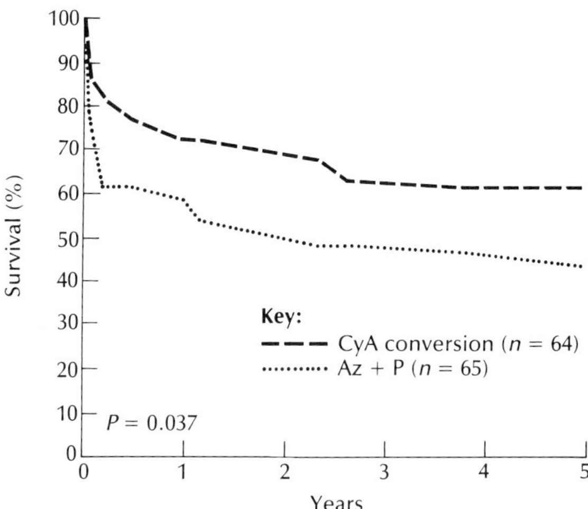

Fig. 89.5. Long-term survival of cadaveric grafts in patients given either azathioprine and prednisolone (AZ + P) or cyclosporin for 90 days, at which time they were converted to azathioprine and prednisolone (Cy A conversion) in the second Oxford conversion trial.

(double therapy) and this also appears to be an effective combination. Another protocol which is being used more commonly, especially in the United States, is called sequential therapy, in which the patient is commenced on azathioprine, prednisolone and ALG (or OKT3), and when renal function is well established after 7–10 days cyclosporin is introduced in place of the biological agent (Somner *et al.* 1986). This protocol is attractive in that it avoids the possibility of cyclosporin-induced damage in an ischaemic kidney immediately after transplantation.

Finally, conversion protocols, first introduced by the Oxford group, have proved less popular in the Western world because of the significant risk of acute rejection episodes following conversion at 90 days (Morris *et al.* 1982b, 1987). However, the dramatic improvement in renal function after conversion (Chapman *et al.* 1985) does make it attractive in concept and it is particularly attractive in the developing world where, if cyclosporin is to be used, it will only be used over a relatively short time because of the high cost of the drug. Certainly the long-term survival of grafts in patients managed with the conversion protocol in the second of the Oxford prospective trials remains impressive at 67% at 5 years from the time of transplantation, with all patients now followed for at least 5 years (Fig. 94.5).

It must be said, however, that at this time there is no evidence that any of the above protocols produce better results than the others in terms of patient and graft survival. Their assessment will have to be based on factors other than short- and medium-term graft survival, especially with respect to the development of complications and the quality of renal function.

Enormous effort has been directed at monitoring either serum or whole-blood trough levels of cyclosporin (Holt 1986; Kahan and Grevel 1988). In general, although low levels are associated with acute rejection and high levels with nephrotoxicity, there are many exceptions reported, possibly due to the inherent difficulties of the various assay systems which are used. It is hoped that the development of new assays, using monoclonal antibodies to cyclosporin which measure purely the parent compound, will result in better correlations with the clinical course than hitherto, but this remains to be seen.

Antilymphocyte globulin and monoclonal antibodies

Antilymphocyte or antithymocyte globulin, which is made by immunizing heterologous species with human lymphocytes or thymocytes (rabbits and horses are used most commonly), was first introduced into immunosuppressive protocols in 1967.

It has remained a useful agent ever since, being used either prophylactically from the time of transplantation for 1–2 weeks, or more commonly to treat rejection which is not responding to high-dose steroids (Cosimi 1988b). Although there has been controversy in the past about the efficacy of ALG or ATG, primarily because of the variable batch effect, there is no doubt that if one has an immunosuppressive product then it can be particularly potent in its effect. However, there is no suitable biological assay for immunosuppressive activity (other than skin grafting in rhesus monkeys), and hence, despite the most rigorous controls, there may be a variation not only in immunosuppressive potency but also in side-effects from batch to batch, although pooling of batches does reduce this inconsistency. Nevertheless, ALGs remain a standard reagent in immunosuppressive protocols and are generally used to treat steroid-resistant rejection. Most ALG or ATG preparations produce their effect by inducing a lymphopenia, although this is not essential for immunosuppression.

The advent of monoclonal antibody technology, allowing the production of antibodies to different leucocyte populations, has enabled the second generation of antilymphocyte reagents to be produced. The first group of antibodies to be tested in the clinic were directed against all T lymphocytes, but only one, OKT3, was especially effective in the treatment of steroid-resistant rejection (Cosimi *et al.* 1981; Ortho Multicenter Transplant Study Group 1985). This was undoubtedly due to the fact that the T3 molecule (now known as CD3) on T lymphocytes is intimately associated with the T cell receptor whereas the other pan-T cell markers are not. Following infusion of OKT3, there is a dramatic clearance of T lymphocytes from the circulation within minutes, but after several days of treatment there is a reappearance of T cells expressing other T cell markers but not CD3. Thus the initial effect is probably due to T cell destruction but subsequently there is either modulation of the CD3 molecule or repopulation with immature CD3 −ve cells (Chatenoud and Bach 1984). OKT3 is a very powerful immunosuppressive reagent and if used in preference to high-dose steroids will reverse virtually all first acute rejection episodes. When used for salvage in steroid-resistant rejection it will save around 80% of kidneys. However, it has to be said that at this time there is is no convincing evidence that OKT3 is more effective than a good immunosuppressive ATG. Both the ATGs and OKT3 are being used prophylactically, usually as part of a sequential protocol including cyclosporin.

A number of other monoclonal antibodies have been used clinically with evidence of efficacy. Campath I, an antibody directed at mononuclear leucocytes, has been used prophylactically (Friend *et al.* 1987). It was immunosuppressive but led to an unacceptable rate of serious infections and is now being tested as a treatment of steroid-resistant rejection. Another very interesting prophylactic monoclonal antibody therapy has been the use of an anti-IL-2 receptor antibody in the first 14 days after transplantation. This seems to have resulted in a low level of subsequent rejection episodes and also impressive graft survival in the short term (Soullilou *et al.* 1988). Certainly there is good evidence from experimental models of transplantation in the rodent to suggest that the use of antibodies against the IL-2 receptor, which is expressed by activated T cells in the rejection reaction, is an appropriate approach to more specific immunosuppression, provided that the antibody recognizes an appropriate epitope such that the functional reaction between IL-2 and the receptor is blocked (Diamenstein *et al.* 1987; Tellides *et al.* 1989).

Total lymphoid irradiation

Total lymphoid irradiation (TLI) has been used for years in the treatment of Hodgkin's disease and was noted by the Stanford group to produce a marked depression of cellular immunity (Fuks *et al.* 1976). It was then shown in a murine model to be able to induce tolerance to skin allografts when combined with pretreatment with donor bone marrow (Strober *et al.* 1979). Total lymphoid irradiation has been explored in clinical renal transplantation by several groups (Waer and Strober 1988), the largest experience being that of Myburgh in Johannesburg. He has in fact used an expanded field of radiation which really represents subtotal body irradiation rather than TLI (Myburgh *et al.* 1987). The results from all these groups are encouraging in that many patients have needed no immunosuppression or very low doses of immunosuppression after transplantation. Indeed, several patients in the Johannesburg experience might be considered to be truly tolerant, in that they have normal renal function and are not receiving immunosuppressive drugs. However, the TLI regimens are difficult to combine with dialysis and the logistics of finding a suitable graft soon after completing the fractionated course of TLI also presents problems. It is unlikely now to supplant cyclosporin protocols unless a large number of patients can be shown to be truly tolerant, requiring no or very little maintenance immunosuppression.

Blood transfusion

It had been noted in 1968 that multiple transfusions before transplantation did not have a deleterious effect on graft outcome (Morris *et al.* 1968). Then in 1974 Opelz and Terasaki first observed that patients who had never had a transfusion before transplantation had a poorer graft survival than transfused patients. This phenomenon became fairly firmly established over the next 10 years. However, with the advent of cyclosporin, it is no longer clear that the transfusion effect still exists (Opelz 1988). Although an increasing number of units are dispensing with blood transfusions in non-transfused male and nulliparous female recipients, there is a body of opinion which still favours deliberate transfusions of non-transfused patients before transplantation.

There is no doubt that, in the experimental animal, transfusion can produce donor-specific immunosuppression, and indeed it is probable that the random blood transfusion effect seen in cadaveric renal transplantation is also a specific immunological effect. This is based on experiments in the rodent, where it has been shown that pre-treatment with a single incompatible antigen shared with the donor can produce specific suppression of all the incompatible histocompatibility antigens in the subsequent donor organ (Hutchinson and Morris 1986; Madsen *et al.* 1988). The mechanism of this blood transfusion effect remains controversial. In the rodent model, certainly, the tolerance it induces is maintained by a suppressor cell mechanism but the method by which it induces this state of specific immunosuppression is unclear. It appears to be due to an altered regulation of IL-2 production (Dallman *et al.* 1991). In man there are data supporting the induction of both suppressor cells and anti-idiotypic responses as a result of prior blood transfusions (Reed *et al.* 1987).

Complications

Technical complications

The majority of the serious technical complications are either vascular or urological (Belzer *et al.* 1988). Renal artery or vein thrombosis occurs within the first week after transplantation and generally within the first 48 hours. Although it is now a relatively uncommon complication, there is a suggestion that it may be occurring more frequently with the use of cyclosporin (Jones *et al.* 1988b). Renal artery stenosis occurs anywhere from 3 months to years after transplantation, and although this may be technical in origin, especially after an end-to-end internal iliac to renal artery anastomosis, usually the stenosis is distal to the anastomosis, the reasons for this being unclear, but perhaps reflecting intimal damage during the nephrectomy or perfusion. Renal artery stenosis is not uncommon but establishing that the lesion is functionally significant may be difficult, for the majority of transplant patients are hypertensive. In general the patient with a functional stenosis will present with hypertension and deteriorating renal function, with a biopsy showing no or only modest evidence of chronic rejection. The first approach is to attempt balloon angioplasty, which will be successful in 50–70% of patients, and which can be repeated as necessary (Belzer *et al.* 1988). If unsuccessful, reconstructive surgery is then required, and in experienced transplant and vascular hands the results are excellent, but there is a risk of loss of the graft in inexperienced hands.

The urological complications comprise either a urinary leak or ureteric obstruction. Urine leaks generally occur from the lower end of the ureter which has necrosed due to ischaemia. This ischaemia is almost inevitably related to damage to the blood supply to the ureter during removal of the kidney (Belzer *et al.* 1988). Most examples of ureteric stenosis are also probably due to low-grade ischaemia of the lower end of the ureter, resulting in subsequent stenosis. Urine leaks should be repaired promptly, rather than adopting a conservative approach which will eventually lead to infection, making surgery more difficult. However, ureteric obstruction may be treated by balloon dilatation and stenting, at least in the first instance (Belzer *et al.* 1988).

Infectious complications

Infection used to be the commonest cause of death after transplantation but with modern immunosuppressive protocols death from infection is now relatively uncommon, although infection remains a significant and often serious problem after transplantation. During the first month after transplantation, infections are mostly conventional bacterial infections and include wound infections, pneumonia and urinary tract infections (Rubin *et al.* 1981), the only viral infection occurring during this time being due to herpes simplex virus.

However, after the first month the more exotic viral, fungal and protozoal infections occur (Cohen *et al.* 1988). The most frequent of these infections is that due to cytomegalovirus (CMV). This infection may be primary when it occurs in a patient who is CMV-seronegative and receives a kidney from a seropositive donor. A primary CMV infection runs a febrile course for approximately 2 weeks and is often associated with a leucopenia. A minority of cases will develop a pneumonitis which may result in death. For this reason it is important to attempt to give seronegative recipients a kidney from a seronegative donor, after which it is rare to see a primary CMV infection (Table 89.2). Treatment of CMV infection is expectant but if a pneumonitis develops then either CMV-specific hyperimmune globulin or the new antiviral agent ganciclovir (DHPG) should be introduced (Cohen *et al.* 1988). Vaccination trials of CMV are in progress in seronegative recipients at this time, which may prove to be of value in providing protection against subsequent infection. More recent experience suggests that prophylactic use of ganciclovir in high-risk patients, e.g., seronegative, recipients who have received a seropositive kidney, prevents the subsequent development of a severe CMV infection.

Table 89.2. The effect of donor CMV status on CMV infection in 306 recipients of renal allografts in the Oxford unit

Donor	CMV+	CMV−	CMV+	CMV−
Recipient	CMV+	CMV+	CMV−	CMV−
No.	84	98	60	64
No. infected	52 (62%)	52 (53%)	38 (63%)	0 (0%)

The next most common opportunistic infection is that caused by *Pneumocystis carinii* and this does seem to have become more common with the use of more potent immunosuppressive cyclosporin protocols. For this reason many units use prophylactic septrin for 6 months to a year after transplantation in a single daily dose of 0.5 g. Other less common infections include those due to *Legionella*, *Listeria*, *Aspergillus*, *Nocardia* and *Cryptococcus*. Infections with *Mycobacterium tuberculosis* are also not uncommon, especially in patients who have had previously untreated or poorly treated tuberculosis, and these patients should be given prophylactic chemotherapy for a year after transplantation.

Patients with a fever are assumed to have an infection until proved otherwise, and require thorough viral and microbiological investigation. If there is a pulmonary infiltrate on radiological assessment, and the clinical features are compatible with a diagnosis of bacterial pneumonia then antibiotics are given, but if the radiological picture is uncertain or there is no response to antibiotics then bronchoscopic alveolar lavage is mandatory, going on to an open lung biopsy if necessary to establish a diagnosis (Cohen *et al.* 1988).

Cardiovascular complications

Hypertension is common after transplantation and the prevalence of hypertension has increased with the use of cyclosporin such that something like 70% of all patients are on hypersensitive medication at 1 year after transplantation (Raine 1988). As so many more patients now survive with functioning grafts for 5–10 years, the incidence of cardiovascular morbidity has become far more prominent, and indeed is now the major cause of death after renal transplantation. This is due to the high prevalence of hypertension as well as hypercholesterolaemia, but is also probably related in ways that are not clear at the moment to the immunosuppressive protocols themselves. In patients with poorly controlled hypertension, it is important to exclude renal artery stenosis as a cause, as this is correctable, as mentioned earlier.

Cancer

The prevalence of all types of cancer is increased in patients on immunosuppressive therapy after renal transplantation but the cancers that have an enormous increase in prevalence are squamous cell cancers of the skin, lymphomas and to a lesser extent cervical cancers (Sheil 1988). These more commonly occurring cancers may be associated with viral infection — human papilloma virus in the case of skin and cervical cancers and the Epstein–Barr virus in the case of lymphomas.

Results of renal transplantation

Living donor transplantation

Living related donors include transplant between identical twins and siblings who are HLA-identical, as well as between siblings who share one or no HLA haplotypes, and parent to child where again one haplotype is shared between the donor and recipient. With modern immunosuppressive protocols the graft survival in patients receiving one- and two-haplotype-disparate living related transplants has improved markedly, approaching that, at least in the medium term, of HLA-identical sibling transplants (Morris 1988c). However, as time passes, the HLA-identical sibling transplant results remain superior, confirming the importance of HLA as the major histocompatibility complex in man. Donor-specific transfusions have been used successfully in the past in one-haplotype-disparate living related donor recipients but with current immunosuppressive protocols the risks of sensitization by deliberate donor-specific transfusions probably no longer justify their use.

Living unrelated donor recipients are also being used with success, but the results cannot be better than unrelated cadaveric transplantation. Nevertheless, there is a limited place for this type of transplantation, but it is of critical importance to ensure that the unrelated donor recipients are emotionally related in some way, as might be the case in transplants between husband and wife (Council of the Transplantation Society 1985).

Cadaver donor transplantation

Again, there has been a steady improvement both in patient survival and graft survival over the last 15 years and now for first cadaver grafts one expects 1-year graft survival to be between 75 and 85%. More striking, perhaps, are the results of regrafts which in the azathioprine–prednisolone days were much poorer than those for first grafts, for now regraft survival rates are not inferior to those of first grafts.

Many factors influence the outcome of patient and graft survival and obviously these include the type of immunosuppression, HLA matching and possibly blood transfusions before transplantation. Age also influences graft outcome but, interestingly, although graft survival in the elderly is identical to that of the younger patient, there is a

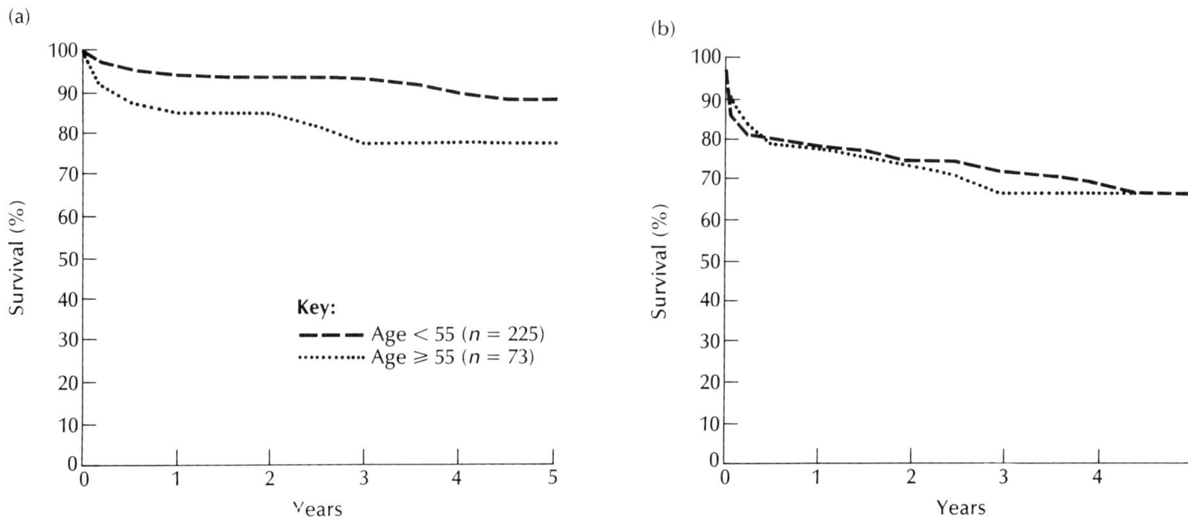

Fig. 89.6. The influence of age (<55 years or ≥55 years) on (a) patient survival and (b) first cadaver graft survival in the cyclosporin era in Oxford.

much poorer patient survival in the former, implying that fewer grafts are lost from rejection in the elderly recipient (Fig. 89.6). Other factors which have been shown to possibly influence graft outcome have been the sex of donors and recipients, the blood groups of donors and recipients, the time spent on dialysis, the race of the donor and recipient and the presence or absence of immediate function of the transplanted kidney (Morris 1988c). However, one of the most important factors influencing graft outcome in all national or regional registries is the centre effect, for reasons that are not entirely clear (Gilks *et al.* 1986; Mickey 1986). Nevertheless, the wide disparity in the results of individual centres both in Europe and in North America has become far less striking since cyclosporin protocols have been generally adopted.

Without question a successful transplant produces a dramatic rehabilitation of the patient and restores a patient to a relatively normal existence (Jacobs *et al.* 1977). It is this that makes renal transplantation so attractive as the preferable form of treatment for end-stage and renal failure. At present one can expect some 80% of transplant patients to function at nearly normal levels after transplantation (Evans *et al.* 1985). This compares with about 50% of patients who are being treated on dialysis. Furthermore, some 75% of transplant recipients are able to work compared with between 25 and 60% of patients on dialysis. Nevertheless, there are many problems to be resolved and it must be realized that 10-year graft survivals are relatively poor, and even with current immunosuppressive protocols the predicted 10-year cadaveric graft survival is likely to be around only 40–50%. Furthermore, with increasing time after transplantation there is a steady morbidity, especially cardiovascular, which decreases the quality of life.

Thus, although there have been enormous achievements in renal transplantation over these past 25 years, there is room for considerable improvement still, especially in long-term outcome. This is likely to be achieved by better and more specific immunosuppressive protocols.

References

Belzer, F.O., Glass, N. and Sollinger, H. (1988). Technical complications after renal transplantation. In *Kidney Transplantation: Principles and Practice*, 3rd edn, ed. P.J. Morris, pp. 511–32, W.B. Saunders, Philadelphia.

Borel, J.F. (1982). The history of cyclosporin A and its significance. In *Cyclosporine A*, ed. D.J. White, pp. 5–17, Elsevier Biomedical, Amsterdam.

Borel, J.F., Feurev, C., Gubler, H.U. and Stahelia, H. (1976). Biological effects by cyclosporine A: a new antilymphocyte agent. *Agents Actions* **6**, 468–75.

Briggs, J.D. (1988). The recipient of a renal transplant. In *Kidney Transplantation: Principles and Practice*, 3rd edn, ed. P.J. Morris pp. 71–92, W.B. Saunders, Philadelphia.

Calne, R.Y., Rolles, K, White, D.J. *et al.* (1979). Cyclosporine A initially as the only immunosuppressant in 34 recipients of cadaveric organs: 30 kidneys, 2 pancreases, and 2 livers. *Lancet* **ii**, 1033–6.

Cameron, J.S. (1982). Glomerulonephritis in renal transplants (overview). *Transplantation* **34**, 237–45.

Chan, L., French, M.E., Beare, J., Oliver, D.O. and Morris, P.J. (1980). Prospective trial of high-dose versus low-dose prednisolone in renal transplant patients. *Transplant. Proc.* **12**, 323–6.

Chapman, J.R., Griffiths, D., Harding, N.G. and Morris, P.J. (1985). Reversibility of cyclosporine nephrotoxicity after three months treatment. *Lancet* **i**, 128–30.

Chatenoud, L. and Bach, J.E. (1984). Antigenic modulation—a major mechanism of antibody action. *Immunol. Today* **5** (1), 20–5.

Cohen, J., Hopkin, J. and Kurtz, J. (1988). Infectious complications after renal transplantation. In *Kidney Transplantation: Principles and Practice*, 3rd edn, ed. P.J. Morris, pp. 532–73. W.B. Saunders, Philadelphia.

Cosimi, A.B. (1988a). The donor and donor nephrectomy. In *Kidney Transplantation: Principles and Practice*, 3rd edn, ed. P.J. Morris, pp. 93–121, W.B. Saunders, Philadelphia.

Cosimi, A.B. (1988b). Antilymphocyte globulin and monoclonal antibodies. In *Kidney Transplantation: Principles and Practice*, 3rd edn, ed. P.J. Morris, pp. 343–69, W.B. Saunders, Philadelphia.

Cosimi, A.B., Colvin, R.B., Burton, R.C. *et al.* (1981). Use of monoclonal antibodies to T-cell subsets for immunologic monitoring and treatment in recipients of renal allografts. *N. Engl. J. Med.* **305**, 308–14.

Council of the Transplantation Society (1985). Commercialisation in transplantation: the problems and some guidelines for practice. *Lancet* **ii**, 715–16.

Cupps, T.R. and Fauci, A.S. (1982). Corticosteroid-mediated immunoregulation in man. *Immunol. Rev.* **65**, 132–55.

d'Apice, A.J., Becker, G.J., Kincaid-Smith, P. *et al.* (1984). A prospective randomized trial of low-dose versus high-dose steroids in cadaver renal transplantation. *Transplantation* **37**, 373–7.

Dallman, M., Shiho, O., Page, T.H., Wood, K.J. and Morris, P.J. (1991) Peripheral tolerance to alloantigen results from altered regulation of the interleukin 2 pathway. *J. Exp. Med.* **173**, 79–87.

Diamenstein, T., Osawa, H., Kirkman, R.L. *et al.* (1987). Interleukin 2 receptor — a target for immunosuppression. *Transplant. Rev.* **1**, 177–96.

Dunnill, M.S. (1988) Histopathology of rejection in renal transplantation. In *Kidney Transplantation: Principles and Practice*,

3rd edn, ed. P.J. Morris, pp. 439–72, W.B. Saunders, Philadelphia.

Evans, R.W., Manninea, D.L., Garrison, L.P. *et al.* (1985). The quality of life of patients with end-stage renal disease. *N. Engl. J. Med.* **312**, 553–9.

Fehrman, I., Widstam, V. and Lundgren, G. (1986). Long-term consequences of renal donation in humans. *Transplant. Proc.* **18**, 102–5.

Friend, P., Calne, R.Y., Hale, G. *et al.* (1987). Prophylactic use of an antilymphocyte monoclonal antibody following renal transplantation: a randomized controlled trial. *Transplant. Proc.* **19** (1), 1898–900.

Fries, D., Hiesse, C., Charpentier, B. *et al.* (1987). Triple combination of low-dose cyclosporine, azathioprine and steroids in first cadaver donor renal allografts. *Transplant. Proc.* **19**, 1911–14.

Fuks, Z., Strober, S., Bobrove, A.M., Sasazuki, T., McMichael, A. and Kaplan, H.S. (1976). Long term effects of radiation on T and B lymphocytes in peripheral blood of patients with Hodgkin's disease. *J. Clin. Invest.* **58**, 803–14.

Gilks, W.R., Selwood, N. and Bradly, B.A. (1986). The variation among transplant centres' results in the United Kingdom and Ireland from 1977 to 1981. *Transplantation* **38**, 235–9.

Holt, D.W. (1986). Clinical interpretation of cyclosporine measurements. In *Progress in Transplantation*, vol. III, ed. P.J. Morris and N.L. Tilney, pp. 32–54, Churchill Livingstone, Edinburgh.

Hutchinson, I.V. and Morris, P.J. (1986). The role of major and minor histocompatibility antigens in active enhancement of rat kidney allograft survival by blood transfusion. *Transplantation* **41**, 166–70.

Jacobs, C., Brunner, F.P., Chantler, C. *et al.* (1977). Registry report: *Proc. Eur. Dialysis Transplant. Assoc.* **14**, 3–69.

Jones, R.M., Murie, J.A., Allen, R.D., Ting, A. and Morris, P.J. (1988a). Triple therapy in cadaver renal transplantation. *Br. J. Surg.* **75**, 4–8.

Jones, R.M., Murie, J.A. and Morris, P.J. (1988b). Renal vascular thrombosis of cadaveric renal allografts in patients receiving cyclosporine, azathioprine and prednisolone triple therapy. *Clin. Transplant.* **2**, 122–6.

Kahan, B. and Grevel, J. (1988). Optimization of cyclosporine therapy in renal transplantation by a pharmacokinetic strategy. *Transplantation* **46**, 631–44.

Lee, H.M. (1988). Surgical techniques of renal transplantation. In *Kidney Transplantation Principles and Practice*, 3rd edn, ed. P.J. Morris, pp. 215–34, W.B. Saunders, Philadelphia.

McGeown, M.G., Kennedy, J.A., Loughbridge, W.G. *et al.* (1977). One hundred kidney transplants in the Belfast City Hospital. *Lancet* **ii**, 648–51.

Madsen, J., Superina, R., Wood, K.J. and Morris, P.J. (1988). Immunological unresponsiveness induced by recipient cell transfected with donor MHC genes. *Nature* **332**, 161–4.

Maizel, S.E., Simmons, R.L., Kjellstrand, S. and Fryd, D.S. (1981). Ten year experience in renal transplantation for Fabry's disease. *Transplant. Proc.* **13** (1), 57–9.

Marshall, V.C., Jablonski, P. and Scott, D.F. (1988). Renal preservation. In *Kidney Transplantation: Principles and Practice*, 3rd edn, ed. P.J. Morris, pp. 151–82, W.B. Saunders, Philadelphia.

Mickey, M.R. (1986). Centre effect. In *Clinical Transplants 1986*, ed. P.I. Teraski, pp. 165–73, UCLA Tissue Typing Laboratory, Los Angeles.

Morris, P.J. (1981). Cyclosporine: overview. *Transplantation* **32**, 349–54.

Morris, P.J. (ed.) (1988a). *Kidney Transplantation: Principles and Practice*, 3rd edn. W.B. Saunders, Philadelphia.

Morris, P.J. (1988b). Cyclosporine. In *Kidney Transplantation: Principles and Practice*, 3rd edn, ed. P.J. Morris, pp. 285–317, W.B. Saunders, Philadelphia.

Morris, P.J. (1988c). Results of renal transplantation. In *Kidney Transplantation: Principles and Practice*, 3rd edn, ed. P.J. Morris, pp. 737–58, W.B. Saunders, Philadelphia.

Morris, P.J., Ting, A. and Stocker, J. (1968) Leukocyte antigens in renal transplantation. I. The paradox of blood transfusions in renal transplantation. *Med. J. Aust.* **2**, 1088–90.

Morris, P.J., Chan, L., French, M.E. and Ting, A. (1982a). Low dose oral prednisolone in renal transplantation. *Lancet* **i**, 525–7.

Morris, P.J., French, M.E, Ting, A., Frostick, S. and Hunniset, A. (1982b). A controlled trial of cyclosporine A in renal transplantation. In *Cyclosporine A*, ed. D.J. White, pp. 355–64, Elsevier Biomedical, Amsterdam.

Morris, P.J., Chapman, J.R., Allen, R.D. *et al.* (1987). Cyclosporine conversion versus conventional immunosuppression: long-term follow-up and histological evaluation. *Lancet* **i**, 586–91.

Myburgh, J.A., Meyers, A.M. and Botha, J.R. (1987). Wide field low-dose total lymphoid irradiation in clinical kidney transplantation. *Transplant. Proc.* **19**, 1974–7.

Opelz, G. (1988). Blood transfusions and renal transplantation. In *Kidney Transplantation: Principles and Practice*, 3rd edn, ed. P.J. Morris, pp. 417–38, W.B. Saunders, Philadelphia.

Opelz, G. and Terasaki, P.I. (1974). Poor kidney transplant survival in recipients with frozen-blood transfusions or no transfusions. *Lancet* **ii**, 696–8.

Ortho Multicenter Transplant Study Group (1985). A randomized clinical trial of OKT3 monoclonal antibody for acute rejection of cadaveric renal transplants. *N. Engl. J. Med.* **313**, 337–42.

Pallis, C. (1988). Brainstem death: the evolution of a concept. In *Kidney Transplantation: Principles and Practice*, 3rd edn, ed. P.J. Morris, pp. 123–50, W.B. Saunders, Philadelphia.

Pasternack, A., Ahonen, J. and Kuhlback, B. (1986). Renal transplantation in 45 patients with amyloidosis. *Transplantation* **42**, 598–601.

Raine, A.E.G. (1988). Cardiovascular complications after renal transplantation. In *Kidney Transplantation: Principles and Practice*, 3rd edn, ed. P.J. Morris, pp. 575–601, W.B. Saunders, Philadelphia.

Reed, E., Hardy, M. and Benvenitsky F. (1987). Effect of antiidiotypic antibodies to HLA on graft survival in renal allograft recipients. *N. Engl. J. Med.* **316**, 1450–5.

Richardson, A.J., Higgins, R.M., Liddington, M., Murie, J., Ting, A. and Morris, P.J. (1989). Antithymocyte globulin for steroid resistant rejection in renal transplant recipient immunosuppressed with triple therapy. *Transplant. Int.* **2**, 27–32.

Rubin, R.H., Wolfson, J.S., Cosimi, A.B. and Tolkoff-Rubin, W.E. (1981). Infection in the renal transplant recipient. *Am. J. Med.* **70**, 405–11.

Scheinman, J.E., Najarian, J.S. and Mauer, S.M. (1984). Successful strategies for renal transplantation in primary oxalosis. *Kidney Int.* **25**, 804–11.

Sheil, A.G.R. (1988). Cancer in dialysis and transplant patients. In *Kidney Transplantation: Principles and Practice*, 3rd edn, ed. P.J. Morris, pp. 603–18, W.B. Saunders, Philadelphia.

Simmons, R.L., Carafax, D.M., Fry, D.S. *et al.* (1986). New immunosuppressive drug combinations for mismatched related and cadaveric renal transplantation. *Transplant. Proc.* **18** (suppl. 1), 76–81.

Somner, B.G., Henry, M.L. and Ferguson, R.M. (1986). Sequential conventional immunotherapy with maintenance cyclosporine following renal transplantation. *Transplant. Proc.* **18** (suppl. 1), 69–75.

Soullilou, J.P., Le Mauff, B. and Cantarovitch, D. (1988). Use of a monoclonal antibody directed agent IL2-receptor in recipients of kidney allografts. *Transplant. Proc.* **20** (suppl. 6), 84–6.

Strober, S., Slavia, S., Gottlieb, M. *et al.* (1979). Allograft tolerance after total lymphoid irradiation (TLI). *Immunol. Rev.* **46**, 87–112.

Tellides, G., Dallman, M.J. and Morris, P.J. (1989). Mechanism of action of interleukin-2 receptor (IL-2R) monoclonal antibody (MAb) therapy: target cell depletion or inhibition of function. *Transplant. Proc.* **21**, 997–8.

Ting, A. (1988). HLA matching and crossmatching in renal transplantation. In *Kidney Transplantation: Principles and Practice*, 3rd edn, ed. P.J. Morris, pp. 183–213, W.B. Saunders, Philadelphia.

Ting, A. and Morris, P.J. (1978). Matching for B-cell antigens of the HLA-DR series in cadaver renal transplantation. *Lancet* **i**, 575–7.

Waer, M. and Strober, S. (1988). Total lymphoid irradiation (TLI). In *Kidney Transplantation: Principles and Practice*, 3rd edn, ed. P.J. Morris, pp. 371–82, W.B. Saunders, Philadelphia.

Wahlberg, J.A., Love, R., Landegaard, L., Southard, J.H. and Belzer, F.O. (1987). 72-hour preservation of the canine pancreas. *Transplantation* **43**, 5–8.

Walker, R.G. and d'Apice, A.J. (1988). Azathioprine and steroids. In *Kidney Transplantation: Principles and Practice*, 3rd edn, ed. P.J. Morris, pp. 319–41, W.B. Saunders, Philadelphia.

Williams, G.M., Hume, D.M., Hudson, R., Morris, P.J., Kyoichi, K. and Milgrom, F. (1968). 'Hyperacute' renal-homograft rejection in man. *N. Engl. J. Med.* **279**, 611–18.

Williams, S.L., Dler, J. and Jorkusky, D.K. (1986). Long-term renal function in kidney donors: a comparison of donors and their siblings. *Ann. Intern. Med.* **105**, 1–8.

90: Liver and Pancreas Transplantation

R.Y. Calne

The development of clinical transplantation of the liver and of the pancreas has been very different for a number of reasons:

1 The liver is a vital organ and its function cannot be replaced artificially; therefore liver transplantation has been offered to patients with no alternative treatment. On the other hand, pancreas transplantation must be justified as better than replacement treatment with insulin. There have been no attempts to replace the exocrine function in the pancreas by grafting.

2 Liver transplantation is an extremely major procedure for the patient and can be technically difficult; therefore surgical aspects have predominated. The pancreas would, however, appear to be a straightforward organ to transplant surgically but, as will be considered later, this has not proved to be the case in clinical practice.

3 The results of liver transplantation in various disease categories are now emerging and are very similar in different centres throughout the world. The success rate justifies its therapeutic use. These positive features are not yet apparent in pancreas transplantation.

Liver

From the late 1950s and early in the next decade, those interested in liver transplantation were mainly concerned with the technique of accessory liver grafting, it being attractive to transplant an extra liver to avoid the dangerous recipient hepatectomy, and leave any residual native liver function to fall back on should the graft fail. The results of experimental accessory or extra liver allografts were, however, dismal, for the following reasons:

1 The irregular, large mass of the liver was not easily accommodated in the abdomen and the vascular connections were particularly vulnerable to kinking and twisting, so that primary technical failure was likely.

2 When successfully accomplished, an accessory liver allograft very rapidly underwent atrophy to a remarkable degree, unless the animal's own liver was severely damaged. This observation led to a series of interesting and important studies on hepatotrophic factors, of which there are probably a number present in the portal blood. These need to be directed to the allograft in preference to the animal's own liver; otherwise the transplant will suffer from metabolic disadvantage and atrophy, often to a minute nub of tissue within a few weeks.

These observations are not only theoretically important but probably represent a serious hurdle to the application of liver cell grafting, which would otherwise be an attractive concept for the treatment of enzyme deficiencies and other inborn errors of metabolism, where a normally structured bile-secreting liver might not be necessary. The hepatotrophic factors in portal blood may not be taken up by the patient's own liver if it is diseased, as in severe cirrhosis. These factors will then be available to the graft and a few heterotopic allografts in cirrhotic patients have functioned well for years. However, heterotopic grafting would be of no value in treating malignancy of the liver, and the patient's own cirrhotic liver would presumably be susceptible to malignant change, as are all patients with cirrhosis. Hepatoma developing in the patient's own liver was the cause of death in one of the long-term survivors from Paris with an otherwise successful heterotopic liver allograft.

Most surgical endeavour, therefore, became focused on the orthotopic liver transplants pioneered by Moore *et al.* (1959) at the Peter Bent Brigham Hospital and Starzl *et al.* (1959, 1960) in Denver. Both groups of workers found that clamping of the portal vein and vena cava, which was required to perform a transplant, often resulted in death, which could be avoided if blood were shunted from the inferior vena cava and portal venous systems to the superior vena cava. Once a reliable technique became available experimentally, application to man was the next step, which was first taken by Starzl *et al.* (1963). Predictably the early results were very bad, there being no method of support for the patients dying from liver disease comparable to dialysis in patients with renal failure. Thus very sick people were submitted to a surgical operation with a high operative and perioperative mortality. However, some patients did well despite the difficulties. An important observation made by Starzl was that artificial shunting of blood to the superior caval systems from the inferior vena cava and portal system was usually not necessary in man.

The Cambridge/King's College Hospital series of liver allografts began in 1968 and for a decade there was little interest in the procedure outside Denver and Cambridge. In 1984, however, a number of long-term survivors were reported to a Consensus Meeting held in Washington. It was concluded that liver transplantation was the treatment of choice for certain end-stage liver diseases. Since then, more than 70 liver transplant units have been established in the United States and probably nearer 100 in Europe and Australia.

The statistics collected in the European Transplant Registry show a steady increase in numbers of liver allografts and improvements in results (Figs 90.1 and 90.2). As confidence in liver transplantation has progressed, so the indications have been widened and fall into five categories.

Chronic cirrhotic disease

In chronic cirrhotic disease primary biliary cirrhosis and chronic active hepatitis are the commonest indications; alcoholic cirrhosis forms about 10% of the total. In children, biliary atresia is the commonest disease requiring grafting.

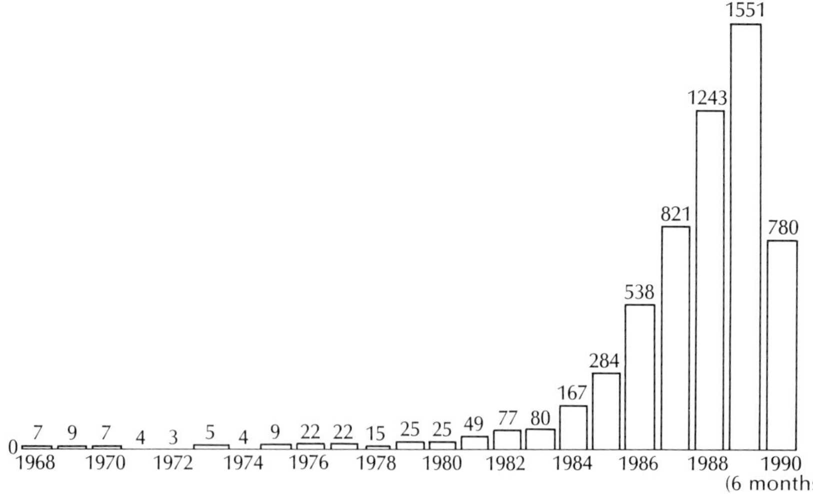

Fig. 90.1. Evolution of liver transplantation. By courtesy of the European Liver Transplant Registry.

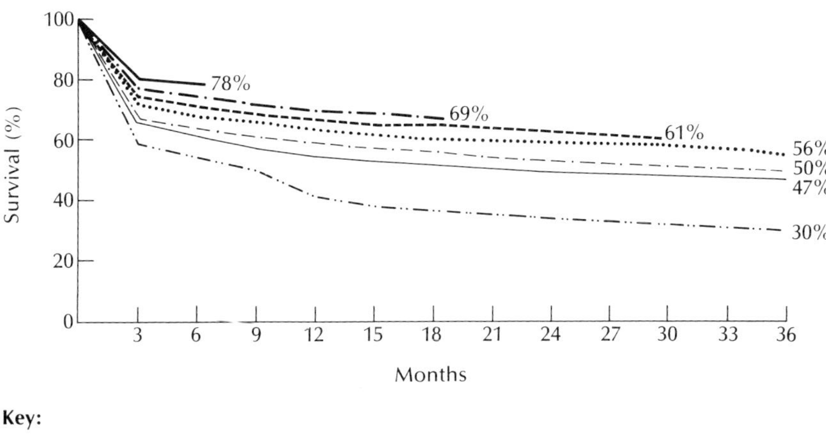

Key:

——— 1990: n = 676
—·—·— 1989: n = 1369
------- 1988: n = 1084
·········· 1987: n = 734
— — · — — 1986: n = 476
——— 1985: n = 263
— ·· — ·· — 1984: n = 154

Fig. 90.2. Evolution of survival in liver transplantation. By courtesy of the European Liver Transplant Registry.

Primary malignancy of the liver

Primary malignancy of the liver may be with or without underlying cirrhosis. If the patient has good residual liver function, the early results of liver grafting for malignancy are good but the recurrence rate is high; approximately 60% of patients develop metastatic tumour in cases of hepatoma, and an even higher recurrence rate has followed grafting for cholangiocarcinoma. The results of liver transplantation for secondary tumour have been very bad. There is a widespread belief that immunosuppression results in rapid and aggressive growth of microscopical malignant deposits.

Inborn errors of metabolism

Inborn errors of metabolism may be (i) with or (ii) without underlying liver disease. The most common indications have been α1-antitrypsin deficiency and Wilson's disease in the first category, and severe forms of oxalosis and haemophilia in the second. In oxalosis it is usually necessary to transplant a kidney together with a liver.

Multiple organ transplants have been performed for a number of indications, the commonest being kidney and pancreas for diabetic renal failure. When the liver is transplanted together with other organs, the allograft reaction seems to have been milder and more easily controlled than when the other organs, for example kidney, pancreas or heart, have been transplanted alone. Moreover, control of rejection of liver allografts in man has been easier to manage than with other organ allografts. These clinical observations are consistent with a large body of experimental work showing that liver allografts are less severely rejected than grafts of other organs and tissues and that the establishment of a successful liver allograft will often permit acceptance of other tissues and organs from the same donor source. Under certain circumstances the liver is able to induce an 'operational immunological tolerance' in the pig and the rat with fully mature immune systems (Calne *et al.* 1969; Kamada *et al.* 1981). This is accomplished without any immunosuppressive agents being given.

Acute and subacute fulminating liver failure

The cause of acute and subacute fulminating liver failure (often in children) is most commonly viral hepatitis, poisoning or idiosyncratic reaction to drugs. In these cases the main difficulty has been timing of the operation, since more than 50% of patients with severe acute liver failure will recover if given specialist intensive care. Those who die tend to deteriorate very quickly and it is only by means of widespread collaboration with those interested in liver grafting that a donor can now usually be found in time to save these patients before irreversible brain damage has occurred.

Acute and chronic graft failure

In acute and chronic graft failure, the only available treatment is a retransplant.

A worry in liver transplantation is recurrence of the patient's original disease, an obvious risk in malignancy, alcoholism, viral hepatitis and to a lesser extent autoimmune liver disease. Patients with congenital abnormalities, such as biliary atresia and inborn errors of metabolism, can be cured by a successful liver transplant, without any danger of recurrence.

The operation

The details of the operation are outside the scope of this article. Very skilled anaesthesia and intensive care management are necessary, together with dedicated, properly trained surgeons prepared to spend many hours in the operating theatre at unsocial times (Calne 1987).

Donor organ removal is usually performed outside the institution where the liver transplant will be done. A major recent advance in liver transplantation, introduced by Jamieson and his colleagues (1989a, b) in experiments performed in the University of Wisconsin, has resulted in a preservation fluid containing lactobionate and raffinose as impermeable ions. This solution will permit cold storage of livers for 36 hours. This has had a major impact on the logistics of liver grafting. No longer is the time element of overriding importance, interfering with other clinical decisions, and it is possible to transport organs long distances by air, thus greatly widening the pool from which donors can be obtained, an especially important consideration in the treatment of patients with fulminating hepatic failure.

In most countries there is a shortage of donor livers, which is more serious for children than for adults because of the size limitations. Although it is possible to transplant a small liver into a large adult, a large liver cannot be accommodated in a small space. Bismuth and Houssin (1984) introduced the idea of lobar transplants of large livers for small recipients and this has proved to be an important advance. When a small liver, or liver segment, is grafted into a large recipient, the size of the vena cava may be inappropriate and in these circumstances the vena cava of the recipient is left intact (Calne *et al*. 1968). Shortage of donor organs and the development of lobar transplants have inevitably led to the utilization of living donors for liver lobes and, although successful cases have been reported, the danger to the donor and the ethical aspects of the procedure will be debated for some time.

Immunosuppression and immunological considerations

There is a consensus now that for all allografts a cocktail of immunosuppression can provide an additive effect with a decrease in the side-effects. In most centres, initial treatment is with three drugs — azathioprine, corticosteroids and cyclosporin. High steroid doses are used to treat rejection crises and antilymphocyte preparations, both polyclonal and monoclonal, are given for steroid-resistant rejection. Prophylactic use of monoclonal antibodies has not been generally adopted due to the increased incidence of infection and the fact that the period of treatment is limited by the development of anti-species antibodies against the animal in which the antilymphocyte globulin was prepared.

Progress in removing the foreign animal protein to produce so-called 'humanized' monoclonal antibodies may widen the scope for the use of monoclonal antibodies and enable a variety of lymphocyte specificities to be targets at different times in relation to the allograft procedure.

Due to the shortage of donors, human leucocyte antigen (HLA) tissue typing has not in general been used to select donors for liver allografts. Transgressing the ABO barrier can sometimes be successful but severe rejection is likely. Grafting an O donor liver to an A or B recipient can result in graft-versus-host disease, in which lymphocytes, transferred with the liver, can attack the recipient, causing haemolysis. A more severe graft-versus-host disease can occur which is similar to the syndrome in bone marrow recipients, especially in recipients with impaired immune systems. Fortunately this potentially fatal complication is rare. A retrospective analysis of tissue matching in liver transplant patients from the two most experienced centres suggests a negative correlation between tissue match and outcome (Donaldson *et al*. 1987; Gordon *et al*. 1986). This phenomenon is now being investigated prospectively in a European multicentre trial. If the phenomenon is real, a variety of factors might be responsible — for example, susceptibility to viral disease and autoimmune liver disease can be expected to be more common when the match is relatively good.

In conclusion, the hazards of liver transplantation are great but certainly less than the inevitable fatal outcome in patients not transplanted. Following liver grafting, many patients are fully restored and rehabilitated in the community. The first patient to receive multiple transplants of liver, heart and lung is alive and well 5 years after the operation, without at any time having evidence of rejection in any of the grafts.

Pancreas

Pancreas grafting has had a much more chequered career than grafting of the liver. First attempted clinically by Kelly *et al.* (1967), the pancreas has proved to be a difficult organ surgically and indications for transplantation are disputed. The idea of transplanting islet or even β cells without the encumbrance of the exocrine pancreas is attractive and in animals short-term success of islet transplants has been regularly reported, especially in rodents. Long-term survival of grafted islets has been more difficult to demonstrate, even with auto- or isografts. Particularly disappointing was the observation of Sutton *et al.* (1987), in Oxford, of eventual failure of long-lasting islet autografts in higher primates. In humans there has been no long-term success with islet allografts. In addition to the difficulty of successfully establishing functioning vascularized islet grafts for long periods, there is the additional worry that the autoimmune process causing diabetes might affect the grafted islets. This has certainly been observed in vascularized pancreas organ allografts when there has been no other immunological barrier, namely in grafts between identical twins and where the barrier has been minimal in grafts between HLA-identical siblings. In these situations the susceptibility to diabetes is presumably present in the donated tissue. We know little of how far the diabetic immune process can cross-react against β cells of differing major histocompatibility complexes (MHCs). Another major obstacle in clinical pancreas grafting has been diagnosis of rejection while it is still treatable, since detectable impairment of glucose metabolism may not occur until the graft is irreversibly damaged. This is probably the reason why results of pancreas grafting alone have been much worse than grafting of pancreas and kidney, since rejection of the kidney and therefore presumably the pancreas can be diagnosed early with the prospect of successful treatment.

There is at present great enthusiasm in the United States for treating end-stage diabetic renal failure by combined pancreas and kidney grafting. The pancreas grafting technique that is favoured is grafting of the pancreas with a segment of duodenum as a patch to the wall of the bladder (Corry *et al.* 1986). This has the advantage of being easy surgically and the estimation of amylase in the urine is a useful indicator of impending rejection. This, taken in relation to the function of the renal allograft from the same donor source, gives the clinician a chance to treat rejection before it becomes too severe. The bladder would seem theoretically to be an unlikely and unsatisfactory place to drain pancreatic exocrine secretion. One might fear activation to trypsinogen with disastrous consequences. This has been an uncommon occurrence. To date there have been no reports of malignancy occurring in the bladder, duodenum or pancreas in patients with grafts using this technique, although one patient suffered sloughing of his penis from activation of trypsinogen (Tom *et al.* 1987).

Over the past decade there has been much argument concerning the best technique for pancreas grafting. When such controversy exists, the usual conclusion to be drawn is that there is as yet no satisfactory technique. The results of pancreas grafting collected throughout the world have been analysed by Dr Sutherland and there has been an increase in enthusiasm over the past few years as results have improved. In the best centres, the pancreas seems to fare nearly as well as the kidney. The patient is cured of his diabetes, requiring no exogenous insulin and is free from the danger of developing recurrent glomerulopathy in the transplanted kidney, although eye changes and macroangiopathy have progressed. Transplantation of half the pancreas, namely the body and tail vascularized by the splenic vessels, being a surgically suitable specimen to graft, was initially popular but troubles with pancreatic exocrine secretion, whether the pancreatic duct was drained into the intestinal tract or an attempt was made to stop exocrine secretion by injecting occlusive glue into the pancreatic duct system, led to a preference to transplant the whole pancreas. This requires both splenic and superior mesenteric blood supply and maintaining intact the segment of duodenum into which the pancreas drains. At present this remains the most acceptable technique. The delivery of insulin is into the systemic venous system rather than the portal system. Whether this is an important disadvantage has not yet been established.

A variety of techniques with good results have been achieved and patients have been fully rehabilitated. For the lucky ones, curing long-standing diabetes and renal failure in one operative procedure has been an enormous advantage. As with the liver, donor organ shortage has led some clinicians to use living volunteer donors and the morbidity in those losing half a pancreas is not negligible. A hemipancreatectomy is a major operation and a diabetic state has resulted after removal of half the pancreas.

It is argued that a controlled trial of diabetic patients being treated by kidney transplantation compared with those given a kidney and pancreas should be made, but so far such a prospective trial has not been performed. In view of the large number of pancreas grafts that have been performed in the last 3 years, especially in North America, long-term appraisal of the value of this treatment should soon be available for analysis. We use pancreas transplantation in selected cases, usually where the patient has specifically requested both a pancreas and kidney.

References

Bismuth, H. and Houssin, D. (1984). Reduced-sized orthotopic liver graft in hepatic transplantation in children. *Surgery* **95**, 367–70.

Calne, R.Y. (1987). *Liver Transplantation*, 2nd edn, Grune Stratton, London.

Calne, R.Y. and Williams, R. (1968). Liver transplantation in man — 1. Observations on technique and organisation in five cases. *Brit. Med. J.* **4**, 535–8.

Calne, R.Y., Sells, R.A., Pena, J.R. *et al.* (1969). Induction of immunological tolerance by porcine liver allografts. *Nature* **233**, 472–6.

Corry, R.J., Nghiem, D.D., Schulak, J.A., Bentel, W.D. and Gonwa, T.A. (1986). Surgical treatment of diabetic nephropathy with simultaneous pancreatic duodenal and renal transplantation. *Surg. Gynecol. Obstet.* **162**, 547–55.

Donaldson, P.T., Alexander, G.J., Nevberger, J. *et al.* (1987). Evidence for an immune response to HLA class I antigens in the vanishing bile duct syndrome after liver transplantation. *Lancet* **i**, 945–8.

Gordon, R.D., Fung, J.J., Markus, B. *et al.* (1986). The antibody crossmatch in liver transplantation. *Surgery* **100**, 705–15.

Jamieson, N.V., Lindell, S., Sundberg, R., Southard, J.H. and Belzer, F.O. (1989a). Evaluation of simplified variants of the VW solution using the isolated perfused rabbit liver. *Transplant. Proc.* **21**, 1294–5.

Jamieson, N.V., Sundberg, R., Lindell, S. *et al.* (1989b). 24–48 hour preservation of the canine liver by simple cold storage using VW lactobionate solution. *Transplant. Proc.* **21**, 1292–3.

Kamada, N., Davies, H.ff.S. and Roser, B. (1981). Reversal of transplantation immunity by liver grafting. *Nature* **292**, 830–42.

Kelly, W.D., Lillehei, R.C., Merkel, F.K. *et al.* (1967). Allotransplantation of the pancreas and duodenum along with the kidney in diabetic nephropathy. *Surgery* **61**, 827–37.

Moore, F.D., Smith, L.L., Burnap, T.K. *et al.* (1959). One-stage homotransplantation of the liver following total hepatectomy in dogs. *Transplant. Bull.* **6**, 103–7.

Starzl, T.E., Berhard, V.M., Cortes, N. and Benvenuto, R. (1959). A technique for one-stage hepatectomy in dogs. *Surgery* **46**, 880–6.

Starzl, T.E., Kaupp, H.A., Brock, D.R., Lazarus, R.E. and Johnson, R.V. (1960). Reconstructive problems in canine liver homotransplantation with special reference to the postoperative role of hepatic venous flow. *Surg. Gynecol. Obstet.* **3**, 733–43.

Starzl, T.E., Marchioro, T.L., Von Kaulla, K.N., Hermann, G., Brittain, R.S. and Waddell, W.R. (1963). Homotransplantation of the liver in humans. *Surg. Gynecol. Obstet.* **117**, 659.

Sutton, R., Gray, D.W.R., McShane, P., Peters, M. and Morris, P.J. (1987). The metabolic efficiency and long-term fate of intraportal islet grafts in the *Cynomolgus* monkey. *Transplant. Proc.* **19** (5), 3575.

Tom, W.W., Munda, R., First, M.R. and Alexander, J.W. (1987). Physiologic consequences of pancreatic allograft exocrine drainage into the urinary tract. *Transplant. Proc.* **19** (1), 2339–42.

Section 11
Tumour Immunology

91: The Immunological Significance of Oncogenes and their Products

G.I. Evan

Introduction

Why should immunologists be concerned about oncogenes and oncoproteins? Principally for three reasons. The first, unrelated to the other two, is something of a legacy from the earlier days of tumour immunology. It arises because antibodies raised against tumour cells in syngeneic or autochthonous hosts occasionally show major specificities for particular polypeptides, some of which are the products of oncogenes. The second reason is that oncogenes encode proteins that are components of signal transduction pathways in lymphoid cells and are therefore responsible for mediating lymphocyte differentiation and activation. The third, clearly linked to the second, is that these same oncogenes are important molecular components of lymphoid carcinogenesis. Indeed, the mechanisms by which oncogenes cause neoplastic transformation are especially well understood in haemopoietic malignancies. This chapter will therefore discuss the known and presumed roles of oncogenes and oncoproteins in both normal and neoplastic lymphoid cell growth and differentiation.

Oncogenes and oncoproteins

Most oncogenes were originally identified as novel genetic elements in various retroviruses that conferred the ability to induce rapid neoplastic changes in specific tissues of infected animals (Bishop 1985). Seminal work in the 1970s demonstrated that the novel oncogenic elements of these 'acutely transforming retroviruses' had been acquired from their hosts via a heterogeneous series of unlikely biological accidents (Bishop 1987). This led to the startling conclusion that normal cells harbour genes with the potential to induce neoplastic change. Such normal cellular genes with oncogenic potential were dubbed 'proto-oncogenes' to distinguish them from their viral counterparts. Given that cancer is an abnormal and pathological state and that oncogenes are unlikely to have evolved just to cause cancer, two self-evident questions arise. First, what are the normal functions of proto-oncogenes? Second, what turns a proto-oncogene into an active oncogene, a process commonly referred to as 'oncogene activation'? The realization over the past decade that all proto-oncogenes encode proteins that are components of the signal transduction pathways effectively answers the first question. Proto-oncogenes and their products comprise part of the machinery by which normal cells receive and interpret signals that regulate growth and differentiation. Detailed molecular analysis of the properties of activated oncogenes provides answers to the second. Activated oncogenes are proto-oncogenes that have sustained mutations that cause inappropriate expression or activation of their encoded proteins. Typically, oncogenically activating mutations involve either damage to genetic elements regulating expression of the oncogene or lesions in regulatory regions of the encoded protein. Such deregulatory mutations presumably result in sustained or inappropriate mitogenic signals that override normal growth control and drive promiscuous cell proliferation.

Growth control in lymphoid cells

In the adult, lymphocyte proliferation is confined either to immature progenitor cells or to mature cells responding to specific antigen. Mature lymphocytes typically spend long periods in a quiescent state, and yet they must retain the ability to respond and proliferate rapidly upon activation of their idiotypic antigen receptor. Lymphoid tumours are presumed to arise either by a block in lymphocyte differentiation, thereby locking the affected cell and its progeny in a self-renewing compartment, or by inappropriate and sustained activation of the mature lymphocyte's mitogenic pathway.

Given the fundamental roles of known proto-oncogenes in signal transduction in lymphocytes, it is not surprising that inappropriate expression or activation of many proto-oncogenes can interfere with growth control of lymphoid cells. Indeed, lesions in many oncogenes have been detected in both human and non-human lymphoid and haemopoietic malignancies. The nature of such lesions and how they lead to neoplastic transformation are perhaps best understood in terms of the roles of proto-oncogenes and their products in normal lymphocyte proliferation and differentiation. This task has been facilitated by our current detailed knowledge of signal transduction in T and B cells.

T cell activation — a paradigm for the role of proto-oncogene products in signal transduction

The T cell antigen receptor

The molecular basis of T lymphocyte activation has received much attention, fostered by the acknowledged pivotal role of the T cell in immune response and immunomodulation. Elucidation of the complete structure of the T cell receptor (TCR) complex and the genes that encode each component has, however, only recently been realized. The clonotypic TCR itself determines antigenic specificity and comprises a disulphide-linked heterodimer of α and β chains, both members of the immunoglobulin (Ig) superfamily. The TCR exists in tight association with the CD3 complex, which consists of three closely related polypeptides, γ, δ and ε, and two other proteins, ζ and η. ζ and η chains are now known to be translated from differentially spliced messenger ribonucleic acids (mRNAs) derived from the same gene and are present as either homo- or heterodimers. Although all TCR–CD3 polypeptides are transmembrane proteins, the TCR α and β chains have very short (9 residue) intracellular tails. It is only the ζ and η chains, which possess extensive cytoplasmic domains, that are thought to mediate the receptor complex's interactions with intracellular effectors. Both ζ and η chains possess potential sites for tyrosine phosphorylation and ζ is rapidly phosphorylated upon engaging the TCR–CD3 complex. The TCR–CD3–$\zeta\eta$ complex associates with either the CD4 or the CD8 glycoprotein, transmembrane polypeptides that recognize monotypic determinants on the Class II and Class I major histocompatibility complex (MHC) molecules respectively. The combined interaction of both TCR–CD3 and CD4/8 results in stabilization and increase in avidity in the interaction between TCR and target antigen–MHC and potentiates the intracellular signal so generated. Several other polypeptides on the T cell surface provide accessory signals that greatly potentiate the TCR–CD3–CD4/8 signal. Perhaps the best characterized of these are CD28 and CD2. CD28 binds the B1/B7 receptor on target cells and this signal leads directly to activation of the interleukin 2 (IL-2) gene (Fraser *et al.* 1991). Interleukin 2 is absolutely required for progression through the cell cycle and effective proliferation. CD2 interacts with another receptor on target cells, called lymphocyte function-associated antigen (LFA)-3. In addition, many other surface polypeptides appear able to provide analogous accessory functions.

Protein kinases

In order for the TCR–CD3 complex to pass information on to appropriate targets within the cell it must be coupled to appropriate intracellular effectors. Coupling occurs by direct activation of tyrosine protein kinases (TPKs) that are associated with the TCR complex. The cytoplasmic domain of CD4/8 interacts with a TPK of about 56 kD encoded by the *lck* gene (Rudd 1990; Sefton 1990). $p56^{lck}$ is a member of the same family of TPKs as $pp60^{src}$, first identified as the protein encoded by the oncogene of the Rous sarcoma virus. The interaction between CD4/8 and $p56^{lck}$ is quite tight, allowing co-immunoprecipitation of one with the other, and it is mediated by a defined helical region in the cytoplasmic tails of CD4/8, which is cysteine-rich and may require metal ions. The CD4/8–$p56^{lck}$ complex thus resembles many other cytokine receptors, for example the epidermal growth factor (EGF), platelet-derived growth factor (PDGF) and insulin receptors, all of which possess intracellular protein kinase effector domains, but it differs in that ligand receptor and catalytic domain reside on different molecules.

The TCR–CD3 complex is associated with its own TPK, encoded by the *fyn* gene (Rudd 1990). *fyn* is widely expressed in many cell types, but T cells possess a uniquely spliced form, yielding a 59 kD protein. The overall structure of $p59^{fyn}$ is very similar to that of $p56^{lck}$. Both contain a C-terminal catalytic domain with high homology to other *src* family kinases (Hunter 1989). Both contain a conserved C-terminal catalytic kinase domain with a conserved lysine residue involved in adenosine triphosphate (ATP) binding, a conserved tyrosine residue that is autophosphorylated in the active protein, and a C-terminal tyrosine (Tyr 505 in $p56^{lck}$ and Tyr 531 in $p59^{fyn}$) whose phosphorylation inactivates kinase activity. Loss of this C-terminal tyrosine results in a permanently active kinase with oncogenic properties (see below). N-terminal to the catalytic domain lie two *src* homology regions (SH2 and SH3), whose functions are to modulate kinase activity, presumably by interaction with other molecules. The N-terminal regions of both $p59^{fyn}$ and $p56^{lck}$ are unique and contain specific sites for interaction with TCR–CD3–ζη and CD4/8 respectively. Both $p59^{fyn}$ and $p56^{lck}$ are N-terminally myristilated and thereby attached to the inner surface of the plasma membrane.

Quite how engaging the TCR–CD3–ζη and CD4/8 receptors leads to activation of the *fyn* and *lck* proteins is unclear. Evidence suggests that such activation is very rapid, preceding and, probably, initiating other signal transductive events. It is suggested that antigen binding induces aggregation of the TCR–CD3–ζη and CD4/8 receptors, which therefore induces concomitant intracellular aggregation of the associated *fyn* and *lck* proteins (Rudd 1990; Sefton 1990). Potentially, this might allow $p59^{fyn}$ and $p56^{lck}$ to phosphorylate and activate each other. Another factor regulating *lck* kinase activity is the membrane-associated phosphotyrosine phosphatase CD45 (leucocyte common antigen). CD45 is absolutely required for $p56^{lck}$ activity and may act by dephosphorylating the inhibitory C-terminal tyrosine 505 on $p56^{lck}$ (Mustelin *et al.* 1989).

Downstream signalling in the cytoplasm and nucleus

A number of candidate targets for the *fyn* and *lck* kinases exist. These include the TCR ζ protein itself, several serine–threonine protein kinases, such as RAF-1 and the microtubule-associated protein-2 kinase (MAP-2K), the guanosine triphosphatase (GTPase)-activating protein (GAP) and phospholipase C_γ (PLC_γ). Activated PLC_γ cleaves membrane inositol phospholipids to generate the two second messengers inositol-1,4,5-triphosphate (IP_3) and diacylglycerol (DAG). Inositol triphosphate initiates release of intracellular CA^{2+}, which in turn activates the serine/threonine calmodulin-dependent protein kinases as well as a host of other intracellular processes. Diacylglycerol activates protein kinase C (PKC), which also exerts complex and pleiotropic effects and may directly phosphorylate and regulate some transcription factors.

Several other well-characterized TPKs and serine/threonine protein kinases are found in lymphocytes in addition to the *fyn* and *lck* proteins (Altman *et al*. 1990) (Table 91.1). All are presumably involved in some aspect of signal transduction pathways because inappropriate activation of many of them is oncogenic (see below). However, their precise roles and positions in the signalling hierarchy are at present unclear.

Within 1 hour of mitogenic activation via the TCR and accessory receptors, at least 60 new cellular genes are induced. The complexity of this 'immediate early' genetic response has recently been analysed by subtractive complementary deoxyribonucleic acid (cDNA) cloning (Zipfel *et al*. 1989). Many of the immediate early T cell genes are also induced in other cell types in response to mitogenic stimuli; others appear to be restricted to haemopoietic or lymphoid cells. Although most immediate early genes are poorly defined and of unknown function, some have been characterized. They include genes encoding cytoskeletal proteins (e.g. β-actin), genes encoding cytokines and their receptors (e.g. IL-2 and IL-2R), and genes encoding transcription factors (e.g. the c-*fos*, c-*myc*, c-*myb*, c-*rel*, c-*ets*-2 and *egr-1/NGFIA* proteins). Members of this latter group are of particular interest for two reasons. First, they are presumed to be responsible for mediating and maintaining the genetic changes that occur when T cells proliferate and differentiate in response to antigen. Thus, elucidation of which genes they regulate, and in what manner, should shed light on the biology of the T cell response. Second, many immediate early transcription factors have been shown to possess oncogenic properties when expressed inappropriately (see below).

B cell activation

Details of the molecular events following B cell activation are less well defined than in T cells (Reth 1991). The B cell antigen receptor comprises a membrane-associated idiotypic IgM associated with at least two other disulphide-linked polypeptides, the 34 kD α and 39 kD β chains. Antigen binding leads to the rapid intracellular activation of an undefined TPK, possibly the *lyn* protein. This, in turn, leads to activation of PLC_{γ} and PKC, with pleiotropic effects analogous to those seen in activated T cells. Many protein kinases and transcription factors are shared between T and B cells (and most other cells also). In general, it is reasonable to assume that the B cell shares many common signal transductive components with T cells, although it clearly utilizes the transduced information in its own unique way.

Table 91.1. Protein kinases in lymphocytes

Gene	Protein	Expression in lymphocytes	Function
lck	p56	T cells	Tyrosine kinase
fyn	p59	T cells	Tyrosine kinase
fyn	p72	B cells	Tyrosine kinase
fps	p92	B cells	Tyrosine kinase
tkl	p52	B and T cells	Tyrosine kinase
abl	p120–140	B and T cells	Tyrosine kinase
ltk	p52	B and T cells	Tyrosine kinase
Insulin receptor-β	p90	B and T cells	Tyrosine kinase
kit	p145	B and T cells	Tyrosine kinase
ret	p96	B and T cells	Tyrosine kinase
pim-1	p33	B and T cells	Tyrosine kinase
PKC	p80	B and T cells	Ser/Thr kinase
raf-1	p74	B and T cells	Ser/Thr kinase
Microtubule-associated protein-2 kinase (MAP-2K)	p42 and p45	B and T cells	Ser/Thr kinase

The oncogenic potential of components of the lymphocyte signal transduction pathways

Many of the signal transduction components of T and B cells can act as oncogenes in a variety of cell types when inappropriately expressed or inappropriately activated by mutation (Fig. 91.1). Some of the known mutations activating oncogenes in lymphocytes are discussed below; they are summarized in Table 91.2.

Tyrosine kinases

Both *lck* and *fyn* kinases are oncogenically activated by loss of their C-terminal tyrosine phosphorylation sites, presumably because this site is important in the negative regulation of kinase activity. In addition, a variety of mutations within the kinase and SH2–SH3 modulatory domains of the *lck* and *fyn* polypeptides are oncogenic. The *lck* protein was first identified in the LSTRA murine lymphoma cell line, in which it is expressed at an abnormally high level. Detailed analysis reveals that this over-expression is a result of the integration of the Moloney murine leukaemia virus (Mo MuLV) upstream of *lck*. As the coding sequence of the *lck* protein in LSTRA is normal, this suggests that simple over-expression of *lck* is sufficient to contribute to the lymphomagenic process.

The *fps* proto-oncogene is the cellular homologue of the viral oncogene of two retroviruses, the Fujinami avian sarcoma virus and the Snyder–Theiler feline sarcoma virus, and encodes a TPK expressed in all lymphoid cells. Like the *fyn* and *lck* proteins, the *fps* protein possesses a C-terminal tyrosine phosphorylation site that negatively modulates the kinase activity. As in the *fyn* and *lck* proteins, loss of this site leads to oncogenic activation.

The *abl* oncogene was first identified as the transforming gene of the Abelson leukaemia retrovirus, which induces pre-B cell leukaemias in mice. c-*abl* encodes a cytoplasmic TPK of unknown specificity and function, which is widely expressed in haemopoietic cells. Like the *src* kinases the *abl* protein contains two *src* homology regions, SH2 and SH3, N-terminal to the catalytic kinase domain. The SH2 and SH3 domains respectively exert a positive and negative modulatory function on the *abl* kinase. In the Abelson leukemia virus, retrovirus *gag* sequences have replaced the SH3 domain, thereby presumably comprising essential negative regulation of the kinase activity. A similar SH3 deletion is common in chronic myelogenous leukaemia (CML) in man, where it occurs as a result of chromosomal translocation (see below).

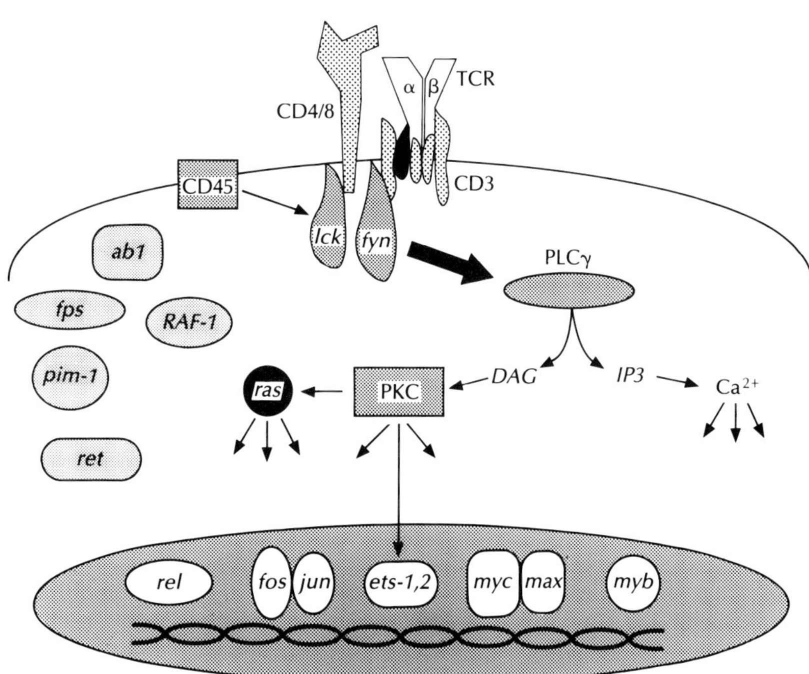

Fig. 91.1. Some key proto-oncogene products in T cell signalling. Known proto-oncogenes are labelled in italics.

Table 91.2. Examples of proto-oncogene activation in lymphoid cells

Mechanism	Lesion	Effect	Examples
Mutation	Point mutation	Loss of self-inactivating function	*ras* oncogenes
	Truncation	Loss of negative regulatory domain	C-terminal deletions in *src*, *fyn*, *lck* and *fps*
	Substitution	Replacement of negative regulatory domain by other sequence	*bcr–abl* fusion in CML *gag–abl* fusion in Abelson B cell leukaemia virus
Deregulated expression	Provirus insertion	Integration of virus promoter/enhancer disrupts normal regulation	Avian leucosis virus and *myc* Moloney MuLV in LSTRA and *lck*
	Chromosomal translocation	Normal regulation disrupted by novel adjacent regulatory elements	*myc* in BL *bcl-1* and *bcl-2* in human B lymphoma *TCL-3* in T lymphoma
	Virus infection	Promiscuous activation of proto-oncogenes by viral transcription factors	HTLV-1 *tax* protein EBV *EBNA-1*, 2 and *LMP* genes

raf-1, *kit*, *pim-1* and *ret* all encode related serine/threonine kinases found in normal lymphocytes, *raf-1* and *kit* are homologues of the oncogenes of the 3611 murine sarcoma virus and the HZ4 feline sarcoma virus respectively. *pim-1* is the site of integration of the Mo MuLV in many murine T lymphomas. *ret* was identified by its oncogenic properties during transfection of human T cell lymphoma DNA into NIH 3T3 fibroblasts. The precise functions of these four protein kinases in lymphocyte signal transduction are currently unknown, but the fact that all have oncogenic potential when functionally deregulated indicates their importance.

ras proteins

Both N-*ras* and c-K-*ras* are expressed in lymphocytes and both are presumed to play important roles in relaying and modulating signal transduction (McCormick 1989). *ras* proteins are oncogenically activated by mutations that knock out their intrinsic GTPase activity and such mutations are found in some 10% of human tumours. Inactivation of the GTPase leaves *ras* proteins in a permanently active state, resulting in sustained and deregulated mitogenic signals. Activated N-*ras* and K-*ras* genes are common in acute lymphoblastic and myeloid leukaemia but very rare in B lymphoma. *ras* gene activation may play an important auxiliary role in the genesis of human CML (see below).

Nuclear proteins — transcription factors

Both c-*fos* and c-*jun* were originally identified as retroviral oncogenes, in the FBJ and FBR murine osteosarcoma viruses and the avian sarcoma virus 17 respectively. They are members of a family of genes encoding transcription factors, a family which includes c-*jun*, *jun*-B, *jun*-D, c-*fos*, *fos*-B and *fra*-1 (Abate and Curran 1990). Expression of c-*fos* and c-*jun* is not limited to lymphocytes; both are rapidly induced in many cell types by a variety of external signals, including (where relevant) mitogenic growth factors, differentiation factors and neurotransmitters (Greenberg and Ziff 1984; Hunt *et al*. 1987; Ryseck *et al*. 1988). The c-*fos* and c-*jun* proteins, FOS and JUN, are components of the AP-1 transcription factor activity. AP-1 was originally isolated from nuclear extracts by its specificity for the common TGACTCA DNA motif and it confers inducibility by the phorbol ester, 12-*O*-tetradecanoylphorbol 13-acetate (TPA). The various FOS and JUN proteins function as a variety of homo- and heterodimers (Jones 1990).

The c-*myc* gene, like *fos* and *jun*, is rapidly induced in cells by mitogenic stimuli (Kelly *et al.* 1983) and has been shown to have an essential role in enabling and regulating cell proliferation (Heikkila *et al.* 1987). C-*myc* is homologous to an oncogene found in several avian and feline tumour viruses. It encodes a nuclear phosphoprotein, MYC, which is active as a heterodimer with another cellular polypeptide called MAX and which specifically binds the DNA sequence CACGTG (Blackwell *et al.* 1990; Blackwood and Eisenman 1991). Although MYC is thought to be a transcription factor, it is not known which genes it regulates or to what biological end.

c-*myb* was first identified as the transforming gene of the avian myeloblastic leukaemia virus. The cellular counterpart of the viral *myb* gene, c-*myb*, encodes a ~70 kD nuclear phosphoprotein with sequence-specific DNA-binding activity (Biedenkapp *et al.* 1988) and the ability to activate transcription (Weston and Bishop 1989). Expression of c-*myb* is confined to haemopoietic tissues, although other members of the *myb* gene family have a more widespread distribution. One gene has so far been identified as a target for c-*myb*, the *mim*-1 gene, which encodes a specifically expressed, secretable protein contained in the granules of promyelocytes (Ness *et al.* 1989).

The *ets* oncogene was isolated from the E26 avian myeloblastosis virus and comprises part of that virus's oncogene. The cellular *ets* gene is a member of a family which includes *ets*-2, *erg*, *elk-1* and *elk-2*, PU.1 and the *Drosophila* homologue E74 (Ghysdael and Yaniv 1991). All *ets* proteins share a region of about 85 amino acids which contains the DNA-binding domain and determines binding specificity (Karim *et al.* 1990). The consensus binding site for *ets* proteins is the DNA sequence $^{A}/_{C}$GGAA, which is present in the enhancer elements of the TCR α and β gene as well as the long terminal repeat (LTR) regulatory element of human T lymphotropic virus-1. *ets-1* and *ets-2* are reciprocally expressed in T cells: *ets-1* is present in quiescent T cells and is rapidly phosphorylated and inactivated upon T cell activation. In contrast, *ets-2* is induced and stabilized by phosphorylation upon T cell activation and appears to play a role in the mitogenic response. Consistent with this, ectopic induction of *ets-2* is mitogenic and oncogenic in mouse 3T3 fibroblasts. PU-1, a homologue of *ets*, is specifically expressed in B cells. The PU-1 gene lies at the common site of integration of the Friend erythroleukaemia virus in murine erythroleukaemias. Consequently its expression is disrupted and this is presumed to be in part responsible for the neoplasm.

The c-*rel* oncogene is the homologue of the oncogene of the avian reticuloendotheliosis virus T, which induces pre-B and T cell lymphomas in chickens. C-*rel* is a member of a family that includes nuclear factor (NF)κ-B and the *Drosophila* homoeotic gene *dorsal* (Gilmore 1990). All encode transcription factors that are maintained in an inactive state by complexing with a cytoplasmic polypeptide IκB. Phosphorylation of IκB by PKC causes dissociation of the NFκ-B–IκB complex, so freeing NFκ-B, and is thought to be the principal mechanism regulating NFκ-B/*rel* activities (Gilmore 1990).

Nuclear proteins — anti-oncogenes or tumour suppressor genes

Within the past few years, it has become clear that many human tumours arise by loss of specific genes. By inference, the functions of such genes must be to provide antiproliferative or growth-restraining regulatory functions in normal cells. Two such 'anti-oncogenes', encoding the nuclear proteins p53 and RB, play a pivotal role in current models of oncogenesis. p53 was first identified as a polypeptide co-immunoprecipitating with the transforming proteins of several DNA tumour viruses. Lesions in the p53 gene are found in some 30% of all human malignancies. RB is the protein product of a gene always deleted or inactivated in human retinoblastoma cells. The RB protein is also involved in complexes with various DNA tumour virus-transforming proteins. The molecular functions of both p53 and RB are unknown, but both appear to function as regulators of the G1/S transition in the mammalian cell cycle. Current models propose that both RB and p53 functions must be actively suppressed for cells to progress through their cycles. Consistent with this idea, there is evidence that some antiproliferative cytokines (chalones) may act through RB and p53 to force cells out of cycle. No evidence has yet been found to suggest a role for p53 or RB in lymphoid malignancies. None the less, the ubiquitous expression of both anti-oncogenes in lymphocytes argues for their importance in the regulation of lymphocyte proliferation.

In addition to p53 and RB, several other candidate anti-oncogenes have been recently identified and found to be deleted in various tumours. It is likely that lesions in anti-oncogenes will eventually be found to play as important a role in human carcinogenesis as do mutations in dominant oncogenes (Levine 1990).

Oncogenes at sites of chromosomal abnormalities in human haemopoietic tumours

Chromosomal abnormalities in human tumours include deletions, translocations (both reciprocal and non-reciprocal), inversions and amplifications. Although extensive and apparently random chromosomal abnormalities are a common feature of aggressive and advanced neoplastic cells, specific types of chromosomal lesion are characteristic of certain malignancies and mark the positions of genes important in that tumour's carcinogenic process.

Burkitt's lymphoma (BL) is a tumour of immature B cells which occurs in endemic and sporadic forms. There is a clear epidemiological association between endemic BL and infection by Epstein–Barr virus (EBV), although the molecular basis for the association is not understood. Virtually all instances of BL show characteristic reciprocal chromosome translocations between chromosome 8 and chromosome 14, 2 or 22. The site of translocation on chromosome 8 (q24) maps to the site of the c-*myc* proto-oncogene, whilst the sites on chromosome 14 (q32), 2 (p13) and 22 (q11) map to the sites of the Ig heavy, κ and λ genes respectively. These various translocations appear to damage the normal regulatory machinery of the c-*myc* gene and hence lead to its inappropriate expression. It is presumed that the translocations are the result of the same enzymatic machinery that is responsible for recombination and generation of diversity of both Ig and TCRs. Thus, lymphoid cells may be peculiarly prone to this type of oncogenic activation.

Almost 90% of all cases of chronic myeloid leukaemia (CML) demonstrate the characteristic Philadelphia chromosome translocation t(9;22)(q34;q11) (Bishop 1989). A similar translocation sometimes also occurs in acute lymphocytic leukaemia. Mapping studies revealed that the q34 site on chromosome 9 is the location of the c-*abl* proto-oncogene, which encodes a cytoplasmic TPK and which had already been identified as the transduced transforming gene of the Abelson B cell leukaemia virus. The site of the reciprocal translocation, 22q11, maps to the location of another gene, christened BCR, for break-point cluster region, whose function is unknown. The effect of the translocation is to fuse a truncated ABL protein kinase on to the C-terminal end of the BCR protein resulting in an ABL protein that has an enhanced or deregulated kinase activity and a different subcellular distribution.

Many human B cell tumours carry either t(14;11)(q32;q13) or t(14;18)(q32;q21) translocations. Once again, the 14q32 locus is the site of the Ig heavy chain. 11q13 and 18q21 are the sites of the BCL1 and BCL2 genes respectively. The BCL2 protein has recently been identified as a mitochondrial protein whose sustained expression blocks programmed cell death (apoptosis) (Hockenbery *et al.* 1990). Apoptosis is an important regulatory component of T and B cell differentiation and the principal mechanism for the deletion of clones reactive with self antigens. It is presumed that, as in the case of the c-*myc* translocation in BL, translocation to the Ig region upsets the normal control of the BCL2 gene. The resultant sutained expression of *bcl-2* suppresses the normal deletion of self-reactive lymphocytes, thus allowing them to mature into an environment in which they are being continuously stimulated to proliferate. In T cell lymphomas, the T cell receptor genes are also occasionally involved in reciprocal translocations. As yet, however, the genes present at the reciprocal breakpoints have not been characterized.

Gross cytogenetic abnormalities have, therefore, allowed identification of several proto-oncogenes as important components in lymphoid carcinogenesis. In all of the above cases, however, activation of each of the oncogenes present at the sites of translocation is not by itself sufficient for full neoplastic transformation. For example, in BL it is clear that EBV plays an essential accessory role in generation of the tumour. ABL–BCR fusion is occasionally observed in the cells of completely normal individuals and therefore cannot be solely responsible for the tumour — indeed, substantial evidence now suggests that mutational activation of a *ras* proto-oncogene is also required for full malignancy. Finally, it is clear that although deregulated expression of BCL2 promotes cell survival it has no direct disruptive effect on the regulation of growth control. Epidemiological data have long suggested that carcinogenesis comprises the protracted and sequential acquisition of multiple oncogenic mutations. This concept is supported by a number of seminal *in vitro* studies which demonstrate that activation of single oncogenes is insufficient for neoplastic transformation and concerted activation of co-operating oncogenes is necessary.

To be or not to be (an oncogene)

Identifying potential oncogenes by mapping the sites of gross chromosomal lesions is a useful strategy. However, many of the lesions that oncogenically activate oncogenes are microscopic point mutations, frame-shifts and deletions and therefore unlikely to involve gross alterations in chromatin. Given our knowledge of signal transduction pathways in T and B lymphocytes, two questions become paramount. Are all genes that are involved in lymphocyte activation potential oncogenes? Which, if any, proto-oncogenes are involved in human lymphoid neoplasias?

Historically, our knowledge of most oncogenes comes from the study of acute retroviruses and their fortuitous acquisition of cellular proto-oncogenes (Table 91.3). One approach to identifying new oncogenes, therefore, is simply to screen more acute retroviruses for novel oncogenic elements. The difficulties with this approach are threefold. First, not all proto-oncogenes may be susceptible to retroviral transduction — for example, it may not be possible for a retrovirus to transduce a very large or complex, alternatively spliced, cellular gene. Second, most acute retroviruses arose in highly inbred and genetically defined host populations. Not only are very few retroviruses found in man but there is, obviously, no possibility of breeding and selecting optimal human hosts. Thus, retroviral oncogenes will only represent genes with oncogenic potential in animal models and can never provide a direct source of human oncogenes. Third, retroviral oncogenes are always dominant oncogenes: that is, they act to induce neoplastic changes in normal cells. As discussed above, however, many human malignancies are associated with loss-of-function mutations in anti-oncogenes or tumour suppressor genes. Clearly, such genes will never appear in a retroviral screen.

Two especially powerful strategies have been employed to identify potential oncogenes not found in retroviruses. One is to transfer DNA from tumour cells into a normal indicator cell, select for transformants in the indicator population, and clone out the exogenous DNA responsible for the neoplastic change. The *ret* gene is an example of a proto-oncogene identified by this strategy (see above). Transfection can also be used to assay the oncogenic potential of genes isolated by their homology to known oncogenes. The *fyn* kinase, closely related to the *src* and *lck* kinases, was tested in this way and found to have oncogenic potential. Similar analyses have revealed the proto-oncogenic nature of individual members of several proto-oncogene families (Table 91.4). The second approach involves the use of transgenic mice. These are animals into whose germlines specific genes, driven by defined tissue-specific regulatory elements, are stably introduced. Any hyperplasias or neoplasias that appear are then subjected to a detailed molecular forensic examination to determine the role of the transgene. Using this approach it has been possible to systematically assay many of the components of the lymphocyte signal transduction pathways for their oncogenic potential when expressed in an inappropriate or deregulated manner. Such studies have clearly demonstrated the co-operative effects of various combinations of oncogenes, cytokines and cytokine receptors (Adams and Cory 1991).

Conclusion

Molecular and cell biology have provided us with many new insights into the mechanisms by which lymphoid cells respond to signals that regulate their growth, death and differentiation. We now know that many of the major components in lymphocyte signal transduction pathways are encoded by proto-oncogenes and, although we have rather less idea of how each of these components is integrated and regulated, we do know that gross deregulation of many of these oncoproteins can lead to neoplastic changes in an

Table 91.3. Oncogenes transduced by retroviruses

General type	Retrovirus	Oncogene	Function	Tumour
Cytokine agonists/ligands	Simian sarcoma	*sis*	PDGF subunit	Sarcoma
	Murine spleen focus-forming	gp55 spike glycoprotein	binds erythropoietic receptor	Erythroleukaemia
Receptor kinases	Avian erythroblastosis	*erb*-B	EGF receptor	Erythroleukaemia
	SM feline sarcoma	*fms*	M-CSF receptor	Sarcoma
	HZ4 feline sarcoma	*kit*	?	Sarcoma
	UR2 chicken sarcoma	*ros*	?	?
Non-receptor kinases	Rous sarcoma	*src*	TPK	Sarcoma
	Fujinami sarcoma	*fps*	TPK	Sarcoma
	Y73/ESV	*yes*	TPK	Sarcoma
	S13	*sea*	TPK	Erythroleukaemia
Cytoplasmic kinases	Abelson leukaemia	*abl*	TPK	Pre-B-cell lymphoma
	Murine sarcoma 3611	*raf*	S/TPK	Sarcoma
	Moloney sarcoma	*mos*	S/TPK	Sarcoma
ras G protein	Harvey sarcoma	H-*ras*	Signal modulation	Sarcoma
	Kirsten sarcoma	K-*ras*	Signal modulation	Sarcoma
Nuclear	FBJ osteosarcoma	*fos*	Transcription factor AP-1	Osteosarcoma
	Avian sarcoma 17	*jun*	Transcription factor AP-1	Sarcoma
	SK57 sarcoma	*ski*	Transcription factor	Sarcoma
	Avian myeloblastosis	*myb*	Transcription factor	Myeloblastic leukaemia
	Avian myelocytic	*myc*	Transcription factor	Myelocytic leukaemia Carcinoma
	E26 avian myeloblastosis	*myb/ets*	Transcription factor	Myeloblastic leukaemia
	Avian erythroblastosis	*erb*-A	Thyroid hormone receptor	Erythroleukaemia
	Reticulo-endotheliosis virus T	*rel*	Transcription factor	Pre-B and T cell leukaemia

affected cell. For the first time it is possible to view the molecular basis of cancer in terms of dysfunction in normal regulatory pathways in cells. Given the rapid advances made within the last decade, it is perhaps not too optimistic to speculate that rational and effective therapies for lymphoid neoplasias may become available within the next.

Table 91.4. Oncogene families and their effects on haemopoietic cells

Parent gene	Family members	Effect on haemopoietic lineages	Tumour association in man
EGF receptor		Erythroblastosis	None known
	neu	Pre-B lymphoma	Breast carcinoma
	ros	NDA	None known
	sea	NDA	None known
	trk	NDA	None known
	met	NDA	None known
src	*src*	Erythroleukaemia lymphoma	None known
	lck	Lymphoma	None known
	fyn	NDA	None known
	fps	Lymphoid hyperplasia	None known
	yes	Lymphoma	None known
	lck	NDA	None known
abl	*abl*	B/T lymphoma myeloid/lymphoblastic leukaemia	CML and ALL
PKC	*raf*	NDA	None known
	mos	Myeloproliferative disease	None known
	pim-1	T lymphoma	None known
ras	H-*ras*	Pre-B/T lymphoma	Diverse
	K-*ras*	Pre-B/T lymphoma	Diverse
	N-*ras*	T lymphoma macrophage tumour	Diverse
fos	*fos*	None observed	None known
	fos B	NDA	None known
	fra-1	NDA	None known
	c-jun	NDA	None known
	jun B	NDA	None known
rel	*rel*	Pre-B and T lymphoma	None known
	NFκ-B	NDA	None known
ets	*ets-1*	NDA	None known
	ets-2	NDA	None known
	PU-1	NDA	None known
	elk	NDA	None known
	erg	NDA	None known
myb	c-*myb*	Myeloblastosis	Colon carcinoma?
	B-*myb*	NDA	None known
myc	c-*myc*	Pre-B/T lymphoma	Diverse
	N-*myc*	myelocytic leukaemia	
		Pre-B and B lymphoma	Neuroblastoma
	L-*myc*	T lymphoma	Small-cell lung cancer
p53	*p53*	—	Diverse
RB	*RB*	—	Retinoblastoma

NDA = no data available.

Data on effects on haemopoietic, cells compiled from various sources (e.g. Pierce 1989; Adams and Cory 1991), including transgenic and transfection experiments and the effects of relevant acute retroviruses.

References

Abate, C. and Curran, T. (1990). Encounters with *fos* and *jun* on the road to AP-1. *Semin. Cancer Biol.* **1**, 19–26.

Adams, J.M. and Cory, S. (1991). Transgenic models for haemopoietic malignancies. *Biochem. Biophys. Acta* **1072**, 9–31.

Altman, A., Coggeshall, K.M. and Mustelin, T. (1990). Molecular events mediating T cell activation. *Adv. Immunol.* **48**, 227–360.

Biedenkapp, H., Borgmeyer, U., Sippel, A.E. and Klempnauer, K.H. (1988). Viral *myb* oncogene encodes a sequence-specific DNA-binding activity. *Nature* **335**, 835–7.

Bishop, J.M. (1985). Viral oncogenes. *Cell* **42**, 23–38.

Bishop, J.M. (1987). The molecular genetics of cancer. *Science* **235**, 305–11.

Bishop, J.M. (1989). Oncogenes and clinical cancer. In *Oncogenes and the Molecular Origins of Cancer*, ed. R. Weinberg, Cold Spring Harbour Laboratory Press.

Blackwell, T.K., Kretzner, L., Blackwood, E.M., Eisenman, R.N. and Weintraub, H. (1990). Sequence-specific DNA binding by the c-Myc protein. *Science* **250**, 1149–51.

Blackwood, E.M. and Eisenman, R.N. (1991). Max: a helix–loop–helix zipper protein that forms a sequence-specific DNA-binding complex with Myc. *Science* **251**, 1211–17.

Fraser, J.D., Irving, B.A., Crabtree, G.R. and Weiss, A. (1991). Regulation of interleukin-2 gene enhancer activity by the T cell accessory molecule CD28. *Science* **251**, 313–16.

Ghysdael, J. and Yaniv, M. (1991). Nuclear oncogenes. *Curr. Biol.* **3**, 484–92.

Gilmore, T. (1990). NF-κB, KBF1, *dorsal* and *rel*ated matters. *Cell* **62**, 841–3.

Greenberg, M.E. and Ziff, E.B. (1984). Stimulation of 3T3 cells induces transcription of the c-*fos* proto-oncogene. *Nature* **311**, 433–8.

Heikkila, R., Schwab, G., Wickstrom, E. *et al.* (1987). A c-*myc* antisense oligodeoxynucleotide inhibits entry into S phase but not progress from G0 to G1. *Nature* **328**, 445–9.

Hockenbery, D., Nunez, G., Milliman, C., Schreiber, R.D. and Korsmeyer, S.J. (1990). *Bcl*-2 is an inner mitochondrial membrane protein that blocks programmed cell death. *Nature* **348**, 334–6.

Hunt, S.P., Pini, A. and Evan, G.I. (1987). Induction of c-*fos*-like protein in spinal cord neurons following sensory stimulation. *Nature (London)* **328**, 632–4.

Hunter, T. (1989). Protein kinase oncogenes. In *Oncogenes and the Molecular Origins of Cancer*, ed. R. Weinberg, pp. 147–73, Cold Spring Harbour Laboratory Press.

Jones, N. (1990). Transcriptional regulation by dimerization: two sides to an incestuous relationship. *Cell* **61**, 9–11.

Karim, F., Urness, L.D., Thummel, C.S. *et al.* (1990). The ETS-domain: a new DNA-binding motif that recognizes a purine-rich core DNA sequence. *Genes Dev.* **4**, 1451–3.

Kelly, K., Cochran, B.H., Stiles, C.D. and Leder, P. (1983). Cell specific regulation of the c-*myc* gene by lymphocyte mitogens and platelet-derived growth factor. *Cell* **35**, 603–10.

Levine, A.J. (1990). Tumor suppressor genes. *Bioessays* **12**, 60–6.

McCormick, F. (1989). *Ras* oncogenes. In *Oncogenes and the Molecular Origins of Cancer*, ed. R. Weinberg, pp. 125–45, Cold Spring Harbour Laboratory Press.

Mustelin, T., Coggeshall, K.M. and Altman, A. (1989). Rapid activation of the T-cell tyrosine protein kinase pp56^{lck} by the CD45 phosphotyrosine phosphatase. *Proc. Nat. Acad. Sci. (USA)* **86**, 6302–6.

Ness, S.A., Marknell, A. and Graf, T. (1989). The v-*myb* oncogene product binds to and activates the promyelocyte-specific *mim*-1 gene. *Cell* **59**, 1115–25.

Pierce, J. (1989). Oncogenes, growth factors and haematopoietic transformation. *Biochem. Biophys. Acta* **989**, 179–208.

Reth, M. (1991). Signal transduction in B cells. *Curr. Biol.* **3**, 340–4.

Rudd, C. (1990). CD4, CD8 and the TCR-CD3 complex: a novel class of protein–tyrosine kinase receptor. *Immunol. Today* **11**, 400–5.

Ryseck, R.P., Hirai, S.I., Yaniv, M. and Bravo, R. (1988). Transcriptional activation of c-*jun* during the G0/G1 transition in mouse fibroblasts. *Nature* **334**, 535–7.

Sefton, B. (1990). The *lck* tyrosine protein kinase. *Oncogene* **6**, 683–6.

Weston, K. and Bishop, J.M. (1989). Transcriptional activation by the v-myb oncogene and its cellular progenitor, c-myb. *Cell* **58**, 85–93.

Zipfel, P.F., Irving, S.G., Kelly, K. and Siebenlist, U. (1989). Complexity of the primary genetic response to mitogenic activation of human T cells. **9**, 1041–8.

92: Tumour-associated Antigens

N.D. James and K. Sikora

Introduction

The concept that the immune system is involved in defence against cancer is not a new one, dating back to ideas first put forward by Ehrlich in 1909. These concepts were reinforced by observations of dramatic reductions in advanced cancer using bacterial extracts by William Coley — possibly the earliest example of immunotherapy in the literature. The concept of tumour surveillance has had a chequered history. It is based on two lines of evidence. Animal data clearly show that the immune system has the ability to identify and reject experimental tumours. The human data are more conflicting, coming from patients with either congenital or acquired immunodeficiency states. Such patients do not have an increased incidence of the common epithelial malignancies, but do have a marked excess of certain rare cancers, in particular, poorly differentiated lymphomas. Until recently this was taken as evidence that tumour surveillance was not a significant factor in the common human tumours. More recently, however, the use of the recombinant cytokine interleukin 2 (IL-2) (Rosenberg 1986) has demonstrated that the immune system, with manipulation, does have the capacity to recognize and eliminate advanced cancers in humans, once more raising the possibility that the immune system does have a central role in the control of tumour development. Ehrlich's dream of effective immunotherapy of cancer may still be feasible.

The antigens found on tumour cells may be considered under two main headings:

1 Antigens not normally expressed in the 'host' animal such as virus antigens, e.g. hepatitis B, Epstein–Barr virus (EBV) and tumour neoantigens, termed tumour-specific transplantation antigens (TSTAs). The latter can be detected in experimental systems by rejection assays. They are not normally present in the 'host' cells. Although viral deoxyribonucleic acid (DNA) may be integrated into the host DNA and be present in cells other than the tumour, it cannot be considered part of the normal genetic material.

2 Normal cellular antigens, expressed either appropriately, such as prostate-specific antigen, or inappropriately, for example differentiation antigens such as the common acute lymphatic leukaemia antigen (CALLA) or embryonic antigens such as carcinoembryonic antigen (CEA). In addition an antigen may be present in the correct tissue but in abnormally high amounts (e.g.

epidermal growth factor receptor (EGFR) in breast cancer). Alternatively, a normal cell antigen such as adrenocorticotrophic hormone (ACTH) may be detected in an inappropriate site such as small-cell lung cancer. The essential feature of these antigens is that the DNA coding for it is normal cellular DNA.

The first group comprises the group of tumour antigens on which most of the 'classical' tumour immunology has been performed. The latter group has become increasingly important with the advent of monoclonal antibodies as a means of diagnosis and of classifying tumours. In addition, they shed valuable light on tumour biology, for example, the process of leukaemogenesis.

Neoantigens — tumour-specific transplantation antigens

Tumour-specific transplantation antigens are defined in rejection assays, which involve the immunization of groups of syngeneic animals with tumour cell extracts or inactivated whole cells. These immunized animals are subsequently challenged with viable cells from the same tumour, the end-points being the cell dose necessary to establish the tumour or the reduction of tumour growth rate in the immune animals as compared with the non-immune animal (Fig. 92.1). Such experiments are clearly not possible in man so no direct evidence on the existence or otherwise of TSTAs in man exists. Indirect evidence, for example, immune infiltrates in tumours, spontaneous regressions of tumours and more recently responses to adoptive immunotherapy with IL-2 and lymphokine-activated killer (LAK) cells suggest that they do exist in human tumours. In the next section, the animal models of TSTAs will be examined and their relationship to human cancers discussed.

Chemically induced tumours

Several points have emerged from experiments involving chemically induced tumours. The first is that for a given animal model, the TSTAs induced by a carcinogen are highly polymorphic, to the extent that each tumour can be regarded as expressing a unique TSTA (Prehn and Main 1957). The TSTAs induced vary in immunogenicity from very strong to very weak (Table 92.1) according to the carcinogen and the tumour induced. It is of interest that spontaneous tumours, in general, tend to be poorly immunogenic. This suggests that the model may be not of general applicability to spontaneously arising human tumours. On the other hand, many human cancers do arise under the influence of known chemical carcinogens; in particular, cigarette smoke contains a variety of polycyclic hydrocarbons similar to those producing strongly immunogenic tumours in animal models.

The chemical nature of carcinogen-induced tumour antigens has proved elusive. This is due to a general failure to raise antibodies of the relevant specificity. Tumour-specific monoclonal antibodies have not helped to characterize the molecular nature of the disparate antigenic determinants evoked.

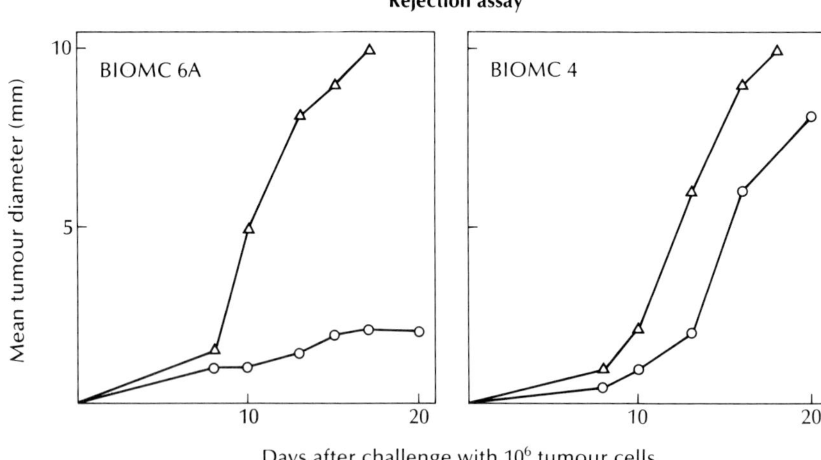

Fig. 92.1. Growth rate reduction of a tumour by immunization.

Table 92.1. Relative strength of tumour-specific transplantation antigens in various experimental murine tumours

Oncogenic agent	Tumour type	TSTA
Chemical carcinogens		
Methylcholanthrene	Sarcoma	Strong to weak
	Squamous cell carcinoma	Strong to weak
	Bladder carcinoma	Strong
	Mammary carcinoma	Weak
	In vitro transformed	Weak
Other polycylic hydrocarbons	Sarcoma	Strong
	Squamous cell carcinoma	Strong
Amino azo dyes, e.g. dimethylaminoazobenzene	Hepatoma	Strong
Aromatic amines, e.g. 2-acetylaminofluorene	Mammary carcinoma	Weak
Alkylnitrosamines, e.g.	Hepatoma	Weak
diethylnitrosamine	Hepatoma	Strong to weak
Inert plastic film	Sarcoma	Weak
	Squamous cell carcinoma	Weak
UV light	Sarcoma	Strong
	Squamous cell carcinoma	Strong
Ionizing radiation	Sarcoma	Weak
	Squamous cell carcinoma	Weak
Spontaneous	Various	Weak or undetectable

There have been several exceptions where tumour-specific antibodies have been prepared (De Leo *et al*. 1977). In addition, without the benefit of completely specific serology, some attempt has been made on the partial purification of these antigens. In one case, a comparison was made of the lectin-binding properties of tumour antigens solubilized from membranes of two non-cross-reacting tumours of a B10 mouse by using a classical transplantation assay. These antigens were alike in not binding to concanavalin A sepharose but in binding specifically to wheat germ agglutinin sepharose. In this regard, they were both unlike H_2 antigens, which have the opposite binding characteristics (Sikora *et al*. 1979). In another case, a partially purified TSTA from a murine tumour, Meth A, was used to prepare an antiserum in rabbits, which after extensive absorption by injection into a normal mouse was specific for the immunizing tumour. By following Meth A-specific transplantation activity and reaction with Meth A-specific antiserum during extensive purification, the protein with TSTA activity was characterized as one of about 60 000 daltons with the electrophoretic mobility of an α-globulin.

So far, there has been no similar isolation of an antigen from another independent tumour. The main source of 'noise' in studying the serology of TSTAs has been the presence of antibodies to ribonucleic acid (RNA) tumour viruses, which are ubiquitous in the host animal. To avoid confusing antiviral specificities with specificities due to TSTAs, it is essential to know the virus status of tumours as well as the presence of various allo-antigens and differentiation antigens. Attempts to raise monoclonal antibodies to specific TSTAs has produced reagents which react to glycoprotein 70 (GP70) (Lennox 1980). Since it is now known that these glycoproteins found so frequently on murine tumour cells may exhibit antigenic variation due to genetic recombination, it is tempting to speculate that the variety of TSTAs arises in a similar way. If recombination in RNA tumour virus genes is the source of variety in the tumour-specific antigens of murine tumours, this variety may be absent from human cancer, for there is no evidence that they display similar proteins.

Virus-induced tumours

Tumours induced by viruses also express antigens that are not found in the uninfected host cells. The tumour antigens expressed are consistent within a given system and are virally encoded. As with chemically induced tumours, the immunogenicity of the virus-induced tumour varies between different models. Since the viral antigens expressed are the same whether the tumour is of high or low immunogenicity, the difference between strongly and weakly immunogenic model systems must lie not with the TSTAs, in this case the viral antigens, but in the host response to them. The virally induced tumours thus provide a means of studying the host factors which determine the immunogenicity of a tumour.

An example of such a system is the induction of tumour formation in mouse cells by simian virus 40 (SV40). Infection of mouse cells *in vitro* results in transformation of the cell line. However, when the transformed cells are introduced into immunocompetent animals they are rejected and fail to establish tumours (Gooding 1982). The cells responsible for rejecting the tumours are cytotoxic T lymphocytes. Further experiments showed that these cells exhibit Class I major histocompatibility complex (MHC)-restricted killing. More specifically, the capacity to respond to the SV40 antigens on the transformed cells is restricted to the K^k MHC antigen.

If SV40-transformed cells are passaged repeatedly in immunosuppressed animals, in which tumour formation can occur, they eventually acquire the ability to form tumours readily in the immunocompetent animals in which they were formerly rejected. These non-immunogenic transformed cells are not lysed *in vitro* by anti-SV40-specific T cells (Gooding 1982). These immunoselected cells consistently fail to express the K^k antigen due to a rearrangement in the region of the K^k gene locus (Rogers *et al*. 1983).

No human tumour induced by SV40 has been described. However, the closely related human papillomaviruses (HPVs) are strongly implicated in the aetiology of cervical cancer (reviewed by Munoz *et al*. 1988). Viral antigens can be detected immunologically on the cell membrane. Interestingly, only HPV 16 and 18 are thought to be involved in carcinogenesis; other serotypes, notably HPV 6 and 11, are detected more frequently than would be expected in abnormal smears but do not appear to be premalignant (Munoz *et al*. 1988). This suggests that differences in antigenicity determine the clinical behaviour in this human tumour system, a finding in keeping with the above observations in animal systems.

Another human virus which can produce both benign and malignant cellular proliferations is EBV. Infection with the virus can be asymptomatic or produce infectious mononucleosis with a non-malignant mononuclear cell proliferation. Epstein–Barr virus is strongly implicated in two human cancers — nasopharyngeal carcinoma (Miller 1983) and Burkitt's lymphoma (d'The *et al*. 1983). In both diseases, the virus becomes integrated into the cellular DNA and viral capsid antigens are not detectable in the cells. However, EBV-specific surface antigens are detectable in the majority of cells (Klein 1972) and may thus be regarded as TSTAs for these tumours.

The role of major histocompatibility complex antigens

Similar results to those outlined above have been obtained in a variety of other tumour systems (reviewed by Tanaka *et al*. 1988b). This strongly suggests that the reason that tumours are not identified and rejected lies not in the absence of TSTAs but in the lack of expression of the appropriate MHC antigen necessary for T cell recognition and killing. Further evidence for this comes from studies in which the induced expression of an MHC antigen reverses the metastatic phenotype of a cell line. Plaksin *et al*. (1988), working with the murine Lewis lung carcinoma, showed that highly metastatic clones expressed greatly reduced levels of the $H\text{-}2K^b$ Class I MHC antigen, whilst weakly metastasizing clones expressed high levels of this antigen. The $H\text{-}2K^b$ gene was then transfected into highly metastatic clones, which became converted into weakly metastasizing clones. Furthermore, immunization of animals with these $H\text{-}2K^b$ +ve clones protected the animal from subsequent challenge with $H\text{-}2K^b$ −ve clones from the highly metastasic cell lines and also brought about the rejection of established tumours. This suggests that, once the relevant T cell clone has identified the abnormal cell antigen and expanded, a process facilitated by the appropriate Class I MHC antigen, other cells expressing the same abnormal antigen can be identified and lysed even in the absence of significant amounts of the MHC antigen necessary for the initial recognition process.

Similar results have been obtained by Tanaka *et al.* (1988a) using the poorly immunogenic B16 melanoma cell line, which readily establishes tumours in immunocompetent animals. In this case, transfection into the tumour cells of a Class I MHC H-2K antigen but not a Class II MHC I-A antigen abrogated the tumorigenic potential of the tumour. Immunization with the H-2K-transfected cells brought about the rejection of established tumours and prevented the establishment of new tumours. As in the previous example, these results suggest that the tumour does express a TSTA but that it is not recognized because of the lack of expression of the appropriate MHC antigen. These results show that a spontaneously occurring, poorly immunogenic tumour can be rendered immunogenic by an *in vitro* manipulation and that, once recognition of the tumour by the appropriate T cell has occurred, expression of the relevant MHC antigen is not necessary for recognition of other tumour cells.

The immunogenicity of a cell — and thus its ability to establish tumours in immunocompetent animals — is determined not only by its TSTAs but by whether or not the cell expresses the MHC antigen necessary for T cell recognition of the TSTA. If this applies to human cancers it would be expected that human tumours would express low levels of Class I MHC human leucocyte antigens (HLA). This does appear to be the case, with many human tumours expressing low levels of Class I MHC HLA (Travers *et al.* 1980). Various lung tumours (Doyle *et al.* 1985), breast tumours (Fleming *et al.* 1981), neuroblastomas (Lampson *et al.* 1983) and skin tumours have been examined. Furthermore, a series of benign epidermal lesions showed normal Class I MHC antigen expression whereas a series of 15 basal cell carcinomas lacked both Class I MHC antigens and β-microglobulin (Holden *et al.* 1983). Similar results have been obtained with squamous cell carcinomas of the skin.

It has been known for some time that the interferons modulate the expression of Class I MHC antigens (Wallach *et al.* 1982). The effect of interferon appears to be at the level of gene transcription. This effect appears to be mediated via an interferon response sequence in the region of the MHC gene (Friedman and Stark 1985). Other cytokines such as tumour necrosis factor (TNF) have also been shown to induce MHC gene expression (Collins *et al.* 1986). Amplification of the N-myc oncogene also induces down-regulation of Class I MHC antigens in neuroblastoma cell lines (Bernards *et al.* 1986). N-myc amplification strongly correlates with prognosis and stage in neuroblastoma with the exception of Evans stage IV-S disease, which presents with advanced-stage disease but which regresses spontaneously and in which N-myc amplification is not found (Brodeur *et al.* 1984).

Tumour-infiltrating lymphocytes

Further evidence that tumours express unique antigens that can be recognized as foreign comes from work done by Rosenberg *et al.* (1986, 1988) with tumour-infiltrating lymphocytes (TILs). In experimental systems, lymphocytes contained within the tumour can be expanded in tissue culture with IL-2. These TILs are 50–100 times as potent in lysing target tumour cells than are IL-2-expanded peripheral blood lymphocytes (LAK cells). In experimental systems, both LAK cells and TILs are effective in eliminating advanced tumours; however, the TILs will effectively treat tumours that do not respond to LAK cells, in keeping with the differences in *in vitro* cytotoxicity.

The above lines of evidence suggest that, even when no TSTAs can be demonstrated by conventional means, they are likely to be present in a significant number of tumours. In addition, manipulation of other aspects of the target cells — the expression of MHC antigens — allows the recognition of these hitherto 'silent' TSTAs even in spontaneous human cancers. Taken as a whole, these results suggest not only that effective immunotherapy is a possibility, but also that the tools necessary for it to work clinically, such as gene transfer and therapeutic quantities of cytokines, are now becoming available.

Host-derived antigens

Parent-tissue-derived differentiation antigens

Parent-tissue-derived differentiation antigens may be further subdivided into antigens found on mature cells of the parent tissue and antigens expressed transiently during differentiation. The best studied example of the latter group are the lymphocyte antigens. Monoclonal antibodies to CD45, the leucocyte common antigen (LCA), distinguish lymphoid from non-lymphoid proliferations (Warnke *et al.* 1983). The availability of monoclonal antibodies directed against various lymphocyte antigens enables subpopulations of morphologically similar cells to be distinguished by immunohistological means. For example, antibodies to T, B and natural killer (NK) cells, plus a variety of T cell differentiation antigens, allow extensive subclassification of malignant lymphomas and leukaemias as well as distinguishing between reactive and malignant lymphoid infiltrates (reviewed by Bobrow and Norton 1987). This information has shed valuable light on the biology of leukaemias and lymphomas as well as being a valuable tool for the pathologist.

Monoclonal antibodies may also be used to shed light on the histogenesis of non-lymphoid tumours. Antibodies recognizing epithelial antigens such as low-molecular-weight cytokeratins (CAM5.2) or epithelial membrane antigen (HMFG2) are reliable indicators of epithelial origin in morphologically undifferentiated tumours (Bobrow and Norton 1987). Similarly, antibodies to intermediate filaments, such as vimentin, which are present in mesenchymal tissues can serve as sarcoma markers. The use of panels of such antibodies is proving of great value in classifying specimens whose tissue of origin cannot be determined on morphological grounds alone, e.g. undifferentiated tumours and aspirates from various sites, and in the assessment of micrometastases, for example in the bone marrow. At present, there are few antigens which indicate the precise tissue of origin as opposed to its broad lineage. Perhaps the best current examples are prostate-specific antigen and thyroglobulin.

Aberrently expressed differentiation antigens

A variety of antigens can be expressed on tumour cells that are not normally expressed in the parent tissue. Tumours that produce ectopic hormones, for example small-cell lung carcinoma (SCLC), can be shown by immunohistological means to be expressing the ectopic hormone on the cell surface. Indeed, a higher proportion of SCLC cases have immunologically detectable adrenocorticotrophic hormone (ACTH) than produce clinically significant quantities of the hormone (Gewirtz and Yalow 1974). Here the abnormal antigen is a marker for an underlying abnormal process, namely inappropriate hormone production, rather than a cell surface antigen in its own right.

Similarly, the expression of oncogene products can be detected by immunological means. A range of oncogene products can be detected in this way (Table 92.2). In some cases, e.g. c-myc, the gene product is nuclear-acting and thus its detection at the cell surface by monoclonal antibodies, like the ACTH example above, reflects an underlying abnormality. In other cases, however, the oncogene product is a cell surface component, for example the c-erbB gene product is EGFR. This is expressed in abnormal amounts in a variety of malignancies, including breast and bladder cancer. In breast cancer, EGFR expression correlates with poor prognosis better than other more traditional markers, such as oestrogen receptor (ER) status (Sainsbury *et al.* 1987). Furthermore, unlike ER status, where initial progress is different but ultimate survival is the same in both groups, EGFR +ve patients have a consistently poorer prognosis than those with EGFR −ve tumours. This suggests that the presence of the EGFR allows the tumour cell to be 'driven' to divide more aggressively.

Another oncogene product with considerable prognostic potential is the protein encoded by c-

Table 92.2. Conditions associated with a raised CEA

Carcinoma
Gastrointestinal tract
Lung
Breast
Kidney
Testes
Glioma
Benign
Colonic polyp
Inflammatory ulcerative colitis
Peptic ulcer
Pancreatitis
Hepatitis
Other
Pernicious anaemia
Ataxia telangiectasia
Heavy cigarette smoking

erbB2. This is also a transmembrane molecule, similar in structure to EGFR. It almost certainly acts as a receptor for an as yet unknown ligand. The expression of c-erbB2 has been clearly correlated with poor prognosis in breast cancer. Indeed, even after patients relapse with local or distant metastases, there is a marked difference in eventual outcome depending on the original tumour's c-erbB2 status. This implies that the expression of this gene is important in determining the natural history of a tumour in an individual (reviewed by Gullick and Venter 1988).

Oncogenes have the potential to act as tumour antigens in other ways. Gene amplification has been detected for a variety of oncogenes and this results in increased expression of their products. In addition rearrangements and differences in intron–exon splicing could result in new sequences becoming available in the encoded proteins. This could result in novel antigenic determinants being expressed which may be recognized as tumour-associated antigens. No such novel structures have been found so far on the external surface of the cell membrane.

The above examples indicate how antigens detectable at the cell surface can provide information about events occurring at a nuclear level. Such information is useful as the techniques required to demonstrate the presence of these antigens are simple to use and reproducible.

Embryonic antigens

One of the earliest tumour antigens described was CEA (Gold and Freeman 1956). This is present on fetal colon and colorectal carcinomas in addition to a range of other malignancies (Table 92.2). It can also be detected in the serum and it was initially hoped that CEA could be used as a tumour marker. Its use as a screening test is precluded by lack of specificity for malignant disease. It can be used to follow the course of an individual patient's disease when the CEA is raised at presentation; unfortunately, however, the early detection of recurrence does not necessarily aid management in the absence of effective measures for metastatic disease.

Alpha-fetoprotein (AFP), which is in fact an embryonic equivalent of albumen, and beta human chorionic gonadotrophin (β-HCG) can also be detected on the cells and in the serum in a variety of malignancies, including germ cell tumours and hepatocellular carcinomas. Again they are not specific enough for use as screening tests but are invaluable as part of the follow-up for germ cell tumours, where it is now practice to treat rising levels of AFP and β-HCG as indicative of recurrence in the absence of any other clinical evidence (reviewed by Lange and Fraley 1982). Alpha-fetoprotein and β-HCG expression on the cell surface can be demonstrated by immunohistology and can thus be used as an aid to diagnosis in marker −ve patients. As with the ectopic ACTH example above, AFP and β-HCG do not have to be detectable in the serum to be present on the cell membrane.

In a sense, embryonic antigens are similar to transiently expressed differentiation antigens in that their expression is appropriate to the tissue. They differ in that differentiation antigens are present in the adult whereas embryonic antigens are not.

The importance of all tumour antigens of host origin lies in the light they shed on the underlying pathological processes. This can vary from indicating the tissue of origin of a tumour when this is not apparent on morphological grounds, to revealing aspects of cell function, e.g. ectopic hormone production, to providing insights into oncogene expression. Thus the study of tumour antigens can be useful both as a research tool and as an aid to diagnosis and management.

Clinical relevance of tumour-associated antigens

The detection and characterization of human tumour-associated antigens have wide implications for both the diagnosis and the therapy of cancer.

Diagnosis

The use of antibodies to determine the lineage of a cell has already been discussed. Although the light-microscopic appearance of tissue sections is sufficient in most cases to provide an unequivocal diagnosis, this is not always the case. An undifferentiated carcinoma and a lymphoma may have similar appearances to the histopathologist; yet the choice of therapy and the prognosis for the two diseases are radically different. Furthermore, the recognition of variants of major diseases is also vital if our understanding of tumour biology is to be used in devising new approaches to treatment (Plate 92.1, between pages 1930 and 1931). In the case of non-Hodgkins lymphoma, for example, at least 15 different varieties can be recognized with a wide spectrum of clinical outcome. Highly purified conventional polyclonal antibodies reacting against certain tumour types can be labelled with specific reagents in order to make the identification of subpopulations within the tumour more readily visible. Monoclonal antibodies have added to the usefulness of immunohistology by increasing the specificity and reliability of the antibodies available. In addition to recognizing cell types, subpopulations can also be identified. This has proved useful in distinguishing different types of B and T cell lymphoma.

The development of metastatic disease is the main cause of treatment failure in the management of patients with solid tumours. The accurate detection of metastases would be a great advantage. Although some tumours shed reliable tumour markers, these are the minority. Extensive studies looking for tumour-associated antigens shed into the blood have identified new glycoprotein markers for ovarian, lung and gastrointestinal cancer (Fig. 92.3). Here again, the advent of the monoclonal technology has increased the potential of novel assays for tumour markers.

Antibodies to tumour-associated antigens may also be useful in the localization of malignant disease. If an antigen is expressed in high quantity on a tumour cell surface, it should be possible to produce an antibody that binds to the tumour cell with higher affinity than to other tissues present in the body. When injected into a patient with cancer, such an antibody will ultimately bind to tumour cell membranes. If prior to injection the antibody is labelled with a radio-isotope such as ^{131}I, then conventional nuclear medicine techniques can be used to scan the patient externally and locate areas of relatively high uptake. Such areas will correspond to areas of tumour deposits. Several groups have now shown that suitably labelled monoclonals can localize colorectal and ovarian cancer and melanoma as well as a variety of other tumours (Plate 92.2, between pages 1930 and 1931).

Most techniques involve giving a very small dose of antibody, usually 1 mg, most of which continues to circulate in the blood pool. With most anti-tumour antibodies, less than 0.5% actually deposit on neoplastic cells, the rest being cleared by the liver and the reticuloendothelial system. This has led to the use of labelled secondary blood pool imaging agents, such as serum albumen, which allow computerized subtraction of the circulating component. This further detracts from image clarity and can introduce considerable artefact.

Recently, there have been some remarkable advances in the technology of antibody design by a combination of gene shuffling and protein engineering. Molecules with high affinity for their target

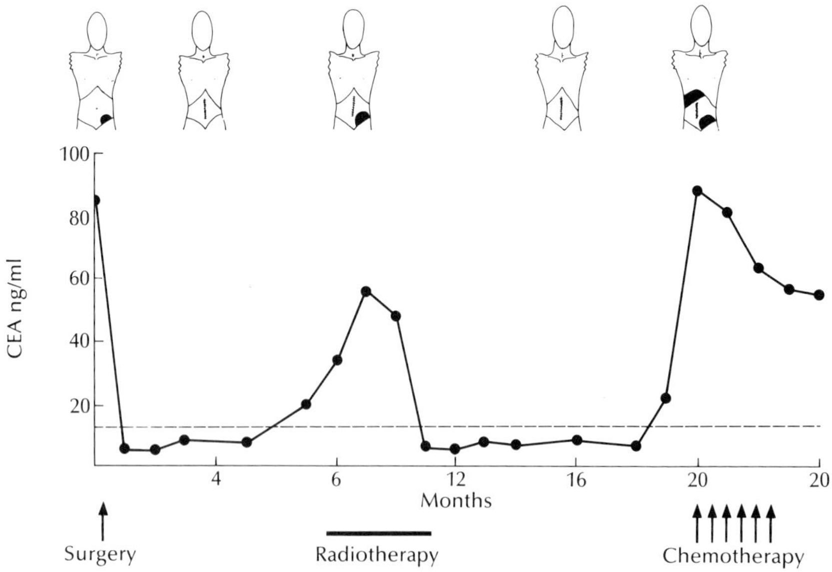

Fig. 92.2. The use of a monoclonal antibody assay for carcinoembryonic antigen (CEA) in a patient with colorectal carcinoma. The CEA level is high at the time of initial presentation, declines following surgery but rises with subsequent relapses.

Table 92.3. Antibody availability to human oncoproteins

Oncoprotein	Antibody	Immunohistology	Manufacturer
pan myc	Sheep PCA	+	CRB
c-myc	Sheep PCA	+	CRB
	Mouse MCA	+	CRB
	Sheep PCA	?	BIOTX
	Sheep PCA	?	ONCOR
N-myc	Sheep PCA	+	CRB
L-myc	Sheep PCA	?	CRB
K-ras	Mouse MCA	+	CETUS
N-ras	Mouse MCA	+	CETUS
H-ras	Mouse MCA	+	CETUS
	Sheep PCA	?	BIOTX
	Sheep PCA	?	ONCOR
C-ras	Mouse MCA	+	CETUS
	Sheep PCA	?	BIOTX
C-ras ser12	Mouse MCA	?	CETUS
C-ras val12	Mouse MCA	?	CETUS
C-ras arg12	Mouse MCA	?	CETUS
C-ras asp12	Mouse MCA	?	CETUS
pan-fos	Sheep PCA	+	CRB
c-fos	Sheep PCA	+	CRB
	Sheep PCA	+	BIOTX
c-src	Mouse MCA	?	ONCOR
c-myb	Sheep PCA	?	CRB
c-fms	Rabbit PCA	?	CRB
c-mos	Rabbit PCA	?	CRB
c-erbB1	Mouse MCA	?	AMERSHAM
c-erbB1	Mouse MCA	?	ONCOR
c-erbB1	Rabbit PCA	+	CRB

PCA = polyclonal antibody; MCA = monoclonal antibody.

antigen can be designed. Hybridoma cell lines producing an antibody of moderate activity can be specifically engineered to produce a much improved version. The molecule can be made smaller so it can easily penetrate the extravascular space surrounding its target. Foreign species determinants can be replaced by human counterparts, thus humanizing a mouse or rat product and reducing the risk of a secondary response. These newer agents are currently undergoing extensive clinical trials.

Therapy

The immunotherapy of cancer has a chequered history and is considered in detail in Chapter 94. The immunological development of specific active therapy requires a detailed understanding of the structure and configuration of tumour-associated antigens. So far, most therapeutic attempts have been based on empirical observations using antibodies or cell-mediated cytotoxicity.

Serotherapy for cancer using conventional antibodies raised against tumour-associated antigens was attempted 50 years ago. Most sera have poor specificity and low titre against their putative antigens. Monoclonals can overcome some of these problems and have the added advantage of consistency in production. Drugs, toxins and radionuclides can be coupled to monoclonals in such a way that their immunological activity remains unaltered. The antibody therefore provides the targeting mechanism whilst the coupled agent acts as the warhead. An agent suitable for cancer therapy must be expected to destroy any cell with which it comes into contact and therefore the unselected destruction of normal tissue would be dangerous. This requires considerable selectivity on the part of the antibody. A variety of antibodies have now been used for therapy, so far with only limited success.

Another approach has been bone marrow purging. The response of normal bone marrow to many conventionally available cytotoxic agents is often critical in determining the amount of chemotherapy that can be employed in a particular patient. One therapeutic tactic to overcome marrow toxicity is to store the patient's bone marrow in the laboratory prior to giving a normally supralethal dose of cytotoxic drug. The patient then receives an autologous bone marrow transplant (ABMT). Unfortunately, if their marrow harvested prior to chemotherapy contains malignant cells, these will be reintroduced into the patient. A variety of intriguing systems have been developed to utilize monoclonal antibodies to destroy tumour cells in the bone marrow. Such bone marrow-purging techniques do not require a high degree of specificity necessary for systemic administration of antibody. In breast cancer, for example, antibodies that react with all epithelial cells can be used effectively to purge the marrow. The major limitation to ABMT with purging is the paucity of evidence that chemotherapy dose escalation results in a significant increase in cure.

Although the antigens recognized by antibodies currently in clinical trial for therapy can be relatively well defined biochemically, those seen by cellular targets are less well characterized. Indeed, the current biological approaches to cancer, whilst producing intriguing clinical results, have little molecular background. This explains the difficulty in understanding and quantitating some of the recent observations.

The further molecular characterization of tumour-associated antigens may well assist in the development of logical therapeutic strategies in the future.

References

Bernards, R., Dessain, S.K. and Weinberg, R.A. (1986). N-myc amplification causes down-modulation of MHC class 1 antigen expression in neuroblastoma. *Cell* **47**, 667–74.

Bobrow, L.G. and Norton, A.J. (1987). Immunohistology in the identification of tumour types. *Cancer Surv.* **6** (2), 209–25.

Brodeur, G.M., Seeger, R.C., Schwab, M., Varmus, H.E. and Bishop, J.M. (1984). Amplification of N-myc in untreated neuroblastoma correlates with advanced disease stage. *Science* **224**, 1121–4.

Collins, T., Lapierre, L.A., Fiers, W., Strominger, J.L. and Pober, J.S. (1986). Recombinant human tumour necrosis factor increases mRNA levels and surface expression of HLA-A,B antigens in vascular endothelial cells and dermal fibroblasts *in vitro*. *Proc. Nat. Acad. Sci. (USA)* **83**, 446–50.

De Leo, A.B., Shiku, H., Takahashi, T., John, M. and Old, L.J. (1977). Cell surface antigens of chemically induced sarcomas of the mouse. *J. Exp. Med.* **146**, 720–9.

d'The, G., Ho, J.H.C. and Muir, C.S. (1983). Nasopharyngeal carcinoma. In *Viral Infections of Humans*. ed. A.F. Evans, pp. 621–52, Plenum Medical Book Company, New York.

Doyle, A., Martin, W.J., Funa, K. *et al.* (1985). Markedly decreased expression of class I histocompatibility antigens, protein and mRNA in human small cell lung cancer. *J. Exp. Med.* **161**, 1135–51.

Fleming, K.A., McMichael, A., Morton, J.A., Woods, J.K. and McGee, J.O.D. (1981). Distribution of HLA class 1 antigens in normal human tissue and in mammary cancer. *J. Clin. Pathol.* **34**, 779–84.

Friedman, R.L. and Stark, G.R. (1985). Alpha-interferon induced transcription of HLA and meta-althionein genes containing homologous upstream sequences. *Nature* **314**, 637–9.

Gewirtz, G. and Yalow, R.S. (1974). Ectopic ACTH production in carcinoma of the lung. *J. Clin. Invest.* **53**, 1022–32.

Gold, P. and Freeman S.O. (1956). Specific carcinoembryonic antigens of the human digestive system. *J. Exp. Med.* **122**, 467–75.

Gooding, L.R. (1982). Characterisation of a progressive tumour from C3H fibroblasts transformed *in vitro* with SV40 virus: immunoresistance *in vivo* correlates with phenotypic loss of H-2K^k. *J. Immunol.* **129**, 1306–12.

Gullick, W.J. and Venter, D.J. (1988). The c-erbB2 gene and its expression in human tumours. In *The Molecular Biology of Cancer*, ed. K. Sikora and J. Waxman, Blackwell Scientific Publication, Oxford.

Holden, C.A., Sanderson, A.R. and MacDonald, D.M. (1983). Absence of human leukocyte antigen molecules in skin tumours and some cutaneous appendages: evidence using monoclonal antibodies. *J. Am. Acad. Dermatol.* **9**, 867–71.

Klein, G. (1972). Herpesviruses and oncogenesis. *Proc. Nat. Acad. Sci. (USA)* **69**, 1056–64.

Lampson, L.A., Fisher, C.A. and Whelan, J.P. (1983). Striking paucity of HLA-A,B,C and beta$_2$-microglobulin on human neuroblastoma cell lines. *J. Immunol.* **130**, 2471–8.

Lange, P.H. and Fraley, E.E. (1982). Use and misuse of tumour markers in testicular cancer. In *Recent Advances in Clinical Oncology*, ed. C.J. Williams and J.M.A. Whitehouse, pp. 95–107, Churchill Livingstone, Oxford.

Lennox, E.S. (1980). The antigens of chemically induced tumours. In *Immunology 1980 — Progress in Immunology IV*, ed. M. Fougereau, p. 658, Academic Press, London.

Miller, G. (1983). Burkitt lymphoma. In *Viral Infections of Humans*, ed. A.F. Evans, pp. 599–619, Plenum Medical Book Company, New York.

Munoz, N., Bosch, X. and Kaldor, K.M. (1988). Does human papilloma virus cause cervical cancer? The state of the epidemiological evidence. *Br. J. Cancer* **57**, 1–5.

Plaksin, D., Gelber, C., Feldman, M. and Eisenbach, L. (1988). Reversal of the metastatic phenotype in Lewis lung carcinoma cells after transfection with syngeneic H-2K^b gene. *Proc. Nat. Acad. Sci. (USA)* **85**, 4463–7.

Prehn, R. and Main, J.M. (1958). Immunity to methyl cholanthrene-induced sarcomas. *J. Nat. Cancer Inst.* **18**, 769–78.

Rogers, M., Gooding, L.H., Margulies, D.H. and Evans, G.A. (1983). Analysis of a defect in the H-2 genes of SV40 transformed C3H fibroblasts that do not express H-2K^k. *J. Immunol.* **130**, 2418–22.

Rosenberg, S.A., Lotze, M.T., Munt, L.M. *et al.* (1987). A progress report on the treatment of 157 patients with advanced cancer using lymphokine activated killer cells and interleukin-2 or high dose interleukin-2 alone. *N. Engl. J. Med.* **316**, 889–97.

Rosenberg, S.A., Speiss, P. and Lafreniere, R. (1986). A new approach to the adoptive immunotherapy of cancer with tumour-infiltrating lymphocytes. *Science* **233**, 1318–21.

Rosenberg, S.A., Packard, B.S., Aebersold, P.M. *et al.* (1988). Use of tumour-infiltrating lymphocytes and interleukin-2 in immunotherapy of patients with metastatic melanoma. *N. Engl. J. Med.* **319** (25), 1676–80.

Sainsbury, J.R.C., Faraden, J.R., Needham, G.K. (1987). Epidermal growth factor status as predictor of early recurrence of and death from breast cancer. *Lancet* **i**, 1398–402.

Sikora, K., Koch, G., Brenner, S. and Lennox, E. (1979). Partial purification of tumour specific transplantation antigens from methylcholanthrene induced murine sarcomas by immobilised lectins. *Br. J. Cancer* **40**, 8–19.

Tanaka, K., Gorelick, E., Watanabe, M., Hozumi, N. and Jay, G. (1988a). Rejection of B16 melanoma induced by expression of a transfected major histocompatibility complex class 1 gene. *Mol. Cell Biol.* **8** (4), 1857–61.

Tanaka, K., Yoshioka, T., Bieberich, C. and Jay, G. (1988b). Role of the major histocompatibility complex class 1 antigens in tumour growth and metastasis. *Ann. Rev. Immunol.* **6**, 359–80.

Travers, P.J., Arklie, J.L., Trowsdale, J., Patillo, R.A. and Bodmer, W.F. (1980). Lack of expression of HLA-A,B,C antigens in choriocarcinoma and other human tumour cells lines. *Nat. Cancer Inst. Monog.* **60**, 175–80.

Wallach, D., Fellous, M. and Revel, M. (1982). Preferential effect of gamma-interferon on the synthesis of HLA antigens and their mRNAs in human cells. *Nature* **299**, 833–6.

Warnke, R.A., Gatter, K.C., Falini, B. *et al.* (1983). Diagnosis of human lymphoma with monoclonal anti-leucocyte antibodies. *N. Engl. J. Med.* **309**, 1275–81.

93: Immune Responses to Tumours

J.P. Johnson and G. Riethmüller

Introduction

Since its foundation at the turn of the last century, tumour immunology has been inspired by the theory of immune surveillance which was first proposed by Paul Ehrlich and later extended and popularized by Lewis Thomas and Sir MacFarlane Burnet (reviewed in Möller and Möller, 1976). According to this theory, the development of a malignant tumour is associated with changes in the genetic material which lead to the expression of altered molecules. These altered molecules are recognized as foreign by the immune system and the malignant cells are destroyed in the same manner as, for example, virus-infected cells. Since such altered cells presumably arise frequently, the presence of a tumour reflects those rare situations in which immunosurveillance has failed.

In the decades since this theory was proposed, a great deal has been learned about the nature of the malignant cell and about how cells are recognized by the immune system. Much of our understanding of the interaction between tumour cells and the immune system continues to come from animal models, where tumours and lymphocytes can be manipulated and where the end result of this interaction, that is, rejection or progressive growth of the tumour, can be assessed. However, the development of procedures for the long-term culture and cloning of antigen-reactive T lymphocytes has opened up the possibility of studying this interaction in human cancer patients also. Although such studies are still in their early stages and have been applied to relatively few tumours, it appears that most tumour patients produce both CD4 and CD8 T lymphocytes which specifically recognize their tumours. However, the origin and nature of the antigens recognized and the interaction between these immune cells *in vivo* remain elusive.

The demonstration of tumour-specific immunity in chemically induced rodent tumours

With the elucidation of the fundamental laws of transplantation immunity and the development of inbred strains of mice in the 1950s, it became possible to transplant tumours and lymphocytes between individuals of the same species and to evaluate tumour immunity. In a now classic study, Prehn and Main (1957) demonstrated that mice bearing methylcholanthrene (MCA)-induced sarcomas specifically recognize their tumours (Fig. 93.1). If tumours are removed at an early stage, these mice recover and are resistant to a second transplant of the same tumour. However, they do not reject normal skin or transplantation of a second tumour arising independently in the same donor mouse. This resistance to tumour growth can be transferred to naïve syngeneic mice with spleen cells of the immune mice but not with their serum, indicating that cell-mediated immunity is responsible for this antitumour activity. An analysis of 25 different tumours induced by MCA in the same inbred mouse strain showed that each tumour was recognized as distinct by the immune system and thus the diversity of tumour-specific antigens appeared endless. These experiments led to the concept that there are tumour-specific transplantation antigens (TSTAs) which are unique to each individual tumour, and which can induce specific immunity leading to tumour rejection. Tumour-specific transplantation antigens have also been demonstrated in rodent tumours induced by other chemicals and by ultraviolet (UV) irradiation. Effector T lymphocytes isolated either from tumour-bearing or from immunized mice have been extensively studied *in vitro*. In MCA-induced tumours both CD8 +ve cytotoxic T lymphocytes (CTL) and CD4 +ve T helper cells can be isolated and shown to be directed against antigens unique to each individual tumour (Howie and

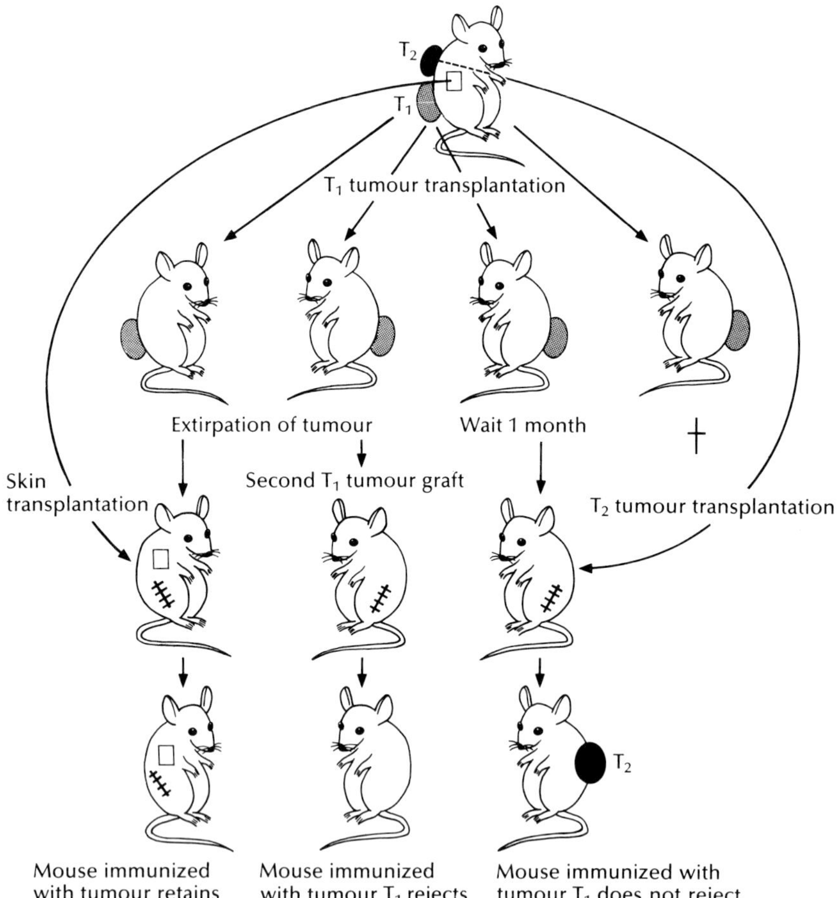

Fig. 93.1. The demonstration of tumour-specific transplantation antigens (TSTAs) in methylcholanthrene-induced sarcomas. T1, T2 are two independently arising tumours in the same mouse.

McBride 1982; Barth *et al.* 1990). Using cloned CTL to select antigen-loss tumour variants in a UV sarcoma also revealed a further level of molecular complexity, namely that individual tumours express multiple independent tumour-unique antigens (Ward *et al.* 1989).

Although TSTAs were long thought to be restricted to certain 'highly immunogenic' experimentally induced tumours, tumour-unique antigens as defined by CTL have now been identified on spontaneously arising murine tumours and on human tumours (Ward *et al.* 1989; Wölfel *et al.* 1989).

The evidence for immune responses against tumours in man

Antibodies

In the 1960s Old and his colleagues demonstrated that approximately 75% of patients with solid tumours have antibodies in their serum which react with their tumours *in vitro* (reviewed in Old 1981). By combining absorption and indirect binding assays they were able to identify antibodies with different specificities. Although most antibodies were reactive with many different autologous and allogeneic cells, some seemed to be reactive only with tumour cells. Most of these antibodies bound to a number of related tumour cell lines but occasionally antibodies were identified which bound only to the patient's own tumour. More recently, it has been possible to analyse antibodies of cancer patients in greater detail by immortalizing the antibody-producing cells through Epstein–Barr virus transformation or cell fusion, thereby providing a source of monoclonal antibody. These analyses have essentially confirmed the original observations. The majority of antibodies are directed against self components which are found in normal as well as malignant cells and many are specific for molecules located within the cytoplasm (Cote *et al.* 1986). Some antibodies are indeed directed against differentiation antigens and tumour-associated molecules which are more restricted in their expression (reviewed in Lloyd and Old 1989). However, in both cases, antibodies with similar specificities are obtained when monoclonal antibodies are produced from normal individuals (Cote *et al.* 1986) and thus their relationship to the presence of a tumour remains unclear.

Cell-mediated immunity

The earliest studies which examined the cellular response of patients to their tumours *in vitro* indicated that most patients recognized their own tumours as well as a range of allogeneic tumours but failed to recognize normal cells (Hellström *et al.* 1968). With the discovery of natural killer (NK) cells and the realization that T cell recognition involves MHC restriction, the interpretation of these data was brought into question. It now seems clear that NK cells are responsible for a major component of the anti-tumour reactivity of lymphocytes of both tumour patients and normal individuals. The cloning of tumour-reactive lymphocytes has revealed, however, that patients also have tumour-specific, generally major histocompatibility complex (MHC)-restricted, T lymphocytes. Many of these studies have been carried out with the cells of melanoma patients, where tumour-specific CTL can be cloned either from the tumour-infiltrating cells or the peripheral blood in more than 70% of patients (reviewed in Parmiani *et al.* 1990). Most of these CTL can be inhibited by antibodies directed to the CD3 complex or to the αβ T cell receptor (TCR) and can be divided into two types: those reactive with human leucocyte antigen (HLA)-matched allogeneic tumours (Darrow *et al.* 1989) and those reactive only with the autologous tumour. These latter CTL appear to recognize unique tumour antigens which are very similar to the TSTAs identified in carcinogen-induced rodent tumours. Analysis of independent CTL clones generated against the same tumour reveal that, like the rodent tumour-unique antigens, individual human tumours also express multiple independent antigens (van den Eynde *et al.* 1989). Using antibody-blocking and HLA-loss variants, the reactivity of these CTL has been shown to be HLA-restricted (Wölfel *et al.* 1989).

What is the nature of the tumour antigens which induce an immune response?

Monoclonal antibodies and cloned CTL are reagents which can be used in a variety of approaches to identify and characterize the antigens which they recognize on tumour cells. Combining these with the technology for expressing foreign deoxyribonucleic acid (DNA) in either prokaryotic or eukaryotic cells has allowed the genes encoding the target antigens that are recognized by antibodies or CTL to be isolated and characterized.

Tumour antigens recognized by antibodies

The antigens recognized by several patient antibodies have been identified. Antibodies directed against tumour-associated antigens with a restricted tissue distribution have been isolated from melanoma and lung cancer patients. Surprisingly, these antibodies are nearly always directed against carbohydrate structures on gangliosides or neutral glycolipids (Lloyd and Old 1989). Tumour cells frequently show a dysregulation in the glycosyl/galactosyl transferases, which leads to the generation of carbohydrate moieties that are not normally expressed by the individual (Hakomori 1985; Metoki *et al.* 1989). Carbohydrate-specific antibodies are common in normal individuals (Castronovo *et al.* 1989) and the presence of malignant cells bearing these epitopes may stimulate their production.

While tumour-unique antigens are most commonly defined by autologous CTL, patient antibodies reacting only with the autologous tumour have also been observed. In one case the molecule recognized by such an antimelanoma antibody has been identified as melanotransferrin, a cell surface iron-binding protein expressed in high amounts on melanoma cells (Furukawa *et al.* 1989). This molecule is not known to be polymorphic and the fact that the antibody does not react with melanotransferrin on allogeneic tumour cells suggests that the molecule is structurally altered (i.e. mutated) in this particular tumour and is recognized as foreign by the patient's immune system.

Tumour antigens recognized by cytotoxic T lymphocytes

Cytotoxic T lymphocytes which lyse allogeneic pancreatic and breast carcinoma cells in an HLA-independent manner can be isolated from pancreatic cancer patients. These cells are CD8 +ve, do not express NK markers, and use αβTCR. By testing the ability of pancreatic carcinoma-reactive monoclonal antibodies to inhibit lysis of such CTL, the target antigen has been identified as a mucin (Barnd *et al.* 1989). Mucins are characteristic of secretory epithelia and are high-molecular-weight molecules with repeated epitopes that are frequently altered in malignant cells so that new epitopes which stimulate antibody production and T cell immunity are created or exposed.

Without question, the most intriguing antigens are the TSTAs and tumour-unique antigens defined by patient CTLs. The fact that these antigens are recognized by T cells which have all the characteristics of classical CTLs and that this recognition requires HLA or H-2 molecules, suggests that the antigens represent peptides that are presented by MHC molecules. It is the diversity of these antigens which is bewildering — not only does each individual tumour have a unique antigen but each tumour has an unknown number of distinct antigens. How such exceedingly diverse antigens might arise is suggested from the analysis of a murine mastocytoma which was exposed to a mutagen *in vitro* and then examined for its *in vivo* growth characteristics (Fig. 93.2; Boon *et al.* 1989). Some of the mutagenized clones lost the ability to produce tumours in syngeneic mice and were therefore called tum −ve. These cells were found to express a new antigen which was recognized by MHC-restricted CTL and led to tumour destruction *in vivo*. The genes encoding these new antigens have been cloned from three independent tum −ve clones. In each case the 'tumour antigen' has been created by a single amino acid change in a different cytoplasmic protein.

The importance of this study is that it indicates that point mutations in any of a variety of cellular proteins can generate new peptides which bind to autologous MHC molecules and induce T cell responses. These tumour antigens were generated by exposure of cells to a mutagen, a step which is generally considered to be involved in human carcinogenesis as well (Weinberg 1989). In any case, DNA analyses indicate that multiple genetic changes characterize malignant tumours of both experimental and spontaneous origin. While many of these changes may be unique to a given tumour (and perhaps even to tumour cell subpopulations), some may be common to allogeneic tumours of related types since genetic changes typical of certain tumours can be identified (Vogelstein *et al.* 1989). Thus it is possible that genetic changes occurring during tumour development can lead to the generation of both unique and shared tumour antigens. The identification of an antibody-defined tumour-unique

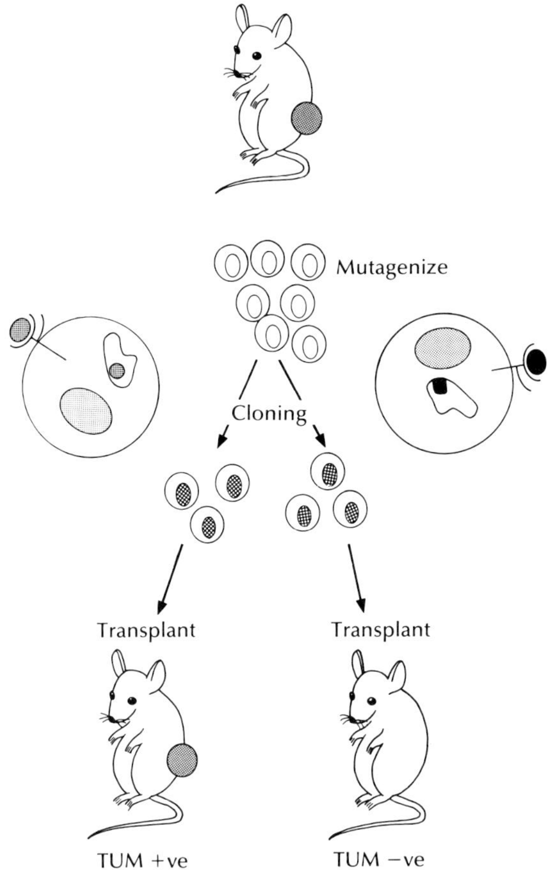

Fig. 93.2. The tum −ve mutations. Exposure of tumour cells to a mutagen *in vitro* followed by cloning and transplantation into syngeneic mice. Mutation of some tumour clones results in cells which no longer form a tumour *in vivo* (tum −ve). These cells have a mutation in a cellular protein (shown in black, as opposed to the normal self peptide in the tum +ve cells, shown as striped), which is presented by the cell's MHC molecules and which induces CTL to destroy the tumour.

antigen as an altered melanotransferrin provides direct evidence that structural changes in normal cellular proteins not only occur in tumours but can lead to immune recognition *in vivo*.

Although T cell-defined tumour-unique antigens in man have not yet been isolated, TSTAs of several carcinogen-induced rodent tumours have been identified. Surprisingly these have not turned out to be unrelated molecules, as predicted from the tum −ve model. Rather they have been shown to be related either to the Class I MHC molecules or to members of the heat-shock protein (HSP)-90 family.

In MCA-induced sarcomas of BALB/c mice, TSTA activity has been localized to an 86 kD cytoplasmic protein (Ullrich *et al*. 1986) and to a 96 kD cell surface protein (Srivastava and Old 1988, 1989). In both cases biochemically related but distinct molecules were isolated from non-cross-reacting tumours of the same mouse strain and shown to be targets of TSTA activity. Although the relationship between the 86 kD and 96 kD molecules remains unclear, both show amino acid sequence homology to the yeast HSP-90 and related molecules. The localization of TSTA activity to the same family of molecules in three different tumours may reflect a peculiarity of the carcinogen; alternatively it may reflect the way in which these antigens were defined. In all cases the TSTAs were identified by assessing the ability of various cytosolic fractions to immunize animals against that specific tumour. In order to induce T cell-dependent tumour cell rejection (generally Class I MHC-restricted), soluble molecules would have to be taken up by cells and processed in the pathway which is primarily important for presentation by Class II MHC molecules. The HSP-90 molecules may be particularly prone to be detected by such a protocol — for example, they may efficiently bind to the Class I MHC molecule peptide groove either from outside of the cell or from the exogenous pathway. The most serious reservation in the evaluation of these studies lies in the fact that the tumours were induced more than 20 years ago and have been passaged by transplantation through many recipients. This may well select for particular mutations which are not related to the original TSTA.

A clearer example of the dangers inherent in the analysis of tumours which have been passaged for years *in vivo* is seen in the identification of TSTAs as MHC molecules. Through gene cloning, the TSTAs of the *N*-ethyl-nitrosourea-induced lung carcinoma LT85 and the UV-induced fibrosarcoma 1591 have been identified as H-2 Class I MHC molecules which are distinct from those of the host mouse strain (reviewed in Parham 1989). These observations appeared to confirm a popular hypothesis which suggested that the diversity of TSTAs reflects structural alterations of these highly polymorphic molecules. However, as more H-2 alleles were sequenced, it became clear that these tumour-associated MHC molecules were simply 'alien antigens' — that is, the products of allogeneic MHC genes which had contaminated the tumours during the years of *in vivo* propagation (Linsk *et al*. 1989).

The question of whether TSTAs and tumour-unique antigens represent structural alterations in random gene products or in common target molecules must await their identification in tumours which have not been carried either *in vivo* or *in vitro* for long periods of time.

The paradox of concomitant immunity and progressing tumours

A major puzzle is presented by the observations that malignant cells express altered molecules capable of inducing an immune response, and that most tumour-bearing individuals can be shown to possess tumour-reactive cells and/or antibodies. Why is this immunity not effective in eliminating the tumour? Experimental studies and clinical observations and suggest two general pathways by which tumour cells may escape specific immune destruction: active effector cells may not be generated *in vivo*, or the tumour cells may down-regulate target antigens or accessory molecules required for effective killing.

The tumour cells may inhibit effector cell development

The tumour-reactive CTL which can be isolated from tumour patients always require restimulation with the tumour cells *in vitro* before activity can be detected, an observation which is consistent with a pre-effector status of these cells *in vivo*. These cells do not appear to be tolerant or specifically anergic since such cells cannot be activated by cytokines or antigen stimulation *in vitro* (Rammensee *et al*. 1989). The development or activation of effector cells *in vivo* may be inhibited by cytokines or other products produced by the tumour cells themselves. For example, the transforming growth factor β (TGF-β), which is produced by many different types of tumour cells, is a potent inhibitor of the development of active CTL (Wahl *et al*. 1989). A demonstration of the effectiveness of this cytokine *in vivo* has recently been reported (Torre-Amione *et al*. 1990). Transfection of the murine TGF-β complementary DNA (cDNA) into a UV-induced sarcoma which is normally rejected by immunocompetent mice completely prevented the development of immune effector cells and this resulted in progressive growth of the tumour.

Immunological mechanisms may prevent effector cell development

The development of active effector cells may also be prevented by specific immunological mechanisms. Essentially all of our knowledge about the cells which play a role in the destruction of autologous tumour cells has come from studies on experimentally induced rodent tumours. Using adoptive transfer experiments in syngeneic recipients, leucocytes from animals which have rejected a tumour can be tested for their capacity to prevent the outgrowth of tumours (when leucocytes and tumour cells are injected together in the Winn assay) or to lead to rejection of an already established tumour. In all cases the destruction of tumours has been found to be mediated by T lymphocytes. Both tumour-reactive CD4 +ve cells, shown to function as helper cells in classical helper assays *in vitro* (e.g. Romerdahl and Kripke 1988), and CD8 +ve CTLs can be isolated from mice which have rejected their tumours. The relative importance of CD4 +ve and CD8 +ve cells in transferring tumour resistance seems to vary from tumour to tumour. In UV-induced fibrosarcomas, CD4 +ve helper cells transferred resistance while the CD8 +ve cells could not (Romerdahl and Kripke 1988). In contrast, tumour-specific CD8 +ve CTL isolated from mice bearing lymphomas (North 1985) and MCA-induced tumours (Barth *et al*. 1990) effectively transfer tumour resistance.

Adoptive transfer has also been used to assess the status of lymphocytes present in mice with progressively growing tumours and has shed some light on the reasons for the ineffective immune response. In several different tumours, a T cell-mediated suppression of effector cell generation has been observed. One system is exemplified by the studies of North and his colleagues on transplantable lymphomas (reviewed in North 1985). As presented schematically in Fig. 93.3, immune effector and suppressor cells can be distinguished when T lymphocytes are transferred from a tumour-bearing mouse into T cell-deficient syngeneic mice bearing the same tumour in an early stage of growth. The CD8 +ve immune effector cells, which are able to reject the small tumour, can only be detected in the donor during the early stages of tumour growth. With progressive tumour growth, these effector cells disappear and, at the same time, CD4 +ve cells appear which are

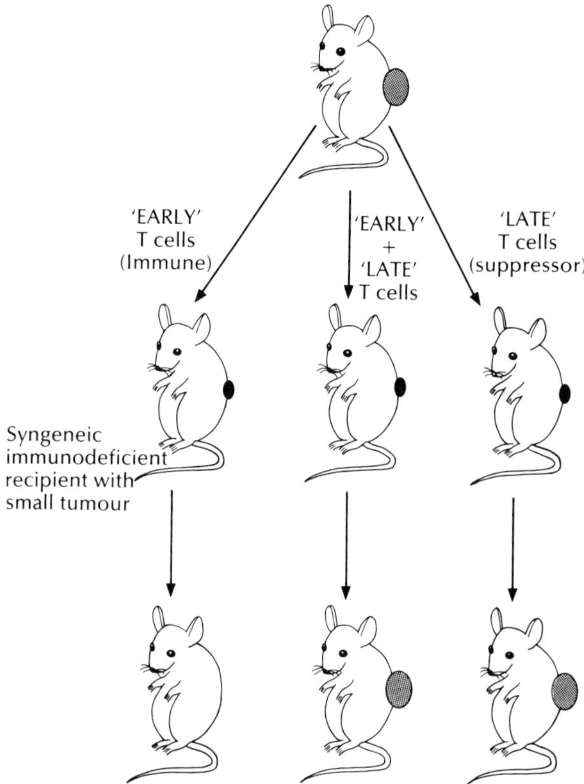

Fig. 93.3. Demonstration of immune and suppressor T lymphocytes in tumour-bearing mice. T cells removed early during tumour growth are able to cause rejection of the same tumour growing in a syngeneic T cell-deficient mouse. T cells removed late cannot. Injection of early and late T cells together does not result in tumour destruction, indicating the 'suppressor' nature of the late T cells.

capable of suppressing effector cell function in the test mouse. Recent experiments have shown that treatment of the tumour-bearing mice with an anti-CD4 monoclonal antibody prevents the development of this suppression and leads to rejection of the tumour (Awwad and North 1988). These suppressor lymphocytes are, like the effector CTL, specific for the individual tumour. This temporal relationship between effector and suppressor T cells is reproducibly observed in a number of different tumours, although the mechanisms controlling it remain unknown.

In UV-induced skin fibrosarcomas, suppressor cells can be detected prior to the appearance of the primary tumour and are thought to be important in the earliest stages of tumour growth. Kripke and her colleagues (Kripke 1981) have shown that the appearance of primary tumours depends not only on the carcinogenic effect of UV irradiation but on its induction of a systemic immunological suppression. This suppression is mediated by T cells which are able to prevent the development of TSTA-specific effector T cells to a wide variety of UV-induced tumours (that is, they are not directed at TSTAs).

Exactly how these cells mediate their suppressive effect is not known for either of these tumour systems. While the lymphoma suppressors appear to develop when the tumours have reached a certain size, the UV-induced suppressors appear to be the result of antigen presentation by UV-damaged antigen-presenting cells in the skin. Recent studies on the mechanism of immunological tolerance have provided evidence for the existence *in vivo* of specific anergic or tolerant CD4 lymphocytes (Mueller 1989; Rammensee *et al.* 1989). These cells respond to antigen by expressing interleukin 2 (IL-2) receptors but cannot produce IL-2 and are unable to proliferate, a defect which exogenous IL-2 cannot overcome. Based on *in vitro* studies, this unresponsiveness seems to be induced when antigen is presented to specific CD4 cells by an 'altered' antigen-presenting cell. The establishment of the unresponsive or anergic state is an active process which is accompanied by intracellular calcium mobilization and which can be prevented by the presence of functional antigen-presenting cells. Such specifically tolerant or anergic CD4 cells could explain the suppression observed in tumour-bearing animals if, as seems likely, CD4 helper cells are required for the development of effector cells. As many tumours express Class II MHC molecules, the tumour cells themselves could be the 'altered' antigen-presenting cells. Recent studies on tumour cells transfected with the IL-2 gene provide some support for this hypothesis (Fearon *et al.* 1990). The secretion of IL-2 converted several different murine tumours from progressively growing to tumours which induced specific CD8 +ve CTL responses in their hosts and were rejected. From these data Fearon *et al.* speculate that the lack of tumour-specific helper cells may be a common cause of the inability of the host to develop active effector cells.

The existence of anergic or suppressive tumour-specific lymphocytes in human cancer patients and the analysis of their interaction with effector cells remain difficult to come to grips with. Only recently has it been possible to clone tumour-reactive CD4 cells and begin to analyse function (Parmiani *et al.* 1990). And, although cells with 'suppressor activity' have been repeatedly isolated from tumour patients (for example, Cozzolino *et al.* 1987), it has remained difficult to show any specificity. It is impossible to overestimate the difficulty of establishing completely *in vitro* systems in which the interactions between a patient's immune cells and his tumour cells can be reliably evaluated. Nevertheless the advances which have been made in the past few years in the cloning and characterization of various lymphocyte populations make it likely that such systems can be established.

The tumour cells can escape from immune effectors

TUMOUR HETEROGENEITY

Even if active effector cells are generated *in vivo*, the majority of tumour cells may escape destruction by a variety of ways. The cloning of tumour cells has provided evidence for heterogeneity in the expression of antigens recognized by CTL (Anichini *et al.* 1989), making it highly unlikely that any single CTL clone can destroy all tumour cells. In fact, *in vitro* studies have demonstrated that CTL can be used to select antigen-loss variants from cloned tumour lines, suggesting that CTL themselves exert a selective pressure which may result in the outgrowth of antigen-negative tumour cells *in vivo*.

ALTERATIONS IN THE EXPRESSION OF MAJOR HISTOCOMPATIBILITY COMPLEX MOLECULES

A down-regulation in the level of MHC molecules which is essential for CTL recognition appears to be an important mechanism by which a tumour cell can escape cell-mediated destruction. This has been directly demonstrated for a highly metastatic rodent tumour which had lost expression of one H-2 Class I MHC allelic product (Wallich *et al.* 1985). Re-expression of this product, induced by transfection of the cloned gene, led to a tumour which grew very slowly and failed to metastasize. This change in growth characteristics was only observed in immunocompetent hosts, and was associated with the development of specific CTL.

Loss of HLA Class I MHC molecules is frequently observed on human tumours examined *in situ* using immunohistochemical methods (Natali *et al.* 1989) and may arise by several mechanisms. Using *in situ* hybridization, the lack of expression of all Class I MHC molecules, which is fairly common in colorectal carcinomas, has been shown to be due to the absence of messenger ribonucleic acid (mRNA) for β2 microglobulin (Momburg and Koch 1989). In the absence of this protein, the heavy chain of the Class I MHC molecules cannot be transported to and expressed on the cell surface. In melanomas and neuroblastomas, the down-regulation of Class I MHC molecules seems to be due to over-expression of the oncogenes c-myc and n-myc respectively. In melanomas, c-myc expression results in a selective down-regulation of mRNAs for the HLA-B and HLA-C loci whereas the mRNA for HLA-A is not affected (Versteeg *et al.* 1989). Although the mechanism by which c-myc expression regulates Class I MHC expression has not been elucidated, n-myc expression has been shown to prevent the binding of a transcriptional factor to one of the Class I MHC enhancers in a cell-specific manner (Lenardo *et al.* 1989).

Although CD8 +ve CTLs have been shown to function as effector cells in tumour destruction in several rodent tumours, tumour-specific CD4 +ve cells are also generated in these animals. As discussed above, these cells appear to play an important role in the generation of effector cells and may demonstrate either a helper or a suppressor function (reviewed in Hamaoka and Fujiwara 1987). CD4 +ve cells require Class II MHC molecules for antigen recognition and in this context it is notable that HLA Class II MHC expression is frequently observed on human tumours derived from Class II MHC −ve tissues. These Class II MHC +ve tumour cells have also been shown to process and present antigen to Class II MHC-restricted T cell clones (Alexander *et al.* 1989), indicating that they may present their own antigens *in vivo*. The expression of Class II MHC molecules by human tumours often appears to have a prognostic significance, which can be either favourable (signifying the induction of helper T cells? (Esteban *et al.* 1989)) or unfavourable (signifying the induction of suppressor T cells? (Bröcker *et al.* 1985)), depending on the type of tumour.

EXPRESSION OF ADHESION MOLECULES

A number of accessory adhesion molecules contribute to the stabilization of effector cell–target cell interactions and their absence on the tumour cells could contribute to the ineffectiveness of immune effectors. The two most important interactions appear to involve lymphocyte function-associated antigen 1 (LFA-1) on the lymphocyte with intercellular adhesion molecule 1 (ICAM-1) on the target, and the T cell CD2 molecule with LFA-3 on the target cell. While LFA-3 is constitutively expressed on nearly all cells of the body, ICAM-1 is regulated by inflammatory cytokines and can be expressed on virtually every cell type in the presence of these mediators. In lymphomas the down-regulation of LFA-1 as well as ICAM-1 and LFA-3 has been associated with high-grade and relapsing tumours and with the loss of the ability of tumour cells to stimulate both autologous and allogeneic T cell proliferation (Clayberger *et al.* 1987; Gregory *et al.* 1988). Little is known about the expression of these molecules on solid tumours, although the occasional loss of LFA-3 expression on colorectal carcinomas has recently been reported (Smith *et al.* 1989). Surprisingly ICAM-1 expression by solid tumours *in situ* is relatively rare even in the presence of a heavy mononuclear cell infiltrate which would be expected to produce inductive cytokines (Vogetseder *et al.* 1989). A notable exception is cutaneous melanoma, where ICAM-1 is found on more than 50% of primary tumours and where, in contrast to all expectation, its expression is associated with advanced tumours which have a poor prognosis (Johnson *et al.* 1989).

While observations on the expression of immunologically relevant molecules (such as HLA and adhesion molecules) by human tumours *in situ* cannot, in the final analysis, tell us anything about the interactions which are occurring between the tumour and the immune system, they can provide a starting-point for *in vitro* experiments.

Non-specific effector cells may also contribute to tumour destruction

In vitro, tumour cells can be killed by cells other than classical antigen-specific CTLs, in particular by activated monocytes and NK cells. Both types of cells are activated by inflammatory cytokines and may contribute to tumour destruction *in vivo*, particularly in the locality of an ongoing T cell response. The tumoricidal activity demonstrated *in vitro* by activated monocytes is mediated through a number of different factors, including tumour necrosis factor alpha (TNF-α), IL-1 and oxygen radicals. The role that cytotoxic monocytes play in tumour defence is documented by the observation that tumour destruction can occur near an area of a bacterial-induced granuloma which is rich in activated monocytes. Such observations led to the discovery and naming of TNF (Oettgen and Old 1987). In fact, the injection of bacillus Calmette-Guérin (BCG) mycobacteria into the vicinity of tumours is effective in inducing regression of local tumours, presumably in part through the activation of cytotoxic monocytes.

Natural killer cells detectable in the peripheral blood of normal as well as tumour patients and they are able to kill a wide variety of tumour cell lines and fresh tumour cells without the requirement for restimulation *it vitro*. Their relatively high levels in athymic nude mice suggested that they may protect these mice against tumours and some evidence in support of such a role has in fact come from studies of the beige mutant, which lacks NK cells (Woodruff 1989). Morphologically NK cells are large granular lymphocytes; they are CD3 –ve, do not rearrange their TCR genes, and usually express the CD56 antigen (recently shown to be the neural cell adhesion molecule (NCAM)) and a low-affinity Fc receptor for immunoglobulin (Ig), CD16. As in MHC-restricted T cells, the adhesion molecules ICAM-1 : LFA-1 and CD2 : LFA-3 contribute to target effector interaction, as does CD56 when NCAM +ve target cells are involved. Whether specific target-receptor structures are involved in NK killing remains unclear. Recently a novel molecular complex consisting of CD16, the TCR-associated zeta chain and an unknown protein has been identified on NK cells (Anderson *et al.* 1990). Given the role of the zeta chain in signal transduction in T cells, it is speculated that this complex may be capable of signal transmission and may represent the NK receptor. Natural killer cells are very sensitive to lymphokine activation and they comprise the majority of lymphokine-activated killer (LAK) cells which are generated *in vitro* (Ortaldo and Longo 1988).

Cells of the immune system may also contribute to tumour growth and progression

Most solid tumours demonstrate, at some time in their development, a heavy infiltration of mononuclear leucocytes. Although initially taken to be a sign of an active antitumour reactivity by the host, there is at present considerable debate about the role of these cells. Examination of the infiltrates using monoclonal antibodies directed against differentiation antigens has shown that they consist primarily of T lymphocytes and macrophages with very few B lymphocytes or cells with NK phenotypes. The T cells frequently express activation markers (HLA-D region products, IL-2 receptor) and more frequently are CD8 than CD4, although this may vary from tumour to tumour and with tumour progression. As more function-associated differentiation markers are defined, analysis of the leucocyte infiltrates of tumours may well provide more information on the interaction between tumour and host. From the studies which are already available, it is clear that this interaction is very complex. Cutaneous melanoma is one tumour in which the composition of the infiltrate has been analysed in different stages of tumour progression (Bröcker *et al.* 1988). Among the changes observed during tumour progression is a shift from CD1 +ve Langerhans/dendritic cells to a predominance of macrophages bearing the 25F9 marker, whose functional significance is not yet clear. In addition, with increasing tumour progression the T lymphocytes change from a predominantly CD4 population to a predominantly CD8 population; at the same time the tumour cells begin to express HLA-DR and the LFA-1 adhesion ligand ICAM-1. The association between infiltrates of CD8 +ve lymphocytes and HLA-DR expression on the tumours has also been observed in breast and colorectal carcinomas. It is difficult to decide whether the infiltrate or the tumour initiates these changes. However, the expression of the interferon-γ-inducible molecules HLA-DR and ICAM-1 by early melanomas has been shown to be strongly correlated with the presence of interferon-γ-containing cells in the infiltrate. These results suggest that the cytokines produced by the cellular infiltrate can alter the phenotype of the tumour cells; as HLA-DR and ICAM-1 are molecules which mediate interaction with the immune system, this may have important functional consequences.

That the tumour-infiltrating cells may actually contribute to the growth and progression of malignant tumours has been discussed for some time. As in the inflammatory process, infiltrating cells produce growth factors, angiogenesis factors and basement membrane-degrading enzymes which facilitate tumour growth and spread (Dvorak 1986). Macrophages in particular have been postulated to directly contribute to tumour development and progression (Munzarova and Kovarik 1987). In experimental rodent tumours there is evidence that fusion between the tumour cells and host macrophages can occur *in vivo* and that this leads to the formation of cells with increased invasive and metastatic potential (Fortuna *et al.* 1989). In addition, activated macrophages can induce chromosomal changes in neighbouring cells (Weitberg *et al.* 1983). Both of these events could directly contribute to the progression of tumours. Based on many years of observation of the interaction between tumour growth and immunity in experimental carcinogenesis in inbred mice, Prehn and Prehn (1987) have in fact promoted the heretical view that a tumour-specific immune response which provides the necessary microenvironment for successful tumour growth may even be a requirement for the development of progressing tumours.

Immunosurveillance?

Nearly a century after it was first proposed, most of the predictions made by the theory of immunosurveillance have been shown to be true. Malignant cells have multiple genetic changes as well as epigenetic alterations in cell metabolism, which lead to the expression of altered molecules. These altered molecules can be detected by the cellular immune system and this recognition can, in rodent models, lead to destruction of the tumour cells. Cloning and analysis of tumour-reactive T lymphocytes indicate that most tumour patients do indeed have cells which are able to specifically recognize their own tumour cells *in vitro*. The reasons why these cells are not able to destroy the tumour cells *in vivo* are undoubtedly multiple and complex, and understanding them presents the greatest challenge to tumour immunologists today.

But what about immunosurveillance itself? Is there any evidence that the immune system plays a crucial role in destroying genetically altered cells which would otherwise develop into malignant tumours? The extensive clinical follow-ups of thousands of organ transplant recipients given immunosuppressive drugs to prevent rejection provide a unique opportunity to examine this question (Penn 1988). While these individuals show an overall threefold increase in malignancies as compared with age-matched controls, this reflects a very great increase in the incidence of a small number of tumour types: squamous cell carcinoma of the skin and lips (7–21-fold increase), non-Hodgkins lymphoma (28–49-fold increase), Kaposi's sarcoma (400–500-fold increase), cervix carcinoma (14-fold increase), carcinomas of the vulva and perineum (100-fold increase), and hepatobiliary carcinomas (30-fold increase). A similar picture emerges from studies of non-transplant recipients treated with immunosuppressive drugs and from patients with immunodeficiencies such as acquired immune deficiency syndrome (AIDS). All of the tumours which show such a dramatic increase in immunosuppressed individuals have been associated with viruses (Epstein–Barr, herpes simplex, papilloma, hepatitis B), suggesting that immunosurveillance does function to prevent the outgrowth of transformed viral-infected cells.

The most common cancers, such as lung, prostate, colon and breast, are not, however, more frequent in immunodeficient individuals, and this would seem to indicate that no significant immunosurveillance exists against malignancies in general.

Conclusions

The demonstration that malignant cells can be recognized as foreign by cells of cancer patients *in vitro* is encouraging because it means that it may eventually become possible to manipulate the patient's own immune response *in vivo*, directing it towards his tumour. Examples of the potential of such manipulations can be seen in some of the responses observed to treatment with LAK cells (Rosenberg *et al.* 1987). It can be hoped that the use of tumour-specific cytotoxic cells, together with the local production of cytokines, may eventually make immunotherapy a reality.

References

Alexander, M.A., Bennicelli, J. and Guerry, D. (1989). Defective antigen presentation by human melanoma cell lines cultured from advanced, but not biologically early, disease. *J. Immunol.* **142**, 4070–8.

Anderson, P., Caligiuri, M., O'Brien, C., Manley, T., Ritz, J. and Schlossman, S.F. (1990). Fc gamma receptor type III (CD16) is included in the zeta NK receptor complex expressed by human natural killer cells. *Proc. Nat. Acad. Sci. (USA)* **87**, 2274–8.

Anichini, A., Mazzocchi, A., Fossati, G. and Parmiani, G. (1989). Cytotoxic T lymphocyte clones from peripheral blood and from tumour site detect intratumor heterogeneity of melanoma cells. *J. Immunol.* **142**, 3692–701.

Awwad, M. and North, R.J. (1988). Immunologically mediated regression of a murine lymphoma after treatment with anti-L3T4 antibody. *J. Exp. Med.* **168**, 2193–206.

Barnd, D.L., Lan, M.S., Metzgar, R.S. and Finn, O.J. (1989). Specific, major histocompatibility complex-unrestricted recognition of tumor-associated mucins by human cytotoxic T cells. *Proc. Nat. Acad. Sci. (USA)* **86**, 7159–63.

Barth, R.J., Jr, Bock, S.N., Mule, J.J. and Rosenberg, S.A. (1990). Unique murine tumor-associated antigens identified by tumor infiltrating lymphocytes. *J. Immunol.* **144**, 1531–7.

Boon, T., Van Pel, A. and De Plaen, E. (1989). Tum – transplantation antigens, point mutations, and antigenic peptides: a model for tumor-specific transplantation antigens? *Cancer Cells* **1**, 25–8.

Bröcker, E.B., Sutrer, L., Brüggen, J., Ruiter, D.J., Macher, E. and Sorg, C. (1985). Phenotypic dynamics of tumor progression in human malignant melanoma. *Int. J. Cancer* **36**, 29–35.

Bröcker, E.B., Zwaldo, G., Holzmann, B., Macher, E. and Sorg, C. (1988). Inflammatory cell infiltrates in human melanoma at different stages in tumor progression. *Int. J. Cancer* **41**, 562–7.

Castronovo, V., Colin, C., Parent, B., Foidart, J.-M., Lambotte, R. and Mahieu, P. (1989). Possible role of human natural anti-gal antibodies in the natural antitumour defense system. *J. Nat. Cancer Inst.* **81**, 212–16.

Clayberger, C., Wright, A., Medeiros, L.J. *et al.* (1987). Absence of cell surface LFA-1 as a mechanism of escape from immunosurveillance. *Lancet* **ii**, 533–6.

Cote, R.J., Morrissey, D.M., Houghton, A.N. *et al.* (1986). Specificity analysis of human monoclonal antibodies reactive with cell surface and intracellular antigens. *Proc. Nat. Acad. Sci. (USA)* **83**, 2959–63.

Cozzolino, F., Torcia, M., Carossino, A.M. *et al.* (1987). Characterization of cells from invaded lymph nodes in patients with solid tumours. *J. Exp. Med.* **166**, 303–18.

Darrow, T.L., Slingluff, C.L., Jr, Seigler, H.F. (1986). The role of HLA class I antigens in recognition of melanoma cells by tumor specific cytotoxic T lymphocytes: evidence for shared tumor antigens. *J. Immunol.* **142**, 3329–35.

Dvorak, H.F. (1986). Tumors: wounds that do not heal. *N. Engl. J. Med.* **315**, 1650–9.

Esteban, F., Concha, A., Huelin, C. *et al.* (1989). Histocompatibility antigens in primary and metastatic squamous cell carcinoma of the larynx. *Int. J. Cancer* **43**, 436–42.

Fearon, E.R., Pardoll, D.M., Itaya, T. *et al.* (1990). Interleukin-2 production by tumor cells bypasses T helper function in the generation of an antitumor response. *Cell* **60**, 397–403.

Fortuna, M.B., Dewey, M.J. and Furmanski, P. (1989). Cell fusion in tumor development and progression: occurrence of cell fusion in primary methylcholanthrene-induced tumorigenesis. *Int. J. Cancer* **44**, 731–7.

Furukawa, K.S., Furukawa, K., Real, F.X., Old, L.J. and Lloyd, K.O. (1989). A unique antigenic epitope of human melanoma is carried on the common melanoma glycoprotein gp95/97. *J. Exp. Med.* **169**, 585–9.

Gregory, C.D., Murray, R.J., Edwards, C.F. and Rickinson, A.B. (1988). Downregulation of cell adhesion molecules LFA-3 and ICAM-1 in Epstein–Barr virus positive Burkitts lymphoma underlies tumour cell escape from virus-specific T cell surveillance. *J. Exp. Med.* **167**, 1811–24.

Hakomori, S.-I. (1985). Aberrant glycosylation in cancer cell membranes as focused on glycolipids: overview and perspectives. *Cancer Res.* **45**, 2405–14.

Hamaoka, T. and Fujiwara, H. (1987). Phenotypically and functionally distinct T-cell subsets in anti-tumor responses. *Immunol. Today* **8**, 267–9.

Hellström, I., Hellström, K.E., Pierce, G.E. and Yang, J.P.S. (1968). Cellular and humoral immunity to different types of human neoplasms. *Nature* **220**, 1352–4.

Howie, S. and McBride, W.H. (1982). Tumor specific T helper activity can be abrogated by two distinct suppressor cell mechanisms. *Eur. J. Immunol.* **12**, 671–5.

Johnson, J.P., Stade, B.G., Holzmann, B., Schwaeble, W. and Riethmüller, G. (1989). *De novo* expression of intercellular adhesion molecule 1 in melanoma correlates with increased risk of metastasis *Proc. Nat. Acad. Sci. (USA)* **86**, 641–4.

Kripke, M.L. (1981). Immunologic mechanisms in UV radiation carcinogenesis. *Adv. Cancer Res.* **34**, 69–106.

Lenardo, M., Rustgi, A.K., Schievella, A.R. and Bernards, R. (1989). Suppression of MHC class I gene expression by N-*myc* through enhancer inactivation. *EMBO J.*, **8**, 3351–5.

Linsk, R., Watts, S., Fischer, A. and Goodenow, R.S. (1989). The tumor rejection antigens of the 1591 ultraviolet fibrosarcoma: potential origin and evolutionary implications. *J. Exp. Med.* **169**, 1043–58.

Lloyd, K.O. and Old, L.J. (1989). Human monoclonal antibodies to glycolipids and other carbohydrate antigens: dissection of the humoral immune response in cancer patients. *Cancer Res.* **49**, 3445–51.

Metoki, R., Kakudi, K., Tsuji, Y., Teng, N., Clausen, H. and Hakomori, S.-I. (1989). Deletion of histo-blood group A and B antigens and expression of incompatible A antigen in ovarian cancer. *J. Nat. Cancer Inst.* **81**, 1151–7.

Möller, G. and Möller, E. (1976). The concept of immunological surveillance against neoplasia. *Transplant. Rev.* **28**, 3–24.

Momburg, F. and Koch, S. (1989). Selective loss of β2 microglobulin mRNA in human colon carcinoma. *J. Exp. Med.* **169**, 309–14.

Mueller, D.L. (1989). Do tolerant T cells exist? *Nature* **339**, 513–14.

Munzarova, M. and Kovarik, J. (1987). Is cancer a macrophage-mediated autoaggressive disease? *Lancet* **i**, 952–4.

Natali, P.G., Nicotra, M.R., Bigotti, A. *et al.* (1989). Selective changes of HLA class I polymorphic determinants in human solid tumours. *Proc. Nat. Acad. Sci. (USA)* **86**, 6719–23.

North, R.J. (1985). Down-regulation of the antitumor immune response. *Adv. Cancer Res.* **45**, 1–43.

Oettgen, H.F. and Old, L.J. (1987). Tumor necrosis factor. In *Important Advances in Oncology*, ed. V.T. DeVita, S. Hellman and S.A. Rosenberg, pp. 105–30, Lippincott, Philadelphia.

Old, L.J. (1981). Cancer immunology: the search for specificity. *Cancer Res.* **41**, 361–75.

Ortaldo, J.R. and Longo, D.L. (1988). Human natural lymphocyte effector cells: definition, analysis of activity and clinical effectiveness. *J. Nat. Cancer Inst.* **80**, 999–1010.

Parham, P. (1989). Alien antigens return to the fold. *Immunol. Today* **10**, 206–11.

Parmiani, G., Anichini, A. and Fossati, G. (1990). Cellular immune response against autologous human malignant melanoma: are *in vitro* studies providing a framework for a more effective immunotherapy? *J. Nat. Cancer Inst.* **82**, 361–70.

Penn, I. (1988). Tumours of the immunocompromised patient. *Ann. Rev. Med.* **39**, 63–73.

Prehn, R.T. and Main, J.M. (1957). Immunity to methylcholanthrene-induced sarcomas. *J. Nat. Cancer Inst.* **18**, 769–78.

Prehn, R.T. and Prehn, L.M. (1987). The autoimmune nature of cancer. *Cancer Res.* **47**, 927–32.

Rammensee, H.G., Kroschewski, R. and Frangoulis, B. (1989). Clonal anergy induced in mature Vβ6+ T lymphocytes on immunizing Mls-1b mice immunized with Mls-1a expressing cells. *Nature* **339**, 541–4.

Romerdahl, C.A. and Kripke, M.L. (1988). Role of helper T-lymphocytes in rejection of UV-induced murine skin cancers. *Cancer Res.* **48**, 2325–8.

Rosenberg, S.A., Lotze, M.T., Muul, L.M. *et al.* (1987). A progress report on the treatment of 157 patients with advanced cancer using lymphokine-activated killer cells and interleukin-2 or high dose interleukin-2 alone. *N. Engl. J. Med.* **316**, 889–97.

Smith, M.E.F., Marsh, S.G.E., Bodmer, J.G., Gelsthorpek, K. and Bodmer, W.F. (1989). Loss of HLA-A,B,C, allele products and lymphocyte function-associated antigen 3 in colorectal neoplasia. *Proc. Nat. Acad. Sci. (USA)* **86**, 5557–61.

Srivastasa, P.K. and Old, L.J. (1988). Individually distinct transplantation antigens of chemically induced mouse tumors. *Immunol. Today* **8**, 78–83.

Srivastava, P.K. and Old, L.J. (1989). Identification of a human homologue of the murine tumor rejection antigen gp96. *Cancer Res.* **49**, 1341–3.

Torre-Amione, G., Beauchamp, R.D., Koeppen, H. *et al.* (1990). A highly immunogenic tumor transfected with a murine transforming growth factor type β1 cDNA escapes immune surveillance. *Proc. Nat. Acad. Sci. (USA)* **87**, 1486–90.

Ullrich, S.J., Robinson, E.A., Law, L.W., Willingham, M. and Appella, E. (1986). A mouse tumor-specific transplantation antigen is a heat shock-related protein. *Proc. Nat. Acad. Sci. (USA)* **83**, 3121–5.

Van den Eynde, B., Hainaut, P., Knuth, A. *et al.* (1989). Presence on a human melanoma of multiple antigens recognized by autologous CTL. *Int. J. Cancer* **44**, 634–40.

Versteeg, R., Krüse-Wolters, K.M., Plomp, A.C. *et al.* (1989). Suppression of class I human histocompatibility leukocyte antigen by c-*myc* is locus specific. *J. Exp. Med.* **170**, 621–35.

Vogelstein, B., Fearon, E.R., Kern, S.E. *et al.* (1989). Allelo-types of colorectal carcinomas. *Science* **244**, 207–11.

Vogetseder, W., Feichtinger, H., Schulz, T.F. *et al.* (1989).

Expression of 7F7-antigen, a human adhesion molecule identical to intercellular adhesion molecule-1 (ICAM-1) in human carcinomas and their stromal fibroblasts. *Int. J. Cancer* **43**, 768–73.

Wahl, S.M., McCartney-Francis, N. and Mergenhagen, S.E. (1989). Inflammatory and immunomodulatory roles of TGFβ. *Immunol. Today* **10**, 258–61.

Wallich, R., Bulbue, N., Hämmerling, G.J., Katzav, S., Segal, S. and Feldman, M. (1985). Abrogation of metastatic properties of tumour cells by *de novo* expression of H-2K antigens following H-2 gene transfection. *Nature* **315**, 301–5.

Ward, P.L., Koeppen, H., Hurteau, T. and Schreiber, H. (1989). Tumor antigens defined by cloned immunological probes are highly polymorphic and are not detected on autologous normal cells. *J. Exp. Med.* **170**, 217–32.

Weinberg, R.A. (1989). Oncogenes, antioncogenes and the molecular bases of multistep carcinogenesis. *Cancer Res.* **49**, 3713–21.

Weitberg, A.C., Weitzman, S.A., Destrempes, M., Latt, S.A. and Stossel, T.P. (1983). Stimulated human phagocytes produce cytogenetic changes in cultured mammalian cells *N. Engl. J. Med.* **308**, 26–30.

Wölfel, T., Klehmann, E., Müller, C., Schütt, K.-H., Meyer zum Büschenfelde, K.-H. and Knuth, A. (1989). Lysis of human melanoma cells by autologous cytolytic T cell clones: identification of human histocompatibility leukocyte antigen A2 as a restriction element. *J. Exp. Med.* **170**, 797–810.

Woodruff, M.F.A. (1989). Immunosurveillance *Curr. Opinion Immunol.* **1**, 910–12.

94: Immunotherapy of Tumours

G.T. Stevenson

Introduction

In developed countries about one person in three receives a diagnosis of cancer during his lifetime and almost one in four dies from it. So it is hardly surprising that physicians have long been tantalized by the prospect of directing immunological weapons against rampant cancer cells. The major problem is simply stated: these cells resemble closely the normal lineages from which they arise, whereas the immune response is geared to microbial parasites of quite different nature. Thus the cancer cells display a paucity of antigenic targets and share with their normal counterparts a set of defences against immunological attack. Yet mammalian tissues can be destroyed immunologically, as witness the fates of allografts and targets of autoimmunity. To turn this destructive power effectively against cancer is a great scientific challenge.

For those unfamiliar with neoplastic disease a few definitions might be helpful. A tumour or neoplasm is a population of cells which grows without regard to normal bodily requirements. In its extreme form the independence appears complete, the growth 'purposeless, progressive and parasitic'. A malignant neoplasm or cancer is one which threatens life by invading and destroying adjacent tissue and/or by seeding (metastasizing) to distant sites. For convenience malignant neoplasms are often divided into carcinomas (arising from epithelia, including skin) and sarcomas (from other tissues). A benign neoplasm neither metastasizes nor invades adjacent tissues (although it can dangerously compress them), and is sometimes delimited by a capsule. There is no clear distinction between malignant and benign neoplasms, nor between benign neoplasms and various non-neoplastic cellular accumulations (hyperplasias, dysplasias, rests and others), but a frankly malignant neoplasm differs from normal tissue in a striking and catastrophic manner. A classical description of neoplastic behaviour has been provided by Foulds (1969) while recent years have seen a considerable improvement in our understanding of the genetic basis of such behaviour (Weinberg 1989).

Vaccination against cancer

At present the only major impact which immunology has on the management of cancer lies in prevention. Vaccination against virus with an aetiological role in tumour has been strikingly successful in veterinary medicine. Marek's disease, a commercially important T cell lymphoma of chickens associated with a horizontally transmitted herpes virus, can be prevented completely by vaccination with either attenuated oncogenic virus (Churchill *et al.* 1969) or a related turkey herpes virus (Biggs 1975). Prototype viral vaccines for feline leukaemia (Osterhaus *et al.* 1985) and marmoset lymphoma (Laufs and Steinke 1975) have followed. In man there is promise of a major reduction in primary hepatocellular carcinoma, a tumour of high incidence in much of Africa and eastern Asia, with the implementation of vaccination against hepatitis B virus (Blumberg and London 1985). It should be noted that such vaccination is justified on the grounds of the direct hepatic damage caused by the virus, quite apart from the appearance of tumour at a low prevalence in those infected. For other viruses with probable aetiological roles in human cancer — human T cell lymphotrophic viruses I and II, certain of the human papillomaviruses, and Epstein–Barr virus (EBV) — cancer is also a relatively rare sequel to infection, but the other possible sequels are largely minor: so one faces the problems entailed in vaccinating and perhaps putting slightly at risk an entire population for the sake of preventing serious disease in a few. Nevertheless vaccination against EBV is being seriously contemplated (Epstein 1987).

The concept of immunotherapy

In comparison with the achievements and promise of vaccination, the deployment of immunology against established tumour — immunotherapy — has been less rewarding. It has been contemplated for about a century. Currie (1972) records a description by Hericourt and Richet in 1895 of 50 patients treated with antitumour sera raised in dogs and donkeys. Tumour regression and symptomatic benefit were sometimes seen but cures were not. Similar variegated results, often lacking reproducibility, have plagued immunotherapy to the present day, so that it has not yet earned a major role in the treatment of any common form of tumour. But the last ten years or so have witnessed a vast improvement in the precision of tumour immunology, due largely to increasing application of monoclonal antibody and recombinant genetic technologies. Therapeutic antibodies are now for the most part molecularly homogeneous, available in indefinitely large amounts, and transferable from group to group so as to confirm results. Cytokines are available as recombinant preparations of defined structure instead of often evanescent activities in biological extracts. Both target and effector cells are better understood, particularly with regard to surface molecular structure, and more readily fractionated. All these developments have led to a resurgent interest in the immunotherapy of cancer, and a need to discuss principles despite the sparseness of clinical results.

The literature to be reviewed expands vastly if one permits inclusion of many therapeutic forays which, although usually lacking a clear immunological rationale, subject the tumour to a variety of para-immunological reagents shown to disadvantage neoplastic cells *in vitro* and/or in animal models. Such agents have included bacteria, toxins, adjuvants, cytokines and lymphoid cell populations. When unencumbered by difficult protocols they have on occasion led to an avalanche of therapeutic trials. Thus in 1975 the National Cancer Institute had on register over 300 trials of bacillus Calmette-Guérin (BCG) inoculation for breast cancer. Such a response to what was merely a glimmer of hope from the laboratory (Old *et al.* 1961) is a reminder of the scale and urgency of the clinical problem posed by disseminated neoplasm. Similar enthusiasm is being displayed currently for treatment with cytokines. The traditional association of such agents with immunotherapy and their suitability for use in combination with frank immunological protocols dictate that they be considered in this chapter.

Immunotherapy has often been divided into three types: active, the stimulation of the patient's own immune response to his tumour; passive, the infusion of tumour-specific antibody which has been raised in another subject; and adoptive, the infusion of cells, either autologous or from another subject, designed and manipulated to attack the tumour. Unfortunately the application of these terms has often been tendentious. Thus 'active immunotherapy' has been applied to the use of BCG or other substances with immunological adjuvant properties to treat a variety of cancers, in the vaguely articulated belief that a host immune response to tumour antigens is being stimulated. Again, the reinfusion of autologous lymphokine-activated blood lymphocytes has been referred to as 'adoptive immunotherapy' despite the lack of any evidence that the cells possess antitumour specificity. Recognizing that the degree of empiricism common in immunotherapeutic schedules does not lend itself to a terminology based on mechanisms, we shall discuss the subject under headings reflecting simply the main therapeutic manipulation carried out: antibody therapy, cytokine therapy, cellular therapy and active immunization.

Antibody therapy (serotherapy)

Although the use of xenogeneic antibody to attack tumour can be regarded as the best characterized class of immunotherapy, there are important aspects that continue to elude understanding — in particular the natures of the relevant effector mechanisms recruited by antibody and of the tumour cell's defences against them.

With the advent of monoclonal antibodies the number of potential antigenic targets on tumours and the number of clinical trials of antibody therapy rapidly increased. The first major lesson to emerge was a confirmation of the impression, gained earlier with polyclonal antibodies, that *unmodified xenogeneic antibody is an inefficient killer of neoplastic cells*. Antibody therapy of leukaemias, lymphomas, gastrointestinal carcinoma and melanoma has usually yielded negligible, or only partial and transient, regressions of tumour (Ritz and Schlossman 1982; Miller *et al.* 1982 and 1983; Dillman *et al.* 1984; Gordon *et al.* 1984; Houghton *et al.* 1985; Meeker *et al.* 1985b; Rankin *et al.* 1985; Sears *et al.* 1985; Press *et al.* 1987; LoBuglio *et al.* 1988; Waldmann *et al.* 1988; Brown *et al.* 1989; Dyer *et al.* 1989). The antibody has always been given intravenously, with varied doses and schedules; total doses have often exceeded 2 g and have reached 15 g. Some of the studies quoted are only preliminary (phase I), and an occasional description of apparently complete regression of tumour is included, but the overall impression of the inadequacy of xenogeneic antibody is overwhelming. It will emerge shortly that some reasons for this problem are apparent and that some remedial action is available. First we begin a discussion of the mechanisms of antibody attack on tumour by considering the cell surface antigens involved.

Target antigens

Tumour-associated antigens are discussed in detail in Chapter 92 of this book. In recent years there has been a move away from an insistence that target molecules for antibody therapy be essentially tumour-specific. The more pragmatic requirement is simply for a useful tumour antigen, which may be defined (somewhat tautologically) as one capable of mediating a useful removal of tumour while damage to normal tissue remains within acceptable limits. To discuss potentially useful tumour antigens we shall consider just three functional categories: tumour-specific transplantation antigens, virus-specified antigens and differentiation antigens. All three are feasible targets for antibody but to date only the third has served this function to any significant extent.

Tumour-specific transplantation antigens are defined by T cell-mediated rejection of small tumour challenges in syngeneic animals sensitized to that particular tumour. They have been described for the most part on chemically induced animal tumours, but are sometimes detectable on apparently spontaneous tumours (Baldwin 1966). The molecular nature of these antigens (or of the parent molecules yielding the peptides actually presented to T cells) has proved elusive and the presence on them of antibody-defined epitopes of the same exquisite specificity as those seen by T cells remains problematical (e.g. Srivastava *et al.* 1986).

In virus-associated tumours two types of *virus-specified antigen* have been identified on the cell surfaces. Both have at least the potential to provide a therapeutic target for antibody, but no such antibodies are yet available for human tumours. Deoxyribonucleic acid (DNA) oncogenic viruses can induce cell surface antigens, not detectable on the virions, which are unique to the particular virus and shared by all tumours associated with it. On this basis African Burkitt lymphoma and

Chinese nasopharyngeal carcinoma (both associated with EBV), primary hepatoma (hepatitis B virus) and cervical carcinoma (certain human papillomaviruses) are candidate neoplasms. Tumours associated with ribonucleic acid (RNA) oncogenic viruses (oncornaviruses) sometimes exhibit virus-specified antigens on their cell surfaces, in this case proteins present also in the virions. Only one such group of viruses is presently known to afflict man, human T cell lymphotrophic viruses (HTLV-I and -II). The T cell neoplasms concerned show only a very low titre of virus, in contrast to many oncornavirus-associated animal tumours.

Differentiation antigens account for the vast majority of epitopes recognized on tumour cells by monoclonal antibodies. Indeed most of the surface molecules concerned have only been recognized as a result of surface mapping of normal, transformed and neoplastic cells by monoclonal technology. The term 'differentiation' is here used broadly, to encompass all antigens restricted to a limited number of cell lineages or to certain stages of development: thus it includes oncofetal, improper lineage (vicarious) and activation antigens.

The cataloguing of differentiation antigens is best developed for myeloid and lymphoid cell lineages, with regular meetings collating the activities of monoclonal antibodies from many laboratories (Knapp *et al.* 1989). Wherever two or more antibodies appear to be reacting with a single surface structure a 'cluster of differentiation' (CD) is defined and allocated a number; generally such a cluster is soon found to represent either a discrete surface molecule or a constituent peptide chain. At the time of writing the number of leucocyte clusters is approaching 80 while some unclustered antibodies remain: so we may soon have catalogued 100 surface molecules. There is no clear reason why a large proportion of these need not be therapeutic targets, alone or in combinations.

The most specific of known differentiation antigens are the idiotypic epitopes on surface immunoglobulin (Ig) of B cell lymphomas, and on the antigen receptor (TCR) of T cell lymphomas. Each tumour displays a set of such epitopes (the idiotype), among which there is a spectrum of specificity (discussed by Stevenson and Glennie 1985). It has been the practice to date to raise a separate antibody or set of antibodies for each tumour to be attacked. However, the possibility of building a library of antibodies against 'semi-public' idiotypic epitopes, with an appropriate selection of such antibodies available for use in individual cases, has often been discussed. One problem with such an approach is that the greater the number of lymphocytic clones sharing a given epitope, the greater the probability that that epitope will be represented on normal plasma Ig to an extent which represents a serious extracellular antigenic barrier.

A class of differentiation antigens which could assume particular importance for antibody therapy comprises those coded by cellular oncogenes (Weinberg 1989). Some of these are surface receptors for growth factors, so that blocking by antibody might be growth-inhibiting even in the absence of cytotoxicity: Drebin *et al.* (1985) have reported such a result for the action of antibody *in vitro* on the surface molecule encoded by the *neu* oncogene. If the continued expression of an oncogene is necessary to maintain neoplastic behaviour, one need not be concerned about mutational escape from antibody specific for the oncogene product.

Some other receptors for growth factors are not currently regarded as oncogene products, but are still attractive targets for antibody on the basis that their continued expression might be necessary for cell division. Following this reasoning a therapeutic trial of antibody directed against the α chain of the interleukin-2 (IL-2) receptor has been undertaken in T cell lymphoma (Waldmann *et al.* 1988). Most of the patients failed to show a significant response: possibly antibody did not achieve a sufficient occupancy of the receptor, possibly the tumour cells had attained independence of IL-2. We discuss in the next section the worrying possibility that an anti-receptor antibody can itself initiate mitosis.

Many differentiation antigens defined on normal epithelia and their tumours by monoclonal antibodies, including some of oncofetal distribution, are carbohydrate moieties on glycoproteins or glycolipids (Feizi 1985). Such antigens may present a particular problem of heterogeneity of expression (Edwards 1985), a point to be noted if they are to be used as therapeutic targets.

Clearly most opportunities for antibody therapy are arising with target molecules which are not strictly tumour-specific. The loss of normal cells bearing these molecules would be acceptable were the tissue involved dispensable in the context of life-threatening disease (breast, prostate, thyroid, etc.) or capable of regeneration from antigen-negative precursors (as is frequently the case with myeloid and lymphoid lineages). A full histological survey for reactivity with the therapeutic antibody is mandatory, as 'lineage jumping', in which the differentiation antigen appears on a tissue not clearly related to the primary target, is well known: for example the murine T lymphoid antigen Thy-1 is present on brain, and the human B lymphoid antigen CD10 (common acute lymphoblastic leukaemia antigen, probably an endopeptidase) is on glomeruli and renal proximal tubules. The potential for serious untoward damage is obvious.

With the number of defined differentiation antigens increasing rapidly it is worth setting out some important questions relating to the suitability of a given molecule as a target for antibody, despite some of the topics involved not yet having been broached. Is the molecule on all the tumour cells? What is its surface density (or, better, density distribution throughout the cellular population)? Is it secreted to form an extracellular antigenic barrier? Does it modulate readily? Do antigen −ve mutants arise with significant frequency? Will engagement of the molecule by antibody activate the cell? On what normal tissues is the molecule present, and with what risk of serious damage from antibody attack?

Metabolic effects of antibody

Only rarely has it been recorded that antibody alighting on a cell surface proves directly harmful: usually damage occurs only as a result of an effector such as complement being recruited. An interesting exception is provided by examples of antibody inducing a series of cellular changes which terminate in a type of death (apoptosis) marked by extensive fragmentation of nuclear DNA. This has been seen in immature thymocytes in organ culture when engaged by antibody to the surface molecule CD3 (Smith *et al.* 1989), and among a variety of human lymphocytes engaged by antibody to a hitherto uncharacterized 52 kD surface molecule (Trauth *et al.* 1989). Among targets susceptible to the latter antibody were some freshly drawn leukaemic cells, and a human tumour xenografted into nude mice. So undoubtedly there exist some antigens through which antibody can transmit a signal for cellular suicide, although common experience with cytotoxicity assays *in vitro* suggests that the phenomenon is unusual.

On the other hand antibodies alone frequently alter the metabolic activities of target cells without apparently harming them. A large literature is concerned with antibody mimicking or blocking the actions of the physiological ligands for various surface antigens. In the worst case the cells could be propelled into increased mitotic activity, and many observations *in vitro* attest to such a possibility (Shearer *et al.* 1975; Baeker and Rothstein 1985; Cambier *et al.* 1987). However, upon confining our attention to lymphoid cells, on which for technical reasons most of the observations have been made, no clear rules emerge even for surface Ig, the best studied antigen. The subject is complicated by the concomitant presence or absence of cytokines and other growth factors, ancillary cells, and, possibly, unsuspected endotoxin (a potent stimulator of cytokine release). Tumours frequently do not mimic the responses of normal cells, and, among the lymphomas, chronic lymphocytic leukaemic cells tend to be notably more indolent than those of follicular lymphoma (Allebes *et al.* 1988; Beiske *et al.* 1988; Hivroz *et al.* 1988). There is evidence from a study of T lymphocytes that simultaneous engagement of two surface antigens (in this case CD3 or CD5 linked to one of a variety of other antigens) by bispecific antibody is particularly apt to impart an activating signal (Ledbetter *et al.* 1989) — a point to be borne in mind if contemplating the therapeutic use of similar antibodies.

In our present state of knowledge a stimulatory activity by antibody cannot be predicted with any confidence but must be feared. Although an accelerated tumour growth following administration of antibody has not been recorded clinically, it might on occasion have been obscured amid the complexity of natural tumour progression and cytotoxic effects of the therapy.

Under some circumstances antibody can impede cell growth *in vitro* without being cytotoxic (Warner and Scott 1988). One report already alluded to describes such a result following the interaction of antibody with the surface protein encoded by a transforming oncogene (Drebin *et al.* 1985).

When used against lymphoid tumours, especially the better differentiated ones, antibody might trigger immunological pathways which secondarily retard tumour growth. Thus Garcia *et al.* (1985) investigated the lymphoid histology in 10 patients with B cell lymphoma who had shown variable responses to treatment with anti-idiotype antibody: clinical remission seemed more likely the greater the number of infiltrating CD4+ve T cells and CD57+ve (natural killer (NK)) cells, and the greater the incidence of positivity for CD25 (IL-2 receptor α chain) among these cells. With only sketchy knowledge of normal regulatory pathways we cannot predict with any confidence an antitumour response by normal lymphoid tissue following an intervention of antibody.

One common metabolic consequence of antibody attaching to a cell surface is antigenic modulation, the clustering and clearing of surface antigen–antibody complexes. The recruitment of effectors by the antibody is thereby impeded — and in that context we consider modulation later.

Recruitment of effectors by antibody

As already discussed, native antibody must in general recruit natural effectors in order to damage its target cells. Many antibody derivatives to be described later work similarly. With antibody attached to its target the outwardly protruding Fc regions combine with effectors via weak interactions: thus K_A for union of Fc_γ with a complement C1q head has been reported at about $5 \times 10^4\ \text{M}^{-1}$; and for union with Fc_γ receptor III (Fc_γRIII), initiating antibody-dependent cellular cytotoxicity (ADCC), at about $5 \times 10^5\ \text{M}^{-1}$ (Hughes-Jones and Gardner 1979; Simmons and Seed 1989). It follows that effective recruitment requires multiple simultaneous interactions — provided by a sufficiently dense array of properly oriented antibody, of appropriate isotype, on the cell surface. This requirement represents a safety factor additional to antibody specificity: it will be appreciated that sparse antibody attaching to normal cells or antigen–antibody complexes taken up by a cell's Fc receptors are unlikely to yield an effective Fc array.

The well-known effectors are complement, macrophages and those lymphocytes which mediate ADCC. The last group might constitute a distinct cellular class, the NK cells or large granular lymphocytes (LGL). Possible consequences of activating these effector systems are set out in Table 94.1, but it must be understood that the tumour cells have antigenic modulation and other defences available as means of escape. In addition to the cells in Table 94.1, others with Fc receptors — neutrophils, eosinophils and platelets — have been suggested as candidates for damaging antibody-coated tumour.

Given samples of the antibody and its cellular targets, complement activation and lymphocytic ADCC can be assessed fairly readily in the test tube, macrophage cytotoxicity somewhat more problematically. Tables 94.2 and 94.3 set out a consensus of which isotypes are capable of invoking the various effector functions (Ralph and Nakoinz 1983; Hale *et al.* 1985; Kipps *et al.* 1985; Anasetti *et al.* 1987; Ortaldo *et al.* 1987; Mellman *et al.* 1988; Unkeless *et al.* 1988; Fanger *et al.* 1989; Walker *et al.* 1989). Isotypes are given for mouse and rat, the sources of the vast majority of monoclonal antibodies; and for man because human Fc regions are available for constructing rodent/human chimeric antibodies.

Table 94.3 overlaps Table 94.2 but moves back a step in the effector process by showing which IgG isotypes will bind to the various Fc_γ receptors. Such information is more readily available than

Table 94.1. Possible consequences of effector activation by antibody to tumour

Effector	Possible consequences
Complement	Opsonization Lysis Promotion of inflammation (anaphylatoxins)
Macrophages	Phagocytosis ADCC (extracellular lysis) Antibody-dependent cellular cytostasis[a] Cellular sequestration[b]
Natural killer (NK) cells[c]	ADCC

a Defined *in vitro* by the tumour cell ceasing to synthesize DNA after being in contact with the macrophage (Pasternack *et al.* 1978).

b Circulating tumour cells may be sequestered on fixed macrophages (e.g. Kupffer cells), with one of the other macrophage-induced fates possibly following.

c Defined by simultaneous possession of the surface antigens CD16 and CD57, and constitute a major component of the morphologically defined large granular lymphocytes.

Table 94.2. Effectors recruited by antibodies

Antibody isotype	Recruitment of human effectors: For complement lysis (via the classical pathway)	Recruitment of human effectors: For lymphocytic ADCC
Human		
IgM	+	−
IgG-1	+	+
IgG-2	±	±
IgG-3	+	+
IgG-4	−	−
Mouse		
IgM	+	−
IgG-1	−	(−)
IgG-2a	+	(+)
IgG-2b	+	(+)
IgG-3	+	+
Rat		
IgM	+	−
IgG-1	−	−
IgG-2a	+	−
IgG-2b	+	+
IgG-2c	+	−

± = Weak or inconsistent; ( ) = disparate reports from different groups.

Table 94.3. Antibody attachments to human Fc_γ receptors

	Fc_γ receptors and cells exhibiting high densities		
	$Fc_\gamma RI^a$	$Fc_\gamma RII^{b,c}$	$Fc_\gamma RIII^b$
Antibody isotype	Monocytes Macrophages	Monocytes Macrophages Neutrophils Eosinophils Platelets B lymphocytes	Macrophages Neutrophils NK cells
Human			
IgG-1	+	+	+
IgG-2	−	±	−
IgG-3	+	+	+
IgG-4	±	±	−
Mouse			
IgG-1	−	±	(±)
IgG-2a	+	−	(+)
IgG-2b	−	+	(−)
IgG-3	+	−	+

± = Weak or inconsistent; ( ) = disparate reports.

a High affinity.

b Low affinity.

c A widespread receptor with at least two subtypes and a fairly catholic binding spectrum.

One can infer from the table which effector cells are likely to adhere to tumour coated with antibody of the given isotype — or, in the case of chimeric antibodies, displaying Fc_γ belonging to the indicated isotype. The consequences of such adherence vary: see text.

subsequent effector performances of the receptor-bearing cells. All of these cells are apt to adhere to target cells coated with an antibody of an appropriate isotype. Among possible consequences for the target are cytostasis, extracellular lysis (ADCC), phagocytosis — or no apparent harm at all. Our predictive ability in this area is sadly deficient, but it seems that engagement of the receptor must activate the effector cell in some way as a minimum requirement for damaging the target. In this context it might be relevant that Fc_γRIII on neutrophils is phospholipid-linked to the cell membrane and will not mediate ADCC, whereas in NK cells it exists as a transmembrane protein and does perform this function (Scallon *et al*. 1989).

The references given for Tables 94.2 and 94.3 contain many contradictions, especially for ADCC. This is not surprising as terms other than antibody isotype enter the equation, sometimes in an uncertain manner — the nature of the surface antigen, its density, its tendency to modulate, the nature of the target cell, even given a non-modulating antigen of high density (Lesley *et al*. 1974), and the source of the effector. A well-known example of the last is the large variation in achievable ADCC using blood lymphocytic effectors from different normal donors.

The performance of effector cells engaging tumour targets could also be modulated by engagement of receptors other than those for Fc_γ: for example, the complement receptors CR1 and CR3 on macrophages — with these receptors in turn subjected to regulation by other signals (Wright and Silverstein 1986).

EFFECTORS RELEVANT *IN VIVO*

The performance of an effector function *in vitro* might not correlate well with that *in vivo*, particularly in the case of cellular effectors where we cannot mimic well in the test-tube the proper metabolic and anatomical environs of interacting cells. This leads to a major conundrum: which effectors are involved in those therapeutic effects of antibody that have been recorded in animals and man? The available evidence is of only limited help.

Even in what might be considered a relatively simple case, the dependence on complement of antibody suppression of animal leukaemia/lymphoma, one is confronted by contradictory results. Reports from two centres using anti-idiotype antibodies suggest that complement is irrelevant, since the therapeutic effects seen in recipients grossly deficient in complement were similar to those occurring in recipients with normal levels (Lanier *et al*. 1980; Stevenson and Glennie 1985). In contrast there are reports of antibody suppression of leukaemia being depressed when complement was depleted by pretreatment of the recipients with cobra venom factor (Johnson *et al*. 1985), or being enhanced by supplementation with exogenous complement (Kassel *et al*. 1973; Bernstein *et al*. 1980). At face value these results imply that the significance of complement varies widely under different circumstances. Individual tumour cells will always be apt to escape direct membrane damage by it because of their multiple lines of defence: antigenic modulation, convertase inactivators and inhibitors, inactivators of the membrane attack complex and excision of the complexes. But complement might enhance ADCC (Lustig and Bianco 1976), and its ability to promote local inflammation could be useful when dealing with tumour masses.

In some animal tumours the therapeutic efficacy of antibody has shown some correlation with its ability to promote ADCC *in vitro* (Hersey 1973; Denkers *et al*. 1985; Kaminski *et al*. 1986). Similarly, in the treatment of human lymphoma with isotypic variants of a rat antibody (Campath-1) directed against the lymphocytic/monocytic antigen CDw52, antibodies which activated complement (IgM and IgG-2a) had a much less pronounced lympholytic effect than an IgG-2b antibody which both activated complement and invoked ADCC (Dyer *et al*. 1989). These findings are consistent with ADCC having a useful role *in vivo* — a matter potentially of considerable practical importance, since the administration of IL-2 might enhance the ADCC activity of NK cells (Shiloni *et al*. 1987).

A role for macrophages in disposing of antibody-coated tumour has been suggested by Seto *et al*. (1986), working with an ascitic mouse mammary carcinoma. Antibody-coated cells implanted subcutaneously invoked a heavy mononuclear, largely macrophage, infiltration, while antibody-induced suppression of the tumour was impaired when the recipients were treated with agents toxic to macrophages (carrageenan or silica particles). In both animals and man many groups have reported the rapid disappearance of leukaemic cells from blood upon infusing antibody reactive with their cell surfaces. Sequestration by macrophages in liver and spleen might be a major mechanism involved here. Whether cells so sequestered are necessarily killed is not clear. *In vitro* the adherence of antibody-coated tumour cells to macrophages need not be followed by either phagocytosis or extracellular killing, but there may be an abrupt cessation of DNA synthesis (antibody-dependent cellular cytostasis (Pasternack *et al.* 1978; Lawson and Stevenson 1983)). The relevance of this phenomenon for events *in vivo* is not known.

The useful recruitment of effectors by antibody *in vivo* is likely to be a complex problem. Optimal recruitment could still leave a heavy dependence on strictly local variables. Such dependence occurs in the context of animals mounting immune responses to tumour challenges, the tumour sometimes being suppressed at sites of secondary challenge while continuing to grow at the primary site (Gorelik 1983).

Factors impeding antibody therapy

The factors can be discussed under the headings set out in Table 94.4.

Cellular seedings in sites such as the central nervous system and testis — both notorious as havens for leukaemic cells in the face of chemotherapy — are likely to be difficult to reach with either antibody or its effectors. There must exist a continuum of accessibility from such areas up to cells sited in the bloodstream itself and thus bathed immediately in infused antibody. The interior of relatively avascular solid tumour is often posed as a problem, but antibody has been shown to penetrate lymphomatous masses (Meeker *et al.* 1985b), and in the worst case there remains the possibility of whittling away solid tumour from the periphery inwards. An interesting discussion of the factors likely to influence antibody permeation of solid tumour has been provided by Cobb (1989).

Some cell surface antigens might not qualify as targets for antibody plus natural effectors because their average density is too low to yield a satisfactory array of antibody Fc. Others, with a satisfactory average density, can exhibit at a given moment within a cellular population a wide range of non-heritable variation (Taupier *et al.* 1983), which could permit a significant proportion of the tumour cells to survive an attack by antibody over a limited period of time.

Any form of chemotherapy or immunotherapy can be thwarted by phenotypic change in the target cells, and antibody treatment is clearly vulnerable to mutations affecting cell surface antigens. In the well-studied case of surface Ig idiotype on neoplastic B lymphocytes, animal tumours under immunological attack have been seen to escape either by Ig chain deletion (the commonest means) or by point mutations affecting the idiotype (Lynch *et al.* 1972; Glennie *et al.* 1987a). It might be supposed that such a problem would arise only rarely with the much more slowly growing human lymphomas, but in fact clonal variants unreactive with a therapeutic monoclonal anti-idiotype antibody have become apparent after a mere 2 months of treatment (Meeker *et al.* 1985a). In the human neoplasms there is evidence to suggest that clonal variation due to idiotype mutation is more often apparent in follicular lymphomas than in chronic lymphocytic leukaemias (Cleary *et al.* 1988; Kipps *et al.* 1988).

The possible evasion of antibody by either mutation or non-heritable variation of antigen presents a strong case for attacking two or more antigens simultaneously, a prospect improving with continuing mapping of cell surfaces.

Antigenic modulation, defined originally as antibody-induced resistance to the cytotoxic action of antibody plus complement (Boyse and Old 1969), is associated with redistribution of antigen–antibody complexes on the cell surface (Stackpole *et al.* 1974). The antigen, tethered by antibody, moves over the surface to form patches and sometimes a cap at one pole of the cell. Simultaneously the complexes are removed by pinocytosis at the patches and cap until the surface is cleared of the target molecules. Clearance can be perpetuated by delayed delivery of further antigen to the surface, perhaps an important contribution to chronic

Table 94.4. Factors impeding antibody therapy of tumour

Inaccessibility of cells
Sparseness of surface antigen, including mutational loss
Modulation of surface antigen
Extracellular antigen
Inadequate recruitment of effectors, including effector exhaustion
Immune response to the antibody

modulation *in vivo* (Sidman and Unanue 1975; Glennie *et al*. 1979). The whole process appears to be triggered by cross-linking of the surface Ig by bivalent antibody: so it is hardly surprising that monoclonal antibodies, with fewer opportunities for crosslinking, are much poorer modulators than polyclonal (Elliott *et al*. 1987). Slow internalization of antigen complexed with univalent (Fab) antibody has been reported (Lamm *et al*. 1968) but it is not clear how this might differ from constitutive turnover of the antigen concerned. Resistance to complement lysis does not require complete clearing of the antigen–antibody from the cell surface: the initial patching process can confer considerable resistance, and in the case of surface Ig can occur with a rapidity sufficient to provide some protection for cells confronted simultaneously by antibody and complement (Gordon and Stevenson 1981). Given this fact it is unfortunate that the term antigenic modulation is often used synonymously with surface clearing: antibody-induced, non-heritable resistance to antibody-mediated killing is closer to the original definition.

Modulation has been recognized as a problem with a variety of surface antigens (e.g. Ritz and Schlossman 1982). The ease with which it occurs varies with different antigens: there appears to be a spectrum from the rapidly modulating surface Ig down to molecules reported not to modulate at all, such as Class I and II major histocompatibility complex (MHC) antigens and the lymphocytic/monocytic Campath-1 target (Hale *et al*. 1983). It should be noted, however, that modulation is probably much more efficient *in vivo* that *in vitro* (Chatenoud *et al*. 1982; Hamblin *et al*. 1987). One mechanism accounting for this could be reflected in the observation that modulation is enhanced by contacts between target cells and monocytes (Schroff *et al*. 1985), the Fc_γ receptors of the latter presumably engaging bound antibody and thereby conveying a further signal to the target cell.

Extracellular antigen will clearly impede the access of antibody to the tumour cell surface. At the same time the immune complexes formed by antibody and extracellular antigen will be a source of toxicity, and may seriously deplete effector capacity.

In the well-studied case of lymphoid cells many surface proteins have not been reported in plasma, their turnover on the cell presumably being associated with internalization followed by either recycling or intracellular degradation. Immunoglobulin appears in extracellular fluid due to the existence of a secretory pathway which accompanies the membrane insertion pathway. Some proteins (e.g. CD8, CD23, CD25) may be released from the surface into the environs by hydrolytic cleavage. Still others may be associated with vesicles or other fragments shed from the plasma membrane. The problem of shedding from cell surfaces is difficult (Black 1980) and its prevalence may have been exaggerated by the behaviour of cells in less than ideal conditions *in vitro*.

In the anti-idiotype approach to lymphoma it was a disappointment to find that most examples of human B cell lymphoma and lymphocytic leukaemia — simplistically regarded as having tumour idiotypic Ig confined to their cell surfaces — have sufficient secretory pathway activity to provide a variable but often significant extracellular antigenic barrier (Stevenson *et al*. 1980). Clinical experience showed that sufficient antibody had to be given to eliminate this barrier before any tumour response was noted (Meeker *et al*. 1985b). Plasmaphaeresis has had a rather variable effect in lowering the level of plasma idiotype prior to antibody infusion (Gordon *et al*. 1984; Meeker *et al*. 1985b).

By activating complement and promoting release of cytokines, immune complexes formed by extracellular antigen during antibody infusion probably contribute substantially to the immediate toxicity (fever, flushing, bronchospasm) which is sometimes troublesome. Transient thrombocytopenia might arise from the same cause (Meeker *et al*. 1985b). The symptoms can generally be avoided by giving the infusion slowly (e.g. 100 mg over 4 hours). The physician should also be alert to the possibility of renal damage and other long-term problems arising from immune complexes.

Inadequate recruitment of effectors could be due to an inappropriate antibody isotype, or to a locally inadequate effector concentration. We have already seen that assessments here are clouded by incomplete knowledge of the effectors and of their relevance. Skilled use of antibody might eventually have to take account of effector capacity: thus both Nadler *et al*. (1980) and Gordon *et al*. (1984) observed the transient persistence of dead leukaemic cells in the blood after antibody treatment, suggesting exhaustion of phagocytic capacity.

Perhaps more than half of cancer patients treated

with mouse monoclonal antibody have exhibited a significant immune response to the xenogeneic Ig. Continued infusion in the face of anti-antibody will lead to hazards from immune complexes similar to those discussed for extracellular antigen, with the aggravation that the anti-antibody will not melt away: so the appearance of an immune response will generally terminate the antibody therapy. It is not clear how rapid the response need be, or whether it is inevitable at all. Foreign serum proteins given intravenously can be tolerogenic if carefully freed of aggregates (Dresser 1962), and there is a suspicion that some early antibody preparations were contaminated not merely by aggregates but also by endotoxin, which could serve as an adjuvant (Amerding and Katz 1974). One experienced group has recorded a lower incidence of anti-antibody responses with the advent of purer antibody preparations (Brown *et al.* 1989). However, the possibility of keeping therapeutic antibody completely tolerogenic must be compromised by the fact that, by its very nature, the antibody is likely to form immune complexes with its target antigen and so assume an immunogenic form.

Anticancer drugs tend to be cytotoxic for dividing cells and hence incidentally immunosuppressive. On this basis chemotherapy can be scheduled with therapeutic antibody so as to reduce the tendency for an anti-antibody response. The use of the specialized immunosuppressant cyclosporin, in conjunction with careful deaggregation of the therapeutic antibody, has also been reported (Ledermann *et al.* 1988).

Chimeric antibodies in which much of the xenogeneic molecule is replaced with human Ig sequences (described below) can be expected to be less immunogenic than the original in man. However, the possibility of an anti-idiotype response to the variable domains on the antibody must always remain.

It has been pointed out that under certain circumstances an immune response to therapeutic antibody could enhance its antitumour effect. An anti-idiotypic response could yield host antibody in which the combining sites sterically resemble the tumour epitope, so that it could in turn evoke a further round of anti-idiotypic response capable of damaging the tumour (Wettendorff *et al.* 1989). Another possibility is for therapeutic antibody to be internalized by the tumour cell, processed and displayed in conjunction with Class II MHC antigens, and thereby to bring down upon the cell cytotoxic T cells which have emerged with anti-Ig specificity (Lanzavecchia *et al.* 1988). The feasibility of both of the above mechanisms has been demonstrated — provided in each case that a fairly selective type of anti-antibody response emerges.

Antibody plus other agents

It may well emerge that antibody administered with another antitumour agent such as a drug or radiotherapy proves more effective than either alone, and this possibility is being explored clinically. Sometimes there is a clear rationale behind the combination, as recorded above in the use of a cytotoxic drug to inhibit the anti-antibody response. Another combination receiving attention is that of antibody plus a cytokine, usually one of the interferons or IL-2 which could activate effector cells and thereby enhance their attack on antibody-coated targets (Shiloni *et al.* 1987; Dearman *et al.* 1988; Brown *et al.* 1989). As both the antibody and cytokine used singly can display antitumour activity, it might not be easy to evaluate the benefits and mechanisms of the combination.

Antibody derivatives

Even before the monoclonal era therapeutic disappointment with native antibody prompted investigation of derivatives with enhanced cytotoxic potential (Mathé *et al.* 1958). In recent years this activity has become widespread. No clear case for any derivative has yet been demonstrated clinically, so the account here will simply survey the underlying principles.

Table 94.5 sets out a list of derivatives which is not exhaustive. It can be seen that they are divisible into two broad categories according to whether they utilize natural or exogenous effectors.

DERIVATIVES UTILIZING NATURAL EFFECTORS

As discussed above the recruitment of complement and cellular effectors is dependent on an effective Fc array on the target cell. Chimeric, univalent and multi-Fc antibodies are all designed ultimately to improve the quality of this array.

In chimeric derivatives, constructed either gen-

Table 94.5. Some antibody derivatives designed to attack neoplastic cells

Utilizing natural effectors
1 Recruiting via Fc
Chimeric antibody
Univalent antibody
2 Recruiting via antibody sites
Bispecific antibody-recruiting effectors
Utilizing exogenous effectors
Radiolabelled antibody
Drug–antibody conjugates
Toxin–antibody conjugates (immunotoxins)
Bispecific antibody-recruiting drug or toxin
Enzyme-antibody activating pro-drug

etically or chemically, the Fc zone of the monoclonal antibody and often parts of the Fab as well are replaced by human sequences to yield rodent/human molecular chimeras. Usually the Fc from the human subclass IgG1 is chosen. The chimerism confers three advantages: (i) the recruitment of human effectors is improved by having an array of human rather than rodent Fc (see Tables 94.2 and 94.3); (ii) the catabolism of the antibody, also dependent on its Fc moiety, is slowed from the rapid rate seen for xenogenic IgG, to attain ideally the half-life of about 20 days characteristic of human IgG (Spiegelberg and Weigle 1965; Waldmann and Strober 1969); (iii) the immunogenicity of the antibody, towards which the Fc makes a major contribution, is reduced.

Chimeric antibodies have been constructed genetically by (i) assembling *in vitro* recombinant heavy and light chain genes in which sequences for mouse variable domains have been combined with those for human constant domains; (ii) transfecting these genes into a suitable expressing cell, often a lymphoid cell (Morrison *et al.* 1984). Even greater representation of human sequences has been achieved by inserting only the hypervariable sequences of a mouse antibody into an IgG molecule otherwise completely human (Riechmann *et al.* 1988). It is reasonable to suppose that the greater the human content of the chimeric molecule the less immunogenic it will be, and in the construction of Riechmann *et al.* only the idiotypic epitopes, and possibly one or more allotypic epitopes, will be foreign to a human recipient. Preliminary accounts of clinical use of genetic chimeras have been published (Hale *et al.* 1988; LoBuglio *et al.* 1989).

Chimeric antibodies may be constructed chemically in a variety of ways. Frequently advantage is taken of sulph-hydryl groups — the most reactive groups found on proteins — released by reduction of Ig interchain disulphide bonds. These may be utilized for example to join Fab'_γ from mouse monoclonal antibody to Fc_γ from human normal Ig, the linkage being by either disulphide or thioether bonds (Rybarska *et al.* 1982; Stevenson *et al.* 1989). The latter bonds can be expected to be the more stable *in vivo*. This approach lacks the convenience of a cell line synthesizing the final product, as is yielded by genetic engineering, but the technology is readily adaptable to formation of chimeras with other features such as univalency or bispecificity of antibody function, or with multiple Fc_γ (Stevenson *et al.* 1989).

Univalent antibody with an intact Fc_γ region was introduced by Glennie and Stevenson (1982) as a means of killing mammalian cells more effectively by avoiding antigenic modulation. Rabbit IgG antibody with anti-idiotypic specificity for lymphoma cells was rendered univalent by limited digestion with papain, removing one Fab arm. The residual molecule (Fab/c) displayed no antigenic modulation *in vitro*, and was clearly superior to its parent IgG both in invoking complement lysis *in vitro* and in immunotherapy of guinea-pig lymphoma. Functionally similar univalent antibodies have subsequently been produced by chemically joining mouse Fab'_γ and human Fc_γ (Watts *et al.* 1985); and by taking advantage of the functional univalency of asymmetric IgG molecules which can be produced by hybrid hybridomas, or can arise in conventional hybridomas when one light chain from the myeloma fusion partner is incorporated per molecule (Milstein and Cuello 1983; Cobbold and Waldmann 1984; Clark *et al.* 1989).

Limited clinical applications of univalent antibodies have been reported (Hamblin *et al.* 1987; Clark *et al.* 1989). It is of some interest that Hamblin *et al.* observed antigenic modulation of lymphoma cells exposed to the univalent antibody *in vivo* but not *in vitro*, possibly reflecting the role of Fc receptor-bearing cells in promoting modulation (Schroff *et al.* 1985). No measurements could be made of the briskness of modulation *in vivo*.

Bispecific antibody and redirected cellular cytotoxicity

An entirely different strategy for recruiting natural effectors entails the construction of bispecific antibody, one arm of which engages the target cell while the other engages an effector. Thus the effector is brought to the target by capture at an antibody site rather than by capture at Fc, and several features follow immediately: the binding of the effector is apt to be tighter than its normal binding to Fc; the bispecific antibody will be restricted to a single effector in contrast to the multiple recruiting capabilities of Fc; but the bispecific antibody can be tailored to effectors such as cytotoxic T cells, which are unavailable to Fc. Although some studies of recruitment of complement components have been reported, the application of bispecific antibodies to natural effectors has usually enlisted cells such as T and NK cells and monocytes. Such recruitment has been called redirected cellular cytotoxicity.

Bispecific antibodies can be prepared by either chemical or genetic methods. For the former a convenient starting-point is the Fab'_{γ} yielded by sequential peptic digestion and reductive cleavage of IgG antibodies. These fragments contain readily utilizable SH groups on their γ chain hinges. Nisonoff and Mandy (1962) noted the formation of bispecific $F(ab')_2$ when Fab'_{γ} from two antibodies were allowed to dimerize by oxidative formation of inter-γ SS, the yield indicating that the dimerization was random. Higher yields, in principle approaching 100%, are obtainable by using directed disulphide interchange or by using the SH to form a tandem thioether linkage between the Fab'_{γ} (Glennie *et al.* 1987b). The latter type of linkage is likely to be more stable than SS bonds *in vivo*. To produce bispecific products without the need for a preliminary enzymic digestion, monoclonal IgG antibodies have simply been aggregated by lysine-reactive/SH-reactive cross-linkers, and the various products fractionated (Karpovsky *et al.* 1984).

Genetic production of bispecific IgG has been accomplished by fusing the two hybridomas which secrete the selected parental antibodies (Milstein and Cuello 1983). In successful hybrid hybridomas the four polypeptide chains involved (two heavy, two light) will be co-dominantly expressed, but problems arise with the variety of chain pairings available. Preservation of good antibody activity requires in general that the homologous heavy–light pairings be preserved, and fortunately it appears that such pairings are often favoured energetically. Given correct heavy–light pairings, bispecificity requires heterologous heavy–heavy (usually γ–γ) union: such pairing should be random, given the same isotypes, and it is not clear whether a mere subclass difference between γ chains will carry a significant energy penalty for their union. Altogether it is clear that the hybrid hybridoma can put out a wide range of products and that the problem of isolating the required species might be difficult.

Redirected cellular cytotoxicity works well *in vitro* and, since the effectors are enlisted highly selectively, it has considerable potential for studying cytotoxic mechanisms (Segal *et al.* 1988). The bispecific antibody may be aimed at any molecule of sufficient specificity and density on the target cell, but the molecule engaged on the effector cell presents the additional requirement that it be suitable for activating that cell for cytotoxicity. Sometimes untoward effects can intrude, as in the demonstration by Clark and Waldmann (1987) that effector cells recruited by Fc-displaying bispecific antibodies can themselves fall victim to NK-mediated ADCC. Such an occurrence argues for bispecific derivatives of the $F(ab')_2$ type, but these are likely to have shorter metabolic survivals than Fc-containing derivatives.

Demonstrations of the effectiveness of redirected cellular cytotoxicity *in vivo* have been restricted to two situations: firstly, Winn-type assays, where antibody-laden effector cells are mixed with tumour cells before inoculation into mice; secondly, treatment of human tumour xenografts localized to the peritoneal cavity in nude mice and treated with intraperitoneal injections of antibody-laden human lymphocytes (Segal *et al.* 1988). Its general application to the treatment of established tumour, by simply injecting the bispecific antibody, will face kinetic problems in that the antibody must neither be consumed by effector cells before reaching the tumour (remembering that it has a higher affinity for the effectors than is conferred normally by Fc), nor be in such excess as to block the bridging of effector and target cells.

DERIVATIVES UTILIZING EXOGENOUS EFFECTORS

A variety of potentially damaging agents have been conjugated to antibody in order that they be delivered to tumour. Radio-isotopes, drugs and toxins have been the most popular, but the list extends to enzymes, complement components, cytokines and others. Related approaches include the recruitment of exogenous effector by bispecific antibody (antitumour/anti-effector), and the activation of a pro-drug by antibody-enzyme conjugate at the site of tumour.

Antibodies conjugated to exogenous agents have often proved much more potent *in vitro* than native antibody, but their use *in vivo* has been attended by problems of complexity and toxicity. A major problem is the limited extent to which systemically injected antibody localizes in tumour (Glennie and Wyeth 1986). Conjugates delivered to the wrong areas have considerable potential for toxicity. We have seen that antibody relying on natural effectors will damage a cell only if it builds up on it a sufficient and correctly oriented Fc array. In contrast antibody conjugated to a potent toxin or radio-isotope offers no such safety factor to complement the specificity of delivery. The problem of systemic toxicity has led to considerable interest in local delivery of antibody/exogenous effector, as into the peritoneal cavity or subarachnoid space: in such sites the natural effectors are likely to be in short supply, whereas the exogenous agent remains effective and is delivered with greater precision than when given by the systemic route.

Radiolabelled antibody

Conjugates of antibody and radioactive isotope offer the attractive possibility of dual function — both locating and therapeutically irradiating tumour deposits. Radio-imaging usually involves external scintigraphy of a γ-emitting isotope carried by antibody to tumour deposits. With the localizing capability thus demonstrated a conjugate suitable for radio-immunotherapy can be administered. The isotope involved may be the same as used for imaging (at perhaps up to 100 times the dose) or different, with the cytotoxic effect dependent on α or β emission.

An advantage of radio-immunotherapy of special relevance to solid tumours is that it is not necessary to deliver a critical dose of antibody to each cell. The isotope, to an extent dependent on its emission characteristics, can be relied upon to irradiate vicinal cells. By the same argument the targeted molecules in solid tumours can include not only those on cell surfaces but also any which are at relatively high concentrations in the tumour interstitial fluid.

The isotope iodine-131 (^{131}I) has been the most widely used for both imaging and therapy. It can be coupled to antibody, over a wide range of activity, by a well-studied substitution on tyrosine. Its γ emission, although more energetic than desirable, permits external scintigraphy. The therapeutic effect relies upon its β emission: the electrons damage cells by virtue of the energy transferred at the point of arrest, and a distribution of path lengths up to a maximum of about 2 mm appears suitable for irradiating tumour masses. A theoretical discussion of this subject has been provided by McGaughey (1974). For over 40 years the isotope has been used in the form of Na^{131}I for the treatment of hyperthyroidism and thyroid cancer, so the distribution and toxicity of ^{131}I released from antibody are well understood.

Recently there has been a move towards the use of antibodies labelled with technetium-99 (^{99}Tc) or indium-111 (^{111}In) for imaging, neither isotope having an emission suitable for therapy. There has been no similar replacement of ^{131}I for therapeutic conjugates although a number of possibilities (including the β emitters ^{90}Y, ^{47}Sc and ^{67}Cu, and the α emitters ^{212}Bi and ^{211}At) have been discussed (Schlom 1986; Goldenberg 1989). The chemistry involved in isotope coupling has been summarized by Glennie and Wyeth (1986).

The Achilles' heel of radiolabelled antibody is the quality of its delivery. Clearly this is a critical factor in determining whether ablative radiation can be delivered to a neoplasm without incurring unacceptable damage to normal tissue such as marrow or gut. Radiolocalization indices have been defined as the ratio of counts per gram of tumour to counts per gram of well-vascularized normal tissue. Values greater than 3 derived from biopsies are 'arbitrarily considered as positive for MAb [monoclonal antibody] localization' (Schlom 1989) — hardly a stringent criterion. Much of the investigation and success in radio-imaging has involved target molecules which are secreted by tumour: carcinoembryonic antigen in various carcinomas, α-fetoprotein in hepatoma, and chorionic gonadotrophin in trophoblastic and germ cell tumours (Bagshawe and Searle 1977; Mach *et al.* 1981; Deland and Goldenberg 1985). Surprisingly little difficulty seems to have been posed by plasma antigen, although in some cases it might be necessary to provide sufficient antibody to complex it all before good access to tumour is attained (Larson 1985). There is convincing evidence that a variable and sometimes large element in the localization of antibody in solid tumour derives simply from leakiness of tumour vasculature. Labelled albumin will sometimes localize in tumours (Busch and Greene 1955). Further, in a project aimed at detecting focal infection, Rubin *et al.* (1989) scanned the distribution of ^{111}In-labelled non-specific IgG and found the label localized in neoplasms in 13 of 16 cancer patients investigated.

Local injection of antibody into the peritoneal cavity, in cases of metastatic ovarian carcinoma confined to this region, was superior to intravenous injection in labelling ascitic but not solid tumour (Ward *et al.* 1987); in some of the patients concerned the intravenous labelling of solid tumour was no better with specific than with irrelevant antibody.

Evidently tumour localization of the radiolabelled antibodies investigated to date can reflect their attaching to cell surfaces, their forming immune complexes locally with secretory molecules present in high concentration, or simply a tendency for leaky blood vessels to allow extravasation of antibody or immune complexes. The multiplicity of mechanisms could compromise reproducibility and reinforces the case for imaging before undertaking therapy with large doses of isotope.

Results of radio-immunotherapy have on the whole been inconsistent and disappointing. The therapeutic use of intraperitoneal ^{131}I–antibody yielded no benefit with solid tumour but showed some promise for controlling malignant ascites (Ward *et al.* 1988), a finding in keeping with the same group's assessment of labelling by antibody. The use of systemic radiolabelled antibody in very large doses has been tried, keeping purged autologous marrow in reserve to treat myelosuppression: complete remissions occurred in four of five cases of refractory non-Hodgkin's lymphoma with moderate tumour burdens who received up to 608 mCi ^{131}I (Press *et al.* 1989). Despite its modest results, radio-immunotherapy can be characterized in depth and enjoys a continually improving technology; not surprisingly it continues to attract a strong band of devotees.

Drug–antibody conjugates

The covalent linking of an anticancer drug to antibody is intended to deliver it more accurately to tumour targets. If successful, the procedure should confer on the drug concerned a higher therapeutic index than it exhibits in the free state. No conjugate has been shown convincingly to have fulfilled this requirement in a clinical setting. The subject is obviously complex. The simplicity of the concept of using antibody to concentrate a drug in the vicinity of tumour vanishes on closer scrutiny: one must consider the quality of antibody localization, the intracellular route of the complex (possibly often lysosomal), its intracellular fate, and the mode of action and efficacy of the drug when delivered thus. A surprising item of background information is that anticancer drugs have sometimes been seen to gain in potency upon conjugation to a macromolecule with no specific homing characteristics: examples are daunomycin conjugated to dextran (Bernstein *et al.* 1978) and a bivalent alkylating agent conjugated to fibrinogen (Wade *et al.* 1967).

Despite all problems, the targeted drug concept has aroused sufficient enthusiasm for conjugates to have been prepared between monoclonal antibodies and virtually all classes of anticancer drugs. Thus the list includes alkylating agents such as chlorambucil and (with an action similar to alkylating agents) cisplatin; DNA-binding antibiotics such as daunomycin and doxorubicin; the vinca alkaloids, which interfere with microtubular function; and antimetabolites such as methotrexate and 5-fluorouracil. A large amount of data exists on actions of the conjugates on transplanted syngeneic murine tumours and on human tumour xenografts in nude mice. A recent comprehensive review of these results, from which no group of conjugates emerges as clearly superior, has been provided by Pimm (1988). Some clinical trials have been started.

Other strategies for guidance of drugs by antibody

Drugs may be targeted to tumour by being enclosed in antibody-coated liposomes, with the caveat that binding of the liposomes to the cell does not necessarily ensure incorporation of their contents (Weinstein *et al.* 1978): the capacity to mediate internalization is a criterion to be used in selecting the target molecule. A comparison of two targets for delivery to leukaemic T lymphocytes has recently been reported by Hege *et al.* (1989).

Another interesting concept, ADEPT (antibody-directed enzyme pro-drug therapy (Bagshawe 1987)), envisages a two-stage approach to selective drug delivery. First an antibody–enzyme conjugate is administered and allowed to accumulate preferentially in tumour. A second injection delivers a pro-drug which can be cleaved and thereby activated by the antibody enzyme. Drug/enzyme combinations being investigated include an alkylating agent activated upon removal of glutamate by a carboxypeptidase (Bagshawe *et al.* 1988); and phosphorylated derivatives of mitomycin C and etoposide activated by an alkaline phosphatase (Senter *et al.* 1989).

Toxin–antibody conjugates (immunotoxins)

The toxins which dominate this field are ribosome-inactivating proteins (RIP), distributed widely in the plant world and with three well-known bacterial representatives. The plant proteins catalytically inactivate eukaryotic 60S ribosomes, rendering them incapable of binding elongation factor 2 (Endo *et al.* 1987). They are divisible into types I and II (Stirpe and Barbieri 1986). Type I plant RIP (e.g. saporin, gelonin) exist naturally as single-chain proteins which have no ready means of entry into cells and are therefore normally innocuous. The type II proteins, of which ricin and abrin are well-known examples, consist of two disulphide-bonded chains: A (ribosome-inactivating) and B (attaching to cell surfaces). With entry into cells mediated by their B chains these are potent toxins.

The recognized bacterial RIP are diphtheria toxin, *Pseudomonas* (exo)toxin and *Shigella* (neuro)toxin. The *Shigella* protein appears to have attracted little attention in this field. The other two have as their mode of action a catalytic inactivation of elongation factor 2. Diphtheria toxin possesses A and B chains analogous to those of the type II plant proteins. *Pseudomonas* toxin is a single-chain protein with three identified domains, serving cellular attachment, translocation from endocytic vesicles into cytosol and toxicity (Fitzgerald and Pastan 1989).

Immunotoxins consisting of antibody linked to RIP are the most potent of the antibody conjugates now being contemplated for use in cancer. Their mode of action can be appreciated by considering ricin and its derivatives (reviewed by Vitetta *et al.* 1987; Blakey and Thorpe 1988). The intact toxin binds via its B chain to galactosyl residues present in large numbers in cell surface glycoproteins and glycolipids. Thence the A chain is translocated into the cytosol by processes poorly understood. Apparently that fraction which is to exert the cytotoxic effect is endocytosed and, with the B chain playing a facilitatory role, passes through the trans-Golgi network before passing into the cytosol (Youle and Colombatti 1987). The efficiency of catalytic ribosomal inactivation means that in principle one ricin molecule can kill a cell, but the inefficiency of translocation might require many molecules to attach to the cell to yield an average of one which becomes catalytically active.

In ricin immunotoxins the cell-attaching role of the B chain is usurped by monoclonal antibody. Most preparations consist of a ricin A chain disulphide-bonded to an antibody molecule. The S of this bond contributed by the A chain derives from the single disulphide bond which linked it originally to the B chain, while the S contributed by the antibody is from thiol groups introduced on lysine residues. Thioether-bonding the two constituents yields a much less cytotoxic conjugate, consistent with the notion that the A chain needs to be reductively cleaved from its carrier protein in the cytosol to attain full catalytic activity.

The cytotoxic activity *in vitro* of the disulphide-bonded A chain immunotoxins, usually measured by inhibition of leucine uptake, has faithfully reflected the antibody specificity but has been variable in extent. It is notably less than that of immunotoxins in which whole ricin molecules are bonded to antibody. Such conjugates can be restricted to antibody specificity *in vitro* by blocking the B chain binding site with a high concentration of lactose: their continued superiority over the A chain immunotoxins therefore presumably reflects the promotion of translocation by the B chain. To produce whole ricin immunotoxins suitable for use *in vivo*, attaching only to cells specified by the antibody, efforts are being made to obtain a recombinant B chain lacking galactose binding but still active in translocation.

A variety of immunotoxins have been made using other RIP, none emerging with a clear superiority. The action of diphtheria toxin is better understood than that of ricin but its clinical use is ruled out by widespread immunization of the populace with toxoid. A promising *Pseudomonas* immunotoxin has been produced using toxin containing just the translocating and toxic domains (Fitzgerald and Pastan 1989). The concept has also been extended to produce conjugates in which RIP is linked to a growth factor (transferrin, IL-2 and others), aimed at targets with a high density of corresponding receptors (Raso 1988).

Clinical trials of immunotoxins have begun. There appear to be three major problems: first, the degree of toxicity, which in one trial included a severe peripheral neuropathy not predicted by animal studies (Gould *et al.* 1989); secondly, the immunogenicity of the toxin component, which has led to early antibody responses by the recipients; thirdly, the fact that human tumours have simply not responded as well as have their animal counterparts. Presumably the latter reflects the relative indolence of the human tumours, which commonly have more than 90% of their cells out of mitotic cycle. Clear evidence that susceptibility to immunotoxin is related to rates of mitosis and protein synthesis is seen among human T lymphocytes, with resting normal cells much less sensitive to ricin A chain immunotoxin than are activated cells or T cell lines (Preijers *et al.* 1988). Indeed the most conspicuous clinical success of immunotoxins has been in the suppression of graft-vs.-host disease by a ricin A–anti-T cell immunotoxin (Kernan *et al.* 1988): here the differential effect on activated cells could be invaluable.

Bispecific antibody-recruiting drug or toxin

An approach related to immunotoxin is the use of a bispecific antibody (antitumour/antitoxin) to deliver a toxin (Glennie *et al.* 1988). The type I plant RIP are suitable for use here. Immunotherapy of an animal leukaemia with anti-idiotype/anti-saporin $F(ab'_{\gamma})_2$ was most successful when the antibody and saporin were combined, in antibody excess, before injection. A similar device has been used to deliver interferon alpha (IFN-α) and has been shown to be effective *in vitro* (Alkan *et al.* 1988). The bispecific strategy offers flexibility in dosage schedules and good control over levels of circulating exogenous effector.

Use of antibody to purge tissue *in vitro*

The use of antibody to purge tissue *in vitro* is a subject peripheral to immunotherapy. Purging or 'laundering' by antibody has been applied to marrow grafts in two situations: the removal of neoplastic cells from autologous grafts and the depletion of T cells from allogeneic grafts. Various effector systems have been tried, including complement (Janossy 1984; Bast *et al.* 1985), immunotoxin (Preijers *et al.* 1989) and mechanical removal on antibody-coated microspheres (Treleaven *et al.* 1984). The efficacy of removal of neoplastic cells is a particularly vexed question: when autologous marrow is used for haemopoietic rescue after ablative conventional therapy, resurgent tumour could have sprung from a residuum either in the body or in the graft. No convincing evidence of the value of purging, or of the method to be used, is available.

Cytokine therapy

The cytokines (Table 94.6) are a densely interconnected system of protein messengers which help regulate cellular activities in inflammation, immune responses, tissue repair and ontogeny. The term, not strictly defined, has been found convenient for embracing the overlapping peptide sets of interleukins, lymphokines, monokines, interferons and miscellaneous growth factors (see Chapters 14–18). Each cytokine acts on its target cells via surface receptors, which are sparse but of high affinity. They interact among each other by exercising additive or antagonistic effects on a given cell, by influencing each other's synthesis, and by influencing each other's receptors. Their activities are for the most part localized to the vicinity of secretion but some (e.g. IL-1 and tumour necrosis factor (TNF)) can have important systemic effects.

It has become apparent that intrusions into this intricate network, as by the administration of large doses of an exogenous cytokine, can sometimes be more damaging to neoplastic than to normal tissues. In this way some notable remissions of disseminated neoplasm have been achieved. If classifiable as immunotherapy, the empirical administration of cytokines is by far the most popular

Table 94.6. Cytokines used or proposed for tumour therapy

Name	Abbreviation	Synonyms
Interleukin 1	IL-1	Lymphocyte activating factor
Interleukin 2	IL-2	T cell growth factor
Interleukin 3	IL-3	Multi-colony-stimulating factor (multi-CSF)
Interleukin 4	IL-4	B cell stimulatory factor 1 (BSF-1)
Interleukin 6	IL-6	BSF-2; IFN-β2
Tumour necrosis factor	TNF	TNF-α; cachectin
Lymphotoxin	LT	TNF-β
Interferon α	IFN-α	Leucocyte interferon
Interferon β	IFN-β	Fibroblast interferon
Interferon γ	IFN-γ	Immune interferon
Granulocyte/macrophage colony-stimulating factor	GM-CSF	CSF-α
Granulocyte colony-stimulating factor	G-CSF	CSF-β

Cytokines recognized at the time of writing which have not been included in the above list are IL-5, IL-7, IL-8, macrophage CSF, transforming growth factor β and (arguably called a cytokine) erythropoietin.

form of this craft being practised. Production for therapy is by recombinant genetic technology, backed by a sizeable element of commercial speculation.

Perhaps the major practical problem which plagues cytokine therapy is that experience remains generally inadequate for predicting responses in individual cases. The major theoretical problem is ignorance of mechanism. Do interferons and IL-2 — currently the most popular cytokines — directly suppress some tumour cells? Or do they promote an inflammatory, vascular or other environment inimical particularly to tumour cell survival? Or do they promote an attack on tumour as an immunological or NK target? No clear answers are available to these questions.

On approaching the physiology of this subject one has the benefit of recent reviews containing plentiful data on the multifarious activities of cytokines (e.g. Balkwill 1989). However, these data refer largely to actions of isolated agents on homogeneous cell populations *in vitro*, far removed from the body's elaborate networks of cytokines, enzymes and cells. Correlations with the clinical effects of exogenous cytokines are often obscure. A variety of observations initiated modern cytokine therapy: in the case of TNF, the finding that it is the factor, demonstrable in serum, which mediates endotoxin-induced haemorrhagic necrosis of certain animal tumours (Carswell *et al.* 1975); in the case of interferons, quite early observations that they can inhibit the proliferation of some cell lines *in vitro* and of some animal tumours *in vivo* (reviewed by Gresser 1972); in the case of IL-2, its ability to expand T lymphocytes *in vitro* and to activate blood lymphocytes for broad cytotoxic activity against certain tumour cells and cell lines (Grimm *et al.* 1982). Some early clinical successes have given impetus to the uses of IL-2 and interferons, while mechanisms have remained obscure. But even considerable insights into the antitumour actions of cytokines would leave rational therapy having to contend with their interdigitating activities and critical dependence upon uncertain local concentrations. Toxicity outside the lymphoid and haemopoietic systems compounds the difficulties: the cytokines have more widespread actions than first suspected, and a given molecule can be used for disparate purposes in different tissues (e.g. myelopoietic and nervous (Yamamori *et al.* 1989)).

In the face of these complexities the commonest clinical approach to cytokine therapy has been simply to monitor the therapeutic and toxic consequences of maximum tolerated doses of an agent which has appeared promising in the laboratory. Trials of biologically active doses well below the maximum tolerated level have been uncommon (e.g. Gastl *et al.* 1989).

Quasi-adjuvants

The antecedents of cytokine preparations, with a history dating back to the late nineteenth century, were a variety of agents whose use was often prompted by a desire to enhance a hypothetical immune response to tumour. Most are known to act as immunological adjuvants under suitable circumstances, while for others such an activity seems often to have been assumed, so they will be gathered together here as 'quasi-adjuvants'.

The first such agents were Coley's toxins (streptococcal and other vaccines), inspired in this case by the observation that cancer sometimes regressed following severe intercurrent infection. Some notable successes were documented (Nauts *et al.* 1953) but toxicity and poor reproducibility presented severe problems. More recent agents have included BCG (attenuated *Mycobacterium tuberculosis* available as several different strains), dead *Corynebacterium parvum*, various preparations of bacterial lipopolysaccharides, double-stranded ribonucleotides, muramyl dipeptides and the antihelminthic drug levamisole. These substances can be presumed to intrude on the cytokine network by stimulation of mononuclear phagocytes and other means. Sometimes, as a further measure to promote an antitumour immune response, they were combined with autologous or allogeneic tumour cell vaccines. Protocols combining them with chemotherapy were also popular.

Enthusiasm for the quasi-adjuvants reached a peak in the 1970s. A good review of their use at that time is provided by Cochran (1978), under the heading 'active non-specific immunotherapy'. It is likely that some remissions of tumour were induced. However, one enterprise which received considerable attention, inoculation of BCG in acute lymphoblastic leukaemia, eventually revealed no benefit in randomized prospective trials (for example, Stryckmans *et al.* 1983).

With the advent of the much more precise recombinant cytokines, dwindling numbers of trials of the quasi-adjuvants are percolating through to the literature. One interesting residue depends upon the ability of locally applied BCG to ablate local tumour by inducing intense granulomatous inflammation in which tumour cells fare poorly (Lieberman *et al.* 1975). Intralesional BCG can be strikingly effective in dealing with cutaneous metastases in melanoma (Morton *et al.* 1976). Similarly, and with potentially greater impact on management, repeated intravesical BCG is reported to yield a high therapeutic response rate in superficial bladder cancer (Kavoussi *et al.* 1988), at the very least postponing the need for cystectomy.

Cytokines from mononuclear phagocytes (monocytes and macrophages)

Many stimuli (including bacterial endotoxins, immune complexes, IFN-γ and IL-2, adjuvants) induce mononuclear phagocytes to release a set of cytokines which includes IL-1 (α and β forms), TNF and IL-6. The overlapping functions of these agents include prominent systemic effects: fever, malaise, anorexia, increased capillary permeability, activation of granulocytes, hepatic secretion of acute-phase proteins and hyperlipaemia (Balkwill 1989; Beutler and Cerami 1989; Kishimoto 1989). Although IL-1 and IL-6 can arise from many other cells, and a variant of TNF (lymphotoxin or TNF-β) is secreted by lymphocytes, the major source of these cytokines — as judged by cells mediating the host response to endotoxins (Beutler and Cerami 1989) — is the mononuclear phagocyte lineage.

Tumour necrosis factor differs from IL-1 and IL-6 in having a direct toxic effect on some tumour cells, and is the only one of the three to have been widely considered for immunotherapy of cancer. However, the combined actions of the whole group intrude repeatedly, with regard to both antineoplastic and toxic effects, when considering cytokine therapy and related topics: endotoxic shock; therapy with quasi-adjuvants such as BCG; therapy with TNF, interferons and IL-2; and both the graft-versus-host (Piguet *et al.* 1987) and antileukaemic effects (Weiden *et al.* 1979) of marrow allografts. The mechanisms involved in these actions have been reviewed by Balkwill (1989) and Beutler and Cerami (1989).

Fever and other symptoms listed above have arisen repeatedly in cytokine therapy, and it is reasonable to suspect that the macrophage products are a major common pathway for systemic toxicity exhibited by cytokines in general. There is also evidence to suggest that TNF has a paramount role: Fraker *et al.* (1989) were able to raise the lethal dose of IL-2 in mice by pre-infusing them with rabbit antibody to murine recombinant TNF, and Dinarello *et al.* (1986) have shown that TNF can act as a pyrogen both by a direct effect on the hypothalamus and by inducing the synthesis of IL-1 to act as a second pyrogen.

THERAPY WITH TUMOUR NECROSIS FACTOR

Two antitumour mechanisms have been demonstrated for TNF. Some cells — all possessing surface receptors for it — are susceptible to a direct toxic effect. Approximately one-third of transformed cell lines studied *in vitro* by Sugarman *et al.* (1985) were killed or growth-inhibited by TNF. A warning is sounded by the same authors recording that some cell lines actually responded with enhanced growth. The second mechanism, to which possibly all vascularized tumours are susceptible at a sufficient dose, entails damage to the tumour blood vessels with consequent haemorrhage and thrombosis. Effects are initiated by changes in the endothelial surface leading to pro-coagulant activity and increased adhesiveness for neutrophils, and a parallel increased adhesiveness of the neutrophils themselves (Nawroth and Stern 1986; Palladino *et al.* 1987). The fact that these changes need not be restricted to tumour vasculature is illustrated by the similar haemorrhagic necrosis which can occur in the adrenals, kidneys and pancreas in severe endotoxic shock.

Unfortunately optimism aroused by promising results with animal tumours and human tumour xenografts (Haranaka *et al.* 1984) has not been borne out in the clinic, where it has been found that the therapeutic and toxic dose ranges of TNF are close or overlapping. Selby *et al.* (1987) were concerned by hypotension (life-threatening in one case), leucopenia, abnormal liver enzymes and mild renal impairment, following doses that yielded only partial regressions of tumour in 3 of 18 patients with advanced cancer. Acute febrile reactions were well controlled by steroids and indomethacin. Spriggs *et al.* (1988) recorded a similar experience with 50 patients and defined hypotension as the dose-limiting toxicity.

At present there is considerable interest in combinations of TNF and IFN-γ, following demonstrations of their synergistic cytotoxicity *in vitro* for cell lines (Williamson *et al.* 1983) and leukaemic blasts (Price *et al.* 1987). Clinical trials have begun.

Interferons

Based on their primary sequences and cell surface receptors the interferons fall into two families: on the one hand IFN-α (multiple species) and IFN-β, on the other IFN-γ. They all appear to use the same antiviral mechanisms (Clemens and McNurlan 1985). Their actions on growth and differentiation of host cells are complex and characterized by rapid changes in patterns of messenger RNA and protein synthesis (Revel and Chedbath 1986). Tumour cells *in vitro*, animal tumours passaged *in vivo* and human tumour xenografts in mice are often growth-inhibited but the effects are quite variable (Dron and Tovey 1983; Clemens and McNurlan 1985; Balkwill 1989). Interferon-γ has additional properties which reflect its role as a T cell lymphokine, including the activation of macrophages, stimulation of antibody synthesis by B lymphoid cells and enhancement of expression of Class II MHC antigens on a range of cells. The higher promise of IFN-γ arising from these activities has not been reflected to date by a better clinical performance against cancer.

The most frequently used of the interferons for treating cancer has been IFN-α. Its most notable successes have occurred in hairy cell (atypical B lymphocytic) and chronic myelocytic leukaemias, with some 95 and 80% of cases respectively undergoing good but not permanent remissions (Quesada *et al.* 1984; Roth and Foon 1986). The response is slow, occurring over a period of several months rather than the 2 weeks or so characteristic of a good response to chemotherapy. Smaller percentages of remissions have been recorded in non-Hodgkin's lymphoma, cutaneous T cell lymphoma and multiple myeloma. Epithelial tumours have in general proved the least responsive but irregular successes have been reported in disseminated or recurrent renal carcinoma, melanoma, malignant carcinoid, and acquired immune deficiency syndrome (AIDS)-related Kaposi sarcoma. The variegated reports of clinical trials with IFN-α have been tabulated by Foon (1989).

Current trials with IFN-β appear to be yielding results similar to those above, but IFN-γ is proving less rewarding. Trials in which interferons are combined with chemotherapy, TNF, IL-2 or antibody, or with more than one of these agents, are also proceeding.

Rigors, fever, myalgia and anorexia have been prominent among side-effects accompanying interferon therapy. These may reflect raised levels of macrophage cytokines, although only IFN-γ is known to stimulate their release by a direct action on macrophages. Occasionally more serious toxicity such as acute renal failure (Ault *et al.* 1988) has emerged.

There have been several reports of antibodies to recombinant interferons arising in the course of therapy, and a minority of such cases may show some resistance to the antineoplastic effect of the preparation concerned (Steis *et al.* 1988). The antibody response might be encouraged by sequence differences between recombinant and natural products, as in the study cited the antibodies sometimes neutralized the antiviral activity of the recombinant IFN-α2a *in vitro*, but never that of natural IFN-α. No toxicity has been attributed to the presence of the antibodies.

Interleukin 2

Interleukin 2 is secreted by T lymphocytes in response to a variety of stimuli, including presentation with antigen plus macrophage cytokines. Originally designated T cell growth factor, it was found later to have broader activities, promoting mitosis and differentiation among all classes of lymphocytes (T, B, NK), and activating macrophages, endothelial and other cells (e.g. Cotran *et al.* 1987). Some of these activities may be promoted indirectly via the release of T cell cytokines and thence macrophage cytokines. Those cells stimulated directly display, when activated, an IL-2 receptor consisting of at least two peptide chains, p55 and p75. Natural killer cells and some T cell subsets express p75 constitutively, when it can act as a low-affinity receptor to initiate activation in the presence of IL-2, leading then to transient expression of p55 and formation of a dimeric high-affinity receptor (Smith 1988; Yagita *et al.* 1989).

The therapeutic use of IL-2 has arisen from the hope that one or both of two lymphocytic populations potentially lethal for tumour cells can be expanded by it: specific cytotoxic T cells (Tc) comprising part of an immune response to the tumour, and lymphokine-activated killer (LAK) cells with a broad antineoplastic activity (Rosenberg 1985).

Lymphokine-activated killer cells emerge when blood lymphocytes from a normal or tumour-bearing subject are cultured *in vitro* for 2 or more days in the presence of IL-2 (Grimm *et al.* 1982). They are defined by their cytotoxic activity against a variety of cells: cell lines susceptible to NK killing; certain cell lines not susceptible to NK killing (e.g. the B lymphocytic line Daudi); and many types of fresh tumour cells — which can include those from autologous tumour. (Authors in this field use 'fresh' to mean non-cultured, the cells being either truly fresh or resurrected from frozen.) Normal lymphocytes are not killed. The susceptible targets can be killed across allogeneic and sometimes even xenogeneic barriers.

The provenance of LAK cells appearing *in vitro* is not settled but the available evidence, particularly the occurrence on their surfaces of the molecules CD16 (Fc_{γ}RIII) and CD56 (NKH-1, Leu-19), suggests that they arise predominantly from NK cells (Phillips and Lanier 1986; Lotzova and Herberman 1987). A minor contribution to LAK activity could arise from T cells rendered broadly cytotoxic in culture (Ortaldo *et al.* 1986). Cancer patients receiving IL-2 therapy can reveal circulating lymphocytes with LAK activity, and these again, although heterogeneous with regard to the CD16 marker, appear from their possession of CD56 to arise from NK cells (McMannis *et al.* 1988). It must be conceded that NK targets are more restricted than LAK targets, but it has been argued that this could simply reflect activation lifting the NK cytotoxic performance against many cells above a previously low level (Lotzova and Herberman 1987).

Following the discovery of the LAK phenomenon Rosenberg's group conducted a series of experiments in which mice bearing minimally immunogenic metastatic sarcoma were treated in one of three ways: with an infusion of syngeneic LAK cells; with recombinant IL-2; or with a combination of these agents. In general tumour suppression was minimal after LAK cells alone; modest and dose-dependent after IL-2; and striking after the combination (Mulé *et al.* 1985; Rosenberg 1985). The result contained a clear message for an initial clinical trial but is not easily interpreted in terms of mechanism. The infused lymphocytic cultures could have contained much else beside LAK cells, and it was not shown that LAK cells were actually killing tumour cells. The experiments described by Mulé *et al.* involved the suppression of pulmonary 'micrometastases' when treatment was begun 3 days after injection of tumour cells, and of visible 'macrometastases' when treatment was begun after 10 days. Curiously IL-2 suppressed macrometastases at a dose which did not effect micrometastases, a finding inconsistent with its acting via the stimulation of endogenous LAK activity. The authors suggest that a host immune response might have been available for stimulation at day 10, but there are other possible explanations independent of any lymphocytic cytotoxicity — such as disturbance of incipient tumour vasculature.

The clinical use of IL-2 with or without concurrent autologous LAK cell infusions has been reviewed by Oliver (1988) and Rosenberg *et al.* (1989). In general maximum tolerated doses of IL-2 have been given, generally as 8-hourly intravenous boluses for 1–3 weeks. It has been claimed (West *et al.* 1987) that continuous infusion is associated with less toxicity, and there is reason to hope that with this approach incipient toxicity should be rapidly reversible, as IL-2 survives only briefly in plasma: Lotze *et al.* (1985) report a half-life of about 7 minutes after intravenous injection in man. When LAK cells have accompanied IL-2, a common protocol has been 5 days of IL-2; a week of rest from IL-2 while four or five leukaphereses are carried out and the blood lymphocytes are cultured in IL-2; and finally intravenous infusions of the cells, after 3–4 days in culture, during a second round of IL-2 injections. Sometimes second and third such courses of treatment have been given. The LAK infusions have not been associated with added toxicity. Nor is it yet apparent whether they have conferred added benefit.

The toxicity of IL-2 therapy has been formidable and deaths have occurred. Non-toxic doses have been associated with fewer tumour responses. A comprehensive table of problems has been provided by Rosenberg *et al.* (1989). Commonly there is fever, malaise, vomiting and diarrhoea, myelosuppression sufficient to require transfusion, and — probably the major problem — capillary leakage with consequent hypotension, severe fluid retention and oliguria. Cotran *et al.* (1987) suggest that widespread endothelial activation underlies the capillary leak syndrome, having observed the appearance of three endothelial activation antigens in skin biopsies of patients undergoing therapy. As IL-2 has not been observed to induce such changes in endothelial cells in culture, they put forward the possibility of secondary release of other cytokines being responsible. In contrast to the severity of all this acute toxicity, and in significant contrast to the record of cytotoxic drugs, no long-term untoward effects of IL-2 have been recorded.

Most successes with IL-2 therapy have been recorded in cases of malignant melanoma and metastatic renal cancer. In these patients, all of whom can be assumed to have been resistant to conventional therapy, response rates of around 20–35% have been recorded, the majority being partial responses. Rates among miscellaneous other cancers have been lower but there has been some benefit in colorectal cancer and lymphoma. Interleukin 2 given as 'adjuvant' treatment, an attempt to deal with microscopic residua after all overt tumour has been removed by conventional means, appears to have been completely unsuccessful.

The possibility of using IL-2 locally for tumours such as bladder carcinoma has some support from animal models and is being assessed clinically (Bubenik 1989).

The striking benefit accruing to a minority of patients receiving IL-2 arises from unknown mechanisms. There is no good evidence that LAK cells, generated endogenously or reinfused, have any role. The degree of LAK cell activity in the blood has not correlated with tumour responses (Ghosh *et al.* 1989), and LAK cells have not been seen to be infiltrating regressing tumour. Cohen *et al.* (1987) describe sequential tumour biopsies undertaken during treatment of nine patients, five of whom had remissions. The responding tumours, and these alone, developed a pronounced infiltration of T cells, mainly T8. Some macrophages also appeared but cells of NK phenotype were virtually absent. Whether the T8 cells were fulfilling a cytotoxic function was not apparent. Another interesting dichotomy reported by these workers was that responding tumours displayed Class II MHC antigens while the non-responding ones did not. The vascular endothelium in the tumours became Class II MHC +ve in all cases, but no evidence was presented of vascular leakage having an antitumour role.

Clinical trials are now proceeding in which IL-2 is combined with another antitumour agent: TNF, IFN-α, granulocyte–macrophage colony-stimulating factor (GM-CSF), monoclonal antibody and cyclophosphamide are all being tried. It is too early to judge results. The combination of IL-2 with tumour-infiltrating lymphocytes, more in line with the older concept of 'adoptive immunotherapy', is dealt with under 'Cellular therapy'.

Other interleukins

Reports of other interleukins being assessed clinically for antitumour activity have been only sporadic, although some promise has emerged from animal work. Interleukin 1 has been shown to promote rejection of mouse tumours against which concomitant immunity can be demonstrated (North *et al.* 1988). Interleukin 4 has proved active against a variety of tumours in a murine model in which malignant cells transfected with the IL-4 gene were mixed with non-transfected tumour and inoculated into syngeneic or nude mice. The presence of the transfected cells promoted local inflammation and tumour rejection (Tepper *et al.* 1989).

The finding that recombinant colony-stimulating factors (CSF) can promote blood cell production in both normal and myelosuppressed subjects has led to a number of applications in cancer and other diseases (reviewed by Laver and Moore 1989). These uses are not usually classified as immunotherapy but bear an obvious kinship. Granulocyte–macrophage CSF and granulocyte CSF (G-CSF) are being evaluated for their abilities to shorten neutropenic periods following chemotherapy or radiotherapy, particularly when an autologous marrow or stem cell graft is used to reconstitute an ablated marrow. Granulocyte–macrophage CSF can dramatically improve the white cell count, and sometimes the platelet count, in the myelodysplastic syndrome. A potential problem in haematological malignancies is that the neoplastic cells themselves can be stimulated to proliferate (Griffin *et al.* 1986), although it has been proposed that leukaemic cells can thereby be sensitized to cycle-specific chemotherapy. Yet another field of investigation is the use of growth factors to induce terminal differentiation in leukaemic cells.

Cellular therapy

Cellular therapy has derived much of its inspiration from experiments starting in the 1950s which demonstrated that mice sometimes mount significant immune responses against autologous tumours, and that lymphocytes from such a mouse can confer upon syngeneic recipients the ability to reject a challenge of the tumour involved (Klein *et al.* 1960; Rouse *et al.* 1972). The antigens concerned are the T cell-defined tumour-specific transplantation antigens (TSTA), which for the most part have proved highly specific to individual tumours.

We have considered the use of LAK cells in the previous section, leaving tumour-infiltrating lymphocytes (TIL) as the only clinical application of cellular therapy presently being tried on a significant scale. Tumour-infiltrating lymphocytes are removed from a tumour biopsy, expanded *in vitro* and reinfused into the donor in combination with other therapeutic measures. Some useful remissions have followed these manoeuvres, but their relationship to the T cell responses to TSTA seen in mice is quite unclear.

Experiments in mice encouraged the TIL approach by demonstrating that these lymphocytes were therapeutically more efficient than LAK cells (Rosenberg *et al.* 1988). Unfortunately the successful protocols entailed the complications of pretreating the tumour-bearing animal with either cyclophosphamide or total body irradiation, plus the administration of IL-2 simultaneously with the reinfused TIL. In the first reported clinical trial (Rosenberg *et al.* 1988), remissions were recorded in 11 of 20 patients with metastatic melanoma. The protocol first entailed resecting tumour samples (10–30 g), teasing out the TIL and expanding them in culture for 4–8 weeks. Thirty-six hours prior to starting infusions the patients were given a large (25 mg/kg) intravenous dose of cyclophosphamide. One to seven infusions of up to 2×10^{11} cells were given over 1–2 days, accompanied by toxicity-limiting doses of IL-2. Acute toxicity was severe but there were no deaths and no long-term problems.

Preliminary reports to hand at the time of writing indicate that — as in treatment with IL-2 ± LAK cells — clinical responses to the TIL regime are being seen mainly in cases of melanoma and renal carcinoma. Trials of TIL infusions in combination with other types of treatment have also begun.

How do TIL work? Several recent reports indicate that human melanoma and some other tumours can yield infiltrating lymphocytes exhibiting cytotoxicity specific for the autologous neoplastic cells (Itoh *et al.* 1988; Okada *et al.* 1989; Topalian *et al.* 1989; Wright *et al.* 1989). Furthermore the majority of the expanded TIL population has been found to be of T8 phenotype (Belldegrun *et al.* 1988). These facts support the notion that the cells' therapeutic performance represents a highly specific T cell phenomenon reminiscent of the murine immune response to TSTA. However, examination of the cytotoxic activity among expanded TIL populations lends little support to this idea. The cells were found by Belldegrun *et al.* to lyse autologous tumour cells in 4-hour chromium-release assays in most cases, but allogeneic targets were equally well lysed. Heo *et al.* (1987) examined cultured TIL separated from squamous carcinomas and found after cytofluorometric sorting that the major cytotoxic activity resided among a minor population of cells which were of large granular morphology and CD3 −ve/CD56 +ve or CD3 +ve/CD56 +ve; these findings are consistent with the cells arising from NK cells and a T cell subset respectively. It seems possible that much of the cytotoxic activity among lymphocytic infiltrates and their expanded descendants is associated with the NK lineage, and specific for the elusive NK molecular target(s).

Active immunization against established tumour

It would be highly desirable to initiate an immune response against established tumour and have the host's own lymphoid system relentlessly hunt down the wayward cells. The immune response probably deals thus with certain virus-associated neoplasms at a subclinical stage, as immunosuppressed mice and men show an enhanced susceptibility to polyoma- and EBV-associated tumours respectively. However, here the lymphoid system is not faced with tumour antigens in large and potentially tolerizing amounts. For clinically apparent tumour a better precedent exists in the organ-specific autoimmune diseases. The destruction of target cells in states such as type I diabetes and Hashimoto's thyroiditis tends to proceed to completion, and perhaps such a conclusion of the autoimmune process is inevitable if life persists.

Can an effective autoimmune process be invoked against cancer cells? It can be invoked against normal thyroid by a tolerance-breaking immunization schedule (Rose and Witebsky 1956; Weigle 1980). This oft-repeated demonstration contains two vital ingredients: a well-defined antigen (thyroglobulin) and a powerful adjuvant (Freund's complete). Useful tumour antigens, as previously defined, are increasingly available for man. However, a powerful adjuvant acceptable for clinical use remains elusive. Two further ingredients of the Rose–Witebsky model emerge when one considers an extension to tumour. The first is an efficient lymphoid system, sometimes lacking in patients due to the depredations of disease or therapy. The second is a compliant target. Thyroid cells do not multiply vigorously nor seek ectopic sites. The contrasting behaviour of tumour can lead to mutational escape, and also to the phenomena of 'concomitant immunity' and 'sneaking through', where an effective immune response can be thwarted by rapid growth or an unfavourable site (Old and Boyse 1964). Some tumours also gain local protection from the production of immunosuppressive factors (Nelson *et al.* 1989). The impression that active immunization is feasible in principle but accompanied by formidable difficulties summarizes the present position.

Animal models for immunization suffer the disadvantage that the common experimental tumours have a mitotic rate comparable with the most vigorous lymphoid expansion, so that established tumour will tend to outpace the immune response. In a mouse lymphoma immunization with a tumour-specific antigen (lymphoma idiotypic IgM) could protect against a small tumour inoculum given 3 days earlier, but such protection was only partial when the inoculum reached 10^4 cells (George *et al.* 1988).

Sporadic evidence has emerged of immune responses against autologous human melanoma: we have referred above to one important item, the isolation of tumour-infiltrating cytotoxic lymphocytes. So it is of some interest that possibly the best evidence for a clinical response to active immunization has occurred in this condition (Hollinshead *et al.* 1982; Mitchell *et al.* 1988). Mitchell *et al.* immunized patients with allogeneic tumour homogenate (from two melanoma cell lines) plus a novel bacterial adjuvant. Major remissions occurred in 5 of 17 patients with measurable lesions, all five exhibiting independent evidence of an immune response. Such work might benefit considerably from precise identification of the antigens concerned.

Several approaches have been made towards rendering tumour cell vaccines more immunogenic by modifying the cell surfaces, with the intention that a strong immune response to the vaccine include an enhanced response to epitopes shared by vaccine and original tumour. Simmons and Rios (1971) reported that established methylcholanthrene sarcomas in mice disappeared after the hosts were immunized with neuraminidase-treated tumour cells. Lachmann's group (Vyakarnam *et al.* 1981; Sia *et al.* 1984) 'heterogenized' tumour cells by coupling the highly immunogenic PPD (purified protein derivative of tuberculin) to the surfaces, and immunized tumour-bearing animals previously primed to tuberculin. In this way the rejection of unmodified tumour cells was enhanced. Adoptive experiments revealed that the enhancement was associated with tuberculin-specific T helper cells in the primed animals. In an interesting variation of this approach, vaccines of tumour cells heterogenized by viral infection are being investigated by Schirrmacher *et al.* (1989).

When one has available a monoclonal antibody (antibody 1) reactive against a useful tumour antigen, that antigen can in principle be isolated by immunosorption on to antibody and used in pure form as an immunogen. But difficulties often intrude, not the least being that the antigen might be poorly immunogenic. So there is much interest in using as a surrogate antigen an anti-idiotype antibody (antibody 2) raised against antibody 1 (Kennedy *et al.* 1987). It should be noted that some but not all antibody 2 bear a significant steric resemblance to antigen (Jerne *et al.* 1982). Herlyn *et al.* (1987) immunized 30 patients, all suffering from advanced colorectal carcinoma, with goat polyclonal antibody 2; all developed antibody 3, which reacted with cultured tumour cells and could compete with antibody 1 in so doing. In six patients this immune response was accompanied by partial remission of disease.

In all the above reports of clinical trials, immunizations have been followed by shrinkage of tumour in only a minority of patients. So although the approaches show some promise they are clearly a long way from the efficacy and reproducibility of the autoimmune thyroiditis model.

Conclusion

The four major approaches to immunotherapy — antibody, cytokines, cells, active immunization — are all benefiting from insights into the molecular core of immunology. With better understanding of what we are about, there may be fewer blind alleys than have blighted the subject in the past. However, I hesitate to guess how closely the immunotherapy chapter in the next edition of this book will resemble the present one.

References

Alkan, S.S., Towbin, H. and Hochkeppal, H.K. (1988). Enhanced anti-proliferative action of interferon targeted by bispecific monoclonal antibodies. *J. Interferon Res.* **8**, 25–33.

Allebes, W.A., Wetzels, R.H.W. and Capel, P.J.A. (1988). Heterogeneous responses of B-cell tumours to anti-Ig and anti-idiotypic antibodies. *Scand. J. Immunol.* **28**, 95–103.

Amerding, D. and Katz, D.H. (1974). Activation of T and B lymphocytes *in vitro*. I. Regulatory influence of bacterial lipopolysaccharide (LPS) on specific T-cell helper function. *J. Exp. Med.* **139**, 24–43.

Anasetti, C., Martin, P.J., Morishita, Y., Badger, C.C., Bernstein, I.D. and Hansen, J.A. (1987). Human large granular lymphocytes express high affinity receptors for murine monoclonal antibodies of the IgG3 subclass. *J. Immunol.* **138**, 2979–81.

Ault, B.H., Stapleton, F.B., Gaber, L., Martin, A., Roy, S. and Murphy, S.B. (1988). Acute renal failure during therapy with recombinant human gamma interferon. *N. Engl. J. Med.* **319**, 1397–400.

Baeker, T.R. and Rothstein, T.L. (1985). Proliferation of human malignant lymphocytes induced by anti-IgM independent of B cell growth factor. *J. Immunol.* **134**, 3532–8.

Bagshawe, K.D. (1987). Antibody directed enzymes revive anti-cancer prodrugs concept. *Br. J. Cancer* **56**, 531–2.

Bagshawe, K.D. and Searle, F. (1977). Tumour markers. *Essays Med. Biochem.* **3**, 25–73.

Bagshawe, K.D., Springer, C.J., Searle, F. *et al.* (1988). A cytotoxic agent can be generated selectively at cancer sites. *Br. J. Cancer* **58**, 700–3.

Baldwin, R.W. (1966). Tumour-specific immunity against spontaneous rat tumours. *Int. J. Cancer* **1**, 257–64.

Balkwill, F.R. (1989). *Cytokines in Cancer Therapy*. Oxford University Press, Oxford.

Bast, R.C., de Fabritis, P., Lipton, J. *et al.* (1985). Elimination of malignant clonogenic cells from human bone marrow using multiple monoclonal antibodies and complement. *Cancer Res.* **45**, 499–503.

Beiske, K., Clark, E.A., Holte, H., Ledbetter, J.A., Smeland, E.B. and Godal, T. (1988). Triggering of neoplastic B cells via surface IgM and the cell surface antigens CD20 and CDw40: responses differ from normal blood B cells and are restricted to certain morphological subsets. *Int. J. Cancer* **42**, 521–8.

Belldegrun, A., Muul, L.M. and Rosenberg, S.A. (1988). Interleukin 2 expanded tumor infiltrating lymphocytes in human renal cell cancer: isolation, characterization and antitumor activity. *Cancer Res.* **48**, 206–14.

Bernstein, A., Hurwitz, E., Maron, R., Arnon, R., Sela, M. and Wilchek, M. (1978). Higher antitumor efficacy of daunomycin when linked to dextran: *in vivo* and *in vitro* studies. *J. Nat. Cancer Inst.* **60**, 379–86.

Bernstein, I.D., Tan, M.R. and Nowinski, R.C. (1980). Mouse leukemia: therapy with monoclonal antibodies against a thymus differentiation antigen. *Science* **207**, 68–71.

Beutler, B. and Cerami, A. (1989). The biology of cachectin/TNF — a primary mediator of the host response. *Ann. Rev. Immunol.* **7**, 625–55.

Biggs, P.M. (1975). Marek's disease — the disease and its prevention by vaccination. *Br. J. Cancer* **31** (suppl. 2), 152–5.

Black, P.H. (1980). Shedding from the cell surface of normal and cancer cells. *Adv. Cancer Res.* **32**, 76–199.

Blakey, D.C. and Thorpe, P.E. (1988). An overview of therapy with immunotoxins containing ricin or its A-chain. *Antibody Immunoconjugates Radiopharmaceuticals* **1**, 1–16.

Blumberg, B.S. and London, W.T. (1985). Hepatitis B virus and the prevention of primary cancer of the liver. *J. Nat. Cancer Inst.* **74**, 267–73.

Boyse, E.A. and Old, L.J. (1969). Some aspects of normal and abnormal cell surface genetics. *Ann. Rev. Genet.* **3**, 269–90.

Brown, S.L., Miller, R.A., Horning, S.J. *et al.* (1989). Treatment of B-cell lymphomas with anti-idiotype antibodies alone and in combination with alpha interferon. *Blood* **73**, 651–61.

Bubenik, J. (1989). Local immunotherapy of cancer with interleukin 2. *Immunol. Lett.* **21**, 267–74.

Busch, H. and Greene, H.S.N. (1955). Studies on metabolism of plasma proteins in tumor-bearing rats. *Yale J. Biol. Med.* **27**, 339–49.

Cambier, J.C., Justement, L.B., Newell, M.K. *et al.* (1987). Transmembrane signals and intracellular 'second messengers' in the regulation of quiescent B-lymphocyte activation. *Immunol. Rev.* **95**, 37–57.

Carswell, E.A., Old, L.J., Kassel, R.L., Green, S., Fiore, N. and Williamson, B. (1975). An endotoxin-induced serum factor that causes necrosis of tumors. *Proc. Nat. Acad. Sci. (USA)* **72**, 3666–71.

Chatenoud, L., Baudrichaye, M.F., Kreis, H., Goldstein, G., Schindler, J. and Bach, J.F. (1982). Human *in vivo* antigenic modulation induced by the anti-T cell OKT3 monoclonal antibody. *Eur. J. Immunol.* **12**, 979–82.

Churchill, A.E., Payne, L.N. and Chubb, R.C. (1969). Immunization against Marek's disease using a live attenuated virus. *Nature* **221**, 744–7.

Clark, M.R., Bindon, C., Dyer, M. *et al.* (1989). The improved lytic function and *in vivo* efficacy of monovalent monoclonal CD3 antibodies. *Eur. J. Immunol.* **19**, 381–8.

Clark, M.R. and Waldmann, H. (1987). T-cell killing of target cells induced by hybrid antibodies: comparison of two bispecific monoclonal antibodies. *J. Nat. Cancer Inst.* **79**, 1393–401.

Cleary, M.L., Galili, N., Trela, M., Levy, R., Sklar, J. (1988). Single cell origin of bigenotypic and biphenotypic B cell proliferation in human follicular lymphomas. *J. Exp. Med.* **167**, 582–97.

Clemens, M.J. and McNurlan, M.A. (1985). Regulation of cell proliferation and differentiation by interferons. *Biochem. J.* **226**, 345–60.

Cobb, L.M. (1989). Intratumour factors influencing the access of antibody to tumour cells. *Cancer Immunol. Immunother.* **28**, 235–40.

Cobbold, S.P. and Waldmann, H. (1984). Therapeutic potential of monovalent monoclonal antibodies. *Nature* **308**, 460–2.

Cochran, A.J. (1978). *Man, Cancer and Immunity*. Academic Press, London,

Cohen, P.J., Lotze, M.T., Roberts, J.R., Rosenberg, S.A. and Jaffe, E.S. (1987). The immunopathology of sequential tumor biopsies in patients treated with interleukin-2. *Am. J. Pathol.* **129**, 208–16.

Cotran, R.S., Pober, J.S., Gimbrone, M.A. *et al.* (1987). Endothelial activation during interleukin 2 immunotherapy. *J. Immunol.* **140**, 1883–8.

Currie, G.A. (1972). Eighty years of immunotherapy: a review of immunological methods used for treatment of human cancer. *Br. J. Cancer* **26**, 141–53.

Dearman, R.J., Stevenson, F.K., Wrightham, M., Hamblin, T.J., Glennie, M.J. and Stevenson, G.T. (1988). Lymphokine-activated killer cells from normal and lymphoma subjects are cytotoxic for cells coated with antibody derivatives displaying human Fc gamma. *Blood* **72**, 1985–91.

Deland, F.H. and Goldenberg, D.M. (1985). Diagnosis and treatment of neoplasms with radionuclide-labeled antibodies. *Semin. Nuclear Med.* **15**, 2–11.

Denkers, E.Y., Badger, C.C., Ledbetter, J.A. and Bernstein, I.D. (1985). Influence of antibody isotype on passive serotherapy of lymphoma. *J. Immunol.* **135**, 2183–6.

Dillman, R.O., Shawler, D.L., Dillman, J.B. and Royston, I. (1984). Therapy of chronic lymphocytic leukemia and cutaneous T-cell lymphoma with T101 monoclonal antibody. *J. Clin. Oncol.* **2**, 881–91.

Dinarello, C.A., Cannon, J.G., Wolff, S.M. *et al.* (1986). Tumor necrosis factor (cachectin) is an endogenous pyrogen and induces production of interleukin 1. *J. Exp. Med.* **163**, 1433–50.

Drebin, J.A., Link, V.C., Stern, D.F., Weinberg, R.A. and Greene, M.I. (1985). Down-modulation of an oncogene protein product and reversion of the transformed phenotype by monoclonal antibodies. *Cell* **41**, 697–706.

Dresser, D.W. (1962). Specific inhibition of antibody production. II. Paralysis induced in mice by small quantities of protein antigen. *Immunology* **5**, 378–88.

Dron, M. and Tovey, M.G. (1983). Isolation of Daudi cells with reduced sensitivity to interferon. I. Characterization. *J. Gen. Virol.* **64**, 2641–7.

Dyer, M.J., Hale, G., Hayhoe, F.G.H. and Waldmann, H. (1989). Effects of CAMPATH-1 antibodies *in vivo* in patients with lymphoid malignancies: influence of antibody isotype. *Blood 73*, 1431–9.

Edwards, P.A. (1985). Heterogeneous expression of cell-surface antigens in normal epithelia and their tumours, revealed by monoclonal antibodies. *Br. J. Cancer* **51**, 149–60.

Elliott, T.J., Glennie, M.J., McBride, H.M. and Stevenson, G.T. (1987). Analysis of the interaction of antibodies with immunoglobulin idiotypes on neoplastic B lymphocytes: implications for immunotherapy. *J. Immunol.* **138**, 981–8.

Endo, Y., Mitsui, K., Motizuki, M. and Tsurugi, K. (1987). The mechanism of action of ricin and related toxic lectins on eukaryotic ribosomes. *J. Biol. Chem.* **262**, 5908–12.

Epstein, M.A. (1987). The Florey Lecture, 1986. Vaccine prevention of virus-induced human cancers. *Proc. Roy. Soc. (London) Biol.* **230**, 147–61.

Fanger, M.W., Li Shen, Graziano, R.F. and Guyre, P.M. (1989). Cytotoxicity mediated by human Fc receptors for IgG.

Immunol. Today **10**, 92–9.

Feizi, T. (1985). Demonstration by monoclonal antibodies that carbohydrate structures of glycoproteins and glycolipids are onco-development antigens. *Nature* **314**, 53–7.

Foon, K.A. (1989). Biological response modifiers: the new immunotherapy. *Cancer Res.* **49**, 1621–39.

Fitzgerald, D. and Pastan, I. (1989). Targeted toxin therapy for the treatment of cancer. *J. Nat. Cancer Inst.* **81**, 1455–63.

Foulds, L. (1969). *Neoplastic Development*, vol. I, Academic Press, London.

Fraker, D.L., Langstein, H.N. and Norton, J.A. (1989). Passive immunization against tumor necrosis factor partially abrogates interleukin 2 toxicity. *J. Exp. Med.* **170**, 1015–20.

Garcia, C.F., Lowder, J., Meeker, T.C., Bindl, J., Levy, R. and Warnke R.A. (1985). Differences in 'host infiltrates' among lymphoma patients treated with anti-idiotype antibodies: correlation with treatment response. *J. Immunol.* **135**, 4252–60.

Gastl, G., Werter, M., de Pauw, B. *et al.* (1989). Comparison of clinical efficacy and toxicity of conventional and optimum biological response modifying doses of interferon-alpha-2C in the treatment of hairy cell leukemia: a retrospective analysis of 39 patients. *Leukemia* **3**, 453–60.

George, A.J.T., Folkard, S.G., Hamblin, T.J. and Stevenson, F.K. (1988). Idiotypic vaccination as a treatment for a B cell lymphoma. *J. Immunol.* **141**, 2168–74.

Ghosh, A.K., Dazzi, H., Thatcher N., Moore, M. (1989). Lack of correlation between peripheral blood lymphokine-activated killer (LAK) cell function and clinical response in patients with advanced malignant melanoma receiving recombinant interleukin 2. *Int. J. Cancer* **43**, 410–14.

Glennie, M.J. and Stevenson, G.T. (1982). Univalent antibodies kill tumour cells *in vitro* and *in vivo*. *Nature* **295**, 712–14.

Glennie, M.J. and Wyeth, P. (1986). Radiolabelled antibody imaging and therapy: theoretical considerations. *Clin. Oncol.* **5**, 51–78.

Glennie, M.J., Stevenson, F.K., Stevenson, G.T. and Virji, M. (1979). Cross-linking of lymphocytic surface immunoglobulin inhibits its production via a cyclic nucleotide mechanism. *Nature* **281**, 305–7.

Glennie, M.J., McBride, H.M., Stirpe, F., Thorpe, P.E., Worth, A.T. and Stevenson G.T. (1987a). Emergence of immunoglobulin variants following treatment of a B cell leukemia with an immunotoxin composed of anti-idiotypic antibody and saporin. *J. Exp. Med.* **166**, 43–62.

Glennie, M.J., McBride, H.M., Worth, A.T. and Stevenson, G.T. (1987b). Preparation and performance of bispecific $F(ab'\gamma)_2$ antibody containing thioether-linked Fab'γ fragments. *J. Immunol.* **139**, 2367–75.

Glennie, M.J., Brennand, D.M., Bryden, F. *et al.* (1988). Bispecific $F(ab'\gamma)_2$ antibody for the delivery of saporin in the treatment of lymphoma. *J. Immunol.* **141**, 3662–70.

Goldenberg, D.M. (1989). Future role of radiolabeled monoclonal antibodies in oncological diagnosis and therapy. *Semin. Nuclear Med.* **19**, 262–81.

Gordon, J. and Stevenson, G.T. (1981). Antigenic modulation of lymphocytic surface immunoglobulin yielding resistance to complement-mediated lysis. II. Relationship to redistribution of the antigen. *Immunology* **42**, 13–17.

Gordon, J., Abdul-Ahad, A.K., Hamblin, T.J., Stevenson, F.K. and Stevenson, G.T. (1984). Mechanisms of tumour cell escape encountered in treating lymphocytic leukaemia with anti-idiotypic antibody. *Br. J. Cancer* **49**, 547–57.

Gorelik, E. (1983). Concomitant tumour immunity and the resistance to a second tumour challenge. *Adv. Cancer Res.* **39**, 71–120.

Gould, B.J., Borowitz, M.J., Groves, E.S. *et al.* (1989). Phase I study of an anti-breast cancer immunotoxin by continuous infusion: report of a targeted toxic effect not predicted by animal studies. *J. Nat. Cancer Inst.* **81**, 775–81.

Gresser, I. (1972). Antitumor effects of interferon. *Adv. Cancer Res.* **16**, 97–140.

Griffin, J.D., Young, D., Herrmann, F., Wiper, D., Wagner, K. and Sabbath, K.D. (1986). Effects of recombinant human GM-CSF on proliferation of clonogenic cells in acute myeloblastic leukemia. *Blood* **67**, 1448–53.

Grimm, E.A., Mazumder, A., Zhang, H.Z. and Rosenberg, S.A. (1982). Lymphokine-activated killer cell phenomenon. *J. Exp. Med.* **155**, 1823–39.

Hale, G., Bright, S., Chumbley, G. *et al.* (1983). Removal of T cells from bone marrow for transplantation: a monoclonal antilymphocyte antibody that fixes human complement. *Blood* **62**, 873–82.

Hale, G., Clark, M.R. and Waldmann, H. (1985). Therapeutic potential of rat monoclonal antibodies: isotype specificity of antibody-dependent cell-mediated cytotoxicity with human lymphocytes. *J. Immunol.* **134**, 3056–61.

Hale, G., Clark, M.R., Marcus, R. *et al.* (1988). Remission induction in non-Hodgkin lymphoma with reshaped human monoclonal antibody CAMPATH-1H. *Lancet* **ii**, 1394–9.

Hamblin, T.J., Cattan, A.R., Glennie, M.J. *et al.* (1987). Initial experience in treating human lymphoma with a chimeric univalent derivative of monoclonal anti-idiotype antibody. *Blood* **69**, 790–7.

Haranaka, K.H., Satomi, N. and Sakurai, A. (1984). Antitumor activity of murine tumor necrosis factor (TNF) against transplanted murine tumors and heterotransplanted human tumors in nude mice. *Int. J. Cancer* **34**, 263–7.

Hege, K.M., Daleke, D.L., Waldmann, T.A. and Matthay, K.K. (1989). Comparison of anti-Tac and anti-transferrin receptor-conjugated liposomes for specific drug delivery to adult T-cell leukemia. *Blood* **74**, 2043–52.

Heo, D.S., Whiteside, T.L., Johnson, J.T., Chen, K., Barnes, E.L. and Herberman, R.B. (1987). Long-term interleukin 2-dependent growth and cytotoxic activity of tumor–infiltrating lymphocytes from human squamous carcinomas of the head and neck. *Cancer Res.* **47**, 6353–62.

Herlyn, D., Wettendorff, M., Schmoll, E. *et al.* (1987). Anti-idiotype immunization of cancer patients: modulation of the immune response. *Proc. Nat. Acad. Sci. (USA)* **84**, 8055–99.

Hersey, P. (1973). New look at antiserum therapy of leukaemia. *Nature N. Biol.* **244**, 22–4.

Hivroz, C., Grillot-Courvalin, C., Labaume, S., Miglierina, R. and Brouet, J.-C. (1988). Cross-linking of membrane IgM on B CLL cells: dissociation between intracellular free Ca^{2+} mobilization and cell proliferation. *Eur. J. Immunol.* **18**, 1811–17.

Hollinshead, A., Arlen, M., Yonemoto, R. *et al.* (1982). Pilot studies using melanoma tumor-associated antigens (TAA) in specific-active immunochemotherapy of malignant melanoma. *Cancer* **9**, 1387–404.

Houghton, A.N., Mintzer, D., Cordon-Cardo, C. *et al.* (1985). Mouse monoclonal IgG3 antibody detecting G_{D3} ganglioside: a phase I trial in patients with malignant melanoma. *Proc. Nat. Acad. Sci. (USA)* **82**, 1242–6.

Hughes-Jones, N.C. and Gardner, B. (1979). Reaction between the isolated globular sub-units of the complement component C1q and IgG-complexes. *Mol. Immunol.* **16**, 697–701.

Itoh, K., Platsoucas, C.D. and Balch, C.M. (1988). Autologous tumor-specific cytotoxic T lymphocytes in the infiltrate of human metastatic melanomas: activation by interleukin 2 and autologous tumor cells, and involvement of the T cell receptor. *J. Exp. Med.* **168**, 1419–41.

Janossy, G. (1984). 'Purging' of bone marrow and immunosuppression. *Br. Med. Bull.* **40**, 247–53.

Jerne, N.K., Roland, J. and Cazenave, P.A. (1982). Recurrent idiotypes and internal images. *EMBO J.* **1**, 243–7.

Johnson, R.J., Kaizer, H., Massey, A.G. and Shin, H.Y. (1985). Role of endogenous complement in monoclonal IgM antibody-dependent leukemia suppression *in vivo*: participation of C3b. *J. Immunol.* **134**, 3497–503.

Kaminski, M.S., Kitamura K., Maloney, D.G., Campbell, M.J. and Levy, R. (1986). Importance of antibody isotype in monoclonal anti-idiotype therapy of a murine B cell lymphoma: a study of hybridoma class switch variants. *J. Immunol.* **136**, 1123–30, 1986.

Karpovsky, B., Titus, J.A., Stephany, D.A. and Segal, D.M. (1984). Production of target-specific effector cells using hetero-cross-linked aggregates containing anti-target cell and anti-Fc receptor antibodies. *J. Exp. Med.* **160**, 1686–701.

Kassel, R.L., Old, L.J., Carswell, E., Fiore, N. and Hardy, W.D. (1973). Serum-mediated leukemia cell destruction in AKR mice. Role of complement in the phenomenon. *J. Exp. Med.* **138**, 925–38.

Kavoussi, L.R., Torrence, R.J., Gillen, D.P. *et al.* (1988). Results of six weekly intravesical bacillus Calmette-Guérin installations on the treatment of superficial bladder tumors. *J. Urol.* **139**, 935–40.

Kennedy, R.C., Zhou, E.-M., Lanford, R.E., Chanh, T.C. and Bona, C.A. (1987). Possible role of anti-idiotypic antibodies in the induction of tumour immunity. *J. Clin. Invest.* **80**, 1217–24.

Kernan, N.A., Byers, V., Scannon, P.J. *et al.* (1988). Treatment of steroid-resistant acute graft-vs-host disease by an *in vivo* administration of an anti-T-cell ricin A chain immunotoxin. *JAMA* **259**, 3154–7.

Kipps, T.J., Parham, P., Punt, J. and Herzenberg, L.A. (1985). Importance of immunoglobulin isotype in human antibody-dependent, cell-mediated cytotoxicity directed by murine monoclonal antibodies. *J. Exp. Med.* **161**, 1–17.

Kipps, T.J., Tomhave, E., Chen, P.P. and Carson, D.A. (1988). Autoantibody-associated κ light chain variable region gene expressed in chronic lymphocytic leukemia with little or no somatic mutation. *J. Exp. Med.* **167**, 840–52,

Kishimoto, T. (1989). The biology of interleukin-6. *Blood* **74**, 1–10.

Klein, G., Sjogren, H.O., Klein, E. and Hellstrom, K.E. (1960). Demonstration of resistance against methylcholanthrene-induced sarcomas in the primary autochthonous host. *Cancer Res.* **20**, 1561–72.

Knapp, W., Dorken, B., Gilks, W.R. *et al.* (1989). *Leucocyte Typing IV: White Cell Differentiation Antigens*. Oxford University Press, Oxford.

Lamm, M.E., Boyse, E.A., Old, L.J., Lisowska-Bernstein, B. and Stockert, E. (1968). Modulation of TL (thymus-leukemia) antigens by Fab-fragments of TL antibody. *J. Immunol.* **101**, 99–103.

Lanier, L.L., Babcock, G.F., Raybourne, R.B., Arnold, L.W., Warner, N.L. and Haughton, G. (1980). Mechanisms of B cell lymphoma immunotherapy with passive xenogeneic anti-idiotype serum. *J. Immunol.* **125**, 1730–6.

Lanzavecchia, A., Abrignani, S., Scheidegger, D., Obrist, R., Dorken, B. and Moldenhauer, G. (1988). Antibodies as antigens: the use of monoclonal antibodies to focus human T cells against selected targets. *J. Exp. Med.* **167**, 345–52.

Larson, S.M. (1985). Radiolabeled monoclonal anti-tumor antibodies in diagnosis and therapy. *J. Nuclear Med.* **26**, 538–45.

Laufs, R. and Steinke, H. (1975). Vaccination of non-human primates against malignant lymphoma. *Nature* **253**, 71–2.

Laver, J. and Moore, M.A.S. (1989). Clinical use of recombinant human hematopoietic growth factors. *J. Nat. Cancer Inst.* **81**, 1370–82.

Lawson, A.D.G. and Stevenson, G.T. (1983). Macrophages induce antibody-dependent cytostasis but not lysis in guinea-pig leukaemic cells. *Br. J. Cancer* **48**, 227–37.

Ledbetter, J.A., Norris, N.A., Grossmann, A. *et al.* (1989). Enhanced transmembrane signalling activity of monoclonal antibody heteroconjugates suggests molecular interactions between receptors on the T cell surface. *Mol. Immunol.* **26**, 137–45.

Ledermann, J.A., Begent, R.H.J., Bagshawe, K.D. *et al.* (1988). Repeated anti-tumour antibody therapy in man with suppression of the host response by cyclosporin-A. *Br. J. Cancer* **58**, 654–7.

Lesley, J., Hyman, R. and Dennert, G. (1974). Effect of antigen density on complement-mediated lysis, T-cell mediated killing and antigen-induced modulation. *J. Nat. Cancer Inst.* **53**, 1759–65.

Lieberman, R., Wybran, J. and Epstein, W. (1975). The immunologic and histopathologic changes of BCG mediated tumor regression in patients with malignant melanoma. *Cancer* **35**, 756–77.

LoBuglio, A.F., Saleh, M.S., Lee, J., Khazaeli, M.B., Carrano, R., Holden, H. and Wheeler, R.H. (1988). Phase I trial of multiple large doses of murine monoclonal antibody CO17-1A. I. Clinical aspects. *J. Nat. Cancer Inst.* **80**, 932–6.

LoBuglio, A.F., Wheeler, R.H., Trang, J. *et al.* (1989). Mouse/human chimeric monoclonal antibody in man: kinetics and immune response. *Proc. Nat. Acad. Sci. (USA)* **86**, 4220–4.

Lotze, M.T., Matory, Y.L., Ettinghausen, S.E. *et al.* (1985). *In vivo* administration of purified interleukin 2. *J. Immunol.* **135**, 2865–75.

Lotzova, E. and Herberman, R.B. (1987). Reassessment of LAK phenomenology: a review. *Nat. Immun. Cell Growth Regulation* **6**, 109–15.

Lustig, H.J. and Bianco, C. (1976). Antibody-mediated cell cytotoxicity in a defined system: regulation by antigen, antibody, and complement. *J. Immunol.* **116**, 253–60.

Lynch, R.G., Graff, R.J., Sirisinha, S., Simms, E.S. and Eisen, H.N. (1972). Myeloma proteins as tumor-specific transplantation antigens. *Proc. Nat. Acad. Sci. (USA)* **69**, 1540–4.

McGaughey, C. (1974). Feasibility of tumor immunoradiotherapy using radioiodinated antibodies to tumor-specific cell membrane antigens with emphasis on leukemias and early metastases. *Oncology* **29**, 302–19.

Mach, J.-P., Buchegger, F., Forni, M. *et al.* (1981). Use of radiolabelled monoclonal anti-CEA antibodies for the detection of human carcinomas by external photoscanning tomoscintigraphy. *Immunol. Today* **2**, 239–49.

McMannis, J.D., Fisher, R.J., Creekmore, S.P., Braun, D.P., Harris, J.E. and Ellis, T.M. (1988). *In vivo* effects of recombinant IL-2. I. Isolation of circulating Leu-19+ lymphokine-activated killer effector cells from cancer patients receiving recombinant IL-2. *J. Immunol.* **140**, 1335–40.

Mathé, G., Tran, B.L. and Bernard, J. (1958). Effect sur la leucémie 1210 de la souris d'une combination par diazotation d'améthopterine et de γ-globulines de hamsters porteurs de cette leucémie par hétérogreffe. C. R. Acad. Sci. **246**, 1626–8.

Meeker, T.C., Lowder, J., Cleary, M.L. *et al.* (1985a). Emergence of idiotype variants during treatment of B-cell lymphoma with anti-idiotype antibodies. *N. Engl. J. Med.* **312**, 1658–65.

Meeker, T.C., Lowder, J., Maloney, D.G. *et al.* (1985b). A clinical trial of anti-idiotype therapy for B cell malignancy. *Blood* **65**, 1349–63.

Mellman, I., Koch, T., Healey, G. *et al.* (1988). Structure and function of Fc receptors on macrophages and lymphocytes. *J. Cell Sci.* **9** (suppl.), 45–65.

Miller, R.A., Maloney, D.G., Warnke, R. and Levy, R. (1982). Treatment of B-cell lymphoma with monoclonal anti-idiotype antibody. *N. Engl. J. Med.* **306**, 517–22.

Miller, R.A., Oseroff, A.R., Stratte, P.T. and Levy, R. (1983). Monoclonal antibody therapeutic trials in seven patients with T-cell lymphoma. *Blood* **62**, 988–95.

Milstein, C. and Cuello, A.C. (1983). Hybrid hybridomas and their use in immunohistochemistry. *Nature* **305**, 537–40.

Mitchell, M.S., Kan-Mitchell, J., Kempf, R.A., Harel, W., Shau, H. and Lind, S. (1988). Active specific immunotherapy for melanoma: phase I trial of allogeneic lysates and a novel adjuvant. *Cancer Res.* **48**, 5883–93, 1988.

Morrison, S.L., Johnson, M.J., Herzenberg, L.A. and Oi, V.T. (1984). Chimeric human antibody molecules: mouse antigen-binding domains with human constant region domains. *Proc. Nat. Acad. Sci. (USA)* **81**, 6851–5.

Morton, D.L., Eilber, F.R., Holmes, E.C., Sparks, F.C. and Ramming, K.P. (1976). Present status of BCG immunotherapy of malignant melanoma. *Cancer Immunol. Immunother.* **1**, 93–8.

Mulé, J.J., Shu, S. and Rosenberg, S.A. (1985). The anti-tumor efficacy of lymphokine-activated killer cells and recombinant interleukin 2 *in vivo*. *J. Immunol.* **135**, 646–52.

Nadler, L.M., Stashenko, P., Hardy, R. *et al.* (1980). Serotherapy of a patient with monoclonal antibody directed against a human lymphoma-associated antigen. *Cancer Res.* **40**, 3147–54.

Nauts, H.C., Fowler, G.A. and Bogatko, F.H. (1953). A review of the influence of bacterial infection and of bacterial products (Coley's toxins) on malignant tumors in man. *Acta Med. Scand. (Suppl.)* **145**, 29–97.

Nawroth, P.P. and Stern, D.M. (1986). Modulation of endothelial cell hemostatic properties by tumor necrosis factor. *J. Exp. Med.* **163**, 740–5.

Nelson, M., Nelson, D.S., Cianciolo, G.J. and Snyderman, R. (1989). Effects of CKS-17, a synthetic retroviral envelope peptide, on cell-mediated immunity *in vivo*: immunosuppression, immunogenicity, and relation to immunosuppressive tumor products. *Cancer Immunol. Immunother.* **30**, 113–18.

Nisonoff, A. and Mandy, W.J. (1962). Quantitative estimation of the hybridization of rabbit antibodies. *Nature* **194**, 355–9.

North, R.J., Neubauer, R.H., Huang, J.J.H., Newton, R.C. and Loveless, S.E. (1988). Interleukin 1-induced, T cell-mediated regression of immunogenic murine tumors: requirement for an adequate level of already acquired host concomitant immunity. *J. Exp. Med.* **168**, 2031–44.

Okada, Y., Yahata, G., Takeuchi, S., Seidoh, T. and Tanaka, K. (1989). A correlation between the expression of CD8 antigen and specific cytotoxicity of tumor-infiltrating lymphocytes. *Jap. J. Cancer Res.* **80**, 249–56.

Old, L.J. and Boyse, E.A. (1964). Immunology of experimental tumours. *Ann. Rev. Med.* **15**, 167–86.

Old, L.J., Benacerraf, B., Clarke, D.A., Carswell, E.A. and Stockert, E. (1961). The role of the reticuloendothelial system in the host reaction to neoplasia. *Cancer Res.* **21**, 1281–300.

Oliver, R.T.D. (1988). The clinical potential of interleukin-2. *Br. J. Cancer* **58**, 405–9.

Ortaldo, J.R., Mason, A. and Overton, R. (1986). Lymphokine-activated killer cells: analysis of progenitors and effectors. *J. Exp. Med.* **164**, 1193–205.

Ortaldo, J.R., Woodhouse, C., Morgan, A.C., Herberman, R.B., Cheresh, D.A. and Reisfeld, R. (1987). Analysis of effector cells in human antibody-dependent cellular cytotoxicity with murine monoclonal antibodies. *J. Immunol.* **138**, 3566–72.

Osterhaus, A., Weijer, K., Uytdehaag, F., Jarrett, O., Sundquist, B. and Morein, B. (1985). Induction of protective immune response in cats by vaccination with feline leukemia virus iscom. *J. Immunol.* **135**, 591–6.

Palladino, M.A., Jr, Shalaby, M.F., Kramer, S.M. *et al.* (1987). Characterization of the antitumor activities of human tumor necrosis factor-α and the comparison with other cytokines: induction of tumor-specific immunity. *J. Immunol.* **138**, 4023–32.

Pasternack, G.R., Johnson, R.J. and Shin, H.S. (1978). Tumor cell cytostasis by macrophages and antibody *in vitro*. I. Resolution into contact-dependent and contact-independent steps. *J. Immunol.* **120**, 1560–6.

Phillips, J.H. and Lanier, L.L. (1986). Dissection of the lymphokine-activated killer phenomenon. *J. Exp. Med.* **164**, 814–25.

Piguet, P.F., Grau, G.E., Allet, B. and Vassalli, P. (1987). Tumor necrosis factor/cachectin is an effector of skin and gut lesions of the acute phase of graft-vs-host disease. *J. Exp. Med.* **166**, 1280–9.

Pimm, M.V. (1988). Drug-monoclonal antibody conjugates for cancer therapy: potentials and limitations. *CRC Crit. Rev. Ther. Drug Carrier Systems* **5**, 189–227.

Preijers, F.W.M.B., Tax, W.J.M., Wessels, J.M.C., Capel, P.J.A., de Witte, T. and Haanen, C. (1988). Different susceptibilities of normal T cells and T cell lines to immunotoxins. *Scand. J. Immunol.* **27**, 533–40.

Preijers, F.W.M.B., De Witte, T., Wessels, J.M.C. *et al.* (1989).

Autologous transplantation of bone marrow purged *in vitro* with anti-CD7-(WT1-) ricin A immunotoxin in T-cell lymphoblastic leukemia and lymphoma. *Blood* **74**, 1152–8.

Press, O.W., Appelbau, F., Ledbetter, J.A. *et al.* (1987). Monoclonal antibody 1F5 (anti-CD20) serotherapy of human B cell lymphomas. *Blood* **69**, 584–91.

Press, O.W., Eary, J.F., Badger, C.C. *et al.* (1989). Treatment of refractory non-Hodgkin's lymphoma with radiolabeled MB-1 (anti-CD37) antibody. *J. Clin. Oncol.* **7**, 1027–38.

Price, G., Brenner, M.K., Prentic, H.G., Hoffbrand, A.V. and Newland, A.C. (1987). Cytotoxic effects of tumour necrosis factor and gamma-interferon on acute myeloid leukaemia blasts. *Br. J. Cancer* **55**, 287–90.

Quesada, J.R., Reuben, J., Manning, J.T., Hersh, E.M. and Gutterman, J.U. (1984). α-Interferon for induction of remission in hairy-cell leukemia. *N. Engl. J. Med.* **310**, 15–18.

Ralph, P. and Nakoinz, I. (1983). Cell-mediated lysis of tumor targets directed by murine monoclonal antibodies of IgM and all IgG isotypes. *J. Immunol.* **131**, 1028–31.

Rankin, E.M., Hekman, A. and ten Bokkel Huinink, W. (1985). Treatment of two patients with B cell lymphoma with monoclonal anti-idiotype antibodies. *Blood* **65**, 1373–81.

Raso, V. (1988). Growth factors and other ligands. In *Immunotoxins*, ed. Frankel, A.E., pp. 297–320, Kluwer Academic Publications, Norwell, Mass.

Revel, M. and Chedbath, J. (1986). Interferon-activated genes. *Trends Biochem. Sci.* **11**, 166 70.

Riechmann, L., Clark, M., Waldmann, H. and Winter, G. (1988). Reshaping human antibodies for therapy. *Nature* **332**, 323–7.

Ritz, J. and Schlossman, S.F. (1982). Utilization of monoclonal antibodies in the treatment of leukemia and lymphoma. *Blood* **59**, 1–11.

Rose, N.R. and Witebsky, E. (1956). Studies on organ specificity. V. Changes in the thyroid glands of rabbits following active immunization with rabbit thyroid extracts. *J. Immunol.* **76**, 417–27.

Rosenberg, S.A. (1985). Lymphokine-activated killer cells: a new approach to immunotherapy of cancer. *J. Nat. Cancer Inst.* **75**, 595–603.

Rosenberg, S.A., Packard, B.S., Aebersold, P.M. *et al.* (1988). Use of tumor-infiltrating lymphocytes and interleukin-2 in the immunotherapy of patients with metastatic melanoma. *N. Engl. J. Med.* **319**, 1676–80.

Rosenberg, S.A., Lotze, M.L., Yang, J.C. *et al.* (1989). Experience with the use of high-dose interleukin-2 in the treatment of 652 cancer patients. *Ann. Surg.* **210**, 474–84.

Roth, S.M. and Foon, K.A. (1986). α-Interferon in the treatment of hematologic malignancies. *Am. J. Med.* **81**, 871–82.

Rouse, B.T., Rollinghoff, M. and Warner, N.L. (1972). Anti-θ serum-induced suppression of the cellular transfer of tumour-specific immunity to syngeneic plasma cell tumour. *Nature N. Biol.* **238**, 116–17.

Rubin, R.H., Fischman, A.J., Callahan, R.J. *et al.* (1989). ^{111}In-labelled nonspecific immunoglobulin scanning in the detection of focal infection. *N. Engl. J. Med.* **321**, 935–40.

Rybarska, J., Konieczny, I., Bobrzecka, K. and Laidler, P. (1982). The hemolytic activity of (Fab-Fc) recombinant immunoglobulins with specificity for the sheep red blood cells. *Immunol. Lett.* **4**, 279–84.

Scallon, B.J., Scigliano, E., Freedman, V.H. *et al.* (1989). A human immunoglobulin G receptor exists in both polypeptide-anchored and phosphatidylinositol-glycan-anchored forms. *Proc. Nat. Acad. Sci. (USA)* **86**, 5079–83.

Schirrmacher, V., von Hoegen, P. and Heicappell, R. (1989). Virus modified tumor cell vaccines for active specific immunotherapy of micrometastases: expansion and activation of tumor-specific T cells. *Prog. Clin. Biol. Res.* **288**, 391–9.

Schlom, J. (1986). Basic principles and applications of monoclonal antibodies in the management of carcinomas. *Cancer Res.* **46**, 3225–38.

Schlom, J. (1989). Innovations in monoclonal antibody tumour targeting. *JAMA* **261**, 744–6.

Schroff, R.W., Farrell, M.M., Klein, R.A., Stevenson, H.C. and Warner, N.L. (1985). Induction and enhancement by monocytes of antibody-induced modulation of a variety of human lymphoid cell surface antigens. *Blood* **66**, 620–6.

Sears, H.F., Herlyn, D., Steplewski, Z. and Koprowski, H. (1985). Phase II clinical trial of a murine monoclonal antibody cytotoxic for gastrointestinal adenocarcinoma. *Cancer Res.* **45**, 5910–13.

Segal, D.M., Garrido, M.A., Perez, P. *et al.* (1988). Targeted cytotoxic cells as a novel form of cancer immunotherapy. *Mol. Immunol.* **25**, 1099–103.

Selby, P., Hobbs, S., Viner, C. *et al.* (1987). Tumour necrosis factor in man: clinical and biological observations. *Br. J. Cancer* **56**, 803–8.

Senter, P.D., Schreiber, G.J., Hirschberg, D.L., Ashe, S.A., Hellström, K.E. and Hellström, I. (1989). Enhancement of the *in vitro* and *in vivo* antitumor activities of phosphorylated mitomycin C and etoposide derivatives by monoclonal antibody–alkaline phosphatase conjugates. *Cancer Res.* **49**, 5789–92.

Seto, M., Takahashi, T., Nakamura, S., Saito, M., Hara, T. and Nishizuka, Y. (1986). Effector mechanism in antitumor activity of monoclonal antibodies produced against an ascitic mouse mammary tumor. *Cancer Res.* **46**, 2056–61.

Shearer, W.T., Philpott, G.W. and Parker, C.W. (1975). Increased nucleoside incorporation, DNA synthesis, and cell growth in L cells treated with anti-L cell antibody. *Cell. Immunol.* **17**, 447–62.

Shiloni, E., Eisenthal, A., Sachs, D. and Rosenberg, S.A. (1987). Antibody-dependent cellular cytotoxicity mediated by murine lymphocytes activated in recombinant interleukin 2. *J. Immunol.* **138**, 1992–8.

Sia, D.Y., Lachmann, P.J. and Leung, K.N. (1984). Studies on the enhancement of tumour immunity by coupling strong antigens to tumour cells ('heterogenisation of tumours'): helper T cell clones against PPD help other T cells mount anti-tumour responses to PPD-coupled tumour cells. *Immunology* **51**, 755–63.

Sidman, C.L. and Unanue, E.R. (1975). Receptor-mediated inactivation of early B lymphocytes. *Nature* **257**, 149–51.

Simmons, D. and Seed, B. (1989). The Fcγ receptor of natural killer cells is a phospholipid-linked membrane protein. *Nature* **333**, 568–9.

Simmons, R.L. and Rios, A. (1971). Immunotherapy of cancer: immunospecific rejection of tumors in recipients of neuraminidase-treated tumor cells plus BCG. *Science* **174**, 591–3.

Smith, C.A., Williams, G.T., Kingston, R., Jenkinson, E.J. and Owen, J.J.T. (1989). Antibodies to CD3/T-cell receptor complex induce death by opoptosis in immature T cells in thymic cultures. *Nature* **337**, 181–4.

Smith, K.A. (1988). The interleukin 2 receptor. *Adv. Immunol.* **42**, 165–79.

Spiegelberg, H.L. and Weigle, W.O. (1965). The catabolism of homologous and heterologous 7S gamma globulin fragments. *J. Exp. Med.* **121**, 323–38.

Spriggs, D.R., Sherman, M.L., Michie, H. *et al.* (1988). Recombinant human tumor necrosis factor administered as a 24-hour intravenous infusion: a phase I and pharmacologic study. *J. Nat. Cancer Inst.* **80**, 1039–44.

Srivastava, P.K., De Leo, A.B. and Old, L.J. (1986). Tumor rejection antigens of chemically induced sarcomas of inbred mice. *Proc. Nat. Acad. Sci. (USA)* **83**, 340–11.

Stackpole, C.W., Jacobson, J.B. and Lardis, M.P. (1974). Antigenic modulation *in vitro*. I. Fate of thymus-leukemia (TL) antigen-antibody complexes following modulation of TL antigenicity from the surfaces of mouse leukemia cells and thymocytes. *J. Exp. Med.* **140**, 939–53.

Steis, R.G., Smith, J.W., Urba, W.J. *et al.* (1988). Resistance to recombinant interferon alfa-2a in hairy-cell leukemia associated with neutralizing anti-interferon antibodies. *N. Engl. J. Med.* **318**, 1409–13.

Stern, D.M. and Nawroth, P.P. (1986). Modulation of endothelial cell hemostatic properties of tumor necrosis factor. *J. Exp. Med.* **163**, 740–5.

Stevenson, F.K., Hamblin, T.J., Stevenson, G.T. and Tutt, A.L. (1980). Extracellular idiotypic immunoglobulin arising from human leukemic B lymphocytes. *J. Exp. Med.* **152**, 1484–96.

Stevenson, G.T. and Glennie, M.J. (1985). Surface immunoglobulin of B-lymphocytic tumours as a therapeutic target. *Cancer Surv.* **4**, 213–44.

Stevenson, G.T. and Stevenson, F.K. (1975). Antibody to a molecularly-defined antigen confined to a tumour cell surface. *Nature* **254**, 714–16.

Stevenson, G.T., Pindar, A. and Slade, C.J. (1989). A chimeric antibody with dual Fc regions (*bis*FabFc) prepared by manipulations at the IgG hinge. *Anti-Cancer Drug Design* **3**, 219–30.

Stirpe, F. and Barbieri, L. (1986). Ribosome-inactivating proteins up to date. *FEBS Lett.* **195**, 1–8.

Stryckmans, P.S., Otten, J., Delbeke, J. *et al.* (1983). Comparison of chemotherapy with immunotherapy for maintenance of acute lymphoblastic leukemia in children and adults. *Blood* **62**, 606–15.

Sugarman, B.J., Aggarwal, B.B., Hass, P.E., Figari, I.S., Palladino, M.A. and Shepard, H.M. (1985). Recombinant human tumor necrosis factor-alpha: effect on proliferation of normal and transformed cells *in vitro*. *Science* **230**, 943–5.

Taupier, M.A., Kearney, J.F., Leibson, P.J., Loken, M.R. and Schreiber, H. (1983). Nonrandom escape of tumor cells from immune lysis due to intraclonal fluctuations in antigen expression. *Cancer Res.* **43**, 4050–6.

Tepper, R.I., Pattengale, P.K. and Leder, P. (1989). Murine interleukin-4 displays potent anti-tumor activity *in vivo*. *Cell* **57**, 503–12.

Topalian, S.L., Solomon, D. and Rosenberg, S.A. (1989). Tumor-specific cytolysis by lymphocytes infiltrating human melanomas. *J. Immunol.* **142**, 3714–25.

Trauth, B.C., Klas, C., Peters, A.M.J. *et al.* (1989). Monoclonal antibody-mediated tumor regression by induction of apoptosis. *Science* **245**, 301–5.

Treleaven, J.G., Gibson, F.M., Ugelstad, J. *et al.* (1984). Removal of neuroblastoma cells from bone marrow with monoclonal antibodies conjugated to magnetic microspheres. *Lancet* **i**, 70–3.

Unkeless, J.C., Scigliano, E. and Freedman, V.H. (1988). Structure and function of human and murine receptors for IgG. *Ann. Rev. Immunol.* **6**, 251–81.

Vitetta, E.S., Fulton, R.J., May, R.D., Till, M. and Uhr, J.W. (1987). Redesigning nature's poisons to create anti-tumor reagents. *Science* **238**, 1098–104.

Vyakarnam, A., Lachmann, P.J. and Sikora, K. (1981). The heterogenization of tumour cells with tuberculin. II. Studies of the antigenecity of tuberculin-heterogenized murine tumour cells in syngeneic BCG positive and BCG negative mice. *Immunology* **42**, 337–48.

Wade, R., Whisson, M.E. and Szekerke, M. (1967). Some serum protein nitrogen mustard complexes with high chemotherapeutic selectivity. *Nature* **215**, 1303–4.

Waldmann, T.A. and Strober, W. (1969). Metabolism of immunoglobulins. *Prog. Allergy* **13**, 1–110.

Waldmann, T.A., Goldman, C.K., Bongiovanni, K.F. *et al.* (1988). Therapy of HTLV-I-induced adult T-cell leukaemia with mo mcl a Tac, an AbG2a vs IL-2 receptor. *Blood* **72**, 1805–16.

Walker, M.R., Woof, J.M., Brüggemann, M., Jefferis, R. and Burton, D.R. (1989). Interaction of human IgG chimeric antibodies with the human FcRI and FcRII receptors: requirements for antibody-mediated host cell–target cell interaction. *Mol. Immunol.* **26**, 403–11.

Ward, B.G., Mather, S.J., Hawkins, L.R. *et al.* (1987). Localization of radioiodine conjugated to the monoclonal antibody HMFG2 in human ovarian carcinoma: assessment of intravenous and intraperitoneal routes of administration. *Cancer Res.* **47**, 4719–23.

Ward, B., Mather, S., Shepherd, J. *et al.* (1988). The treatment of intraperitoneal malignant disease with monoclonal antibody guided ^{131}I radiotherapy. *Br. J. Cancer* **58**, 658–62.

Warner, G.L. and Scott, D.W. (1988). Lymphoma Models for B-cell activation and tolerance. VII. Pathways in anti-Ig-mediated growth inhibition and its reversal. *Cell Immunol.* **115**, 195–203.

Watts, H.F., Anderson, V.A., Cole, V.M. and Stevenson, G.T. (1985). Activation of complement pathways by univalent antibody derivatives with intact Fc zones. *Mol. Immunol.* **22**, 803–10.

Weiden, P.L., Flournoy, N., Thomas, E.D. *et al.* (1979). Antileukemic effect of graft-versus-host disease in human recipients of allogeneic-marrow grafts. *N. Engl. J. Med.* **300**, 1068–73.

Weigle, W.O. (1980). Analysis of autoimmunity through experimental models of thyroiditis and allergic encephalomyelitis. *Adv. Immunol.* **30**, 159–273.

Weinberg, R.A. (1989). Oncogenes, antioncogenes, and the molecular basis of multistep carcinogenesis. *Cancer Res.* **49**, 3713–21.

Weinstein, J.N., Blumenthal R., Sharrow, S.O. and Henkart, P.A. (1978). Antibody-mediated targeting of liposomes:

binding to lymphocytes does not ensure incorporation of vesicle contents into the cells. *Biochem. Biophys. Acta* **509**, 272–88.

West, W.H., Tauer, K.W., Yannelli, J.R. *et al.* (1987). Constant-infusion recombinant interleukin-2 in adoptive immunotherapy of advanced cancer. *N. Engl. J. Med.* **316**, 898–905.

Wettendorf, M., Iliopoulos, D., Tempero, M. *et al.* (1989). Idiotypic cascades in cancer patients treated with monoclonal antibody CO17–1A *Proc. Nat. Acad. Sci. (USA)* **86**, 3787–91.

Williamson, B.D., Carswell, E.A., Rubin, B.Y., Prendergast, J.S. and Old, L.J. (1983). Human tumor necrosis factor produced by human B-cell lines: synergistic cytotoxic interaction with human interferon. *Proc. Nat. Acad. Sci. (USA)* **80**, 5397–401.

Wright, A., Lee, J.E., Link, M.P. *et al.* (1989). Cytotoxic T lymphocytes specific for self tumor immunoglobulin express T cell receptor with chain. *J. Exp. Med.* **169**, 1557–64.

Wright, S.D. and Silverstein, S.C. (1986). Overview: the function receptors in phagocytosis. In *Cellular Immunology*, ed. D.M. Weir, Vol. II, pp. 41.1–41.14, Blackwell Scientific Publications, Oxford.

Yagita, H., Nakata, M., Azuma, A. *et al.* (1989). Activation of peripheral blood T cells via the p75 interleukin 2 receptor. *J. Exp. Med.* **170**, 1445–50.

Yamamori, T., Fukada, K., Aebersold, R., Korsching, S., Fann, M.-J. and Patterson, P.H. (1989). The cholinergic neuronal differentiation factor from heart cells is identical to leukemia inhibitory factor. *Science* **246**, 1412–16.

Youle, R.J. and Colombatti, M. (1987). Hybridoma cells containing intracellular anti-ricin antibodies show ricin meets secretory antibody before entering the cytosol. *J. Biol. Chem.* **262**, 4676–82.

Section 12
Organ-based Immunology

95: Blood

W.H. Ouwehand, A.H. Waters, A.G. Hadley and N.C. Hughes-Jones

Autoimmune haemolytic anaemia

Autoimmune haemolytic anaemia (AIHA) is a rare disease in adults, usually with a late onset in the fifth to seventh decades (Dacie 1962; Dacie and Worlledge 1969), but it is seldom observed in children (Habibi *et al.* 1974). In patients with an acquired haemolytic anaemia of the normochromic normocytic type, the haemolysis can be caused by autoantibodies directed against antigenic structures on the red cell membrane. The clinical presentation of AIHA can vary from a mild, well-compensated haemolysis to an acute and severe condition requiring immediate treatment in order to protect the patient from cardiovascular complications caused by a rapid fall in haemoglobin concentration (Dacie and Worlledge 1969).

Classification of the syndromes

It is useful to classify the AIHA by the temperature at which the autoantibodies react with suitable red cells, because this correlates with the distinct clinical syndromes. These syndromes are:
1 AIHA associated with warm-reactive autoantibodies (37°C);
2 AIHA associated with cold-reactive antibodies (below 37°C).
Within each division there are both complement- and non-complement-activating antibodies. The warm immunoglobulin (Ig)G antibodies are the most common and they are predominantly non-complement-activating; in contrast, the warm IgM antibodies are complement-activating. The cold-reacting antibodies, on the other hand, are predominantly IgM and also complement-activating. Table 95.1 shows the distribution based on the serological profile of the autoantibodies of 2400 patients (Engelfriet *et al.* 1987). These results are in accordance with the data obtained in three other smaller series (Petz and Garratty 1980; Vroclans-Deiminas and Boivin 1980; Sokol *et al.* 1981).

Clinical features

Autoimmune haemolytic anaemia can present as a primary disease (46% of the patients) or secondary

Table 95.1. Distribution of antibody type in a series of 2400 patients

Type of antibody	Number of patients
Warm autoantibodies	
Non-lytic, IgG and IgA	1649
IgM, lytic + enzyme-treated cells	259
IgM, lytic + native cells	4
Combination of above	77
Cold autoantibodies	
IgM (CHAD)	325
IgG (PCH)	59
IgM + IgG	7
Warm + cold autoantibodies	
IgG (warm, non-lytic) + IgM (cold)	7
IgG (warm, lytic) + IgM (cold)	3

Source: Engelfriet *et al.* (1987).

to other organ-specific or generalized disorders (Table 95.2). On physical examination, the classical signs of anaemia are present in combination with jaundice and splenomegaly, although the last two are not essential. There is a great variation between patients in the rate of red cell destruction. On the one hand, there may be only a small increase in the rate of red cell destruction and, as a result, the haemoglobin concentration may be almost within normal limits. Such patients are frequently diagnosed during routine investigation or during screening for irregular antibodies. On the other hand, a very rapid rate of destruction may be found, sometimes in combination with haemoglobinuria, requiring immediate intervention by transfusion of red cell concentrates in combination with a high dose of corticosteroids.

In cold haemagglutinin disease (CHAD), two different syndromes are found. First, there is a long-continued chronic form which is caused by a monoclonal IgM autoantibody. In these patients, the severity of the haemolysis is related to the concentration and the temperature range of the antibody produced by the monoclonal B cells. Patients present with acrocyanosis of the extremities (Raynaud's phenomenon) and haemoglobinuria, both symptoms being precipitated by exposure to a cold environment. Second, AIHA caused by cold autoantibodies is also seen as a transient and self-limiting form in the presence of a *Mycoplasma* infection or infectious mononucleosis; the cold autoantibodies are polyclonal and transient and the haemolysis is caused by an increase in the concentration and temperature amplitude of the normal cold autoantibodies.

Table 95.2. Distribution of patients between primary and secondary aetiology

	Number of patients
Primary	245 (46.6%)
Secondary (total)	292 (54.4%)
Lympho/myeloproliferative	130 (44.5%)
Autoimmune-related	141 (48.3%)
Solid tumours	12 (4.1%)
Miscellaneous	9 (3.1%)

Source: Engelfriet *et al.* (1987).

In paroxysmal cold haemoglobinuria (PCH), the manifestations are also precipitated by cold but they are clearly distinct from those seen in CHAD. The syndrome results from the presence of the Donath–Landsteiner (D–L) antibody, whose serological characteristics are also distinct. Most patients suffer from a single attack of haemoglobinuria, whereas some may have repeated attacks whenever the weather is cold. The clinical picture resembles that seen in an acute haemolytic transfusion reactions due to anti-A or anti-B antibodies. Paroxysmal cold haemoglobinuria is now a rare disease; formerly, it was seen in association with tertiary syphilis but now there is a closer association to viral infections. The extent of red cell destruction in patients is often considerable during the acute phase but is self-limiting.

Laboratory investigations

The peripheral blood picture in AIHA is almost always normochromic and normocytic; spherocytes are obligatory. Reticulocyte numbers are usually raised and occasionally erythrophagocytosis and erythroblastosis can be observed. The peripheral blood and the bone marrow should be carefully examined for signs of lympho- or myeloproliferative disorders. Lactate dehydrogenase is increased, haptoglobin levels are reduced and both free and conjugated bilirubin levels in the plasma are increased. Conjugated bilirubin is demonstrable in the urine but haemoglobinuria is only seen when there is a considerable amount of intravascular red cell destruction. As autoantibodies against red cells are often accompanied by auto-

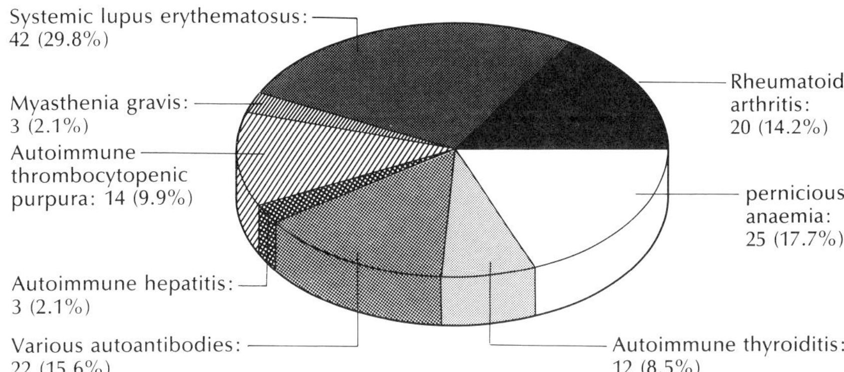

Fig. 95.1. Autoimmune diseases in which AIHA is a feature. Data from 141 patients. From Engelfriet *et al.* (1987).

antibodies against other blood cells or other organs (Fig. 95.1), a routine investigation for the presence of these against a panel of autoantigens should be carried out. It is important to distinguish between a primary idiopathic AIHA and a secondary condition due to underlying disease, such as the lymphoproliferative disorders, since treatment with corticosteroids can mask the latter.

The crucial screening test in AIHA is the direct antiglobulin test, using an anti-human Ig reagent containing anti-C3d antibodies. If the antiglobulin test is positive, a further analysis should be performed using class- and subclass-specific antisera. This is of importance if transfusion is required and to enable the appropriate therapy to be applied. There is no simple direct correlation between the intensity of the antiglobulin reaction with either a polyvalent reagent or a class-specific reagent and the clinical severity of red cell destruction.

WARM ANTIBODIES

Immunoglobulin G non-complement-activating autoantibodies

In most cases of AIHA due to warm antibodies, the Ig is of the IgG class (Table 95.3). The subclass of the IgG autoantibodies can be determined with subclass-specific reagents. The majority of IgG autoantibodies are of the IgG1 (74%) and IgG3 subclasses, either on their own or in combination (Table 95.4). Immunoglobulin G2 or IgG4 autoantibodies, which are not capable of shortening the red cell lifespan, are infrequent and are usually found by chance during screening procedures for other reasons in patients without evidence of haemolysis. The presence of IgG1 antibodies is often associated with the use of α-methyldopa. The clinical importance of subclass typing results from the differences in the efficiency of different IgG subclasses in their ability to bring about red

Table 95.3. Distribution of immunoglobulin class in a series of 1825 patients

Antibody class	Number of patients
Total	1825
IgG	1770
IgM	8
IgA	4
IgG + IgM	20
IgG + IgA	13
IgG + IgA + IgM	7
IgM + IgA	3

Source: Engelfriet *et al.* (1987).

Table 95.4. Distribution of immunoglobulin G subclasses amongst warm antibodies

IgG subclass	Number of patients
Total	745
IgG1	552
IgG2	5
IgG3	16
IgG4	7
IgG1+2	65
IgG1+3	57
IgG1+4	7
IgG2+4	1
IgG3+4	1
IgG1+2+3	14
IgG1+2+3+4	6
No classification	14

Source: Engelfriet *et al.* (1987).

cell destruction. Autoantibodies of the IgG1, IgG2 and IgG4 subclasses are often responsible for the phenomenon of a positive direct antiglobulin test without signs of haemolysis (see above), while IgG3 autoantibodies always cause significant red cell destruction *in vivo*.

It is generally accepted that incomplete warm autoantibodies of the IgG and IgA class are non-complement-binding. Nevertheless, it is not uncommon to find that a positive test is obtained using an anti-C3d antiserum, especially when the AIHA is of secondary origin. Immunoglobulin G autoantibodies present in the patient's serum or in an eluate prepared from the red cells do not fix complement *in vitro*. Further, a positive test for complement components was found in 50% of the patients who only had IgA antibodies, which do not fix complement (Engelfriet *et al.* 1987). It is generally believed that the presence of complement factors on the red cells is due to the absorption of immune complexes associated with the primary disease.

Immunoglobulin A autoantibodies

Immunoglobulin A-mediated haemolytic anaemia is relatively rare (Table 95.3). The severity of the haemolysis can be life-threatening, but mild cases are also observed. It is not known whether this difference in clinical presentation is dependent on the subclass of the IgA antibody, on the density of the antibody on the red cells or on a combination of both.

Specificity of warm antibodies

Warm autoantibodies can be eluted from the patient's red cells and specificity can be determined with a panel of donor red cells of known antigenic constitution. The warm autoantibodies frequently show a broad reactivity with such a panel. Autoantibodies reacting optimally at 37°C are directed against a variety of autoantigens (Fig. 95.2), whose biochemical structure is mostly unknown and can only be defined serologically. It is not infrequent to find autoantibodies specific for epitopes associated with the Rhesus (Rh) system. Only occasionally are these antibodies identical in specificity with the Rh alloantibodies. Sometimes the specificity is similar, e.g. anti-e-like, but it is more usual for the antibody to recognize an epitope common to all the Rh polypeptides (C, c, D, E and e) and this type of antibody is only recognized by its inability to react with Rh_{null} cells.

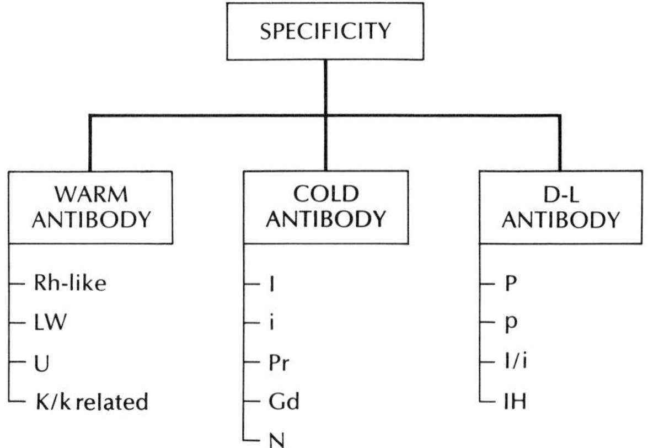

Fig. 95.2. Specificity of blood group autoantibodies that have been detected in AIHA.

An interesting feature concerning the Kell blood group system is that the antigens can be depressed or absent in the presence of autoantibodies with specificities associated with this system. The patient's phenotype is $Kell_{null}$ during the acute episode of the disease and the antibody is therefore defined incorrectly as an alloantibody. Infrequently IgG autoantibodies with other specificities are described in patients with AIHA, e.g. anti-A, -Jk^a, -N, -S, -Vel, -I^t, -Ge, -Sd^x -Kx (Issitt *et al.* 1976; Petz and Garratty 1980; Becton and Kinney 1986; Ciaffoni *et al.* 1987, Sander *et al.* 1987; Reid *et al.* 1988). Wakui *et al.* (1988) showed that the autoantibodies can be directed also against the erythrocyte membrane protein 4.1.

Free antibodies in the serum

Autoantibodies can be detected in the serum of the majority of patients who have a positive direct antiglobulin test with anti-IgG (Petz and Garratty 1980). The antibodies are often present at low concentrations and it is frequently necessary to enhance the antiglobulin test. Using polyethylene glycol as a potentiator, the indirect antiglobulin test is positive in almost all patients who have

IgG autoantibodies on the red cell surface (M.A.M. Overbeeke, pers. comm.).

Warm complement-activating autoantibodies

Warm complement-activating antibodies have a low affinity for their antigen and are thus only detected by a haemolysin test or indirectly by the finding of complement factors on the red cells. Warm antibodies with lytic activity resulting from activation of the complement system belong to the IgM class and fall into two categories, namely, those that only lyse enzyme-treated cells and those that lyse normal cells. The former are by far the most common (259 of the 263 patients; see Table 95.1). The auto-antibodies in only four out of the 2000 patients were able to lyse normal cells. These latter patients have a severe form of the disease which is nearly always fatal (Shirley *et al.* 1987). Patients whose antibodies only lyse enzyme-treated cells usually have a mild degree of red cell destruction (Atkinson and Frank 1974), with a haemoglobin concentration often lying within the normal range due to the increase in red cell production.

COLD AUTOANTIBODIES

Cold haemagglutinin disease

Cold autoantibodies associated with CHAD are capable of both agglutinating red cells suspended in saline and of haemolysing untreated red cells *in vitro*. They are almost always IgM and occur as a monoclonal antibody population. The antibody is usually only active up to 30–32°C and the temperature in the exposed skin may well be within this range. When the antibody is bound to red cells, the complement cascade is activated. On rewarming to 37°C, the antibody elutes off but complement components remain and are present in sufficient quantity on some of the red cells to lead to lysis. On the remainder of the cells, activated C3 is broken down to the haemolytically inactive C3d form. It is this form that is responsible for giving the positive antiglobulin reaction (due to the anti-C3d antibody contained in the reagent).

Free cold antibody is always present in the serum of a CHAD patient, resulting in high agglutination titres. It is often present in sufficient amounts to be detected as an abnormal band on electrophoresis. These antibodies fix complement *in vitro* and this is best demonstrated at a pH of 6.5–7.0 using enzyme-treated cells. The lytic titre usually parallels the clinical severity.

Donath–Landsteiner antibody

The D–L antibody belongs to the IgG class and is able to lyse normal red cells when present in low concentrations. It is also known as a biphasic haemolysin, as cooling to 4°C, followed by incubation at 37°C, is often necessary to demonstrate lysis *in vitro*. The reason for this is that the upper limit of the antibodies' thermal range is about 15°C. The positive direct antiglobulin reaction is only seen when the antiserum contains anti-C3d antibodies. Unless the test is carried out at low temperature, no IgG is detectable on the red cell surface. The test becomes negative shortly after the attack.

Specificity of cold antibodies

Both the D–L antibody and the cold antibody associated with CHAD are examples of autoantibodies with well-defined specificities. The D–L antibody usually reacts specifically with the blood group antigen P but other specificities are occasionally found (Fig. 95.2). Potent, naturally occurring, cold autoantibodies (IgM) or monoclonal IgM cold autoantibodies may be confused with biphasic haemolysins; however, the Ig class (IgG), the non-agglutinating character and the anti-P specificity of the biphasic haemolysins help to distinguish the D–L antibody from others.

The majority of high-titred cold autoantibodies associated with CHAD have the specificity anti-I. Occasionally high-titred anti-i is found; in low titre, anti-i is associated with Epstein–Barr virus (EBV) infections. Those antibodies associated with *Mycoplasma pneumoniae* infections are invariably I-specific.

Serum complement

In CHAD the serum complement concentrations are often reduced or even absent in the presence of high-titre cold autoantibodies. This protects the patient from the worst effects of the disease. Infusion of fresh frozen plasma can trigger severe haemolysis.

Harmless cold autoantibodies

Cold autoantibodies are normally present in low titre in the serum of most human subjects. These cold autoagglutinins almost always have anti-I specificity. Other examples of target antigens for harmless cold autoantibodies are i, Pr, A, A_1, B, BI, Bi, HI, Hi, M, N and LW. Since their reactivity with red cells is restricted to a low temperature (below 32°C) and as they are present in very low concentrations, these autoagglutinins do not cause red cell destruction *in vivo*. If the titre of this type of cold autoantibody increases acutely as a consequence of a viral infection, the temperature amplitude of the antibodies can alter and a self-limiting haemolysis can occur.

Treatment

The choice of treatment is determined by many factors. In the case of secondary AIHA, the treatment of the primary disease is essential. When haemolysis causes unacceptable symptoms, the main task should be to lower the extent of cell destruction, and transfusion may be necessary. The ability to reduce the erythrocyte destruction is dependent on the type of immune mechanism which is operative. A serological investigation is thus of the greatest value.

The methods of treatment are twofold; first, a broad non-specific drug-induced immunosuppressive therapy and, secondly, in the case of IgG autoantibodies, the inhibition of the Fc receptor (FcR)-mediated red cell destruction. In CHAD and PCH avoidance of cold can protect the patient from haemolysis. Either plasmaphaeresis or autoantibody absorption (Besa *et al.* 1981) can be life-saving when there is considerable haemolysis.

WARM NON-COMPLEMENT-ACTIVATING AUTOANTIBODIES

Corticosteroids

Prednisone orally in a dose of 1 mg/kg bodyweight brings about both a reduction in the intensity of red cell destruction and in antibody production. The effect on red cell survival is immediate whereas the reduction of antibody production takes a few weeks or months to appear (Rosse 1971). The mechanism which is responsible for the decline in red cell destruction is not fully understood, but the extracellular cytotoxic lysis and phagocytosis of IgG-coated erythrocytes by monocytes *in vitro* is diminished, resulting from a reduced release of lysosomal enzymes (Fleer *et al.* 1978a). In most patients the amount of antibody on the red cells decreases in the first weeks or months of prednisone therapy. Changes in the IgG subclass profile of the autoantibodies have also been described. After the initial high-dose therapy, the reduced rate of formation of autoantibodies can be maintained at a much lower dose, e.g. 2.5–10 mg/day. However, 50% of the patients relapse and in these cases other therapy should be considered or the dose of corticosteroids should be increased.

Cyclophosphamide and azathioprine

Cyclophosphamide and azathioprine can also be effective in suppression of antibody production but are not the drugs of first choice (Hitzig and Massimo 1966).

Splenectomy

In most patients with warm-type AIHA the destruction of red cells is mainly confined to the spleen. Survival studies with ^{51}Cr-labelled autologous red cells can be performed before splenectomy takes place. Even when sequestration is restricted to the spleen, removal of this organ will not always be effective, as destruction can relocalize to the liver. This relocalization cannot be predicted. Splenectomy is usually followed by a fall in autoantibody production.

Intravenous immunoglobulin therapy

Administration of large amounts of IgG intravenously (IVIgG; 1–5 g/kg body-weight/day, on 5 consecutive days) reduces the red cell destruction in about 40–60% of the patients (Macintyre *et al.* 1985; Mueller-Eckhardt *et al.* 1985; Hilgartner and Bussel 1987; Besa 1988; Newland 1989). The effect lasts only 2–3 weeks and repeated administration is usually required. The administered IgG probably acts by competitive blocking of the FcRs for IgG on the macrophages (see later). It is also possible that anti-idiotype antibodies (Masouredis *et al.* 1987) present in the IgG preparations bring about a reduction in autoantibody production. As the effectiveness of IVIgG is low and the costs are high, IVIgG therapy should only be considered when other therapy has been ineffective or is contraindicated. Children may benefit from IVIgG therapy since it does not interfere with normal development.

Blocking of the FcRs with monoclonal antibodies seems to be a promising development; however, our understanding of the interaction of the macrophage FcRs and the IgG-coated erythrocytes is still limited. There is one report of the effect of FcR blocking using monoclonal antibody against FcRIII (CD16) in a patient with autoimmune thrombocytopenia (AIT) (Clarkson *et al.* 1986).

Vinblastin

Another method of reducing the destruction of IgG- or IgA-coated erythrocytes by macrophages is to selectively damage the macrophages with vinca-loaded platelets. Autologous or ABO-compatible donor platelets have been incubated with vinca alkaloids, usually vinblastin, together with plasma from patients with AIT and subsequently infused into patients (Ahn *et al.* 1978, 1983; Gertz *et al.* 1981). In three splenectomized patients remission of haemolysis was observed, lasting from several months to 3 years (Ahn *et al.* 1983). The results of studies obtained with vinblastin alone are conflicting (Ahn *et al.* 1978, 1983).

Plasma exchange and autoantibody absorption appear to be most useful during episodes of acute haemolysis to gain time for other forms of therapy (Bernstein *et al.* 1981; Besa *et al.* 1981; Brooks *et al.* 1982).

COLD HAEMAGGLUTININ DISEASE

Therapy is aimed at reducing the activation of complement by preventing the antibody from binding to its antigen. The most effective way to do this is by the avoidance of cold, such as the use of warm clothing and well-heated rooms or moving to a milder climate in the cold months. Prophylaxis is thus the primary aim. Reduction of autoantibody production with alkylating agents or the use of corticosteroids (Lahav *et al.* 1989) and interferon-α can be helpful (O'Connor *et al.* 1989). When cold AIHA is secondary to a lymphoproliferative process, therapeutic success largely depends on the effectiveness of the treatment for the neoplasm. Patients with life-threatening haemolysis due to cold autoantibodies can also benefit from plasmaphaeresis. This should be accompanied by replacement with albumin, as plasma rich in complement factors will reactivate the haemolysis.

PAROXYSMAL COLD HAEMOGLOBINURIA

The clinical symptoms in the acute phase of PCH can be severe. Avoidance of exposure to cold improves the clinical condition. The transfusion of complement-rich plasma products should be avoided. At the present time, PCH is a self-limiting post-viral condition.

Relationship between antibody structure and function

There is ample evidence that the binding of red cell autoantibodies to its target antigen on the red cell membrane does not damage the red cell (Jandl 1965; Palek *et al.* 1968; von dem Borne *et al.* 1971; Atkinson and Frank 1974); thus other mechanisms must be responsible for the shortened survival of the red cells. The two pathways which are available for the removal of immune complexes are through activation of the complement cascade or by involvement of macrophages through the FcR mechanism. The Ig class of the antibody, its temperature amplitude and the nature of the antigen determine which of these paths is activated.

THE COMPLEMENT PATHWAY

The activation of the complement system can be complete, leading to the penetration of the membrane attack complex (MAC, C5–9) into the red cell membrane, or incomplete, when the process is limited to C3 and C4 deposition and subsequent adherence of the complement-coated cells to receptors on phagocytic cells.

Receptors for C4b/C3b and iC3b

The reason why some antibodies do not always lead to the deposition of the MAC and thus to complement lysis of the red cell is not clear. It may be the result of an interruption in the activation of the complement cascade by regulatory proteins such as decay-accelerating factor (DAF), which is a powerful regulator of C3/C5 convertase (Pangburn *et al*. 1983; Medof *et al*. 1984) or it may result from the inactivation of the membrane attack complex by homologous restriction factor or C8-binding protein (Schonermark *et al*. 1986). The membrane inhibitor of reactive lysis (CD59) could also play a role in this respect (Holguin *et al*. 1990). Red cells which remain intact after complement activation are coated with C4b, C3b and iC3b and will therefore adhere to the complement receptors CR1 and CR3. Attachment may lead to phagocytosis of the adherent red cell or to its cytotoxic destruction outside the membrane of the cell, as shown by the experiments of Brown *et al*. (1970), Schreiber and Frank (1972) and Atkinson and Frank (1974). On the other hand, the adherent cells may be detached from the receptor on the phagocyte before damage has taken place, probably as a result of the conversion of C4b and C3b into the inactive C3d and C4d forms. Red cells coated with these complement factors appear to be protected against haemolysis by further complement activation (Evans *et al*. 1968; Engelfriet *et al*. 1972; Jaffe *et al*. 1976). Removal of C3/C4-coated red cells occurs mainly in the liver, as shown by Mollison and Cutbush (1955) and Cutbush and Mollison (1958).

THE FC RECEPTOR PATHWAY

The number of IgG molecules on red cells from patients with a warm-type AIHA can vary between 200 and 20000 per red cell. Red cells sensitized with IgG antibodies at this level are usually not lysed by complement *in vivo*, but they will adhere to cells with receptors (FcR) for the constant part of the IgG molecule (Berken and Benacerref 1966; LoBuglio *et al*. 1967; Huber and Fudenberg 1968; Abramson *et al*. 1970; Huber *et al*. 1971). This adherence may be followed either by cytotoxic lysis or by phagocytosis (Fleer *et al*. 1978a, b), the particular mechanism involved depending on both the density of antibody molecules on the cells (Fleer *et al*. 1978a, b; Engelfriet *et al*. 1981; Ouwehand 1984) and on the IgG subclass of the molecules (Abramson *et al*. 1970; Huber *et al*. 1971; Hay *et al*. 1972; Engelfriet *et al*. 1981; Zupanska *et al*. 1986, 1987; Wiener *et al*. 1987, 1988; Ouwehand *et al*. 1990).

Immunoglobulin G-mediated red cell destruction is mainly confined to the spleen (Cutbush and Mollison 1958) and it is evident from histological observations made on spleens from patients with a warm-type AIHA that macrophages are the effector cells (Rappaport and Crosby 1957). Studies *in vitro* have shown that IgG-sensitized red cells (EAIgG) adhere to monocytes, macrophages, granulocytes and a subset of lymphocytes (Urbaniak 1976; Fleer *et al*. 1978a; Engelfriet *et al*. 1981; Ouwehand 1984; Zupanska *et al*. 1986; Klaassen *et al*. 1990) but it is only the adherence to monocytes and macrophages that leads to extracellular cytotoxic lysis or phagocytosis (Fleer *et al*. 1978a). Granulocytes can only process EAIgG *in vitro* if the FcRI (CD64) is also expressed on the cell surface (see later) and FcRIII (CD16)+ve lymphocytes will lyse red cells sensitized with IgG antibodies if the target cells have been pretreated with proteolytic enzymes (Urbaniak 1976; Ouwehand 1984). The adherence to monocytes and macrophages *in vitro* can easily be inhibited by low concentrations of free IgG (Fleer *et al*. 1978b; Ouwehand 1984). However, the inhibitory effect of IgG is dependent both on the number (Fleer *et al*. 1978b) and subclass of the antibodies bound to the red cells and on the state of functional activity of the effector cells (Ouwehand 1984). Immunoglobulin G3-coated red cells interact with a higher efficiency than IgG1-coated cells (see later).

The family of Fc receptors

All the FcRs so far defined on peripheral blood cells, (FcRI (CD64), FcRII (CD32) and FcRIII (CD16)), are glycoproteins (GPs) and all are members of the Ig supergene family (Huizinga *et al*. 1990). The tissue distribution of a particular member of this family is either restricted (FcRI, CD64) or widely distributed (FcRII, CD32) (Fig. 95.3). Not all cells expressing FcRs will interact with EAIgG anti-D (e.g. B lymphocytes and platelets); moreover, those FcR+ve cells to which EAIgG anti-D does adhere will not necessarily bring about red cell destruction (e.g. granulocytes and FcRIII+ve killer (K) lymphocytes). The variation in the repertoire of the FcRs expressed on the cells is probably the basis for the differences in functional activity. The structural basis for this functional heterogeneity of the FcRs is mainly based on divergency in the intramembrane and intracytoplasmic domains, and not in the ligand-

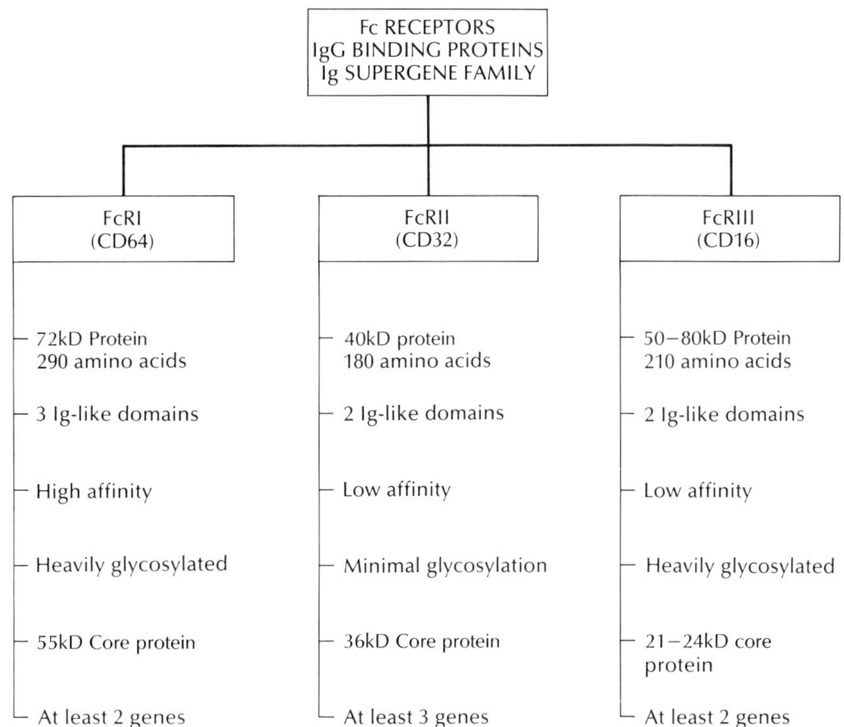

Fig. 95.3. Characteristics of the three Fc receptors, FcRI, FcRII and FcRIII.

binding domains. However, in humans the high-affinity FcRI (CD64) has three Ig-like domains, compared with two in the low-affinity FcRs, CD16 and CD32 (Brooks *et al.* 1989).

The Fc receptor expression on different effector cells

Monocytes and macrophages It is only those effector cells which express the FcRI (CD64) that are capable of inducing destruction of EAIgG *in vitro* at a reasonable level of efficiency. Experiments performed by Klaassen *et al.* (1990) showed that selective blocking of the FcRI on cultured monocytes (which are positive for FcRI, FcRII and FcRIII) results in complete inhibition of the extracellular cytotoxic lysis of cells sensitized with IgG anti-D (about 12 000 IgG molecules/erythrocyte). The FcRII on monocytes also plays a role in lysis but only when the number of antibody molecules/cell is increased to about 500 000 (Klaassen *et al.* 1990).

Granulocytes The role of the CD16/CD32 +ve neutrophilic granulocytes in the destruction of EAIgG in AIHA patients seems to be minimal under normal conditions. However, it is known that a bacterial infection can precipitate a haemolytic episode in AIHA patients. Van der Meulen *et al.* (1978) showed that neutrophils from patients with acute bacterial infection were as effective in lysing EAIgG anti-D *in vitro* as monocytes from normal healthy donors. Interferon-γ treatment of neutrophils *in vitro* induces FcRI (CD64) expression and these primed cells are capable of causing extracellular cytotoxic lysis of EAIgG anti-D. Thus, increased red cell destruction in AIHA patients with bacterial infection may be the result of an increase in FcRI on neutrophil membranes.

FcRIII-positive lymphocytes The subset of FcRIII (CD16) +ve K lymphocytes can form rosettes with enzyme-treated red cells sensitized with IgG anti-D. At high effector-to-target cell ratios this will result in target cell killing (Urbaniak 1976; Ouwehand 1984). Due to the low efficiency of this pathway, it is unlikely that it will play a major role in the *in vivo* destruction of EAIgG. Histological observations on splenic material obtained from AIHA patients do not give any evidence that lymphocytes are involved in the destruction of EAIgG (Rappaport and Crosby 1957).

Subclass of immunoglobulin G autoantibodies and Fc receptor interaction

Observations on a cohort of AIHA patients have shown that the degree of red cell destruction *in vivo* not only is a function of the density of the autoantibodies bound to the red cells, but is also dependent on the subclass of the antibodies (van der Meulen *et al.* 1978, 1980). Table 95.4 shows results that were obtained from subclass studies performed in patients with IgG-mediated AIHA. All patients except one having IgG3 autoantibodies had a severe haemolytic process; on the other hand, when IgG1 autoantibodies were present alone, only 50% of the patients had marked red cell destruction. Patients with IgG2 or IgG4 autoantibodies did not show any signs of haemolysis and ^{51}Cr survival studies with IgG2- or IgG-4-coated autologous cells showed a normal survival (von dem Borne *et al.* 1977; W.H. Ouwehand, pers. obs.). This difference in clinical severity is based on differences in the affinity of the IgG subclasses for the different FcRs. In general the relative strength of the interaction between IgG and its receptors on monocytes and granulocytes is in the following order: IgG1 = IgG3 ≫ IgG2 = IgG4 (Anderson and Looney 1987). Van der Meulen *et al.* (1980) performed elegant experiments which showed that, in patients with IgG1 autoantibodies only, the extent of haemolysis is related to the amount of antibody on the red cells. Studies by other groups have confirmed this, and Zupanska *et al.* (1987) measured the number of IgG1 autoantibodies bound to the patient's red cells and showed that red cell destruction only took place when the number of antibody molecules exceeded 1200/red cell, whereas in the case of IgG3 antibodies haemolysis occurred at levels that are barely detectable with the antiglobulin test (i.e. about 200 antibody molecules per red cell). There are also differences between IgG1 and IgG3 human monoclonal IgG anti-D antibodies of the Rh system in their ability to bring about attachment and phagocytosis of red cells by monocytes *in vitro* (Zupanska *et al.* 1986; Armstrong *et al.* 1987; Wiener *et al.* 1987, 1988). Thomson *et al.* (1990) also demonstrated that *in vivo* IgG3 is much more potent than IgG1 in destroying autologous red cells in humans. Lalezari *et al.* (1982) surprisingly found that in patients with AIHA due to α-methyldopa there is a relation between cell-bound IgM and haemolysis.

Extracellular cytotoxic lysis and phagocytosis In vitro studies with monoclonal anti-D antibodies have shown that IgG1 and IgG3 antibodies are both capable of inducing adherence of the IgG-coated erythrocytes to monocytes. However, experiments show that the ratio between phagocytosis and extracellular cytotoxic lysis is related to the subclass of the sensitizing antibody and the number of antibodies actually bound to the erythrocyte membrane (Ouwehand 1984). Wiener *et al.* (1988) found that IgG3 was superior to IgG1 in bringing about adherence (only 100 IgG3 molecules/red cell are required as opposed to 10 000 IgG1 molecules), but that IgG1 was superior in promoting phagocytosis. However, Hadley and Kumpel (1989) found that IgG3 is efficient in bringing about phagocytosis *in vitro* provided that the monocytes are presented with only a few red cells. The relative roles of IgG1 and IgG3 in red cell destruction require further elucidation.

It is probable that both phagocytosis and extracellular lysis of red cell destruction take place in patients with warm IgG-mediated AIHA. Cytotoxically damaged red cells are probably released after primary interaction with effector cells and are present in the peripheral blood as spherocytes with a lowered resistance to hypotonic stress. This type of sublytic cell damage can be induced *in vitro* by incubating IgG-sensitized red cells with monocytes (Fleer *et al.* 1978b; Ouwehand 1984). Heavily damaged spherocytes are probably phagocytosed by macrophages in the spleen.

STRUCTURAL STUDIES ON AUTOANTIBODIES

Initial studies have been made on the amino acid sequences and genetic origin of red cell autoantibodies. Silberstein *et al.* (1988, 1989) have determined the amino acid sequences of the variable regions of anti-Pr2 autoantibodies obtained from a patient with CHAD. They found a high degree of homology between the sequences derived from different B cell clones obtained from this patient and suggested that the frequency of somatic mutations in this type of B cell malignancy is low. They relate this low mutation frequency to the developmental stage of the B cells producing these anti-Pr2 antibodies. In autoimmune-prone mice considerable evidence has been obtained for a restricted use of the genes which are coding for the variable regions of the heavy and light chains

(Eilat *et al.* 1989). Members of the family of heavy-chain variable (V_H) genes situated in the genome in close proximity to the heavy-chain joining (J_H) gene cluster are over-represented in B cells producing autoantibodies. A restricted repertoire of V_H genes has been found in EBV-transformed human B cell clones producing IgM autoantibodies against a panel of autoantigens (Logtenberg *et al.* 1989; Sanz *et al.* 1989; Pascual *et al.* 1990). Dersimonian *et al.* (1989) have shown that autoreactive anti-deoxyribonucleic acid (DNA) autoantibodies from different patients have a very high degree of homology in their amino acid sequences, and Bailey *et al.* (1989) have produced convincing data that V_H families at the 3′ end of the V_H gene area on the genome are more frequently used in autoantibody-producing B cells compared with B cells producing normal antibodies.

CELL LINEAGES

There is some uncertainty whether there is a particular subset of B cells involved in the formation of autoantibodies. The CD5 +ve B cells, which are a minor subset *in vivo*, have attracted much attention (Casali and Notkins 1989; Herzenberg *et al.* 1989; van Rooijen 1989). This subset is considered to represent a separate cell lineage which can be expanded in autoimmune mice and in patients suffering from rheumatoid arthritis. It has been found that the production of rheumatoid factor by CD5 +ve B cells is higher than that of CD5 −ve cells (Werner-Favre *et al.* 1989).

Autoimmune thrombocytopenia

Autoimmune thrombocytopenia (AIT) is more common than its red cell counterpart, AIHA. There are three distinct clinical syndromes:

1 *Idiopathic thrombocytopenic purpura (ITP)*, a chronic AIT of insidious onset without any antecedent or associated illness, which typically affects young and middle-aged adults, predominantly women (3F : 1M).

2 *Secondary AIT* resembles ITP clinically, but is associated with other autoimmune diseases, malignancy or a variety of other disorders (Table 95.5), which have in common a postulated imbalance of the immune system.

3 *Acute post-viral AIT*, an acute self-limiting thrombocytopenic purpura, which typically affects young children within about 3 weeks of an acute viral infection; it is also described as acute or childhood ITP. The alternative terminology is confusing and unsatisfactory; it fails to link the acute viral infection with the subsequent thrombocytopenia; furthermore, ITP, as described above, may occasionally occur in children and should be differentiated from the post-viral condition because of its different clinical course.

Table 95.5. Conditions associated with autoimmune thrombocytopenia

Post-viral infection
Acute AIT of childhood (see text)
Specific viral infections (1)[a]
Other autoimmune diseases
Blood (e.g. Evans syndrome) (2, 3)
Generalized (e.g. SLE, rheumatoid arthritis) (3, 4)
Organ-specific (e.g. thyroid) (3, 5)
Lymphoproliferative disorders (3, 6)
Chronic lymphocytic leukaemia
Lymphoma
Cancer
Solid tumours (3, 7)
Immune system imbalance
HIV[b] infection (8, 9)
Chemo/radiotherapy (10)
Bone marrow transplantation (11, 12)

a (1) Chapman *et al.* (1984). (2) Pegels *et al.* (1982b). (3) von dem Borne *et al.* (1986). (4) Kaplan (1988). (5) Hymes *et al.* (1981). (6) Kaden *et al.* (1979). (7) Schwartz *et al.* (1982). (8) Karpatkin (1987). (9) van der Lelie (1987). (10) Chapman *et al.* (1986). (11) Minchinton *et al.* (1984a). (12) First *et al.* (1985).
b Human immunodeficiency virus.

For a detailed description of the three AIT syndromes the reader is referred to reviews by Lusher and Iyer (1977), McWilliams and Maurer (1979), Karpatkin and Karpatkin (1981), McMillan (1983), Karpatkin (1985) and von dem Borne (1987).

Clinical features

Thrombocytopenia is responsible for the clinical signs and symptoms, which are not specific for AIT and may occur in thrombocytopenia from other causes. Patients usually present with cutaneous purpura (petechiae, ecchymoses, easy bruising), with or without mucosal bleeding. It is important to differentiate 'dry' from 'wet' purpura

(Crosby 1975). 'Dry' purpura is synonymous with cutaneous purpura. 'Wet' purpura is a more serious clinical condition in which the patient may have active mucosal bleeding (oozing from gums, 'blood' blisters in the mouth, epistaxis, haematuria, menorrhagia, positive faecal occult blood tests or melaena) and fundal haemorrhages. These patients are at risk from more serious haemorrhage, including intracranial bleeding (although rare), and require urgent treatment (see Management). Splenomegaly is not a feature of AIT and, if present, would suggest an associated disease or another diagnosis.

In secondary AIT the clinical features of the associated disease will also be apparent. However, AIT is sometimes the first manifestation of systemic lupus erythematosus (SLE) and this possibility should be considered in the laboratory investigation of the patient.

Laboratory diagnosis

The characteristic haematological features of AIT are isolated thrombocytopenia (platelet count usually $<80 \times 10^9$/litre) and normal or increased numbers of megakaryocytes in the bone marrow. With modern electronic cell counting and particle sizing, the reduced platelet count is accompanied by an increase in mean platelet volume and platelet distribution width, indicating an increased population of large platelets.

Other conditions (e.g. disseminated intravascular coagulation, thrombotic thrombocytopenic purpura) which may produce a similar haematological picture should be excluded. If anaemia is also present (without obvious bleeding), the possibility of associated AIHA, i.e. Evans syndrome, should be investigated. Diagnosis is supported by the demonstration of platelet autoantibodies (see below) and a shortened platelet lifespan, using ^{111}In-labelled platelets (Kiefel *et al.* 1985; Waters and Minchinton 1985), although this additional information is not mandatory.

Three other immunological conditions may mimic AIT and should always be considered:

1 Drug-induced immune thrombocytopenia: a drug history is essential (Murphy and Kelton 1988; Mueller-Eckhardt and Salama 1990).

2 Post-transfusion purpura (PTP): a blood transfusion within 2 weeks will suggest this (Waters 1989).

3 Pseudo-thrombocytopenia: the patient has an ethylenediamine tetra-acetic acid (EDTA)-dependent platelet antibody which is active only *in vitro*. The antibody (either IgG or IgM or both) reacts with hidden (cryptic) antigens on platelet GPIIb/IIIa, which are exposed due to conformational changes in the complex caused by the removal of Ca^{2+} by EDTA (Pegels *et al.* 1982a). The antibody causes platelet agglutination in the EDTA blood sample associated with large platelet clumps on the blood film or platelet satellitism around neutrophils, both of which lead to a false low platelet count. These effects are not seen when a citrate anticoagulant is used.

Failure to recognize these conditions may lead to a false diagnosis of AIT by the unwary, but platelet serology will help to differentiate a platelet autoantibody from the various antibodies responsible for the above conditions

Immunological investigations

It can be misleading, when looking for platelet autoantibodies, to test only the patient's serum against normal platelets, as positive reactions may be due to the presence of alloantibodies (e.g. human leucocyte antigen (HLA) or platelet-specific) induced by previous transfusion or pregnancy. On the other hand, autoantibody may not be detectable in the patient's serum even though present on the patient's platelets (von dem Borne *et al.* 1986). Ideally a direct antiglobulin test (e.g. platelet immunofluorescence test (PIFT)) should be performed before treatment is given, to detect antibody bound to the patient's platelets *in vivo*. Where severe thrombocytopenia exists, it may not be possible to harvest enough platelets for the tests; nevertheless, serum samples should be stored frozen and tested retrospectively against the patient's platelets when the peripheral platelet count has increased in response to treatment.

For routine diagnostic investigations, methods based on the antiglobulin technique are widely used — radioimmunoassay (Soulier *et al.* 1975), immunofluorescence (von dem Borne *et al.* 1978) and enzyme-linked immunosorbent assay (ELISA) (Horai *et al.* 1981). Quantitative modifications of these assays have been criticized on the grounds that they detect not only platelet autoantibody, but also Ig non-specifically trapped or bound to platelets and platelet fragments (Shulman *et al.*

1982), and are therefore generally non-specific in the diagnosis of AIT (see review, von dem Borne 1984; Mueller-Eckhardt 1988). A valuable development in platelet serology is the application of methods to study antibody binding at the level of membrane GPs (Kiefel *et al.* 1987; McMillan *et al.* 1987). This approach is relevant to investigating the target antigens for autoantibodies in AIT (see below).

Using the PIFT to study 75 patients with ITP, von dem Borne *et al.* (1986) found a weak positive direct PIFT in 60% of patients and strong reactions in 26% of patients. These results suggest that the amount of platelet-bound autoantibodies in ITP is low in most patients, and negative in a variable proportion of patients (10–20%). In the same study, the indirect PIFT was positive with the patient's serum in 66% of cases who had a positive direct PIFT, and with an ether eluate of the patient's platelets in 94% of the same cases. While these results may be a reflection of the relative insensitivity of the method, they may nevertheless be due to a low-affinity antibody that is easily eluted during the assay procedure (Shulman *et al.* 1982), or indicate an alternative immune mechanism for thrombocytopenia in some cases.

The Ig class of platelet autoantibodies is similar in idiopathic and secondary AIT, and mostly IgG (92%), but often IgM (42%) and sometimes IgA (9%) (von dem Borne *et al.* 1986). All IgG subclasses may occur: IgG-1 (82%), IgG-2 (11%), IgG-3 (50%) and IgG-4 (29%).

The target antigen for platelet autoantibodies from patients with ITP appears to be the platelet GPIIb/IIIa complex. This conclusion is based on the observation that in most cases the autoantibody does not react with platelets of patients with type I Glanzmann's disease, which are deficient in GPIIb/IIIa (van Leeuwen *et al.* 1982; Ribera *et al.* 1983). Subsequent immunochemical studies with isolated platelet GPs have confirmed this observation in some, but not all, cases, suggesting that the autoantibodies may be directed against conformational determinants only present on the native GPs or that the autoantibodies in ITP are more heterogeneous than previously thought (Rosa *et al.* 1984; McMillan *et al.* 1987; von dem Borne 1987; Beardsley 1988; Mueller Eckhardt 1988).

More precise definition of the immunochemical properties of the platelet autoantibody in AIT in terms of Ig class/subclass and GP target antigen may provide useful diagnostic and prognostic information.

Pathogenesis

In AIT platelets are sensitized with autoantibodies, which are predominantly both IgG and IgM. Platelet destruction by IgG autoantibodies is thought to be similar to IgG-mediated extravascular phagocytosis of red cells in the spleen, which is also an important site of platelet autoantibody production (Firkin *et al.* 1969; McMillan *et al.* 1974a, b; Tavasoli and McMillan 1975). However, unlike AIHA, the mode of action of IgM autoantibodies in AIT is uncertain, as the relative importance of complement is controversial. It has been assumed that increased platelet destruction in AIT is accompanied by a compensatory increase in platelet production by megakaryocytes. However, recent observations suggest that platelet production may actually be depressed, especially in more severely affected patients (Grossi *et al.* 1983; Stoll *et al.* 1985; Heyns *et al.* 1986; Ballem *et al.* 1987).

In addition to promoting platelet destruction, the autoantibody may also inhibit the function of platelet membrane GPs and cause an acquired thrombocytopathy (Clancy *et al.* 1972; Lackner and Karpatkin 1975; Heyns *et al.* 1978; Stuart *et al.* 1981; Greaves *et al.* 1982; Stricker *et al.* 1985; Di Minno *et al.* 1986; Niessner *et al.* 1986). Furthermore, the autoantibody may affect primary haemostasis by reacting with a GPIIb/IIIa complex on the surface of endothelial cells similar to that on the platelet membrane (Leeksma *et al.* 1986, 1987; George 1987).

Acute post-viral thrombocytopenia, which predominantly affects young children, also appears to be autoantibody-mediated (van Leeuwen *et al.* 1981). In contrast to ITP, the autoantibody is predominantly IgM, which could be a reflection of the short duration of the illness, and may be related to its spontaneous remission (von dem Borne 1984, 1987). The autoantibody may be a cross-reacting antibody due to molecular mimicry between virus and platelets, an anti-idiotype antibody to the anti-viral antibody produced in the wake of the viral infection (Plotz 1983), or the product of virus-induced immune system dysfunction in which interferons may play a part (von dem Borne 1984, 1987; McLaughlin *et al.* 1985; Abdi *et al.* 1986). The sequence of events would seem to exclude a mechanism involving an immune complex of virus and antibody as the cause of severe thrombocytopenia during the convalescent phase.

Management

CHRONIC AUTOIMMUNE THROMBOCYTOPENIA

Chronic AIT includes ITP and secondary AIT. The aim of treatment is to restore the platelet count to safe, but not necessarily normal, levels and to maintain remission. The principles of treatment will be discussed and the reader is referred to reviews for details of therapeutic regimens (Rosse 1983; Firkin *et al.* 1988; Berchtold and McMillan 1989). Steroids (e.g. oral prednisolone), followed by splenectomy if necessary, are standard treatment for chronic AIT, and can be expected to achieve a remission in over 80% of patients. A review of experience with high-dose IVIgG (Bussel and Pham 1987; Newland 1988) suggests that the addition of IVIgG may improve the response rate to steroids; in those patients who proceed to splenectomy, the use of IVIgG immediately prior to surgery not only raises the platelet count, so making surgery safer, but may also increase the likelihood of remission (Newland *et al.* 1983).

In secondary AIT the primary underlying disease should be treated. Splenectomy is less likely to benefit patients with SLE (Hall *et al.* 1985); these patients also appear to be less responsive to IVIgG (Firkin *et al.* 1987).

The mechanism of action of steroids is complex, and is thought to involve suppression of macrophage function (Fries *et al.* 1983; Gernsheimer *et al.* 1989). High-dose IVIgG appears to have similar effects and may also suppress antibody production (Mueller-Eckhardt 1988; Newland 1988). Splenectomy not only removes the main site of platelet destruction, but also a major site of autoantibody production.

Immunosuppression by drugs other than steroids should be used only if steroids, splenectomy and IVIgG are ineffective or cannot be used (see reviews, Firkin *et al.* 1988; Berchtold and McMillan 1989).

IDIOPATHIC THROMBOCYTOPENIA IN PREGNANCY

The occurrence of pregnancy during the course of ITP requires special consideration. In the absence of a previous history of ITP, it may be difficult to distinguish ITP appearing for the first time during pregnancy from mild thrombocytopenia associated with pre-eclamptic toxaemia (Giles and Inglis 1981) or 'benign' thrombocytopenia of pregnancy (Fay *et al.* 1983; Burrows and Kelton 1988).

Two important aspects of the maternofetal relationship require consideration: (i) the effect of maternal treatment on the welfare of the fetus; and (ii) the extent of fetal thrombocytopenia, if any, due to the maternal platelet autoantibody.

Treatment of the mother should be as conservative as possible and based on a combination of steroids and IVIgG; splenectomy, if indicated, should be postponed until after delivery (Tchernia 1988).

Fetal thrombocytopenia is due to placental transfer of the maternal platelet IgG autoantibody. There is no reliable way of predicting the fetal platelet count from the platelet serology of the mother. However, increasing expertise in fetal blood sampling (FBS) by cordocentesis under ultrasound guidance will make it possible to measure the fetal platelet count and to study the natural course of the disease in the fetus in relation to maternal therapy. Pre-delivery FBS provides an opportunity to transfuse platelets to a thrombocytopenic fetus in order to safeguard against the risk of intracranial haemorrhage (ICH) due to birth trauma. Much will be learnt from similar developments in the prenatal management of alloimmune neonatal thrombocytopenia, where the risk of ICH appears to be much greater (Editorial 1989).

ACUTE POST-VIRAL AUTOIMMUNE THROMBOCYTOPENIA

Acute post-viral AIT primarily affects young children (>90% of cases), although occasional young adults may also have a similar acute post-viral AIT. It is essential to exclude acute leukaemia by examination of the blood film and bone marrow.

The majority of patients recover spontaneously within 3 months, though a few may have further relapses. Although usually benign, the condition has a mortality of about 1%, due mainly to ICH, which is most likely to occur during the first 2 weeks.

Management is controversial with respect to how much treatment is required (Lilleyman 1983; Buchanan 1985; Imbach *et al.* 1985). The major consideration is the risk of ICH, and there is general agreement that severely thrombocytopenic children with the clinical signs of 'wet' purpura should be urgently treated to raise the platelet count and reduce capillary bleeding. A multicentre trial has demonstrated the superiority of a combination of steroids and high-dose IVIgG over either therapy alone (Imbach *et al.* 1985). Outside this high-risk group of children, the same clinical trial showed that steroids or IVIgG were equally effective in raising the platelet count in 62% of children who responded to the initial course of treatment, a group where treatment is probably not necessary. However, in those children requiring more than the initial course of treatment, response was more durable in those randomized to receive IVIgG.

About 10% of children fail to recover within 6 months and are considered to be suffering from chronic AIT, similar to ITP in adults. Steroids and IVIgG are important therapeutic options for such children (Bussel 1985; Imbach *et al.* 1985); splenectomy, if indicated, should be deferred to as late an age as possible, because of risk of serious infection following the procedure in children (Lusher and Iyer 1977; Hosea *et al.* 1981).

Autoimmune neutropenia

Patients with autoimmune neutropenia may be considered in two groups: those whose neutropenia is primary (or idiopathic), and those whose neutropenia is secondary and associated with diseases such as rheumatoid arthritis or SLE.

Primary autoimmune neutropenia is a rare illness which occurs most frequently in infants. Bone marrow aspiration reveals granulocytic hyperplasia and a decrease in segmented neutrophils. Infectious illnesses, particularly otitis media and skin and upper respiratory tract infections, are common (Madyastha *et al.* 1982). Recovery of neutrophil count usually occurs spontaneously within 3 years; transient increases in neutrophil levels have been reported after prednisolone or intravenous gamma globulin therapy (Boxer *et al.* 1975; Bussel *et al.* 1983). Autoantibodies are usually IgG and specific for the neutrophil alloantigens NA1 or NA2 (Lalezari *et al.* 1975; Madyastha *et al.* 1982). There is generally good correlation between the presence of autoantibodies and episodes of neutropenia. Leucoagglutination (Lalezari *et al.* 1975) and immunofluorescence tests (Verheugt *et al.* 1978) have most frequently been used to demonstrate autoantibodies in these patients.

In adults, autoimmune neutropenia is usually associated with other autoimmune disorders. These include SLE (Starkebaum and Arend 1979), rheumatoid arthritis (Felty's syndrome) (Starkebaum *et al.* 1980a), AIHA and ITP (Evan's syndrome) (Pegels *et al.* 1982b) and Graves' disease (Weitzman *et al.* 1985). Acquired immune deficiency syndrome (AIDS) (Murphy *et al.* 1985) and various lymphoproliferative disorders (Verheugt *et al.* 1978; Hunter *et al.* 1982) have also been associated with autoimmune neutropenia. Autoimmune neutropenia after bone marrow transplantation has also been described (Minchinton *et al.* 1984b). In allografted patients, antibodies reactive with engrafted donor cell antigens were shown to be of donor origin. Corticosteroid therapy (Cines *et al.* 1982) or splenectomy (Logue 1976) may increase neutrophil counts in some patients with secondary autoimmune neutropenia.

Numerous techniques have been employed to demonstrate anti-neutrophil antibodies in these patients. Most depend on the binding to neutrophils of fluorescein-labelled (Verheugt *et al.* 1978) or radiolabelled (Cines *et al.* 1982) antiglobulin reagent or staphylococcal protein A (McCallister *et al.* 1979). These tests detect Ig on the patient's neutrophils (direct tests), or on normal donor neutrophils after sensitization in serum from the patient (indirect tests). The use of HL-60 cells in indirect tests may permit the detection of antibodies to granulocyte precursors (Currie *et al.* 1987). Complement-mediated (Drew and Terasaki 1978) and lymphocyte-mediated cytotoxicity assays (Logue *et al.* 1978) have also been developed.

Despite the many reports describing anti-neutrophil antibodies in sera from patients with secondary neutropenia, the clinical significance of these antibodies is uncertain. For example, in patients with SLE or Felty's syndrome, there is no inverse correlation between the level of neutrophil-associated IgG and neutrophil count (Starkebaum and Arend 1979; Starkebaum *et al.* 1980a) and cytotoxic antibodies have been detected in non-neutropenic patients (Drew and Terasaki 1978).

There may be several explanations why these assays fail to discern clinically significant antibodies. Low sensitization temperatures are frequently used in cytotoxicity assays to overcome the tendency of viable neutrophils to internalize membrane-bound antibody (Weitzman *et al*. 1979). This may result in the detection of IgM antibodies present in many normal individuals. Anti-neutrophil antibodies may also vary in their functional activity; Rustagi *et al*. (1985) reported an association between the ability of IgG antibodies to fix complement and the severity of neutropenia.

The nature of neutrophil-binding IgG in sera from these patients may also affect its clinical significance. Fc receptor-mediated binding of immune complexes in sera from patients with SLE or Felty's syndrome may contribute, entirely in some cases, to the increased level of neutrophil-binding IgG (Petersen and Wiik 1983; Starkebaum *et al*. 1980b). Neutropenia in these patients may result from immune complex-induced margination (shift neutropenia), and this may be one explanation for the lack of recurrent infections in some patients (van der Veen *et al*. 1986). Finally, the maturational specificity of autoantibodies may affect their clinical significance. Since over 90% of neutrophils are present in the bone marrow reserve, antibodies reactive with precursor cells may cause neutropenia more effectively than antibodies directed against circulating cells (Harmon *et al*. 1984). The finding that sera from some neutropenic patients with myeloid hypoplasia contain HL-60-binding antibodies which may inhibit colony-forming unit, granulocyte–monocyte (CFU-GM) colony formation suggests that anti-precursor antibodies may promote neutropenia by inhibiting granulopoiesis (Fitchin and Cline 1980; van der Veen *et al*. 1986; Currie *et al*. 1987). Unlike patients with immune complex-induced 'shift' neutropenia, recurrent infections are common in neutropenic patients with precursor cell-reactive antibodies (van der Veen *et al*. 1986).

A separate class of neutrophil autoantibodies reacting with cytoplasmic antigen(s) occurs in patients with certain forms of vasculitis and is not associated with leucopenia.

Haemolytic disease of the new-born

Haemolytic disease of the new-born (HDN) results from maternal IgG with specificity for fetal red cell antigens crossing the placenta and bringing about premature destruction of the erythrocytes. The commonest antibody to be involved is anti-D of the Rh system, which accounted for about 93% of cases of HDN (Giblett 1964). Before the introduction in 1967–70 of prophylactic administration of anti-D, about 6% of the remaining cases resulted from anti-c, -E, or -Ce, of the Rh system, and approximately 1% was caused by a wide variety of antibodies involving most of the other blood group systems. Transfer of antibody is slow during the first 22 weeks of pregnancy but thereafter increases rapidly and thus the fetus is most usually affected from the 22nd week onwards.

Mechanisms

Apart from the ABO antibodies, maternal antibody usually arises as the result of fetomaternal haemorrhage in the first pregnancy, although mismatched transfusion now plays an increasingly significant role. The D antigen is a fairly potent immunogen; two injections of 0.5–1.0 ml of D +ve red cells into D −ve individuals usually results in over 50% of the recipients being immunized. Immunization against the D antigen has been seen with only approximately 0.03 ml of cells (Jakobowicz *et al*. 1972). Other antigens in the Rh system are much less potent, c being estimated to be only about 2–4% as potent as D (Giblett 1964).

Very few red cells cross the placenta during the first two trimesters, more are found in the third trimester, but the greatest transfer is at labour, and about 5–10% of women have more than 0.5 ml of fetal cells in their circulation at this time (Mollison *et al*. 1987). This late transfer of red cells during pregnancy is the reason why immunization is uncommon during the first pregnancy and hence HDN in the first-born is relatively rare.

Approximately 47% of the D −ve women in a Caucasian population (17% of the population are D −ve) carry two D +ve fetuses in succession but only about one in eight of these women who have the potential to be immunized actually are immunized. There are probably three main reasons for the failure to be immunized. First, an insufficient volume of red cells crosses the placenta, second, there is ABO incompatibility between fetus and mother, whereby the rapid destruction of the fetal red cells by anti-A or -B prevents immunization with the D antigen (Clarke 1989), and, third, about 10% of people fail to make anti-D even after repeated immunization (Mollison *et al.* 1987).

Incidence

There has been a dramatic reduction in deaths from HDN during the four decades from 1950. This has been due partly to a reduction in the number of children born to individual women, partly to the development of treatment by exchange transfusion and partly to the prophylactic use of anti-D. In the UK, the mortality has been about 4–5/100 000 births each year since 1983 (Clarke and Mollison 1989); other countries using similar therapies have similar values. The occurrence of HDN is now mainly due either to its appearance in the first-born child, or to mismatched transfusion or to a failure of prophylaxis because too small a dose of anti-D has been given (usually the result of a transplacental haemorrhage of over 4 ml of red cells).

Antenatal prediction of severity

It is well recognized that estimations of antibody concentration by manual agglutination titres are very inaccurate and hence it is not surprising that the titre of anti-D in the plasma only weakly correlates with severity. Titres carried out with machines such as the Autoanalyzer, however, give a better correlation. Bowell *et al.* (1982) found that, in 78 cases where the maternal antibody concentration was below 0.8 μg/ml, only three infants required exchange transfusion whereas, when the level was above this value, 79 out of 106 infants required exchange. The failure to make an accurate assessment of the severity from maternal antibody levels reflects the fact that other factors play a large part in determining severity, namely, the rate of placental transfer of IgG, the IgG subclass of the antibody, the ability of the fetal marrow to respond to anaemia and the ability of the liver to conjugate and excrete bilirubin in the immediate postnatal period.

The results of antibody-dependent cell-mediated cytotoxicity (ADCC) tests using monocytes as effectors also correlate well with severity. Ouwehand *et al.* (1990) found that a strongly positive result at the end of pregnancy was frequently associated with severe disease, whereas a weakly positive test was always associated with mild disease. This result is surprising, since the destruction of red cells, at least in adults, is mainly by phagocytosis and not through extracellular lysis. The explanation could be that the factors which bring about ADCC *in vitro* are also those that result in phagocytosis *in vivo*.

Assessment of severity in the new-born

Diagnosis of disease in the infant is primarily dependent on finding a direct antiglobulin test with the infant's cells. The best single criterion of severity is the cord haemoglobin concentration, the normal range being 13.6–19.6 g/dl. Most infants with haemoglobin concentration within the normal range do not require transfusion. Cord plasma bilirubin levels correlate less well but a value of 4 mg/dl (70 μmol/litre) or more is a good indicator that the disease will be severe.

It had been hoped that an estimate of the amount of antibody on cord red cells would give a reliable indication of severity but this has proved not to be so. In general, the higher the amount, the more severe the disease, so that in one series all infants with more than 8 μg/ml of red cells required treatment, but at lower levels the value was a poor indicator of severity (Hughes-Jones *et al.* 1967).

Subclass of immunoglobulin and severity

Anti-D belongs predominantly to the IgG1 and IgG3 subclasses but the relative proportion varies widely between individuals. The IgG1 and IgG3 subclasses are the only subclasses actively involved in red cell destruction through phagocytosis, but there are clearly differences in their functional ability (see above) and there is evidence that the two subclasses can act synergistically (Hadley and Kumpel 1989). The idea that the subclasses play different roles is supported by the finding that the concentration of IgG1 antibody in the maternal serum bears a linear relationship to severity whereas the concentration of IgG3 anti-D is poorly related (Schanfield *et al.* 1980).

Prophylaxis

The idea that the post-partum passive administration of anti-D into D −ve mothers giving birth to D +ve infants would prevent active immunization was developed in Liverpool (Finn *et al.* 1961; Clarke *et al.* 1963) and New York (Freda *et al.* 1964). With the former authors, the rationale was based on the recognition that the presence of anti-A or -B in the mother would protect (Clarke 1989) and therefore it seemed possible that anti-D would do the same. In New York, the rationale was the well-established observation in animals that immune complexes were not as potent as immunogens as the antigen alone. The Liverpool group established that only IgG anti-D was effective, not IgM, and the Medical Research Council trials in the UK (Medical Research Council 1974) established the dose as 100 μg, unless the transplacental haemorrhage exceeded about 4 ml of red cells, in which case a proportionally larger dose is required; the recommended dose is 25 μg anti-D/ml of red cells. The volume of fetal red cells in the mother post-partum can be determined by the Kleihauer technique, in which fetal red cells can be differentiated from maternal cells in a maternal blood smear by the failure of fetal haemoglobin to be eluted from the cells at an acid pH (Betke and Kleihauer 1958). A transplacental haemorrhage of more than 4 ml occurs in about 0.7% of women. Passive immunization with anti-D carried out post-partum is effective in reducing active immunization: without prophylaxis, about 17% of D −ve women with ABO-compatible D +ve infants become immunized, but this rate drops to 1.5% with prophylaxis. The failures are mainly due to primary immunization occurring during pregnancy, and the incidence of anti-D arising in this way is about 0.7% of all Rh −ve women carrying an Rh +ve child.

The mechanism of prophylaxis is uncertain. The most likely explanation is that the destruction of the red cells by phagocytosis in the spleen (Jandl 1965) is followed by the rapid destruction of the D antigen. It is known that the D epitope is extremely labile and is lost when the integrity of the lipid membrane is disturbed (Hughes-Jones *et al.* 1975). This explanation is supported by the finding that passive administration of anti-Kell prevents active immunization to anti-D by Kell +ve D +ve red cells (Woodrow *et al.* 1975).

References

Abdi, A.E., Brun, W. and Venner, P.M. (1986). Autoimmune thrombocytopenia related to interferon therapy. *Scand. J. Haematol.* **36**, 515–19.

Abramson, N.E., Gelfand, W., Jandl, J.H. and Rosen, F.S. (1970). The interaction between human monocytes and red cells: binding characteristics. *J. Exp. Med.* **132**, 1191–206.

Ahn, J.S., Byrnes, J.J. and Brunskill, D.E. (1978). Selective injury to macrophages: a new treatment for idiopathic autoimmune hemolytic anaemia. *Clin. Res.* **26**, 340.

Ahn, J.S., Harrington, W.J., Byrnes, J.J., Pall, L. and McCraime, J. (1983). Treatment of autoimmune hemolytic anaemia with vinca-loaded platelets. *JAMA* **249**, 2189–94.

Anderson, C.L. and Looney, R.J. (1987). Immunoglobulin G Fc receptors of human leucocytes. *Methods Enzymol.* **150**, 524–36.

Armstrong, S.S., Wiener, E., Garner, S.F., Urbaniak, S.J. and Contreras, M. (1987). Heterogeneity of IgG1 monoclonal anti-Rh(D): an investigation using ADCC and macrophage binding assays. *Br. J. Haematol.* **66**, 257–62.

Atkinson, J.P. and Frank, M.M. (1974). Studies on the *in vivo* effects of antibody: interaction of IgM antibody and complement in the immune clearance and destruction of erythrocytes in man. *J. Clin. Invest.* **54**, 339–48.

Bailey, N.C., Fidanza, V., Mayer, R., Mazza, G., Fougereau, M. and Bona, C. (1989). Activation of clones producing self-reactive antibodies by foreign antigen and antiidiotype antibody carrying the internal image of the antigen. *J. Clin. Invest.* **84**, 744–56.

Ballem, P.J., Segal, G.M., Stratton, J.R., Gernsheimer, T., Adamson, J.W. and Slichter, S.J. (1987). Mechanisms of thrombocytopenia in chronic autoimmune thrombocytopenic purpura. *J. Clin. Invest.* **80**, 33–40.

Beardsley, D.S. (1988). Target antigens for platelet autoantibodies. *Curr. Studies Hematol. Blood Transfusion* **54**, 64–70.

Becton, D.L. and Kinney, T.R. (1986). An infant girl with severe autoimmune hemolytic anaemia: apparent anti-Vel specificity. *Vox Sang.* **51**, 108–10.

Berchtold, P. and McMillan, R. (1989). Therapy of chronic idiopathic thrombocytopenic purpura in adults. *Blood* **74**, 2309–17.

Berken, A. and Benacerref, B. (1966). Properties of antibodies cytophilic for macrophages. *J. Exp. Med.* **123**, 119–44.

Bernstein, M.L., Schneider, E.A. and Naiman, J.C. (1981). Plasma exchange in refractory acute autoimmune hemolytic anaemia. *J. Pediatr.* **98**, 774–5.

Besa, E.C. (1988). Rapid transient reversal of anaemia and long-term effects of maintenance intravenous immunoglobulin for autoimmune hemolytic anaemia in patients with lymphoproliferative disorders. *Am. J. Med.* **84**, 691–8.

Besa, E.C., Ray, P.K., Swami, V.K., Idiculla, A. *et al.* (1981). Specific immunoadsorption of IgG antibody in a patient with chronic lymphocytic leukemia and autoimmune hemolytic anemia: a new form of therapy for the acute critical stage. *Am. J. Med.* **71**, 1035–40.

Betke, K. and Kleihauer, E. (1958). Fetaler und bleibender Blutfarbstoff in Erythrozyten und Erythroblasten von menschlichen Feten und Neugeboren. *Blut* **4**, 241–9.

Bowell, P.J., Wainstoat, J.S., Peto, T.E.A. and Gunson, H.S. (1982). Maternal anti-D concentrations and outcome in rhesus haemolytic disease of the newborn. *Br. Med. J.* **285**, 327–9.

Boxer, L.A., Greenberg, M.S., Boxer, G.J. and Stossel, T.P. (1975). Autoimmune neutropenia. *N. Engl. J. Med.* **293**, 748–53.

Brooks, B.D., Steane, E.A., Sheehan, R.G. and Frenkel, E.P.

(1982). Therapeutic plasma exchange in the immune hemolytic anaemias and immunological thrombocytopenic purpura. *Prog. Clin. Biol. Res.* **106**, 317–29.

Brooks, D.G., Qui, W.Q., Luster, A.D. and Ravetch, J.V. (1989). Structure and expression of human IgG FcRII (CD32): functional heterogeneity is encoded by the alternatively spliced products of multiple genes. *J. Exp. Med.* **170**, 1369–85.

Brown, D.L., Lachmann, P.J. and Dacie, J.V. (1970). The *in vivo* behaviour of complement-coated red cells: studies in C6-deficient, C3-depleted and normal rabbits. *Clin. Exp. Immunol.* **7**, 401–21.

Buchanan, G.R. (1985). Childhood acute idiopathic thrombocytopenic purpura: how many tests and how much treatment required? *J. Paediatr.* **106**, 928–9.

Burrows, R.F. and Kelton, J.G. (1988). Incidentally detected thrombocytopenia in healthy mothers and their infants. *N. Engl. J. Med.* **319**, 142–5.

Bussel, J.B. (1985). Treatment with intravenous immunoglobulin: use in chronic idiopathic thrombocytopenic purpura to avoid splenectomy; and mechanism of action. In *Intravenous Immunoglobulins in Immunodeficiency Syndromes and Idiopathic Thrombocytopenic Purpura*, ed. A.H. Waters and A.D.B. Webster, pp. 83–91, International Congress and Symposium Series 84, Royal Society of Medicine, London.

Bussel, J.B. and Pham, L.C. (1987). Intravenous treatment with gammaglobulin in adults with immune thrombocytopenic purpura: a review of the literature. *Vox Sang.* **52**, 206–11.

Bussel, J.B., Lalezari, P., Hilgartner, J. *et al.* (1983). Reversal of neutropenia with intravenous gammaglobulin in autoimmune neutropenia of infancy. *Blood* **62**, 398–400.

Casali, P. and Notkins, A.L. (1989). CD5+ B lymphocytes, polyreactive antibodies and the human B-cell repertoire. *Immunol. Today* **10**, 364–8.

Chapman, J.F., Metcalfe, P., Murphy, M.F., Burman, J.F. and Waters, A.H. (1984). Sequential development of platelet, neutrophil and red cell autoantibodies associated with measles infection. *Clin. Lab. Haematol.* **6**, 219–28.

Chapman, J.F., Murphy, M.F., Minchinton, R.M., Metcalfe, P., Lister, T.A. and Waters, A.H. (1986). Autoimmune thrombocytopenia and neutropenia after remission induction therapy for acute leukaemia. *Br. J. Haematol.* **63**, 693–702.

Ciaffoni, S., Ferro, I., Potenza, R. and Campo, G. (1987). Evans syndrome: a case of autoimmune thrombocytopenia and autoimmune hemolytic anaemia caused by anti Jk^a. *Haematol. Pavia* **72**, 245–7.

Cines, D.B., Passero, F., Guerry, D., Bina, M., Dusak, B. and Schreiber, A.D. (1982). Granulocyte-associated IgG in neutropenic disorders. *Blood* **59**, 124–32.

Clancy, R., Jenkins, B. and Firkin, B.G. (1972). Qualitative platelet abnormalities in idiopathic thrombocytopenic purpura. *N. Engl. J. Med.* **286**, 622–6.

Clarke, C.A. (1989). Preventing rhesus babies: the Liverpool Research and follow-up. *Arch. Dis. Child.* **64**, 1734–40.

Clarke, C.A. and Mollison, P.L. (1989). Deaths from Rh haemolytic disease of the fetus and newborn 1977 to 1987. *J. Roy. Coll. Physicians (London)* **23**, 181–4.

Clarke, C.A., Donohoe, W.T.A., McConnell, R.B. *et al.* (1963). Further experimental studies on the prevention of Rh haemolytic disease. *Br. Med. J.* **i**, 979–84.

Clarkson, S.B., Bussel, J.B., Kimberley, R.P., Valinsky, J.E., Nachman, R.L. and Unkeless, J.C. (1986). Treatment of refractory immune thrombocytopenic purpura with an anti-Fcγ-receptor antibody. *N. Engl. J. Med.* **314**, 1236–9.

Crosby, W.H. (1975). Wet purpura, dry purpura. *JAMA* **232**, 744–5.

Currie, M.S., Weinberg, J.B., Rustagi, P.K. and Logue, G.L. (1987). Antibodies to granulocyte precursors in selective myeloid hypoplasia and other suspected autoimmune neutropenias: use of HL-60 cells as targets. *Blood* **69**, 529–36.

Cutbush, M. and Mollison, P.L. (1958). Relation between characteristics of blood group antibodies *in vitro* and associated patterns of red cell destruction *in vivo*. *Br. J. Haematol.* **4**, 115–37.

Dacie, J.V. (1962). The auto-immune haemolytic anaemias. In *The Haemolytic Anaemias, Congenital and Acquired*, vol. II, pp. 410–14, Churchill, London.

Dacie, J.V. and Worlledge, S. (1969). Autoimmune haemolytic anaemias. *Prog. Hematol.* **6**, 82–120.

Dersimonian, H., McAdam, K.P.J.W., Mackworth-Young, C. and Stollar, B.D. (1989). The recurrent expression of variable region segments in human IgM anti-DNA autoantibodies. *J. Immunol.* **142**, 4027–33.

Di Minno, G., Coraggio, F., Cerbone, A.M. *et al.* (1986). A myeloma paraprotein with specificity for platelet glycoprotein IIIa in a patient with a fatal bleeding disorder. *J. Clin Invest.* **77**, 157–64.

Drew, S.I. and Terasaki, P.I. (1978). Autoimmune cytotoxic granulocyte antibodies in normal persons and various diseases. *Blood* **52**, 941–52.

Editorial (1989). Management of alloimmune neonatal thrombocytopenia: a reappraisal. *Lancet* **i**, 137–8.

Eilat, D., Hochberg, M., Tron, F., Jacob, L. and Bach, J.F. (1989). The VH gene sequences of anti-DNA antibodies in two different strains of lupus-prone mice are highly related. *Eur. J. Immunol.* **19**, 1241–6.

Engelfriet, C.P., von dem Borne, A.E.G.K., Beckers, T.A.P., Reynierse, E. and van Loghem, J.J. (1972). Autoimmune haemolytic anaemia. V. Studies on the resistance against complement haemolysis of red cells of patients with chronic cold agglutinin disease. *Clin. Exp. Immunol.* **11**, 255–64.

Engelfriet, C.P., von dem Borne, A.E.G.K., van der Meulen, F.W. *et al.* (1981). Immune destruction of red cells. Presented at a Seminar on Immune-mediated Cell Destruction, 34th Annual Meeting for the American Association of Blood Banks, Chicago.

Engelfriet, C.P., van 't Veer, M.B., Maas, N., Ouwehand, W.H., Beckers, D. and von dem Borne, A.E.G.K. (1987). Autoimmune haemolytic anaemias. Baillière's *Clin. Immunol. Allergy* **1**, 251–67.

Evans, R.S., Turner, E., Bingham, M. and Woods, R. (1968). Chronic haemolytic anaemia due to cold agglutinins. II. The role of C in red cell destruction. *J. Clin. Invest.* **47**, 691–701.

Fay, R.A., Hughes, A.O. and Farron, N.T. (1983). Platelets in pregnancy: hyperdestruction in pregnancy. *Obstet. Gynecol.* **61**, 238–40.

Finn, R., Clarke, C.A., Donohoe, W.T.A. *et al.* (1961). Further experimental studies on the prevention of Rh haemolytic disease. *Br. Med. J.* **i**, 1486–90.

Firkin, B.G., Wright, R., Miller, S. and Stokes, E. (1969). Splenic macrophages in thrombocytopenia. *Blood* **33**, 240–5.

Firkin, B.G., Buchanan, R.R.C., Pfueller, S. and Ryan. P. (1987). Lupoid thrombocytopenia. *Aust. NZ J. Med.* **17**, 295–300.

Firkin, B.G., Hunt, H.A. and Jane, S.M. (1988). Management of refractory idiopathic thrombocytopenia. *Blood Rev.* **2**, 149–56.

First, L.R., Smith, B.R., Lipton, J., Nathan, D.G., Parkman, R. and Rappeport, J.M. (1985). Autoimmune thrombocytopenia after allogeneic bone marrow transplantation — existence of transient and chronic thrombocytopenic syndromes. *Blood* **65**, 368–74.

Fitchin, J.H. and Cline, M.J. (1980). Serum inhibitors of myelopoiesis. *Br. J. Haematol.* **44**, 7–16.

Fleer, A., van Shaik, M.L.J., von dem Borne, A.E.G.K. and Engelfriet, C.P. (1978a). Destruction of sensitized erythrocytes by human monocytes *in vitro:* effect of cytochalasin B, hydrocortisone and colchicine. *Scand. J. Immunol.* **8**, 515–24.

Fleer, A., van der Meulen, F.W., Linthout, E., von dem Borne, A.E.G.K. and Engelfriet, C.P. (1978b). Destruction of IgG sensitized erythrocytes by human blood monocytes: modulation of inhibition by IgG. *Br. J. Haematol.* **39**, 425–36.

Freda, V.J., Gorman, J.G. and Pollack, W. (1964). Successful prevention of experimental Rh sensitization in man with an anti-Rh gamma-globulin antibody preparation. *Transfusion* **4**, 26–32.

Fries, L.F., Brickman, C.M. and Frank, M.M. (1983). Monocyte receptors for the Fc portion of IgG increase in number in autoimmune hemolytic anaemia and other hemolytic states and are decreased by glucocorticoid therapy. *J. Immunol.* **131**, 1240–5.

George, J.N. (1987). The role of membrane glycoproteins in platelet function. *Transfusion Med. Rev.* **1**, 34–46.

Gernsheimer, T., Stratton, J., Ballem, P.J. and Slichter, S.J. (1989). Mechanisms of response to treatment in autoimmune thrombocytopenic purpura. *N. Engl. J. Med.* **320**, 974–80.

Gertz, M.A., Petitt, R.M., Pineda, A.A., Wick, M.R. and Burgstaler, E.A. (1981). Vinblastine-loaded platelets for autoimmune hemolytic anaemia. *Ann. Intern. Med.* **95**, 325–6.

Giblett, E.R. (1964). Blood group antibodies causing haemolytic disease of the newborn. *Clin. Obstet. Gynecol.* **7**, 1044–55.

Giles, C. and Inglis, T.C.M. (1981). Thrombocytopenia and macrothrombocytosis in gestational hypertension. *Br. J. Obstet. Gynaecol.* **88**, 1115–19.

Greaves, M., Pickering, C., Porter, N.R., Magee, J.M. and Preston, F.E. (1982). Acquired Glanzmann's thrombasthenia. *Blood* **60**, 209–10.

Grossi, A., Vannuchi, A.M., Caspirini, P. *et al.* (1983). Different patterns of platelet turnover in chronic idiopathic thrombocytopenic purpura. *Scand. J. Haematol.* **31**, 206–14.

Habibi, B., Homberg, J.C., Schaison, G. and Salmon, C. (1974). Autoimmune hemolytic anaemia in children: a review of 80 cases. *Am. J. Med.* **56**, 61–9.

Hadley, A.G. and Kumpel, B.M. (1989a). Phagocytosis by human monocytes with monoclonal IgG1 and IgG3 anti-D. *Vox Sang.* **57**, 150–1.

Hadley, A.G. and Kumpel, B.M. (1989b). Synergistic effect of blending IgG1 and IgG3 monoclonal anti-D in promoting the metabolic response of monocytes to sensitized red cells. *Immunology* **67**, 550–2.

Hall, S., McCormick, J.L. and Grieppe, P.R. (1985). Splenectomy does not cure the thrombocytopenia in systemic lupus erythematosus. *Ann. Intern. Med.* **102**, 325–8.

Harmon, D.C., Weitzman, S.A. and Stossel, T.P. (1984). The severity of immune neutropenia correlates with the maturational specificity of antineutrophil antibodies. *Br. J. Haematol.* **58**, 209–15.

Hay, F.C., Torrigiani, G. and Roitt, J.M. (1972). The binding of human IgG subclass to human monocytes. *Eur. J. Immunol.* **2**, 257–61.

Herron, R., Clark, M., Young, D. and Smith, D.S. (1986). Correlation of mononuclear phagocyte assay results and *in vivo* haemolytic rate in subjects with a positive direct antiglobulin test. *Clin. Lab. Haematol.* **8**, 199–207.

Herzenberg, L.A., Lalor, P.A. and Stall, A.M. (1989). Are Ly-1 B cells important in autoimmune disease? *J. Autoimmunity* **2**, 225–31.

Heyns, A. du P., Fraser, J. and Retief, F.P. (1978). Platelet aggregation in chronic idiopathic thrombocytopenic purpura. *J. Clin. Pathol.* **31**, 1239–43.

Heyns, A. du P., Badenhorst, P.N., Lotter, M.G., Pieters, H., Wessels, P. and Kotze, H.F. (1986). Platelet turnover and kinetics in immune thrombocytopenic purpura: results with autologous In-labelled platelets and homologous Cr-labelled platelets differ. *Blood* **67**, 86–92.

Hilgartner, M.W. and Bussel, J. (1987). Use of intravenous gamma globulin for the treatment of autoimmune neutrophenia of childhood and autoimmune hemolytic anaemia. *Am. J. Med.* **83**, 25–9.

Hitzig, W.H. and Massimo, L. (1966). Treatment of autoimmune hemolytic anemia in children with azathioprine (Imuran). *Blood* **28**, 840–50.

Holguin, M.H., Wilcox, L.A., Bernshaw, N.J., Rosse, W.F. and Parker, C.J. (1990). Erythrocyte membrane inhibitor of reactive lysis: effects of phosphatidylinositol-specific phospholipase C on the isolated and cell-associated protein. *Blood* **75**, 284–9.

Horai, S., Claas, F.J. and van Rood, J.J. (1981). Detection of platelet antibodies by enzyme-linked immunosorbent assay (ELISA) on artificial monolayers of platelets. *Immunol. Lett.* **3**, 67–72.

Hosea, S.W., Brown, E.J., Hamburger, M.I. and Frank, M.M. (1981). Opsonic requirements for intravascular clearance after splenectomy. *N. Engl. J. Med.* **304**, 245–50.

Huber, H. and Fudenberg, H.H. (1968). Receptor sites of human monocytes for IgG. *Int. Arch. Allergy Appl. Immunol.* **34**, 18–31.

Huber, H., Douglas, S.D., Nusbacher, J., Kockwa, S. and Rosenfield, R.E. (1971). IgG subclass specificity of human monocyte receptor sites. *Nature* **229**, 419–20.

Hughes-Jones, N.C., Hughes, M.I.J. and Walker, W. (1967). The amount of anti-D on red cells in haemolytic disease of the newborn. *Vox Sang.* **12**, 279–85.

Hughes-Jones, N.C., Green, E.J. and Hunt, V.A.M. (1975). Loss of Rh antigen activity following the action of phospholipase A_2 on red cell stroma. *Vox Sang.* **29**, 184–91.

Huizinga, T., Roos, D. and von dem Borne, A.E.G.K. (1990). The Fc receptors: a two way bridge in the immune system. *Blood* **75**, 1211–13.

Hunter, J.D., Logue, G.L. and Joyner, J.T. (1982). Autoimmune neutropenia in Hodgkin's disease. *Arch. Intern. Med.* **142**, 386–8.

Hymes, K., Blum, M., Lackner, H. and Karpatkin, S. (1981). Easy bruising, thrombocytopenia and elevated platelet immunoglobulin G in Graves' disease and Hashimoto's thyroiditis. *Ann. Intern. Med.* **94**, 27–30.

Imbach, P., Berchtold, W. and Hirt, A. (1985). Intravenous immunoglobulin versus oral corticosteroids in acute immune thrombocytopenic purpura in childhood. *Lancet* **ii**, 464–8.

Issitt, P.D., Pavone, B.G., Goldfinger, D. *et al.* (1976). Anti-Wr^b, and other autoantibodies responsible for positive direct antiglobulin tests in 150 individuals. *Br. J. Haematol.* **34**, 5–18.

Jaffe, C.J., Atkinson, J.P. and Frank, M.M. (1976). The role of complement in the clearance of cold agglutinin-sensitized erythrocytes in man. *J. Clin. Invest.* **58**, 942–9.

Jakobowicz, R., Williams, L. and Silberman, F. (1972). Immunization of Rh-negative volunteers by repeated injections of very small amounts of Rh-positive blood. *Vox Sang.* **23**, 376–81.

James, P., Rowe, G.P. and Tozzo, G.G. (1988). Elucidation of alloantibodies in autoimmune haemolytic anaemia. *Vox Sang.* **54**, 167–71.

Jandl, J.H. (1965). Mechanism of antibody-induced red cell destruction. *Series Haematol.* **9**, 35–46.

Kaden, B.R., Rosse, W.F. and Hauch, T.W. (1979). Immune thrombocytopenia in lymphoproliferative diseases. *Blood* **53**, 545–51.

Kaplan, C. (1988). Antiplatelet antibodies in systemic lupus erythematosus: an overview: *Curr. Studies Hematol. Blood Transfusion* **55**, 90–3.

Karpatkin, M. and Karpatkin, S. (1981). Immune thrombocytopenia in children. *Am. J. Pediatr. Hematol. Oncol.* **3**, 213–19.

Karpatkin, S. (1985). Autoimmune thrombocytopenia. *Semin. Hematol.* **22**, 260–88.

Karpatkin, S. (1987). Immunologic thrombocytopenic purpura in patients at risk for AIDS. *Blood Rev.* **1**, 119–25.

Kiefel, V., Becker, T., Mueller-Eckhardt, G., Grebe, S. and Mueller-Eckhardt, C. (1985). Platelet survival determined with Cr versus In. *Klin. Wochenschr.* **63**, 84–9.

Kiefel, V., Santoso, S., Weisheit, M. and Mueller-Eckhardt, C. (1987). Monoclonal antibody specific immobilisation of platelet antigens (MAIPA): a new tool for the identification of platelet reactive antibodies. *Blood* **70**, 1722–6.

Klaassen, R.J.L., Ouwehand, W.H., Huizinga, T.W.J., Engelfriet, C.P. and von dem Borne, A.E.G.K. (1990). The Fc-receptor III of cultured human monocytes structural similarity with FcRIII of natural killer cells and role in the extracellular lysis of sensitized erythrocytes. *J. Immunol.* **144**, 599–606.

Lackner, H. and Karpatkin, S. (1975). On the 'easy bruising' syndrome with normal platelet count: a study of 75 patients. *Ann. Intern. Med.* **83**, 190–4.

Lahav, M., Rosenburg, I. and Wysenbeek, A.J. (1989). Steroid-responsive idiopathic cold agglutinin disease: a case report. *Acta Haematol. (Basel)* **81**, 166–8.

Lalezari, P., Jiang, A.F., Yegen, L. and Santorineou, M. (1975). Chronic autoimmune neutropenia due to anti-NA2 antibody. *N. Engl. J. Med.* **293**, 744–7.

Lalezari, P., Louie, J.E. and Fadlallak, N. (1982). Serological profile of alpha methyldopa-induced hemolytic anaemia: correlation between cell-bound IgM and hemolysis. *Blood* **59**, 61–8.

Leeksma, O.C., Zandbergen-Spaargaren, J., Giltay, J.C. and van Mourick, J.A. (1986). Cultural human endothelial cells synthesise a plasma membrane protein complex immunologically related to the platelet glycoprotein IIb/IIIa complex. *Blood* **67**, 1176–80.

Leeksma, O.C., Giltay, J.C., Zandbergen-Spaargaren, J., Modderman, P.W., van Mourick, J.A. and von dem Borne, A.E.G.K. (1987). The platelet alloantigen Zw^a or Pl^{a1} is expressed by cultured endothelial cells. *Br. J. Haematol.* **66**, 369–73.

Lilleyman, J.S. (1983). Management of childhood idiopathic thrombocytopenic purpura. *Br. J. Haematol.* **54**, 11–14.

LoBuglio, A.F., Cotran, R.S. and Jandl, J.H. (1967). Red cells coated with immunoglobulin G: binding and sphering by mononuclear cells in man. *Science* **158**, 1582–5.

Logtenberg, T., Young, F.M., van Es, J.H., Gmelig-Meyling, F.H.J. and Alt, F.W. (1989). Autoantibodies encoded by the most JH proximal human immunoglobulin heavy chain variable region gene. *J. Exp. Med.* **170**, 1347–55.

Logue, G.L. (1976). Felty's syndrome: granulocyte-bound immunoglobulin G and splenectomy. *Ann. Intern. Med.* **85**, 437–42.

Logue, G.L., Kurlander, R., Pepe, P., Davis, W. and Silberman, H. (1978). Antibody-dependent lymphocyte-mediated granulocyte cytotoxicity in man. *Blood* **51**, 97–108

Lusher, J.M. and Iyer, R. (1977). Idiopathic thrombocytopenic purpura in children. *Semin. Thrombosis Hemostasis* **3**, 175–98.

McCallister, J.A., Boxer, L.A. and Baehner, R.L. (1979). The use and limitation of labelled staphylococcal protein A for study of anti-neutrophil antibodies. *Blood* **54**, 1330–7.

Macintyre, E.A., Linch, D.C., Macey, M.G. and Newland, A.C. (1985). Successful response to intravenous immunoglobulin in autoimmune haemolytic anaemia. *Br. J. Haematol.* **60**, 387–8.

McLaughlin, P., Talpaz, M., Quesada, J.R., Salem, A., Barlogie, B., Gutterman, J.U. (1985). Immune thrombocytopenia following α-interferon therapy in patients with cancer. *JAMA* **254**, 1353–4.

McMillan, R. (1983). Immune thrombocytopenia. *Clin. Haematol.* **12** (1), 69–89.

McMillan, R., Longmire, R.L., Tavasoli, M., Armstrong, S. and Yelenosky, R. (1974a). *In vitro* phagocytosis by splenic leucocytes in idiopathic thrombocytopenic purpura. *N. Engl. J. Med.* **290**, 249–51.

McMillan, R., Longmire, R.L., Yelenosky, R., Donnell, R.L. and Armstrong, S. (1974b). Quantitation of platelet-binding IgG produced *in vitro* by spleens from patients with idiopathic thrombocytopenic purpura. *N. Engl. J. Med.* **291**, 812–17.

McMillan, R., Tani, P., Millard, F., Berchtold, P., Renshaw, L. and Woods, V.L., Jr (1987). Platelet-associated and plasma anti-glycoprotein antibodies in chronic ITP. *Blood* **70**, 1040–5.

McWilliams, N.B. and Maurer, H.M. (1979). Acute idiopathic thrombocytopenic purpura in children. *Am. J. Hematol.* **7**, 87–96.

Madyastha, P.R., Fudenberg, H.H., Glassman, A.B., Madyastha, K.R. and Smith, C.L. (1982). Autoimmune neutropenia in early infancy: a review. *Ann. Clin. Lab. Sci.* **12**, 356–67.

Masouredis, S.P., Branks, M.J. and Victoria, E.J. (1987). Anti-idiotypic IgG crossreactive with Rh alloantibodies in red cell autoimmunity. *Blood* **70**, 710–15.

Medical Research Council (1974). Working Party report of controlled trial of various anti-D dosages in suppression of Rh sensitisation following pregnancy. *Br. Med. J.* **2**, 75–80.

Medof, M.E., Kinoshita, T. and Nussenzweig, V. (1984). Inhibition of complement activation on the surface of cells after incorporation of decay-accelerating factor (DAF) into their membranes. *J. Exp. Med.* **160**, 1558–78.

Minchinton, R.M., Waters, A.H., Malpas, J.S., Gordon Smith, E.C. and Barrett, A.J. (1984a). Selective thrombocytopenia and neutropenia occurring after bone marrow transplantation — evidence of an autoimmune basis. *Clin. Lab. Haematol.* **6**, 157–63.

Minchinton, R.M., Waters, A.H., Malpas, J.S., Starke, I., Kendra, J.R. and Barrett, A.J. (1984b). Platelet- and granulocyte-specific antibodies after allogenic and autologous bone marrow grafts. *Vox Sang.* **46**, 125–35.

Mollison, P.L. and Cutbush, M. (1955). The use of isotope labelled red cells to demonstrate incompatibility *in vivo*. *Lancet* **i**, 1290–5.

Mollison, P.L., Engelfriet, C.P. and Contreras, M. (1987). *Blood Transfusion in Clinical Medicine*. Blackwell Scientific Publications, Oxford.

Mueller-Eckhardt, C. (1988). Autoimmune thrombocytopenic purpura: diagnostic and therapeutic actualities: *Curr. Studies Hematol. Blood Transfusion* **55**, 69–80.

Mueller-Eckhardt, C. and Salama, A. (1990). Drug-induced immune cytopenias: a unifying pathogenetic concept with special emphasis on the role of drug metabolites. *Transfusion Med. Rev.* **4**, 69–77.

Mueller-Eckhardt, C., Salama, A., Mahn, J., Kiefel, V., Neuzner, J. and Graubner, M. (1985). Lack of efficacy of high-dose intravenous immunoglobulin in autoimmune haemolytic anaemia: a clue to its mechanism. *Scand. J. Haematol.* **34**, 394–400.

Murphy, M.F., Metcalfe, P., Linch, D.C., Cheingsong-Popov, R., Carne, C. and Weller, I.V.D. (1985). Immune neutropenia in homosexual men. *Lancet* **i**, 225–6.

Murphy, W.G. and Kelton, J.G. (1988). Idiosyncratic drug-induced thrombocytopenia. *Curr. Studies Hematol. Blood Transfusion* **54**, 71–88.

Newland, A.C. (1988). Clinical use of intravenous immunoglobulin in blood disorders. *Blood Rev.* **2**, 157–67.

Newland, A.C. (1989). The use and mechanisms of action of intravenous immunoglobulin: an update. *Br. J. Haematol.* **72**, 301–5.

Newland, A.C., Treleavan, J.G., Minchinton, R.M. and Waters, A.H. (1983). High-dose intravenous IgG in adults with autoimmune thrombocytopenia. *Lancet* **i**, 84–7.

Niessner, H., Clemetson, K.J., Panzer, S., Mueller-Eckhardt, C., Santoso, S. and Bettelheim, P. (1986). Acquired thrombasthenia due to gpIIb/IIIa specific platelet autoantibodies. *Blood* **68**, 571–6.

O'Connor, B.M., Clifford, J.S., Lawrence, W.D. and Logue, G.L. (1989). Alpha-interferon for severe cold agglutinin disease. *Ann. Intern. Med.* **111**, 255–6.

Ouwehand, W.H. (1984). The activity of IgG1 and IgG3 antibodies in immune mediated destruction of red cells. Academic thesis, University of Amsterdam, The Netherlands, pp. 65–114.

Ouwehand, W.H., Mallens, T.E.J.M., Huiskes, E. *et al.* (1990). Predictive value of a monocyte-driven cytotoxicity assay for the severity of rhesus (D) haemolytic disease of the newborn: a comparison with two other techniques. *Br. J. Haematol.* (in press).

Palek, J., Mircevova, L., Brabec, V., Friedmann, B. and Majsky, A. (1968). The effect of anti-A antibody on red cell organic phosphates and adenosine triphosphatase activity *in vitro*. *Scand. J. Haematol.* **5**, 191–210.

Pangburn, M.K., Schreiber, R.D. and Mueller-Eckhardt, H.J. (1983). Deficiency of an erythrocyte membrane protein with complement regulatory activity in paroxysmal nocturnal hemoglobinuria. *Proc. Nat. Acad. Sci. (USA)* **80**, 5430–4.

Pascual, V., Randen, I., Thompson, K. *et al.* (1990). The complete nucleotide sequences of the heavy chain variable regions of six monospecific rheumatoid factors derived from EBV transformed B cells isolated from the synovial tissue of patients with rheumatoid arthritis: further evidence that some autoantibodies are unmutated copies of germline genes. *J. Clin. Invest.* **86** (4), 1320–8.

Pegels, J.G., Bruynes, E.C.E., Engelfriet, C.P. and von dem Borne, A.E.G.K. (1982a). Pseudothrombocytopenia: an immunologic study on platelet antibodies dependent on ethylene diamine tetra-acetate. *Blood* **59**, 157–61.

Pegels, J.G., Helmerhorst, F.M., van Leeuwen, F.F., van de Plas-van Dalen, C., Engelfriet, C.P. and von dem Borne, A.E.G.K. (1982b). The Evans syndrome: characterization of the responsible autoantibodies. *Br. J. Haematol.* **51**, 445–50.

Petersen, J. and Wiik, A. (1983). Lack of evidence for granulocyte specific membrane-directed autoantibodies in neutropenic cases of rheumatoid arthritis and in autoimmune neutropenia. *Acta Pathol. Microbiol. Immunol. Scand. (Section C)* **91**, 15–22.

Petz, L.D. and Garratty, G. (1980). *Acquired Immune Hemolytic Anemias*. Churchill-Livingstone, New York.

Plotz, P.H. (1983). Autoantibodies are anti-idiotype antibodies to antiviral antibodies. *Lancet* **ii**, 824–6.

Rappaport, H. and Crosby, W.H. (1957). Autoimmune hemolytic anaemia. 2. Morphological observations and clinical pathologic correlations. *Am. J. Pathol.* **33**, 429–57.

Reid, M.E., Vengelen-Tyler, V., Shulman, I. and Reynolds, M.V. (1988). Immunochemical specificity of autoanti-Gerbich from two patients with autoimmune haemolytic anaemia and concomitant alteration in the red cell membrane sialoglycoprotein β. *Br. J. Haematol.* **69**, 61–6.

Ribera, A., Martin-Vega, C., Massuet, L., Angelagues, E., Tornos, C. and Triginer, J. (1983). Autoimmune thrombocytopenia: serological behaviour of platelet antibodies. *Vox Sang.* **45**, 438–9.

Rosa, J.P., Kieffer, N., Didry, D., Picard, D., Kunicki, T.J. and Nurden, A.T. (1984). The human platelet membrane glycoprotein complex IIb/IIIa expresses antigenic sites not exposed on the dissociated glycoproteins. *Blood* **64**, 1246–53.

Rosse, W.F. (1971). Quantitative immunology of immune hemolytic anaemia II. The relationship of cell-bound antibody to hemolysis and the effect of treatment. *J. Clin. Invest.* **50**, 734–43.

Rosse, W.F. (1983). Management of chronic immune thrombocytopenia. *Clin. Hematol.* **12** (1), 267–84.

Rustagi, P.K., Currie, M.S. and Logue, G.L. (1985). Complement-activating antineutrophil antibody in systemic lupus erythematosus. *Am. J. Med.* **78**, 971–7.

Sander, R.P., Hardy, N.M. and Van-Meter, S.A. (1987). Anti-Jk[a] autoimmune hemolytic anaemia in an infant. *Transfusion* **27**, 58–60.

Sanz, I., Casali, P., Thomas, J.W., Notkins, A.L. and Capra, J.D. (1989). Nucleotide sequences of eight human natural autoantibody VH regions reveals apparent restricted use of VH families. *J. Immunol.* **142**, 4054–61.

Schanfield, M.S., Schoepner, S.L. and Stevens, J.O. (1980). New approaches to detecting clinically significant antibodies in the laboratory. In *Immunobiology of the Erythrocyte*, ed. S.G. Sandler, J. Nusbacher and M.S. Schanfield. Alan R. Liss, New York.

Schonermark, S., Rauterberg, E.W., Shin, M.L., Loke, S., Roelcke, D. and Hansch, G.M. (1986). Homologous species restriction in lysis of human erythrocytes: a membrane-derived protein with C8-binding capacity functions as an inhibitor. *J. Immunol.* **136**, 1772–6.

Schreiber, A.D. and Frank, M.M. (1972). The role of antibody and complement in the immune clearance and destruction of erythrocytes: *in vivo* effect of IgG and IgM complement fixing sites. *J. Clin. Invest.* **51**, 575–82.

Schwartz, K.A., Slichter, S.J. and Harker, L.A. (1982). Immune-mediated platelet destruction and thrombocytopenia in patients with solid tumours. *Br. J. Haematol.* **51**, 17–24.

Shirley, R.S., Kickler, T.S., Bell, W., Little, B., Smith, B. and Ness, P.M. (1987). Fatal immune hemolytic anaemia and hepatic failure associated with a warm-reacting IgM autoantibody. *Vox Sang.* **52**, 219–22.

Shulman, N.R., Leissinger, C.A., Hotchkiss, A.J. and Kautz, C.A. (1982). The non-specific nature of platelet associated IgG. *Trans. Assoc. Am. Physicians* **95**, 213–20.

Silberstein, L.E., Goldman, J., Kant, J.A. and Spitalnik, S.L. (1988). Comparative biochemical and genetic characterization of clonally related human B-cell lines secreting pathogenic anti-Pr2 cold agglutinins. *Arch. Biochem. Biophys.* **264**, 244–52.

Silberstein, L.E., Litwin, S. and Carmack, C.E. (1989). Relationship of variable region genes expressed by a human B cell lymphoma secreting pathologic anti-Pr2 erythrocyte autoantibodies. *J. Exp. Med.* **169**, 1631–43.

Sokol, R.J., Hewitt, S. and Stamps, B.K. (1981). Autoimmune haemolysis: an 18-year study of 865 cases referred to a regional transfusion centre. *Br. Med. J.* **282**, 2023–7.

Soulier, J.P., Patereau, C. and Drouet, J. (1975). Platelet indirect radioactive Coombs' test: its utilization for Pl^{A1} grouping. *Vox Sang.* **29**, 253–68.

Starkebaum, G. and Arend, W.P. (1979). Neutrophil-binding immunoglobulin G in systemic lupus erythematosus: evidence for the presence of both soluble immune complexes and immunoglobulin G antibodies to neutrophils. *J. Clin. Invest.* **64**, 902–12.

Starkebaum, G., Singer, J.W. and Arend, W.P. (1980a). Humoral and cellular mechanisms of neutropenia in patients with Felty's syndrome. *Clin. Exp. Immunol.* **39**, 307–14.

Starkebaum, G., Arend, W.P., Nardella, F.A. and Gavin, S.E. (1980b). Characterization of immune complexes and immunoglobulin G antibodies reactive with neutrophils in the sera of patients with Felty's syndrome. *J. Lab. Clin. Med.* **96**, 238–51.

Stoll, D.B., Cines, D.B., Aster, R.H. and Murphy, S. (1985). Platelet kinetics in patients with idiopathic thrombocytopenic purpura and moderate thrombocytopenia. *Blood* **65**, 584–8.

Stricker, R.B., Wong, D., Saks, S.R., Corash, L. and Shuman, M.A. (1985). Acquired Bernard–Soulier syndrome: evidence for the role of a 210 000 molecular weight protein in the interaction of platelets with von Willebrand factor. *J. Clin. Invest.* **76**, 1274–8.

Stuart, M.J., Kelton, J.G. and Allen, J.B. (1981). Abnormal platelet function and arachidonate metabolism in chronic idiopathic thrombocytopenic purpura. *Blood* **58**, 326–9.

Tavasoli, M. and McMillan, R. (1975). Structure of the spleen in idiopathic thrombocytopenic purpura. *Am. J. Clin. Pathol.* **64**, 180–91.

Tchernia, G. (1988). Immune thrombocytopenic purpura and pregnancy. *Curr. Studies Hematol. Blood Transfusion* **55**, 81–9.

Thomson, A., Contreras, M., Gorick, B. *et al.* (1990). Clearance of Rh D-positive red cells with monoclonal anti-D. *Lancet* **336**, 1147–50.

Urbaniak, S.J. (1976). Lymphoid cell dependent (K-cell) lysis of human erythrocytes sensitized with rhesus alloantibodies. *Br. J. Haematol.* **33**, 409–15.

van der Lelie, J. (1987). Immune cytopenias in human immunodeficiency virus infection. *Baillière's Clin. Immunol. Allergy* **1** (2), 487–96.

van der Meulen, F.W., van der Hart, M., Fleer, A., von dem Borne, A.E.G.K., Engelfriet, C.P. and van Loghem, J.J. (1978). The role of adherence to human mononuclear phagocytes in the destruction of red cells sensitized with non-complement binding IgG antibodies. *Br. J. Haematol.* **38**, 541–9.

van der Meulen, F.W., de Bruin, H.G., Goosen, P.C.M. *et al.* (1980). Quantitative aspects of the destruction of red cells sensitized with IgG1 autoantibodies: an application of flow cytofluorometry. *Br. J. Haematol.* **46**, 47–56.

van der Veen, J.P.W., Hack, C.E., Engelfriet, C.P., Pegels, J.G. and von dem Borne, A.E.G.K. (1986), Chronic idiopathic and secondary neutropenia: clinical and serological investigations. *Br. J. Haematol.* **63**, 161–71.

van Leeuwen, E.F., von dem Borne, A.E.G.K., van der Plas-van Dalen, C.M. and Engelfriet, C.P. (1981). Idiopathic thrombocytopenic purpura in children: detection of platelet autoantibodies by immunofluorescence. *Scand. J. Haematol.* **26**, 285–91.

van Leeuwen, E.F., van der Veen, J.P.W., Engelfriet, C.P. and von dem Borne, A.E.G.K. (1982). Specificity of autoantibodies in autoimmune thrombocytopenia. *Blood* **59**, 23–6.

van Rooijen, N. (1989). Are bacterial endotoxins involved in autoimmunity by CD5+(Ly-1+) B cells? *Immunol. Today* **10**, 334–6.

Verheugt, F.W.A., von dem Borne, A.E.G.K., van Noord-Bokhorst, J.C. and Engelfriet, C.P. (1978). Autoimmune granulocytopenia: the detection of granulocyte autoantibodies with the immunofluorescence test. *Br. J. Haematol.* **39**, 339–50.

von dem Borne, A.E.G.K. (1984). Autoimmune thrombocytopenia. *Res. Monog. Immunol.* **5**, 222–56.

von dem Borne, A.E.G.K. (1987). Autoimmune thrombocytopenia. *Baillière's Clin. Immunol. Allergy* **1** (2), 269–302.

von dem Borne, A.E.G.K., Engelfriet, C.P., Beckers, D. and van Loghem, J.J. (1971). Autoimmune haemolytic anaemias. IV.

Biochemical studies of red cells from patients with autoimmune haemolytic anaemia with incomplete warm autoantibodies. *Clin. Exp. Immunol.* **8**, 377–88.

von dem Borne, A.E.G.K., Beckers, D., Meulen, F.W. and Engelfriet, C.P. (1977). IgG4 autoantibodies against erythrocytes, without increased haemolysis: a case report. *Br. J. Haematol.* **37**, 137–40.

von dem Borne, A.E.G.K., Verheugt, F.W.A., Oosterhof, F., von Riesz, E., Brutel de la Rivière, A. and Engelfriet, C.P. (1978). A simple immunofluorescence test for the detection of platelet antibodies. *Br. J. Haematol.* **39**, 195–207.

von dem Borne, A.E.G.K., Vos, J.J.E., van der Lelie, J., Bossers, B. and van Dalen, C.M. (1986). Clinical significance of positive platelet immunofluorescence test in thrombocytopenia. *Br. J. Haematol.* **64**, 767–76.

Vroclans-Deiminas, M. and Boivin, P. (1980). Analyse des résultats observés au cours de la recherche d'une autosensibilisation anti-érythrocytaire chez 2400 malades. *Rev. Fr. Transfusion Immunohematol.* **23**, 105–17.

Wakui, H., Imai, H., Kobayashi, R. *et al.* (1988). Autoantibody against erythrocyte protein 4.1 in a patient with autoimmune haemolytic anaemia. *Blood* **72**, 408–12.

Waters, A.H. (1989). Post-transfusion purpura. *Blood Rev.* **3**, 83–7.

Waters, A.H. and Minchinton, R.M. (1985). Immune thrombocytopenia and neutropenia. *Recent Adv. Haematol.* **4**, 309–31.

Weitzman, S.A., Desmond, M.C. and Stossel, T.P. (1979). Antigenic modulation and turnover in human neutrophils. *J. Clin. Invest.* **64**, 321–5.

Weitzman, S.A., Stossel, T.P., Harmon, D.C., Daniels, G., Maloof, F. and Ridgway, E.C. (1985). Antineutrophil autoantibodies in Graves' disease: implications for thyrotropin binding to neutrophils. *J. Clin. Invest.* **75**, 119–24.

Werner-Favre, C., Vischer, T.L., Wohlwend, D. and Zubler, R.H. (1989). Cell surface antigen CD5 is a marker for activated human B cells *Eur. J. Immunol.* **19**, 1209–13.

Wiener, E., Atwal, A., Thompson, K.M., Melamed, M.D., Gorick, B. and Hughes-Jones, N.C. (1987). Differences between the activities of human monoclonal IgG1 and IgG3 subclasses of anti-D (Rh) antibody in their ability to mediate red cell-binding to macrophages. *Immunology* **62**, 401–4.

Wiener, E., Jollifer, V.M., Scott, H.C.F. *et al.* (1988). Differences between the activity of human monoclonal IgG1 and IgG3 anti-D antibodies of the Rh blood group system in their abilities to mediate effector functions of monocytes. *Immunology* **65**, 159–63.

Woodrow, J.C., Clarke, C.A., Donohoe, W.T.A. *et al.* (1975). Mechanism of Rh prophylaxis: an experimental study on specificity of immunosuppression. *Br. Med. J.* **2**, 57–9.

Zupanska, B., Thomson, E.E. and Merry, A.H. (1986). Fc receptors for IgG1 and IgG3 on human mononuclear cells: an evaluation with known levels of erythrocyte-bound IgG. *Vox Sang.* **50**, 97–103.

Zupanska, B., Brojer, E., Thomson, E.E., Merry, A.H. and Seyfried, H. (1987). Monocyte erythrocyte interaction in autoimmune haemolytic anaemia in relation to the number of erythrocyte-bound IgG molecules and subclass specificity of autoantibodies. *Vox Sang.* **52**, 212–18.

96: Immunological Aspects of Skin Diseases

D.W. Shaw and I. Gigli

Although diseases of the skin are easily observed morphologically, until recently little was known about their aetiology. This may be partially attributed to the fact that a single pathogenic mechanism may be manifested in the skin by a number of superficially dissimilar lesions. Moreover, being exposed to the outside world, a lesion in the skin is often the result of a combination of internal and external factors.

Skin diseases thought to be immunological in nature can be divided into two major categories: primarily antibody-mediated or primarily cell-mediated. However, as is the case in other organ systems, there is often simultaneous participation of these two systems. Certain bullous diseases are primarily antibody-mediated. Urticaria is in some cases an immunoglobulin E (IgE)-mediated immediate hypersensitivity reaction while allergic contact dermatitis is an example of a primarily cell-mediated disease. Vasculitis usually occurs secondary to deposition of circulating immune complexes but may also occur as a result of cell-mediated immunity.

Bullous diseases

The observation by Beutner and Jordon (1964) that sera of patients with pemphigus contained antibodies directed against normal epidermal cell surface antigens provided the initial evidence that immunoglobulins may play a role in the pathogenesis of bullous disorders. Since then, autoantibodies directed against different normal structural constituents of the epidermis and its basement membrane zone (BMZ) have been shown in many of the bullous diseases. This has permitted the development of serological criteria for their diagnosis. However, the deposition of immunoglobulins and complement seen by immunofluorescent techniques may not necessarily be the primary event in each disease. Only in pemphigus vulgaris and pemphigus foliaceus is the pathogenicity of the autoantibodies widely accepted. Some evidence also supports the pathogenicity of the autoantibodies in bullous pemphigoid and epidermolysis bullosa acquisita.

Pemphigus

Pemphigus is a group of diseases all of which have autoantibodies directed against normal intercellular or cell surface peptides of squamous epithelium. Based on the level of blister formation in the epidermis, pemphigus is divided into superficial and deep forms. The superficial forms are pemphigus foliaceus and pemphigus erythematosus while the deep forms are pemphigus vulgaris and its rare variant pemphigus vegetans.

Pemphigus vulgaris

Pemphigus vulgaris (PV), by far the most common form, is a chronic bullous disease found principally in patients between 40 and 60 years of age, although occasional cases have been reported in children. It occurs in all races and ethnic groups, but is most common among people of Jewish or Mediterranean origin. Coexistence with thymoma and myasthenia gravis has been frequently reported in PV and in other types of pemphigus (Chorzelski *et al.* 1987a). The characteristic lesions are thin, flaccid blisters or erosions appearing on normal or erythematous skin (Lever 1965). Patients almost always develop mucous membrane lesions, often as the initial disease manifestation. The blisters extend peripherally when pressure is applied to the blister (Nikolsky's sign). The lesions have little tendency to heal and the disease is usually fatal without treatment. Therapy consists of systemic corticosteroids, frequently in conjunction with azathioprine or cyclophosphamide.

Pemphigus vulgaris is associated with the human leucocyte antigen (HLA) phenotypes DR4/DQw3 and DRw6/DQw1 (Szafer *et al.* 1987), the latter strongly associated with the rare allele *DQB1.3*, which differs from the common DQ β-chain *DQB1.1* by a single amino acid (Scharf *et al.* 1988). The presence of *DQB1.3* in Israelis gives an estimated relative risk for disease of greater than 100 compared with a relative risk of only 2.6 for DRw6.

The histology of PV shows separation of epidermal cells from one another (acantholysis) immediately above the basal layer. Direct immunofluorescence shows intercellular IgG (Beutner *et al.* 1970; Jordon *et al.* 1971) and complement proteins (van Joost *et al.* 1972) at all levels of the epidermis. Indirect immunofluorescence with normal skin substrate demonstrates deposition of IgG with the same intercellular pattern (Beutner *et al.* 1965). Titres of these autoantibodies correlate with disease severity (Krasny *et al.* 1987). Both direct (Kelly *et al.* 1989a) and indirect (Jones *et al.* 1988; Yamada *et al.* 1989) methods have shown that the predominant immunoglobulin subclass is IgG4, although one direct immunofluorescence study showed IgG1 to be slightly more common than IgG4 during active disease (David *et al.* 1989). Electron microscopy shows early dissolution of intercellular cement with subsequent desmosomal separation (Hashimoto and Lever 1967). The PV antigen has been identified as a 130 kD polypeptide (Eyre and Stanley 1988) covalently bound to the 85 kD peptide plakoglobin (Korman *et al.* 1989), a constituent of desmosomes and adherens junctions (Cowin *et al.* 1986; Iwatsuki *et al.* 1989).

Pemphigus foliaceus

Pemphigus foliaceus (PF) is less common than PV. Superficial vesicles or bullae are present early, but these quickly rupture, leaving erosions, scales and crusting. The scalp, face, upper chest, abdomen and back are typical areas of involvement, but the disease may generalize. As in PV, Nikolsky's sign is positive. In contrast to PV, oral lesions are rare, the prognosis is good, topical therapy may be effective and systemic therapy can be used in low doses.

Certain drugs, particularly penicillamine (Tan and Rowell 1976), may induce PF or a PF-like disease. An endemic form of PF, termed fogo selvagem, is widespread in rural areas of Brazil that border rivers. Epidemiological studies strongly implicate an environmental factor as the cause of the autoantibody production (Diaz *et al.* 1989). Brazilian PF is positively associated with HLA-DR1 and DR4 and negatively associated with HLA-DR7 (Petzl-Erler and Santamaria 1988).

Acantholysis in PF occurs immediately above or below the granular layer of the epidermis. Direct and indirect immunofluorescence is identical to that seen in PV. In PF the autoantibodies are directed against the 160 kD desmosomal core glycoprotein desmoglein 1 (Eyre and Stanley 1987). As is the case with the PV antigen, the PF antigen is covalently bound to plakoglobin (Korman *et al.* 1989). It is unclear why acantholysis occurs at different levels of the epidermis in PV and PF when the respective antigens appear to be present at all levels of the epidermis.

Pemphigus erythematosus

Pemphigus erythematosus (Senear–Usher syndrome) is a rare form of pemphigus with features of lupus erythematosus and PF. Erythematous, scaly, crusted plaques occur most often on the trunk and the malar area. In addition to the histological and immunofluorescence findings of PF, patients have deposits of immunoglobulins and complement at the dermal–epidermal junction as seen in cutaneous lupus (Chorzelski *et al.* 1968). Antinuclear antibodies are present in some cases (Jablonska *et al.* 1977). However, the presence of systemic lupus erythematosus (SLE) is rare (Chorzelski *et al.* 1987a).

PATHOGENESIS

Pemphigus vulgaris and pemphigus foliaceus are the only skin diseases where the pathogenic role of the autoantibody is unquestioned. When IgG from serum of patients with PV (Anhalt *et al.* 1982) or from rabbits immunized with PV antigen (Peterson and Wuepper 1984) is injected into neonatal mice, the clinical, histological and immunopathological features of PV are reproduced. In PF, only IgG4 can passively transfer the disease to mice (Rock *et al.* 1989). Consistent with the inability of IgG4 to fix complement, murine C3 is not detected in the lesions in mice after disease transfer.

The mechanism of PV antibody-induced acantholysis is controversial. Although PV IgG in the absence of complement can induce acantholysis in skin culture (Schiltz and Michel 1976; Barnett *et al.* 1977), there is evidence *in vivo* of activation of the classical pathway of complement (Jordon 1980). Lesional, but not normal skin, contains in addition to early complement proteins, the membrane attack complex (MAC) C5b-9 (Kawana *et al.* 1989). Moreover, complement enhances PV IgG-induced epidermal cell detachment, both in skin culture (Kawana *et al.* 1985) and in animal passive transfer experiments (Anhalt *et al.* 1986).

A role for plasminogen activator in PV has been postulated, based on experiments showing that acantholysis is totally inhibited by antibodies against plasminogen activator (Morioka *et al.* 1987) and by purified plasminogen activator inhibitor (Hashimoto *et al.* 1989). This supports the hypothesis that PV IgG stimulates endogenous epidermal plasminogen activator, causing conversion of plasminogen to plasmin, which could degrade adhesive cell surface molecules (Hashimoto *et al.* 1983).

It is possible that complement and plasmin as well as other proteolytic enzymes each may play a role in PV acantholysis.

Bullous pemphigoid

In contrast to the flaccid blisters and erosions seen in pemphigus, bullous pemphigoid (BP) is characterized by the formation of tense bullae on erythematous or normal-appearing skin (Lever 1965). The flexor areas of the body are common sites of involvement, but the disease is often generalized. Mucous membrane lesions are found in only about one-third of BP patients but, in contrast to PV, are rarely the presenting lesions. Although BP occurs mostly in patients between 50 and 70 years, it has been reported in all age-groups, including children (Bean and Jordon 1974). Statistically significant HLA associations have not been demonstrated (Ahmed *et al.* 1984; Venning *et al.* 1989). Unlike PV, untreated BP has a low mortality rate due to its tendency for spontaneous healing. Therapy is similar to pemphigus, but lower doses of corticosteroids and immunosuppressive agents are required.

Skin biopsy shows a subepidermal blister, with a prominence of eosinophils in the upper dermis. Direct immunofluorescence almost always demonstrates a homogeneous linear deposition of C3 and IgG along the epidermal BMZ (Jordon *et al.* 1971). Most patients have circulating anti-BMZ autoantibodies (Beutner *et al.* 1970), usually capable of complement fixation (Jordon 1976). While nearly all BP sera contain some anti-BMZ IgG4, this is the only subclass present in non-complement-fixing sera (Yamada *et al.* 1989). In contrast to PV, there is not a close correlation between antibody titre and disease activity (Sams and Jordon 1971). Direct immunoelectron microscopy of BP skin biopsies shows immune deposits and blister formation in the lamina lucida of the BMZ (Fig. 96.1, Table 96.1; Holubar *et al.* 1975; Schmidt-Ullrich *et al.* 1975).

Using cultured skin as the substrate for indirect immunoelectron microscopy, BP IgG binds to the extracellular lamina lucida, directly beneath hemidesmosomes (Mutasim *et al.* 1989). However, with normal frozen skin substrate, BP IgG binds predominantly to the intracellular hemidesmosomes of basal layer keratinocytes (Fig. 96.1; Mutasim *et al.* 1985; Westgate *et al.* 1985), apparently due to increased cell membrane permeability produced by freezing. It is hypothesized that the larger intracellular pool of antigen is less accessible *in vivo* to BP antibodies than is the smaller extracellular pool, accounting for the predominance of *in vivo* deposits in the lamina lucida (Mutasim *et al.* 1989).

Sera from BP patients bind specifically to a hemidesmosomal glycoprotein of 230 kD (Mueller *et al.* 1989). Other molecular-weight antigens have been identified less commonly, including a 180 kD molecule (Labib *et al.* 1986). A complementary deoxyribonucleic acid (cDNA) encoding the immunogenic carboxy terminus of the 230 kD BP antigen has been cloned and sequenced (Stanley *et al.* 1988).

PATHOGENESIS

Lymphocytes and hypogranulated mast cells appear in early lesions, along with mast cell-derived chemotactic factors for eosinophils and neutrophils (Baba *et al.* 1976; Wintroub *et al.* 1978). Morphological evidence of eosinophil degranulation is also present (Dvorak *et al.* 1982).

There is local deposition of classical and alternative pathway complement proteins (Jordon *et al.* 1975). The presence of the membrane attack complex indicates that complement activation proceeds to completion (Dahl *et al.* 1984). In addition, blister fluid contains complement-derived chemotactic activity and decreased total haemolytic complement (Jordon *et al.* 1973; Diaz-Perez and Jordon 1976).

Circulating complement-fixing BP antibodies can mediate recruitment, attachment and activation of neutrophils at the BMZ *in vitro* on frozen skin sections, with subsequent subepidermal blister formation (Gammon *et al.* 1982). Deletion of antibodies, complement or leucocytes inhibits blister formation. However, variations of these experiments demonstrate that leucocyte attachment does not occur unless injury of the basal-layer keratinocytes has already occurred (Gammon

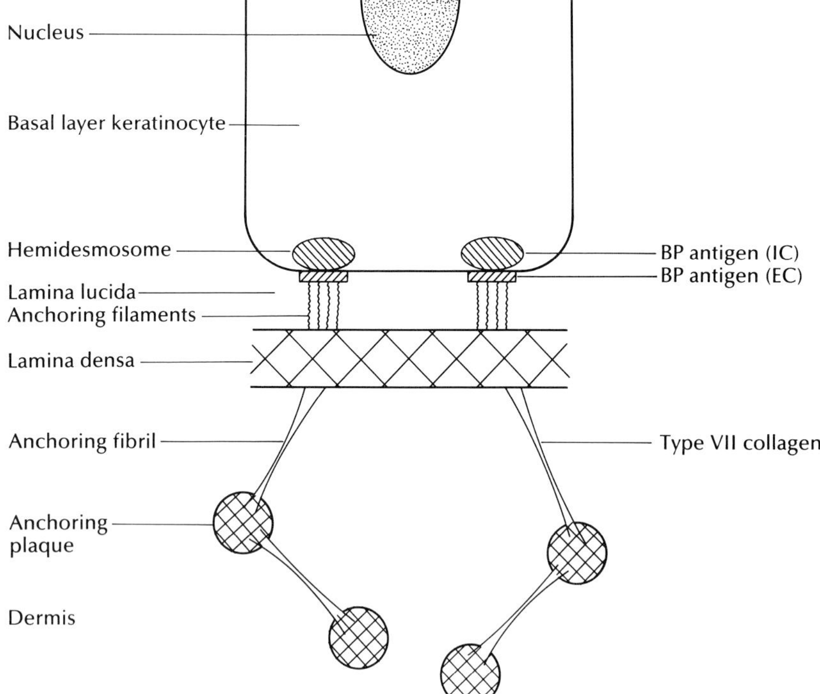

Fig. 96.1. The epidermal basement membrane zone. The bullous pemphigoid (BP) antigen is associated predominantly with the intracellular (IC) portion of hemidesmosomes. However, a smaller pool of BP antigen may be present on the extracellular (EC) surface of hemidesmosomes. Type VII collagen is the backbone of a network of interconnecting anchoring fibrils which anchor the lamina densa to the dermis via anchoring plaques.

Table 96.1. Summary of bullous diseases

Disease	Immunofluorescence pattern; major immunoglobulin	Antigen location	Antigen identity
Keratinocyte cell surface diseases			
Pemphigus vulgaris	Intercellular IgG4, IgG1	Desmosomes	130 kD
Pemphigus foliaceus	Intercellular IgG4	Desmosomes	Desmoglein I (160 kD)
Epidermal BMZ diseases (lamina lucida)			
Bullous pemphigoid	Linear IgG4, IgG1	Hemidesmosomes Lamina lucida	220–240 kD 180 kD
Herpes gestationis	Linear IgG1 (C3)	Lamina lucida, BCPM	180 kD
Cicatricial pemphigoid	Linear IgG (or IgA)	Lamina lucida	240 kD
LABD CBDC	Linear IgA	Lamina lucida	Unknown
Epidermal BMZ diseases (sub-lamina densa)			
EBA	Linear IgG	Sub-LD, anchoring fibrils	Type VII collagen
Bullous SLE	Linear IgG	Sub-LD, anchoring fibrils	Type VII collagen
Bullous SLE	Granular IgG	Sub-LD	Unknown
LABD CBDC	Linear IgA	Sub-LD	Unknown
Dermatitis herpetiformis	Granular IgA1	Papillary dermis	Unknown

BCPM = basement cell plasma membrane; LABD = linear IgA bullous dermatosis; CBDC = chronic bullous dermatosis of childhood; LD = lamina densa.

1987). This suggests that complement activation may be a secondary phenomenon.

While subepidermal blisters have been induced in guinea-pigs after intradermal injection of BP sera (Naito *et al*. 1982, 1984), these results could not be duplicated by other investigators (Gammon and Briggaman 1988). Passive transfer has also been unsuccessful in neonatal mice (Roscoe *et al*. 1987) and in rabbit skin (Anhalt *et al*. 1981), but successful in rabbit cornea (Anhalt *et al*. 1981). Thus, while some evidence points to the pathogenicity of BP antibodies, in contrast to pemphigus, passive transfer experiments to prove this hypothesis are not conclusive.

Cicatricial pemphigoid

Cicatricial pemphigoid (CP) is a subepidermal blistering disorder characterized by blistering and scarring of mucosa, particularly conjunctival and oral. Blindness often results. Cutaneous bullae that may or may not scar occur in about 25% of cases with a predilection for the face, neck and scalp (Ahmed and Hombal 1986). The usual treatment is systemic steroids, although conjunctival disease may sometimes be treated with intralesional steroids. One large study of ocular CP demonstrated an association with the HLA antigens DR4, DR5, DQw3, A2, B8, B35 and B49 (Zaltas *et al*. 1989).

Histology is usually indistinguishable from BP. As in BP, direct immunofluorescence demonstrates a homogeneous linear deposition of IgG and C3 at the epidermal BMZ. In contrast to BP, patients with CP have detectable circulating anti-BMZ antibodies in their sera in only 20% of cases when normal skin substrate is used (Ahmed and Hombal 1986). Immunoglobulin A may be present without IgG (Wojnarowska *et al*. 1984; Peters and Rogers 1989); in these cases, there may be clinical overlap with linear IgA bullous dermatosis. Electron microscopy shows the same findings as seen in BP, with blister formation and immune deposits occurring in the lamina lucida (Table 96.1; Fine *et al*. 1984). Attempts to more precisely localize the antigen by the use of split-skin immunofluorescence have provided inconsistent results (Fine

1985; Kelly and Wojnarowska 1988), although, in at least some cases, the antigen appears to be located in the lower lamina lucida (Fine *et al.* 1984). Autoantibodies are directed against an epidermal protein with a molecular weight the same as or close to that of the BP antigen (220–240 kD) (Labib *et al.* 1986).

When compared with normal controls, CP patients have hyperproliferative conjunctival fibroblasts in tissue culture (Roat *et al.* 1989). Since this persists through multiple cell divisions and media changes, there is an apparent change in phenotype. This is presumed to be a secondary effect of the antibody-induced inflammatory infiltrate.

Herpes gestationis

Herpes gestationis (HG), also referred to as pemphigoid gestationis, is an uncommon vesiculobullous disease, unrelated to herpes virus infection. It generally appears during the second or third trimester of pregnancy and usually recurs in subsequent pregnancies. The disease is generally self-limited but exacerbations are often noted in the post-partum period, during menstrual periods or with subsequent oral contraceptive use. The lesions of HG may be erythematous papules, vesicles or large and tense blisters that often begin at the umbilicus but usually spread to cover large areas of the body (Hertz *et al.* 1976). Mucosal involvement is unusual. Treatment with systemic corticosteroids will relieve the intense pruritus and blister formation, although, in some mild cases, disease can be controlled with topical steroids and antihistamines.

Histology shows a subepidermal blister, large numbers of eosinophils in the upper dermis and basal cell necrosis (Hertz *et al.* 1976). By direct immunofluorescence, IgG is present in a homogeneous linear pattern at the epidermal BMZ in 40% of perilesional biopsies, while indirect IF testing shows only 20% positive sera in the same pattern (Lawley *et al.* 1978). However, in a recent study using monoclonal anti-IgG1 antiserum, all cases demonstrated this immunoglobulin by direct and indirect immunofluorescence, with only occasional deposition of other IgG subclasses (Kelly *et al.* 1989a.) Heavy C3 BMZ deposition is a hallmark of this disease (Provost and Tomasi 1973). Initially, complement fixation was thought to be mediated by an antibody-independent serum factor termed the HG factor (Provost and Tomasi 1973). However, later studies showed it to be a complement-fixing IgG with apparent anti-BMZ specificity (Jordon *et al.* 1976; Katz *et al.* 1976b).

Western blot analysis of epidermal extracts shows that nearly all HG sera recognize a 180 kD antigen (Morrison *et al.* 1988). This may be the same protein recognized by a minority of BP sera (see 'Bullous pemphigoid' and Table 96.1). Direct immunoelectron microscopy shows that the deposition of IgG and C3 is very similar to that noted in BP (Yaoita *et al.* 1976). The use of saline split skin as a substrate for indirect immunofluorescence shows that both HG sera and BP sera bind to the epidermal side of the BMZ (Gammon *et al.* 1984a). While this is consistent with a hemidesmosomal localization of the HG antigen, the absence of indirect immunoelectron microscopic studies using normal frozen skin and HG sera precludes any definite conclusion (see 'Bullous pemphigoid').

PATHOGENESIS

Complement-fixing antibodies from HG sera bind to the BMZ of normal amnion (Kelly *et al.* 1988) or amnion and chorion laeve (Ortonne *et al.* 1987). As noted in the skin, the most common immunoglobulin subclass is IgG1 (Kelly *et al.* 1989a). Abnormal expression of Class II major histocompatibility complex (MHC) antigens is observed predominantly in the villous stroma of chorionic villi adjacent to the maternal decidua (Borthwick *et al.* 1988; Kelly *et al.* 1989b). It has been proposed that this could initiate a local allogeneic response to paternal MHC antigens in the fetal placenta, with a subsequent autoimmune response against normal placental basement membrane antigens. These antibodies cross-react with normal epidermal BMZ antigens and could account for the skin disease. Consistent with this concept is the observation that HG patients have anti-paternal MHC antibodies at a significantly higher rate than do normal pregnant women (Shornick *et al.* 1983b). Hormonal alterations also appear to be important in disease expression (Holmes *et al.* 1983).

Compared with BP, HG occurs in a much younger age-group and has much lower titres of circulating antibodies, more intense complement fixation, more basal cell damage and an association with HLA-DR3 and DR4 (Shornick *et al.* 1981).

Herpes gestationis antibodies are almost exclusively IgG1 while BP antibodies are more heterogeneous and IgG4 is the predominant subclass (Kelly *et al.* 1989a). Thus, even though HG sera may possibly be directed against the same antigen as some BP sera, other factors clearly influence disease expression.

Epidermolysis bullosa acquisita

The term epidermolysis bullosa (EB) refers to a heterogeneous inherited group of disorders characterized by extreme skin fragility. Epidermolysis bullosa acquisita (EBA) refers to an acquired, non-hereditary disease with some features similar to inherited EB. The following criteria have been proposed for the diagnosis of EBA (Yaoita *et al.* 1981): (i) trauma-induced bullae that heal with scarring and milia; (ii) no family history; (iii) subepidermal blister; (iv) linear IgG at the epidermal BMZ; and (v) IgG deposition beneath the lamina densa. Patients with this classical presentation tend to have an acral distribution of lesions that may closely mimic porphyria cutanea tarda. In addition, some of these patients may have scarring alopecia and nail dystrophy.

The use of immunological techniques to further define EBA leads to a broader clinical scope of the disease. In addition to the classical trauma-induced bullae, patients may have widespread inflammatory bullous disease very similar to BP (Gammon *et al.* 1984b) or CP (Rubenstein *et al.* 1987). A number of systemic diseases have been reported in association with EBA. These include inflammatory bowel disease, diabetes mellitus, multiple endocrinopathies syndrome and rheumatoid arthritis (Raab *et al.* 1983; Gammon *et al.* 1984b; Burke *et al.* 1986). There is an increased frequency of the HLA-DR2 haplotype (Gammon *et al.* 1988).

Epidermolysis bullosa acquisita tends to be a chronic disease that seldom remits spontaneously (Woodley 1988). Systemic steroids alone or in combination with dapsone, azathioprine, gold or methotrexate have minimal therapeutic effect, although cyclosporin A may be of benefit in some cases (Connolly and Sander 1987).

In the classical form of the disease, a sparse mononuclear infiltrate is present, while in the inflammatory form there is an upper dermal infiltrate of mononuclear cells and neutrophils. The occasional presence of many eosinophils (Gammon and Briggaman 1987) can cause confusion with BP. Direct immunofluorescence shows linear IgG at the epidermal BMZ, usually with C3, and often with IgA or IgM. Indirect immunofluorescence demonstrates linear BMZ binding of a complement-fixing IgG antibody in 20–50% of cases (Gammon *et al.* 1984b). Although routine immunofluorescence results cannot distinguish EBA from BP, a recently developed saline split-skin immunofluorescence technique, which splits skin through the lamina lucida of the epidermal BMZ, has shown that EBA sera bind to the dermal side of the split while BP sera bind predominantly to the epidermal side (Gammon *et al.* 1984a).

Immunoglobulins in sera from both classical and inflammatory types of EBA recognize specifically the carboxyl terminus, non-collagenous, globular domain of type VII collagen (Woodley *et al.* 1988). This type of collagen is the backbone of anchoring fibrils which anchor the lamina densa to the papillary dermis (Fig. 96.1; Keene *et al.* 1987). Consistent with this observation, anchoring fibrils in this entity are disordered or decreased in number (Richter and McNutt 1979) and immune deposits occur beneath the lamina densa (Gibbs and Minus 1975). Blistering usually occurs in this location as well, although lamina lucida blisters have also been reported (Fine *et al.* 1989).

PATHOGENESIS

In vivo and *in vitro* leucocyte attachment assays indicate a possible pathogenic role for EBA antibodies. When normal human skin is cultured in the presence of EBA sera, neutrophils and fresh serum as a source of complement, activation of complement induces neutrophil migration to the BMZ with subsequent dermal–epidermal separation (Gammon *et al.* 1984c). However, since classical EBA often occurs in the absence of clinical or histological evidence of inflammation, other mechanisms may also be operative.

Bullous systemic lupus erythematosus

Vesicles and/or bullae are a rare cutaneous manifestation of SLE (Hall *et al.* 1982). The lesions may clinically resemble bullous pemphigoid (Olansky *et al.* 1982) or dermatitis herpetiformis. Severity of skin involvement may or may not correlate with systemic disease exacerbations.

As opposed to the lymphocytic infiltrate of a typical lesion of cutaneous lupus erythematosus, skin biopsy shows a dense infiltrate of neutrophils in the upper dermis of bullous SLE. As is common in normal SLE skin, about half of reported cases have a granular pattern of IgG and C3 at the BMZ (Camisa 1988). In contrast, half have a homogeneous linear pattern as seen in BP or EBA (Gammon *et al.* 1985). Some of the patients showing a linear deposition have circulating anti-BMZ antibodies, demonstrated by indirect immunofluorescence, which, as in EBA, bind to the dermal side of saline split skin. By Western blot analysis these are shown to be directed against the EBA antigen (Gammon *et al.* 1985), now known to be type VII collagen (Woodley *et al.* 1988). Immunoelectron microscopy demonstrates that the immune deposits in both the granular and the linear forms are located on and beneath the lamina densa (Gammon *et al.* 1985).

Even though both EBA and some bullous SLE patients have autoantibodies against type VII collagen and an association with HLA-DR2 (Gammon *et al.* 1988), there are significant clinical differences between the two diseases. Unlike EBA, bullous SLE patients usually respond to dapsone and seldom develop skin fragility, trauma-induced blisters or healing with scars and milia (Gammon *et al.* 1985). Thus, as seen in other bullous diseases, factors in addition to antigenic specificity of autoantibodies play a role in disease expression.

Dermatitis herpetiformis

Dermatitis herpetiformis (DH) is characterized by small groups of tense vesicles on an erythematous base, involving primarily extensor surfaces. There are intense burning and pruritus, which often appear before the eruption of a lesion. It may occur at any age, but is most common in middle life. Biopsies of the small intestine have revealed a patchy jejunal atrophy indistinguishable from adult coeliac disease, but signs and symptoms of malabsorption are only occasionally seen (Marks *et al.* 1966; Fry *et al.* 1967). There is a positive association with HLA antigens B8 (Katz *et al.* 1977b), DR3 and DQw2, the latter being present in 95–100% of cases (Sachs *et al.* 1986; Hall *et al.* 1989) and a negative association with HLA-DPw2 (Hall *et al.* 1989).

Skin biopsies show subepidermal bullae with neutrophilic microabscesses in the dermal papillae. Direct immunofluorescence of perilesional or uninvolved skin shows a characteristic granular deposition of IgA (almost exclusively IgA-1) and C3 in the dermal papillae (van der Meer 1969; Hall and Lawley 1985). Some patients with DH-like lesions have a homogeneous linear IgA band at the BMZ. This group is now considered to represent a separate disease, linear IgA bullous dermatosis (see next section). Indirect immunofluorescence using DH sera shows no binding of immunoglobulins to normal skin (Provost and Tomasi 1974).

Patients often have circulating antibodies against gliadin, reticulin and gastrointestinal tract smooth-muscle endomysium. However, IgA class anti-endomysial antibodies have the highest frequency and specificity for DH (Beutner *et al.* 1986; Kumar *et al.* 1987; Reunala *et al.* 1987).

PATHOGENESIS

The relationship between the gut and skin disease is unknown. Gluten (gliadin)-free diet causes resolution of skin and gut lesions in DH, and gut lesions in coeliac disease, with a very slow disappearance of dermal IgA deposits. After gluten is reintroduced into the diet, there is a recurrence of antibodies (Beutner *et al.* 1986) and of gut and skin disease (Fry *et al.* 1982; Leonard *et al.* 1983). Treatment with dapsone will control the skin lesions but has no effect on the gut lesions or the presence of dermal IgA and complement (Katz *et al.* 1976a).

One theory of pathogenesis suggests that, in genetically predisposed individuals, dietary gluten forms IgA-containing immune complexes in the small intestine, producing patchy jejunal atrophy. The immune complexes may re-enter the circulation and deposit in the skin. However, antigliadin activity has not been detected in these circulating immune complexes (Hall and Lawley 1985) nor has gliadin been detected in DH skin (Pehamberger *et al.* 1979). While the exact mechanism is still elusive, information so far available supports a central role for IgA and gluten/gliadin.

Of interest is the recent observation that coeliac disease patients have a high incidence of neutralizing antibodies to adenovirus 12 (Kagnoff *et al.* 1984). The homology between a region of A-gliadin and the Elb adeno 12 protein suggests the possibility of environmental factors in this disease, which may also be relevant in patients with DH.

Linear immunoglobulin A bullous dermatosis

Linear IgA bullous dermatosis (LABD) is a post-adolescent, subepidermal blistering disorder which may clinically mimic DH or BP or may have features of both (Leonard *et al*. 1982; Mobacken *et al*. 1983). There is a tendency to form arciform, polycyclic, target or annular lesions. Blisters are commonly seen at the edge of annular lesions, the 'string of pearls' sign. Mucosal involvement is common and mucosal scarring may occur (Leonard *et al*. 1984; Wojnarowska *et al*. 1988). While skin lesions respond rapidly to dapsone or sulphonamides, mucosal lesions do not respond as well.

Dermatitis herpetiformis (defined by granular IgA deposits in the dermal papillae) differs from LABD in several respects: LABD rarely has gluten-sensitive enteropathy (Lawley *et al*. 1980; Leonard *et al*. 1987), does not have a gluten-sensitive skin eruption (Leonard *et al*. 1987), has an increased frequency of HLA-DQw1 rather than DQw2 (Sachs *et al*. 1988), may have detectable anti-BMZ antibodies and lacks anti-endomysial antibodies (Chorzelski *et al*. 1984).

The histology shows a subepidermal blister with an upper dermal infiltrate of neutrophils, sometimes contained in papillary microabscesses. By definition, direct IF demonstrates homogeneous linear IgA at the BMZ of the dermal–epidermal junction, with C3 detected in about 20–30% of cases (Wojnarowska *et al*. 1988). Indirect IF is positive for circulating IgA anti-BMZ antibodies in only 20% of cases.

Controversy exists regarding classification of cases with coexistent linear deposits of IgG. If IgG deposits are weaker than IgA, C3 is lacking and circulating IgG anti-BMZ antibodies are not detected, most authors would label such cases as LABD (Chorzelski *et al*. 1987b). Although direct and indirect immunoelectron microscopy demonstrates immunoreactants beneath the lamina densa in most patients (Bhogal *et al*. 1987), in others they are noted in the lamina lucida (Yaoita and Katz 1976) or in both locations simultaneously (Prost *et al*. 1989). These ultrastructural distinctions are not associated with consistent clinical differences.

Chronic bullous dermatosis of childhood

Chronic bullous dermatosis of childhood (CBDC) is very similar clinically and immunopathologically to LABD. However, it differs by its predominant involvement of perineal and perioral skin, higher frequency of detectable circulating IgA anti-BMZ antibodies and higher HLA-B8 frequency (Wojnarowska *et al*. 1988). Some authors (Wojnarowska *et al*. 1988), but not others (Chorzelski *et al*. 1987c), have found that CBDC has a slightly greater tendency for spontaneous resolution than does LABD.

Cutaneous vasculitis

Clinical disorders in which there are inflammation and necrosis of the blood-vessels are termed necrotizing vasculitis or angiitis. A definition of clinical syndromes includes criteria based on the dimension of the blood-vessels involved (Table 96.2; Zeek 1953; Copeman and Ryan 1970; Lie 1989), the type of cell infiltrating the vessel walls, the pattern of systemic involvement and the presence of serological abnormalities. This section will concentrate on small-vessel cutaneous necrotizing vasculitis, but will briefly summarize the cutaneous findings seen in vasculitides of large and medium-sized vessels. It should be noted that there is a great deal of overlap among the different categories and that no system of classification is entirely satisfactory.

Clinical and histological findings

SMALL-VESSEL VASCULITIS

Involvement primarily of venules, but also of capillaries and arterioles, has been termed hypersensitivity vasculitis, allergic vasculitis or cutaneous necrotizing vasculitis. In a large majority of cases, the vessel wall is infiltrated by neutrophils which typically demonstrate fragmented nuclei, referred to as 'nuclear dust'. This type of necrotizing vasculitis is often referred to as leucocytoclastic vasculitis. Occasional cases of vasculitis may demonstrate a predominantly mononuclear infiltrate (Soter *et al*. 1976a). In either type of necrotizing vasculitis, vessel damage is manifested by fibrin deposition in and around vessel walls and degenerative or necrotic endothelium, usually

Table 96.2. Classification of necrotizing vasculitis

Small-sized vessels
Infectious
Hepatitis B
Cytomegalovirus
Streptococci
Staphylococci
Rickettsia
Human immunodeficiency virus
Leprosy
Erythema nodosum leprosum
Lucio's reaction
Associated with collagen–vascular diseases
Rheumatoid arthritis
Systemic lupus erythematosus
Sjögren's syndrome
Dermatomyositis
Urticarial vasculitis
Drug-induced reactions
Cryoglobulinaemia
Hypergammaglobulinaemic purpura
Lymphoproliferative malignancies
Myeloproliferative malignancies
C2 or C4 deficiency
Intestinal bypass surgery
Idiopathic
Henoch–Schönlein syndrome
Erythema elevatum diutinum
Degos' disease
Microscopic polyarteritis
Medium-sized vessels
Polyarteritis nodosa
Polyangiitis overlap syndrome
Kawasaki's disease
Wegener's granulomatosis
Churg–Strauss vasculitis
Behçet's disease
Nodular vasculitis
Large and medium-sized vessels
Giant cell (temporal) arteritis
Takayasu's arteritis

with accompanying erythrocyte extravasation. Although cutaneous necrotizing vasculitis may affect a variety of organs, the skin is usually the most evident primary target.

The principal diagnostic lesions in small-vessel cutaneous necrotizing vasculitis are erythematous purpuric papules that do not blanch when pressed, which are called palpable purpura (Braverman 1970; Soter *et al*. 1974a). This palpable quality is important since it distinguishes these lesions clinically from non-inflammatory purpura. Haemorrhagic vesicles and bullae, pustules and urticaria are also found. (See the following section 'Urticaria and angio-oedema' for a discussion of urticarial vasculitis.) Nodules, ulcers, livedo reticularis and gangrene may also be seen but are more typical of medium-vessel vasculitis. The lesions appear at irregular intervals, most often over the lower extremities, but the eruption may be seen on any part of the body. Individual lesions last from 1 to 4 weeks and may be accompanied by burning or pain. Post-inflammatory hyperpigmentation may occur after healing. Fever, malaise, arthralgias or myalgias may occur, irrespective of a defined underlying or associated disease.

Cutaneous necrotizing vasculitis has been associated with a number of infectious agents (Table 96.2), including hepatitis B, cytomegalovirus, streptococci, staphylococci, leprosy, certain rickettsial infections and the human immunodeficiency virus. Hepatitis B virus has been associated with polyarteritis nodosa (Sergent *et al*. 1976), urticarial vasculitis and the small-vessel vasculitis seen in mixed cryoglobulinaemia (Levo *et al*. 1977). Direct roles for both hepatitis B (Gower *et al*. 1978) and cytomegalovirus (Bulpitt and Brahn 1989) are supported by their presence in vasculitic vessel walls. During the course of lepromatous leprosy, vasculitis may occur in two different forms: erythema nodosum leprosum or Lucio's reaction (Rea and Ridley 1979).

Cutaneous vasculitis is also seen in a variety of connective tissue diseases, notably rheumatoid arthritis, Sjögren's syndrome, SLE and dermatomyositis. These diseases are sometimes also associated with vasculitis of muscular arteries. Commonly incriminated medications are β-lactam antibiotics, sulphonamides, thiazides and heterologous serum (serum sickness). Vasculitis is associated with lymphoproliferative and myeloproliferative malignancies much more often than with other malignancies (Greer *et al*. 1988). Other reported associations include hypergammaglobulinaemic purpura, cryoglobulinaemias (associated with a variety of diseases in addition to hepatitis B) and congenital C2 or C4 deficiency. Rarely reported causes include intestinal bypass surgery, inflammatory bowel disease and primary biliary cirrhosis.

A large group of patients exists with cutaneous necrotizing vasculitis of unknown cause. In these individuals the vascular lesions may involve a variety of organ systems or may remain restricted to the skin. The most widely recognized idiopathic disorder is the *Henoch–Schönlein syndrome*, in which the skin, joints, gastrointestinal tract and kidneys are characteristically affected (Cream *et al.* 1970). This syndrome occurs predominantly in children. However, a clinically characteristic form may occur in adults, with plaques of palpable purpura containing areas of hemorrhage in a livedoid pattern (Piette and Stone 1989).

Erythema elevatum diutinum is an idiopathic, chronic, small-vessel necrotizing vasculitis mainly involving the skin. It is clinically unique and is characterized by red, purple or yellow papules, nodules and plaques located on the buttocks and extensor surfaces (Katz *et al.* 1977a). There is often accompanying arthralgia.

In *atrophie blanche*, also referred to as livedoid vasculitis, painful purpuric macules and papules develop into ulcers on the lower legs that heal with ivory-white, slightly depressed, scar-like plaques surrounded by telangiectases. Livedo reticularis is present in some cases (Milstone *et al.* 1983). Early lesions show fibrin plugs occluding superficial vessels, with the subsequent development of vessel wall necrosis. However, since vascular leucocyte infiltration is rarely seen at any stage of lesion development, this is no longer considered a true vasculitis by most authors (Shornick *et al.* 1983a).

Skin lesions of *malignant atrophic papulosis* (Degos' disease) start as pink dome-shaped papules that heal with a porcelain-white centre. While this disease may be limited to the skin, it is usually a systemic vasculitis, with death occurring due to gastrointestinal or neurological involvement (Degos 1979). Necrosis and fibrosis of dermal arterioles and venules with subsequent focal infarction may occur due to a lymphocyte-mediated vasculitis (Soter *et al.* 1982; Su *et al.* 1985).

Microscopic polyarteritis, originally described as a form of polyarteritis nodosa, is a systemic vasculitis affecting arterioles and capillaries, with prominent skin and musculoskeletal involvement. There is focal necrotizing glomerulonephritis, often causing renal failure. These patients share some features of polyarteritis nodosa and Wegener's granulomatosis (Savage *et al.* 1985; Savage 1989).

MEDIUM-VESSEL VASCULITIS

Medium-vessel vasculitis principally involves medium and small muscular arteries, although most of the vasculitides in this category also involve venules, capillaries and arterioles. Involvement of the skin by medium-sized vessel vasculitis is typically manifested by nodules, ecchymotic plaques, ulcers, livedo reticularis or gangrene.

Classic *polyarteritis nodosa* is a systemic vasculitis involving medium- and small-sized muscular arteries, which frequently involves the subcutaneous tissue, giving clinically apparent skin lesions in approximately 40% of cases (Cupps and Fauci 1981). Occasionally, the arteritis may involve the muscle, subcutaneous tissue and, rarely, the lower dermis without apparent systemic involvement; this is referred to as cutaneous polyarteritis nodosa (Diaz-Perez and Winkelmann 1974). The most common skin lesions of the classic form are non-specific macules and papules, purpura or urticaria. In both the classic and the cutaneous forms, nodules, livedo reticularis and ulcers are found most frequently on the lower extremities. The histological findings in involved arteries include neutrophils, nuclear dust and fibrin, as seen in small-vessel vasculitis. The *polyangiitis overlap syndrome* has features of different distinct vasculitic syndromes, usually including polyarteritis nodosa. In most cases, coexistent cutaneous vasculitis is present, involving vessels of any size (Leavitt and Fauci 1986).

Wegener's granulomatosis involves the skin in approximately 40–50% of cases, affecting both medium and small vessels. Lesions include ulcers, papules, vesicles and subcutaneous nodules (Cupps and Fauci 1980). The histology may show typical necrotizing (leucocytoclastic) vasculitis, granulomatous vasculitis or extravascular necrotizing granulomas.

In *allergic angiitis and granulomatosis* (Churg–Strauss syndrome), skin involvement occurs in the majority of cases. Nodules, often on the scalp or the extensor aspects of the extremities, are the most common lesions, followed by papules, vesicles and purpura. Livedo reticularis occurs infrequently. Histology may show extravascular 'Churg–Strauss' granulomas, vasculitis of muscular arteries with vascular infiltration by varying proportions of neutrophils, lymphocytes and histiocytes, or typical small-vessel leucocytoclastic vasculitis (Crotty *et al.* 1981). Large numbers of eosinophils are seen in all of these histological patterns.

Nodular vasculitis presents as chronic, recurrent, tender, subcutaneous nodules or plaques that often ulcerate and heal with an atrophic scar. It is usually seen on the calves of women. Systemic vasculitis is unusual. In some cases, this entity may represent a hypersensitivity reaction to tuberculosis elsewhere in the body, although this is a subject of great controversy (Eberhartinger 1963). The tuberculosis-associated cases are sometimes referred to as erythema induratum. Histological examination demonstrates vasculitis of subcutaneous arteries and veins, associated with severe granulomatous panniculitis.

LARGE- AND MEDIUM-VESSEL VASCULITIS

Takayasu's arteritis has a strong predilection for the aortic arch and its branches. Patients occasionally have skin lesions demonstrating granulomatous or necrotizing vasculitis (Perniciaro *et al.* 1987). These are typically lower-extremity nodules and ulcers clinically simulating erythema nodosum or pyoderma gangrenosum (diseases which seldom show vasculitis).

Giant-cell (temporal) arteritis is a systemic vasculitis with predominant involvement of the extracranial branches of the carotid artery. The most common cutaneous manifestations include tenderness, erythema, nodules, ulceration and necrosis along the path of the temporal artery; similar changes may affect the tongue (Hitch 1970). As in Takayasu's arteritis, lower-extremity vasculitic nodules may clinically simulate erythema nodosum (Goldberg *et al.* 1987). Raynaud's phenomenon (Klein *et al.* 1975) and leg gangrene (Greene *et al.* 1986) occur rarely.

Laboratory abnormalities

The most common laboratory finding in the broad spectrum of vasculitides is an elevated erythrocyte sedimentation rate. Additional laboratory data are consistent with the underlying disorders or may reflect the involvement of additional organ systems, most importantly the kidneys.

Patients with cutaneous necrotizing venulitis and associated collagen–vascular disease have been found to have an increased prevalence of the HLA antigen pair A11/Bw35, suggesting that genetic factors may play a role in these patients (Glass *et al.* 1976). An increased frequency of the HLA-B8/DR3 phenotype has been seen in rheumatoid arthritis patients with vasculitis compared with those without (Cunningham *et al.* 1982). However, this was not confirmed in a later study (Gladman and Anhorn 1986).

Studies of the complement system in cutaneous vasculitis may show low, normal or elevated plasma component concentrations (Soter *et al.* 1976a). In patients with palpable purpura, hypocomplementaemia and concomitant collagen–vascular diseases, the complement abnormalities reflect the associated disease or the existence of cryoglobulins (Soter *et al.* 1974a). For example, in patients with rheumatoid arthritis having high levels of rheumatoid factor, the hypocomplementaemia is consistent with classical pathway activation (Soter *et al.* 1974a). In SLE patients with or without vasculitis, classical pathway activation occurs with profound depletion of C1q, often in the presence of anti-C1q autoantibodies (Uwatoko and Mannik 1988). In addition, SLE patients with vasculitis may occasionally lack individual classical pathway components due to genetic deficiencies. In primary Sjögren's syndrome, hypocomplementaemia and high titres of Ro and La autoantibodies are associated with the typical neutrophilic type of cutaneous necrotizing vasculitis. In contrast, these findings are absent in Sjögren's syndrome patients with a mononuclear cell vasculitis (Molina *et al.* 1985). A similar dichotomy in complement levels between the neutrophilic and mononuclear types of vasculitis has been previously observed (Soter *et al.* 1976a). Significantly elevated levels of activated terminal complement components (C5b–9) are also observed in Sjögren's syndrome patients with peripheral (usually cutaneous) vasculitis and/or central nervous system disease (Alexander *et al.* 1988). This study, however, did not separate the neutrophilic from the mononuclear type of vasculitis.

Immune complexes have been demonstrated in serum and in fresh lesional tissue. In the latter case, they have been detected by electron microscopy as electron-dense subendothelial deposits (Braverman 1970) and by immunofluorescence as granular deposits of immunoglobulins and the complement protein C3 (Sams *et al.* 1975).

The immune complexes and complement proteins are rarely detectable in lesions that have lasted more than 24 hours, but they may be induced by local injection of histamine (Braverman and Yen 1975; Gower *et al.* 1977). It is of interest that the serum of Henoch–Schönlein syndrome patients contains circulating immune complexes and vascular deposits that are predominantly IgA, but which often contain IgG as well. This may be explained by the finding that the IgA-containing immune complexes often contain IgA rheumatoid factor activity (Saulsbury 1987).

Numerous studies have been performed in an attempt to serologically classify vasculitis or to assess disease activity. Anti-neutrophil cytoplasmic autoantibodies are present in Wegener's granulomatosis (van der Woude *et al.* 1985), microscopic polyarteritis (Lockwood *et al.* 1987) and Kawasaki's disease (Savage *et al.* 1989); they are useful diagnostically and in monitoring disease activity. Several non-specific markers of vascular damage have also been examined. For example, serum concentrations of a basement membrane antigen, laminin fragment P1, roughly correlate with extent of disease activity in patients with essential cryoglobulinaemia associated with vasculitis (Gabrielli *et al.* 1988). The endothelial cell marker factor VIII-related antigen (von Willebrand factor) is elevated in systemic necrotizing arteritis and large-vessel arteritis but not in small-vessel vasculitis, which is usually confined to the skin (Woolf *et al.* 1987). However, these markers of basement membrane and vascular damage are also elevated in various other diseases.

Pathophysiological mechanisms

The exact pathogenic mechanism by which patients develop necrotizing vasculitis lesions has not been clearly elucidated, but the evidence indicates that the leucocytoclastic form of vasculitis is an immune complex disease (type III immunological reaction), although the nature of the antigen is usually unknown. Complexes are formed in the circulation, which, when present in slight antigen excess, remain soluble. Under the appropriate stimulus they may become lodged within vessel walls. The finding of hypogranulated mast cells in lesional skin biopsies (Soter *et al.* 1976a) and the local induction of vasculitis with histamine injections suggests that increased vascular permeability due to the effects of mast cell mediators may be important in the early pathogenesis of the lesion. The deposited immune complexes activate complement to completion (Boom *et al.* 1987). Furthermore, the immunoelectron microscopic localization of membrane attack complex to areas of endothelial swelling suggests that it may play a role in vessel wall damage (Boom *et al.* 1989). Liberated anaphylatoxins formed during complement activation can degranulate mast cells as well as attract neutrophils which release their lysosomal enzymes, destroying the integrity of the vessel wall and leading to extravasation of erythrocytes, fibrin deposition and vessel necrosis.

Early endothelial injury and exposure of vascular subendothelial collagen set in motion a series of procoagulant actions, including activation of intrinsic and extrinsic coagulation pathways. In addition, patients with many types of vasculitis demonstrate decreased cutaneous fibrinolytic activity (Cunliffe and Menon 1971; Sun *et al.* 1976), which could inhibit clot degradation. This appears to be due to decreased tissue plasminogen activator release by blood-vessels (Jordan *et al.* 1987). Decreased tissue plasminogen activator activity is most extreme in atrophie blanche (Jordan *et al.* 1987), a cutaneous vasculopathy characterized by microvascular thrombosis.

While tissue deposition of circulating immune complexes appears to play a major role in neutrophil-mediated (leucocytoclastic) necrotizing vasculitis, other mechanisms may also cause vasculitis. For example, a recent study demonstrated a cytotoxic, complement-fixing autoantibody with specificity for vascular endothelial cells in most patients with a variety of systemic vasculitides (Brasile *et al.* 1989). However, of the four patients with small-vessel vasculitis, only one individual, a patient with SLE, possessed this circulating autoantibody. It was also present in one of 10 SLE control patients without vasculitis. It is not clear what role, if any, these autoantibodies play in the pathogenesis of vasculitis.

The presence of a perivenular infiltrate rich in activated lymphocytes suggests that cell-mediated immunity may also play a role in some cases of necrotizing vasculitis, particularly in normocomplementaemic patients (Soter *et al.* 1976a). It may also be largely responsible for the vasculitis seen in Degos' disease (Soter *et al.* 1982) and some rickettsial diseases (Walker *et al.* 1981). Both cell-mediated (O'Duffy *et al.* 1971; Bang *et al.* 1987) and immune complex-mediated (Jorizzo *et al.* 1984) mechanisms have been proposed to contribute to the vasculitis of Behçet's disease.

Therapy

Identification and removal or treatment of known causes of vasculitis should be attempted. If there is evidence of progressive renal disease, steroid and cytotoxic therapy is indicated (see Chapter 62). The presence of extrarenal systemic vasculitis involving small or medium-sized muscular arteries is also an indication for the addition of cytotoxic agents such as cyclophosphamide (Fauci *et al.* 1978).

Vasculitis limited to the skin may require treatment due to discomfort and pain but need not be as aggressive as in systemic vasculitis. Numerous agents have been used but controlled studies are lacking. In one large study, colchicine, corticosteroids and azathioprine were effective in most patients while non-steroidal anti-inflammatory drugs, antihistamines and antimalarials were usually ineffective (Callen and Ekenstam 1987). Patients with erythema elevatum diutinum respond to dapsone (Katz *et al.* 1977a).

Urticaria and angio-oedema

Urticaria (hives) is an intensely pruritic, cutaneous eruption characterized by transient, circumscribed, pale red, raised areas of oedema (weals) caused by excessive leakage of fluid from blood-vessels of the upper dermis. Individual lesions usually persist for only a few hours, but new lesions may continue to appear for an indefinite period. When the process involves the deep dermis and/or subcutaneous tissue, it is known as angio-oedema. These lesions are larger and paler than urticaria and do not usually itch. While angio-oedema may involve any part of the body, the most common sites are the face, extremities and genitalia. Gastrointestinal and respiratory tract involvement may occasionally occur. Angio-oedema, with the exception of the hereditary type, is frequently associated with urticaria.

Approximately one-fifth of the population of the United States develops urticaria or angio-oedema at some time in their lives. The lesions appear most frequently after adolescence, although persons of any age may experience urticaria and/or angio-oedema. Urticaria is classified as either acute or chronic; a duration of more than 6 weeks is arbitrarily considered chronic.

In about 75% of cases, the cause of urticaria/angio-oedema cannot be identified in spite of extensive investigation (Warin and Champion 1974). Likewise, the mechanism of urticaria production is unknown. However, in some cases the mechanism is immunological while in others it is clearly non-immunological (Table 96.3).

Associated with immunological processes

IMMUNOGLOBULIN E-MEDIATED

In many cases, urticaria/angio-oedema is due to a type I (immediate hypersensitivity) reaction mediated by IgE antibodies capable of causing the release of biologically active factors from mast cells and basophils (Holgate *et al.* 1988). Urticaria or angio-oedema appearing in individuals with a family history of asthma, rhinitis or atopic dermatitis is thought to be IgE-mediated. Similarly, IgE-dependent reactions appear to be involved in symptoms produced by bee stings, inhalants such as pollens, drugs such as penicillin, and foods such as eggs, milk, nuts and crustacea (Halmepuro *et al.* 1987). Other possible examples include helminth infestations and reactions to therapeutic hormones of non-human origin such as porcine insulin. Some cases of contact urticaria, for example those due to latex products (rubber gloves, balloons and contraceptives), are IgE-mediated and may be associated with non-cutaneous anaphylactic symptoms (Wrangsjo *et al.* 1988; Slater 1989). Physical urticarias that appear to be IgE-mediated in many cases include dermatographism and cold, solar and cholinergic urticarias.

IMMUNE COMPLEX-MEDIATED

Patients presenting with episodes of chronic urticaria or angio-oedema, arthralgias, abdominal pain and, rarely, glomerulonephritis (McDuffie *et al.* 1973; Soter *et al.* 1974b) have been recognized histologically as having necrotizing vasculitis. In contrast to common urticaria, individual skin lesions often persist longer than 24 hours and may contain occasional foci of purpura. This syndrome is termed *urticarial vasculitis*.

Table 96.3. Classification of urticaria/angio-oedema

Immunological
Immediate hypersensitivity (IgE)
Drugs (penicillin)
Foods (nuts, shellfish, eggs)
Infections (helminths)
Inhalants (pollens)
Bee stings
Therapeutic hormones, non-human
Vaccines (egg sensitivity)
Contactants (latex)
Physical (dermatographism, cold, solar, cholinergic)
Immune complex reactions
Urticarial vasculitis
SLE, Sjögren's syndrome, hepatitis B, serum sickness, drugs, IgM gammopathy
Blood products
C1 inhibitor deficiencies
Genetic (hereditary angio-oedema)
Acquired (malignancies)
Non-immunological
Changes in eicosanoid metabolism
Aspirin and related drugs
Direct mast cell activators
Radiocontrast media?
Drugs (opiates, curare, polymyxin)
Contactants?
Presumed alterations in kinin metabolism
Angiotensin-converting enzyme inhibitors
Idiopathic
Miscellaneous
Thyroid autoimmunity
Menses-associated
Episodic angio-oedema with eosinophilia
Hypereosinophilic syndrome
Physical urticarias (heat, vibratory, pressure, aquagenic, exercise)

Many of these patients have serum hypocomplementaemia with reduced levels of the early classical pathway complement proteins, particularly C1q (Agnello 1986). The majority of patients with hypocomplementaemia have a circulating C1q precipitin (Agnello 1986), which has been demonstrated to be IgG (Marder *et al*. 1978). While it was originally thought that the C1q precipitin function was mediated by the Fc portion of IgG, recent evidence implicates the action of autoantibodies with antigenic specificity for the collagen-like portion of C1q (Wisnieski and Naff 1989). These autoantibodies have also been demonstrated in SLE (Uwatoko and Mannik 1988). The group of urticarial vasculitis patients with hypocomplementaemia (hypocomplementaemic urticarial vasculitis syndrome) may have an increased incidence of systemic involvement when compared with patients with normocomplementaemia (Sanchez *et al*. 1982).

The detection of circulating immune complexes by a variety of techniques (Monroe 1981), along with the occasional detection of cryoglobulins, 7S IgM, rheumatoid factor and perivascular deposits of immunoglobulins and complement proteins (Sanchez *et al*. 1982), suggests an immune complex-mediated pathogenesis, at least in some cases. The mast cell degranulation sometimes observed (Soter *et al*. 1976a) could result from immune complex-generated anaphylatoxins or from the anti-IgE autoantibodies recently described in this condition (Gruber *et al*. 1988).

Vasculitis expressed clinically as urticaria may also be seen in patients with SLE (Provost *et al*. 1980), Sjögren's syndrome (Alexander and Provost 1983), serum sickness, drug reactions, the preicteric phase of hepatitis B (Dienstag *et al*. 1978), monoclonal IgM gammopathy (Clauvel *et al*. 1982) and, under certain conditions, physical urticarias (Eady *et al*. 1981; Armstrong *et al*. 1985).

Urticaria/angio-oedema associated with blood or blood product transfusions is often accompanied by immune complex formation with IgG antibodies directed against transfused IgA (Schmidt *et al*. 1969), especially in IgA-deficient patients. In some patients, gamma globulin replacement therapy may lead to episodes of urticaria or anaphylaxis. In these cases, complement activation may be responsible for disease pathogenesis.

For a discussion of angio-oedema associated with deficiencies of C1 inhibitor, see Chapter 67.

Physical urticarias and angio-oedemas

Physical urticarias and angio-oedemas are elicited by physical agents (Casale *et al*. 1988). Different types of physical urticarias may coexist in the same individual.

Dermatographism refers to a rapidly appearing weal and flare where skin has been firmly stroked, usually fading within 15–30 minutes. This exaggerated form of the classic 'triple response of Lewis' occurs in 2–5% of the population. A subgroup with concomitant pruritus is referred to as having *symptomatic dermatographism* (Breathnach *et al.* 1983). The sera of some affected individuals can transfer this response to normal individuals (passive transfer), supporting the view that this is an IgE-mediated reaction (Newcomb and Nelson 1973).

Acquired *cold urticaria* is usually a local urticarial response, beginning within minutes after challenge with cold water, ice, cold air and cold drinks or foods. The reaction may evolve into angio-oedema. Some patients may develop cold-induced hypotension, most often due to aquatic activities. The elicitation of an urticarial weal after the local application of ice is the easiest diagnostic test. The disease is most commonly idiopathic, but may be associated with the presence of cryoglobulins, vasculitis, infections and/or cold agglutinins. Passive transfer of cold urticaria to normal individuals can occur due to the presence in serum of IgE (Houser *et al.* 1970) or IgG anti-IgE autoantibodies (Gruber *et al.* 1988). In contrast to the acquired idiopathic form, the familial cold urticarias (Tindall *et al.* 1969; Soter *et al.* 1977) do not have an immunological mechanism.

In *solar urticaria*, sun exposure is followed within minutes by a weal-and-flare reaction, usually limited to areas of exposure. The lesions are typically confluent and resolve within half an hour to 3 hours. The reaction may be induced by various portions of the solar spectrum. Passive transfer experiments are often positive (Kojima *et al.* 1986) and are thought to be due to IgE transfer (Sams 1970). It has been suggested that patient sera contain photoallergen(s) which are activated upon irradiation (Horio 1978; Kojima *et al.* 1986). Interestingly, weals induced by wavelengths within the light spectrum causing urticaria may sometimes be inhibited by irradiation of the skin or serum with a significantly different, well-defined portion of the solar spectrum (Hasei and Ichihashi 1982; Leenutaphong *et al.* 1988). Most commonly, the irradiation causing inhibition must be given immediately after the urticaria-inducing exposure, suggesting that it inactivates or interferes with the action of the presumed photoallergen rather than its precursor (Horio *et al.* 1984).

Patients with *cholinergic urticaria* develop small (1–2 mm), pruritic, papular weals surrounded by extensive erythema, although the eruption may also appear as typical urticaria. The lesions develop after an increase in core body temperature, often as a result of exercise or a hot bath. The injection of cholinergic agents often reproduces the eruption while anticholinergic agents may prevent it. Passive transfer has been successfully accomplished (Illig and Heinicke 1967).

In the *exercise-induced anaphylactic syndrome*, urticaria and angio-oedema are accompanied by a range of anaphylactic symptoms. In contrast to cholinergic urticaria, the hives are usually larger than 1 cm in diameter, the reaction is independent of body temperature and it is not reproduced by cholinergic agonists (Casale *et al.* 1986).

In *localized heat urticaria*, local heat application causes lesions at the site of exposure, ranging from small papular weals with large flares to angio-oedema (Atkins and Zweiman 1981). Neither exercise nor increased core body temperature causes a similar reaction.

Vibratory angio-oedema can be precipitated by activities such as motor-cycling and lawn-mowing (Ting *et al.* 1983). There is typically an early oedematous component but angio-oedema may peak several hours after challenge and last up to 24 hours (Keahey *et al.* 1987).

Delayed pressure urticaria/angio-oedema typically occurs 4–6 hours after application of sustained or repeated pressure, for example after prolonged sitting or walking. Deep painful swelling and urticaria may occur together or separately, the intensity being related to the degree and duration of pressure applied (Estes and Yung 1981). Delayed dermatographism is commonly present (Dover *et al.* 1988). Associated malaise, arthralgias, chills, leucocytosis and elevated erythrocyte sedimentation rate may occur.

Morphological and biochemical analysis of mast cell activation has been extensively carried out in the physical urticarias, due to the ease with which these lesions can be reproduced. After provocative challenge, mast cell degranulation has been observed in many of the physical urticarias and may occur in ultrastructurally distinctive patterns, suggesting different mechanisms of degranulation (Murphy *et al.* 1987). Increased serum and/or skin levels of histamine have been demonstrated in each of the urticarias in this group (Casale *et al.* 1988).

In many of the physical urticarias, increased levels of other mast cell mediators have also been observed. For example, levels of prostaglandin D_2

(PGD_2), the major cyclo-oxygenase pathway product in cutaneous mast cells, increase after provocative challenge in cold (Heavey *et al.* 1986) and heat (Koro *et al.* 1986) urticarias. However, the concentrations measured are less than that required experimentally to induce erythema and oedema. Furthermore, PGD_2 causes only a very modest augmentation of experimental histamine-induced wealing (Maurice *et al.* 1987), although it may enhance the weal formation produced by intracutaneous injection of leukotriene B-4 (Soter *et al.* 1983). After cold challenge, increases in leukotriene E-4 (Maltby *et al.* 1989), platelet-activating factor (Grandel *et al.* 1985) and the platelet-derived mediator, platelet factor 4 (Wasserman and Ginsberg 1984), have also been observed, although the latter finding was not confirmed in a subsequent study (Ormerod *et al.* 1988). When injected into the skin, leukotrienes cause weal formation of longer duration than that induced by histamine or PGD_2 (Soter *et al.* 1983), but their relative pathogenic importance has not been determined. In delayed pressure urticaria, in which the lesions are of long duration, the leukotriene levels in skin exudates do not increase significantly (Lawlor *et al.* 1989).

Neutrophil and eosinophil chemotactic factors have also been observed in several of the physical urticarias (Soter *et al.* 1976b, 1980). Consistent with this observation, eosinophils and neutrophils have been observed histologically, usually in the absence of vasculitis. In addition, eosinophil major basic protein has been noted in the dermis of patients with pressure (Peters *et al.* 1987) and solar (Leiferman *et al.* 1989) urticarias. In chronological studies, a transition from a neutrophil-rich to a predominantly mononuclear infiltrate has been demonstrated in some cases of dermatographism (Winkelmann 1985) and pressure (Winkelmann *et al.* 1986) and solar (Norris *et al.* 1988) urticarias.

Non-immunological urticaria and angio-oedema

Aspirin often exacerbates urticaria. Patients may have similar reactions to a variety of other structurally unrelated cyclo-oxygenase inhibitors (Samter and Beers 1967) and lack anti-salicyloyl IgE antibodies (Krilis *et al.* 1981). Thus it is assumed that alterations in arachidonic acid metabolism may account for the urticaria (Szczeklik 1987). Rare cases may be due to a specific IgE mechanism (Blanca *et al.* 1989). Urticaria may also be aggravated by food additives, especially tartrazine. As with aspirin, this is probably not due to an allergic mechanism (Warin and Smith 1982).

A variety of other therapeutic agents can cause urticaria and angio-oedema in the absence of specific antibodies. For example, the intravenous use of *radiocontrast media* frequently results in a spectrum of anaphylactoid symptoms. It has been proposed that this may result from direct mast cell activation, but the mechanism remains uncertain (Greenberger and Patterson 1988). *Opiates*, *curare* and *polymyxin* are other examples of urticaria-inducing agents that directly degranulate mast cells. In addition, the *neuropeptides*, substance P, somatostatin and vasoactive intestinal peptide, can each induce direct degranulation of human cutaneous mast cells (Lowman *et al.* 1988). The electron microscopic observation that human skin mast cells may be found in direct contact with nerve-endings (Wiesner-Menzel *et al.* 1981) is consistent with the hypothesis that mast cell degranulation, and thus possibly urticaria, may be regulated in part by neural input (Foreman 1987). It should be noted, however, that mast cells, eosinophils, macrophages and lymphocytes also produce and release several peptide mediators identical or similar to these neuropeptides (Goetzl *et al.* 1988), complicating the interpretation of these experiments.

Most cases of *contact urticaria* are non-immunological. In contrast to IgE-mediated contact urticaria (discussed earlier), this type gives only a local reaction, develops in most exposed persons and occurs without prior exposure (Lahti and Maibach 1989). Common causes include benzoic acid, sorbic acid and cinnamic acid. In some cases, e.g. stinging nettle, the pathogenesis of the reaction may include direct inoculation of vasoactive substances into the dermis and/or direct mast cell activation (Saxena *et al.* 1965; Kulze and Greaves 1988).

Angiotensin-converting enzyme inhibitors such as captopril and enalapril are associated with angio-oedema in one in 1000 persons (Slater *et al.* 1988). These drugs interfere with the degradation of bradykinin and significantly increase the weal-and-flare reaction to intradermal injections of bradykinin (Fuller *et al.* 1987). Thus it has been postulated that the mechanism of this process may involve increased activity of the kallikrein–kinin system.

Idiopathic urticaria and angio-oedema

In most cases, a specific cause for urticaria is not found. Likewise, the pathogenesis of these cases is unknown. However, the observation of elevated skin histamine levels (Kaplan *et al.* 1978; Phanuphak *et al.* 1980) is consistent with a final common pathway of mast cell degranulation. While some patients have IgG anti-IgE autoantibodies, their functional importance in disease pathogenesis is unknown (Gruber *et al.* 1988). Releasability of mast cell mediators has been shown to be increased or decreased, depending on the particular releasing agent and its concentration (Brunet *et al.* 1988). Peripheral blood basophils may show decreased releasability (Greaves *et al.* 1974; Kern and Lichtenstein 1976), possibly due to a state of desensitization.

In the involved skin, mast cells may be increased in number (Natbony *et al.* 1983) while monocytes and a large percentage of T lymphocytes with variable ratios of helper and suppressor cell phenotyes are often present (Elias *et al.* 1986). As in the physical urticarias, some cases of chronic idiopathic urticaria may have a predominantly neutrophilic infiltrate in the absence of any evidence of vasculitis (Winkelmann *et al.* 1988). It is not clear how many of these represent early lesions that will subsequently develop a predominance of mononuclear cells. Eosinophil major basic protein has also been found in the dermis of these patients (Peters *et al.* 1983).

Miscellaneous causes of urticaria and angio-oedema

Certain diseases or syndromes that do not fit well in the above mechanism-based classification are included in this section.

Thyroid autoimmunity is found in urticaria/angio-oedema patients at a rate two to three times that of the normal population. These patients are distinguished by the severe, relentless course and the usual presence of angio-oedema (Leznoff and Sussman 1989). Patients are most commonly euthyroid, but may be hypothyroid or hyperthyroid.

Menses-associated urticaria occurs most often at the beginning of the menstrual period. It appears to be related to increased progesterone sensitivity (Farah and Shbaklu 1971), although the mechanism for this sensitivity is not understood (Slater and Kaliner 1987). One case of urticaria beginning at the end of menses associated with hypereosinophilia has been described. The hives and the eosinophilia were ameliorated by progesterone (Mittman *et al.* 1989).

A syndrome termed *episodic angio-oedema with eosinophilia* is characterized by recurrent attacks of angio-oedema, urticaria, fever, 10–18% weight gain and marked eosinophilia (Gleich *et al.* 1984). Similarly, about 10% of patients with the *hypereosinophilic syndrome* develop angio-oedema (Fauci *et al.* 1982). It has been postulated that eosinophil products may promote angio-oedema by direct mast cell activation. Support for this view is the observation that eosinophil major basic protein can activate rat mast cells (O'Donnell *et al.* 1983).

Patient evaluation

Underlying associated diseases should be sought by history and physical examination and should direct further laboratory evaluation. Screening laboratory procedures include a complete blood count with differential, urinalysis and erythrocyte sedimentation rate (ESR). Provocative tests in suspected physical urticarias should be performed. If the history or elevated ESR suggests urticarial vasculitis, a skin biopsy should be performed, which, if positive, should focus diagnostic effort on the known causes of urticarial vasculitis. Tests of thyroid function and anti-thyroid antibodies may be of value. Any suggestion of infection should be pursued, including stool examination for ova and parasites. Evaluation of the role of foods and food additives is difficult but involves elimination diets and double-blind challenges with suspected agents (Bock *et al.* 1988). When specific antigens are suspected of causing IgE-mediated urticaria, the use of prick skin testing or, in special circumstances, the radioallergosorbent test (RAST) may be of value.

Therapy

When a cause for urticaria cannot be identified and removed, treatment with H_1 antihistamines may cause substantial symptomatic improvement. In patients non-responsive to an H_1 antihistamine, the addition of an H_2 antihistamine is usually beneficial (Bleehen *et al.* 1987). The calcium channel antagonist nifedipine may be an effective adjunctive treatment in patients non-responsive to H_1 and H_2 antihistamines (Bressler *et al.* 1989). Finally, ketotifen (Kamide *et al.* 1989) and doxepin (Greene *et al.* 1985) may be more effective than some H_1 antihistamines. Aspirin and other non-steroidal anti-inflammatory drugs should be avoided due to their propensity to exacerbate urticaria.

In the physical urticarias, avoidance of the provoking stimulus is the ideal form of therapy. When this is impossible, induction of tolerance by repetitive exposure is sometimes successful in cold (Bentley-Phillips *et al.* 1976), solar (Ramsay 1977), heat (Leigh and Ramsay 1975), cholinergic and vibratory (Ting *et al.* 1983) urticarias. This approach, however, is often impractical due to the frequency of exposure required to maintain tolerance (Kobza Black *et al.* 1979). Many of the physical urticarias improve with H_1 antihistamines. Several double-blind studies have demonstrated the value of combined H_1 and H_2 antihistamine therapy in dermatographism (Matthews *et al.* 1979). Isolated cases of cold (Duc and Pecoud 1986) and solar (Irwin *et al.* 1985) urticarias have also been reported to respond to this combined therapy. Doxepin is also effective in cold urticaria (Neittaanmaki *et al.* 1984). In addition, ketotifen, which may act in part by preventing mast cell degranulation, may be effective in some types of physical urticarias (Huston *et al.* 1986). However, in delayed pressure urticaria, systemic steroids are usually required for disease management.

Allergic contact dermatitis

Clinical considerations

Allergic contact dermatitis (ACD) represents an altered acquired reactivity of the skin which is the result of exposure to a variety of allergens. This reaction may develop at any age but is less common in children and the elderly. It is responsible for common allergic skin diseases in man caused by contact with substances such as nickel, chromates, poison-ivy, topical medications, cosmetics and numerous other environmental and industrial chemicals. Sensitization can occur from 7 to 10 days after initial contact with a potent allergen or sensitizer but, more often, it may require repeated exposure to the allergen. Once contact allergy is established, and as long as it persists, subsequent encounters with the allergen will produce dermatitis within 24–48 hours. Some sensitivities, such as poison-ivy and poison-oak, may last most of the patient's life.

The first signs of ACD are redness, swelling and papulovesicle formation. These may burst and result in an acute weeping dermatitis. Intense pruritus is usual. Initially, the dermatitis is confined to the site of allergen contact and its distribution pattern may suggest its cause. In severe cases the dermatitis may spread to cover wide areas of the body. Once the reaction is initiated the intensity of the dermatitis increases for 4–7 days. The entire process may take a month or longer to resolve, although healing often occurs within 1–2 weeks. In the chronic phase, it may be very difficult to separate a possible irritant dermatitis from ACD, both clinically and histologically. In both cases the skin is pruritic and is red, thickened, scaly and fissured. Occasionally, ACD may have an urticarial appearance (discussed in the section 'Urticaria and angio-oedema'). Pre-existing skin disease may predispose to ACD, possibly by allowing easier access of sensitizing materials into the living portion of the epidermis. Resolution of ACD may be hastened by the use of topical or systemic steroids.

In North America, poison-ivy/oak is the most common clinical cause of ACD and is a frequent cause of occupational disability. Partial tolerance has been induced to these plants by prolonged oral ingestion of urushiol, the allergenic chemical. However, due to the side-effects and short duration of tolerance, this is not usually a practical approach (Epstein *et al.* 1982). A different strategy for prevention of poison-ivy/oak dermatitis involves the use of topical prophylaxis with barrier creams. Promising examples include the use of polyamine salts of a linoleic acid dimer (Orchard *et al.* 1986) and an organoclay preparation (Epstein 1989).

Diagnostic techniques

The technique of greatest value in the diagnosis of

ACD is the patch test. This is performed by applying both suspect allergens and screening batteries of known allergens to intact skin in an effort to reproduce the dermatitis at the test site. A positive test implies contact allergy to the tested substance. The test substance is prepared in non-irritating concentrations, mixed with appropriate vehicles and applied under semi-occlusive dressings.

Ready-to-use patch test systems of the most common allergens are being developed for commercial use. The one that has been the most widely tested is the thin-layer rapid-use epicutaneous test (TRUE test). This system incorporates standard allergens into a flexible, solid hydrophilic polymer (Fischer and Maibach 1989). It solves the problems of time-consuming application, uncertain dosage and uneven distribution that are common with traditional patch testing. However, interpretation of patch test results still remains difficult, particularly the differentiation of marginally irritant reactions from allergic reactions. In addition, strongly positive patch test reactions may sometimes cause other concomitantly tested, otherwise weakly reacting substances, to give false positive reactions (Bruynzeel and Maibach 1986). The presence of active dermatitis elsewhere on the body may do likewise, while the use of steroids at the time of testing may result in a false negative result. For this reason, patch testing should be performed when the dermatitis is quiescent and the patient is not using immunosuppressive medications.

A technique of supplemental value to patch testing is provocative usage testing (Fisher 1986). Suspect topical medications or cosmetics are applied twice daily for 1 week to a small area behind the ear or on antecubital or forearm skin. Development of dermatitis can provide evidence that a particular product is the cause of a dermatitis or can be used to provide confirmation of the accuracy of regular patch testing. This technique, however, does not determine which constituent of a given product is the relevant allergen. In addition, false negative reactions are common.

Pathophysiological mechanisms

Allergic contact dermatitis is an example of a type IV delayed hypersensitivity reaction. It can be divided into an inductive or sensitization phase when sensitivity is developed to an allergen and a later elicitation phase when re-exposure to the allergen causes development of clinically apparent skin disease. The Langerhans' cell (LC) is the antigen-presenting cell and the helper T lymphocyte is the principal effector cell.

In the *inductive or sensitization phase*, a small foreign substance (hapten) enters the epidermis, eventually gaining access to an LC. Numerous observations have confirmed the role of this cell in the sensitization phase of ACD. For example, purified hapten-coupled LC injected intravenously induce hapten-specific contact sensitization (Sullivan *et al.* 1986) while systemic introduction of hapten alone induces hapten-specific tolerance. Diminished LC number or function is also usually associated with induction of tolerance or diminished sensitization (Toews *et al.* 1980). Finally, hapten-modified LC are able to generate hapten-specific helper T cell lines *in vitro* (Hauser and Katz 1988). While activation of LC by hapten appears to be important in T cell activation (Kolde and Knop 1987), immunoelectron microscopic studies show that the actual uptake of hapten occurs in a passive, non-specific fashion by both LC and keratinocytes (Kolde and Knop 1988). This finding is in contrast with earlier histochemical observations that contact sensitizers have a specific affinity for LC (Shelley and Juhlin 1977).

After an allergen is processed by the LC, it is presented to a helper T lymphocyte, which must have receptors able to recognize the antigen as well as the immune response-associated marker (Ia/DR) present on the LC surface (Stingl *et al.* 1978). The T lymphocyte must also be activated by interleukin 1 (IL-1), a lymphokine secreted by LC (Sauder *et al.* 1984) and keratinocytes (Luger *et al.* 1981; Kupper *et al.* 1986). The activated T cell produces IL-2 allowing further amplification of the T cell response. The demonstration of antigen-bearing LC in dermal lymphatics and regional lymph nodes (Silberberg-Sinakin *et al.* 1976; Macatonia *et al.* 1987) suggests that antigen presentation may also occur in lymph nodes, where LC may change to the phenotype of the Ia-bearing dendritic cells of lymphoid organs (Schuler *et al.* 1985). Activated helper T lymphocytes then undergo further proliferation and propagation in regional lymph nodes, with release of memory and effector cells. These circulate to lymph nodes throughout the body.

The *elicitation phase* occurs after re-exposure

anywhere on the skin to an allergen that has previously induced sensitization. Within 4 hours after rechallenge with dinitrochlorobenzene, mast cell degranulation is observed around the venules of the superficial dermis (Lewis *et al.* 1989). The stimulus for this is unknown. It is likely that mast cells, through cytokine-dependent pathways, induce the appearance of endothelial leucocyte adhesion molecule 1 (ELAM-1), an endothelial antigen important for leucocyte adhesion to dermal venules (Klein *et al.* 1989).

Within 24–48 hours there is homing of antigen-specific as well as antigen-non-specific T cells from regional lymph nodes to the specific cutaneous areas of hapten exposure. Modulation of this inflammatory response occurs due to secretion of various cytokines. T cells may undergo further clonal expansion as a result of re-exposure to a Class II MHC-bearing antigen-presenting cell. While the evidence is not as certain as it is in the sensitization phase, this cell is probably an LC. Activation of this cell type is observed by electron microscopy during the elicitation phase (Kolde and Knop 1987).

Several *in situ* immunohistological studies of the elicitation phase have shown the lymphocytic dermal infiltrate to have a predominance of helper T cells (Wood *et al.* 1986) and the epidermal infiltrate to have a predominance of helper (Wood *et al.* 1986) or suppressor (Smolle *et al.* 1988) cells. Many of these lymphocytes express the activation markers HLA-DR and IL-2 receptor (Wood *et al.* 1986). In comparison, normal skin contains approximately equal small numbers of perivascular helper and suppressor cells in the dermis and mainly suppressor cells in the epidermis (Bos *et al.* 1987). Using an antigen-independent technique, T cells have been cloned from human skin undergoing positive patch test reactions to nickel. In agreement with the above immunohistological studies, most of the clones are CD4 +ve (helper) rather than CD8 +ve (suppressor). While 7–15% of the CD4 +ve CD8 −ve T lymphocyte clones proliferate only in response to nickel, none of the CD4 −ve CD8 +ve clones do so (Kapsenberg *et al.* 1987). This confirms a specific role for hapten-specific helper T cells in the elicitation phase of ACD. The observation in guinea-pigs that some of these cells may remain at sites of previous ACD reactions (Scheper *et al.* 1983) presumably accounts for the accelerated contact sensitivity observed in retest reactions or in flare-up at sites of previous dermatitis following systemic exposure to an antigen.

Acknowledgements

This work was supported by grant number AI20067 from the National Institutes of Health.

References

Agnello, V. (1986). Lupus diseases associated with hereditary and acquired deficiencies of complement. *Springer Semin. Immunopathol.* **9**, 161–78.

Ahmed, A.R. and Hombal, S.M. (1986). Cicatricial pemphigoid. *Int. J. Dermatol.* **25**, 90–6.

Ahmed, A.R., Konqui, A., Park, M.S., Tiwari, J.L. and Terasaki, P.I. (1984). DR antigens in bullous pemphigoid. *Arch. Dermatol.* **120**, 795.

Alexander, E.L. and Provost, T.T. (1983). Cutaneous manifestations of primary Sjögren's syndrome: a reflection of vasculitis and association with anti-RO(SSA) antibodies. *J. Invest. Dermatol.* **80**, 386–91.

Alexander, E.L., Provost, T.T., Sanders, M.E., Frank, M.M. and Joiner, K.A. (1988). Serum complement activation in central nervous system disease in Sjögren's syndrome. *Am. J. Med.* **85**, 513–18.

Anhalt, G.J., Bahn, C.F., Labib, R.S., Voorhees, J.J., Sugar, A. and Diaz, L.A. (1981). Pathogenic effects of bullous pemphigoid autoantibodies on rabbit corneal epithelium. *J. Clin. Invest.* **68**, 1097–101.

Anhalt, G.J., Labib, R.S., Voorhees, J.J., Beals, T.F. and Diaz, L.A. (1982). Induction of pemphigus in neonatal mice by passive transfer of IgG from patients with the disease. *N. Engl. J. Med.* **306**, 1189–96.

Anhalt, G.J., Till, G.O., Diaz, L.A., Labib, R.S., Patel, H.P. and Eaglstein, N.F. (1986). Defining the role of complement in experimental pemphigus vulgaris in mice. *J. Immunol.* **137**, 2835–40.

Armstrong, R.B., Horan, D.B. and Silvers, D.N. (1985) Leukocytoclastic vasculitis in urticaria induced by ultraviolet irradiation. *Arch. Dermatol.* **121**, 1145–8.

Atkins, P.C. and Zweiman, B. (1981). Mediator release in local heat urticaria. *J. Allergy Clin. Immunol.* **68**, 286–9.

Baba, T., Sonozaki, H., Seki, K., Uchiyama, M., Ikesawa, Y. and Torisu, M. (1976). An eosinophil chemotactic factor present in blister fluids of bullous pemphigoid patients. *J. Immunol.* **116**, 112–16.

Bang, D., Honma, T., Saito, T., Nakagawa, S., Ueki, H. and Lee, S. (1987). The pathogenesis of vascular changes in erythema nodosum-like lesions of Behçet's syndrome: an electron microscopic study. *Hum. Pathol.* **18**, 1172–9.

Barnett, M.L., Beutner, E.H. and Chorzelski, T.P. (1977). Organ culture studies of pemphigus antibodies. II. Ultrastructural comparison between acantholytic changes *in vitro* and human pemphigus lesions. *J. Invest. Dermatol.* **68**, 265–71.

Bean, S.F. and Jordon, R.E. (1974). Chronic nonhereditary blistering disease in children. *Arch. Dermatol.* **110**, 941–4.

Bentley-Phillips, C.B., Black, A.K. and Greaves, M.W. (1976). Induced tolerance in cold urticaria caused by cold-evoked histamine release. *Lancet* **ii**, 63–6.

Beutner, E.H. and Jordon, R.E. (1964). Demonstration of skin antibodies in sera of pemphigus vulgaris patients by indirect immunofluorescent staining. *Proc. Soc. Exp. Biol. Med.* **117**, 505–10.

Beutner, E.H., Lever, W.F., Witebsky, E., Jordon, R.E. and Chertock, B. (1965). Autoantibodies in pemphigus vulgaris: response to an intercellular substance of epidermis. *JAMA* **192**, 682–8.

Beutner, E.H., Chorzelski, T.P. and Jordon, R.E. (1970). *Autosensitization in Pemphigus and Bullous Pemphigoid*. Charles C. Thomas, Springfield, Illinois.

Beutner, E.H., Chorzelski, T.P., Kumar, V., Leonard, J. and Krasny, S. (1986). Sensitivity and specificity of IgA-class antiendomysial antibodies for dermatitis herpetiformis and findings relevant to their pathogenic significance. *J. Am. Acad. Dermatol.* **15**, 464–73.

Bhogal, B., Wojnarowska, F., Marsden, R.A., Das, A., Black, M.M. and McKee, P.H. (1987). Linear IgA bullous dermatosis of adults and children: an immunoelectron microscopic study. *Br. J. Dermatol.* **117**, 289–96.

Blanca, M., Perez, E., Garcia, J.J. *et al.* (1989). Angioedema and IgE antibodies to aspirin: a case report. *Ann. Allergy* **62**, 295–8.

Bleehen, S.S., Thomas, S.E., Greaves, M.W. *et al.* (1987). Cimetidine and chlorpheniramine in the treatment of chronic idiopathic urticaria: a multi-centre randomized double-blind study. *Br. J. Dermatol.* **117**, 81–8.

Bock, S.A., Sampson, H.A., Atkins, F.M. *et al.* (1988). Double-blind, placebo-controlled food challenge (DBPCFC) as an office procedure: a manual. *J. Allergy Clin. Immunol.* **82**, 986–97.

Boom, B.W., Out-Luiting, C.J., Baldwin, W.M., Westedt, M.-L., Daha, M.R. and Vermeer, B.-J. (1987). Membrane attack complex of complement in leukocytoclastic vasculitis of the skin: presence and possible pathogenetic role. *Arch. Dermatol.* **123**, 1192–5.

Boom, B.W., Mommaas, M., Daha, M.R. and Vermeer, B.-J. (1989). Complement-mediated endothelial cell damage in immune complex vasculitis of the skin: ultrastructural localization of the membrane attack complex. *J. Invest. Dermatol.* **89**, 68S–72S.

Borthwick, G.M., Holmes, R.C. and Stirrat, G.M. (1988). Abnormal expression of class II MHC antigens in placentae from patients with pemphigoid gestationis: analysis of class II MHC subregion product expression. *Placenta* **9**, 81–94.

Bos, J.D., Zonneveld, I., Das, P.K., Krieg, S.R., van der Loos, C.M. and Kapsenberg, M.L. (1987). The skin immune system (SIS): distribution and immunophenotype of lymphocyte subpopulations in normal human skin. *J. Invest. Dermatol.* **88**, 569–73.

Brasile, L., Kremer, J.M., Clarke, J.L. and Cerilli, J. (1989). Identification of an autoantibody to vascular endothelial cell-specific antigens in patients with systemic vasculitis. *Am. J. Med.* **87**, 74–80.

Braverman, I.M. (1970). The angiitides. In *Skin Signs of Systemic Disease*, p. 199, W.B. Saunders, Philadelphia.

Braverman, I.M. and Yen, A. (1975). Demonstration of immune complexes in spontaneous and histamine-induced lesions and in normal skin of patients with leukocytoclastic angiitis. *J. Invest. Dermatol.* **64**, 105–12.

Breathnach, S.M., Allen, R., Ward, A.M. and Greaves, M.W. (1983). Symptomatic dermographism: natural history, clinical features, laboratory investigations and response to therapy. *Clin. Exp. Dermatol.* **8**, 463–76.

Bressler, R.B., Sowell, K. and Huston, D.P. (1989). Therapy of chronic idiopathic urticaria with nifedipine: demonstration of beneficial effect in a double-blinded, placebo-controlled, crossover trial. *J. Allergy Clin. Immunol.* **83**, 756–63.

Brunet, C., Bedard, P.M. and Hebert, J. (1988). Analysis of compound 48/80-induced skin histamine release and leukotriene production in chronic urticaria. *J. Allergy Clin. Immunol.* **82**, 398–402.

Bruynzeel, D.P. and Maibach, H.I. (1986). Excited skin syndrome (angry back). *Arch. Dermatol.* **122**, 323–8.

Bulpitt, K.J. and Brahn, E. (1989). Systemic lupus erythematosus and concurrent cytomegalovirus vasculitis: diagnosis by antemortem skin biopsy. *J. Rheumatol.* **16**, 677–80.

Burke, W.A., Briggaman, R.A. and Gammon, W.R. (1986). Epidermolysis bullosa acquisita in a patient with multiple endocrinopathies syndrome. *Arch. Dermatol.* **122**, 187–9.

Callen, J.P. and Ekenstam, E. (1987). Cutaneous leukocytoclastic vasculitis: clinical experience in 44 patients. *South. Med. J.* **80**, 848–51.

Camisa, C. (1988). Vesiculobullous systemic lupus erythematosus. *J. Am. Acad. Dermatol.* **18**, 93–100.

Casale, T.B., Keahey, T.M. and Kaliner, M. (1986). Exercise-induced anaphylactic syndromes: insights into diagnostic and pathophysiologic features. *JAMA* **255**, 2049–53.

Casale, T.B., Sampson, H.A., Hanifin, J. *et al.* (1988). Guide to physical urticarias. *J. Allergy Clin. Immunol.* **82**, 758–63.

Chorzelski, T., Jablonska, S. and Blaszczyk, M. (1968). Immunopathological investigations in the Senear–Usher syndrome (coexistence of pemphigus and lupus erythematosus), *Br. J. Dermatol.* **80**, 211–17.

Chorzelski, T.P., Beutner, E.H., Sulej, J. *et al.* (1984). IgA anti-endomysium antibody: a new immunological marker of dermatitis herpetiformis and coeliac disease. *Br. J. Dermatol.* **111**, 395–402.

Chorzelski, T.P., Jablonska, S. and Beutner, E.H. (1987a). Relationship of autoimmunity to clinical findings in pemphigus. In *Immunopathology of the Skin*, ed. E.H. Beutner, T.P. Chorzelski and V. Kumar, pp. 249–68, John Wiley & Sons, New York.

Chorzelski, T.P., Jablonska, S. and Beutner, E.H. (1987b). Bullous pemphigoid: relationship of immunopathology to clinical findings. In *Immunopathology of the Skin*, ed. E.H. Beutner, T.P. Chorzelski and V. Kumar, pp. 337–54, John Wiley & Sons, New York.

Chorzelski, T.P., Jablonska, S., Beutner, E.H. and Wilson, B.D. (1987c). Linear IgA bullous dermatosis. In *Immunopathology of the Skin*, ed. E.H. Beutner, T.P. Chorzelski and V. Kumar, pp. 407–20, John Wiley & Sons, New York.

Clauvel, J.-P., Brouet, J.C., Danon, F., Leibowitch, M. and Seligmann, M. (1982). Chronic urticaria with monoclonal IgM — a report of five cases. *Clin. Immunol. Immunopathol.* **25**, 348–53.

Connolly, S.M. and Sander, H.M. (1987). Treatment of

epidermolysis bullosa acquisita with cyclosporine. *J. Am. Acad. Dermatol.* **16**, 890.

Copeman, P.W.M. and Ryan, T.J. (1970). Angiitis: the problems of classification of cutaneous angiitis with reference to histopathology and pathogenesis. *Br. J. Dermatol.* **82** (suppl. 5), 2–14.

Cowin, P., Kapprell, H.-P., Franke, W.W., Tamkun, J. and Hynes, R.O. (1986). Plakoglobin: a protein common to different kinds of intercellular adhering junctions. *Cell* **46**, 1063–73.

Cream, J.J., Gumpel, J.M. and Peachey, R.D.G. (1970). Schönlein–Henoch purpura in the adult: a study of 77 adults with anaphylactoid or Schönlein–Henoch purpura. *Quart. J. Med.* **39**, 461–84.

Crotty, C.P., DeRemee, R.A. and Winkelmann, R.K. (1981). Cutaneous clinicopathologic correlation of allergic granulomatosis. *J. Am. Acad. Dermatol.* **5**, 571–81.

Cunliffe, W.J. and Menon, I.S. (1971). The association between cutaneous vasculitis and decreased blood fibrinolytic activity. *Br. J. Dermatol.* **84**, 99–105.

Cunningham, T.J., Tait, B.D., Mathews, J.D. and Muirden, K.D. (1982). Clinical rheumatoid vasculitis associated with the B8 DR3 phenotype. *Rheumatol. Int.* **2**, 137–9.

Cupps, T.R. and Fauci, A.S. (1980). Wegener's granulomatosis. *Int. J. Dermatol.* **19**, 76–80.

Cupps, T.R. and Fauci, A.S. (1981). The vasculitides. In *Major Problems in Internal Medicine*, vol. XXI, pp. 26–49, W.B. Saunders Co., Philadelphia.

Dahl, M.V., Falk, R.J., Carpenter, R. and Michael, A.F. (1984). Deposition of the membrane attack complex of complement in bullous pemphigoid. *J. Invest. Dermatol.* **82**, 132–5.

David, M., Katzenelson, V., Hazaz, B., Ben-Chetrit, A. and Sandbank, M. (1989). Determination of IgG subclasses in patients with pemphigus with active disease and in remission. *Arch. Dermatol.* **125**, 787–90.

Degos, R. (1979). Malignant atrophic papulosis. *Br. J. Dermatol.* **100**, 21–35.

Diaz, L.A., Sampaio, S.A.P., Rivitti, E.A. *et al.* (1989). Endemic pemphigus foliaceus (fogo selvagem). II. Current and historic epidemiologic studies. *J. Invest. Dermatol.* **92**, 4–12.

Diaz-Perez, J.L. and Jordon, R.E. (1976). The complement system in bullous pemphigoid. IV. Chemotactic activity in blister fluid. *Clin. Immunol. Immunopathol.* **5**, 360–70.

Diaz-Perez, J.L. and Winkelmann, R.K. (1974). Cutaneous periarteritis nodosa. *Arch. Dermatol.* **110**, 407–14.

Dienstag, J.L., Rhodes, A.R., Bhan, A.K., Dvorak, A.M., Mihm, M.C., Jr and Wands, J.R. (1978). Urticaria associated with acute viral hepatitis type B: studies of pathogenesis. *Ann. Intern. Med.* **89**, 34–40.

Dover, J.S., Black, A.K., Ward, A.M. and Greaves, M.W. (1988). Delayed pressure urticaria: clinical features, laboratory investigations, and response to therapy of 44 patients. *J. Am. Acad. Dermatol.* **18**, 1289–98.

Duc, J. and Pecoud, A. (1986). Successful treatment of idiopathic cold urticaria with the association of H1 and H2 antagonists: a case report. *Ann. Allergy* **56**, 355–7.

Dvorak, A.M., Mihm, M.C., Jr, Osage, J.E., Kwan, T.H., Austen, K.F. and Wintroub, B.U. (1982). Bullous pemphigoid, an ultrastructural study of the inflammatory response: eosinophil, basophil and mast cell granule changes in multiple biopsies from one patient. *J. Invest. Dermatol.* **78**, 91–101.

Eady, R.A.J., Keahey, T.M., Sibbald, R.G. and Black, A.K. (1981). Cold urticaria with vasculitis: report of a case with light and electron microscopic, immunofluorescence and pharmacological studies. *Clin. Exp. Dermatol.* **6**, 355–66.

Eberhartinger, C. (1963). Das Problem des Erythema induratum bazin. *Arch. Klin. Exp. Dermatol.* **217**, 196–254.

Elias, J., Boss, E. and Kaplan, A.P. (1986). Studies of the cellular infiltrate of chronic idiopathic urticaria: prominence of T-lymphocytes, monocytes, and mast cells. *J. Allergy Clin. Immunol.* **78**, 914–18.

Epstein, W.L. (1989). Topical prevention of poison ivy/oak dermatitis. *Arch. Dermatol.* **125**, 499–501.

Epstein, W.L., Byers, V.S. and Frankart, W. (1982). Induction of antigen specific hyposensitization to poison oak in sensitized adults. *Arch. Dermatol* **118**, 630–3.

Estes, S.A. and Yung, C.W. (1981). Delayed pressure urticaria: an investigation of some parameters of lesion induction. *J. Am. Acad. Dermatol.* **5**, 25–31.

Eyre, R.W. and Stanley, J.R. (1987). Human autoantibodies against a desmosomal protein complex with a calcium-sensitive epitope are characteristic of pemphigus foliaceus patients. *J. Exp. Med.* **165**, 1719–24.

Eyre, R.W. and Stanley, J.R. (1988). Identification of pemphigus vulgaris antigen extracted from normal human epidermis and comparison with pemphigus foliaceus antigen. *J. Clin. Invest.* **81**, 807–12.

Farah, F.S. and Shbaklu, Z. (1971). Autoimmune progesterone urticaria. *J. Allergy Clin. Immunol.* **48**, 257–61.

Fauci, A.S., Haynes, B.F. and Katz, P. (1978). The spectrum of vasculitis: clinical, pathologic, immunologic, and therapeutic considerations. *Ann. Intern. Med.* **89**, 660–76.

Fauci, A.S., Harley, J.B., Roberts, W.C., Ferrans, V.J., Gralnick, H.R. and Bjornson, B.H. (1982). The idiopathic hypereosinophilic syndrome: clinical, pathophysiologic, and therapeutic considerations. *Ann. Intern. Med.* **97**, 78–92.

Fine, J.-D. (1985). Cicatricial pemphigoid, bullous pemphigoid, and epidermolysis bullosa acquisita antigens: differences in organ and species specificities and localization in chemically-separated human skin of three basement membrane antigens. *Collagen Relat. Res.* **5**, 369–77.

Fine, J.-D., Neises, G.R. and Katz, S.I. (1984). Immunofluorescence and immunoelectron microscopic studies in cicatricial pemphigoid. *J. Invest. Dermatol.* **82**, 39–43.

Fine, J.-D., Trying, S. and Gammon, W.R. (1989). The presence of intra-lamina lucida blister formation in epidermolysis bullosa acquisita: possible role of leukocytes. *J. Invest. Dermatol.* **92**, 27–32.

Fischer, T. and Maibach, H.I. (1989). Easier patch testing with TRUE test. *J. Am Acad. Dermatol.* **20**, 447–53.

Fisher, A.A. (1986). The role of patch testing. In *Contact Dermatitis*, 3rd edn, ed. A.A. Fisher, pp. 9–29, Lea and Febiger, Philadelphia.

Foreman, J.C. (1987). Neuropeptides and the pathogenesis of allergy. *Allergy* **42**, 1–11.

Fry, L., Keir, P., McMinn, R.M.H., Cowan, J.D. and Hoffbrand, A.V. (1967). Small-intestinal structure and function and haematological changes in dermatitis herpetiformis. *Lancet* **ii**, 729–733.

Fry, L., Leonard, J.N., Swain, F. *et al.* (1982). Long term follow-up of dermatitis herpetiformis with and without dietary gluten withdrawal. *Br. J. Dermatol.* **107**, 631–40.

Fuller, R.W., Warren, J.B., McCusker, M. and Dollery, C.T. (1987). Effect of enalapril on the skin response to bradykinin in man. *Br. J. Clin. Pharmacol.* **23**, 88–90.

Gabrielli, A., Marchegiani, G., Rupoli, S. *et al.* (1988). Assessment of disease activity in essential cryoglobulinemia by serum levels of a basement membrane antigen, laminin. *Arthritis Rheum.* **31**, 1558–62.

Gammon, W.R. (1987). Immune complex-mediated complement activation in bullous pemphigoid. *Clin. Dermatol.* **5**, 110–16.

Gammon, W.R. and Briggaman, R.A. (1987). Functional heterogeneity of immune complexes in epidermolysis bullosa acquisita. *J. Invest. Dermatol.* **89**, 478–83.

Gammon, W.R. and Briggaman, R.A. (1988). Absence of specific histologic changes in guinea pig skin treated with bullous pemphigoid antibodies. *J. Invest. Dermatol.* **90**, 495–500.

Gammon, W.R., Merritt, C.C., Lewis, D.M., Sams, W.M., Jr, Carlo, J.R. and Wheeler, C.E., Jr (1982). An *in vitro* model of immune complex-mediated basement membrane zone separation caused by pemphigoid antibodies, leukocytes, and complement. *J. Invest. Dermatol.* **78**, 285–90.

Gammon, W.R., Briggaman, R.A., Inman, A.O., Queen, L.L. and Wheeler, C.E. (1984a). Differentiating anti-lamina lucida and anti-sublamina densa anti-BMZ antibodies by indirect immunofluorescence in 1.0 M sodium chloride-separated skin. *J. Invest. Dermatol.* **82**, 139–44.

Gammon, W.R., Briggaman, R.A., Woodley, D.T., Heald, P.W. and Wheeler, C.E., Jr. (1984b). Epidermolysis bullosa acquisita — a pemphigoid-like disease. *J. Am. Acad. Dermatol.* **11**, 820–32.

Gammon, W.R., Inman, A.O., III and Wheeler, C.E., Jr. (1984c). Differences in complement-dependent chemotactic activity generated by bullous pemphigoid and epidermolysis bullosa acquisita immune complexes: demonstration by leukocytic attachment and organ culture methods. *J. Invest. Dermatol.* **83**, 57–61.

Gammon, W.R., Woodley, D.T., Dole, K.C. and Briggaman, R.A. (1985). Evidence that anti-basement membrane zone antibodies in bullous eruption of systemic lupus erythematosus recognize epidermolysis bullosa acquisita autoantigen. *J. Invest. Dermatol.* **84**, 472–6.

Gammon, W.R., Heise, E.R., Burke, W.A., Fine, J.-D., Woodley, D.T. and Briggaman, R.A. (1988). Increased frequency of HLA-DR2 in patients with autoantibodies to epidermolysis bullosa acquisita antigen: evidence that the expression of autoimmunity to type VII collagen is HLA Class II allele associated. *J. Invest. Dermatol.* **91**, 228–32.

Gibbs, R.B. and Minus, H.R. (1975). Epidermolysis bullosa acquisita with electron microscopical studies. *Arch. Dermatol.* **111**, 215–20.

Gladman, D.D. and Anhorn, K.A.B. (1986). HLA and disease manifestations in rheumatoid arthritis — a Canadian experience. *J. Rheumatol.* **13**, 274–6.

Glass, D., Soter, N.A., Gibson, D., Carpenter, C.B. and Schur, P.H. (1976). Association between HLA and cutaneous necrotizing venulitis. *Arthritis Rheum.* **19**, 945–9.

Gleich, G.J., Schroeter, A.L., Marcoux, J.P., Sachs, M.I., O'Connell, E.J. and Kohler, P.F. (1984). Episodic angioedema associated with eosinophilia. *N. Engl. J. Med.* **310**, 1621–6.

Goetzl, E.J., Sreedharan, S.P. and Harkonen, W.S. (1988). Pathogenetic roles of neuroimmunologic mediators. *Immunol. Allergy Clin. North Am.* **8**, 183–200.

Goldberg, J.W., Lee, M.L. and Sajjad, S.M. (1987). Giant cell arteritis of the skin simulating erythema nodosum. *Ann. Rheum. Dis.* **46**, 706–8.

Gower, R.G., Sams, W.M., Jr, Thorne, E.G., Kohler, P.F. and Claman, H.N. (1977). Leukocytoclastic vasculitis: sequential appearance of immunoreactants and cellular changes in serial biopsies. *J. Invest. Dermatol.* **69**, 477–84.

Gower, R.G., Sausker, W.F., Kohler, P.F., Thorne, G.E. and McIntosh, R.M. (1978) Small vessel vasculitis caused by hepatitis B virus immune complexes: small vessel vasculitis and HBsAG. *J. Allergy Clin Immunol.* **62**, 222–8.

Grandel, K.E., Farr, R.S., Wanderer, A.A., Eisenstadt, T.C. and Wasserman, S.I. (1985). Association of platelet-activating factor with primary acquired cold urticaria. *N. Engl. J. Med.* **313**, 405–9.

Greaves, M.W., Plummer, V.M., McLaughlan, P. and Stanworth, D.R. (1974). Serum and cell bound IgE in chronic urticaria. *Clin. Allergy* **4**, 265–71.

Greenberger, P.A. and Patterson, R. (1988). Adverse reactions to radiocontrast media. *Prog. Cardiovasc. Dis.* **31**, 239–48.

Greene, G.M., Lain, D., Sherwin, R.M., Wilson, J.E. and McManus, B.M. (1986). Giant cell arteritis of the legs: clinical isolation of severe disease with gangrene and amputations. *Am. J. Med.* **81**, 727–33.

Greene, S.L., Reed, C.E. and Schroeter, A.L. (1985). Double-blind crossover study comparing doxepin with diphenhydramine for the treatment of chronic urticaria. *J. Am. Acad. Dermatol.* **12**, 669–75.

Greer, J.M., Longley, S., Edwards, N.L., Elfenbein, G.J. and Panush, R.S. (1988). Vasculitis associated with malignancy: experience with 13 patients and literature review. *Medicine* **67**, 220–30.

Gruber, B.L., Baeza, M.L., Marchese, M.J., Agnello, V. and Kaplan, A.P. (1988). Prevalence and functional role of anti-IgE autoantibodies in urticarial syndromes. *J. Invest. Dermatol* **90**, 213–17.

Hall, R.P. and Lawley, T.J. (1985). Characterization of circulating and cutaneous IgA immune complexes in patients with dermatitis herpetiformis. *J. Immunol.* **135**, 1760–5.

Hall, R.P., Lawley, T.J., Smith, H.R. and Katz, S.I. (1982). Bullous eruption of systemic lupus erythematosus. *Ann. Intern. Med.* **97**, 165–70.

Hall, R.P., Sanders, M.E., Duquesnoy, R.J., Katz, S.I. and Shaw, S. (1989). Alterations in HLA-DP and HLA-DQ antigen frequency in patients with dermatitis herpetiformis. *J. Invest. Dermatol.* **93**, 501–5.

Halmepuro, L., Salvaggio, J.E. and Lehrer, S.B. (1987). Crawfish and lobster allergens: identification and structural similarities with other crustacea. *Int. Arch. Allergy Appl. Immunol.* **84**, 165–72.

Hasei, K. and Ichihashi, M. (1982). Solar urticaria: determinations of action and inhibition spectra. *Arch. Dermatol.* **118**, 346–50.

Hashimoto, K. and Lever, W.F. (1967). An electron microscopic study on pemphigus vulgaris of the mouth and the skin with special reference to the intercellular cement. *J. Invest. Dermatol.* **48**, 540–52.

Hashimoto, K., Shafran, K.M., Webber, P.S., Lazarus, G.S. and Singer, K.H. (1983). Anti-cell surface pemphigus autoantibody stimulates plasminogen activator activity of human epidermal cells: a mechanism for the loss of epidermal cohesion and blister formation. *J. Exp. Med.* **157**, 259–72.

Hashimoto, K., Wun, T.-C., Baird, J., Lazarus, G.S. and Jensen, P.J. (1989). Characterization of keratinocyte plasminogen activator inhibitors and demonstration of the prevention of pemphigus IgG-induced acantholysis by a purified plasminogen activator inhibitor. *J. Invest. Dermatol.* **92**, 310–15.

Hauser, C. and Katz, S.I. (1988). Activation and expansion of hapten- and protein-specific T helper cells from non-sensitized mice. *Proc. Nat. Acad. Sci. (USA)* **85**, 5625–8.

Heavey, D.J., Kobza-Black, A., Barrow, S.E., Chappell, C.G., Greaves, M.W. and Dollery, C.T. (1986). Prostaglandin D_2 and histamine release in cold urticaria. *J. Allergy Clin. Immunol.* **78**, 458–61.

Hertz, K.C., Katz, S.I., Maize, J. and Ackerman, A.B. (1976). Herpes gestationis: a clinicopathologic study. *Arch. Dermatol.* **112**, 1543–8.

Hitch, J.M. (1970). Dermatologic manifestations of giant-cell (temporal, cranial) arteritis. *Arch. Dermatol.* **101**, 409–15.

Holgate, S.T., Robinson, C. and Church, M.K. (1988). The contribution of mast cell mediators to acute allergic reactions in human skin and airways. *Allergy* **43** (suppl. 5), 22–31.

Holmes, R.C., Black, M.M., Jurecka, W. *et al.* (1983). Clues to the aetiology and pathogenesis of herpes gestationis. *Br. J. Dermatol.* **109**, 131–9.

Holubar, K., Wolff, K., Konrad, K. and Beutner, E.H. (1975). Ultrastructural localization of immunoglobulins in bullous pemphigoid skin. *J. Invest. Dermatol.* **64**, 220–7.

Horio, T. (1978). Photoallergic urticaria induced by visible light: additional cases and further studies. *Arch. Dermatol.* **114**, 1761–4.

Horio, T., Yoshioka, A. and Okamoto, H. (1984). Production and inhibition of solar urticaria by visible light exposure. *J. Am. Acad. Dermatol.* **11**, 1094–9.

Houser, D.D., Arbesman, C.E., Ito, K. and Wicher, K. (1970). Cold urticaria: immunologic studies. *Am. J. Med.* **49**, 23–33.

Huston, D.P., Bressler, R.B., Kaliner, M., Sowell, L.K. and Baylor, M.W. (1986). Prevention of mast-cell degranulation by ketotifen in patients with physical urticarias. *Ann. Intern. Med.* **104**, 507–10.

Illig, L. and Heinicke, A. (1967). Zur Pathogenese der cholinergischen Urticaria. IV. Zur Frage einer echten Antigen-Antikorperreaktion. *Arch. Klin. Exp. Dermatol.* **229**, 360–71.

Irwin, R.B., Lieberman, P., Friedman, M.M. *et al.* (1985). Mediator release in local heat urticaria: protection with combined H_1 and H_2 antagonists. *J. Allergy Clin. Immunol.* **76**, 35–9.

Iwatsuki, K., Takigawa, M., Imaizumi, S. and Yamada, M. (1989). *In vivo* binding site of pemphigus vulgaris antibodies and their fate during acantholysis. *J. Am. Acad. Dermatol.* **20**, 578–82.

Jablonska, S., Chorzelski, T., Blaszczyk, M. and Maciejewski, W. (1977). Pathogenesis of pemphigus erythematosus. *Arch. Dermatol. Res.* **258**, 135–40.

Jones, C.C., Hamilton, R.G. and Jordon, R.E. (1988). Subclass distribution of human IgG autoantibodies in pemphigus. *J. Clin. Immunol.* **8**, 43–9.

Jordan, J.M., Allen, N.B. and Pizzo, S.V. (1987). Defective release of tissue plasminogen activator in systemic and cutaneous vasculitis. *Am. J. Med.* **82**, 397–400.

Jordon, R.E. (1976). Complement activation in pemphigus and bullous pemphigoid. *J. Invest. Dermatol.* **67**, 366–71.

Jordon, R.E. (1980). Complement activation in pemphigus. *J. Invest. Dermatol.* **74**, 357–9.

Jordon, R.E., Triftshauser, C.T. and Schroeter, A.L. (1971). Direct immunofluorescent studies of pemphigus and bullous pemphigoid. *Arch. Dermatol.* **103**, 486–91.

Jordon, R.E., Day, N.K., Sams, W.M., Jr and Good, R.A. (1973). The complement system in bullous pemphigoid. I. Complement and component levels in sera and blister fluids. *J. Clin. Invest.* **52**, 1207–14.

Jordon, R.E., Schroeter, A.L., Good, R.A. and Day, N.K. (1975). The complement system in bullous pemphigoid. II. Immunofluorescent evidence for both classical and alternate-pathway activation. *Clin. Immunol. Immunopathol.* **3**, 307–14.

Jordon, R.E., Heine, K.G., Tappeiner, G., Bushkell, L.L. and Provost, T.T. (1976). The immunopathology of herpes gestationis: immunofluorescence studies and characterization of 'HG factor'. *J. Clin. Invest.* **57**, 1426–33.

Jorizzo, J.L., Hudson, R.D., Schmalstieg, F.C. *et al.* (1984). Behçet's syndrome: immune regulation, circulating immune complexes, neutrophil migration, and colchicine therapy. *J. Am. Acad. Dermatol.* **10**, 205–14.

Kagnoff, M.F., Austin, R.K., Hubert, J.J., Bernardin, J.E. and Kasarda, D.D. (1984). Possible role for a human adenovirus in the pathogenesis of celiac disease. *J. Exp. Med.* **160**, 1544–57.

Kamide, R., Niimura, M., Ueda, H. *et al.* (1989). Clinical evaluation of ketotifen for chronic urticaria: multicenter double-blind comparative study with clemastine. *Ann. Allergy* **62**, 322–5.

Kaplan, A.P., Horakova, Z. and Katz, S.I. (1978). Assessment of tissue fluid histamine levels in patients with urticaria. *J. Allergy Clin. Immunol.* **61**, 350–4.

Kapsenberg, M.L., Res, P., Bos, J.D., Schootemijer, A., Teunissen, M.B.M. and Schooten, W.V. (1987). Nickel-specific T lymphocyte clones derived from allergic nickel-contact dermatitis lesions in man: heterogeneity based on requirement of dendritic antigen-presenting cell subsets. *Eur. J. Immunol.* **17**, 861–5.

Katz, S.I., Hertz, K.C., Crawford, P.S., Gazze, L.A., Frank, M.M. and Lawley, T.J. (1976a). Effect of sulfones on complement deposition in dermatitis herpetiformis and on complement-mediated guinea-pig reactions. *J. Invest. Dermatol.* **67**, 688–90.

Katz, S.I., Hertz, K.C. and Yaoita, H. (1976b). Herpes gestationis: immunopathology and characterization of the HG factor. *J. Clin. Invest.* **57**, 1434–41.

Katz, S.I., Gallin, J.I., Hertz, K.C., Fauci, A.S. and Lawley, T.J. (1977a). Erythema elevatum diutinum: skin and systemic manifestations, immunologic studies, and successful treatment with dapsone. *Medicine* **56**, 443–55.

Katz, S.I., Hertz, K.C., Rogentine, G.N. and Strober, W. (1977b). HLA-B8 and dermatitis herpetiformis in patients with IgA deposits in skin. *Arch. Dermatol.* **113**, 155–6.

Kawana, S., Geoghegan, W.D. and Jordon, R.E. (1985). Complement fixation by pemphigus antibody. II. Complement enhanced detachment of epidermal cells. *Clin. Exp. Immunol.* **61**, 517–25.

Kawana, S., Geoghegan, W.D., Jordon, R.E. and Nishiyama, S. (1989). Deposition of the membrane attack complex of complement in pemphigus vulgaris and pemphigus foliaceus skin. *J. Invest. Dermatol.* **92**, 588–92.

Keahey, T.M., Indrisano, J., Lavker, R.M. and Kaliner, M.A. (1987). Delayed vibratory angioedema: insights into pathophysiologic mechanisms. *J. Allergy Clin. Immunol.* **80**, 831–8.

Keene, D.R., Sakai, L.Y., Lunstrum, G.P., Morris, N.P. and Burgeson, R.E. (1987). Type VII collagen forms an extended network of anchoring fibrils. *J. Cell Biol.* **104**, 611–21.

Kelly, S.E. and Wojnarowska, F. (1988). The use of chemically split tissue in the detection of circulating anti-basement membrane zone antibodies in bullous pemphigoid and cicatricial pemphigoid. *Br. J. Dermatol.* **118**, 31–40.

Kelly, S.E., Bhogal, B.S., Wojnarowska, F. and Black, M.M. (1988). Expression of a pemphigoid gestationis-related antigen by human placenta. *Br. J. Dermatol.* **118**, 605–11.

Kelly, S.E., Cerio, R., Bhogal, B.S. and Black, M.M. (1989a). The distribution of IgG subclasses in pemphigoid gestationis: PG factor is an IgG1 autoantibody. *J. Invest. Dermatol.* **92**, 695–8.

Kelly, S.E., Fleming, S., Bhogal, B.S., Wojnarowska, F. and Black, M.M. (1989b). Immunopathology of the placenta in pemphigoid gestationis and linear IgA disease. *Br. J. Dermatol.* **120**, 735–43.

Kern, F. and Lichtenstein, L.M. (1976). Defective histamine release in chronic urticaria. *J. Clin. Invest.* **57**, 1369–77.

Klein, L.M., Lavker, R.M., Matis, W.L. and Murphy, G.F. (1989). Degranulation of human mast cells induces an endothelial antigen central to leukocyte adhesion. *Proc. Nat. Acad. Sci. (USA)* **86**, 8972–6.

Klein, R.G., Hunder, G.G., Stanson, A.W. and Sheps, S.G. (1975). Large artery involvement in giant cell (temporal) arteritis. *Ann. Intern. Med.* **83**, 806–12.

Kobza Black, A., Sibbald, R.B. and Greaves, M.W. (1979). Cold urticaria treated by induction of tolerance. *Lancet* **ii**, 964.

Kojima, M., Horiko, T., Nakamura, Y. and Aoki, T. (1986). Solar urticaria: the relationship of photoallergen and action spectrum. *Arch. Dermatol.* **122**, 550–5.

Kolde, G. and Knop, J. (1987). Different cellular reaction patterns of epidermal Langerhans cells after application of contact sensitizing, toxic, and tolerogenic compounds: a comparative ultrastructural and morphometric time-course analysis. *J. Invest. Dermatol.* **89**, 19–23.

Kolde, G. and Knop, J. (1988). Ultrastructural localization of 2,4-dinitrophenyl groups in mouse epidermis following skin painting with 2,4-dinitrofluorobenzene and 2,4-dinitrothiocyanatebenzene: an immunoelectron microscopical study. *J. Invest. Dermatol.* **90**, 320–4.

Korman, N.J., Eyre, R.W., Klaus-Kovtun, V. and Stanley, J.R. (1989). Demonstration of an adhering-junction molecule (plakoglobin) in the autoantigens of pemphigus foliaceus and pemphigus vulgaris. *N. Engl. J. Med.* **321**, 631–5.

Koro, O., Dover, J.S., Francis, D.M. *et al.* (1986). Release of prostaglandin D_2 and histamine in a case of localized heat urticaria, and effect of treatments. *Br. J. Dermatol.* **115**, 721–8.

Krasny, S.A., Beutner, E.H. and Chorzelski, T.P. (1987). Specificity and sensitivity of indirect and direct immunofluorescent findings in the diagnosis of pemphigus. In *Immunopathology of the Skin*, ed. E.H. Beutner, T.P. Chorzelski and V. Kumar, pp. 207–47, John Wiley & Sons, New York.

Krilis, S., Gregson, R.P., Basten, A. and Baldo, B.A. (1981). Investigation of the possible involvement of IgE anti-salicyloyl antibodies in patients with urticaria. *Int. Arch. Allergy Appl. Immunol.* **64**, 293–301.

Kulze, A. and Greaves, M. (1988). Contact urticaria caused by stinging nettles. *Br. J. Dermatol.* **119**, 269–70.

Kumar, V., Hemedinger, E., Chorzelski, T.P., Beutner, E.H., Valeski, J.E. and Kowalewski, C. (1987). Reticulin and endomysial antibodies in bullous diseases. *Arch. Dermatol.* **123**, 1179–82.

Kupper, T.S., Ballard, D.W., Chua, A.O. *et al.* (1986). Human keratinocytes contain mRNA indistinguishable from monocyte interleukin 1α and βmRNA: keratino-cyte epidermal cell-derived thymocyte-activating factor is identical to interleukin 1. *J. Exp. Med.* **164**, 2095–100.

Labib, R.S., Anhalt, G.J., Patel, H.P., Mutasim, D.F. and Diaz, L.A. (1986). Molecular heterogeneity of the bullous pemphigoid antigens as detected by immunoblotting. *J. Immunol.* **136**, 1231–5.

Lahti, A. and Maibach, H.I. (1989). Immediate contact reactions. *Immunol. Allergy Clin. North Am.* **9**, 463–78.

Lawley, T.J., Stingl, G. and Katz, S.I. (1978). Fetal and maternal risk factors in herpes gestationis. *Arch. Dermatol.* **114**, 552–5.

Lawley, T.J., Strober, W., Yaoita, H. and Katz, S.I. (1980). Small intestinal biopsies and HLA types in dermatitis herpetiformis patients with granular and linear IgA skin deposits. *J. Invest. Dermatol.* **74**, 9–12.

Lawlor, F., Barr, R., Kobza-Black, A., Cromwell, O., Isaacs, J. and Greaves, M. (1989). Arachidonic acid transformation is not stimulated in delayed pressure urticaria. *Br. J. Dermatol.* **121**, 317–21.

Leavitt, R.Y. and Fauci, A.S. (1986). Polyangiitis overlap syndrome: classification and prospective clinical experience. *Am. J. Med.* **81**, 79–85.

Leenutaphong, V., von Kries, R., Plewig, G. and Holze, E. (1988). Solar urticaria induced by visible light and inhibited by UVA. *Photodermatology* **5**, 170–4.

Leiferman, K.M., Norris, P.G., Murphy, G.M., Hawk, J.L.M. and Winkelmann, R.K. (1989). Evidence for eosinophil degranulation with deposition of granule major basic protein in solar urticaria. *J. Am. Acad. Dermatol.* **21**, 75–80.

Leigh, I.M. and Ramsay, C.A. (1975). Localized heat urticaria treated by inducing tolerance to heat. *Br. J. Dermatol.* **92**, 191–4.

Leonard, J.N., Haffenden, G.P., Ring, N.P. *et al.* (1982). Linear IgA disease in adults. *Br. J. Dermatol.* **107**, 301–16.

Leonard, J.N., Haffenden, G.P., Tucker, W. *et al.* (1983). Gluten challenge in dermatitis herpetiformis. *N. Engl. J. Med.* **308**, 816–19.

Leonard, J.N., Wright, P., Williams, D.M. *et al.* (1984). The relationship between linear IgA disease and benign mucous membrane pemphigoid. *Br. J. Dermatol.* **110**, 307–14.

Leonard, J.N., Griffiths, C.E.M., Powles, A.V., Haffenden, G.P. and Fry, L. (1987). Experience with a gluten free diet in the treatment of linear IgA disease. *Acta Dermatol. Venereol. (Stockholm)* **67**, 145–8.

Lever, W.F. (1965). *Pemphigus and Pemphigoid*. Charles C. Thomas, Springfield, Illinois.

Levo, Y., Gorevic, P.D., Kassab, H.J., Zucker-Franklin, D. and Franklin, E.C. (1977). Association between hepatitis B virus and essential mixed cryoglobulinemia. *N. Engl. J. Med.* **296**, 1501–4.

Lewis, R.E., Buchsbaum, M., Whitaker, D. and Murphy, G.F. (1989). Intercellular adhesion molecule expression in the evolving human cutaneous delayed hypersensitivity reaction. *J. Invest. Dermatol.* **93**, 672–7.

Leznoff, A. and Sussman, G.L. (1989). Syndrome of idiopathic chronic urticaria and angioedema with thyroid autoimmunity: a study of 90 patients. *J. Allergy Clin. Immunol.* **84**, 66–71.

Lie, J.T. (1989). Systemic and isolated vasculitis: a rational approach to classification and pathologic diagnosis. *Pathol. Ann.* **24**, 25–114.

Lockwood, C.M., Jones, S., Moss, D.W., Bakes, D., Whitaker, K.B. and Savage, C.O.S. (1987). Association of alkaline phosphatase with an autoantigen recognised by circulating antineutrophil antibodies in systemic vasculitis. *Lancet* **i**, 716–20.

Lowman, M.A., Benyon, R.C. and Church, M.K. (1988). Characterization of neuropeptide-induced histamine release from human dispersed skin mast cells. *Br. J. Pharmacol.* **95**, 121–30.

Luger, T.A., Stadler, B.M., Katz, S.I. and Oppenheim, J.J. (1981). Epidermal cell (keratinocyte)-derived thymocyte-activating factor. *J. Immunol.* **127**, 1493–8.

Macatonia, S.E., Knight, S.C., Edwards, A.J., Griffiths, S. and Fryer, P. (1987). Localization of antigen on lymph node dendritic cells after exposure to the contact sensitizer fluorescein isothiocyanate: functional and morphological studies. *J. Exp. Med.* **166**, 1654–67.

McDuffie, F.C., Sams, W.M., Jr, Maldonado, J.E., Andreini, P.H., Conn, D.L. and Samayoa, E.A. (1973). Hypocomplementemia with cutaneous vasculitis and arthritis: possible immune complex syndrome. *Mayo Clin. Proc.* **48**, 340–8.

Maltby, N.H., Ind, P.W., Causon, R.C., Fuller, R.W. and Taylor, G.W. (1989). Leukotriene E_4 release in cold urticaria. *Clin. Exp. Allergy* **19**, 33–6.

Marder, R.J., Burch, F.X., Schmid, F.R., Zeiss, C.R. and Gewurz, H. (1978). Low molecular weight C1q-precipitins in hypocomplementemic vasculitis-urticaria syndrome: partial purification and characterization as immunoglobulin, *J. Immunol.* **121**, 613–18.

Marks, J., Shuster, S. and Watson, A.J. (1966). Small-bowel changes in dermatitis herpetiformis. *Lancet* **ii**, 1280–2.

Matthews, C.N.A., Boss, J.M., Warin, R.P. and Storari, F. (1979). The effect of H_1 and H_2 histamine antagonists on symptomatic dermographism. *Br. J. Dermatol.* **101**, 57–61.

Maurice, P.D.L., Barr, R.M., Koro, O. and Greaves, M.W. (1987). The effect of prostaglandin D_2 on the response of human skin to histamine. *J. Invest. Dermatol.* **89**, 245–8.

Milstone, L.M., Braverman, I.M., Lucky, P. and Fleckman, P. (1983). Classification and therapy of atrophie blanche. *Arch. Dermatol.* **119**, 963–9.

Mittman, R.J., Bernstein, D.I., Steinberg, D.R., Enrione, M. and Bernstein, I.L. (1989). Progesterone-responsive urticaria and eosinophilia. *J. Allergy Clin. Immunol.* **84**, 304–10.

Mobacken, H., Kastrup, W., Ljunghall, K. *et al.* (1983). Linear IgA dermatosis: a study of ten adult patients. *Acta Dermatol. Venereol. (Stockholm)* **63**, 123–8.

Molina, R., Provost, T.T. and Alexander, E.L. (1985). Two types of inflammatory vascular disease in Sjögren's syndrome: differential association with seroreactivity to rheumatoid factor and antibodies to Ro (SS-A) and with hypocomplementemia. *Arthritis Rheum.* **28**, 1251–8.

Monroe, E.W. (1981). Urticarial vasculitis: an updated review. *J. Am. Acad. Dermatol.* **5**, 88–95.

Morioka, S., Lazarus, G.S. and Jensen, P.J. (1987). Involvement of urokinase-type plasminogen activator in acantholysis induced by pemphigus IgG. *J. Invest. Dermatol.* **89**, 474–7.

Morrison, L.H., Labib, R.S., Zone, J.J. Diaz, L.A. and Anhalt, G.J. (1988). Herpes gestationis autoantibodies recognize a 180-kD human epidermal antigen. *J. Clin. Invest.* **81**, 2023–6.

Mueller, S., Klaus-Kovtun, V. and Stanley, J.R. (1989). A 230-kD basic protein is the major bullous pemphigoid antigen. *J. Invest. Dermatol.* **92**, 33–8.

Murphy, G.F., Austen, K.F., Fonferko, E. and Sheffer, A.L. (1987). Morphologically distinctive forms of cutaneous mast cell degranulation induced by cold and mechanical stimuli: an ultrastructural study. *J. Allergy Clin. Immunol.* **80**, 603–11.

Mutasim, D.F., Takahashi, Y., Labib, R.S., Anhalt, G.J., Patel, H.P. and Diaz, L.A. (1985). A pool of bullous pemphigoid antigen(s) is intracellular and associated with the basal cell cytoskeleton–hemidesmosome complex. *J. Invest. Dermatol.* **84**, 47–53.

Mutasim, D.F., Morrison, L.H., Takahashi, Y. *et al.* (1989). Definition of bullous pemphigoid antibody binding to intracellular and extracellular antigen associated with hemidesmosomes. *J. Invest. Dermatol.* **92**, 225–30.

Naito, K., Morioka, S. and Ogawa, H. (1982). The pathogenic mechanisms of blister formation in bullous pemphigoid. *J. Invest. Dermatol.* **79**, 303–6.

Naito, K., Morioka, S., Ikeda, S. and Ogawa, H. (1984). Experimental bullous pemphigoid in guinea pigs: the role of pemphigoid antibodies, complement, and migrating cells. *J. Invest. Dermatol.* **82**, 227–30.

Natbony, S.F., Phillips, M.E., Elias, J.M., Godfrey, H.P. and Kaplan, A.P. (1983). Histologic studies of chronic idiopathic urticaria. *J. Allergy Clin. Immunol.* **71**, 177–83.

Neittaanmaki, H., Myohanen, T. and Fraki, J.E. (1984). Comparison of cinnarizine, cyproheptadine, doxepin, and hydroxyzine in treatment of idiopathic cold urticaria: usefulness of doxepin. *J. Am. Acad. Dermatol.* **11**, 483–9.

Newcomb, R.W. and Nelson, H. (1973). Dermographia mediated by immunoglobulin E. *Am. J. Med.* **54**, 174–80.

Norris, P.G., Murphy, G.M., Hawk, J.L.M. and Winkelmann, R.K. (1988). A histological study of the evolution of solar urticaria. *Arch. Dermatol.* **124**, 80–3.

O'Donnell, M.C., Ackerman, S.J., Gleich, G.J. and Thomas, L.L. (1983). Activation of basophil and mast cell histamine release by eosinophil granule major basic protein. *J. Exp. Med.* **157**, 1981–91.

O'Duffy, J.D., Carney, J.A. and Deodhar, S. (1971). Behçet's disease: report of 10 cases, 3 with new manifestations. *Ann. Intern. Med.* **75**, 561–70.

Olansky, A.J., Briggaman, R.A., Gammon, W.R., Kelly, T.F. and Sams, W.M., Jr (1982). Bullous systemic lupus erythematosus.

J. Am. Acad. Dermatol. **7**, 511–20.

Orchard, S., Fellman, J.H. and Storrs, F.J. (1986). Poison ivy/oak dermatitis: use of polyamine salts of a linoleic acid dimer for topical prophylaxis. *Arch. Dermatol.* **122**, 783–9.

Ormerod, A.D., Kobza Black, A., Dawes, J. *et al.* (1988). Prostaglandin D_2 and histamine release in cold urticaria unaccompanied by evidence of platelet activation. *J. Allergy Clin. Immunol.* **82**, 586–9.

Ortonne, J.-P., Hsi, B.-L., Verrando, P. *et al.* (1987). Herpes gestationis factor reacts with the amniotic epithelial basement membrane. *Br. J. Dermatol.* **117**, 147–54.

Pehamberger, H., Gschnait, F., Menzel, J. and Holubar, K. (1979). Failure to detect gliadin or gliadin binding sites in the skin of patients with dermatitis herpetiformis: immunofluorescence, organ culture and autoradiographic studies. *J. Invest. Dermatol.* **73**, 174–5.

Perniciaro, C.V., Winkelmann, R.K. and Hunder, G.G. (1987). Cutaneous manifestations of Takayasu's arteritis: a clinicopathologic correlation. *J. Am. Acad. Dermatol.* **17**, 998–1005.

Peters, M.S. and Rogers, R.S., III (1989). Clinical correlations of linear IgA deposition at the cutaneous basement membrane zone. *J. Am. Acad. Dermatol.* **20**, 761–70.

Peters, M.S., Schroeter, A.L., Kephart, G.M. and Gleich, G.J. (1983). Localization of eosinophil granule major basic protein in chronic urticaria. *J. Invest. Dermatol.* **81**, 39–43.

Peters, M.S., Winkelmann, R.K., Greaves, M.W., Kephart, G.M. and Gleich, G.J. (1987). Extracellular deposition of eosinophil granule major basic protein in pressure urticaria. *J. Am. Acad. Dermatol.* **16**, 513–17.

Peterson, L.L. and Wuepper, K.D. (1984). Isolation and purification of a pemphigus vulgaris antigen from human epidermis. *J. Clin. Invest.* **73**, 1113–20.

Petzl-Erler, M.L. and Santamaria, J. (1988). Are HLA class II genes controlling susceptibility and resistance to Brazilian pemphigus foliaceus (fogo selvagem)? *Tissue Antigens* **33**, 408–14.

Phanuphak, P., Schocket, A.L., Arroyave, C.M. and Kohler, P.F. (1980). Skin histamine in chronic urticaria. *J. Allergy Clin. Immunol.* **65**, 371–5.

Piette, W.W. and Stone, M.S. (1989). A cutaneous sign of IgA-associated small dermal vessel leukocytoclastic vasculitis in adults (Henoch–Schönlein purpura). *Arch. Dermatol.* **125**, 53–6.

Prost, C., De Leca, A.C., Combemale, P. *et al.* (1989). Diagnosis of adult linear IgA dermatosis by immunoelectronmicroscopy in 16 patients with linear IgA deposits. *J. Invest. Dermatol.* **92**, 39–45.

Provost, T.T. and Tomasi, T.B., Jr (1973). Evidence for complement activation via the alternate pathway in skin diseases. I. Herpes gestationis, systemic lupus erythematosus, and bullous pemphigoid. *J. Clin. Invest.* **52**, 1779–87.

Provost, T.T. and Tomasi, T.B., Jr (1974). Evidence for the activation of complement via the alternate pathway in skin diseases. II. Dermatitis herpetiformis. *Clin. Immunol. Immunopathol.* **3**, 178–86.

Provost, T.T., Zone, J.J., Synkowski, D., Maddison, P.J. and Reichlin, M. (1980). Unusual cutaneous manifestations of systemic lupus erythematosus. I. Urticaria-like lesions: correlation with clinical and serological abnormalities. *J. Invest. Dermatol.* **75**, 495–9.

Raab, B., Fretzin, D.F., Bronson, D.M., Scott, M.J., Roenigk, H.H., Jr and Medenica, M. (1983). Epidermolysis bullosa acquisita and inflammatory bowel disease. *JAMA* **250**, 1746–8.

Ramsay, C.A. (1977). Solar urticaria treatment by inducing tolerance to artificial radiation and natural light. *Arch. Dermatol.* **113**, 1222–5.

Rea, T.H. and Ridley, D.S. (1979). Lucio's phenomenon: a comparative histological study. *Int. J. Leprosy* **47**, 161–6.

Reunala, T., Chorzelski, T.P., Viander, M. *et al.* (1987). IgA anti-endomysial antibodies in dermatitis herpetiformis: correlation with jejunal morphology, gluten-free diet and anti-gliadin antibodies. *Br. J. Dermatol.* **117**, 185–91.

Richter, B.J. and McNutt, N.S. (1979). The spectrum of epidermolysis bullosa acquisita. *Arch. Dermatol.* **115**, 1325–8.

Roat, M.I., Sossi, G., Lo, C. and Thoft, R.A. (1989). Hyperproliferation of conjunctival fibroblasts from patients with cicatricial pemphigoid. *Arch. Ophthalmol.* **107**, 1064–7.

Rock, B., Martins, C.R., Theofilopoulos, A.N. *et al.* (1989). The pathogenic effect of IgG4 autoantibodies in endemic pemphigus foliaceus (fogo selvagem). *N. Engl. J. Med.* **320**, 1463–9.

Roscoe, J.T., Anhalt, G.J., Patel, H. and Diaz, L.A. (1987). Recent advances in passive transfer studies of bullous diseases. In *Immunopathology of the Skin*, ed. E.H. Beutner, T.P. Chorzelski and V. Kumar, pp. 281–94, John Wiley & Sons, New York.

Rubenstein, R., Esterly, N.B. and Fine, J.-D. (1987). Childhood epidermolysis bullosa acquisita. *Arch. Dermatol.* **123**, 772–6.

Sachs, J.A., Awad, J., McCloskey, D. *et al.* (1986). Different HLA associated gene combinations contribute to susceptibility for coeliac disease and dermatitis herpetiformis. *Gut* **27**, 515–20.

Sachs, J.A., Leonard, J., Awad, J. *et al.* (1988). A comparative serological and molecular study of linear IgA disease and dermatitis herpetiformis. *Br. J. Dermatol.* **118**, 759–64.

Sams, W.M., Jr (1970). Solar urticaria: studies of the active serum factor. *J. Allergy* **45**, 295–301.

Sams, W.M., Jr, Claman, H.N., Kohler, P.F., McIntosh, R.M., Small, P. and Mass, M.F. (1975). Human necrotizing vasculitis: immunoglobulins and complement in vessel walls of cutaneous lesions and normal skin. *J. Invest. Dermatol.* **64**, 441–5.

Sams, W.M., Jr and Jordon, R.E. (1971). Correlation of pemphigoid and pemphigus antibody titres with activity of disease. *Br. J. Dermatol.* **84**, 7–13.

Samter, M. and Beers, R.J., Jr (1967). Concerning the nature of intolerance to aspirin. *J. Allergy* **40**, 281–93.

Sanchez, N.P., Winkelmann, R.K., Schroeter, A.L. and Dicken, C.H. (1982). The clinical and histopathologic spectrums of urticarial vasculitis: study of forty cases. *J. Am. Acad. Dermatol.* **7**, 599–605.

Sauder, D.N., Dinarello, C.A. and Morhenn, V.B. (1984). Langerhans cell production of interleukin-1. *J. Invest. Dermatol.* **82**, 605–7.

Saulsbury, F.T. (1987). The role of IgA_1 rheumatoid factor in the formation of IgA-containing immune complexes in Henoch-Schonlein purpura. *J. Clin. Lab. Immunol.* **23**, 123–7.

Savage, C.O.S. (1989). Microscopic polyarteritis: definition and relation to Wegener's granulomatosis. *APMIS* **6** (suppl.), 8–9.

Savage, C.O.S., Winearls, C.G., Evans, D.J., Rees, A.J. and

Lockwood, C.M. (1985). Microscopic polyarteritis: presentation, pathology and prognosis. *Quart. J. Med.* **56**, 467–83.

Savage, C.O.S., Tizard, J., Jayne, D., Lockwood, C.M. and Dillon, M.J. (1989). Antineutrophil cytoplasm antibodies in Kawasaki disease. *Arch. Dis. Child.* **64**, 360–3.

Saxena, P.R., Pant, M.C., Kishor, K. and Bhargava, K.P. (1965). Identification of pharmacologically active substances in the Indian stinging nettle, urtica parviflora (ROXB). *Can. J. Physiol. Pharmacol.* **43**, 869–76.

Scharf, S.J., Friedmann, A., Brautbar, C. *et al.* (1988). HLA class II allelic variation and susceptibility to pemphigus vulgaris. *Proc. Nat. Acad. Sci. (USA)* **85**, 3504–8.

Scheper, R.J., von Blomberg, M., Boerrigter, G.H., Bruynzeel, D., van Dinther, A. and Vos, A. (1983). Induction of immunological memory in the skin: role of local T cell retention. *Clin. Exp. Immunol.* **51**, 141–8.

Schiltz, J.R. and Michel, B. (1976). Production of epidermal acantholysis in normal human skin *in vitro* by the IgG fraction from pemphigus serum. *J. Invest. Dermatol.* **67**, 254–60.

Schmidt, A.P., Taswell, H.F. and Gleich, G.J. (1969). Anaphylactic transfusion reactions associated with anti-IgA antibody. *N. Engl. J. Med.* **280**, 188–93.

Schmidt-Ullrich, B., Rule, A., Schaumburg-Lever, G. and Leblanc, C. (1975). Ultrastructural localization of *in vivo*-bound complement in bullous pemphigoid. *J. Invest. Dermatol.* **65**, 217–19.

Schuler, G., Romani, N. and Steinman, R.M. (1985). A comparison of murine epidermal Langerhans cells with spleen dendritic cells. *J. Invest. Dermatol.* **85**, 99s–106s.

Sergent, J.S., Lockshin, M.D., Christian, C.L. and Gocke, D.J. (1976). Vasculitis with hepatitis B antigenemia: long-term observations in nine patients. *Medicine* **55**, 1–18.

Shelley, W.B. and Juhlin, L. (1977). Selective uptake of contact allergens by the Langerhans cell. *Arch. Dermatol.* **113**, 187–92.

Shornick, J.K., Stastny, P. and Gilliam, J.N. (1981). High frequency of histocompatibility antigens HLA-DR3 and DR4 in herpes gestationis. *J. Clin. Invest.* **68**, 553–5.

Shornick, J.K., Nicholes, B.K., Bergstresser, P.R. and Gilliam, J.N. (1983a). Idiopathic atrophie blanche. *J. Am. Acad. Dermatol.* **8**, 792–8.

Shornick, J.K., Stastny, P. and Gilliam, J.N. (1983b). Paternal histocompatibility (HLA) antigens and maternal anti-HLA antibodies in herpes gestationis. *J. Invest. Dermatol.* **81**, 407–9.

Silberberg-Sinakin, I., Thorbecke, G.J., Baer, R.L., Rosenthal, S.A. and Berezowsky, V. (1976). Antigen-bearing Langerhans cells in skin, dermal lymphatics and in lymph nodes. *Cell. Immunol.* **25**, 137–51.

Slater, E.E., Merrill, D.D., Guess, H.A. *et al.* (1988). Clinical profile of angioedema associated with angiotensin converting-enzyme inhibition. *JAMA* **260**, 967–70.

Slater, J.E. (1989). Rubber anaphylaxis. *N. Engl. J. Med.* **320**, 1126–30.

Slater, J.E. and Kaliner, M. (1987). Effects of sex hormones on basophil histamine release in recurrent idiopathic anaphylaxis. *J. Allergy Clin. Immunol.* **80**, 285–90.

Smolle, J., Soyer, H.-P., Juettner, F.-M., Torne, R., Stettner, H. and Kerl, H. (1988). HLA-DR-positive keratinocytes are associated with suppressor lymphocyte epidermotropism: a biomathematical study. *Am. J. Dermatopathol.* **10**, 128–32.

Soter, N.A., Austen, K.F. and Gigli, I. (1974a). The complement system in necrotizing angiitis of the skin: analysis of complement component activities in serum of patients with concomitant collagen-vascular diseases. *J. Invest. Dermatol.* **63**, 219–26.

Soter, N.A., Austen, K.F. and Gigli, I. (1974b). Urticaria and arthralgias as manifestations of necrotizing angiitis (vasculitis). *J. Invest. Dermatol.* **63**, 485–90.

Soter, N.A., Mihm, M.C., Jr, Gigli, I., Dvorak, H.F. and Austen, K.F. (1976a). Two distinct cellular patterns in cutaneous necrotizing angiitis. *J. Invest. Dermatol.* **66**, 344–50.

Soter, N.A., Wasserman, S.I. and Austen, K.F. (1976b). Cold urticaria: release into the circulation of histamine and eosinophil chemotactic factor of anaphylaxis during cold challenge. *N. Engl. J. Med.* **294**, 687–90.

Soter, N.A., Joshi, N.P., Twarog, F.J., Zeiger, R.S., Rothman, P.M. and Colten, H.R. (1977). Delayed cold-induced urticaria: a dominantly inherited disorder. *J. Allergy Clin. Immunol.* **59**, 294–7.

Soter, N.A., Wasserman, S.I., Austen, K.F. and McFadden, E.R., Jr (1980). Release of mast-cell mediators and alterations in lung function in patients with cholinergic urticaria. *N. Engl. J. Med.* **302**, 604–8.

Soter, N.A., Murphy, G.F. and Mihm, M.C., Jr (1982). Lymphocytes and necrosis of the cutaneous microvasculature in malignant atrophic papulosis: a refined light microscope study. *J. Am. Acad. Dermatol.* **7**, 620–30.

Soter, N.A., Lewis, R.A., Corey, E.J. and Austen, K.F. (1983). Local effects of synthetic leukotrienes (LTC_4, LTD_4, LTE_4, and LTB_4) in human skin. *J. Invest. Dermatol.* **80**, 115–19.

Stanley, J.R., Tanaka, T., Mueller, S., Klaus-Kovtun, V. and Roop, D. (1988) Isolation of complementary DNA for bullous pemphigoid antigen by use of patients' autoantibodies. *J. Clin. Invest.* **82**, 1864–70.

Stingl, G., Katz, S.I., Clement, L., Green, I. and Shevach, E.M. (1978). Immunologic functions of Ia-bearing epidermal Langerhans cells. *J. Immunol.* **121**, 2005–13.

Su, W.P.D., Schroeter, A.L., Lee, D.A., Hsu, T. and Muller, S.A. (1985). Clinical and histologic findings in Degos' syndrome (malignant atrophic papulosis). *Cutis* **35**, 131–8.

Sullivan, S., Bergstresser, P.R., Tigelaar, R.E. and Streilein, J.W. (1986). Induction and regulation of contact hypersensitivity by resident, bone marrow-derived, dendritic epidermal cells: Langerhans cells and Thy-1^+ epidermal cells. *J. Immunol.* **137**, 2460–7.

Sun, N.C.J., Conn, D.L., Schroeter, A.L. and Kazmier, F.J. (1976). Skin fibrinolytic activity in cutaneous and systemic vasculitis. *Mayo Clin. Proc.* **51**, 216–22.

Szafer, F., Brautbar, C., Tzfoni, E. *et al.* (1987). Detection of disease-specific restriction fragment length polymorphisms in pemphigus vulgaris linked to the *DQw1* and *DQw3* alleles of the HLA-D region. *Proc. Nat. Acad. Sci. (USA)* **84**, 6542–5.

Szczeklik, A. (1987). Adverse reactions to aspirin and non-steroidal anti-inflammatory drugs. *Ann. Allergy* **59**, 113–18.

Tan, S.G., and Rowell, N.R. (1976). Pemphigus-like syndrome induced by D-penicillamine. *Br. J. Dermatol.* **95**, 99–103.

Tindall, J.P., Beeker, S.K. and Rosse, W.F. (1969). Familial cold urticaria: a generalized reaction involving leukocytosis. *Arch.*

Intern. Med. **124**, 129–34.

Ting, S., Reimann, B.E.F., Rauls, D.O. and Mansfield, L.E. (1983). Nonfamilial, vibration-induced angioedema. *J. Allergy Clin. Immunol.* **71**, 546–51.

Toews, G.B., Bergstresser, P.R. and Streilein, J.W. (1980). Epidermal Langerhans cell density determines whether contact hypersensitivity or unresponsiveness follows skin painting with DNFB. *J. Immunol.* **124**, 445–53.

Uwatoko, S. and Mannik, M. (1988). Low-molecular weight C1q-binding immunoglobulin G in patients with systemic lupus erythematosus consists of autoantibodies to the collagen-like region of C1q. *J. Clin. Invest.* **82**, 816–24.

van der Meer, J.B. (1969). Granular deposits of immunoglobulins in the skin of patients with dermatitis herpetiformis: an immunofluorescent study. *Br. J. Dermatol.* **81**, 493–3.

van der Woude, F.J., Lobatto, S., Permin, H. *et al.* (1985). Autoantibodies against neutrophils and monocytes: tool for diagnosis and marker of disease activity in Wegener's granulomatosis. *Lancet* **i**, 425–9.

van Joost, T., Cormane, R.H. and Pondman, K.W. (1972). Direct immunofluorescent study of the skin on occurrence of complement in pemphigus. *Br. J. Dermatol.* **87**, 466–74.

Venning, V.A., Taylor, C.J., Ting, A. and Wojnarowska, F. (1989). HLA type in bullous pemphigoid, cicatricial pemphigoid and linear IgA disease. *Clin. Exp. Dermatol.* **14**, 283–5.

Walker, D.H., Gay, R.M. and Valdes-Dapena, V. (1981). The occurrence of eschars in Rocky Mountain spotted fever. *J. Am. Acad. Dermatol.* **4**, 571–6.

Warin, R.P. and Champion, R.H. (1974). *Urticaria*. W.B. Saunders, New York.

Warin, R.P. and Smith, R.J. (1982). Role of tartrazine in chronic urticaria. *Br. Med. J.* **284**, 1443–4.

Wasserman, S.I. and Ginsberg, M.H. (1984). Release of platelet factor 4 into the blood after cold challenge of patients with cold urticaria. *J. Allergy Clin. Immunol.* **74**, 275–9.

Westgate, G.E., Weaver, A.C. and Couchman, J.R. (1985). Bullous pemphigoid antigen localization suggests an intracellular association with hemidesmosomes. *J. Invest. Dermatol.* **84**, 218–24.

Wiesner-Menzel, L., Schulz, B., Vakilzadeh, F. and Czarnetzki, B.M. (1981). Electron microscopical evidence for a direct contact between nerve fibres and mast cells. *Acta Dermatol. Venereol. (Stockholm)* **61**, 465–9.

Winkelmann, R.K. (1985). The histology and immunopathology of dermographism. *J. Cutan. Pathol.* **12**, 468–92.

Winkelmann, R.K., Black, A.K., Dover, J. and Greaves, M.W. (1986). Pressure urticaria — histopathological study. *Clin. Exp. Dermatol.* **11**, 139–47.

Winkelmann, R.K., Wilson-Jones, E., Smith, N.P., English, J.S.C. and Greaves, M.W. (1988). Neutrophilic urticaria. *Acta Dermatol. Venereol. (Stockholm)* **68**, 129–33.

Wintroub, B.U., Mihn, M.C., Jr, Goetzl, E.J., Soter, N.A. and Austen, K.F. (1978). Morphologic and functional evidence for release of mast-cell products in bullous pemphigoid. *N. Engl. J. Med.* **298**, 417–21.

Wisnieski, J.J. and Naff, G.B. (1989). Serum IgG antibodies to C1q in hypocomplementemic urticarial vasculitis syndrome. *Arthritis Rheum.* **32**, 1119–27.

Wojnarowska, F., Marsden, R.A., Bhogal, B. and Black, M.M. (1984). Childhood cicatricial pemphigoid with linear IgA deposits. *Clin. Exp. Dermatol.* **9**, 407–15.

Wojnarowska, F., Marsden, R.A., Bhogal, B. and Black, M.M. (1988). Chronic bullous disease of childhood, childhood cicatricial pemphigoid, and linear IgA disease of adults. *J. Am. Acad. Dermatol.* **19**, 792–805.

Wood, G.S., Volterra, A.S., Abel, E.A., Nickoloff, B.J. and Adams, R.M. (1986). Allergic contact dermatitis: novel immunohistologic features. *J. Invest. Dermatol.* **87**, 688–93.

Woodley, D.T. (1988). Epidermolysis bullosa acquisita. *Prog. Dermatol.* **22**, 1–13.

Woodley, D.T., Burgeson, R.E., Lunstrum, G. *et al.* (1988). Epidermolysis bullosa acquisita antigen is the globular carboxyl terminus of type VII procollagen. *J. Clin. Invest.* **81**, 683–7.

Woolf, A.D., Wakerley, G., Wallington, T.B., Scott, D.G.I. and Dieppe, P.A. (1987). Factor VIII related antigen in the assessment of vasculitis. *Ann. Rheum. Dis.* **46**, 441–7.

Wrangsjo, K., Wahlberg, J.E. and Axelsson, I.G.K. (1988). IgE-mediated allergy to natural rubber in 30 patients with contact urticaria. *Contact Dermatitis* **19**, 264–71.

Yamada, H., Hashimoto, T. and Nishikawa, T. (1989). IgG subclasses of intercellular and basement membrane zone antibodies: the relationship to the capability of complement fixation. *J. Invest. Dermatol.* **92**, 585–7.

Yaoita, H. and Katz, S.I. (1976). Immunoelectronmicroscopic localization of IgA in skin of patients with dermatitis herpetiformis. *J. Invest. Dermatol.* **67**, 502–6.

Yaoita, H., Gullino, M. and Katz, S.I. (1976). Herpes gestationis: ultrastructure and ultrastructural localization of *in vivo*-bound complement. *J. Invest. Dermatol.* **66**, 383–8.

Yaoita, H., Briggaman, R.A., Lawley, T.J., Provost, T.T. and Katz, S.I. (1981). Epidermolysis bullosa acquisita: ultrastructural and immunological studies. *J. Invest. Dermatol.* **76**, 288–92.

Zaltas, M.M., Ahmed, R. and Foster, C.S. (1989). Association of HLA-DR4 with ocular cicatricial pemphigoid. *Curr. Eye Res.* **8**, 189–93.

Zeek, P.M. (1953). Periarteritis nodosa and other forms of necrotizing angiitis. *N. Engl. J. Med.* **248**, 764–72.

97: Psoriasis — a T-lymphocyte-mediated Disease

H. Valdimarsson

Clinical features

Psoriasis is a chronic inflammatory skin disease which affects approximately 2% of Caucasians but is less common in other ethnic groups. The disease begins between puberty and the age of 30 in approximately two-thirds of patients, and it rarely presents before the age of 8 or after the age of 50 years. It affects males and females equally. Disease severity ranges from minor skin lesions confined to the elbows or the scalp to a mutilating condition affecting nearly all the body surface or causing severe joint damage. The disease tends to persist with fluctuating activity in the majority of patients, approximately 50% have disease-free periods of varying duration, but less than 10% of patients can expect permanent remission. Early onset tends to be associated with a severe disease, but patients with late onset may also develop extensive lesions.

Clinical variants

The most common clinical form of the disease is often called psoriasis vulgaris. The skin lesions are sharply demarcated, salmon-pink papules or plaques covered with silvery white scales which leave fine bleeding points when removed. They tend to be symmetrically distributed and occur most commonly on the elbows, knees, scalp and buttocks. Individual lesions may remain small and solitary or may coalesce into large irregular patterns which may have a central area of normal skin because resolution of the disease usually begins at the centre of the plaques. Nails are often affected with numerous small pits; they may also become thickened or lift from the nail-bed.

Many descriptive terms have been invented for clinical variants of the disease as regards distribution, extent and inflammatory activity, but only a few of these are likely to have biomedical or practical significance. The generalized erythrodermic and exfoliative form of the disease is incapacitating. In guttate psoriasis the numerous red papules which appear suddenly all over the body usually resolve spontaneously within a few weeks. The pustular form, generalized or confined to the palms and soles, and characterized by foci of heavy epidermal infiltration by neutrophils, may be an entity with a different aetiology and pathogenic mechanism. Approximately 10% of patients with psoriasis are also affected by one of five forms of arthritis (Table 97.1).

Table 97.1. Different types of psoriatic arthritides

	Percentage of patients
Asymmetrical oligoarticular arthritis	70
Seronegative symmetrical polyarthritis	15
Predominant distal interphalangeal involvement	5
Destructive arthritis mutulans	5
Sacroiliitis and spondylitis	5

Aetiological and precipitating factors

An association between guttate psoriasis and throat infections with β-haemolytic streptococci was reported 40 years ago (Norrlind 1950; Norholm-Pederson 1952), and the existence of this important link is now generally accepted, although frequently overlooked. The psoriatic eruption usually begins about 1 week after the throat infection, but, in contrast to rheumatic fever and glomerulonephritis, guttate psoriasis has not been associated with any particular streptococcal serotypes. Retrovirus-like particles have also been observed both in skin lesions and urine of patients with psoriasis vulgaris (Iversen *et al.* 1983), but it remains to be demonstrated that these particles are disease-specific and not merely secondary to abnormal activation of the immune system. Patients with chronic psoriasis frequently experience deterioration after various types of infections, but no specific infectious agents other than streptococci have been definitely implicated.

Certain drugs, notably lithium, β-blockers, indomethacin and antimalarial drugs, have also been reported to aggravate the disease in some patients.

HEREDITY

A study by Hellgren (1967) on 40 000 individuals in parts of Sweden showed that 6.4% of relatives of patients with psoriasis were affected. Family studies are consistent with polygenic inheritance, but in some families a pattern suggestive of dominant Mendelian transmission has been observed. The disease has a concordance of 65–70% in monozygotic twins and 15–20% in dizygotic twins. It has also been reported that the age of onset, certain clinical features and the prognosis of psoriasis are determined to a large extent by genetic factors (Bandrup *et al.* 1978).

Associations with human leucocyte antigens (HLA)-B13, B17 and B37 were reported in early studies, but these are probably secondary to linkage with CW6 and DR7, which show a five- to six-fold increase in patients with psoriasis. However, patients with pustular psoriasis do not have increased incidence of these HLA antigens, and psoriatic arthropathy is associated with B38 and DR4.

THE KOEBNER PHENOMENON

Approximately 25% of psoriasis patients develop psoriatic lesions at the site of skin injury. This reaction is named after Heinrich Koebner, who first described it in 1872. It is not detectable clinically until 2–3 weeks after the injury is inflicted and is an all-or-none phenomenon. If a patient is positive at one site, the reaction can also be provoked elsewhere on the body at the same point in time. However, patients may vary at different times in whether they are positive or negative, and a positive Koebner reaction is usually associated with periods of increased disease activity. In some patients an area of psoriatic plaque which is removed may heal to give clinically uninvolved skin. This has been called 'reverse Koebner reaction' and is mutually exclusive with Koebner positivity (Eyre and Krueger 1982). This suggests that the response of psoriasis patients to injury and their disease activity are controlled by a systemic factor, which may at least in part affect the traffic of T cell subsets into the skin (see below).

Since no animal model is available for psoriasis, the Koebner reaction is currently the only way to study the early pathogenic mechanisms and changes of a developing psoriasis lesion.

Histopathology

EARLY PIN-POINT LESIONS

Capillary dilatation and oedema in the papillary dermis, with infiltrates of mononuclear leucocytes surrounding the capillaries, are the first microscopic features of a developing psoriasis lesion. Mononuclear leucocytes can also be observed in the lower portion of the epidermis in association with slight oedema. In the upper portion of the epidermis, foci of vacuolated granular cells develop. The granular cells then disappear and heaps of lamellated keratin ('parakeratin') appear above these foci. Already at this stage, neutrophils may be discharged periodically from the dilated papillary capillaries and migrate rapidly towards the top of the parakeratotic mounds to form characteristic microabscesses. The mononuclear leucocytes remain confined to the dermis and the lower layers of the epidermis, which becomes increasingly hyperplastic. Large gaps can be detected in the basement membrane between the dermis and epidermis (Brody 1978).

PERSISTENT LESIONS

The early focal lesions may later become confluent and form the characteristic plaques of chronic psoriasis. The classical histological picture of such lesions consists of a hypertrophic epidermis that has lost its granular layer but is covered by heaps of lamellated parakeratin containing scattered foci of dense neutrophil infiltrates, the Munro microabscesses. These microabscesses are considered to be the histological hallmark of psoriasis, and in pustular psoriasis aggregates of neutrophils are also seen deeper down in the spinous layer of the epidermis. The epidermal hyperplasia accentuates the undulations seen in cross-sections of normal skin between the epidermal rete and the dermis, to the extent that elongated club-shaped columns (rete ridges) of epidermal cells penetrate deep into the dermis. The elongated dermal papillae between the rete ridges are oedematous, with dilated and tortuous capillary loops, and infiltrated with scattered mononuclear leucocytes, while perivascular aggregates of mononuclear leucocytes are present in the deeper layers of the dermis. The epidermal plates above the tips of the dermal papillae are abnormally thin. This explains why capillary bleeding spots tend to appear when the parakeratotic crusts are removed (Auspitz sign).

Cellular features

It has been argued that the inflammatory features of psoriasis are secondary to an innate keratinocyte defect. Conversely, it has been postulated that the epidermal changes are caused by abnormal immune or inflammatory responses in the skin. It should be emphasized that many skin diseases are associated with dermal and epidermal infiltration of leucocytes, but abnormal proliferation and maturation of keratinocytes are a characteristic feature in psoriasis. Any attempt to elucidate the cause of this disease must take this into account.

Epidermal hyperproliferation and abnormal keratinization

The average transit time of cells from the basal epidermal layer to the uppermost row of cells in the squamous layer has been calculated to be 4–5 days in psoriatic lesions, compared with approximately 14 days in normal skin. The shortened transit time is associated with increased mitotic activity in the basal cell layer and an abnormal process of keratinization that includes a substantial decrease in the amount of the 67 kD α chain, which is a major component of normal keratin. It was previously believed that the cell division cycle time was shortened in psoriasis, but it is now thought that an abnormally large proportion of the germinative cells are actively cycling (Weinstein 1971). There is also an increased deoxyribonucleic acid (DNA) synthesis by epidermal cells in clinically uninvolved skin of patients with psoriasis, and this has even been demonstrated in 5-week-old grafts on nude mice (Krueger *et al*. 1981). These observations led to the assumption that abnormal epidermal cell replication is the primary abnormality in psoriasis, and that drugs had to be antimitotic in order to be effective against this disease (Wright and Campeljohn 1983).

However, recent studies have demonstrated that grafts of psoriatic skin on nude mice are infiltrated by Thy 1.2 +ve mouse T cells. It is therefore possible that the psoriatic keratinocytes are responding abnormally to inflammatory cytokines released by mouse lymphocytes that are reacting against the skin grafts (Baker *et al*. 1992).

Inflammatory cells

Heavy epidermal infiltration by neutrophils (Munro microabscesses) is a characteristic feature which is not seen in inflammatory skin diseases other than psoriasis. The observation that psoriasis is exacerbated by ingestion of compounds such as lithium and iodides, which activate neutrophils, has further implicated these cells in the pathogenesis of the disease (Skoven and Thormann 1979; Fernandez and Fox 1980). It has also been reported that circulating neutrophils (Sedgwick *et al*. 1980) and monocytes (Krueger *et al*. 1978) are abnormally activated in patients with psoriasis. Factors that are strongly chemotactic for neutrophils are present in psoriatic lesions, including C5a, 12-hydroxyeicosatetraenoic acid (12-HETE) and the very potent leukotriene B-4 (LTB-4) (reviewed by Tagami *et al*. 1987). Furthermore, the potent neutrophil attractant interleukin 8 (IL-8) has recently been detected in psoriatic scales (Gearing *et al*. 1990). However, the formation of these chemotactic agents and the neutrophil infiltration are a relatively late feature in the development of the psoriasis lesion compared with the mononuclear cell infiltration and the increased keratinocyte mitosis (Braun-Falco and Christophers 1974). Furthermore, repeated topical application of LTB-4 to uninvolved skin of patients with active psoriasis does not give rise to psoriatic lesions, although this procedure induces abundant epidermal microabscesses (Wong *et al*. 1985). Leukotrienes and neutrophils are therefore not likely to be primary pathogenic agents in psoriasis, although they may perhaps contribute to the persistence of established lesions.

Immunocytes

IMMUNOCYTES IN NORMAL SKIN

Normal skin contains large numbers of dendritic antigen-presenting cells (APC) and scattered T lymphocytes, but B lymphocytes are not found in healthy skin. It has been suggested that the epidermis may influence T lymphocyte maturation (Fichtelius *et al*. 1970), and keratinocytes produce mediators which are known to influence lymphocyte function (see below). The concept of skin-associated lymphoid tissue (SALT) was introduced by Streilein (1978) and it has recently been reported that the endothelial cell leucocyte adhesion molecule (ELAM-1) may function as an addressin that enables memory T cells to home selectively in the skin (Picker *et al*. 1991; Shimizu *et al*. 1991). A substantial proportion of the lymphocyte pool normally resides within the skin, and it can be calculated that this largest organ of the body contains at least 2×10^{10} extravascular T cells. Approximately 98% of these cells are in the dermis, largely localized around post-capillary venules. In this location there are about equal numbers of CD4 and CD8 +ve cells, but in normal skin the great majority (80–90%) of the intraepidermal T cells are of the CD8 phenotype (Bos *et al*. 1987). It is surprising that, with the exception of the epidermal T cells, more than 80% of the T cells in the other compartments of normal skin are activated, as judged by expression of the interleukin 2 (IL-2) receptor α chain.

IMMUNOCYTES IN PSORIATIC SKIN

It was first reported in 1977 that the dermis of early pin-point psoriatic lesions was abnormally infiltrated by macrophages and lymphocytes before any definite epidermal changes could be detected (Braun-Falco and Schmoecekel 1977). A study of clinically normal skin of early eruptive guttate psoriasis demonstrated gaps in the basement membrane between the epidermis and dermis, and this was associated with an influx of mononuclear cells into the epidermal compartment, while no neutrophils could be detected at this early stage (Brody 1978). It was further shown that the infiltrating lymphocytes were almost exclusively T cells (Bjerke *et al*. 1978) and that CD4 +ve cells predominated in the dermis, suggesting that psoriasis resulted from persistent stimulation of T cells (Bos *et al*. 1983).

It was also demonstrated that the CD4/CD8 ratio tended to be higher in lesional skin than in the blood of patients with active psoriasis, suggesting a selective recruitment from the blood of CD4 +ve cells into psoriatic lesions (Baker *et al*. 1984a).

Cellular changes were investigated throughout the course of self-limiting lesions in patients with guttate psoriasis. Compared with normal skin, a definite increase in CD8 +ve cells was found in the patients' uninvolved epidermis, but no corresponding increase was observed in CD4 +ve cells. Biopsies from the uninvolved skin were taken at least 1 cm away from the margins of the lesions, and they showed a dermal infiltration by mononuclear leucocytes which was very similar to that of lesional dermis, and in both instances the great majority of the T cells were of the CD4 phenotype and activated, as judged by HLA-DR expression. Eruption of clinical lesions was associated with a marked epidermal influx of CD4 +ve T cells, and these cells were seen in close apposition to Langerhans cells. Conversely, in late or resolving guttate lesions the preponderance of CD8 +ve T cells was restored in the epidermis, and a substantial proportion of these cells was activated (Baker *et al.* 1984b).

In persistent psoriasis plaques the epidermal numbers of CD8 +ve T cells generally exceeded that of CD4 +ve T cells. However, there was a preferential activation of CD4 +ve cells, both in the epidermis and particularly in the dermis of such lesions (Baker *et al.* 1985a). Several reports have now confirmed and extended these findings (Placek *et al.* 1988; Ramirez-Bosca *et al.* 1988; Sackstein *et al.* 1988).

A marked increase in HLA-DR +ve dendritic cells in lesional dermis has been found by most investigators, but data have been conflicting concerning the numbers of such cells in lesional epidermis. While abnormal clustering of these cells has been a consistent finding, some investigators have found decreased numbers of Langerhans and related cells in lesional epidermis (Bos 1988; Placek *et al.* 1988), but others have reported that they are present in increased numbers (Baker *et al.* 1985a). The reason for this discrepancy is likely to be technical. During treatment with topical steroids, dithranol or psoralen ultraviolet A-range (PUVA) therapy, resolution of clinical lesions was always preceded by disappearance of epidermal T lymphocytes, whereas normalization of Langerhans cells did not occur until after the healing was well advanced (Baker *et al.* 1985a, b).

On the basis of these findings it was postulated that psoriasis lesions erupt where epidermal influx of antigen-carrying Langerhans cells and CD4 +ve T cells overrides the normal epidermal suppressor mechanisms. It was further argued that the abnormal epidermal proliferation in psoriasis is triggered by growth factors produced by the activated CD4 +ve T cells and the prediction was made that treatment with cyclosporin A would clear psoriasis lesions (Valdimarsson *et al.* 1986). That prediction has now been confirmed in several trials (Ellis *et al.* 1986; Griffiths *et al.* 1986; Wentzell *et al.* 1987; Joost *et al.* 1986). Indeed, cyclosporin A appears to be the most potent antipsoriatic agent available, although nephrotoxicity limits its use to patients with severe forms of the disease. The drug does not inhibit keratinocyte proliferation in pharmacological concentration, but it has been demonstrated to suppress T lymphocyte activation in psoriatic plaques although the keratinocytes remain abnormally active (Gottlieb *et al.* 1992). This indicates that the therapeutic benefit of cyclosporin A in psoriasis is due to a direct effect on T lymphocytes.

Further support for the notion that eruption of psoriasis lesions is a T-cell-dependent phenomenon came from a prospective study of the development of the Koebner reaction. T cell sub-populations were enumerated in uninvolved epidermis and dermis of psoriasis patients. Low numbers of CD8 +ve relative to CD4 +ve T cells in both skin compartments before the injury was inflicted were found to predispose to a positive Koebner reaction (Baker *et al.* 1988a).

DERMAL FIBROBLASTS

Fibroblasts from both lesional and uninvolved psoriatic skin have been found to have increased proliferative and metabolic activity *in vitro* (Priestley 1983; Priestley and Adams 1983). However, psoriatic fibroblasts did not stimulate abnormal proliferation of normal or psoriatic keratinocytes *in vitro* (Baden *et al.* 1981). More recently keratinocyte proliferation has been studied in full-thickness punch biopsies explanted on to a dermal equivalent *in vitro* (Saiag *et al.* 1985). In this system keratinocyte hyperproliferation was observed when explants of normal skin were cultured on fibroblasts from patients with psoriasis, but keratinocytes in biopsies from psoriatic skin continued to show abnormal proliferation when explanted on to fibroblasts derived from normal skin. These observations and the transplantation studies of Krueger *et al.* (1981) are inconclusive with respect to what cell type is intrinsically abnormal in psoriasis.

ENDOTHELIAL CELLS

The capillary loops in the dermal papillae become dilated and tortuous before other histological evidence of psoriasis can be detected in a developing lesion (Braun-Falco and Christopher 1974) and abnormally dilated capillary loops have even been observed in uninvolved psoriatic skin (Kulka 1964). These vessels have an increased permeability (Aschheim and Farber 1966) and show enhanced endothelial cell proliferation (Ryan 1980) and some features of high endothelial post-capillary venules (Heng *et al.* 1988; Jónsdóttir *et al.* 1990). Furthermore, specific and selective binding was recently demonstrated between CD4 +ve T cells and endothelial cells of lesional but not uninvolved psoriatic dermis (Sackstein *et al.* 1988), supporting the notion that development of psoriasis lesions is dependent upon selective influx of CD4 +ve T cells, first into the dermis and then into the epidermal compartment (Valdimarsson *et al.* 1986). The role of interferon gamma (IFN-γ) in cutaneous traffic of lymphocytes has been reviewed by Nickoloff (1988).

Biochemical features

Early studies on biochemical changes in psoriasis were directed at the cyclic nucleotides, and it was postulated that a defective cyclic adenosine monophosphate (cAMP) cascade might explain the increased proliferation and abnormal maturation of the keratinocytes (Voorhees and Duell 1971). However, variable cAMP levels have been reported in psoriatic epidermis (Voorhees 1982), perhaps reflecting the multifactorial nature of the disease, differences in methodology or, most likely, variable activity of the psoriasis lesions studied. Reported increases in epidermal levels of cyclic guanosine monophosphate (cGMP), calmodulin, phospholipase C, tyrosine kinase activity and epidermal growth factor (EGF) binding are also likely to be secondary to increased turnover of keratinocytes.

These agents are all related to systems that transfer activation signals across cell membranes, and which can be triggered by mediators from mononuclear leucocytes. It has also been pointed out that many of these observations have been made in keratome sections from lesions, which can be heavily infiltrated by immunocytes that could be directly responsible for some of the changes found (Bos 1988). Similarly, elevation of certain polyamines which are associated with cell growth is probably also epiphenomenal. However, the relatively high levels of leukotrienes and hydroxyeicosatetraenoic acids (HETEs) compared with the prostaglandins have led to the proposal that the cyclo-oxygenase pathway is inhibited in psoriatic skin (Penneys *et al.* 1975), whereby more arachidonic acid would be directed to the lipoxygenase system. This might explain the high levels of 12-HETE and LTB-4 in psoriatic scales. In addition to potent chemotactic activity, LTB-4 has been reported to stimulate keratinocyte proliferation *in vitro* (Kragballe *et al.* 1985), although this could not be confirmed *in vivo* (Wong *et al.* 1985). However the 5-lipoxygenase inhibitor benoxaprofen improves psoriasis (Kragballe and Herlin 1983) suggesting that lipoxygenase products may contribute to the pathogenic process. It is of interest in this context that prostaglandins of the E series are immunosuppressive.

Is psoriasis an immunological disease?

Early theories on immunological mechanisms in psoriasis focused on autoantibodies and humoral mechanisms (Beutner *et al.* 1975; Jablonska *et al.* 1979), but Cormane (1981) suggested that both humoral and cellular mechanisms were at play. Disturbance of immune homoeostasis involving dendritic cells was suggested by Bos *et al.* (1983), and Morhenn (1984) proposed that T suppressor cells might provide 'turn-off' signals to basal cells during normal wound healing and that the hyperproliferation of psoriatic keratinocytes might reflect a defect in that mechanism. It was further postulated, on the basis of a series of immunohistological studies (reviewed by Fry 1988), that the inflammation and abnormal keratinocyte proliferation in psoriasis lesions were caused by influx and antigenic activation of CD4 +ve T cells within the epidermal compartment, resulting in the generation of epidermotrophic cytokines (Valdimarsson *et al.* 1986).

There is now compelling evidence for the notion that CD4 + ve T cells play a central role in the pathogenesis of psoriasis. First, two structurally different, potent anti-psoriatic drugs, cyclosporin A and FK 506, both selectively inhibit cytokine production by CD4 +ve T cells. Cyclosporin A not only clears psoriatic skin lesions but is probably equally effective against psoriatic arthritis (Steinsson *et al.* 1990). Second, patients with severe and persistent psoriasis who have been treated with monoclonal antibodies to CD4, have consistently shown a prompt and dramatic improvement. (Nicolas *et al.* 1991; Prinz *et al.* 1991; Poizot-Martin *et al.* 1991). It has further been reported that psoriatic lesions resolve after administration of peptide T that binds selectively to the CD4 molecule (J.A. Marcusson; *Clinical Derma-*

tology in the Year 2000, p. 194, London). However, the evidence for primary involvement of the immune system in the aetiology of psoriasis is more tenuous, although the relationship between guttate psoriasis and streptococcal throat infections may provide an important clue in this respect. An extensive cross-reaction involving multiple epitopes has been demonstrated between β-haemolytic streptococci and human skin components (Swerlick *et al.* 1986; Hermosura *et al.* 1987). An abnormal autoreactivity between epidermal cells and blood lymphocytes has been reported in patients with psoriasis compared to normal individuals and patients with lichen planus, another supposedly T cell mediated skin disease (Steinmuller *et al.* 1988). Blood lymphocytes from patients with persistent psoriasis have been found to be hyper-reactive to β-haemolytic streptococci (Baker *et al.* 1992). It is therefore possible that infections with microorganisms which cross-react with human skin, possibly keratin, may trigger an autoimmune reaction that is characterized by epidermal hyperproliferation in predisposed individuals. However, the psoriatic predisposition may be quite complex and even variable between individuals. It is probably polygenic and could be inherent in more than one cell type, including keratinocytes, synovial cells, immunocytes or fibroblasts. In the skin, the common denominator appears to be abnormal proliferation and maturation of keratinocytes in the presence of inflammatory mediators. Recent data suggest that epidermal growth is controlled by highly complex homoeostatic mechanisms, involving interaction between keratinocytes, Langerhans cells, T lymphocytes and fibroblasts. These are examined in the next section.

Interaction between keratinocytes and immunocytes

There is growing evidence for the existence of a special homoeostatic mechanism involving interaction between keratinocytes and the immune system. Keratinocytes produce a variety of cytokines which can influence the maturation and function of immunocytes. These include epidermal thymocyte-activating factor (ETAF) that is indistinguishable from interleukin 1β (Luger *et al.* 1981) interleukin 3 (IL-3) (Luger *et al.* 1984), interleukin 6 (IL-6) (Kupper *et al.* 1988a), interleukin 8 (IL-8) (Krueger *et al.* 1990; Reusch *et al.* 1990), granulocyte-macrophage colony stimulating factor (GM-CSF) (Kupper *et al.* 1988b) and tumour necrosis factor-α (TNF-α) (Pillai *et al.* 1989, Symington 1989). Interleukin 1 is strongly chemotactic for T lymphocytes (Sauder 1984), and although keratinocyte IL-1β normally remains largely intracellular, significant quantities can probably be released after trauma and during epidermal immune responses. Conversely, IFN-γ induces keratinocytes to express the intercellular adhesion molecule-1 (ICAM-1) and Class II MHC molecules (Griffiths *et al.* 1989). It has been demonstrated that supernatants from both activated and non-activated T cells contain factors that stimulate growth of human keratinocytes *in vitro*, while factors that suppress keratinocyte growth predominate in supernatants of monocyte cultures. The stimulatory activity of T cell cultures has been attributed to IL-3 and GM-CSF (Hancock *et al.* 1988). Recombinant IL-2 has also been found to increase thymidine incorporation by keratinocytes *in vitro* at a concentration which suggests that keratinocytes have high-affinity receptors for this growth factor. However, IL-2 receptors could not be detected *in situ* on basal keratinocytes, but basal cells reacted with a monoclonal antibody which is specific for the IL-4 receptor (Baker *et al.* 1991). Several investigators have reported that IFN gamma inhibits keratinocyte growth (Baker *et al.* 1988b; Hancock *et al.* 1988), and reduced expression of IFN-γ receptors has been observed in lesional although not in uninvolved psoriatic skin (Scheynius *et al.* 1992). Transforming growth fator (TGF)-β and tumour necrosis factor (TNF)-α have also been found to suppress keratinocyte growth (Pillai *et al.* 1989; Symington 1989). Transforming growth factor (TGF)-α which is structurally related to EGF, and binds to the EGF receptor, has been reported to be produced by primary keratinocyte cultures and to stimulate keratinocyte growth, suggesting an autocrine mechanism (Coffey *et al.* 1987). Table 97.2 lists some of the substances which may affect keratinocyte growth.

Psoriasis as a disease of T-cell-mediated hyperproliferation of keratinocytes

Various types of skin rashes frequently occur in association with infections and allergic responses to drugs or food substances. This suggests that

Table 97.2. Some factors which may affect keratinocyte growth

Substance	Source	Effects on KC growth
IL-2	T cells	Stimulation
IL-3	T cells, KC	Stimulation
GM-CSF	T cells, KC	Stimulation
LTB-4	KC	Stimulation
Somatomedin	Fibroblasts	Stimulation
TGF-α	KC	Stimulation
EGF	Fibroblasts	?
IL-6	T cells, KC	?
ETAF (IL-1)	KC, LC	?
TNF-β	T cells	?Suppression
TNF-α	T cells, KC	Suppression
PGE_2	KC	?Suppression
IFN-γ	T cells	Suppression
TGF-β	Fibroblasts, T cells, KC	Suppression

KC = keratinocytes; LC = Langerhans cells; TNF = tumour necrosis factor; PGE_2 = prostaglandin E_2.

antigens or immune complexes tend to accumulate in the dermis during episodes of abnormal antigenic load. The basement membrane of the skin, although largely impermeable to soluble antigens and immune complexes, is frequently penetrated by APCs, which may thereby act as vehicles for transport of antigens from the dermis into the epidermis. It should be emphasized in this context that in psoriasis T cell activation in the dermis is much more widespread than are the clinical lesions (Baker *et al.* 1984b), which may only erupt in foci where sufficient epidermal influx and activation of CD4+ve T cells coincides with that of antigen-carrying dendritic cells. This does not exclude the possibility that psoriatic lesions may sometimes also be initiated by externally derived antigens. It has been suggested that products of activated T cells may enhance keratinocyte proliferation during normal wound healing, and that this regulatory mechanism is malfunctioning in individuals who are predisposed to psoriasis (Morhenn 1988). However, this homoeostatic mechanism, if it exists, is likely to be complicated and involve a variety of both stimulatory and inhibitory signals derived from T cells, keratinocytes, Langerhans cells and fibroblasts. Figure 97.1 illustrates only some of the substances that have been reported and studied in this context and how they could be involved in the generation of the hyperproliferative keratinocyte response that characterizes the

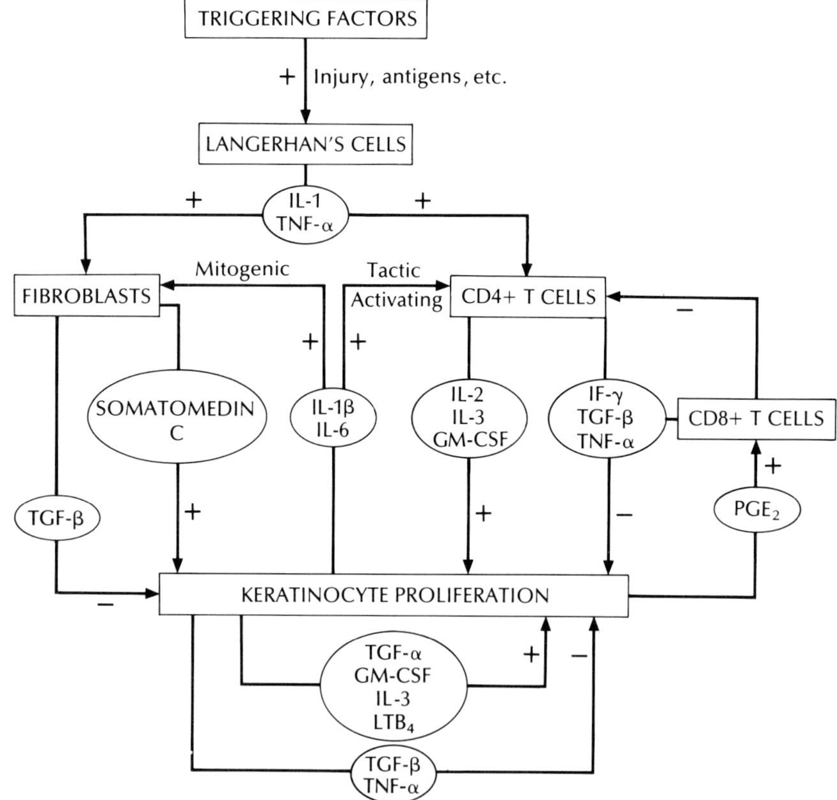

Fig. 97.1. Some factors that could contribute to keratinocyte hyperproliferation in psoriasis.

psoriatic skin. This model predicts that the genetic basis of psoriasis may be complex and vary in different families, the common denominator being a predisposition to keratinocyte hyperproliferation in the presence of cellular immune mediators. This might result from a variety of abnormalities in the signal transduction mechanisms which mediate and control keratinocyte proliferation. An imbalance in the production of immune mediators in favour of those that stimulate rather than inhibit keratinocyte growth is another, not mutually exclusive, possibility. Although psoriasis is a disease that lacks animal models, it is certainly not short of experimental options.

References

Aschheim, E. and Farber, E. (1966). Blood–tissue exchange in psoriatic skin. *Acta Dermatol. Venereol.* **46**, 310–13.

Baden, H.P., Kubilus, J. and MacDonald, M.J. (1981). Normal and psoriatic keratinocytes and fibroblasts compared in culture. *J. Invest. Dermatol.* **76**, 53–5.

Baker, B.S., Swain, A.F., Valdimarsson, H. and Fry, L. (1984a). T-cell subpopulations in the blood and skin of patients with psoriasis. *Br. J. Dermatol.* **110**, 37–44.

Baker, B.S., Swain, A.F., Fry, L. and Valdimarsson, H. (1984b). Epidermal T lymphocytes and HLA-DR expression in psoriasis. *Br. J. Dermatol.* **110**, 555–64.

Baker, B.S., Swain, A.F., Griffiths, C.E.M., Leonard, J.N., Fry, L. and Valdimarsson, H. (1985a). Epidermal T lymphocytes and dendritic cells in chronic plaque psoriasis: the effects of PUVA treatment. *Clin. Exp. Immunol.* **61**, 526–34.

Baker, B.S., Swain, A.F., Griffiths, C.E.M., Leonard, J.N., Fry, L. and Valdimarsson, H. (1985b). The effects of topical treatment with steroids or dithranol on epidermal T lymphocytes and dendritic cells in psoriasis. *Scand. J. Immunol.* **22**, 471–7.

Baker, B.S., Powles, A.V., Lambert, S., Valdimarsson, H. and Fry, L. (1988a). A prospective study of the Koebner reaction and T lymphocytes in uninvolved psoriatic skin. *Acta Dermatol. Venereol.* **68**, 430–4.

Baker, B.S., Powles, A.V., Valdimarsson, H. and Fry, L. (1988b). An altered response by psoriatic keratinocytes to gamma interferon. *Scand. J. Immunol.* **28**, 735–40.

Baker, B.S., Malkani, A.K., Powles, A.V., Valdimarsson, H. and Fry L. (1991). IL-2 stimulates proliferation of human keratinocytes *in vitro*. *J. Invest. Dermatol.* **96**, 1001 (abstract).

Baker, B.S., Brent, L., Valdimarsson, H. *et al.* (1992). Is epidermal cell proliferation in psoriatic skin grafts on nude mice driven by T-cell derived cytokines? *Br. J. Dermatol.* **126**, 105–10.

Baker, B.S., Powles, A.V., Malkani, A.K., Lewis, H., Valdimarsson, H. and Fry, L. (1992). Altered cell mediated immunity to group A haemolytic streptococcal antigens in chronic plaque psoriasis. *Br. J. Dermatol.* **125**, 38–42.

Bandrup, F., Hauge, M., Henningsen, K. and Eriksen, B. (1978). A study of psoriasis in unselected series of twins. *Arch. Dermatol.* **114**, 874–8.

Beutner, E.H., Jablonska, S., Jarzabek-Chorzelska, M., Marciejowska, E., Rzesa, G. and Chorzelski, T.P. (1975). Studies in immunodermatology. IV. IF studies of autoantibodies to the stratum corneum and of *in vivo* fixed IgG in stratum corneum of psoriatic lesions. *Int. Arch. Allergy Appl. Immunol.* **48**, 301–23.

Bjerke, J.R., Krogh, H.K. and Matre, R. (1978). Characterization of mononuclear cell infiltrates in psoriatic lesions. *J. Invest. Dermatol.* **71**, 340–3.

Bos, J.D. (1988). The pathomechanisms of psoriasis: the skin immune system and cyclosporin. *Br. J. Dermatol.* **118**, 141–55.

Bos, J.D., Hulsebosch, H.J., Krieg, S.R., Bakker, P.M. and Cormane, R.H. (1983). Immunocompetent cells in psoriasis: *in situ* immunophenotyping by monoclonal antibodies. *Arch. Dermatol. Res.* **275**, 181–9.

Bos, J.D., Zonneveld, I., Das, P.K., Krieg, S.R., van der Loos, C.M. and Kapsenberg, M.L. (1987). The skin immune system (SIS): distribution and immunophenotype of lymphocytes subpopulations in normal human skin. *J. Invest. Dermatol.* **88**, 569–73.

Braun-Falco, O. and Christophers, E. (1974). Structural aspects of initial psoriatic lesions. *Arch. Dermatol. Forsch.* **251**, 95–110.

Braun-Falco, O. and Schmoeckel, C. (1977). The dermal inflammatory reaction in initial psoriatic lesions. *Arch. Dermatol. Res.* **258**, 9–16.

Brody, I. (1978). Alterations of clinically normal skin of early eruptive guttate psoriasis patients: a light- and electron-microscopic study. *J. Cutan. Pathol.* **5**, 219–33.

Coffey, R.J., Derynck, R., Wilcot, J.N. *et al.* (1987). Production and auto-induction of transforming growth factor-α in human keratinocytes. *Science* **328**, 817–20.

Cormane, R.H. (1981). Immunopathology of psoriasis. *Arch. Dermatol. Res.* **270**, 201–15.

Ellis, C.N., Gorsulowsky, D.C., Hamilton, T.A. *et al.* (1986). Cyclosporin improves psoriasis in a double-blind study. *JAMA* **256**, 3110–16.

Eyre, R.W. and Krueger, G.P. (1982). Response to injury of skin involved and uninvolved with psoriasis, and its relation with disease activity. *Br. J. Dermatol.* **106**, 153–9.

Fernandez, L.A. and Fox, R.A. (1980). Perturbation of the human immune system by lithium. *Clin. Exp. Immunol.* **41**, 527–32.

Fichtelius, K.E., Groth, O. and Liden, S. (1970). The skin, a first level lymphoid organ? *Int. Arch. Allergy. Appl. Immunol.* **37**, 607–20.

Fry, L. (1988). Psoriasis: centenary review. *Br. J. Dermatol.* **119**, 445–61.

Gearing, A.J.H., Fincham, N.J., Bird, C.R. *et al.* (1990). Cytokines in skin lesions of psoriasis. *Cytokine* **1**, 68–75.

Gottlieb, A.B., Grossman, R.M., Khandke, L. *et al.* (1992). Studies on the effect of cyclosporin in psoriasis *in vivo*: combined effects on activated T lymphocytes and epidermal regenerative maturation. *J. Invest. Dermatol.* **98**, 302–9.

Griffiths, C.E.M., Powles, A.V., Leonard, J.N., Fry, L., Baker, B.S. and Valdimarsson, H. (1986). Clearance of psoriasis with low dose cyclosporin. *Br. Med. J.* **293**, 731–2.

Griffiths, C.E.M., Voorhees, J.J. and Nickoloff, B.J. (1989). Gamma interferon induces different keratinocyte cellular patterns of expression of HLA-DR and DQ and intercellular adhesion molecule-1 (ICAM-1) antigens. *Br. J. Dermatol.* **120**, 1–7.

Hancock, G.E., Kaplan, G. and Cohn, Z. (1988). Keratinocyte growth regulated by the products of immune cells. *J. Exp. Med.* **168**, 1395–402.

Hellgren, L. (1967). *Psoriasis*. Almqvist and Wiksell, Stockholm.

Heng, M.C.Y., Allen, S.G. and Chase, D.G. (1988). High endothelial venules in involved and uninvolved psoriatic skin: recognition by homing receptors on cytotoxic T lymphocytes. *Br. J. Dermatol.* **188**, 315–26.

Hermosura, M.C., Jónsdóttir, I. and Valdimarsson, H. (1987). Cross-reaction of monoclonal antibodies against streptococci with normal human tissues. *Scand. J. Immunol.* **26**, 313 (abstract).

Iversen, O.J., Nissen-Meyjer, J. and Dalen, A.B. (1983). Characterization of virus-like particles from psoriatic patients with respect to the possible presence of particle-associated RNA and RNA-directed DNA polymerase. *Acta Pathol. Microbiol. Immunol. Scand.* **91**, 413–17.

Jablonska, S., Beutner, E.H., Binder, L.W., Jarzabeck-Charozelska, M., Rzesa, G. and Chowaniec, O. (1979). Immunopathology of psoriasis. *Arch. Dermatol. Res.* **264**, 65–71.

Jónsdóttir, I., Hermosura, M.C., Fry, L. and Valdimarsson, H. (1990). Cross-reactive epitope on group A streptococci with dendritic cells and endothelium; increased expression in inflammatory skin disease. *Scand. J. Immunol.* **32**, 399 (abstract).

Joost, T., Heule, F., Stolz, E. and Beukers, R. (1986). Short-term use of cyclosporin a in severe psoriasis. *Br. J. Dermatol.* **114**, 615–20.

Kragballe, K. and Herlin, T. (1983). Benoxaprofen improves psoriasis: a double-blind study. *Arch. Dermatol.* **119**, 548–52.

Kragballe, K., Desjarlais, L. and Voorhees, J.J. (1985). Leukotrienes B4, C4 and D4 stimulated DNA synthesis in cultured human epidermal keratinocytes. *Br. J. Dermatol.* **113**, 43–52.

Krueger, G.G., Jederberg, W.W., Ogden, B.E. and Reese, D.L. (1978). Inflammatory and immune cell function in psoriasis. II. Monocyte function, lymphokine production. *J. Invest. Dermatol.* **71**, 195–201.

Krueger, G.G., Chambers, D.A. and Shelby, J. (1981). Involved and uninvolved skin from psoriatic subjects: are they equally diseased? *J. Clin. Invest.* **68**, 1548–57.

Kulka, J.P. (1964). Microcirculatory impairments as a factor in inflammatory tissue damage. *Ann. NY Acad. Sci.* **116**, 1018–44.

Kupper, T.S., May, L., Birchall, N. and Sehgal, P. (1988a). Keratinocytes produce interleukin 6, a cytokine which can provide a second signal in the activation of T cells. *J. Invest. Dermatol.* **90**, 578 (abstract).

Kupper, T.S., Lee, F., Coleman, D., Chodakewitz, J. Flood, P. and Horowitz, M. (1988b). Keratinocyte-derived T-cell growth factor (KTGF) is identical to granulocyte macrophage colony stimulating factor (GM-CSF). *J. Invest. Dermatol.* **91**, 185–8.

Luger, T.A., Stadler, B.M., Luger, B.M. *et al.* (1981). Epidermal cell (keratinocyte) derived thymocyte activating factor (ETAF). *J. Immunol.* **127**, 1493–8.

Luger, T.A., Wirth, U. and Köck, A. (1985). Epidermal cells synthesize a cytokine with interleukin 3 like properties. *J. Immunol.* **154**, 915–19.

Morhenn, V.B. (1984). Is psoriasis a disease of the immune system? *Cutis* **34**, 223–4.

Morhenn, V.B. (1988). Keratinocyte proliferation in wound healing and skin disease. *Immunol. Today* **9**, 104–7.

Nickoloff, B.J. (1988). Role of interferon gamma in cutaneous trafficking of lymphocytes with emphasis on molecular and cellular adhesion events. *Arch. Dermatol.* **124**, 1835–43.

Nicolas, J.F., Chamchick, N., Thivolet, J., Wijdenes, J., Morel, P. and Revillard, J.P. (1991). CD4 antibody treatment of severe psoriasis. *Lancet* **338**, 321 (letter).

Norholm-Pederson, A. (1952). Infections and psoriasis. *Acta Dermato-venereol.* **32**, 159–67.

Norrlind, R. (1950). Psoriasis following infections with haemolytic streptococci. *Acta Dermato-venerol.* **30**, 64–72.

Penneys, N.S., Ziboh, V., Lord, J. and Simon, P. (1975). Inhibitor(s) of prostaglandin synthesis in psoriatic plaque. *Nature* **254**, 351–2.

Picker, L.J., Kishimoto, T.K., Smith, C.W., Warnock, R.A. and Butcher, E.C. (1991). ELAM-1 is an adhesion molecule for skin-homing T cells. *Nature* **349**, 796–9.

Pillai, S., Bikle, D.D., Eessalu, T.E., Aggarwal, B.B. and Elias, P.M. (1989). Binding and biological effects of tumour necrosis factor alpha on cultured human neonatal foreskin keratinocytes. *J. Clin. Invest.* **83**, 816–21.

Placek, W., Haftek, M. and Thivolet, J. (1988). Sequence of changes in psoriatic epidermis. *Acta Dermatol. Venereol. (Stockholm)* **68**, 369–77.

Poizot-Martin, I., Dhiver, C., Mawas, C., Olive, D. and Gastaut, J.A. (1991). Are CD4 antibodies and peptide T new treatment for psoriasis? *Lancet* **337**, 1477 (letter).

Priestley, G.C. (1983). Hyperactivity of fibroblasts cultured from psoriatic skin. II. Synthesis of macromolecules. *Br. J. Dermatol.* **109**, 157–64.

Priestley, G.C. and Adams, L.W. (1983). Hyperactivity of fibroblasts cultured from psoriatic skin. I. Faster proliferation and effect of serum withdrawal. *Br. J. Dermatol.* **109**, 149–56.

Ramirez-Bosca, A., Martinez-Ojeda, A., Valcuende-Cavero, F. and Castellas-Rodellas, A. (1988). A study of local immunity on psoriasis. *Br. J. Dermatol.* **119**, 587–95.

Reusch, M.K., Studtmann, M., Schröder, J.-M., Sticherling, M. and Christophers, E. (1990). NAP/interleukin 8 is a potent mitogen for human keratinocytes *in vitro*. *J. Invest. Dermatol.* **95**, 485 (abstract).

Ryan, T.J. (1980). Microcirculation in psoriasis: blood vessels, lymphatics and tissue fluid. *Pharmacol. Ther.* **10**, 27–64.

Sackstein, R., Falanga, V., Streilein, J.W. and Chin, Y.H. (1988). Lymphocyte adhesion to psoriatic dermal endothelium is mediated by a tissue-specific receptor/ligand interaction. *J. Invest. Dermatol.* **91**, 423–8.

Saiag, P., Coulomb, B., Lebreton, C., Bell, E. and Dabertret, L. (1985). Psoriatic fibroblasts induce hyperproliferation of normal keratinocytes in a skin equivalent model *in vitro*. *Science* **230**, 669–72.

Sauder, D.N. (1984). Epidermal cytokines: properties of epidermal cell thymocyte activating factor (ETAF). *Lymphokine Res.* **3**, 145–51.

Scheynius, A., Fransson, J., Johansson, C. *et al.* (1992). Expression of interferon-gamma receptors in normal and psoriatic skin. *J. Invest. Dermatol.* **98**, 255–8.

Sedgwick, J.B., Bergstresser, P.R. and Hurd, E.R. (1980). Increased granulocyte adherence in psoriasis and psoriatic arthritis. *J. Invest. Dermatol.* **74**, 81–4.

Shimizu, Y., Shaw, S., Graber, N. *et al.* (1991). Activation independent binding of human memory T cells to adhesion molecule ELAM-1. *Nature* **349**, 799–802.

Skoven, I. and Thormann, J. (1979). Lithium compound treatment and psoriasis. *Arch. Dermatol.* **115**, 1185–7.

Steinmuller, D., Zinsmeister, A.R. and Rogers, R.S. (1988). Cellular autoimmunity in psoriasis and lichen planus. *J. Autoimmunity* **1**, 279–98.

Steinsson, K., Jónsdóttir, I. and Valdimarsson, H. (1990). Cyclosporin A for psoriatic arthritis: an open study. *Ann. Rheum. Dis.* **49**, 603–6.

Streilein, J.W. (1978). Lymphocyte traffic, T cell malignancies and the skin. *J. Invest. Dermatol.* **71**, 167–71.

Swerlick, R.A., Cunningham, M.W. and Hall, N.K. (1986). Monoclonal antibodies cross-reactive with group A streptococci and normal and psoriatic human skin. *J. Invest. Dermatol.* **87**, 367–71.

Tagami, H., Iwatsuki, K. and Takematsu, H. (1987). Psoriasis and leukocyte chemotaxis. *J. Invest. Dermatol.* **88** (suppl.), 18–23.

Valdimarsson, H., Baker, B.S., Jónsdóttir, I. and Fry, L. (1986). Psoriasis: a disease of abnormal keratinocyte proliferation induced by T lymphocyte. *Immunol. Today* **7**, 256–9.

Voorhees, J.J. (1982). Psoriasis as a possible defect of the adenyl cyclase–cyclic AMP cascade. *Arch. Dermatol.* **118**, 862–8.

Voorhees, J.J. and Duell, E.A. (1971). Psoriasis as a possible defect of the adenyl cyclase–cyclic AMP cascade: a defective chalone mechanism. *Arch. Dermatol.* **104**, 352–8.

Weinstein, G.D. (1971). Biochemical and pathophysiological rationale for methotrexate in psoriasis. *Ann. NY Acad. Sci.* **186**, 452–66.

Wentzell, J.M., Banghman, R.D., O'Connor, G.T. and Bernier, G.M. (1987). Cyclosporine in the treatment of psoriasis. *Arch. Dermatol.* **123**, 163–5.

Wong, E., Camp, R.D. and Greaves, M.W. (1985). The response of normal and psoriatic skin to single and multiple topical applications of leukotriene LTB4. *J. Invest. Dermatol.* **84**, 421–3.

Wright, N.A. and Campeljohn, R.S. (1983). *Psoriasis: Cell Proliferation*. Churchill Livingstone, London.

98: Lung Disease

A. Newman Taylor, P.J. Cole and R. du Bois

Introduction

In man the lungs are evolved from foregut to mediate gas exchange. Their defences are derived from those previously protecting foregut and a number of pathological conditions in the airways and lungs can be ascribed, at least in part, to a lack of 'custom-built' defences. An obvious example is the origin of the laryngeal and tracheal airway from the lower oropharynx, hazarding it to aspiration of solid and fluid foods passing from the latter into the oesophagus.

During the last 15 years it has become apparent that the lung can mount a sophisticated local immune response and that several inflammatory diseases of unknown origin affecting the lung are mediated at least in part by the lung's own immunological mechanisms. The most obvious examples of this are the acute hypersensitivity conditions such as asthma (see Chapter 54) but there is accumulating evidence of inflammatory immune pathogenesis in interstitial lung disease, collagen vascular disease affecting the lung, chronic lung damage such as fibrosis and emphysema, and chronic airway damage such as bronchiectasis. The humoral and cellular mechanisms (e.g. granulomatous mechanisms) by which such conditions arise are described in detail elsewhere in this book but the evidence for their role in a variety of lung conditions will be cited in this organ-based chapter which, while not pretending to be a comprehensive review of all pulmonary disease, will highlight those conditions in which evidence for inflammatory immune mechanisms is strongest or in which evidence is particularly controversial.

Throughout this chapter runs a theme that the lung's intricate and delicate structure, necessary for successful gas exchange from air to blood, carries with it disadvantages. Exuberant lung defences, required to eliminate particularly noxious material inhaled into the lungs, or poorly controlled such defences, may damage the delicate anatomy of the lung and repair may permanently impair this primary gas-exchanging function. Hence, there is always a two-edged sword to the function of lung defences and there is a thin dividing line between health and disease in this organ as a result.

If the late 1970s and the 1980s were important for their observations of immunological and inflammatory phenomena associated with pulmonary disease, it is of immense importance that the 1990s should produce hard evidence for the definitive role of such *in vitro* or experimental *in vivo* phenomena in human respiratory diseases *in vivo*. The new technologies of molecular medicine together with the accessibility of the respiratory tract should make this possible.

Lung defences

The respiratory tract is a major interface with the environment. During a 24 hour period the approximately 500 m^2 surface area of the conducting airways and alveolar gas-exchanging portions of the adult respiratory tract 'see' organic and inorganic particles, including micro-organisms, inhaled in approximately 7000 litres of air. Such particles must be removed from this arena by the respiratory defence mechanisms if the individual is to remain healthy. Persistence of such matter, either organic or inorganic, living or dead, tends to stimulate a local response in the host which may be harmful. Hence, integrity of the clearance mechanisms of the airways and alveolar regions of the lung is of fundamental importance to maintenance of healthy lungs.

Clearance is achieved by integrated response of physical, protein-mediated and cellular mechanisms. Large particulate material is deposited on the fluid lining of the nose, paranasal sinuses, trachea and bronchi, whereas particles of less than 2.5 μm diameter may penetrate to the peripheral alveolar regions. Physical, protein-mediated and cellular mechanisms act at all these levels but physical and protein-mediated mechanisms are more important higher in the respiratory tract, whereas cellular mechanisms tend to predominate more peripherally. Information about the relative importance of the various defences with respect to specific insults to the lung is still mainly gained by study of nature's experiments (immune deficiency diseases) and of experimental models. And, although it is relatively easy to make observations regarding possible mechanisms for function and dysfunction of lung defences from *in vitro* and *in vivo* experimental models, it is crucial that in future we 'grasp the nettle' and take pains to demonstrate the actual role of such defence mechanisms in human disease *in vivo*.

Physical defences

It is particularly important to outline the principles underlying the operation of physical defences (Clarke 1990) as mechanisms for elimination of inhaled noxious agents from the respiratory tract, because not only are they the first-line defence mechanisms of the respiratory tract, but they also underlie to a large extent the principles of local targetting of particulate and aerosolized medication via the airways to various sites where drug action is required. This is a therapeutic advantage which the lung possesses over less accessible organs.

PARTICLE DEPOSITION

In the upper airways, between the external nares and lower border of the cricoid cartilage, air is filtered of its largest particles by inertial impaction and turbulent airflow via a system of baffles which also assist in humidifying and warming inspired air. The upper airways also participate in swallowing, speech and smell. In the lower airways, airflow patterns determine the sites of deposition of particles and generally, respired air moves by convective flow in the conducting airways where non-linear conditions allow central particle deposition, by axial molecular diffusion in the peripheral respiratory airways where forward flow is low, and by molecular diffusion across the alveolar capillary membrane. Particles less than 2.5 μm may penetrate to the alveolar regions, above this size such particles are deposited in the conducting and respiratory airways.

COUGH AND MUCOCILIARY CLEARANCE

Particles deposited in airways lining fluid (a layer of thicker mucus overlying a pericellular layer of thinner secretions) are removed principally by mucociliary clearance in which the thicker mucus is moved cephalad by coordinated dynein-dependent beating (at 12–15 Hz) of numerous hair-like epithelial lining cell appendages called cilia. Airway mucus originates from submucosal glands, goblet cells, Clara cells and tissue fluid transudate. Abnormality in the composition of the thicker mucus or in the beating of the cilia will disrupt this clearance and any change in underlying thinner secretions may act to disengage or obstruct the engagement of the tips of the beating cilia in the overlying mucus in which particles deposit. Reflex cough and sneeze are back-up mechanisms called into play to clear airways (in the case of cough down to the seventh or eighth bronchial division) by causing high linear airflow which interacts with secretions to cause two phase air–liquid flow transferring energy, from the air to the liquid, to shear it from the airway wall and carry it centrally. Changes in composition of mucus therefore also affect the efficiency of cough in clearing the airways.

ALVEOLAR CLEARANCE

Whereas the majority of particles are cleared from the conducting airways within 6 hours of deposition, alveolar clearance of particles less than 2.5 μm diameter takes much longer (more than 24 hours). It is achieved by transport of particles in surfactant to the ciliated airways for removal by mucociliary clearance, by transport of particles through the epithelium — across or between cells, and by removal of particles in phagocytes to the draining lymphatics or via the ciliated airways. The permeability of the alveolar epithelium is altered by a number of diseases and by cigarette smoking — leading to a tendency for leakage of proteins into the respiratory tract.

Protein-mediated defences

In addition to the physical clearance mechanisms an intricate system of proteins has been evolved within the respiratory tract largely to prevent microbial proliferation but also to reduce the likelihood of systemic spread through microbial invasion of pulmonary tissue (Stockley 1990). A large number of proteins have been demonstrated in respiratory secretions and these are basically concentrated by three routes: plasma-derived proteins (e.g. albumin, transferrin) probably diffusing through intercellular junctions to achieve a local concentration related to molecular size; local production (e.g. lysozyme); and selective transportation (e.g. immunoglobulin A (IgA) which binds to receptors for secretory component on epithelial cells and is actively transported through the cell to be released at the luminal surface). Some proteins enter the secretions by more than one route (e.g. complement components and some proteinase inhibitors present in plasma are also produced by lung cells). These proteins play a protective role in preventing microbial colonization of the respiratory tract and augment this 'static' role by acting to mobilize cellular defences.

ANTIMICROBIAL PROTEINS

These are relatively understudied but examples are the iron-binding proteins, lactoferrin and transferrin, which can prevent iron (required for bacterial growth) from being taken up by bacteria, and lysozyme which damages bacterial membrane carbohydrates leading to their disruption.

SECRETORY IMMUNOGLOBULINS (Burnett 1986)

All classes of immunoglobulins (Ig) are present in plasma and are of a size permitting diffusion into the lung, but the local concentration of these in secretions exceeds that which would be extrapolated from their size. It is thought that the majority of IgA and IgG present in the lung is synthesized locally. In larger airways the bronchial wall contains more plasma cells staining for IgA than IgG, whereas in peripheral airways the reverse is the case. Correspondingly, selective sampling of secretions in the trachea and main bronchi shows them to contain relatively more IgA than IgG, and secretions from bronchioles and alveoli contain relatively more IgG. Immunoglobulin A is present in a different form in the secretions to that in plasma — at least 50% being dimeric. Dimeric IgA is assembled in plasma cells from two monomeric IgA molecules joined by a protein J chain. The dimer when released is bound by a receptor, secretory component (SC), inserted into the basolateral surface of some mucosal epithelial cells. This dimeric IgA–SC complex is taken up by endocytosis, transported in vesicles across the cell and released at the luminal surface as a complete IgA molecule. The two subclasses of IgA are present in secretions in different ratios to their presence in plasma — in secretions 70% is IgA1 whereas in plasma up to 90% is of this subclass. The relevance of this to the ability of certain bacteria containing IgA1 proteinases to cleave IgA1 is uncertain.

Immunoglobulin G subclasses in secretions also differ in proportion to that in plasma in that more IgG3 and IgG4 appear to be synthesized within the lung than IgG1 and IgG2. The mechanisms of transport of IgG from the submucosal plasma cells to the epithelial surface is not known. At any one time the proportion of Ig synthesized locally to that derived from plasma depends on the amount of lung inflammation but it is thought that at least 50% of IgG is locally produced.

The presence of IgA as the major Ig in the proximal airway secretions suggests an important role for it in defence — but its function in this respect is not obvious and therefore it is possible that it is prominent because of a former role in the foregut from which the lung is derived. Nevertheless, binding of SC not only assists its movement into secretions but also protects the heavy chain region of the molecule against IgA1 proteinases (Kilian *et al.* 1980), and excess SC stabilizes one of the IgG2 antibody species (IgAm2) which is resistant to bacterial proteolysis. Dimeric IgA, having four antigen binding sites, could block binding of bacteria and viruses by epithelial cells, but the J chain and SC could interfere with its ability to opsonize and activate complement. Immunoglobulin A could also interfere with specific IgG opsonizing antibodies by preferential binding of antigen (Musher *et al.* 1984). Much of the information about IgA function is indirect — antibodies are known to increase after local but not systemic antigen challenge and have been detected up to 3 years after such challenge, suggesting that a challenged secretory IgA system might provide long-lived protection. Patients with selective IgA deficiency tend to suffer from recurrent respiratory viral infections but on the other hand, blood transfusion donor studies have suggested about one in 700 normal persons to have plasma deficiency of the antibody (although the local secretory IgA antibody status of such persons was not assessed and might be normal, also both IgG and IgM are thought to be able to provide a compensatory mechanism for IgA deficiency). Secretory IgA is suggested to play a role in preventing antigen access across the mucosa and atopy has been ascribed to failure of secretory IgA to provide this role early in life.

The role of IgG in the respiratory tract is somewhat clearer where it is the major local antibody in the peripheral airways and alveoli. Immunoglobulin G3 and IgG4 tend to be the more abundant subclasses locally and this may reflect their importance in opsonization for macrophage phagocytosis — these cells tending to have the appropriate Fc receptors (FcR) for these subclasses (Merrill *et al.* 1985). Nevertheless, polysaccharide antigens (e.g. capsulated bacteria) induce IgG2 responses which are obviously important in defence in the respiratory tract. The important role of IgG in the respiratory tract is suggested by the major featuring of recurrent respiratory bacterial infections in patients with hypogammaglobulinaemia, and by similar infections in patients with more subtle deficiencies of IgG2 alone or in combination with IgA deficiency (Bjorkander *et al.* 1985). It has been suggested that the most important role for IgG in the lung is in secondary defence after initial penetration of antigen and entry to the tissues with resulting inflammation which increases protein transudation (including plasma Igs) and increases local numbers of IgG staining cells. Experimental work has shown that bacterial proliferation in the lung can be prevented by simultaneous administration of IgG systemically (Toews *et al.* 1985) which provides specific antibodies found in the lung secretions. The ability of IgG to opsonize bacteria and activate complement is suggested by observations in cystic fibrosis in which persistence of *Pseudomonas aeruginosa* occurs even in the presence of an exuberant host response. It has been suggested that the micro-organism prevents its own clearance by releasing proteinases which cleave IgG: the Fab fragment is still able to bind bacterial antigen but the loss of the Fc portion prevents binding to complement or phagocyte receptors (Fick *et al.* 1985). It has also been suggested that antigen binding with IgG2 which is predominant in the secretions in this situation might block the binding of other subclasses such as IgG3 and IgG4 which are better opsonins (Fick *et al.* 1986). Both IgA and IgM appear to have potential to be helpful or harmful in protection against micro-organisms depending on the amount and subclass of antibody produced.

Immunoglobulin M, a pentameric molecule with 10 binding sites, is the best complement-fixing Ig. Being the initial Ig to be produced in primary and secondary immune responses it is well placed to neutralize micro-organisms in the vascular compartment. However its role in lung secretions is uncertain. Immunoglobulin D-bearing cells are increased in respiratory tract tissue in selective IgA deficiency and therefore the former antibody could play a compensatory role but its function is unknown. Immunoglobulin E is fully considered in Chapter 52 in relation to its role in type I hypersensitivity and both asthma and parasitic disease.

COMPLEMENT COMPONENTS

The majority of complement components in the lung secretions are derived from plasma during the inflammatory response, but early activation of small amounts of C3 and C5 in the secretions may be crucial to initial inflammation, and it is well recognized that alveolar macrophages can synthesize most complement components. Macrophages, and also bacteria, can cleave C3 and C5 into the chemotactic peptides C3a and C5a which recruit neutrophils, monocytes and eosinophils to the respiratory tract. Complement fragment C3b can also stimulate antibody production, cytokine production and antibody-dependent cell-mediated cytotoxicity, and C5a is an opsonin. Diffusion of other complement components activates the cascade which ultimately lyses bacterial cells by binding the terminal components forming the attack complex. The importance of complement components to defence is demonstrated indirectly by the C5-deficient mouse which cannot clear bacteria from the lung, and C3 deficiency in man in which recurrent respiratory bacterial infections are characteristic. Since activation of C3 results in production of C3b which opsonizes via specific phagocyte receptors and also binds factor B which activates the alternative pathway of complement, it is likely that the latter pathway is of considerable importance in protecting the respiratory tract.

CYTOKINES

Of considerable importance in the respiratory tract are the cytokines, and among them the chemotaxins which recruit and activate inflammatory cells to the site of the initial inflammatory response. Dose-dependent cellular responses to these chemotaxins and presence of inactivators of them suggest intricate homeostatic control processes to enable such cell recruitment to remain beneficial in lung infection and inflammation. Nevertheless, persistent recruitment of inflammatory cells in some situations leads to harmful lung inflammation (e.g. in bronchiectasis).

PROTEINASE INHIBITORS

There are several inhibitors of proteolytic enzymes produced in the lung (e.g. α-1-antichymotrypsin, anti-leukoproteinase) as well as those derived from plasma (α-1-proteinase inhibitor). These proteinase inhibitors are crucial for neutralizing the proteolytic enzymes released from resident alveolar macrophages and recruited inflammatory cells (e.g. neutrophils) during their activation, phagocytosis and non-apoptotic death. In persistent inflammation this anti-proteolytic activity may be overwhelmed, allowing harmful proteolytic enzymes (e.g. neutrophil elastase) to remain free in the secretions.

Cellular defences

Phagocytes, especially macrophages and polymorphonuclear neutrophils (PMN), represent major components of pulmonary inflammatory and immunological responses. They participate in both defensive and injurious processes in the lungs. Macrophages compose the majority of phagocytes in the lower respiratory tract in health and are morphologically and functionally heterogeneous — including alveolar, interstitial, intravascular and airway macrophages — each with characteristic features (reviewed in Sibille and Reynolds 1990). The macrophage is a versatile cell with paradoxical properties — able to release mediators, oxidants and proteolytic enzymes, but also able to secrete inhibitors to cytokines, antioxidants and anti-proteinases. By contrast, polymorphonuclear leucocytes (PMN) compose less than 1% of cells in the lower airways in health but when recruited in inflammatory states can easily outnumber macrophages, and therefore produce a considerable burden of proteolytic enzymes and reactive oxygen species within respiratory tissues. This may be used to the host's advantage but may also be to its disadvantage in some situations. Both these phagocytes however represent only one component of a complete network of interacting humoral and cellular factors in defence, injury and repair. Other cellular components include lymphocytes, eosinophils, fibroblasts, platelets, endothelial and epithelial cells.

ALVEOLAR MACROPHAGES

There is considerable literature of *in vitro* observations concerning the role of alveolar macrophages (AM) in lung defence (reviewed by Sibille and Reynolds 1990) and it is unfortunate that experimental conditions can so easily alter such observed functions. Therefore a crucial question is always the cell's role in *in vivo* human disease — about which there is much less written. *In vivo* evidence of its function from experimental models includes clearance of small numbers (10^5) of aerosol-administered Gram +ve bacteria such as

Staphylococcus aureus without observed inflammation (Rehn *et al.* 1980), and clearance of *Streptococcus sanguis* — which requires a doubling of the macrophage population (Onofrio *et al.* 1981). Experiments with larger numbers of *Staph. aureus* and other pathogens has shown clearance to require recruitment of PMN. In the presence or absence of opsonins, AM clear Gram +ve bacteria and acid-fast mycobacteria on the whole better than they do Gram +ve pathogens (Reynolds 1979).

Although no selective functional defect has been reported in AM their importance in infection is suggested when their function is impaired by factors in their immediate *in vivo* environment. For example, in alveolar proteinosis, in which lipoprotein material from surfactant is not cleared, AM are seen to be full of lipoprotein in the form of lamellar bodies and this is associated with disordered function of these cells when they are tested *in vitro*. Patients with this disorder suffer respiratory infections and their blood monocytes function normally suggesting the acquired environmental alteration of AM function underlies the infections (Nugent and Persanti 1983). Another example is acute smoke inhalation which impairs AM chemotaxis and may be associated with infection (Demarest *et al.* 1979). There are other conditions associated with infection in which *in vitro* functions of AM are impaired, but without an experiment of nature in which AM are specifically defective, the case for the cell as primarily a scavenger cell for killing micro-organisms is weak, and it is likely that the scavenger role of AM is concerned more with antigen presentation to effector cells in the immune response.

Similarly, there is much literature of *in vitro* observations concerning the role of the AM in lung injury, but evidence for an important role for these cells *in vivo* in these conditions is less convincing — again because of the lack of an *in vivo* model with specific AM defect. Preliminary evidence of a contribution of AM to *in vivo* lung injury came from experimental studies in which lung damage was induced by intratracheal administration of phorbol myristate acetate. Here the damage was independent of PMN but was complement dependent and was associated with macrophage activation (Johnson and Ward 1982). Further evidence accrued from the observation that PMN depletion did not prevent lung injury from IgA immune complexes in a model in which increased numbers of AM were found and in which these cells spontaneously released reactive oxygen species when tested *in vitro* (Johnson *et al.* 1984, 1986). This latter model is obviously very artificial, with high levels of intra-alveolar IgA probably never encountered *in vivo*, so interpretation must be cautious. The finding of increased levels of AM secretory products in bronchoalveolar lavage from diseased lungs suggests a role for AM in pathogenesis of such diseases, but is far from conclusive since other cell types are inevitably present. Observations that support a contribution of the macrophage to repair processes are appearing — for instance, Rappolee *et al.* (1988) have shown macrophages in healing wounds of mice produce several growth factors including transforming growth factors alpha and beta, and platelet derived growth factor, as detected by *in situ* hybridization with messenger ribonucleic acid (mRNA).

The role of AM in attracting PMN is suggested by animal studies, by studies in normal volunteers and by studies in interstitial lung diseases all of which have shown release of several chemotaxins and activating factors from AM. Inhibitory factor from PMN chemotaxis has also been demonstrated to be released by AM and suggest that the latter cell can regulate PMN recruitment, activation and control.

POLYMORPHONUCLEAR NEUTROPHILS

The contribution of the PMN to pulmonary defence is inferred, as in the case of AM, mainly from *in vitro* observations of the nature of its adherence, migration and secretory products.

However, there is better evidence of PMN function being important in human disease *in vivo* from the study of natural immunodeficiency in man and in experimental animal models. Patients with profound neutropenia, or with selective defects in PMN function, suffer from recurrent respiratory infections. Examples of this are chronic granulomatous disease (Segal *et al.* 1987) and specific granule deficiency (Gallin 1985), although there are several others described. In chronic granulomatous disease, owing to a genetic defect in cytochrome b and inefficient phosphorylation of a membrane-associated protein, patients cannot mount an oxidative metabolic response in phagocytes and suffer frequent severe infections with catalase +ve bacteria. Acquired disorders of PMN are illustrated by neutropenia associated with myeloproliferative disease induced by irradiation or chemotherapy, or associated with toxic agents, in which respiratory infections may frequently occur.

The evidence for a role of PMN in lung injury unfortunately again rests mainly on *in vitro* observation, but study of these cells in adult respiratory distress syndrome, emphysema, interstitial lung diseases and bronchiectasis lends some support for an active role for the PMN in diseases *in vivo*. In these conditions it is proposed that PMN-derived proteinases and reactive oxygen species are damaging to host tissue. But in most of these conditions there are other hypotheses for the source of lung injury and most evidence points to the fact that the PMN's role is not exclusive and depends on the participation of a number of other cell types.

DENDRITIC CELLS

Schon-Hegrad *et al*. (1991) have recently prepared rat bronchus for microscopy by cutting it tangentially, parallel to the plane of the bronchial lumen. By this technique they have defined a webbed network of cells lining the airways with classical dendritic cell morphology, which they have shown to be responsible for the majority of Ia staining in the rat respiratory tree. These cells number approximately 600–800/mm^2 epithelial surface in large airways and 75/mm^2 epithelial surface in small peripheral airways, co-stain for CD4, and increase in density by up to 50% in large airways with threefold increase in expression of activation markers (including beta chain of CD11/CD18) on stimulation with lipopolysaccharide. The kinetics of changes in this dendritic cell network in response to lipopolysaccharide mirrored those of transient neutrophil influx, suggesting that airway intraepithelial dendritic cells constitute a dynamic population which is rapidly upregulated in response to local inflammation.

LYMPHOCYTES

It is well established that many cells of the lymphoid series are found throughout the lung. They are scattered between epithelial cells and basement membrane, aggregated as follicles and present as loose aggregates. The follicles contain B cells staining for IgA and IgM and both aggregates and follicles are in contact with the epithelium making it likely that this 'bronchus-associated lymphoid tissue' has a role in processing antigen, and providing local antibody and cellular responses. Lymphocytes recovered in bronchoalveolar lavage in normal subjects compose about 10% of total cell yield and, of these, approximately 70% are T cells, 10% B cells and 20% null cells. Further information about the local role of T lymphocytes comes from study of asthma (see Chapter 54) and bronchiectasis (see below).

Lung responses

Helpful versus harmful responses

Elimination of potentially harmful agents, inhaled or arriving in the lung via blood, is the first requirement of the respiratory host defences. Helpful responses in the respiratory tract involve operation of non-specific and immunological defences described above. Should these fail to eliminate such agents even after local responses have been augmented by defences recruited from the systemic circulation, the host response to persistent antigen may become injurious to the host. The nature and severity of such host responses will depend upon the amount of the agent, its quality (size and shape — determining deposition site, solubility, degradability and immunogenicity), its route of arrival in the lung, and the quality of exposure conditions (e.g. single large exposure or continuous/intermittent small exposures).

The function of processes controlling and curtailing normal host responses appear to be of considerable importance because in a number of conditions in which host processes damage the lung there appear to be a lack of such regulation. On the other hand, deficiency of host-defence mechanisms within the respiratory tract may also fail to eliminate living micro-organisms which may then proliferate and either colonize the airways or invade the epithelium to spread elsewhere in the body.

Responses to infection

Host responses allowing acute or recurrent respiratory infection tend to be deficient, whereas chronic respiratory infection tends to be associated with poorly regulated host responses, often giving rise to host-mediated disease even though these host mechanisms are stimulated by presence of persistent micro-organisms.

DEFICIENT IMMUNE RESPONSES AND ACUTE OR RECURRENT INFECTION

There are many immune deficiencies, often rare, which may present in childhood or adult life with respiratory infection and these are described in Chapter 66. However, in this organ-based chapter, it is appropriate to consider the commonest immune deficiencies of adults presenting to respiratory physicians. In a clinic devoted to problematic recurrent-acute and chronic respiratory infections, if patients suffering from human immunodeficiency virus (HIV) infection presenting with recurrent opportunistic infections are first excluded, two major syndromes are seen (Cole 1989). These syndromes are: (i) recurrent-acute respiratory infections (often slow to resolve or to respond to antibiotics) with apparently completely normal periods between episodes; and (ii) persistent purulent infected sputum production daily (i.e. chronic infection). In the first group of patients were found the majority of immune deficiencies, the commonest being selective IgA deficiency (more than 40%). The latter condition is associated with recurrent upper and lower respiratory viral infections and when tested, secretory as well as serum IgA is usually selectively decreased or absent. Such patients rarely progress to chronic (e.g. bronchiectatic) lung disease. Oxelius and her colleagues (1981) demonstrated that symptomatic children with selective IgA deficiency also lack IgG2 and/or IgG4 subclass antibody — but this has not been the general experience in adults, although it is important to identify such patients because of the implication for treatment with Ig reconstitution. It is likely that decreased IgA levels in secretions can be compensated by increased IgG or IgM levels in some patients. Because patients with selective absence of IgA are prone to allergic reactions and anaphylaxis to blood products, it is important to screen such patients for the presence of anti-IgA antibodies before contemplating Ig treatment of associated IgG subclass deficiency as preparations may contain small amounts of IgA.

Recurrent bacterial pneumonias were uncommon in Cole's series (1989) but 25% of those presenting with this pattern of infection were found to have treatable panhypogammaglobulinaemia, making it mandatory to retain a high index of suspicion of this deficiency in such patients. The majority of such patients have common variable immunodeficiency which may represent a spectrum of diseases. No mode of inheritance has been found, males and females are equally affected, and the condition is associated with recurrent bronchial infections or pneumonias with recurrent paranasal sinusitis. As time passes and more permanent damage occurs to the respiratory tract symptoms tend to become more chronic. There may be associated chronic or recurrent diarrhoea, often associated with giardiasis. Hepatosplenomegaly can occur with non-caseating granulomata of lungs, spleen, skin and liver (which may be diagnosed as sarcoidosis) and these may respond to corticosteroids. Biopsy of the gastrointestinal tract shows lymphocytic infiltration of the lamina propria, blunting of the intestinal villi and occasional nodular lymphoid hyperplasia. Neoplasia of the stomach, thymoma and lymphoma may supervene. Associated with the low IgG levels in this condition there are various patterns of IgA and IgM deficiency.

Most patients with common variable immunodefiency have normal or increased numbers of B lymphocytes (in contrast to congenital X-linked agammaglobulinaemia) but these do not develop into mature secreting plasma cells and these are not found in the tissues. The B lymphocytes either fail to proliferate or to synthesize Ig or do synthesize it but fail to secrete it. The role of suppression of B cell function in these patients is probably small. Treatment with intravenous Ig infusions every 2–3 weeks usually results in much improved control of infection but irreversible lung damage influences the final response to treatment. Total serum IgG in such treated patients seems to bear little relation to therapeutic response, but studies measuring the opsonic capacity of treated patients' serum suggest this to be better related to response, and of some use in planning dose and interval between doses (Garbett *et al.* 1989).

RESPONSE TO PERSISTENT BACTERIA: CHRONIC BRONCHIAL INFECTION

The second syndrome seen in the respiratory clinic devoted to infective problems is chronic bronchial sepsis presenting as persistent production of purulent infected (as opposed to eosinophilic) sputum. The majority of patients presenting with this syndrome are never-smokers (occasionally ex-smokers) who can be shown by imaging techniques to have diffuse bronchiectasis (Cole 1990). There is a female preponderance of the condition and 30% of patients have a known cause for this syndrome (e.g. cystic fibrosis, primary ciliary dyskinesia). The 70% of patients with idiopathic bronchiectasis constitute a group of patients in whom much has been recently learned about host–microbial interrelationships in the respiratory tract (Cole and Wilson 1989) — particularly with respect to subversion of host immunological responses by colonizing/infecting micro-organisms.

Bronchiectasis (Cole 1990), irreversibly damaged and dilated bronchi, is a condition often associated with para-nasal sinusitis in which there is less than 10% prevalence of immune deficiency and in which, by contrast, host immune responses are either normal or heightened (Cole 1989). On the other hand the micro-organisms found in the respiratory secretions are not of virulent, tissue-invading type. The various known causes of the condition have in common the ability to impair mucus clearance and it transpires that an insult to the respiratory tract (e.g. viral infection) in the presence of such susceptibility gives rise to a 'vicious circle' of events resulting in progressive lung damage. When mucus clearance is slowed, inhaled micro-organisms loiter within the sino-bronchial tree and those which are able to produce epithelium-injuring exotoxins are selected to colonize the airways (Wilson *et al.* 1987; Steinfort *et al.* 1989). Colonization by such micro-organisms causes direct toxin-mediated damage to the respiratory tract which further impairs clearance (Munro *et al.* 1989) and increases microbial colonization. Two host responses occur in this situation: relentless recruitment of PMN which traverse the bronchial wall (Currie *et al.* 1990) and pass into the bronchial mucus where the majority of bacteria are found, and development of a florid cellular immune response within the bronchial wall. The latter is characterized by a diffuse increase in CD8 +ve lymphocytes (activated with respect to a variety of activation markers) and in both mature and dendritic macrophages with development of discrete follicular collections of mainly activated CD4 +ve lymphocytes (Lapa e Silva 1989a). This sequence of events is interpreted as being bacteria-stimulated but host-mediated and it is postulated that, following initial bacterial stimulus to neutrophil recruitment, the continuous traffic which occurs thereafter may be driven by local cytokine production (interleukin 8 (IL-8) has been found in significant levels in the bronchoalveolar lavage from patients with cystic fibrosis (Wilmott *et al.* 1992)). Since this neutrophil traffic appears to be damaging to the host (released neutrophil elastase damages epithelium and matrix proteins, stimulates mucus gland proliferation and is a potent mucin secretagogue) by causing progressive 'innocent bystander' lung damage, it would appear that this is an example of predominantly host-mediated disease. The continuous PMN traffic in this process contrasts starkly with the apparent switch off of PMN recruitment to alveolar regions about 20 hours into bacterial pneumonia caused by pneumococcus. An experimental model of bronchiectasis in the rat confirms the findings in the human (Lapa e Silva 1989b) and allows manipulation of the host response from which it appears that anti-inflammatory strategies can prevent the onset of tissue damage (Lapa e Silva 1992) — although it is unclear whether this is mediated through effects on the PMN directly or indirectly via the cell-mediated immune response within the bronchial wall.

ACQUIRED IMMUNE DEFICIENCY SYNDROME

The syndrome of acquired immune deficiency syndrome (AIDS) is discussed in Chapter 72. However, it is relevant in this organ-based chapter to comment on one or two aspects particularly related to the lung. First, although HIV infection of alveolar macrophages has been demonstrated (Salahuddin *et al.* 1986) it is thought that the functional impairment of these cells is mainly secondary to reduced T4 cell-derived lymphokines (Murray *et al.* 1985). Secondly, B lymphocytes are normal in number but due to polyclonal activation there is a polyclonal increase in IgG and IgA (also IgM in children). These B cells do not respond to neo-antigens therefore serological diagnosis of opportunistic infections is usually unhelpful. The elevated IgG is mainly IgG1 subclass and the subclasses IgG2–4 may be abnormal and predispose to bacterial infections, particularly with capsulated organisms (e.g. pneumococcus). This disease has a T cell defect as its predominant feature, with associated B cell abnormalities and most of the information about these cells has been gleaned from study of blood cells. Bronchoalveolar lavage cell data from both AIDS-related complex (Venet *et al*. 1985b) and AIDS patients (Young *et al*. 1985) show significantly increased lymphocyte numbers which are mainly CD8 +ve in phenotype (contrasting with the reduced numbers of circulating cells), suggesting either sequestering of these cells in the lung or local expansion of this subpopulation. There is increased IgG and IgA in bronchoalveolar lavage fluid which may arise from transudation or local production (Young *et al*. 1985).

ACUTE RESPIRATORY DISTRESS SYNDROME

This is included in this section because one of its causes is sepsis — although trauma is the important other cause. Acute respiratory distress syndrome (ARDS) or 'shock lung' presents as progressively worsening lung function a few hours or days after an episode of septic shock or severe trauma often remote from the lung. There is interstitial pulmonary oedema, without elevation of pulmonary capillary wedge pressure, progressive difficulty in achieving oxygenation using high concentrations of inspired oxygen, and reduced lung compliance. Mortality is high.

Pathogenesis of the condition remains unclear — the precipitating insults vary and there is evidence for participation of many biological systems. The characteristic delay of 12–72 hours between insult and onset of the syndrome has not been adequately explained. There is considerable literature suggesting a central role for the PMN in pathogenesis with pulmonary microvascular sequestration and translocation, for activation of the complement system, for changes in microvascular permeability and for a role of platelets. However, although this literature heavily incriminates the PMN as effector cell in the lung injury of ARDS, most of it constitutes observations *in vitro* or in experimental models and does not constitute a proven case in the *in vivo* human disease. In addition, there is a subset of causes of ARDS (e.g. caused by oxygen toxicity (Deneke and Fenberg 1980)) in which non-complement-derived stimulation of PMN appears to be important in a pathogenetic sequence that may be intrapulmonary rather than intravascular. The fact that potent oxidizing toxins such as paraquat may damage lung cells in culture in the absence of granulocytes (Martin *et al*. 1981) also suggests that PMN may not always be as essential for the condition to develop as the literature might suggest.

Granulomatous responses

Granulomata are focal accumulations of cells of the mononuclear phagocyte system. Granuloma formation is provoked by stimuli which persist in tissue; these may be inert (e.g. talc) which cause 'foreign body' granulomata or antigenic (e.g. *Mycobacterium tuberculosis*, *Faenia rectivirgula*, beryllium salts) which cause 'hypersensitivity' or immune granulomata. Whereas 'foreign body' granulomata are formed almost solely of mononuclear phagocytes, immune granulomata in addition contain T lymphocytes.

Several lung diseases in which a T-lymphocyte response is believed to play an important role are characterized by granuloma formation in the lungs. These include diseases of known cause such as tuberculosis and farmer's lung and of unknown cause such as sarcoidosis. The immunopathology of these diseases will be considered separately. Other diseases in which granuloma formation occurs (such as Wegener's granulomatosis and allergic granulomatosis — Churg–Strauss syndrome) will be considered with the other forms of vasculitis of the lung.

SARCOIDOSIS

Sarcoidosis is a granulomatous disease of unknown cause which involves many organs of the body and especially the lungs, lymph nodes and liver. Sarcoid granulomata are composed of mononuclear phagocytes with epithelioid and giant cells in their centre, and T lymphocytes. CD4 +ve T lymphocytes are closely associated with the epithelioid cells while both CD4 and CD8 T lymphocytes accumulate at the periphery (Campbell *et al*. 1985b).

The characteristic immunological abnormalities in sarcoidosis are: peripheral blood and bronchoalveolar lavage (BAL) hyper-globulinaemia; depression of 'delayed type' hypersensitivity reactions in the skin to tuberculin and other similar antigens such as Candida and mumps. Peripheral blood lymphocyte numbers are reduced and CD4 : CD8 ratios depressed to approximately 1–1.5 : 1. These are not manifestations of a generalized immune defect, but the consequence of heightened immunological activity which is 'compartmentalized' to sites of disease activity (Hunninghake and Crystal 1981). In patients with pulmonary sarcoidosis the total number of cells recovered by bronchoalveolar lavage is increased five- to tenfold and the proportion of lymphocytes increased from the normal of less than 10–14% to between 15% and 50%. More than 90% of the lymphocytes recovered are T lymphocytes and the CD4 :CD8 ratio has been reported to be increased from the value of 1.8 : 1 in normal controls to 10.5 : 1 (Hunninghake and Crystal 1981). T lymphocytes recovered at BAL from patients with sarcoidosis (but not those circulating in blood of these patients or recovered from 'normal' BAL) spontaneously secrete interleukin-2 (IL-2) contain increased amounts of mRNA for IL-2 and show a tenfold increase in spontaneous replication, consistent with the known biological activity of IL-2 (Pinkston *et al.* 1983; Muller-Quernheim *et al.* 1986). Other T cell surface markers of activation are expressed. Increased percentages of T cells expressing IL-2 receptor (IL-2R) have been noted in studies of T lymphocytes recovered at BAL and in lung tissue, lymph nodes, and conjunctiva of patients with sarcoidosis (Semenzato *et al.* 1984). In the lung, IL-2R expression has been reported both on T lymphocytes and on epithelioid and multinucleate giant cells within granulomata in lung and lymph node specimens from patients with sarcoidosis (Hancock *et al.* 1986). More recently, soluble IL-2R has been found in increased concentration in the blood (four- to fivefold) and in BAL from patients with active sarcoidosis (Lawrence *et al.* 1988). An increased number of T cells bearing HLA-DR class II MHC molecules as well as the VLA-1 marker of late activations are present (Costabel *et al.* 1985; Saltini *et al.* 1988). Bronchoalveolar lavage T lymphocytes from patients with pulmonary sarcoidosis also spontaneously secrete a monocyte chemotactic factor, migration inhibitory factor and interferon-γ (Hunninghake *et al.* 1980b; Robinson *et al.* 1985; Saltini and Crystal 1985). The number of cells recovered at BAL from patients with pulmonary sarcoidosis secreting IgG and IgM is no different from controls despite increases in BAL Igs suggesting that it is in the interstitium that increased Ig synthesis occurs (Hance *et al.* 1988). Furthermore, BAL T lymphocytes from sarcoidosis patients co-cultured with blood mononuclear cells from normal individuals, induce differentiation of Ig secreting cells, whereas T lymphocytes from normal individuals do not exert this effect (Hunninghake and Crystal 1981).

Alveolar macrophages recovered at BAL from patients with pulmonary sarcoidosis although reduced as a proportion of the total cells are increased in number. In addition they have been reported to secrete IL-1 spontaneously (Hunninghake 1984) although this point remains controversial, and TNF-α, a potent inducer of other inflammatory mediator gene expression, as well as inflammatory cell adhesion molecules, particularly after IL-2 stimulation (Strieter *et al.* 1989). Although all macrophages from normal individuals and patients with sarcoidosis express HLA-DR class II molecules, an increased density of class II expression is observed in sarcoidosis (Campbell *et al.* 1986). Consistent with this observation, alveolar macrophages from sarcoid patients are capable of enhanced presentation of recall antigens (Venet *et al.* 1985a). Other studies have shown alveolar macrophages to have reduced available C3b receptor sites and decreased intracellular *N*-acetyl-βd-glucosaminidase, a lysosomal enzyme (du Bois *et al.* 1981).

All available evidence suggests that granuloma formation in sarcoidosis is the consequence of a T cell driven process resulting in the accumulation of mononuclear cells into granulomata. Further evidence which supports the concept that T cells are subjected to persistent antigen stimulation includes: T cells from the lower respiratory tract bear the CD45RO phenotype of the primed memory type T cell (Dominique *et al.* 1990); lung but not blood T cells express reduced surface levels of T cell antigen receptor (TCR) but increased TCR beta chain mRNA (du Bois *et al.* 1992); the presence of a limited bias in TCR V-beta chain usage (Vβ8) in some patients which suggests a specific response to antigen (Moller *et al.* 1988). The nature of the antigen remains unidentified.

BERYLLIUM DISEASE

Chronic beryllium disease is a granulomatous multisystem disease caused by inhaled beryllium probably acting as an immunogenic hapten. Its manifestations are not in any important respect different from sarcoidosis, the major difference being the identifiable extrinsic cause. Like sarcoidosis the number of T lymphocytes recovered at BAL is increased with an increased CD4 : CD8 ratio, they express HLA class II, molecules, IL-2R and release IL-2. A recent study (Saltini *et al.* 1989) has shown the T-lymphocyte response to beryllium to be antigen-specific, IL-2 dependent and MHC class II restricted, consistent with the disease being the outcome of a specific T-lymphocyte response to beryllium. Beryllium-stimulated T-cell clones showed different rearrangements of TCR β chains suggesting that beryllium does not induce a monoclonal population but a T-cell response with different specificities. As in sarcoidosis, lung T cells from patients with chronic beryllium disease express the CD45RO phenotype of primed T cells (Saltini *et al.* 1990). Both lung and blood T cells from patients with chronic beryllium disease transform in response to *in vitro* stimulation with appropriate concentration of beryllium (Rossman *et al.* 1988).

EXTRINSIC ALLERGIC ALVEOLITIS

Concepts of the immunological basis of extrinsic allergic alveolitis (EAA) have undergone considerable change in recent years, particularly since the introduction of BAL has provided direct access to cells from the lungs which may be participating in the immunological response.

The hypothesis that EAA was the outcome of local complement fixing immune complexes, formed between inhaled antigen and circulating antibody, deposited in the lungs, was based on several observations: the presence of specific IgG antibodies (precipitins) in the sera of patients with EAA; the provocation by inhaled antigens of a late alveolar response with a time of onset and duration which parallels the time course of the late 'oedematous' skin reaction; and the finding of Ig and complement by immunofluorescence at the site of late skin responses provoked in the skin (Pepys *et al.* 1968) and in lung tissue of patients with farmer's lung 36 hours after inhalation of *F. rectivirgula* (*M. faeni*) (Ghose *et al.* 1974). However, this explanation of EAA as an immune complex mediated response was unsatisfactory for two major reasons: granuloma formation, a characteristic component of the pathological response in EAA, is more typical of a T lymphocyte than immune complex dependent inflammatory reaction; also, depending on the sensitivity of the assay, IgG antibody can be detected in up to 50% of individuals without disease exposed to causes of EAA.

Investigation of responses to specific antigens of T lymphocytes from the blood of patients with EAA produced conflicting results (Turner-Warwick 1978). The role of the T lymphocyte in EAA and the nature of the immunological response in the disease has been considerably clarified by the study of T lymphocytes recovered from the lungs by lavage. Incubation with pigeon serum of lymphocytes recovered by lavage from the lungs of a patient with pigeon fancier's lung disease stimulated their transformation (Schuyler *et al.* 1978) and stimulation of T cells with specific antigen induces lymphokine secretion. The proportion of lymphocytes recovered at BAL from patients with extrinsic allergic alveolitis may be increased to 60–70% or more; the ratio of CD4 : CD8 T lymphocytes can be normal or low. CD8 +ve T lymphocytes can comprise 40% and CD4 +ve T lymphocytes 30% of the total lymphocytes to give a CD4 : CD8 ratio of less than one (Salvaggio 1987). Patients with extrinsic allergic alveolitis characteristically also have an increase in the number of mast cells recovered at BAL (Haslam *et al.* 1987). The increase in the proportion of lymphocytes recovered at BAL and the reversed CD4 : CD8 T-lymphocyte ratio has, however, also been observed in healthy asymptomatic farmers and pigeon breeders. In one study of 28 farmers with increased BAL lymphocytes, none of 27, all of whom had remained on their farms, studied 2–3 years later, had developed farmer's lung disease (Cormier *et al.* 1987). Pigeon fanciers with extrinsic allergic alveolitis however differ from asymptomatic exposed individuals with similar increases in BAL lymphocytes in a defect in antigen-specific T-lymphocyte suppressor function (Keller *et al.* 1984). This defect may allow inhaled allergen to provoke a T-lymphocyte-dependant inflammatory response; in the asymptomatic person with BAL lymphocytosis, translation of the immunological response into granulomatous inflammation may be inhibited by antigen specific 'suppressor' T lymphocytes.

The risk of developing specific IgG antibody and allergic alveolitis in those exposed to its causes has been consistently reported to be lower in cigarette smokers than in non-smokers (Morgan *et al.* 1975; Warren 1977). This may reflect impaired alveolar macrophage function. Cigarette smoking depresses the expression of class II MHC molecules on the cell surface of alveolar macrophages which could affect antigen presentation to CD4+ve helper/inducer T lymphocytes (Lawrence *et al.* 1983).

Connective tissue inflammatory processes

The term 'connective tissue diseases' is an unsatisfactory name for a heterogeneous group of clinical syndromes of unknown cause, characterized by inflammatory damage in many organs, which is believed to be the outcome of immunological disturbances. The organs particularly involved are the joints, kidneys, skin, lungs and serosal surfaces; the most common immunological abnormalities identified are autoantibodies in blood and circulating immune complexes.

The lungs are involved in several connective tissue diseases; one disease (such as systemic lupus erythematosus (SLE) or rheumatoid arthritis (RA)) may in different individuals be associated with several different patterns of pulmonary pathology and one pathology (fibrosing alveolitis) can occur in several different diseases. Studies of the prevalence of lung disease in the connective tissue diseases have produced extremely variable results which probably reflect differences in referral and investigation patterns in different institutions. There is as yet little knowledge of the relationship between the observed immunological abnormalities and the pathological changes in the lungs.

CRYPTOGENIC FIBROSING ALVEOLITIS

Although cryptogenic fibrosing alveolitis (CFA) is not strictly a connective tissue disease it is a convenient starting point as it is an important manifestation of several connective tissue diseases, is the most studied intrapulmonary manifestation of these diseases, and exhibits many of the features in the lung which are seen in tissues involved in autoimmune processes (such as the synovium in RA).

Cryptogenic fibrosing alveolitis is a progressive disease of the lungs, characterized by infiltration of alveolar walls and alveolar spaces with inflammatory cells, and progressive distortion of lung architecture by fibrosis. Because CFA may be a manifestation of connective tissue diseases (such as RA and scleroderma), and circulating autoantibodies and immune complexes can be identified in some cases, immunological mechanisms are believed to participate in the disease.

The most commonly identified circulating autoantibodies in CFA are rheumatoid factor and antinuclear antibodies. In one group of cases of pulmonary fibrosis, rheumatoid factors were detected in 31.2% and antinuclear antibodies (ANA) in 36.5% of cases of CFA (Turner-Warwick and Haslam 1971). Rheumatoid factor is present more frequently in cases of RA and of CFA with polyarthritis (Turner-Warwick *et al.* 1980). Circulating ANA are more commonly present in sera of cases of CFA associated with Raynaud's phenomenon and digital vasculitis. The types of ANA found in CFA differ from those in SLE. In one study of 53 cases of CFA, 22 of whom had detectable circulating ANA, serum binding of single stranded deoxyribonucleic acid (ss-DNA) was greatly increased in all 53 cases and of double stranded DNA (ds-DNA) in 25% of the cases. The presence of antibodies to ds-DNA was unrelated to disease activity suggesting that, unlike SLE they are not of importance in the pathogenesis of CFA (Holgate *et al.* 1983). In another study of ANAs in CFA, (Chapman *et al.* 1984) identified antibodies to nuclear ribonucleoprotein (nRNP) in some 15% of cases. The presence of nRNP was associated with Raynaud's phenomenon and circulating rheumatoid factor; however, none of the cases in whom it was present fulfilled the criteria of mixed connective tissue disease (Sharp *et al.* 1972).

Two autoantibodies identified in the sera of cases of CFA are directed against ubiquitous intracellular enzymes. Antibodies to DNA topoisomerase II have been found in the sera of some 37% of a group of cases of CFA (Melconi *et al.* 1989). These antibodies seem specific for CFA; although identified in 31% of their cases of SLE, binding was absorbed out in the SLE but not the CFA cases by prior incubation with ds-DNA. Anti-Jo 1 antibody occurs particularly in cases of myositis associated with CFA (Bernstein *et al.* 1984). It has been shown to inhibit the activity of the enzyme histidyl t-RNA synthetase (Matthews and Bernstein 1983). The finding of sequence homologies between *Escherichia coli* histidyl t-RNA synthetase and viral and muscle proteins has been suggested as support for 'molecular mimicry' of viral proteins as a cause of autoimmune diseases (Walker and Jeffrey 1986). Other autoantibodies have been identified in the sera of patients with both myositis and fibrosing alveolitis which have specificity for other amino-acyl (threonyl-, alanyl-, isoleucyl- and glycyl-) t-RNA synthetases (Targoff *et al.* 1988; Targoff 1990; Targoff and Arnett 1990).

Circulating immune complexes have been identified in sera in cases of 'lone' CFA and CFA associated with connective tissue disease. Haslam *et al.* (1979) reported increased C1q binding in one-half of 42 sera from patients with CFA, 35% of 'lone' CFA and 60% of CFA associated with connective tissue disease. Increased C1q binding in this series was associated with the presence of rheumatoid factor and with arthritis, but not with the degree of cellularity or fibrosis of the lung biopsy.

In a later study of this series of cases, Martinet *et al.* (1984) identified circulating immune complexes in cases of CFA of shorter duration but their presence was unrelated to response to treatment or survival.

Dreisen *et al.* (1978) found circulating immune complexes identified by Raji cell radio immunoassay, in 13 of 24 patients with CFA. The presence of immune complexes in this series was associated with a cellular lung biopsy, the presence of granular deposits of IgG and C3 within alveolar walls and capillaries, and response to treatment with corticosteroids. In an earlier study Turner-Warwick *et al.* (1971) identified Ig and complement in alveolar wall capillaries in only six of 33 cases of CFA and its presence was unrelated to the histological appearances of the lungs.

Lavage cell profiles from patients with fibrosing alveolitis commonly consist of an excess of granulocytes. Some patients have a predominantly lymphocyte alveolitis. This is associated with a better treatment response to corticosteroids. The ratio of CD4+ve to CD8+ve T cells is normal (approximately 2 : 1) and this reflects the same ratio observed on immunohistochemical analysis of open lung biopsy material obtained from patients with fibrosing alveolitis (Campbell *et al.* 1985a). Furthermore, such analysis has identified the presence of secondary lymphoid follicles within the lung consistent with active antibody production and class II MHC molecule expression on lung epithelial cells, a feature found in tissues involved in autoimmune processes and consistent with the presence of high levels of interferon-γ in lung lavage fluid from some patients with fibrosing alveolitis (Campbell *et al.* 1985a; Robinson and Rose 1990).

Alveolar macrophages from BAL of patients with CFA but not controls spontaneously secrete two neutrophil chemotactic factors (NCF), the first a small molecular weight lipid (now believed to be LTB_4) and a second, larger, glycoprotein. (Merrill *et al.* 1980; Hunninghake *et al.* 1980). More recently mRNA for IL-8 has been found in AM from patients with fibrosing alveolitis which suggests that IL-8 is the glycoprotein neutrophil chemotactic factor (Carre *et al.* 1991). Immune complexes stimulate alveolar macrophages recovered from normal BAL to release NCF suggesting a role for local immune complexes being involved in stimulating neutrophil influx into sites of disease (Hunninghake *et al.* 1980). The level of spontaneous release of NCF was proportional to the concentration of immune complexes in BAL and alveolar macrophages releasing NCF had suppression of IgG Fc receptor function. du Bois *et al.* (1981) found evidence of C3b receptor occupation on alveolar macrophages in CFA, supporting the concept of local immune complex binding.

Alveolar macrophages can synthesize other cytokines such as IL-1, tumour necrosis factor alpha (TNF-α) and granulocyte colony-stimulating factor (G-CSF) as well as transforming growth factor beta (TGF-β), platelet-derived growth factor (PDGF), insulin-like growth factor (IGF-1) and fibronectin, all of which may play critical roles in adhesion molecule regulation, fibroblast proliferation and collagen secretion. Macrophages from cases of CFA spontaneously secrete fibronectin at a rate of some 20 times normal and fibronectin is found in increased concentrations in BAL. Fibronectin is chemotactic for fibroblasts and acts as a 'competence' factor initiating lung fibroblast replication (Yamauchi *et al.* 1987). Platelet-derived growth factor, secreted spontaneously by alveolar macrophages in CFA but not by normal macrophages, is a progression factor allowing fibroblast replication to progress through G1 and to complete the growth cycle (Martinet *et al.* 1987).

RHEUMATOID ARTHRITIS

Several different patterns of pleuro-pulmonary disease may occur in RA: pleural effusions, necrobiotic nodules, fibrosing alveolitis, obliterative bronchiolitis and vasculitis. The factors determining these manifestations of the disease are obscure although, in contrast to RA generally, they occur more frequently in males than females. The serological features of cases with lung involvement seem similar to those without; titres of rheumatoid factor in the series of Turner-Warwick and Courtney-Evans (1977) were not different from cases of RA without pulmonary involvement.

Pleural effusion

The pleural fluid is typically a lymphocyte exudate with a low glucose content. A low level of C3 has also been reported consistent with the low values found in synovial fluid in the disease. Pleural biopsy may show a lymphocyte infiltration, but occasionally typical rheumatoid nodules have been reported.

Necrobiotic nodules

Necrobiotic nodules in the lungs are now a well documented association of RA. Originally described in the lungs of coal miners with RA (Caplan's syndrome) they have subsequently been reported in the lungs of non-miners. Their histological appearances are identical with subcutaneous nodules of RA. In general the development of intrapulmonary nodules is preceded by joint symptoms. In one report of six cases in whom necrobiotic nodules preceded joint disease, rheumatoid factor was negative until joint symptoms developed (Eraut *et al*. 1978).

Fibrosing alveolitis

In general the pathological changes in the lungs of cases of fibrosing alveolitis in RA are not different from those of 'lone' CFA although in most cases infiltration of lymphocytes and germinal follicle formation may be very prominent. The mean survival of 22 cases followed to death by Turner-Warwick and Courtney-Evans (1977) was 4.9 years. The range of titres of circulating rheumatoid factor has been reported to be no different in such cases from cases of RA without lung involvement. Antinuclear antibody titres of one in 10 and greater were reported in 16 (46%) of 35 cases of RA fibrosing alveolitis and ANA and RF together in 25% of cases (Turner-Warwick and Courtney-Evans 1977). Immunofluorescent studies of lung biopsies have shown deposits of IgG and IgM but not complement in alveolar walls (Turner-Warwick 1967; de Horatius *et al*. 1972).

SYSTEMIC SCLEROSIS

Lung disease is the commonest cause of death in systemic sclerosis (LeRoy 1989). Two forms of lung disease may occur. Patients with more limited disease, especially of the CREST (calcinosis, Raynaud's phenomenon, eosophageal dysfunction, sclerodactyly, and telangiectasia) variant, are at higher risk of developing progressive pulmonary hypertension particularly if gas transfer measurements at presentation are significantly lowered. Secondly, and more commonly, fibrosing alveolitis may occur. The prevalence of fibrosing alveolitis in systemic sclerosis varies with the sensitivity of the test used to make this diagnosis (Alton and Turner-Warwick 1988). Pathological features are identical to those of lone cryptogenic fibrosing alveolitis. Recent studies have demonstrated an immunogenetic component: fibrosing alveolitis associated with systemic sclerosis mainly occurs in patients with a class II major histocompatibility complex (MHC) DR3/DRw 52a haplotype (Briggs *et al*. 1991). Furthermore, 10 of 42 patients with systemic sclerosis involving the lung by comparison with 0/33 without evidence of pulmonary fibrosis demonstrated circulating antibodies against DNA topoisomerase I (anti-Scl 70) (Briggs *et al*. 1991). Bronchoalveolar lavage findings have demonstrated an increase in granulocytes, usually neutrophils, eosinophils or both, but also in some patients, lymphocytes (Harrison *et al*. 1989b). As in lone cryptogenic fibrosing alveolitis, the lymphocytes are also observed on open lung biopsy material both within secondary follicles and within the interstitium. Attempts to show the presence of immune complexes by immunofluorescence have been unsuccessful.

SYSTEMIC LUPUS ERYTHEMATOSUS

The lungs and pleura are among the many organs which may be involved in systemic lupus erythematosus (SLE). The manifestations of pleuropulmonary SLE include pleurisy with or without effusion, pulmonary haemorrhage, 'lupus pneumonitis' recognized as fleeting shadows on the chest radiograph, bilateral elevation of the diaphragms — so called 'shrinking lungs' and fibrosing alveolitis.

In one study of 30 patients with predominant intrathoracic manifestations of SLE, Holgate *et al.* (1975) found antibodies to ss-DNA in 66% but antibodies to ds-DNA by Farr binding technique in only 19%. In keeping with this, few cases had renal involvement and serum C3 levels were normal or elevated in those tested.

The pattern of clinical and immunological changes reported in this series are very similar to those reported in SLE induced by drugs such as procainamide.

POLYMYOSITIS AND DERMATOMYOSITIS

The incidence of pulmonary involvement in these diseases is unknown but is probably uncommon. In a review of the world literature (Schwartz *et al.* 1976) 31 cases with pulmonary disease had been described since 1956. Patients with polymyositis, however, are particularly likely to develop pulmonary fibrosis if they have autoantibodies to the antigen Jo-1 (histidyl t-RNA synthetase) (Matthews and Bernstein 1983). Anti-Jo-1 was found in 77% of cases with both myositis and lung disease but less than 5% of cases with either alone (Bernstein *et al.* 1984).

GOODPASTURE'S SYNDROME (see Chapter 99)

Goodpasture's syndrome is the association of pulmonary haemorrhage and glomerulonephritis with antiglomerular basement membrane (anti-GBM) antibody in serum and deposited linearly along the capillary loops of the glomeruli. It is probable that the pulmonary damage and haemorrhage are also caused by binding of autoantibodies in the lungs. Linear deposits of IgG and complement are found in alveolar septa of involved lungs and IgG eluted from involved lungs and kidneys binds to alveolar basement membrane of lung sections (Koffler *et al.* 1969). The development of pulmonary haemorrhage has been reported in only some two-thirds of cases of glomerulonephritis with anti-GBM antibody. Donaghy and Rees (1983) found that 37 of 39 such patients with lung haemorrhage were cigarette smokers whereas all eight without haemorrhage were non-smokers. In one case lung haemorrhage recurred within 36 hours of resuming cigarette smoking.

Goodpasture's syndrome is strongly associated with human leucocyte antigen (HLA) DR w2. Rees *et al.* (1978) identified this Class II MHC allele in 15 of 17 (88%) of their cases compared with 32% of a group of 100 Caucasian blood donors. Further studies have suggested that the anti-GBM antibodies bind to epitopes located on the carboxy terminal propeptides of type IV collagen (Kefalides 1987).

VASCULITIS AND THE LUNGS

Vasculitis of the blood vessels of the lungs is a major pathological feature of Wegener's granulomatosis and allergic angiitis and granulomatosis (Churg–Strauss syndrome) but may also develop in the connective tissue diseases, such as SLE and RA (see Chapter 62).

Wegener's granulomatosis characteristically involves the upper respiratory tract, the lungs and the kidneys. The pathological changes are vasculitis, extravascular granulomata and tissue necrosis. Allergic angiitis and granulomatosis invariably involves the lungs and also typically involves serosal surfaces (pleural and pericardial). It occurs in patients with a previous history of asthma. The pathological changes in affected tissues are vasculitis, extravascular granulomata and tissue necrosis (similar to Wegener's granulomatosis) with eosinophilic infiltration.

Although it has been suggested that vasculitis in pulmonary blood vessels is a manifestation of immune complex deposition, and granular deposition of IgG and complement has been reported in the lungs of some cases of Wegener's granulomatosis (Shasby *et al.* 1982), evidence of immune complex deposition in this disease has frequently not been found consistent (Shillitoe *et al.* 1974).

Patients with Wegener's granulomatosis (and microscopic polyarteritis) have been found to have serum antibodies which bind to cytoplasmic components of neutrophils — anti-neutrophil cytoplasmic antibodies (cANCA). A bright coarsely granular pattern of cytoplasmic fluorescence pattern is highly specific for Wegener's granulomatosis (Harrison *et al.* 1989a), although the authors also reported finding this pattern of ANCA in one patient with Churg–Strauss granulomatosis. Remissions of Wegener's granulomatosis have also been reported to be associated with reductions in titres of cANCA (Specks *et al*. 1989). Other patterns of anti-neutrophil antibody immunofluorescence have been described in other systemic diseases. Of these, the perinuclear (pANCA) is observed most commonly. This pattern of immunofluorescence is, because of its presence in such a wide range of diseases, much less specific for Wegener's granulomatosis and microscopic polyarteritis. Perinuclear anti-neutrophil cytoplasmic antibodies are thought to represent antibody reacting with myeloperoxidase, whereas cANCA identifies a 29 kD serine protease, protease 3. Problems of interpretation of immunofluorescence may be overcome by ELISA techniques. More recently, studies by Lai *et al*. (1990) using solid phase radioimmunoassay techniques have shown differential binding patterns of sera from patients with various forms of vasculitis to neutrophil antigen. The technique has also shown differences in serum binding pattern between Wegener's granulomatosis and microscopic polyarthritis.

While serial studies of ANCA have been of value in monitoring disease, the role of the antibody in pathogenesis is less clear, certainly the presence of autoantibodies against neutrophils could amplify the autoimmune process, or alternatively may be a reflection of the presence of local inflammation only without their having a pathogenetic role. In either event, measurement of ANCA has become very helpful in diagnosis of the systemic vascular disease.

References

Alton, E., Turner-Warwick, M. (1988). Lung involvement in scleroderma. In *Systemic Sclerosis: Scleroderma*, eds M.I.V. Jayson and C.M. Black, p. 181, John Wiley & Sons, Chichester.

Bernstein, R.N., Morgan, S.H., Chapman, J. *et al*. (1984). Anti-Jo-1 antibody: a marker for myositis with interstitial lung disease. *Br. J. Med.* **289**, 151–2.

Bjorkander, J., Bake, B., Oxelius, V.-A. and Hanson, L.A. (1985). Impaired lung function in patients with IgA deficiency and low levels of IgG_2 or IgG_3. *N. Engl. J. Med.* **313**, 720–4.

Briggs, D.C., Vaughan, R.W., Welsh, K.I., Myers, A., du Bois, R.M. and Black, C.M. (1991). Immunogenetic prediction of pulmonary fibrosis in systemic sclerosis. *Lancet* **338**, 661–2.

Burnett, D. (1986). Immunoglobulins in the lung. *Thorax* **41**, 337–44.

Campbell, D.A., Poulter, L.W., Janossy, G. and du Bois, R.M. (1985a). Immunohistological analysis of lung tissue from patients with cryptogenic fibrosing alveolitis suggesting local expression of immune hypersensitivity. *Thorax* **40**, 405–511.

Campbell, D.A., Poulter, L.W. and du Bois, R.M. (1985b). Immunocompetent cells in bronchoalveolar lavage reflect the cell populations in transbronchial biopsies in pulmonary sarcoidosis. *Am. Rev. Respir. Dis.* **132**, 1300–6.

Campbell, D.A., du Bois, R.M., Butcher, R.G. and Poulter, N.W. (1986). The density of HLA-DR antigen expression on alveolar macrophages is increased in pulmonary sarcoidosis. *Clin. Exp. Immunol.* **65**, 165–71.

Carre, P.C., Mortensen, R.L., King, T.E., Noble, T.W., Sable, C.R. and Riches, D.W.H. (1991). Increased expression of the interleukin-8 gene by alveolar macrophages in idiopathic pulmonary fibrosis. *J. Clin. Invest.* **88**, 1802–10.

Chapman, J.R., Charles, P.J., Venables, P.J.W. *et al*. (1984). Definition and clinical relevance of antibodies to nuclear ribonucleoprotein and other nuclear antigens in patients with cryptogenic fibrosing alveolitis. *Am. Rev. Respir. Dis.* **130**, 439–43.

Clarke, S. (1990). Respiratory defences: physical defences. In *Textbook of Respiratory Medicine*, eds R.A.L. Brewis, G.J. Gibson and D.M. Geddes, pp. 176–89, Bailliere Tindall, London.

Cole, P.J. (1989). Host–microbe relationships in chronic respiratory disease. In *Recent Advances in Infection*, eds D. Reeves and A.M. Geddes, pp. 141–51. Churchill Livingstone, Edinburgh.

Cole, P.J. (1990). Bronchiectasis. In *Textbook of Respiratory Medicine*, eds R.A.L. Brewis, G.J. Gibson and D.M. Geddes, pp. 726–59, Bailliere Tindall, London.

Cole, P.J. and Wilson, R. (1989). Host–microbial interrelationships in respiratory infection. *Chest* **95**, 217s–21s.

Cormier, Y., Belanger, J. and Laviolette, M. (1987). Prognostic significance of bronchoalveolar lymphocytosis in farmer's lung. *Am. Rev. Respir. Dis.* **135**, 692–5.

Costabel, U., Bross, R.J., Ruhler, K.H., Lohr, G.W. and Matthys, H. (1985). Ia-like antigens on T-cells and their subpopulations in pulmonary sarcoidosis and in hypersensitivity pneumonitis. Analysis of bronchoalveolar and blood lymphocytes. *Am. Rev. Respir. Dis.* **131**, 337–42.

Currie, D.C., Peters, A.M., Garbett, N.D. *et al*. (1990). Indium-111-labelled granulocyte scanning to detect inflammation in the lungs of patients with chronic sputum expectoration. *Thorax* **45**, 541–4.

de Horatius, R.J., Abruzzo, J.L. and Williams, R.C., Jr. (1972). Immunofluorescent and immunologic studies of rheumatoid lung. *Arch. Intern. Med.* **129**, 441–6.

Demarest, G.B., Hudson, L.D. and Altman, L.C. (1979). Impaired alveolar macrophage chemotaxis in patients with acute smoke inhalation. *Am. Rev. Respir. Dis.* **119**, 279–86.

Deneke, S.M. and Fenberg, B.L. (1980). Normobaric oxygen toxicity of the lung. *N. Engl. J. Med.* **303**, 76–86.

Dominique, S., Bouchonnet, F., Smiejan, J.-M. and Hance, A.J. (1990). Expression of surface antigens distinguishing 'naive' and previously activated lymphocytes in bronchoalveolar lavage fluid. *Thorax* **45**, 391–6.

Donaghy, M. and Rees, A.J. (1983). Cigarette smoking and lung haemorrhage and glomerulophritis caused by autoantibodies to glomerular basement membrane. *Lancet* **ii**, 1390–2.

Dreisen, N.R.B., Schwartz, M.I., Theofilopoulos, A.N. and Stanford, R.E. (1978). Circulating immune complexes in the idiopathic interstitial pneumonias. *N. Engl. J. Med.* **298**, 353–7.

du Bois, R.M., Townsend, P.J., Cole, P.J., Haslam, P.L. and Turner-Warwick, M. (1981). Bronchoalveolar macrophages in sarcoidosis and cryptogenic fibrosing alveolitis. *Clin. Allergy* **11**, 409–19.

du Bois, R.M., Kirby, M., Balbi, B., Saltini, C. and Crystal, R.G. (1992). T-lymphocytes that accumulate in the lung in sarcoidosis have evidence of recent stimulation of the T-cell antigen receptor. *Am. Rev. Respir. Dis.* **145**, 1205–11.

Eraut, C.D., Evans, J.A. and Caplin, M. (1978). Pulmonary necrobiotic rheumatoid nodules without rheumatoid arthritis. *Br. J. Dis. Chest* **72**, 301–6.

Fick, R.B., Baltimore, R.S., Squier, S.U. and Reynolds, H.Y. (1985). The immunoglobulin-G proteolytic activity of *Pseudomonas aeruginosa* in cystic fibrosis. *J. Infect. Dis.* **151**, 589–98.

Fick, R.B., Olchowski, J., Squier, S.U., Merrill, W.W. and Reynolds, H.Y. (1986). Immunoglobulin-G subclasses in cystic fibrosis. IgG_2 response to *Pseudomonas aeruginosa* lipopolysaccharide. *Am. Rev. Respir. Dis.* **133**, 418–22.

Gallin, J.I. (1985). Neutrophil specific granule deficiency. *Ann. Rev. Med.* **36**, 263–74.

Garbett, N.D., Currie, D.C. and Cole, P.J. (1989). Comparison of the clinical efficacy and safety of an intramuscular and an intravenous immunoglobulin preparation for replacement therapy in idiopathic adult onset panhypogammaglobulinaemia. *Clin. Exp. Immunol.* **76**, 1–7.

Ghose, T., Landrigan, P., Killeen, R. and Dill, J. (1974). Immunopathological studies in patients with farmer's lung. *Clin. Allergy*, **4**, 119–29.

Hancock, W.W., Kobzik, L., Colby, A.J., O'Hara, C.J., Cooper, A.G. and Godleski, J.J. (1986). Detection of lymphokines and lymphokine receptors in pulmonary sarcoidosis. *Am. J. Pathol.* **123**, 1–8.

Hance, A.J., Saltini, C. and Crystal, R.G. (1988). Does de novo immunoglobulin synthesis occur on the epithelial surface of the human lower respiratory tract? *Am. Rev. Respir. Dis.* **137**, 17–24.

Harrison, D.J., Simpson, R., Kharbanda, R., Abernethey, V.E. and Nimmo, G. (1989a). Antibodies to neutrophil cytoplasmic antigens in Wegener's granulomatosis and other conditions. *Thorax* **44**, 373–7.

Harrison, N.K., Glanville, A.R., Strickland, B. *et al.* (1989b) Pulmonary involvement in systemic sclerosis: The detection of early changes by thin section CT scan, bronchoalveolar lavage and 99m Tc DTPA clearance. *Respiratory Med.* **83**, 403–14.

Haslam, P.L., Thompson, B., Mohammed, I. *et al.* (1979). Circulating immune complexes in patients with cryptogenic fibrosing alveolitis. *Clin. Exp. Immunol.* **37**, 318–90.

Haslam, P.L., Deward, A., Butchers, P., Primett, Z.S., Newman Taylor, A.J., Turner-Warwick, M. (1987). Mast cells, atypical lymphocytes and neutrophils in bronchoalveolar lavage in extrinsic allergic alveolitis. *Am. Rev. Respir. Dis.* **135**, 35–47.

Holgate, S.T., Glass, D.N., Haslam, P., Maini, R.N. and Turner-Warwick, M. (1976). Respiratory involvement in systemic lupus erythematosis. A clinical and immunological study. *Clin. Exp. Immunol.* **24**, 385–95.

Holgate, S.T., Haslam, P. and Turner-Warwick, M. (1983). The significance of antinuclear and DNA antibodies in cryptogenic fibrosing alveolitis. *Thorax* **38**, 67–70.

Hunninghake, G.W. (1984). Release of interleukin 1 by alveolar macrophages in patients with active pulmonary sarcoidosis. *Am. Rev. Respir. Dis.* **129**, 569–72.

Hunninghake, G.W. and Crystal, R.G. (1981). Pulmonary sarcoidosis: A disorder mediated by excess helper T-lymphocyte activity at sites of disease activity. *N. Engl. J. Med.* **305**, 429–34.

Hunninghake, G.W., Gadek, G.E., Faith, H.M. and Crystal R.G. (1980a). Human alveolar macrophage derived chemotactic factor for neutrophils. *J. Clin. Invest.* **66**, 473–83.

Hunninghake, G.W., Keogh, B.A., Line, B.R. *et al.* (1980b). Pulmonary sarcoidosis; pathogenesis and therapy. In *Basic and Clinical Aspects of Granulomatous Diseases*, eds D.L. Boros and T. Yoshida, pp. 275–90, Elsevier/North-Holland, Amsterdam.

Johnson, K.J. and Ward, P.A. (1982). Acute and progressive lung injury after contact with phorbol myristate acetate. *Am. J. Pathol.* **107**, 29–35.

Johnson, K.J., Wilson, B.S., Till, G.O. and Ward, P.A. (1984). Acute lung injury in rat caused by immunoglobulin A immune complexes. *J. Clin. Invest.* **74**, 358–69.

Johnson, K.J., Ward, P.A., Kunkel, P.G. and Wilson, B.S. (1986). Mediation of IgA induced lung injury in the rat. Role of macrophages and reactive oxygen products. *Lab. Invest.* **54**, 499–506.

Kefalides, N.A. (1987). The Goodpasture antigen and basement membranes: The search must go on. *Lab. Invest.* **56**, 1–3.

Keller, R.H., Swartz, S., Schlueter, D.P., Bar-Sela, S. and Fink, J.N. (1984). Immunoregulation in hypersensitivity pneumonitis: phenotypic and functional studies of bronchoalveolar lavage lymphocytes. *Am. Rev. Respir. Dis.* **130**, 766–71.

Kilian, M., Mestecky, J. Kulhavy, R., Tomana, M. and Butler, W.T. (1980). IgA proteases from *Haemophilus influenzae*, *Streptococcus pneumoniae*, *Neisseria meningitidis* and *Streptococcus sanguis*: comparative immunochemical studies. *J. Immunol.* **124**, 2596–600.

Koffler, D., Sandson, J., Carr, R. and Kunkel, H.G. (1969). Immunologic studies concerning the pulmonary lesions in Goodpasture's syndrome. *Am. J. Pathol.* **54**, 293–305.

Lai, A.N., Jayne, D.R.W., Brownlee, A. and Lockwood, C.M. (1990). The specificity of anti-neutrophil cytoplasm autoantibodies in systemic vascular disease. *Clin. Exp. Immunol.* **82**, 233–7.

Lapa e Silva, J.R., Jones, J.A.H., Cole, P.J. and Poulter, L.W. (1989a). The immunological component of the cellular inflammatory infiltrate in bronchiectasis. *Thorax* **44**, 668–73.

Lapa e Silva, J.R., Guerreiro, D., Noble, B., Poulter, L.W. and Cole, P.J. (1989b). Immunopathology of experimental bronchiectasis. *Am. J. Respir. Cell Mol. Biol.* **1**, 297–304.

Lapa e Silva, J.R., Munro, N.C., Guerreiro, D., Poulter, L.W. and Cole, P.J. (1992). Immunopathogenesis of experimental bronchiectasis in the rat: effects of prednisolone. *Am. Rev. Respir. Dis.* **145**, A639.

Lawrence, E.C., Fox, T.B., Hall, B.T. and Martin, R.R. (1983). Deleterious effects of cigarette smoking on expression of Ia antigens by human pulmonary alveolar macrophages. *Clin. Res.* **31**, 418a.

Lawrence, E.C., Brousseau, K.P., Berger, M.B., Kurman, C.C., Markon, L. and Nelson, D.L. (1988). Elevated concentrations of soluble interleukin-2 receptors in serum samples and bronchoalveolar lavage in active sarcoidosis. *Am. Rev. Respir.*

Dis. **137**, 759–64.

LeRoy, E.C. (1989). Sentinel signs and symptoms of systemic sclerosis. *Curr. Opin. Rheumatol.* **1**, 499–504.

Martin, W.J., Gadek, J.E., Hunninghake, G.W. and Crystal, R.G. (1981). Oxidant injury of lung parenchymal cells. *J. Clin. Invest.* **68**, 1277–88.

Martinet, Y., Haslam, P. and Turner-Warwick, M. (1984). Clinical significance of circulating immune complexes in 'lone' cryptogenic fibrosing alveolitis and those with associated connective tissue disorders. *Clin. Allergy* **14**, 491–7.

Martinet, Y., Rom, W.N., Grotendost, G.R., Martin, G.R. and Crystal, R.G., (1987). Exaggerated spontaneous release of platelet-derived growth factor by alveolar macrophages from patients with idiopathic pulmonary fibrosis. *N. Engl. J. Med.* **317**, 202–9.

Matthews, M.D. and Bernstein, R.N. (1983). Myositis autoantibody inhibits histidyl-tRNA synthetase: A model of autoimmunity. *Nature* **304**, 177–9.

Melconi, R., Bestagno, M., Sturani, C. *et al.* (1989). Autoantibodies to DNA topoisomerase II. In cryptogenic fibrosing alveolitis and connective tissue disease. *Clin. Exp. Immunol.* **76**, 184–9.

Merrill, W.W., Nagel, G.P., Matthay, R.A. and Reynolds, H.Y. (1980). Alveolar macrophage derived chemotactic factor. Kinetics of *in vitro* production and partial characterisation. *J. Clin. Invest.* **65**, 268–76.

Merrill, W.W., Naegel, G.P., Olchowski, J.J. and Reynolds, H.Y. (1985). Immunoglobulin G subclass proteins in serum and lavage fluid of normal subjects: quantitation and comparison with immunoglobulins A and E. *Am. Rev. Respir. Dis.* **131**, 584–7.

Moller, D.R., Konishi, K., Kirby, M., Balbi, B. and Crystal, R.G. (1988). Bias towards use of a specific T-cell receptor β-chain variable region in a subgroup of individuals with sarcoidosis. *J. Clin. Invest.* **82**, 1183–91.

Morgan, D.C., Smyth, J.T., Lister, R.W. *et al.* (1975). Chest symptoms in farming communities with special reference to farmer's lung. *Br. J. Ind. Med.* **32**, 228–34.

Muller-Quernheim, J., Saltini, C., Sondermeyer, P. and Crystal, R.G. (1986). Compartmentalised activation of the interleukin-2 gene by lung T-lymphocytes in active pulmonary sarcoidosis. *J. Immunol.* **137**, 3475–83.

Munro, N.C., Barker, A., Rutman, A. *et al.* (1989). The effect of pyocyanin and 1-hydroxyphenazine on *in vivo* tracheal mucus velocity. *J. Appl. Physiol.* **67**, 316–23.

Murray, H.W., Gellene, R.A., Libby, D.M., Rothermel, C.D. and Rubin, B.Y. (1985). Activation of tissue macrophages from AIDS patients: *In vitro* response of AIDS alveolar macrophages to lymphokines and interferon-gamma. *J. Immunol.* **135**, 2374–7.

Musher, D.M., Goree, A., Baughn, R.E. and Birdsall, H.H. (1984). Immunoglobulin A from bronchopulmonary secretions blocks bactericidal and opsonising effects of antibody to non-typable *Haemophilus influenzae*. *Infect. Immun.* **45**, 36–40.

Nugent, K.M. and Persanti, E.L. (1983). Macrophage function in pulmonary alveolar proteinosis. *Am. Rev. Respir. Dis.* **127**, 780–1.

Onofrio, M., Shulkin, N., Heidbrink, P.J., Toews, G.B. and Pierce, A.K. (1981). Pulmonary clearance and phagocyte cell response to normal pharyngeal flora. *Am. Rev. Respir. Dis.* **123**, 222–5.

Oxelius, V.-A., Laurell, A.-B., Lindquist, B. *et al.* (1981). IgG subclasses in selective IgA deficiency: the importance of IgG_2–IgA deficiency. *N. Engl. J. Med.* **304**, 1476–7.

Pepys, J., Turner-Warwick, M., Dawson, P.C. and Hinson, K.F.W. (1968). Arthus (type 3) skin test reactions in man. In *Clinical and Immunopathological Features. Allergology*, eds B. Rose, M. Richer, A. Sehon and S.W. Frankland, pp. 221–35, Excerpta Medica, Amsterdam.

Pinkston, P., Bitterman, P.B. and Crystal, R.G. (1983). Spontaneous release of interleukin-2 by lung T-lymphocytes in active pulmonary sarcoidosis. *N. Engl. J. Med.* **308**, 793–800.

Rappolee, D.A., Mark, D., Banda, M.J. and Werb, Z. (1988). Wound macrophages express TGF alpha and other growth factors *in vivo*: analysis by mRNA phenotyping. *Science* **241**, 708–12.

Rees, A.J., Peters, D.K., Compston, D.A.S. and Batchelor, J.R. (1978). Strong association between HLA DRW2 and antibody mediated Goodpasture's syndrome. *Lancet* **i**, 966–8.

Rehn, S.T., Gross, G.N. and Pierce, A.K. (1980). Early bacterial clearance from murine lungs: species-dependent phagocyte response. *J. Clin. Invest.* **166**, 194–9.

Reynolds, H.Y. (1979). Lung host defenses: a status report. *Chest* **75**, S39–S42.

Robinson, B.W.S. and Rose, A.H. (1990). Pulmonary gamma interferon production in patients with fibrosing alveolitis. *Thorax* **45**, 105–8.

Robinson, B.W.S., McLemore, T.L. and Crystal, R.G. (1985). Gamma interferon is spontaneously released by alveolar macrophages and lung T-lymphocytes in patients with pulmonary sarcoidosis. *J. Clin. Invest.* **75**, 1488–95.

Rossman, M.D., Kern, J.A., Elias, J.A. *et al.* (1988). Proliferative response of bronchoalveolar lymphocytes to beryllium: A test for chronic beryllium disease. *Ann. Intern. Med.* **108**, 687–93.

Salahuddin, S.Z., Rose, R.M., Groopman, J.E., Markham, P.D. and Gallo, R.C. (1986). Human T-lymphotropic virus type III infection of human alveolar macrophages. *Blood* **68**, 281–4.

Saltini, C. and Crystal, R.G. (1985). Pulmonary sarcoidosis, pathogenesis, staging and therapy. *Int. Nat. Arch. Allergy Immunol.* **76**(suppl.), 92–100.

Saltini, C., Hemler, M.E. and Crystal, R.G. (1988). T-lymphocytes compartmentalized on the epithelial surface of the lower respiratory tract express the very late activation complex VLA-1. *Clin. Immunol. Immunopathol.* **46**, 221–33.

Saltini, C., Winestock, K., Kirby, M., Pinkston, P. and Crystal, R.G. (1989). Maintenance of the alveolitis in patients with chronic beryllium disease by beryllium-specific helper T-cells. *N. Engl. J. Med.* **320**, 1103–9.

Saltini, C., Kirby, M., Trapnell, B.C., Tamura, N. and Crystal, R.G. (1990). Biased accumulation of T-lymphocytes with 'memory'-type CD45 leucocyte common antigen gene expression on the epithelial surface of the human lung. *J. Exp. Med.* **171**, 1123–40.

Salvaggio, J. (1987). Hypersensitivity pneumonitis. *J. Allergy Clin. Immunol.* **79**, 558–71.

Schon-Hegrad, M.A., Oliver, J., McMenamin, P.G. and Holt, P.G. (1991). Studies on the density, distribution, and surface phenotype of intraepithelial class II major histocompatibility complex antigens(Ia)-bearing dendritic cells (DC) in the conducting airways. *J. Exp. Med.* **173**, 1345–56.

Schuyler, M.R., Thypen, T.P. and Salvaggio, J.E. (1978). Local pulmonary immunity in pigeon breeder's lung. *Am. Intern. Med.* **88**, 55–358.

Schwartz, M.I., Matthay, R.A., Shan, S.A., Stanfold, R.E., Marmorstein, B.L. and Scheinhorn, D.J. (1976). Interstitial lung disease and polymyositis and dermatomyositis: Analysis of 6 cases and review of the literature. *Medicine (Baltimore)* **55**, 89–104.

Segal, A.W., Heyworth, P.G., Cockcroft, S. and Barrowman, M.M. (1987). Stimulated neutrophils from patients with autosomal recessive chronic granulomatous disease fail to phosphorylate a Mr-44 000 protein. *Nature* **316**, 547–9.

Semenzato, G., Agostini, C. and Trentin, L. (1984). Evidence of cells bearing interleukin-2 receptor at the sites of disease activity in sarcoid patients. *Clin. Exp. Immunol.* **57**, 331–7.

Sharp, D.C., Irvin, W.S., Tan, E.M., Gould, R.G. and Holman, H.R. (1972). Mixed connective tissue disease — an apparently distinct rheumatic disease syndrome associated with a specific antibody to an extractable nuclear antigen (ENA). *Am. J. Med.* **52**, 148–59.

Shasby, D.M., Schwartz, M.I., Forstort, A.Z., Theofilopoulos, A.M. and Kassan, S.S. (1982). Pulmonary immune complex deposition in Wegener's granulomatosis. *Chest* **81**, 338–40.

Shillitoe, E.J., Lehner, T., Lessof, M.H. and Harrison, D.F.N. (1974). Immunological features of Wegener's granulomatosis. *Lancet* **i**, 281.

Sibille, Y. and Reynolds, H.Y. (1990). State of the Art: Macrophages and polymorphonuclear neutrophils in lung defense and injury. *Am. Rev. Respir. Dis.* **141**, 471–501.

Specks, U., Wheatley, C.L., McDonald, T.J., Rohrback, M.S. and De Remee, R.A. (1989). Anticytoplasmic autoantibodies in diagnosis and follow up of Wegener's granulomatosis. *Mayo Clin. Proc.* **64**, 28–36.

Steinfort, C., Wilson, R., Mitchell, T. *et al.* (1989). Effect of *Streptococcus pneumoniae* on human respiratory epithelium *in vitro*. *Infect. Immun.* **57**, 2006–13.

Stockley, R.A. (1990). Respiratory defences: cellular and humoral mechanisms. In *Textbook of Respiratory Medicine*, eds R.A.L. Brewis, G.J. Gibson and D.M. Geddes, pp. 189–203, Bailliere Tindall, London.

Strieter, R.M., Remick, D.G., Lynch, J.P., III, Spengler, R.N. and Kunkel, S.L. (1989). Interleukin-2 induced tumour necrosis factor-α (TNF-α) gene expression in human alveolar macrophages and blood monocytes. *Am. Rev. Respir. Dis.* **139**, 335–42.

Targoff, I.N. (1990). Autoantibodies to amino acyl-transfer RNA synthetases for isoleucine and glycine: Two additional synthetases are antigenic in myositis. *J. Immunol.* **144**, 1737–43.

Targoff, I.N. and Arnett, F.C. (1990). Clinical manifestations in patients with antibody to PL-12 antigen (alanyl-tRNA synthetase). *Am. J. Med.* **88**, 241–51.

Targoff, I.N., Arnett, F.C. and Reichlin, M. (1988). Antibody to threonyl-transfer RNA synthetase in myositis sera. *Arthritis Rheum.* **31**, 515–24.

Toews, G.B., Hart, D.A. and Hansen, E.J. (1985). Effect of systemic immunisation on pulmonary clearance of *Haemophilus influenzae* type b. *Infect. Immun.* **48**, 343–9.

Turner-Warwick, M. (1967). Auto, allergy and lung diseases. *J. Roy. Col. Physicians* **2**, 57–66.

Turner-Warwick, M. (1978). *Immunology of the Lung*, pp. 178–9. Edward Arnold, London.

Turner-Warwick, M. and Haslam, P. (1971). Antibodies in some chronic fibrosing lung diseases I. Non-specific autoantibodies. *Clin. Allergy* **1**, 83–95.

Turner-Warwick, M. , Haslam, P. and Weeks, J. (1971). Antibodies in some chronic fibrosing lung diseases. II. Immunofluorescent studies. *Clin. Allergy* **1**, 209–19.

Turner-Warwick, M. and Courtenay-Evans, R. (1977). Pulmonary manifestations of rheumatoid disease. Extra-articular manifestations of rheumatoid arthritis. In *Clinics in Rheumatic Diseases*, vol. 3, pp. 549–64, W.B. Saunders, London.

Turner-Warwick, M., Burrows, B. and Johnson, A. (1980). Cryptogenic fibrosing alveolitis: clinical features and their influence on survival. *Thorax* **35**, 171–80.

Venet, A., Hance, A.J., Saltini, C., Robinson, W.S. and Crystal, R.G. (1985a). Enhanced alveolar macrophage-mediated antigen-induced T-lymphocyte proliferation in sarcoidosis. *J. Clin. Invest.* **75**, 293–301.

Venet, A., Clavel, F., Israel-Biet, D. *et al.* (1985b) Lung in acquired immune deficiency syndrome: infections and immunological status assess by broncho-alveolar lavage. *Bull. Eur. Physio-pathol. Respir.* **21**, 535–43.

Walker, E.J. and Jeffrey, P.D. (1986). Polymyositis and molecular mimicry; a mechanism of autoimmunity. *Lancet* **ii**, 605–7.

Warren, C.P.W. (1977). Extrinsic allergic alveolitis: a disease commoner in non smokers. *Thorax* **32**, 567–9.

Wilmott, R.W., Wood, R.E. and Frenzke, M. (1992). Interleukin-8 concentrations in bronchoalveolar lavage fluid from children with cystic fibrosis and controls. *Am. Rev. Respir. Dis.* **145**, A234.

Wilson, R., Pitt, T., Taylor, G. *et al.* (1987). Pyocyanin and 1-hydroxyphenazine inhibit the beating of human respiratory cilia *in vitro*. *J. Clin. Invest.* **79**, 221–9.

Yamauchi, K., Martinet, Y. and Crystal, R.G. (1987). Modulation of fibronectin gene expression in human mononuclear phagocytes. *J. Clin. Invest.* **80**, 1720–7.

Young, K.R., Rankin, J.A., Naegel, G.P., Paul, E.S. and Reynolds, H.Y. (1985). An immunologic analysis of bronchoalveolar lavage cells and proteins in patients with the acquired immunodeficiency syndrome. *Ann. Intern. Med.* **103**, 522–33.

99: Immunology of Nephritis

C.D. Pusey and D.K. Peters

Introduction

Since the last edition of this work there have been shifts in the emphasis placed upon the role of various mechanisms involved in both the induction of nephritis and the development of renal injury (Pusey *et al.* 1988). These have stemmed from the rapid advances made in the understanding of autoimmunity and inflammation. The production of autoantibodies to renal antigens has been implicated in several forms of nephritis, whereas there has been less work supporting the involvement of circulating immune complexes. Indeed, the previous distinction between antibody-mediated and immune complex-mediated nephritis has become less clear, since there are now examples of 'immune complex' nephritis, with granular deposits of immunoglobulin (Ig) on immunohistochemistry, in which it has been shown that autoantibodies reactive with glomerular antigens are responsible — the best defined is Heymann nephritis, a model of membranous glomerulonephritis (GN) in the rat (Brentjens and Andres 1989).

Since autoimmune disease in man generally shows strong associations with Class II major histocompatibility complex (MHC) genes, it is assumed to depend upon the interaction of peptides derived from self antigens with Class II MHC gene products on antigen-presenting cells, followed by recognition of this complex by the T helper (T_h) lymphocyte receptor and subsequent recruitment of effector T or B cells (Todd *et al.* 1988; Gregersen 1989). Proof that this mechanism operates in human renal disease will depend upon the identification of the respective autoantigens, MHC gene products and autoreactive T cells. Although this has not yet been achieved, there are examples such as anti-glomerular basement membrane (GBM) antibody-mediated nephritis, where considerable advances have been made (Hudson *et al.* 1989; Pusey and Lockwood 1989). In certain other forms of nephritis, associations with MHC genes and/or identification of autoantibodies suggest a similar pathogenesis, whereas in yet others it is possible that different mechanisms are involved.

In respect of renal injury, more evidence has accumulated for the role of macrophages and T lymphocytes, and of the cytokine network which links them and resident renal cells. It is now appreciated that glomerular endothelial and mesangial cells can respond to, and produce, various cytokines and are likely themselves to be involved in the modulation of renal inflammation (Lovett and Sterzl 1986). In addition to the traditional role of complement activation in neutrophil-mediated GN, the direct involvement of the membrane attack complex has been demonstrated in certain models of nephritis — principally those in which immune reactants are localized to the subepithelial space (Salant *et al.* 1989).

In this chapter we shall review selected experimental models of nephritis which illustrate valuable concepts, and consider these in the context of current understanding of the pathogenesis of human nephritis. The dangers implicit in extrapolation from animal models of disease should be remembered. This approach is not intended to be comprehensive, or to duplicate the contents of the previous edition.

Experimental nephritis

We shall consider three separate categories of experimental nephritis: (i) disease resulting from administration of foreign antibody and/or antigen; (ii) induction of autoimmunity by antigen or polyclonal activators; and (iii) nephritis developing spontaneously in certain species.

Nephritis induced by exogenous antibody or antigen

The understanding of pathological mechanisms in nephritis is based upon the use of models such as nephrotoxic nephritis (NTN) and serum sickness. Although these models cannot directly contribute to the elucidation of autoimmune processes, they have provided a valuable test-bed for theories of the mediation of glomerular injury. Their current clinical relevance is in the development of novel anti-inflammatory therapy, such as the use of monoclonal antibodies to, or antagonists of, various cytokines.

NEPHROTOXIC NEPHRITIS

The administration to experimental animals of heterologous antibody raised to renal cortical or GBM preparations results in a biphasic disease known as NTN (Unanue and Dixon 1967). In the first or heterologous phase, there is binding of foreign antibodies to the GBM, followed by polymorph accumulation and proteinuria. This is followed within 2 weeks by the second or autologous phase, in which there is production of host antibodies to the planted Ig on the GBM. This phase leads to more severe pathological changes, with mesangial and endothelial cell proliferation, and macrophage infiltration. The speed and severity of the autologous phase can be increased by preimmunization with the appropriate foreign Ig, resulting in the 'telescoped' model of NTN.

Such models have been used extensively to examine mechanisms of antibody-mediated renal injury, which are most relevant to human anti-GBM disease. It is clear that the amount of antibody bound, the rate of deposition and the characteristics of the antibody (e.g. avidity, complement-fixing ability) are important determinants of injury. Under certain circumstances, antibody binding alone is sufficient to cause injury (Simpson *et al.* 1975). In addition, multiple mediator systems have been identified using variations of the basic model in different species. These include: (i) neutrophil-dependent injury, which is usually mediated via complement C3 but may occur independently of complement (Cochrane *et al.* 1965; Naish *et al.* 1975; Thomson *et al.* 1976; Pilia *et al.* 1983; (ii) complement-dependent injury mediated by the membrane attack complex of complement (Groggel *et al.* 1985; Tipping *et al.* 1989); and (iii) macrophage-dependent injury, which generally requires deposition of fibrin in Bowman's space (Schreiner *et al.* 1978; Thomson *et al.* 1979; Holdsworth *et al.* 1981) — both T cells and antibody may be important in signalling macrophages (Tipping *et al.* 1985; Boyce and Holdsworth 1989).

The mediation of polymorph-dependent injury has been shown to be due, at least in part, to reactive oxygen species (Boyce and Holdsworth 1986). The role of eicosanoids has also been investigated (Lianos *et al.* 1983); both leukotrienes (LTB_4) and hydroxyeicosatetraenoic acids (5-HETE) are produced by glomeruli from rats with heterologous-phase NTN. Their production was complement-dependent, and may represent an important pro-inflammatory stimulus (Lianos 1988). On the other hand, prostaglandin E_1 (PGE_1) has been shown to protect rats with autologous-phase NTN (Kuntel *et al.* 1982; Cattel *et al.* 1990). In the autologous phase, T lymphocytes are important, not only for induction of the humoral response, but also in certain circumstances for tissue injury. For example, infiltration of the glomerulus by T cells precedes (and is necessary for) macro-

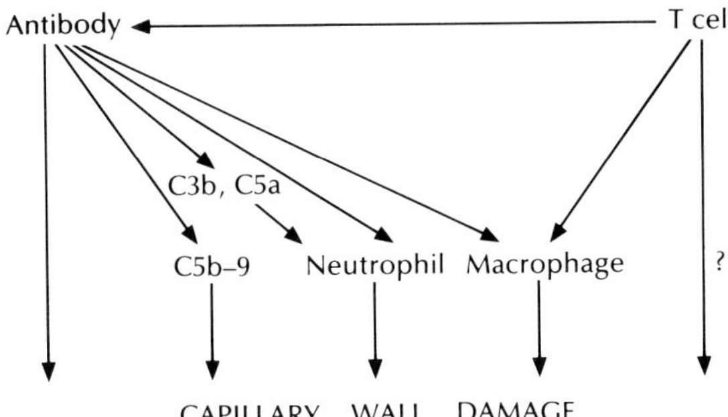

Fig. 99.1. Mechanisms involved in the mediation of glomerular injury in experimental models of nephritis. See text for details of the models concerned.

phage accumulation and renal injury in a telescoped model of NTN in the rat (Tipping *et al.* 1985). Details of these mechanisms are published elsewhere (Couser 1988; Pusey *et al.* 1988) and are summarized in Fig. 99.1.

The mechanisms by which intercurrent infection may enhance renal injury in GN have also been studied, using NTN as a model. The severity of the heterologous phase in the rat can be increased by the administration of subtoxic doses of lipopolysaccharide (LPS), and also by the cytokines, tumour necrosis factor (TNF) and interleukin 1 (IL-1), known to be released following stimulation with LPS (Tomosugi *et al.* 1989). The effects of these cytokines are synergistic, and can be abrogated by concurrent administration of the appropriate anticytokine antibodies. Whether the effects of these mediators are important in antibody-mediated nephritis *per se* is not yet known.

IMMUNE COMPLEX NEPHRITIS

The notion that GN often resulted from the deposition of circulating immune complexes was supported by experiments using serum sickness as a model. Although such complexes are detectable in various human diseases associated with nephritis, the relevance of this observation to the majority of patients with primary GN is now in doubt. In particular, it has been hard to define whether disease is related to 'trapping' of preformed complexes, or initiated by reactions of antigen and/or antibody with renal tissue, followed by formation of immune aggregates.

In acute serum sickness, a single injection of antigen such as bovine serum albumin is followed by the development of proliferative nephritis and vasculitis at the time of immune elimination, when complexes are found in the circulation and deposited in tissue (Germuth 1953). The severity of disease is related to the strength of the immune response, which determines the characteristics of the immune complexes (Wilson and Dixon 1970). Localization to the kidney appears to depend upon reactions between the antigen or complex with sites in the glomerulus — thus even in this classic model of immune complex nephritis there may be a role for 'planted' antigen (see below).

In chronic serum sickness, repeated injections of antigen result in a variety of histological appearances, from membranous to diffuse proliferative nephritis (Dixon *et al.* 1961). Again, variations in immune responsiveness determine the pattern of disease — animals with a low response do not generate complexes, those with a high response clear complexes rapidly, and those with an intermediate response develop potentially injurious complexes. It is clear that the characteristics of the immune complex depend on properties of the antigen (size, number of reactive sites) and antibody (avidity, concentration, Fc function), and on the proportion of antigen to antibody (Germuth *et al.* 1972; Wilson and Dixon 1971).

In addition, several factors determine the disposal of immune complexes, including solubilization and inhibition of precipitation by complement, uptake by the complement receptor CR1 on erythrocytes (in primates), and clearance by the mononuclear phagocytic system. These mechanisms have been reviewed recently (Schifferli and Taylor 1989) and are considered elsewhere in this book. As in the case of NTN, models of serum sickness have been of value in defining mediator systems involved in glomerular injury, and these are summarized in Fig. 99.1.

PLANTED ANTIGENS

The initial localization of antigen, antibody or immune complexes to the glomerulus, by a variety of mechanisms, can provide a nidus for subsequent reactions leading to immune deposits (Mauer *et al.* 1973; Couser and Salant 1980). Indeed, the microscopically visible deposits characteristic of certain types of nephritis could only have arisen in this way. Several experimental models have been described in which the administration of antigen, followed by antibody to that antigen, leads to 'immune complex' nephritis. Of particular interest are experiments using the isolated perfused rat kidney, which excludes effects of the intact immune system; renal accumulation of immune deposits was achieved by alternating perfusion with antigen and antibody (Fleuren *et al*. 1980). Antigens such as lectins, Ig and deoxyribonucleic acid (DNA) can be 'planted' in the glomerulus by virtue of their physicochemical affinity for glomerular components (Izui *et al*. 1976; Golbus and Wilson 1979; Adler *et al*. 1983a). Many cationic macromolecules are localized to the glomerular capillary wall and mesangium by the array of anionic sites on glycosaminoglycans (Border *et al*. 1982; Gauthier *et al*. 1982; Oite *et al*. 1982; Vogt *et al*. 1982; Gallo *et al*. 1983). Neutralization of these sites by positively charged molecules (such as protamine) can prevent localization of positively charged antigens and subsequent development of nephritis (Adler *et al*. 1983b).

The site of localization of immune deposits appears to be relevant to both the initiating mechanism and the inflammatory mediators involved (Salant *et al*. 1985). The reaction of antigen and antibody in the subepithelial space, as in models of membranous nephropathy, generally leads to complement-dependent, leucocyte-independent injury, probably due to the membrane attack complex. These reactions necessarily occur locally, since preformed complexes are generally unable to traverse the intact glomerular capillary barrier. Limitation of the effects of leucocytes may be due to their restricted access to this site and/or due to the inability of chemotaxins to diffuse against the flux of glomerular ultrafiltration. Subendothelial deposits, as seen in models of proliferative nephritis, may contain preformed complexes, and generally result in complement-mediated, leucocyte-dependent injury. It has been shown that immune complexes are rapidly cleared from this site, with resolution of injury, whereas subepithelial deposits and the accompanying noninflammatory injury tend to persist (Fries *et al*. 1988).

IMMUNOGLOBULIN A-DEPENDENT EXPERIMENTAL NEPHRITIS

The role of IgA-containing immune complexes in mesangial nephritis was first examined in mice bearing an IgA myeloma specific for dinitrophenyl (DNP) conjugated with bovine serum albumin (Rifai *et al*. 1979). Passive administration of such complexes demonstrated that polymeric IgA was necessary for development of disease (Rifai and Millard 1985), and that the nature of the antigen was important in complement activation (Rifai *et al*. 1987). Chronic immunization of mice with dextrans produces mesangial nephritis with IgA deposits, and both size and charge of the antigen were shown to relate to complement activation and injury (Isaacs and Miller 1982). Orally administered antigens, including ovalbumin, are also capable of inducing IgA nephritis in mice (Emancipator *et al*. 1983), and reticuloendothelial system blockade with colloidal carbon has been shown to increase mesangial IgA deposition and glomerular injury (Sato *et al*. 1986). However, further experiments in similar models, involving intravenous challenge with the prior oral immunogen, demonstrated that co-deposition of IgG or IgM (or of complement-activating antigens) was necessary for complement deposition and injury (Emancipator *et al*. 1987). The role of liver disease in IgA nephritis was studied by experiments involving bile duct ligation or administration of carbon tetrachloride — mesangial deposits of IgA were observed but there were no major histological changes (Gormly *et al*. 1981; Melvin *et al*. 1983).

ANTIBODIES TO RENAL CELLS

There has been recent interest in the possibility that renal injury may be caused by antibodies against specific glomerular cell types. The best characterized model is that involving antibodies to epithelial cell antigens — 'passive Heymann nephritis' (Feenstra *et al*. 1975). In Heymann nephritis (see below) immunization of rats with homologous renal tubular cell preparations (Fx1A) results in a form of membranous nephropathy with granular immune deposits (Edgington *et al*. 1968). It was believed that these represented complexes formed between renal tubular antigens and antibodies directed against them, which were trapped in the glomerulus. However, it has now been shown that immunized animals produce autoantibodies reactive with antigens (including the glycoprotein, gp330) common to tubular and glomerular epithelial cells (Couser *et al*. 1978; Van Damme *et al*. 1978; Kerjaschki and Farquhar 1982).

Direct administration of heterologous anti-Fx1A or anti-gp330 antibodies reproduces the immunofluorescence pattern of active Heymann nephritis, and to a varying extent the renal injury (Feenstra *et al*. 1975; Bagchus *et al*. 1986b). These antibodies react with gp330 in the clathrin-coated pits of the podocytes, and this is followed by capping and shedding of the complexes formed (Camussi *et al*. 1985; Kerjaschki *et al*. 1987b). This process is illustrated in Fig. 99.2. Proteinuria in the early phase of passive Heymann nephritis depends upon the membrane attack complex of complement, although decomplementation with cobra venom factor (CVF) does not totally abrogate renal injury during the later autologous phase, suggesting a role for other mechanisms (Salant *et al*. 1980; Adler *et al*. 1983a).

The role of anti-endothelial cell antibodies has been investigated following their detection in systemic lupus erythematosus (SLE) (Cines *et al*. 1984) and other forms of systemic vasculitis (Ferraro *et al*. 1990). Heterologous antibodies to angiotensin-converting enzyme (ACE), present on endothelial cells, can cause injury to glomerular endothelium in the rabbit (Matsuo *et al*. 1987). Similarly, the possibility that mesangial cells are the target for autoantibodies in human mesangial proliferative nephritis has been investigated in the rat, using antibodies to the Thy 1.1-like antigen on mesangial cells. Administration of rabbit anti-rat thymocyte antibody resulted in mesangiolysis in recipient animals, followed by mesangial hypercellularity and proteinuria in certain rat strains (Bagchus *et al*. 1986a). The initial lytic lesion was complement-dependent, and shown to involve the membrane attack complex (Yamamoto and Wilson 1987a).

Experimental autoimmune glomerulonephritis

Animal models of autoimmune GN allow the analysis, at a cellular and molecular level, of mechanisms involved in the induction and regulation of renal autoimmunity. Of particular clinical relevance is that these models are suitable for the investigation, *in vivo*, of specific immunotherapeutic approaches aimed at modifying the autoreactivity of T and/or B lymphocytes. The principal features of selected models are shown in Table 99.1.

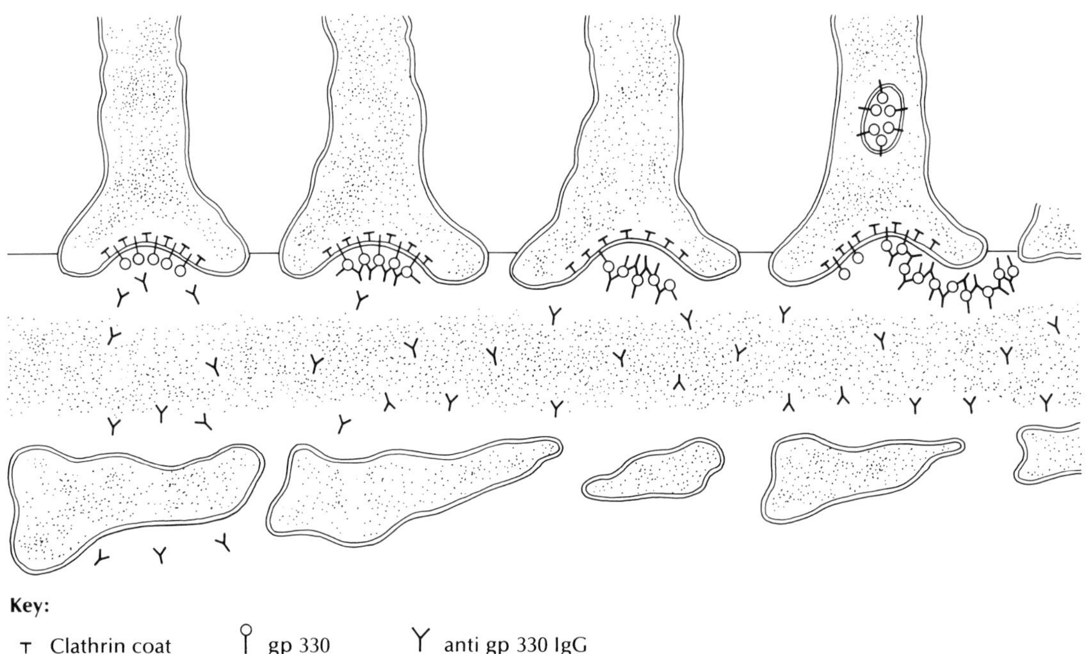

Fig. 99.2. Diagrammatic representation of *in situ* immune complex formation in Heymann nephritis (courtesy of Prof. D. Kerjaschki). Anti-gp330 antibodies bind to gp330 in the coated pits, forming the initial immune complex which becomes attached to the GBM and is partially shed. The immune deposit grows in size by repeated cycles of *in situ* complex formation, until it encroaches on the slit diaphragm. This process requires synthesis of new gp330 molecules by the podocytes.

Table 99.1. Features of experimental autoimmune nephritis

Disease	Stimulus	Species	Strain	Serology	Immunohistology	Pathogenesis	Regulation
Anti-GBM nephritis (Steblay)	GBM + CFA	Sheep	—	Anti-GBM Ab	Linear IgG ± C3 on GMB	Transfer by Ab	—
		Rat	BN, WKY	Anti-GBM Ab	Linear IgG on GBM	Transfer by Ab Priming by MC	CsA
		Chicken	SC (bursectomized)	—	—	Transfer by MC	—
Membranous nephritis (Heymann)	Fx1A + CFA	Rat	LEW, PVG	Anti-brush border Ab Anti-GP330 Ab	Granular IgG ± C3 on GBM	Transfer by Ab	T_s cells Anti-id Ab CsA
Interstitial nephritis	TBM + CFA	Guinea-pig	XIII	Anti-TBM Ab	Linear IgG ± C3 on TBM	Transfer by Ab	Anti-id Ab
		Rat	BN	Anti-TBM Ab	Linear IgG ± C3 on TBM	Transfer by Ab MC required	Anti-id Ab CsA, Cyclo
		Mouse	SJL	Anti-TBM Ab	Linear IgG ± C3 on TBM	Transfer by Tdth cells Mild form by Ab	T_s cells (id and anti-id)
Toxic nephropathy	Hg, Au, penicillamine	Rat	BN	Anti-GBM Ab Common idiotype Polyclonal activation with other auto-Ab	Linear IgG on GBM (later granular IgG)	Transfer by T_h cells	T_s cells Anti-id Ab (*in vitro*) Cyclo, CsA
'Lupus' nephritis	Spontaneous	Mouse	NZB/W, BXSB MRL/lpr	Anti-DNA Ab Polyclonal activation	Granular Ig + C3 on GBM	—	Anti-id Ab Anti-MHC Ab Anti-T cell Ab Anti-IL-2R Ab

Ab = antibody; MC = mononuclear cell; id = idiotype; CsA = cyclosporin A; Cyclo = cyclophosphamide.

STEBLAY NEPHRITIS

An antigen-induced experimental model of anti-GBM disease, Steblay nephritis, was first described by Steblay in 1962, who found that sheep immunized with heterologous or homologous GBM preparations in adjuvant developed linear deposits of IgG and C3 on the basement membrane together with a proliferative (crescentic) nephritis. The role of circulating antibody was demonstrated by both cross-circulation and passive transfer experiments (Steblay and Rudofsky 1968a).

Subsequently, experimental autoimmune GN (EAG) has been induced in numerous species, including mice (Avasthi *et al.* 1971), rats (Stuffers-Heiman *et al.* 1979; Sado *et al.* 1984), rabbits (Unanue *et al.* 1967), guinea-pigs (Couser *et al.* 1973) and monkeys (Steblay 1963). In general, immunization with heterologous GBM in adjuvant has been required, and in this situation the response of T cells to antigens to which the animal is not tolerant could lead to stimulation of autoreactive B cells. The pathogenicity of anti-GBM antibodies in the WKY rat has been confirmed by passive transfer of nephritis (Sado *et al.* 1989). The use of both heterologous and isologous GBM preparations in inbred strains of rat has allowed the demonstration of genetic susceptibility (Stuffers-Heiman *et al.* 1979; Pusey *et al.* 1991), although this has not yet been formally linked to the MHC. Brown Norway (BN) rats given a single injection of isologous GBM in adjuvant developed sustained anti-GBM antibody production, with linear deposits of IgG on the GBM and proteinuria; PVG and DA strains showed a similar but less consistent response, with no real injury; and LEW and WAG strains showed a lower level of circulating antibody, with no glomerular deposits. The role of T cells in the induction of this disease is suggested by the therapeutic effect of cyclosporin A on anti-GBM antibody production and proteinuria in BN rats with EAG (Reynolds *et al.* 1991). More direct evidence for T cell involvement in EAG comes from the experiments of Bolton *et al.* (1984), who found that bursectomized chicks immunized with heterologous GBM in adjuvant developed nephritis in the absence of detectable autoantibodies. This disease could be transferred to naïve syngeneic SC chickens by T lymphocytes (Bolton *et al.* 1988).

The relationship between renal and pulmonary injury, the principal clinical features of Goodpasture's syndrome, has been investigated in various models of EAG. Alveolar basement membrane can be used to induce nephritis (Steblay and Rudofsky 1968b), and GBM can induce lung haemorrhage (Sado *et al.* 1984; Pusey *et al.* 1991). These observations support the immunohistological and immunochemical findings in man (see below), which suggest that the same autoantigen is present in both sites. The development of lung haemorrhage may depend upon the permeability of the alveolar capillary wall, which limits access of antibody to the alveolar antigen. Experimental support for this suggestion is provided by studies of anti-basement membrane antibody binding in animals exposed to toxic concentrations of oxygen (Jennings *et al.* 1981) or gasoline (Yamamoto and Wilson 1987b).

MERCURIC CHLORIDE-INDUCED NEPHRITIS

The administration of various polyclonal activators, including mercuric chloride ($HgCl_2$) and penicillamine, has been found to induce anti-GBM disease in rats (Sapin *et al.* 1977; Donker *et al.* 1984) and rabbits (Roman-Franco *et al.* 1978). Mercuric chloride-induced nephritis in the BN rat is the best characterized. Repeated subcutaneous injections of subnephrotoxic doses of $HgCl_2$ lead to a biphasic disease, in which linear deposits of IgG on the GBM are followed by granular deposits. Proteinuria accompanies the immune response, but histological changes are slight (Druet *et al.* 1978).

Several observations of importance to the mechanisms of induction and regulation of nephritis have been made in this model:

1 The anti-GBM response occurs as part of a polyclonal stimulation of the immune system (Hirsch *et al.* 1982; Pusey *et al.* 1990), which is related to the induction of anti-Ia T lymphocytes (Pelletier *et al.* 1986). Whether this results from direct stimulation of T_h cells, or also depends upon inhibition of T suppressor (T_s) mechanisms, is not yet clear. However, T cells from affected animals can be used to transfer the disease to normal recipients (Pelletier *et al.* 1988). The role of T cells in the induction of the disease is further supported by the beneficial effects of cyclosporin A (Baran *et al.* 1986).

2 Susceptibility to induction of the disease is

strain-dependent, and involves the MHC as well as one or two other genes (Druet *et al.* 1982).

3 The autoimmune response is rapidly self-limiting, with anti-GBM antibody levels peaking at around 2 weeks and becoming undetectable by 4 weeks. This occurs despite continued injection of $HgCl_2$, and treated animals remain resistant to rechallenge for several weeks. There is evidence for the role of both T_s cells (Bowman *et al.* 1984) and anti-idiotypic antibodies (Chalopin and Lockwood 1984) in this resistance.

4 Anti-GBM antibody production and proteinuria can be suppressed by a single high dose of cyclophosphamide given at the start of $HgCl_2$ administration, although a much lower dose was associated with increased antibody levels, perhaps due to selective effects on T_s cells (Pusey *et al.* 1983a). Of possible therapeutic interest is that animals treated with the single high dose of cyclophosphamide remained resistant to further induction of antibodies by $HgCl_2$ for up to a year.

A similar form of GN, occurring as part of a polyclonal B cell response, has been reported in murine experimental graft-versus-host (GVH) disease (Rolink *et al.* 1983) and host-versus-graft (HVG) disease (Goldman *et al.* 1983). In both instances it is believed that this involves semi-allogeneic T–B cell co-operation, with resulting autoimmunity. A similar disease occurs in rats with GVH disease, and recently it has been shown that the anti-GBM antibodies produced in mercury-, gold-, penicillamine- and GVH-induced nephritis share common cross-reactive idiotypes (Guery *et al.* 1990). Thus it seems that similar B cell clones are triggered by anti-Class II MHC T cells generated by different stimuli.

HEYMANN NEPHRITIS

In this model of membranous GN, first described by Heymann *et al.* in 1959, rats immunized with kidney homogenates in adjuvant developed granular deposits of Ig along the glomerular capillary wall, accompanied by proteinuria. The antigen involved was initially described as a fraction (Fx1A) of the cellular membrane of proximal tubular cells (Edgington *et al.* 1968), and at least one component has now been characterized as a glycoprotein (gp330) found on both proximal tubular and glomerular epithelial cells (Kerjaschki and Farquhar 1982). Recently, a cDNA clone encoding the pathogenic domain of gp330 has been isolated, and the resulting fusion protein can induce Heymann nephritis (Pietromonaco *et al.* 1990).

Although this disease was originally thought of as an example of 'immune complex' nephritis, it is now clear that it represents an autoimmune process, in which antibodies to a cell surface antigen react *'in situ'* on the epithelial cell (Camussi *et al.* 1985). The disease can be transferred passively by antibodies to Fx1A (see above), and perfusion of isolated kidneys with such antibodies results in subepithelial immune deposits similar to those seen in the actively induced model. Less proteinuria is found following administration of anti-gp330 antibodies, or active immunization with gp330, than in the original Heymann model, suggesting that more than one antigen–antibody system may be involved (Kamata *et al.* 1985; Bagchus *et al.* 1986b; Ronco *et al.* 1986; Verroust *et al.* 1986; Mendrick and Rennke 1988).

The induction of Heymann nephritis is strain-dependent, and linked to MHC genes (Stenglein *et al.* 1978; Cheng *et al.* 1988). LEW, AS and WG rats are susceptible, whereas BN, DA and BUF strains are resistant. As in EAG, cyclosporin A has a protective effect, suggesting T cell involvement (Gronhagen-Riska *et al.* 1990). In addition, resistance to the disease can be produced by T_s cells (Litwin *et al.* 1979; De Heer *et al.* 1985b; Cheng *et al.* 1988), and by the induction of anti-idiotypic antibodies (Ebert *et al.* 1981). Renal injury is reduced by complement depletion with CVF in the early stages of the disease, but not by neutrophil depletion (Salant *et al.* 1980), and there is indirect evidence for the role of the membrane attack complex of complement (De Heer *et al.* 1985a). This is supported by more direct evidence that terminal components of complement are responsible for glomerular injury in passive models of Heymann nephritis (Parkinson *et al.* 1985; Cybulsky *et al.* 1986; Kerjaschki *et al.* 1989).

INTERSTITIAL NEPHRITIS

Tubulointerstitial nephritis (TIN) can be induced in several species, including mice, rats and guinea-pigs, by the administration of tubular basement membrane (TBM) preparations in adjuvant. The role of autoantibodies, immune complexes and T cells has been illustrated in different models, none of which directly corresponds to drug-induced acute interstitial nephritis in man (McCluskey and Colvin 1978). Steblay and Rudofsky (1971) first established a model of TIN in the guinea-pig, using rabbit TBM in adjuvant, in which there was linear deposition of IgG along the TBM and severe interstitial inflammation with T cells, monocytes and giant cells. The disease could be transferred by anti-TBM antibodies (Steblay and Rudofsky 1973), but not by lymphoid cells, and its severity could be reduced both by complement depletion with CVF (Rudofsky *et al.* 1975) and by leucocyte depletion using irradiation (Rudofsky and Pollara 1976). The disease could be inhibited by heterologous anti-idiotypic sera (Brown *et al.* 1979). Genetic susceptibility has been demonstrated, since strain XIII animals develop TIN more readily than do strain II animals; this susceptibility is inherited as a dominant or co-dominant trait linked to the MHC (Hyman *et al.* 1976).

The use of rat and mouse models of TIN has allowed more detailed examination of immunogenetics and immunoregulation. In BN rats, administration of isologous (Sugisaki *et al.* 1973) or heterologous (bovine) (Lehman *et al.* 1974b) TBM in adjuvant leads to linear deposits of IgG and C3 on proximal TBM within 2–3 weeks — this is initially accompanied by neutrophil infiltration, and later by accumulation of lymphocytes and monocytes. Several weeks after the injection of rat (but not bovine) TBM, granular deposits of IgG are found in the glomerulus, similar to those seen in Heymann nephritis. A mild form of the disease can be passively transferred by anti-TBM antibodies (Sugisaki *et al.* 1973), but not by lymphocytes alone, although cell-mediated mechanisms have been implicated in pathogenesis (Mampaso and Wilson 1983).

Two separate elements determining genetic susceptibility to TIN have been identified. Certain strains (F344, AUG) do not produce sufficient anti-TBM antibody to produce disease, and others (LEW, MAXX) develop circulating antibody but lack immunoreactive antigen in the TBM. Susceptible BN rats develop an adequate immune response and possess the relevant antigen (Lehman *et al.* 1974b; Neilson *et al.* 1983). Transplantation of kidneys from strains possessing the nephritogenic antigen into animals normally lacking it is followed by the development of anti-TBM disease in the allograft (Lehman *et al.* 1974a). Interestingly, immunization of LEW rats with BN TBM induces a cell-mediated form of TIN without deposition of anti-TBM antibodies (Bannister *et al.* 1987).

The development of TIN in the BN rat can be suppressed by the administration of heterologous (rabbit) anti-idiotypic antibodies (Zanetti *et al.* 1983). Protection is also provided by measures leading to generation of auto-anti-idiotypic responses — for example, by immunizing animals with TBM-reactive T lymphoblasts (Neilson and Phillips 1982a). It has been suggested that susceptibility is based upon the failure of development of auto-anti-idiotypic immunity (Neilson *et al.* 1984b). Disease can be suppressed, or at a later stage ameliorated, by high doses of cyclophosphamide, whereas low doses appear to increase severity of disease, as noted in $HgCl_2$-induced nephritis (Agus *et al.* 1986). Cyclosporin A is effective in prevention and amelioration of TIN, supporting the involvement of T cells (Gimenez *et al.* 1987). The stable analogue of PGE_1 was also found to inhibit anti-TBM antibody production and interstitial nephritis (Ulich and Ni 1986) — this is likely to be mediated via effects on the induction of effector T cells (Kelly *et al.* 1987).

In a similar model of TIN in mice, there is a strain-dependent response to injection of rabbit TBM (Rudofsky *et al.* 1980; Neilson and Phillips 1982b). Susceptibility has been shown to depend upon the MHC haplotype (H-2K) and upon Ig genes (Igh-1) (Neilson *et al.* 1985a). The disease can be transferred by T cells with delayed-type hypersensitivity function, and also (in a milder form) by anti-TBM antibodies (Zakheim *et al.* 1984). Amelioration of the disease can be achieved by immunization with tubular antigen-'derivatized' lymphocytes. This has been shown to induce a T_s cell system involving both idiotypic (T_s1) and anti-idiotypic (T_s2) cells, which are functionally restricted by MHC (I-J) and Ig (IgH-V) gene products (Neilson *et al.* 1985b).

The target antigen of the anti-TBM response has been characterized as a glycoprotein of molecular weight 42 kD in the rat and 30 kD in the mouse. It was isolated using a monoclonal antibody reactive with BN but not LEW proximal tubules (Clayman *et al.* 1985) — since it was known that LEW rats did not express the nephritogenic antigen (Lehman *et al.* 1974b). The antigen, known as 3M-1, is localized to the most lateral aspect of the TBM and can be used to induce typical TIN (Clayman *et al.* 1985). Lately, the gene encoding 3M-1 has been cloned from a complementary DNA (cDNA) library derived from a murine tubular epithelial cell line (Neilson *et al.* 1989), and synthetic peptides based on its sequence are being used to examine T cell responses in different strains of mouse.

Spontaneous nephritis

The spontaneous development of GN has been observed in a variety of laboratory and domestic animals. We shall consider briefly what has been learnt from the study of murine SLE and progressive TIN.

MURINE LUPUS NEPHRITIS

Three separate lupus-prone inbred strains have been described: NZB/NZW F_1, BXSB and MRL/lpr. The principal immunological features of these strains have been reviewed elsewhere (see Smith and Steinberg 1983; Theofilopoulous *et al.* 1983; Fournie 1988) and are considered in Chapter 61. Despite the common feature of polyclonal B cell activation, the underlying mechanisms involved appear to be multiple and varied. The role of a specific subpopulation of B cells (responsive to certain T-independent antigens) has been demonstrated in breeding experiments in which susceptible NZB/W or BXSB animals are crossed with CBA/N mice, which lack this subset of cells (Scher 1982). Several genetic and environmental factors influencing the severity of disease have been identified: male chromosomal sex (BXSB); the lymphoproliferative gene (MRL/lpr); female sex hormones (NZB/W); and viral infections (all strains).

The antibody response is of relatively restricted specificity and idiotypy (Andrzejewski *et al.* 1980). Immunization of NZB/W mice with a monoclonal anti-DNA antibody induces an anti-idiotypic response and protects animals from disease (Hahn and Ebling 1983). This model was one of the first to explore the therapeutic use of monoclonal antibodies to various components of the immune system:

1 Administration of monoclonal antibodies to a cross-reaction idiotype in NZB/W mice resulted in transient suppression of disease, although there was subsequent production of anti-DNA antibodies bearing a different idiotype (Hahn and Ebling 1984). This approach was not successful in MRL/lpr mice (Teitlebaum *et al.* 1984).

2 Monoclonal antibodies to T cells or to T_h cells (anti-L3T4) prevented or ameliorated disease in all three strains (Wofsy *et al.* 1985; Wofsy and Seaman 1986). In one series of experiments, the effect was mediated via the $F(ab)_2$ fragment and did not depend upon depletion of T_h numbers (Carteron *et al.* 1989).

3 Monoclonal antibodies to MHC (I-A) gene products suppressed disease in the NZB/W strain (Adelman *et al.* 1983).

4 Recently, monoclonal antibodies to the IL-2 receptor (present on activated T cells) have been shown to limit disease in NZB/W mice (Strom and Kelly 1989).

MURINE TUBULOINTERSTITIAL NEPHRITIS

A spontaneously occurring form of progressive TIN has been described in kdkd mice, a mutant subline of the CDA strain (Lyon and Hulse 1971; Neilson *et al.* 1984a). This disease is inherited in an autosomal recessive pattern, and is considered a model for nephronophthisis. Affected mice developed severe peritubular mononuclear cell infiltrates by around 8 weeks of age, followed by progressive tubular destruction and interstitial fibrosis. No autoantibodies have been identified, but the disease can be transferred by Class I MHC-restricted (H-2K^k) CD8+ve T cells (Kelly *et al.* 1986). T cells from non-disease prone CDA mice can suppress development of TIN in kdkd animals, and susceptibility is thought to depend on the presence of antigen-specific contra-suppressor cells (Kelly and Neilson 1987).

Human nephritis

We shall consider the immunopathology of the various histologically defined types of GN and of acute interstitial nephritis. Understanding of these diseases is incomplete, and still relies heavily upon analogies with experimental models (Pusey *et al.* 1988). For convenience, we shall group the types of glomerulonephritis into: (i) those where there is reasonable evidence for the pathogenic involvement of deposited immune reactants (antibodies and complement); and (ii) those in which there are no (or few) such immune deposits. In the latter group, it remains likely or possible that immune mechanisms are involved, but that immune deposits are not seen because they are rapidly cleared, or that local or distant T-cell-mediated responses are important. A brief and over-simplified summary of the immunology of human nephritis, with and without immune deposits, is given in Table 99.2. The clinical features and natural history of these disorders have been reviewed elsewhere (Glassock 1985; Cameron 1988a), as have the histopathological findings (Heptinstall 1983).

Nephritis with immune deposits

ANTI-GLOMERULAR BASEMENT MEMBRANE DISEASE

Autoantibodies to the GBM are associated with rapidly progressive GN (RPGN), often accompanied by alveolar haemorrhage — the combination of these features is termed Goodpasture's syndrome (Stanton and Tange 1958; Wilson and Dixon 1973). The detection of linear deposits of IgG on the GBM on immunofluorescence, similar to the pattern observed in NTN, prompted the notion that this disease was antibody-mediated (Scheer and Grossman 1964; Duncan *et al.* 1965). The pathogenicity of these antibodies was later demonstrated by Lerner *et al.* (1967), who showed that anti-GBM antibody eluted from patients' kidneys could be used to produce nephritis in monkeys. The diagnosis of Goodpasture's syndrome can now be made by solid-phase immunoassays for circulating anti-GBM antibodies (Mahieu *et al.* 1974; Wieslander *et al.* 1981; Bowman and Lockwood 1985), as well as by direct immunohistology of renal biopsies (Fig. 99.3).

Immunohistological studies, using eluted anti-GBM antibodies and a murine monoclonal antibody (P1) to human GBM, have demonstrated that the same target antigen is present in GBM, distal TBM and alveolar basement membrane — thus the same antibody–antigen interaction accounts for both clinical aspects of the disease (Pusey *et al.* 1987). The Goodpasture antigen is also present in basement membranes of the choroid plexus, retina/choroid, lens capsule, cochlea and certain endocrine glands (Cashman *et al.* 1988; Kleppel *et al.* 1989). Its distribution always coincides with that of type IV collagen, but is considerably more restricted. Western blotting studies have shown that the same antigenic components of GBM, glycoproteins of 26–58 kD, are recognized by all patients and by monoclonal P1, demonstrating the restricted specificity of this autoimmune response (Pusey *et al.* 1987).

The biochemical characterization of the autoantigen is not yet complete, although it is known to form part of the non-collagenous globular domain (NC1) of type IV collagen (Hudson *et al.* 1989). The monomeric and dimeric components recognized on Western blotting represent respectively single or linked C-terminal regions of α(IV) pro-collagen molecules (Wieslander *et al.* 1984; Butkowski *et al.* 1985). Current evidence, based on amino acid sequence data, suggests that the antigenic site is located on one or more novel α(IV) chains, rather than on the well-characterized α1 and α2 chains (Butkowski *et al.* 1987; Saus *et al.* 1988). Recently, cloning of cDNA encoding the autoantigen confirms it to be the NCI domain of the α3 chain of type IV collagen (Turner *et al.* 1992).

Susceptibility to the disease depends upon genetic and environmental factors. Identical twins with anti-GBM disease have been reported (D'Apice *et al.* 1978); there is a strong association with MHC genes (Rees *et al.* 1984b); and there is also a link with Ig allotypes (Rees *et al.* 1984a). Serological techniques revealed that development of anti-GBM disease was associated with human leucocyte antigen (HLA)-DR2, and that patients also possessing B7 developed more severe nephritis (Rees *et al.* 1984b). More recently, techniques of restriction fragment length polymorphism (RFLP) analysis and oligonucleotide subtyping have shown a strong association with the DRw15 (DR2) allele and a weaker association with DR4 (Burns *et al.* 1990). No unique disease-associated sequences have yet been identified, and it remains possible that a normal sequence common to DR2 and DR4 is involved. Environmental factors have proved difficult to define, although there are reports of associations with influenza A2 infection (Benoit *et al.* 1964) and hydrocarbon exposure (Beirne and Brennan 1972). There is a clear relationship between cigarette smoking and the development of lung haemorrhage (Donaghy and Rees 1983).

Although anti-GBM antibodies are known to be pathogenic, the mechanisms of tissue injury are not fully understood. The work of Bonsib (1988) suggests that breaks in the glomerular capillary wall may be fundamental to the crescent formation that characterizes severe disease in man (Fig. 99.4). Immunofluorescence of renal biopsies

Table 99.2. Features of human glomerulonephritis

Disease	MHC association	Serology	Immunohistology	Pathogenesis	Treatment
Anti-GBM disease	DR2, DR4	Anti-GBM Ab	Linear IgG ± C3 on GBM	Auto-Ab to GBM	PE + Pred + Cyclo
Membranous nephropathy	DR 3 (DR2 in Japan)	Variable IC	Subepithelial fine granular IgG ± C3	?Auto-Ab to epithelial cells ?Planted Ag	Pred + chlorambucil
MCGN I	—	Variable IC, low C3	Subendothelial granular IgG + C3 (± IgM)	?IC disease	—
MCGN II	?DR7	NeF, low C3	Linear C3 on GBM	?Auto-Ab to C3bBb	—
IgA nephropathy	DR4 DQw7	Variable raised IgA ± IgA-IC ?Anti-mesangial cell Ab	Mesangial IgA + C3 (± IgG)	?IC disease ?Auto-Ab to mesangial cells	?Cyclo + anticoagulants ?Pred in nephrotic syndrome
Post-streptococcal GN	DR4	Anti-strep Ab Variable raised Ig + IC Low C3 ± C4	Subepithelial IgG + C3 (± other Ig)	?Planted Ag	—
SLE	DR3	Anti-DNA Ab Anti-Sm Ab Polyclonal increase Ig ± IC Low C4 ± C3	Subepithelial, subendothelial and mesangial IgG + IgM + IgA + C3	?Autoimmune ?Planted Ag ?IC disease	Pred ± Cyclo or Aza ?PE or pulse MP (severe)
MEC II	—	Cryoglobulins Paraprotein (IgM) IC + RF Low C4	Subendothelial granular IgM + IgG + C3	IC disease	PE ± Pred ± Cyclo
Minimal change nephropathy	DR7 (DR8 in Japan)	Sometimes raised IgM	Negative or sparse mesangial IgM	Not known ?Role of T cell factors	Pred Cyclo or CsA (relapse)
Focal necrotizing GN	?DR2 DQw7	ANCA Variable raised Ig + IC	Negative or variable scattered IgG ± IgM ± C3	?Autoimmune	Pred + Cyclo (induction) Pred + Aza (maintenance) PE or pulse MP (severe)

Ab = antibody; Ag = antigen; IC = immune complex; Cyclo = cyclophosphamide; Aza = Azathioprine; CsA = cyclosporin A; Pred = prednisolone; PE = plasma
exchange; MP = methyl prednisolone.

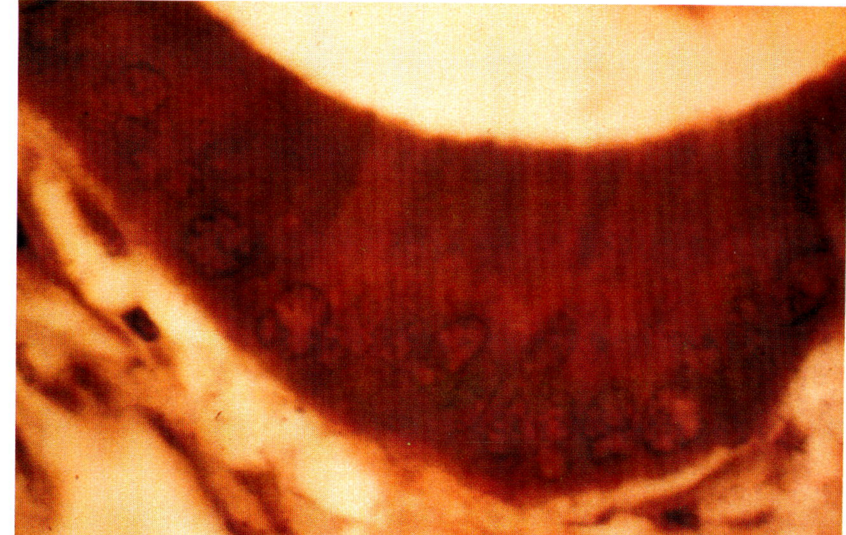

Plate 92.1. The detection by an immunoperoxidase technique of the protein encoded by the c-*myc* oncogene in a colorectal carcinoma section.

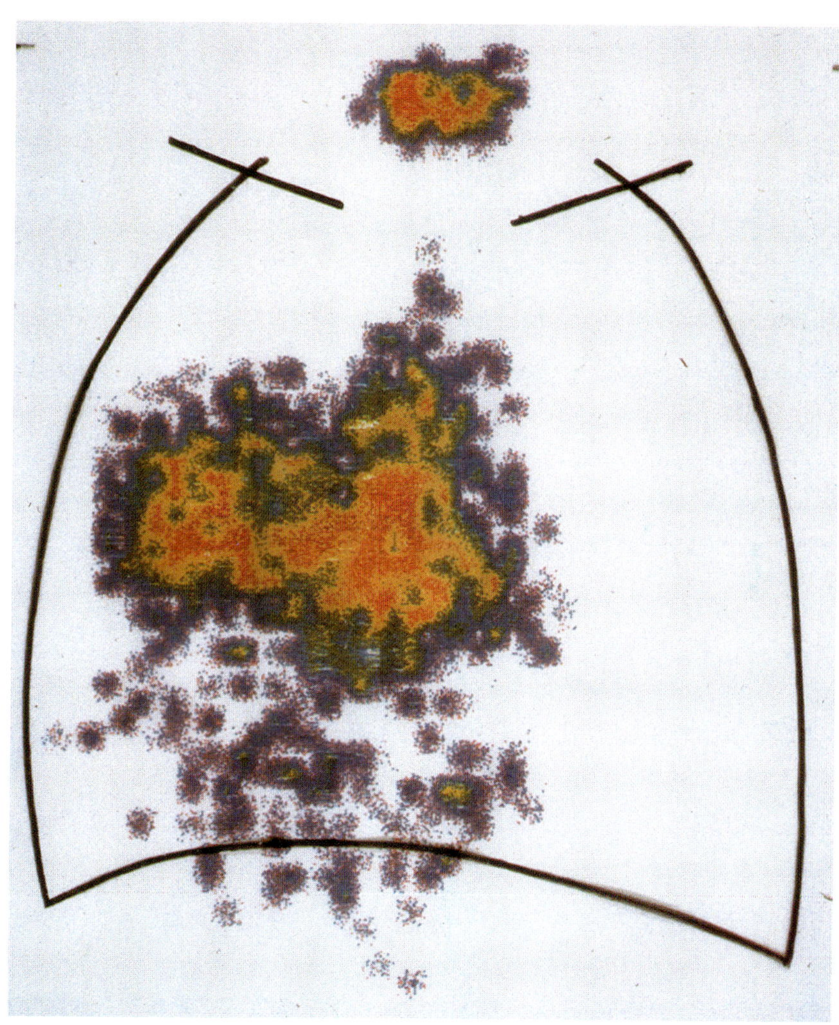

Plate 92.2. The use of a radio-iodinated monoclonal antibody to localize small-cell lung cancer.

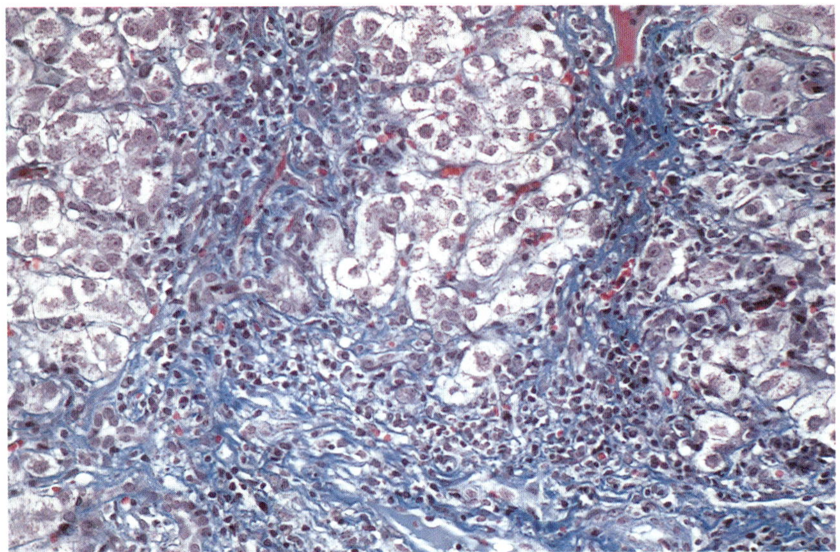

Plate 101.1. The histological features of chronic active hepatitis showing a mononuclear portal tract infiltrate with periportal extension and piecemeal necrosis of periportal hepatocytes.

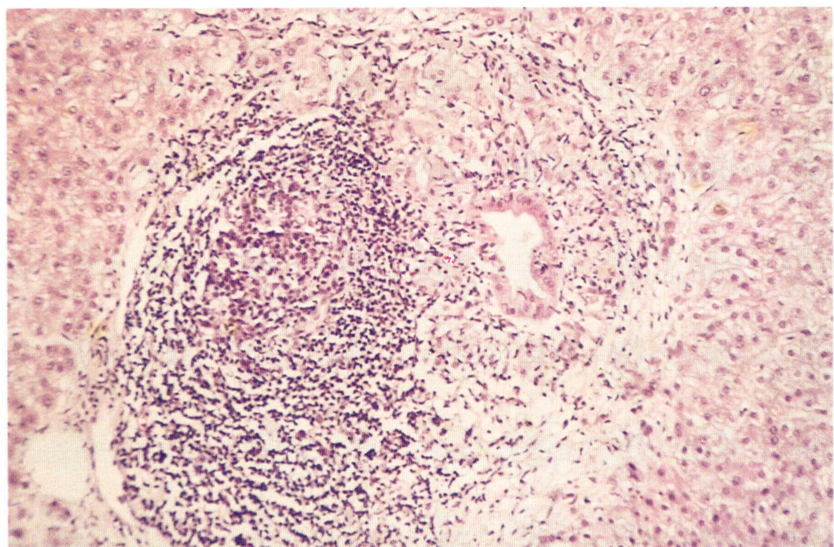

Plate 101.2. The histological features of the granulomatous bile duct destructive lesion in primary biliary cirrhosis.

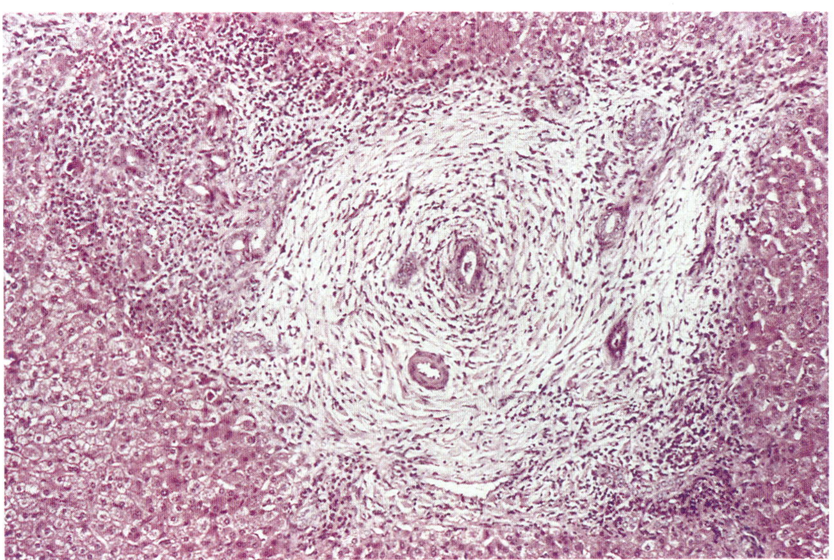

Plate 101.3. The histological features of the fibrotic 'onion skin' lesion surrounding damaged bile ducts in primary sclerosing cholangitis. Photomicrograph courtesy of Dr Bernard Portmann.

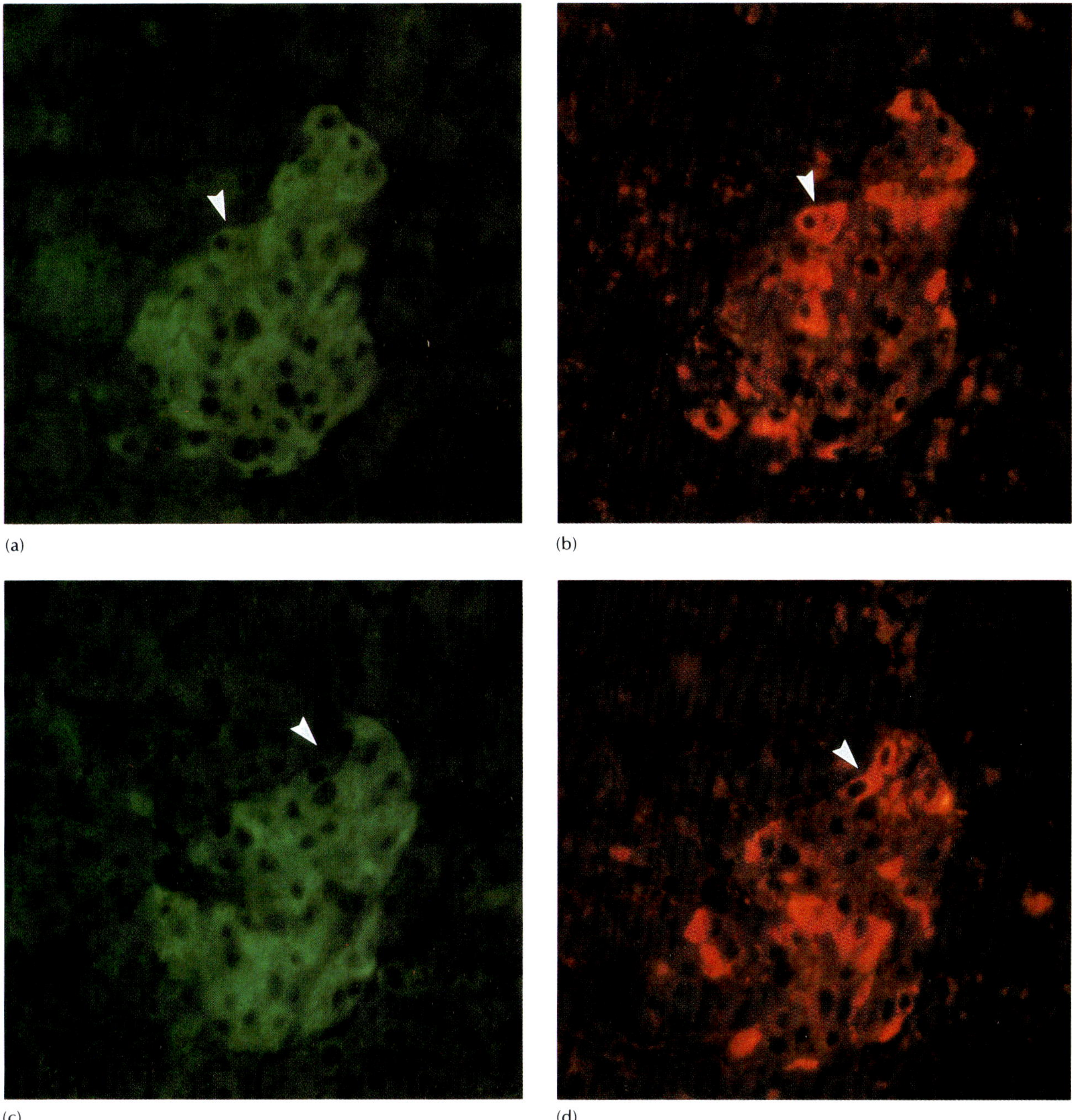

(a) (b) (c) (d)

Plate 103.1. Section of pancreas stained by double immunofluorescence with serum from a diabetic patient (a), together with monoclonal antibodies to glucagon (b). The glucagon cells (arrows) stained in (b) are also stained by the ICA in the diabetic serum. (c) and (d) An islet stained with serum from an ICA +ve non-diabetic endocrine autoimmune patient (c), together with monoclonal antibodies to glucagon (d). In this section the majority of glucagon cells (arrows) are not stained by the serum, indicating a beta cell-selective islet pattern.

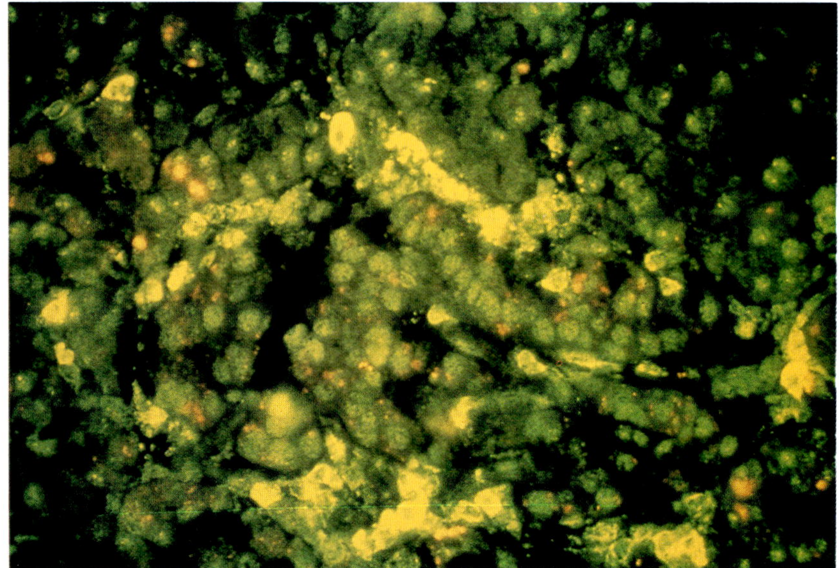

Plate 103.2. Section of pancreas of a newly diagnosed IDDM patient stained with interleukin-2 receptors by indirect immunofluorescence. The strongly stained cells are activated T lymphocytes, which express these molecules on their surface (× 1350). From Bottazzo *et al*. 1985.

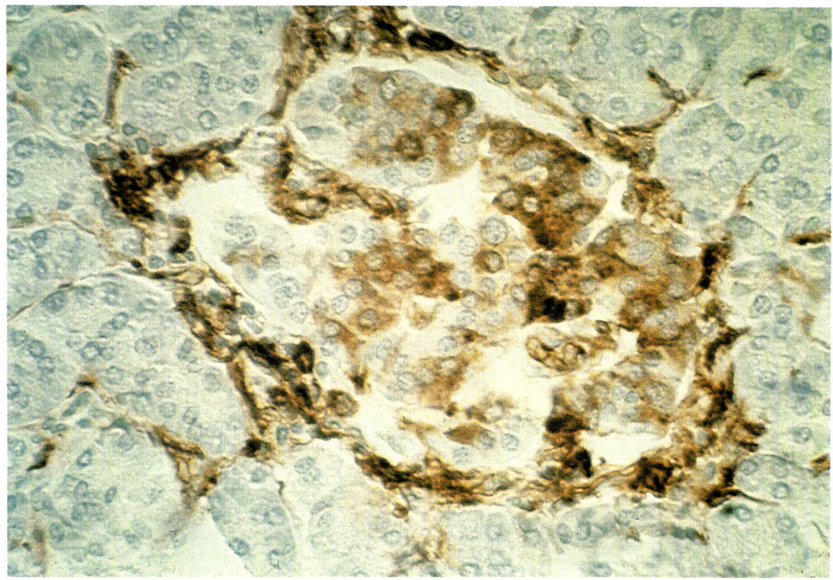

Plate 103.3. Section of pancreas of a newly diagnosed IDDM patient stained with monoclonal antibodies to HLA Class II MHC molecules, by peroxidase–antiperoxidase technique. The strong positive cells in the islet are beta cells expressing Class II molecules. The unstained cells in the islet are glucagon and somatostatin cells, which do not express these molecules. Note also the strong positive reactivity of the crown and capilliary endothelial cells around the islets (× 1350). Illustration courtesy of Dr A. Foulis.

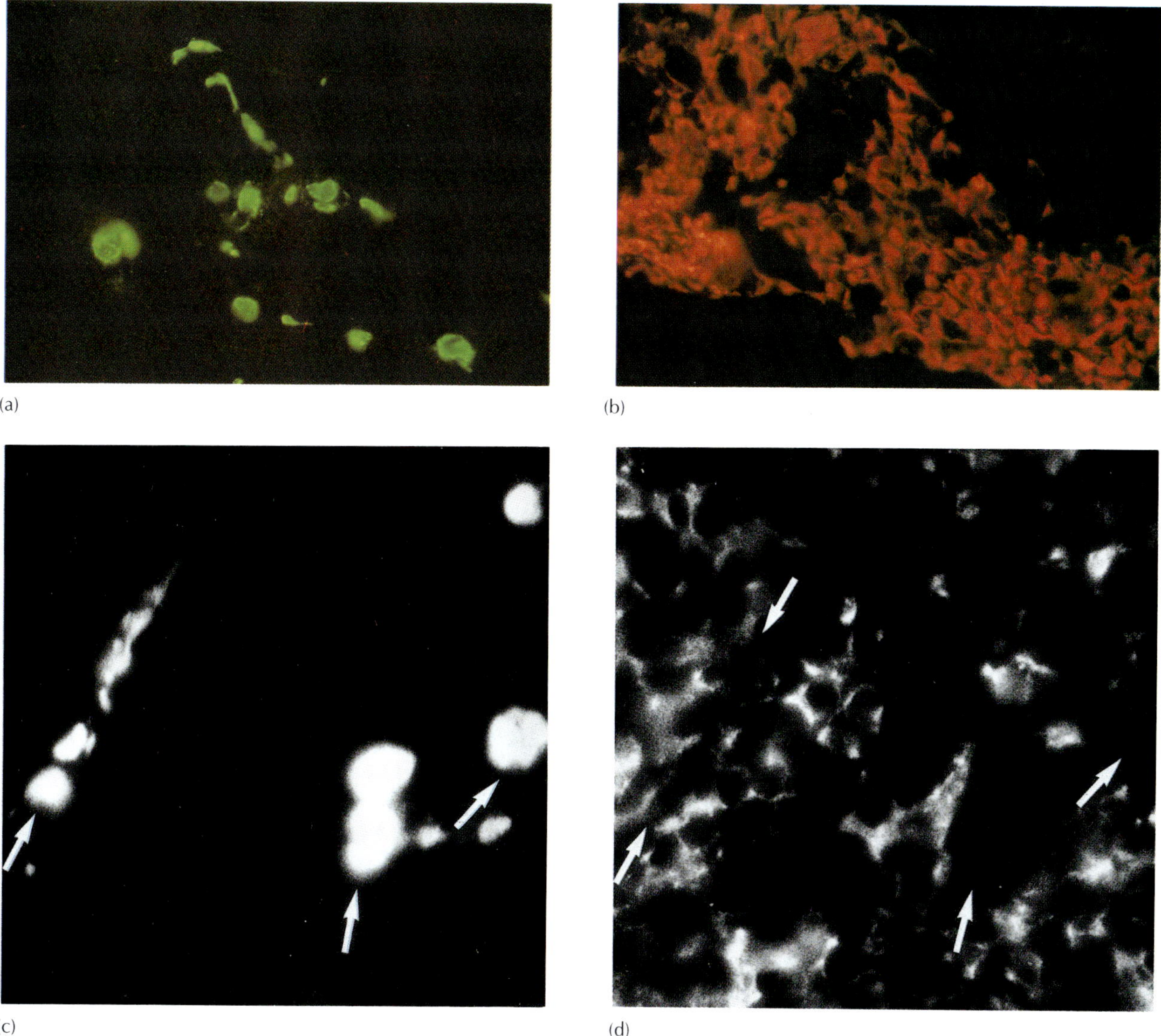

Plate 106.1. Most thymic myoid cells label for AChR ((a), Mab C3, FITC) and are located within or at the edges of the medullary epithelial bands (as in Fig. 106.5(b)), visualised here (b) with MR19 (TRITC). Myoid cells were never seen in the germinal centres (situated above/right and below this particular band). Myoid cells (arrowed) were consistently positive for troponin (not shown) and myosin ((c), FITC) but negative for HLA-DR ((d), TRITC) both in MG and healthy control thymus (Schluep *et al.* 1987). From Schluep *et al.* 1987.

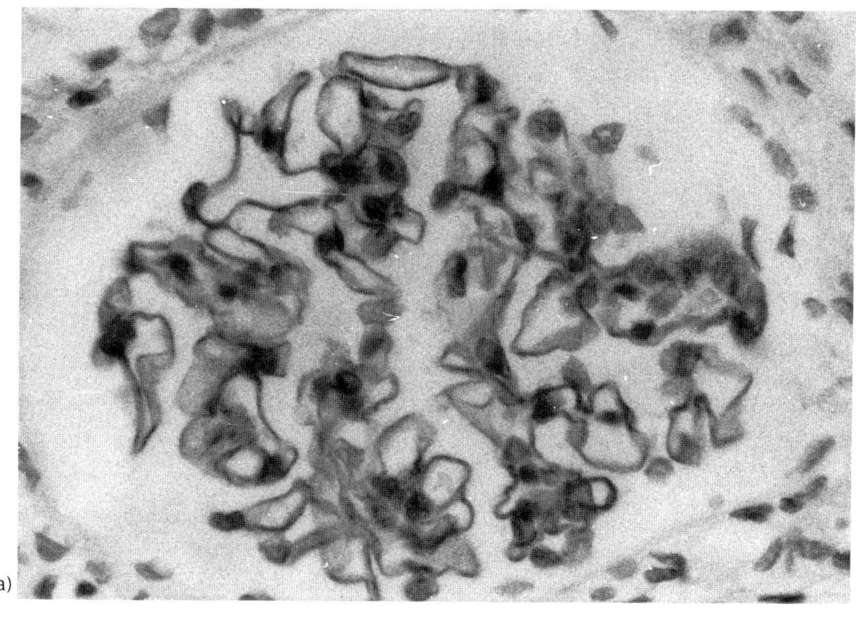
(a)

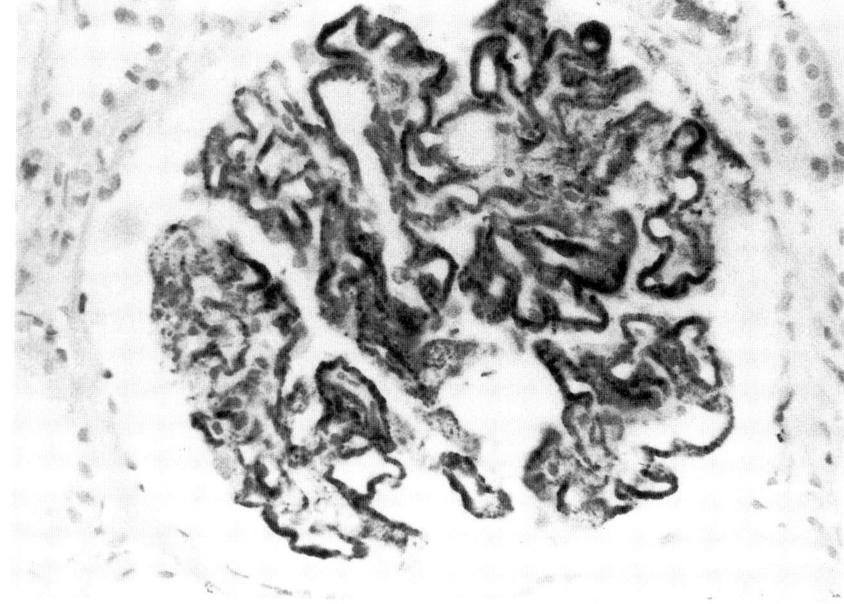
(b)

Fig. 99.3. Patterns of immunoglobulin deposition in glomerulonephritis demonstrated by direct immunoperoxidase staining of renal biopsies: (a) anti-GBM disease — linear deposits of IgG; (b) membranous nephropathy — fine granular deposits of IgG; (c) (*overleaf*) mesangiocapillary nephritis type I — coarse granular deposits of IgG; (d) IgA nephropathy — mesangial deposits of IgA. Courtesy of Dr E.M. Thompson.

almost invariably demonstrates the presence of IgG, with IgM and/or IgA in around 10% of cases (Wilson 1981; Savage *et al.* 1986). Circulating antibodies are mainly of the IgG-1 and IgG-4 subclasses (Bowman *et al.* 1987). Deposition of complement C3 is found in only one-third to one-half of cases, suggesting that non-complement-dependent injury may be important. As in other forms of crescentic nephritis, T cell (Stachura and Whitside 1984) and macrophage (Atkins *et al.* 1976) infiltration of the glomerulus and interstitium has been reported. Most studies reveal a predominance of CD4 +ve T cells, although smaller numbers of CD8 +ve cells can be detected (Bolton *et al.* 1987; Nolasco *et al.* 1987; Neale *et al.* 1988). It has been suggested that infiltration with T cells occurs at an early stage of the disease, preceding macrophage influx. These observations, however, can only provide indirect evidence for participation of the systems concerned.

Treatment with a combination of prednisolone, cyclophosphamide and plasma exchange has been shown to be effective in reducing anti-GBM antibody levels (Peters *et al.* 1982; Pusey *et al.* 1983b).

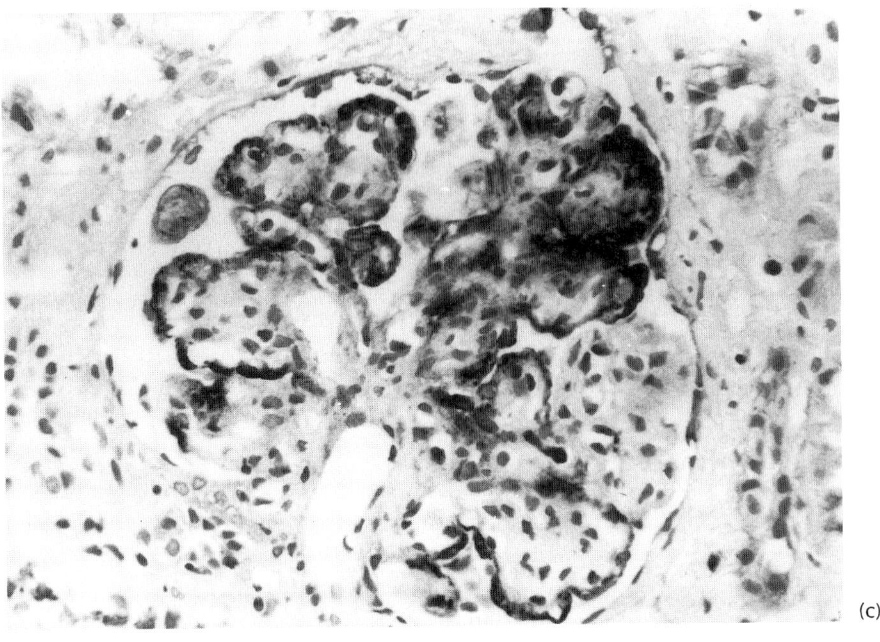

(c)

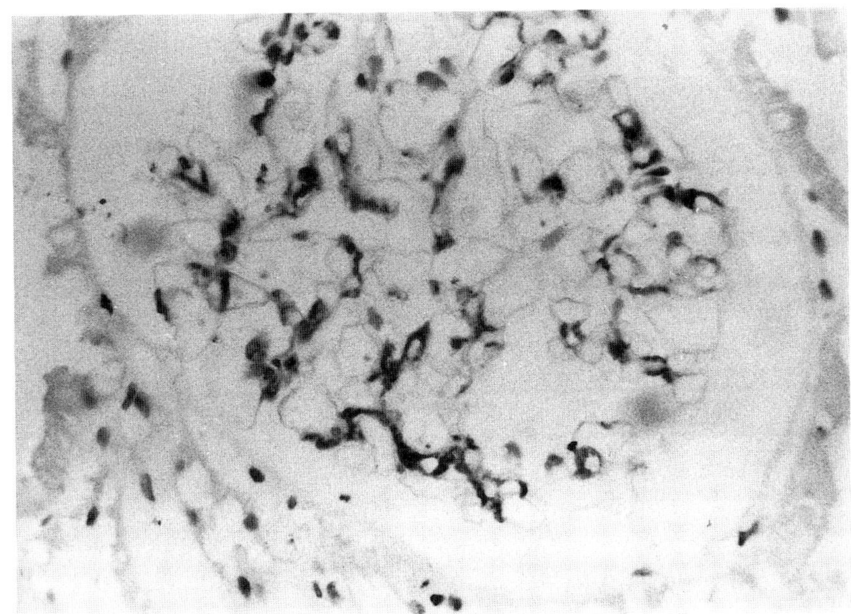

(d) **Fig. 99.3.** (Continued).

Antibody generally becomes undetectable by 8 weeks, whereas it persists for around a year in untreated patients on dialysis. Solid-phase immunoassays for circulating anti-GBM antibodies have proved of value in monitoring treatment, and also allow the selection of dialysis-dependent patients for transplantation. Interestingly, recurrence of anti-GBM antibody after such short-term treatment is exceptional, and maintenance therapy is not required. The clinical outcome depends upon the severity of renal injury at the time of treatment. The great majority of patients treated before reaching dialysis show an improvement in renal function, whereas only a small minority of dialysis-dependent patients improve (Johnson *et al*. 1985; Walker *et al*. 1985; Savage *et al*. 1986). This, none the less, represents a great improvement in the natural history of the disease (Wilson and Dixon 1973).

MEMBRANOUS NEPHROPATHY

Membranous nephropathy commonly presents as isolated proteinuria or as the nephrotic syndrome

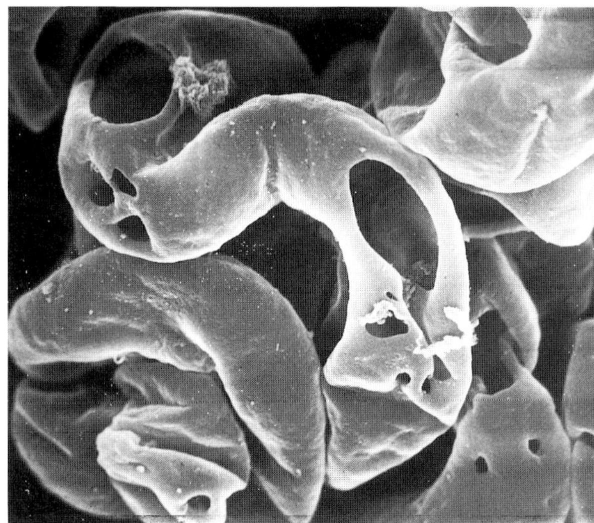

Fig. 99.4. Scanning electron micrograph of an acellular glomerulus from a patient with RPGN demonstrating 'perforations' in the glomerular capillaries. Courtesy of Dr S.M. Bonsib.

and progresses to renal failure in around 50% of cases by 10 years. It was long regarded as an example of 'immune complex' disease because of the characteristic granular deposits of IgG, occasionally with IgM and IgA, and complement C3 along the glomerular capillary wall (Cameron 1979) (Fig. 99.3). Electron microscopy (EM) reveals that these immune deposits are predominantly subepithelial. The similarity to Heymann nephritis has prompted suggestions that they represent '*in situ*' complexes formed between circulating autoantibodies and epithelial cell antigens (Camussi *et al.* 1985; Kerjaschki *et al.* 1987b); however, no such antibody–antigen system has yet been demonstrated convincingly in man. The presence of antibodies to 'brush border' antigens has been reported in isolated patients (Zanetti *et al.* 1981; Naruse *et al.* 1983), but their specificity differs from that in Heymann nephritis (Collins *et al.* 1981). Indeed, a gp330-like molecule has recently been identified in human proximal tubules, but not in the glomerulus (Kerjashki *et al.* 1987a). An alternative explanation is that a 'planted' antigen is involved. There have been several reports of the detection of specific antigens in the deposits of membranous GN, although these findings have not been widely confirmed, and would not provide good evidence for the pathogenicity of these antigens.

The same immunohistological pattern is found in primary membranous nephropathy and in cases occurring in association with other diseases. Secondary cases have been related to: (i) malignancy (Row *et al.* 1975), especially of the lung, gut, breast and kidney; (ii) infection (Levy and Kleinknecht 1980), including hepatitis B and various chronic bacterial and protozoal infections; (iii) drugs (Tornath and Skrifvars 1974), particularly gold, penicillamine and captopril; (iv) autoimmune disease (Baldwin *et al.* 1970), most commonly SLE, and rarely thyroid disorders and anti-GBM nephritis; and (v) sickle-cell anaemia (Pardo *et al.* 1975). Although the 'planted' antigen therapy appears attractive as an explanation, many of these conditions could also lead to disordered regulation of immunity, and hence to an autoantibody-mediated form of the disease.

There is a strong association with HLA-DR3 in Caucasians with both primary membranous nephropathy (Klouda *et al.* 1979) and the secondary form complicating gold and penicillamine therapy (Wooley *et al.* 1980). However, the association is with HLA-DR2 in Japanese (Hiki *et al.* 1984), suggesting either that the MHC gene responsible is in linkage disequilibrium with different alleles in the two populations, or that the diseases involve intrinsically different glomerular antigens. Severity of the disease may also depend upon genetic influences, since one study showed that patients with the haplotype DR3 B18 BfF1 had a worse prognosis than those with DR3 in association with other HLA antigens (Short *et al.* 1983). However, another report does not confirm this finding in a similar group of patients, and suggests that the haplotype DR3 B8 BfS is associated with a worse outcome (Papiha *et al.* 1987).

Recent experience with immunosuppressive drugs has provided further evidence that membranous nephropathy may be immunologically mediated. The use of high-dose steroids alone was of marginal benefit in one study (Coggins 1979). Although the value of steroids remains controversial, the combination of prednisolone with chlorambucil (Ponticelli *et al.* 1984), or cyclophosphamide (West *et al.* 1987), appears to have a considerable effect on the natural history of the disease. Ponticelli *et al.* (1984) reported that both proteinuria and progression of renal impairment could be modified by treatment with alternating months of prednisolone and chlorambucil for 6 months. Most patients in his trial were treated early — i.e. had grossly normal renal function. Mathieson *et al.* (1988) used a modification of this regimen in an uncontrolled study of patients with membranous nephropathy and impaired renal function, and demonstrated a marked improvement.

MESANGIOCAPILLARY (MEMBRANOPROLIFERATIVE) GLOMERULONEPHRITIS

Mesangiocapillary GN (MCGN) usually presents with a combination of haematuria and proteinuria, or with nephrotic syndrome. Progression to renal failure occurs in around 50% of cases by 10 years. There are two principal subtypes with similar appearances on light microscopy, but different immunohistology and EM: in type I there are subendothelial immune deposits and in type II there are linear 'dense deposits' along the GBM (Habib *et al.* 1975). Type I MCGN has therefore been regarded as 'immune complex' disease, which seems reasonable in view of the location of the deposits (Fig. 99.3), whereas the immunopathology of type II remains uncertain.

The majority of cases are idiopathic (Habib *et al.* 1973; Cameron *et al.* 1983), although the appearances of type I MCGN have been noted in association with various infective (Date *et al.* 1983), including subacute infective endocarditis, 'shunt nephritis' and leprosy, and with malignancy. It also forms part of the spectrum of nephritis due to SLE and mixed essential cryoglobulinaemia (MEC) (see below), and occurs in the presence of genetic complement deficiencies (Pickering *et al.* 1971; Kim *et al.* 1977; Pussell *et al.* 1980; Berger *et al.* 1983; Coleman *et al.* 1983). A finding of particular immunological interest is that of a specific autoantibody, nephritic factor (NeF) (Spitzer *et al.* 1969), in association with type II and rarely type I MCGN (Schena *et al.* 1982; Cameron *et al.* 1983). Nephritic factor is an IgG antibody with specificity for determinants on the alternative pathway C3 convertase, C3bBb (Daha *et al.* 1976; Scott *et al.* 1978), and has the effect of rendering this normally labile enzyme resistant to its inhibitors, factors H and I. As a result, there is generally profound lowering of C3, with sparing of the early components of the classical pathway. Nephritic factor is of slightly higher molecular weight than most IgG molecules due to glycosylation, which appears to be important for its activity (Daha *et al.* 1978; Scott *et al.* 1981). The use of sensitive assay systems has allowed the demonstration of NeF even in some normocomplementaemic patients with MCGN type II (Liebowitch *et al.* 1980). It is also found in patients with partial lipodystrophy, who are particularly prone to develop MCGN type II (Sissons *et al.* 1976).

More recently, atypical C3 NeF have been described, which cause weak fluid-phase C3 conversion and yet stabilize cell-bound C3bBb (Ng and Peters 1986). They are associated with decreased levels of C5, and increased activation of the terminal complement pathway *in vivo* (Mollnes *et al.* 1986). The molecular basis for this difference in activity is unknown. Less common than C3 NeF are antibodies which stabilize the classical pathway C3 convertase, C4b2b. These have been described in post-streptococcal GN (Halbwachs *et al.* 1980) and in SLE (Daha *et al.* 1980).

There may be a genetic predisposition to the development of NeF, since there was a predominance of HLA-DR7 in one small series (Rees 1984), and development of MCGN has been related to partial complement deficiency due to hypomorphism of C3f (McLean and Hoefnagel 1980). The relationship between NeF and the development of nephritis is not understood, although there are two categories of explanation: (i) the complement deficiency induced by NeF leads to nephritis by mechanisms similar to those found in genetic complement deficiency; (ii) the persistent activation of complement, under certain circumstances, is nephrotoxic. There is little direct evidence in support of these suggestions; nephritis in complement deficiency generally has features of immune complex disease, and prolonged complement activation in experimental animals has failed to produce nephritis (Verroust *et al.* 1974; Simpson *et al.* 1978). The nature of the dense deposits is not known; they are associated with C3 but not usually with Ig deposition.

Treatment of mesangiocapillary nephritis has generally been unsuccessful. Although there are uncontrolled series in which early steroid therapy was associated with an improved outcome as compared with historical controls (West 1986), controlled trials of steroids and of cyclophosphamide with anticoagulants and anti-platelet drugs (Cattran *et al.* 1985) have failed to demonstrate significant benefit.

IMMUNOGLOBULIN A-ASSOCIATED GLOMERULONEPHRITIS

Mesangial proliferative GN with IgA deposition, also known as Berger's disease (Berger and Hinglais 1968), is now one of the commonest forms of nephritis (D'Amico 1987) — perhaps because of the increased tendency to obtain biopsies from patients with mild disease. Presentation is often with recurrent episodes of macroscopic haematuria, sometimes accompanied by proteinuria, but renal failure develops slowly in around 10–20% of cases over 10–20 years. Very similar histological and immunological findings occur in Henoch–Schönlein purpura (HSP), which has prompted suggestions that IgA nephritis represents a limited form of HSP (Emancipator *et al.* 1985).

The distinctive feature of these conditions is the mesangial deposition of IgA (Fig. 99.3), usually accompanied by IgG and the alternative pathway complement components C3 and properdin (Evans *et al.* 1973; Nakamoto *et al.* 1978). Similar deposits have been reported in skin (Tsai *et al.* 1975). The nature of the IgA in deposits has been extensively studied (Conley *et al.* 1980; Tomino *et al.* 1982b; Lomax-Smith *et al.* 1983; Valentijn *et al.* 1984; reviewed in Feehally 1988; Lai *et al.* 1988); the consensus view is that it is mainly IgA-1, with a predominance of lambda light chains, and is usually polymeric with J chain, but that secretory component is not found. There is usually a high circulating concentration of IgA, and an altered kappa/lambda ratio of light chains in IgA and IgG; IgA-containing immune complexes are reported in one-third to two-thirds of cases (Woodroffe *et al.* 1980; Egido *et al.* 1984).

Considerable efforts have been made to implicate IgA antibodies to dietary and other environmental antigens in the formation of these immune complexes, since IgA forms the majority of antibody in epithelial secretions. Despite some evidence in favour of this notion (Sancho *et al.* 1983; Gallo *et al.* 1985; Fornasieri *et al.* 1988; Nagy *et al.* 1988), there are also many negative reports. An alternative explanation is that there is polyclonal activation of IgA- and IgG-secreting B cells (Hale *et al.* 1986; Schena *et al.* 1986; Van den Wall Bake *et al.* 1989), and that the antibodies produced react directly with mesangial antigens. There are now a number of reports of abnormal regulation of Ig synthesis in IgA nephropathy, but no single coherent mechanism has been defined (Cosio *et al.* 1982; Feehally *et al.* 1986a; Wyatt *et al.* 1988). The proposed autoimmune mechanism has received support from the observations that IgA eluted from renal biopsies recombines with autologous kidney (Tomino *et al.* 1982a), and that IgA from patients' sera binds to various glomerular constituents including collagen, fibronectin and laminin (although this binding was not shown to be $F(ab)_2$-dependent) (Cederholm *et al.* 1986, 1988). More recently IgG autoantibodies reactive with mesangial cells have been reported in IgA nephropathy and HSP (Ballardie *et al.* 1988). The presence of IgA rheumatoid factors has been detected by several groups (Sinico *et al.* 1986; Saulsbury 1987) and it has been suggested that these could react with IgG deposits in the mesangium; this possibility requires further investigation.

The role of genetic factors in susceptibility to IgA nephropathy has proved hard to define. Familial cases have been reported, although family studies did not reveal MHC linkage (Sabatier *et al.* 1979; Katz *et al.* 1980; Julian *et al.* 1985). An association with HLA-DR4 has been reported in both European and Japanese studies (Vignon *et al.* 1980; Hiki *et al.* 1982; Kasahara *et al.* 1982; Egido *et al.* 1987), although other European and American series failed to confirm this. Recently, RFLP analysis has revealed an association with HLA-DQw7 in the UK (Li *et al.* 1991). An association with Ig heavy chain allotypes has been reported (Demaine *et al.* 1988). The possible role of environmental factors, such as food antigens, has been considered above. It is clear that infection, usually of the upper respiratory tract, may provoke episodes of macroscopic haematuria (D'Amico *et al.* 1985), although this could be a non-specific enhancement of immune inflammation. Deposition of IgA in the mesangium also accompanies cirrhosis of the liver (Nochy *et al.* 1976; Sancho *et al.* 1982; Sinniah 1984) and various enteropathies (Katz *et al.* 1979). In these circumstances, however, the nature of the immune deposits is different from that in primary IgA nephritis, and the development of clinically significant renal injury is rare.

The treatment of IgA nephropathies remains generally unsatisfactory and, since many cases pursue a benign course, specific therapy is often unnecessary. The use of steroids alone was reported to induce remission of nephrotic syndrome, but not to alter progression of renal failure (Lai *et al.* 1986). Another uncontrolled study involved the use of steroids for up to 2 years, followed by anti-platelet agents; treatment was reported to reduce proteinuria and the rate of decline of renal function (Kobayashi *et al.* 1986). One controlled trial, involving the use of cyclophosphamide together with anti-platelet agents and warfarin, showed less proteinuria and less decline in renal function in the treated group (Woo *et al.* 1987). In the rare cases where crescentic nephritis develops on a background of IgA disease, there are uncontrolled reports of benefit from immunosuppressive drugs and plasma exchange (Coppo *et al.* 1985).

POST-INFECTIVE NEPHRITIS

Post-streptococcal nephritis was the first form of glomerular disease in which immunological mechanisms were implicated, because of the serum sickness-like latent period followed by hypocomplementaemia and nephritis. The characteristic presentation is with acute nephritis 2–3 weeks after group A streptococcal infection of the respiratory tract or skin. Certain M serotypes are particularly associated with development of the disease (Rodriguez-Iturbe *et al.* 1979). The natural history is of resolution; second attacks and progression to renal failure are rare.

Light microscopy shows diffuse hypercellularity, immunofluorescence reveals discrete deposits of Ig and complement along the capillary walls and EM demonstrates the presence of large subepithelial immune aggregates, sometimes termed 'humps' (Feldmann *et al.* 1966; Hinglais *et al.* 1974). Assays for circulating immune complexes are generally positive, there is often a polyclonal rise in IgG and IgM, and complement levels are reduced (Van de Rijn *et al.* 1978; Rodriguez-Iturbe 1984). The majority of patients show a reduction in C3 levels, whereas reduction in early classical pathway components is less frequent. A raised antibody titre to streptococcal antigens is found in a large proportion of patients.

The disease was considered to be due to deposition of circulating immune complexes. However, early studies of epidemic streptococcal infection weakened this argument, in that haematuria was demonstrated at the onset of infection in those who would later develop the full syndrome — suggesting some affinity of streptococcal antigens for the kidney (Stetson *et al.* 1955). An early notion is now gaining support — namely, that nephritogenic streptococcal antigens act as 'planted' antigens for subsequent local immune complex formation. The precise nature of the antigens concerned is not yet clear, although there are a number of candidates (Villareal *et al.* 1979; Lange *et al.* 1983; Vogt *et al.* 1983). Evidence implicating these antigens includes their isolation from nephritogenic streptococci, their detection in renal biopsies, and the presence of antibodies to them in patients. Recent work supports the role of 'endostreptosin' — a 45 kD molecule extracted from the cytoplasm of group A streptococci — as a major immunogen (Cronin *et al.* 1989). The development of post-streptococcal GN depends upon genetic susceptibility, as well as the characteristics of the organism. This was suggested by family studies (Rodriguez-Iturbe *et al.* 1981), and MHC associations have also been reported, notably with HLA-DR4 in South America (Layrisse *et al.* 1983).

Many other persistent infections — bacterial, viral and protozoal — have been associated with proliferative GN. These have been reviewed elsewhere (Guttman *et al.* 1988) and will not be considered in detail. The best characterized examples are organisms responsible for infective endocarditis (*Staphylococcus albus, Streptococcus faecalis* and *S. viridans, Coxiella burnetti*) (Dathan and Heyworth 1975; McKenzie *et al.* 1980; Schena *et al.* 1983; Neugarten and Baldwin 1984), ventriculoatrial shunt infection (*Staphylococcus albus*) and visceral abscesses (*Staphylococcus aureus, Pseudomonas aeruginosa*) (Beaufils *et al.* 1976).

SYSTEMIC LUPUS ERYTHEMATOSUS

The immunology of SLE is described in detail in Chapter 61. We shall briefly consider renal involvement in this condition, since nephritis is an important clinical feature. The spectrum of lupus nephritis includes most of the histologically defined patterns of primary GN (Grishman *et al.* 1982). Although attempts have been made to classify renal involvement in SLE on a morphological basis, and many patients do indeed show a consistent pattern of histology, in others the pattern may vary between individual glomeruli in a single biopsy and can change considerably between sequential biopsies.

Immunofluorescence generally reveals abundant deposits of IgG, IgM, IgA and complement components C3, C4 and C1q in a subendothelial and/or mesangial distribution in proliferative nephritis (Grishman *et al*. 1982; Roberts *et al*. 1983), and in a subepithelial location in membranous nephritis. The presence of the membrane attack complex of complement has also been reported (Biesecker *et al*. 1981; Falk *et al*. 1983). Although eluted immune deposits have been shown to contain DNA and anti-DNA antibodies, this antigen–antibody system can only account for a small proportion of the immune complexes present (Koffler 1974).

Serological abnormalities are abundant, and include hyperglobulinaemia, a variety of autoantibodies (such as the diagnostic anti-dsDNA and anti-Sm antibodies), hypocomplementaemia involving C1q, C4 and C3, and circulating immune complexes (Koffler *et al*. 1971; Cameron *et al*. 1976; Adu *et al*. 1981; Coppo *et al*. 1982; Morimoto *et al*. 1982). However, the pathogenetic role of autoantibodies and immune complexes and their value in monitoring disease activity remain uncertain. In general, there is a poor correlation of anti-dsDNA antibodies, hypocomplementaemia or titre of immune complexes with severity of nephritis. However, in certain patients the sequential changes in these factors are useful in predicting the course of the disease.

There has been considerable interest in the relationship between development of nephritis and characteristics of anti-dsDNA antibodies. High concentrations and high avidity of precipitating antibodies were linked to proliferative nephritis, and lower levels of non-precipitating antibody to membranous nephritis (Friend *et al*. 1977; Tron and Bach 1977; Asano and Nakamoto 1978). There is, however, no direct evidence for the pathogenicity of anti-DNA antibodies or the immune complexes they form. There are indications that normal immune complex clearance mechanisms are compromised in SLE (Schifferli and Taylor 1989). Abnormalities are present at three major stages of clearance: (i) hypocomplementaemia leads to impaired solubilization and opsonization of complexes (Miller and Nussenzweig 1975; Schifferli *et al*. 1980; Takata *et al*. 1984); (ii) there is depletion of erythrocyte receptors (CR1) for complement-reacted complexes (Miyakawa *et al*. 1981; Kazatchkine *et al*. 1982; Wilson *et al*. 1982; Walport *et al*. 1985a); (iii) there is impairment of the capacity of the mononuclear phagocytic system to clear antibody-coated red cells (Frank *et al*. 1979; Lockwood *et al*. 1979; Walport *et al*. 1985b). It now seems likely that most of these phenomena are acquired rather that of primary pathogenetic importance, although they could none the less contribute towards disease.

Alternative explanations for the development of nephritis in SLE include the 'planting' of various autoantigens in the glomerulus, and direct reactivity of autoantibodies with antigens on glomerular components. It was observed that DNA has an affinity for GBM and for collagen V, and might therefore act as a focus for local immune deposits (Izui *et al*. 1976; Gay *et al*. 1985). On the other hand, monoclonal antibodies to DNA were found to bind directly to normal glomeruli (Madaio *et al*. 1985). Antibodies to endothelial cells have been identified in patients with SLE (Cines *et al*. 1984), although their reactivity with glomerular capillaries has not yet been demonstrated. Another potential target for autoimmunity is the lupus-associated membrane protein (LAMP), found in coated pits of the glomerular epithelial cells (Jacob *et al*. 1987).

Genetic, hormonal and environmental factors are important in the development of lupus (see Chapter 61). There is an increased incidence of disease in relatives of patients (Walport *et al*. 1982), and over 50% of monozygotic (but not dizygotic) twins are concordant for SLE (Block *et al*. 1975; Arnett and Schulman 1976). There are associations with HLA-DR3 (Celada *et al*. 1980; Black *et al*. 1982), and with null alleles of C2 and C4 (Fielder *et al*. 1983). However, the factors which determine whether or not nephritis develops, and which influence its severity, remain to be clarified.

The treatment of lupus nephritis with immunosuppressive drugs has considerably improved the prognosis of this condition. Treatment with steroids was a substantial advance, and the introduction of azathioprine or cyclophosphamide has improved prognosis further (Felson and Anderson 1984). Recent controlled studies of the treatment of diffuse proliferative nephritis from the National Institutes of Health (NIH) have shown a better long-term outcome with cyclophosphamide (particularly given as intravenous boluses) and prednisolone than with prednisolone alone (Austin *et al*. 1986). The addition of azathioprine to prednisolone also appeared to confer benefit, although this was not regarded as significant. In renal lupus it therefore seems reasonable to use steroids alone for mild histological lesions, but to add a second drug for more severe disease. In life-threatening cases, high doses of intravenous prednisolone (Kimberly *et al.* 1981) or plasma exchange (Haworth *et al.* 1985; Leaker *et al.* 1986) has been used successfully, but there are insufficient controlled data to draw firm conclusions about indications or benefit.

CRYOIMMUNOGLOBULINAEMIA

Cryoglobulinaemia is frequently accompanied by nephritis, most often MCGN (Gorevic *et al.* 1980; Tarantino *et al.* 1981; Cordonnier *et al.* 1983). Type I cryoglobulin is due to a paraprotein which has the property of precipitating in the cold; this type is rarely associated with clinically important nephritis and will not be considered further. Mixed cryoglobulins consist of rheumatoid factors (usually IgM) complexed with other Ig and complement. In type II cryoglobulinaemia, the rheumatoid factor is monoclonal, whereas in type III, rheumatoid factors are polyclonal (Brouet *et al.* 1974). The physicochemical basis for cryoprecipitation remains unknown (Winfield 1983), but this phenomenon is presumably a gross reflection of the molecular interactions which lead to *in vivo* immune complex formation.

Mixed essential cryoglobulinaemia is perhaps the best example of human 'immune complex' disease, in which nephritis occurs as part of a systemic vasculitis. There is usually profound lowering of early components of the classical pathway of complement, C1, C4 and C2, but with no (or smaller) changes in C3 levels (Linscott and Kane 1975; Tarantino *et al.* 1978; D'Amico *et al.* 1984). Immunofluorescence of renal tissue reveals granular deposits of the constituents of the cryoglobulin along the capillary wall, and EM in those cases with a monoclonal component reveals subendothelial deposits of material with ultrastructural characteristics of cryoglobulin (Cordonnier *et al.* 1975; Feiner and Gallo 1977).

The monoclonal rheumatoid factors in type II cryoglobulinaemia bear common cross-reactive idiotypes, which are highly conserved and likely to represent Ig gene products in germline configuration (Kunkel *et al.* 1973; Abraham *et al.* 1983; Ono *et al.* 1987). It has been suggested that they result from paraneoplastic changes in B cells which form part of a 'primitive' immune defence system. The products of these cells, by binding to IgG Fc pieces, could enhance opsonization of foreign antigens recognized by the antibody concerned. Type III cryoglobulins are often associated with chronic infection, autoimmune disease and malignancy (Brouet *et al.* 1974; Gorevic *et al.* 1980; Tarantino *et al.* 1981), and the polyclonal rheumatoid factors produced in this disorder could therefore result from antigenic stimulation or abnormalities of immune regulation.

Management of these disorders has proved unsatisfactory, but plasma exchange effectively reduces cryoglobulin levels in association with clinical improvement (Ferri *et al.* 1986). In patients with a rapid rate of resynthesis of the cryoglobulin, cytotoxic drugs have been of value in conjunction with plasmaphaeresis. In view of the generally indolent nature of the nephritis, management by intermittent plasma exchange alone seems the best initial choice for most patients.

Nephritis without immune deposits

MINIMAL CHANGE NEPHROPATHY AND FOCAL GLOMERULOSCLEROSIS

Minimal change nephropathy (MCN) and focal glomerulosclerosis (FGS) generally present with nephrotic syndrome and are much commoner in the young. There are widespread ultrastructural abnormalities of glomerular epithelial cells, notably podocyte fusion, in both disorders. However, light microscopy reveals no change or mild mesangial cell proliferation only in MCN, but focal and segmental areas of sclerosis in FGS (Habib *et al.* 1979). Some authors have adopted an operational approach to these conditions depending upon their responsiveness to steroids, and it has become apparent that there is considerable overlap between the traditionally steroid-sensitive MCN and steroid-resistant FGS (Cameron *et al.* 1978; Arbus *et al.* 1982; Tejani *et al.* 1983). There are also reported cases of evolution from MCN to FGS, but it is impossible to exclude the presence of mild focal lesions at the time of the earlier biopsy.

Although the pathogenesis of these disorders remains uncertain, there is strong circumstantial evidence for an immune aetiology. A number of disease associations have been reported, more frequently in MCN than in FGS. These include atopy, a variety of allergies (including drugs and insect stings) (Wittig and Goldman 1970; Richards *et al.* 1977; Sandberg *et al.* 1977) and, more convincingly, lymphoma, notably Hodgkin's disease (Yum *et al.* 1975; Moorthy *et al.* 1976a; Couser *et al.* 1977). There are reports in which successful treatment of lymphoma, or control of allergy, has led to a favourable response of the renal lesion. Perhaps the best evidence for immunopathogenesis, however, comes from the response to immunosuppressive drugs (see below). Familial cases are well recognized (White 1973), and there is an association with HLA-DR7 in Europe (Alfifer *et al.* 1980; Mouzon-Cambon *et al.* 1981; Nunex-Roldan *et al.* 1982) and HLA-DR8 in Japan (Komori *et al.* 1979).

The lack of immune reactants on renal biopsy prompted the hypothesis, elaborated by Shalhoub (1974), that T cells were important in pathogenesis. The identification of lymphocyte-derived permeability factors has been reported by several investigators in different experimental systems, although the evidence for their role in disease remains incomplete and no 'factor' has yet been fully characterized (Ooi *et al.* 1974; Lagrue *et al.* 1975; Tomizawa *et al.* 1985). However, it seems likely that lymphocytes or monocytes from patients with MCN are responsible for the production of factors which affect the charge of the glomerular capillary wall. Neutralization of glomerular polyanions reduces the 'charge barrier' effect for molecules such as albumin — and may account for the highly selective proteinuria. One group has suggested a generalized abnormality of membrane charge in MCN, following the observation of a reduction in negatively charged sites on erythrocytes and platelets (Levin *et al.* 1985). However, these findings have not been confirmed by others, and there is controversy over the methodology (Feehally *et al.* 1986b).

There are also various reports of abnormalities in lymphocyte function in MCN, including impaired mitogen response *in vitro*, decreased T_s cell activity, and variably raised IgM and lowered IgG concentrations (Giangiacomo *et al.* 1975; Schulte-Wisserman *et al.* 1977; Tomizawa *et al.* 1979). In addition, a variety of effects of sera from patients has been recorded, including inhibition of mitogenic responses and of T_s cell function (Moorthy *et al.* 1976b; Iitaka and West 1979; Martini *et al.* 1981; Taube *et al.* 1981). However, in many instances, similar findings are obtained when studying patients with other causes of nephrotic syndrome, and no clear overall picture has emerged. Of interest is the description of soluble immune response suppressors (SIRS) produced by lymphocytes, the presence of which correlates well with disease activity in MCN (Schnaper and Aune 1985).

The dramatic response of MCN to corticosteroids is well known, but relapse after reduction or withdrawal of therapy is common (Imbasciati *et al.* 1985; Srivasta *et al.* 1986). Cyclophosphamide and chlorambucil are both effective in treating frequently relapsing patients, although their toxicity is a particular anxiety in the young (Barratt *et al.* 1975; Cameron *et al.* 1984; Tejani *et al.* 1985). Of therapeutic and immunological interest are recent reports of the effectiveness of cyclosporin A in MCN (Hoyer *et al.* 1986; Meyrier *et al.* 1986; Tejani *et al.* 1987). Since the main action of cyclosporin is to inhibit the production of IL-1 and IL-2 by activated T cells (by binding to peptidyl–prolyl isomerase), its therapeutic effect provides further indirect support for the role of T lymphocytes in the pathogenesis of MCN.

SYSTEMIC VASCULITIS AND FOCAL NECROTIZING GLOMERULONEPHRITIS

Focal necrotizing GN (FNGN) with crescent formation presents as a rapidly progressive nephritis, and is usually associated with a small-vessel vasculitis such as Wegener's granulomatosis or microscopic polyarteritis (Fauci *et al.* 1983; Pinching *et al.* 1983; Ronco *et al.* 1983; Serra *et al.* 1984; Savage *et al.* 1985) (see Chapter 62). A histologically identical form of GN may occur in isolation, often referred to as idiopathic RPGN (Couser 1982; Balow 1985). There is increasing evidence that isolated FNGN represents a localized form of microscopic polyarteritis, and we shall consider the immunology of this group of disorders together (Pusey and Lockwood 1989).

It may be surprising, in view of the severity of tissue injury, that there is so little evidence for the involvement of humoral immune factors. Sparse, granular deposits of Ig and complement may be found on biopsy in a variable proportion of patients in different series, although these are generally localized to necrotic or sclerosed glomeruli (Ronco *et al*. 1983; Serra *et al*. 1984). American authors have used the terms 'pauci-immune' and 'no immune deposit' GN (Couser 1982), although there is no evidence that the lesion is any different whether or not a few deposits are detected. Because of the presence of vasculitis in classic studies of serum sickness (Rich and Gregory 1943), it was long presumed that immune complex mechanisms were important in primary systemic vasculitis. The lack of detectable immune deposits could be explained by their rapid clearance or digestion at the site of inflammation, or by the insensitivity of methods of detection. However, features such as circulating complexes, raised Ig concentrations and rheumatoid factor are found inconsistently in around one-third to two-thirds of patients (Ronco *et al*. 1983; Serra *et al*. 1984). Despite considerable efforts, evidence for the involvement of immune complexes is generally lacking.

More recently, interest has focused on the presence of antibodies to neutrophil cytoplasmic antigens (ANCA), first described by Davies *et al*. (1982). These are found in the great majority of patients with active Wegener's granulomatosis or microscopic polyarteritis (Van der Woude *et al*. 1985; Savage *et al*. 1987), and have also been identified in idiopathic RPGN (Falk and Jennette 1988). Two different types of ANCA have been described on indirect immunofluorescence of ethanol-fixed normal neutrophils, using patients' sera: (i) diffuse granular cytoplasmic-staining, known as C-ANCA; (ii) predominantly perinuclear-staining, known as P-ANCA. Although there is considerable overlap in most studies, C-ANCA are generally associated with Wegener's granulomatosis, and P-ANCA with microscopic polyarteritis and idiopathic RPGN (Jennette *et al*. 1989; Nolle *et al*. 1989). The antigenic targets of these autoantibodies have not been conclusively identified. However, there is increasing evidence that C-ANCA recognize a neutrophil serine proteinase known as proteinase-3 (Goldschmeding *et al*. 1989; Ludemann *et al*. 1990), and that P-ANCA recognize myeloperoxidase (Falk and Jennette 1988). Whether ANCA have a pathogenic role in systemic vasculitis is unclear, although they are of value in monitoring disease activity (Specks *et al*. 1989; Gaskin *et al*. 1991) and there is a recent report that they can induce neutrophil degranulation and oxygen radical production *in vitro* (Falk *et al*. 1990). Antibodies binding to endothelial cells in enzyme-linked immunosorbent assay (ELISA) systems, apparently not cross-reactive with ANCA (Ferraro *et al*. 1990; Savage *et al*. 1991), and antibodies binding to glomerular endothelial and epithelial cells in culture (Abbott *et al*. 1989), have also been reported.

It has been suggested that T cells are directly involved in glomerular injury in FNGN. Immunohistology using monoclonal antibodies to T cell subsets has revealed the presence of both CD4- and CD8-bearing T lymphocytes in the glomeruli and interstitium (Stachura *et al*. 1984; Bolton *et al*. 1987; Nolasco *et al*. 1987). The CD4 +ve cells could be involved in delayed-type hypersensitivity reactions, leading to the influx of macrophages, which are the predominant inflammatory cells in crescentic nephritis (Magil and Wadsworth 1982; Boucher *et al*. 1987).

Genetic factors are likely to be important in susceptibility. Several pairs of siblings with Wegener's granulomatosis have been described, and in at least one report they had lived apart for many years, making a common environmental cause less likely (Knudsen *et al*. 1988). An association with HLA-DR2 has been reported in both Wegener's granulomatosis (Elkon *et al*. 1983) and idiopathic RPGN (Muller *et al*. 1984). Recently, RFLP analysis has revealed an association with HLA-DQw7 in Wegener's granulomatosis and microscopic polyarteritis (Spencer *et al*. 1992). Environmental factors may also be involved, in particular persistent infection. Polyarteritis has been associated with hepatitis B (Michalak 1978); there is a history of long-standing upper respiratory or pulmonary disease in many patients with Wegener's granulomatosis (Pinching *et al*. 1983); and crescentic nephritis may also be associated with drugs, neoplasia and deep-seated visceral abscesses.

A distinctive feature of this group of disorders is the excellent response to immunosuppressive drugs. Steroids alone may control inflammatory lesions, but did not greatly improve prognosis in Wegener's granulomatosis; however, the introduction of cyclophosphamide led to improvement in the majority of cases (Fauci *et al*. 1983; Balow 1985). Renal disease improves in almost all patients treated with prednisolone and cyclophosphamide orally, unless they are already on dialysis. In this group with advanced disease, the addition of plasma exchange has been shown to lead to improved renal outcome (Hind *et al.* 1983; Pusey and Lockwood 1984). Uncontrolled studies suggest that high-dose intravenous methyl prednisolone may also confer benefit in this situation (Bolton and Sturgill 1989). Reports of the benefit of co-trimoxazole in indolent or limited disease (De Remee *et al.* 1985) require confirmation, since it is possible that such treatment acts by control of infection (known to exacerbate disease) rather than on the underlying disease process. There are isolated reports of the successful use of cyclosporin A (Gremmel *et al.* 1988).

Acute interstitial nephritis

The clinicopathological syndrome of acute interstitial nephritis leads to a generally self-limiting form of acute renal failure, accompanied histologically by interstitial infiltration with lymphocytes, plasma cells, macrophages and sometimes eosinophils. The great majority of cases are now associated with allergic reactions to drugs, most commonly antibiotics (penicillins, sulphonamides and rifampicin), non-steroidal anti-inflammatory agents, diuretics and anticonvulsants (Kleinknecht *et al.* 1978; Pusey *et al.* 1983a; Bender *et al.* 1984; Cameron 1988b). Evidence that these reactions involve allergic mechanisms includes: (i) frequent presence of rash and eosinophilia; (ii) occurrence in only a small minority of patients exposed to normal (non-toxic) doses of the drug; (iii) recurrence on re-exposure to the drug in a few reported cases; and (iv) response to corticosteroid therapy. However, the mechanisms involved have not been identified, and there is no comparable experimental model of TIN (see above).

There are a few reports suggesting the involvement of humoral mechanisms, for example circulating and fixed anti-TBM antibodies (Baldwin *et al.* 1968), and immune deposits consisting of penicillin-derived antigens and Ig (Border *et al.* 1974; Hyman *et al.* 1978), but these have not been detected in many more similar cases. The histological findings suggest a predominant role for cell-mediated mechanisms, and several studies have identified CD4 and CD8 +ve lymphocytes in the interstitial infiltrate (Finkelstein *et al.* 1982; Bender *et al.* 1984; Gimenez and Mampaso 1986). In a few cases, evidence of specific drug sensitivity has been suggested by *in vitro* studies of lymphocyte function (Colvin *et al.* 1974; Sheth *et al.* 1977). Although there are no controlled data, the rapid response to steroids is impressive and provides indirect evidence for involvement of immune mechanisms (Galpin *et al.* 1978; Pusey *et al.* 1983c).

Interstitial nephritis may also occur in association with infections, historically most often streptococcal and diphtherial, but a range of different organisms has now been implicated (Cameron 1988b). In some cases there may be a direct pathogenic effect of the micro-organism, but others could be due to the resulting immune reactions. Several systemic and primary glomerular diseases are associated with immune deposits on the TBM and interstitial nephritis. These include SLE, MEC, Sjögren's syndrome, anti-GBM disease and MCGN (Brentjens *et al.* 1975; Lehman *et al.* 1975; Andres *et al.* 1978; McCluskey and Colvin 1978; Makker 1980). Whether the tubular lesions are due to deposition of antibodies or immune complexes similar to those responsible for the glomerular lesions is not known. There are, however, rare but well-documented instances of 'anti-TBM' disease, in which circulating and fixed anti-TBM antibodies are demonstrated, following renal transplantation or occurring in isolation (Klassen *et al.* 1973; Bergstein and Litman 1975; Paul *et al.* 1979). A granulomatous interstitial nephritis may occur in sarcoidosis (Mac Scarraigh *et al.* 1978; Mignon *et al.* 1984), and there is an uncommon oculorenal syndrome of unknown aetiology comprising acute TIN with uveitis (Steinman and Silva 1984; Vanhaesebrouck *et al.* 1985).

Conclusions

Despite a considerable increase in understanding of immune mechanisms in nephritis over the last 10 years, there have been few important advances in immunotherapy. This reflects our incomplete knowledge of the molecular basis of autoimmune reactions affecting the kidney, as well as a lack of new clinically applicable immunotherapeutic agents. However, what has been learnt points the way to the development of techniques of specific immune intervention. The majority of disorders discussed in this chapter are now perceived as autoimmune, and a critical role for T lymphocytes in their induction, if not in tissue injury, seems highly probable. There is increasing evidence from experimental autoimmune disease, including some models of nephritis, that methods of blocking the interaction between Class II MHC gene products, autoantigenic peptides and the T cell receptor can be therapeutically effective (Wraith *et al.* 1989). The development and application of monoclonal antibodies — 'humanized' by recombinant DNA technology — offer considerable promise for the control of autoimmunity in man, and a successful example of this approach has recently been reported in a patient with vaculitis (Mathieson *et al.* 1990). Knowledge of the effector mechanisms involved in glomerular inflammation, particularly the role of various cytokines, is increasing rapidly. Whether antagonists of pro-inflammatory cytokines would be effective in limiting renal injury, without adverse systemic effects, is not yet known. Application of the rapidly expanding techniques of molecular and cell biology to human renal disease should soon allow the introduction of these new approaches into the treatment of nephritis.

References

Abbott, F., Jones, S., Lockwood, C.M. and Rees, A.J. (1989). Autoantibodies to glomerular antigens in patients with Wegener's granulomatosis. *Nephrol. Dial. Transplant.* **4**, 1.

Abraham, G.N., Podell, D.N., Welch, E.H. and Johnston, S.L. (1983). Idiotypic relatedness of human monoclonal IgG cryoglobulins. *Immunology* **48**, 315.

Adelman, N., Watting, D. and McDevitt, H.O. (1983). Treatment of NZB/W F1 disease with monoclonal anti-I-A antibodies. *J. Exp. Med.* **158**, 1350.

Adler, S.G., Salant, D.J., Dittmer, J.E., Rennke, H.G., Madaio, M.P. and Couser, W.G. (1983a). Mediation of proteinuria in membranous nephropathy due to a planted glomerular antigen. *Kidney Int.* **23**, 807.

Adler, S.G., Wang, H., Ward, H.J., Cohen, A.H. and Border, W.A. (1983b). Electrical charge: its role in the pathogenesis and prevention of experimental membranous nephropathy in the rabbit. *J. Clin. Invest.* **71**, 487.

Adu, D., Dobson, J. and Williams, D.G. (1981). DNA–anti-DNA circulating complexes in the nephritis of systemic lupus erythematosus. *Clin. Exp. Immunol.* **43**, 605.

Agus, D., Mann, R., Clayman, M. *et al.* (1986). The effects of daily cyclophosphamide administration on the development and extent of primary experimental interstitial nephritis in rats. *Kidney Int.* **29**, 635.

Alfifer, C.A., Roy, L.P., Doran, T., Sheldon, A. and Bashir, H. (1980). HLA-DR7 and steroid responsive nephrotic syndrome. *Clin. Nephrol.* **14**, 71.

Andres, G., Brentjens, J., Kohli, R. *et al.* (1978). Histology of human tubulo-interstitial nephritis associated with antibodies to renal basement membranes. *Kidney Int.* **13**, 480.

Andrzejewski, C., Rauch, J., Lafer, E.M., Stollar, B.D. and Schwartz, R.S. (1980). Antigen binding diversity and idiotypic cross-reactions among hybridoma autoantibodies to DNA. *J. Immunol.* **126**, 226.

Arbus, G.S., Poucell, S., Bacheyie, G.S. and Baumal, R. (1982). Focal segmental glomerulosclerosis with idiopathic nephrotic syndrome. *J. Pediatr.* **101**, 40.

Arnett, F.C. and Schulman, L.E. (1976). Studies in familial systemic lupus erythematosus. *Medicine* **55**, 313.

Asano, Y. and Nakamoto, Y. (1978). Avidity of anti-native DNA antibody and glomerular immune complex localisation in lupus nephritis. *Clin. Nephrol.* **10**, 134.

Atkins, R.C., Holdsworth, S.R., Glasgow, E.F. and Matthews, F.E. (1976). The macrophage in human rapidly progressive glomerulonephritis. *Lancet* **i**, 830.

Austin, H.A., Klippel, J.H., Balow, J.E. *et al.* (1986). Therapy of lupus nephritis: controlled trial of prednisolone and cytotoxic drugs. *N. Engl. J. Med.* **514**, 614.

Avasthi, P.S., Avasthi, P., Tokuda, S., Anderson, R.E. and Williams, R.C. (1971). Experimental glomerulonephritis in the mouse. I. The model. *Clin. Exp. Immunol.* **9**, 667.

Bagchus, W.M., Hoedemaeker, P.J., Rozing, J. and Bakker, W.W. (1986a). Glomerulonephritis induced by monoclonal anti-Thy 1.1 antibodies: a sequential histological and ultrastructural study in the rat. *Lab. Invest.* **55**, 680.

Bagchus, W.M., Vos, J.T.W.M., Hoedemaeker, P.J. and Bakker, W.W. (1986b). The specificity of nephritogenic antibodies. III. Binding of anti-FxIA antibodies in glomeruli is dependent on dual specificity. *Clin. Exp. Immunol.* **63**, 639.

Baldwin, D.S., Levine, B.B., McCluskey, R.T. and Gallo, G.R. (1968). Renal failure and interstitial nephritis due to penicillin and methicillin. *N. Engl. J. Med.* **279**, 1245.

Baldwin, D.S., Lowenstein, J., Rothfield, N.F., Gallo, G.R. and McCluskey, R.T. (1970). The clinical course of the proliferative and membranous forms of lupus nephritis. *Ann. Intern. Med.* **73**, 929.

Ballardie, F.W., Brenchley, P.E.C. and Williams, S. (1988). Autoimmunity in IgA nephropathy. *Lancet* **ii**, 598.

Balow, J.E. (1985). Renal vasculitis. *Kidney Int.* **27**, 954.

Bannister, K.M., Ulich, T.R. and Wilson, C.B. (1987). Induction, characterization, and cell transfer of autoimmune tubulo-interstitial nephritis. *Kidney Int.* **32**, 642.

Baran, D., Vendeville, B., Vial, M.C. *et al.* (1986). Effect of cyclosporin A on mercury-induced autoimmune glomerulonephritis in the Brown Norway rat. *Clin. Nephrol.* **25**, 175.

Barratt, T.M., Bercowsky, A., Osofsky, S.G. and Soothill, J.F. (1975). Cyclophosphamide treatment in steroid-sensitive nephrotic syndrome of childhood. *Lancet* **i**, 55.

Beaufils, M., Morel-Maroger, L., Sraer, J.D., Kanfer, A., Kourilsky, O. and Richet, G. (1976). Acute renal failure of glomerular origin during visceral abscesses. *N. Engl. J. Med.* **295**, 185.

Beirne, G.J. and Brennan, J.T. (1972). Glomerulonephritis associated with hydrocarbon solvents. *Arch. Environ. Health* **25**, 365.

Bender, W.L., Whetton, A., Beschormer, W.E., Darwish, M.O., Hall-Craggs, M. and Solez, K. (1984). Interstitial nephritis, proteinuria and renal failure caused by non-steroidal anti-inflammatory drugs. *Am. J. Med.* **76**, 1006.

Benoit, F.L., Rulon, C.B., Theil, G.B., Doolan, P.D. and Watten, R.H. (1964). Goodpasture's syndrome: a clinicopathologic entity. *Am. J. Med.* **37**, 424.

Berger, J. and Hinglais, N. (1968). Les dépôts intercapillaires d'IgA–IgG. *J. Urol. Nephrol.* **74**, 694.

Berger, M., Balow, J.E., Wilson, C.B. and Frank, M.M. (1983). Circulating immune complexes and glomerulonephritis in a patient with congenital absence of the third component of complement. *N. Engl. J. Med.* **308**, 1009.

Bergstein, J. and Litman, N. (1975). Interstitial nephritis with anti-tubular basement membrane antibody. *N. Engl. J. Med.* **292**, 875.

Biesecker, G., Katz, S.M. and Koffler, D. (1981). Renal localization of the membrane attack complex in systemic lupus erythematosus nephritis. *J. Exp. Med.* **154**, 1779.

Black, C.M., Welsh, K.I., Fielder, A., Hughes, G.R.V. and Batchelor, J.R. (1982). HLA antigens and Bf allotypes in SLE: evidence for the association being with specific haplotypes. *Tissue Antigens* **19**, 115.

Block, S.R., Winfield, J.B., Lockshin, M.D., D'Angelo, W.A. and Christian, C.L. (1975). Studies of twins with systemic lupus erythematosus: a review of the literature and presentation of 12 additional sets. *Am. J. Med.* **59**, 533.

Bolton, W.K. and Sturgill, B.C. (1989). Methyl prednisolone therapy for acute crescentic rapidly progressive glomerulonephritis. *Am. J. Nephrol.* **9**, 368.

Bolton, W.K., Tucker, F.L. and Sturgill, B.C. (1984). New avian model of experimental glomerulonephritis consistent with mediation by cellular immunity. *J. Clin. Invest.* **73**, 1263.

Bolton, W.K., Innes, D., Sturgill, B.C. and Kaiser, D.L. (1987). T cells and macrophages in rapidly progressive glomerulonephritis: clinicopathological correlations. *Kidney Int.* **32**, 869.

Bolton, W.K., Chandra, M., Tyson, T.M., Kirkpatrick, P.R., Sadovnic, M.J. and Sturgill, B.C. (1988). Transfer of experimental glomerulonephritis in chickens by mononuclear cells. *Kidney Int.* **34**, 598.

Bonsib, S.M. (1988). Glomerular basement membrane necrosis and crescent organisation. *Kidney Int.* **33**, 966.

Border, W.A., Lehman, D.H., Egon, J.D., Sass, H.J., Glock, J.E. and Wilson, C.B. (1974). Anti-tubular basement membrane antibodies in methicillin-associated interstitial nephritis. *N. Engl. J. Med.* **291**, 381.

Border, W.A., Ward, H.J., Kamil, E.S. and Cohen, A.H. (1982). Induction of membranous nephropathy in rabbits by administration of an exogenous cationic antigen. *J. Clin. Invest.* **69**, 451.

Boucher, A., Droz, D., Adafer, E. and Noel, L.-H. (1987). Relationship between the integrity of Bowman's capsule and the composition of cellular crescents in human crescentic glomerulonephritis. *Lab. Invest.* **56**, 526.

Bowman, C. and Lockwood, C.M. (1985). Clinical application of a radio-immunoassay for auto-antibodies to glomerular basement membrane. *J. Clin. Lab. Immunol.* **17**, 197.

Bowman, C., Mason, D.W., Pusey, C.D. and Lockwood, C.M. (1984). Autoregulation of autoantibody synthesis in mercuric chloride nephritis in the Brown Norway rat. I. A role for T suppressor cells. *Eur. J. Immunol.* **14**, 464.

Bowman, C., Ambrus, K. and Lockwood, C.M. (1987). Restriction of human IgG subclass expression in the population of autoantibodies to glomerular basement membrane. *Clin. Exp. Immunol.* **69**, 341.

Boyce, N.W. and Holdsworth, S.R. (1986). Hydroxyl radical mediation of immune renal injury by desferrioxamine. *Kidney Int.* **30**, 813.

Boyce, N.W. and Holdsworth, S.R. (1989). Macrophage Fc-receptor affinity: role in cellular mediation of antibody initiated glomerulonephritis. *Kidney Int.* **36**, 537.

Brentjens, J.R. and Andres, G. (1989). Interaction of antibodies with renal cell surface antigens. *Kidney Int.* **35**, 954.

Brentjens, J.R., Sepulveda, M., Baliah, T.J. *et al.* (1975). Interstitial immune complex nephritis in patients with systemic lupus erythematosus. *Kidney Int.* **7**, 342.

Brouet, J.-C., Clauvel, J.-P., Danon, F., Klein, M. and Seligmann, M. (1974). Biologic and clinical significance of cryoglobulins: a report of 86 cases. *Am. J. Med.* **57**, 775.

Brown, A.C., Carey, K. and Colvin, R.B. (1979). Inhibition of autoimmune tubulointerstitial nephritis in guinea pigs by heterologous antisera containing anti-idiotype antibodies. *J. Immunol.* **123**, 2102.

Burns, A., So, A., Pusey, C.D. and Rees, A.J. (1990). The susceptibility to Goodpasture's syndrome. *Quart. J. Med.* **77**, 1094.

Butkowski, R.J., Weislander, J., Wisdom, B.J., Barr, J.F., Noelken, M.E. and Hudson, B.G. (1985). Properties of the globular domain of Type IV collagen and its relationship to the Goodpasture antigen. *J. Biol. Chem.* **260**, 3739.

Butkowski, R.J., Langweld, J.P.M., Wieslander, J., Hamilton, J. and Hudson, P.G. (1987). Localisation of the Goodpasture epitope to a novel chain of basement membrane collagen. *J. Biol. Chem.* **262**, 7874.

Cameron, J.S. (1979). Pathogenesis and treatment of membranous nephropathy. *Kidney Int.* **15**, 88.

Cameron, J.S. (1988a). The long-term outcome of glomerular diseases. In *Diseases of the Kidney*, 4th edn, ed. R.W. Schrier and C.W. Gottschalk, p. 2127, Little, Brown and Co., Boston.

Cameron, J.S. (1988b). Allergic interstitial nephritis: clinical features and pathogenesis. *Quart. J. Med.* **66**, 97.

Cameron, J.S., Lessoff, M.H., Ogg, C.S. and Williams, D.G. (1976). Disease activity in the nephritis of systemic lupus erythematosus in relation to serum complement concentrations. *Clin. Exp. Immunol.* **25**, 418.

Cameron, J.S., Turner, D.R., Ogg, C.S., Chantler, C. and Williams, D.G. (1978). The long term prognosis of patients with local segmental glomerulonephritis. *Clin. Nephrol.* **10**, 213.

Cameron, J.S., Turner, D.R., Heaton, J. *et al.* (1983). Idiopathic mesangiocapillary glomerulonephritis. *Am. J. Med.* **74**, 175.

Cameron, J.S., Turner, D.R., Ogg, C.S., Sharpstone, P. and Brown C.B. (1984). The nephrotic syndrome in adults with 'minimal change' glomerular lesions. *Quart. J. Med.* **43**, 461.

Camussi, G., Brentjens, J.R., Noble, B. *et al.* (1985). Antibody-induced redistribution of Heymann antigen on the surface of cultured glomerular visceral epithelial cells: possible role in the pathogenesis of Heymann glomerulonephritis. *J. Immunol.* **135**, 2409.

Carteron, N.L., Schimenti, C.L. and Wofsy, D. (1989). Treatment of murine lupus with $F(ab)_2$ fragments of monoclonal antibody to L3T4. *J. Immunol.* **142**, 1470.

Cashman, S.J., Pusey, C.D. and Evans, D.J. (1988). Extraglomerular distribution of immunoreactive Goodpasture antigen. *J. Pathol.* **135**, 61.

Cattel, V., Smith, J. and Cook, H.T. (1990). Prostaglandin E1 suppresses macrophage infiltration and ameliorates injury in an experimental model of macrophage-dependent glomerulonephritis. *Clin. Exp. Immunol.* **79**, 260.

Cattran, D.C., Cardella, C.J., Roscoe, J.M. *et al.* (1985). Results of a controlled drug trial in membranoproliferative glomerulonephritis. *Kidney Int.* **27**, 436.

Cederholm, B., Wieslander, J. and Bygren, P. (1986). Patients with IgA nephropathy have circulating anti-basement membrane antibodies reacting with structures common to collagen I, II and IV. *Proc. Nat. Acad. Sci. (USA)* **83**, 6151.

Cederholm, B., Wieslander, J. and Bygren, P. (1988). Circulating complexes containing IgA and fibronectin in patients with primary IgA nephropathy. *Proc. Nat. Acad. Sci. (USA)* **85**, 4865.

Celada, A., Barras, C., Benzonana, G. and Jeannet, M. (1980). Increased frequency of HLA-DRw3 in systemic lupus erythematosus. *Tissue Antigens* **15**, 283.

Chalopin, J.M. and Lockwood, C.M. (1984). Auto-regulation of auto-antibody synthesis in mercuric chloride nephritis in the Brown Norway rat. II. Presence of antigen augmentable plaque forming cells in the spleen is associated with humoral factors behaving as auto-anti-idiotypic antibodies. *Eur. J. Immunol.* **14**, 470.

Cheng, I.K.P., Dorsch, S.E. and Hall, B.M. (1988). The regulation of autoantibody production in Heymann's nephritis by T lymphocyte subsets. *Lab. Invest.* **59**, 780.

Cines, D.B., Lyss, A.P., Reeber, M.B. and De Horatius, R.J. (1984). Presence of complement-fixing anti-endothelial cell antibodies in systemic lupus erythematosus. *J. Clin. Invest.* **73**, 611.

Clayman, M., Martinez-Hernandez, A., Michaud, L. *et al.* (1985). Isolation and characterisation of the nephritogenic antigen producing anti-tubular basement membrane disease. *J. Exp. Med.* **161**, 290.

Cochrane, C.G., Unanue, E.R. and Dixon, F.J. (1965). A role of polymorphonuclear leucocytes and complement in nephrotoxic nephritis. *J. Exp. Med.* **122**, 99.

Coggins, C.H. (1979). A controlled study of short-term prednisolone treatment in adults with membranous nephropathy. *N. Engl. J. Med.* **301**, 1301.

Coleman, T.H., Forristal, J., Kosaka, T. and West, C.D. (1983). Inherited complement component deficiencies in membranoproliferative glomerulonephritis. *Kidney Int.* **24**, 681.

Collins, A.B., Andres, G. and McCluskey, R.T. (1981). Lack of evidence for a role of renal tubular antigen in human membranous glomerulonephritis. *Nephron* **27**, 197.

Colvin, R.B., Burton, J.R., Hyslop, M.E., Spitz, L. and Lichtenstein, N.S. (1974). Penicillin-associated interstitial nephritis. *Ann. Intern. Med.* **81**, 404.

Conley, M.E., Cooper, M.D. and Michael, A.F. (1980). Selective deposition of IgA in immunoglobulin A nephropathy, anaphylactoid purpura nephritis and systemic lupus erythematosus. *J. Clin. Invest.* **66**, 1432.

Coppo, R., Bosticardo, G.M., Basoli, B. *et al.* (1982). Clinical significance of the detection of circulating immune complexes in lupus nephritis. *Nephron* **32**, 320.

Coppo, R., Basolo, B. and Grachino, O. (1985). Plasmapheresis in a patient with rapidly progressive idiopathic IgA nephropathy: removal of IgA containing circulating immune complexes and clinical recovery. *Nephron* **40**, 488.

Cordonnier, D., Martin, H., Groslambert, P., Micovin, C., Chenais, F. and Stoebner, P. (1975). Mixed IgG–IgM cryoglobulinaemia with glomerulonephritis. *Am. J. Med.* **59**, 867.

Cordonnier, D., Vialtel, P., Renversez, J.C. *et al.* (1983). Renal diseases in 18 patients with mixed type II IgM–IgG cryoglobulinaemia: monoclonal lymphoid infiltration (2 cases) and membranoproliferative glomerulonephritis (14 cases). *Adv. Nephrol.* **12**, 177.

Cosio, F.G., Lam, S. and Folami, A.O. (1982). Immune regulation of immunoglobulin production in IgA nephropathy. *Clin. Immunol. Immunopathol.* **23**, 430.

Couser, W.G. (1982). Idiopathic rapidly progressive glomerulonephritis. *Am. J. Nephrol.* **2**, 57.

Couser, W.G. (1988). Rapidly progressive glomerulonephritis: classification, pathogenetic mechanisms and therapy. *Am. J. Kidney Dis.* **11**, 449.

Couser, W.G. and Salant, D.J. (1980). *In situ* immune complex formation and glomerular injury. *Kidney Int.* **17**, 1.

Couser, W.G., Stilmant, M. and Lewis, E.J. (1973). Experimental glomerulonephritis in the guinea pig. I. Glomerular lesions associated with antiglomerular basement antibody deposits. *Lab. Invest.* **29**, 236.

Couser, W.G., Badger, A., Cooperband, S. *et al.* (1977). Hodgkin's disease and lipoid nephritis. *Lancet* **i**, 912.

Couser, W.G., Steinmuller, D.R., Stilmant, M.M., Salant, D.J. and Lowenstein, L.M. (1978). Experimental glomerulonephritis in the isolated perfused rat kidney. *J. Clin. Invest.* **62**, 1275.

Cronin, W., Deal, H., Azadegan, A. and Lange, K. (1989). Endostreptosin: isolation of the probable immunogen of acute post-streptococcal glomerulonephritis. *Clin. Exp. Immunol.* **76**, 198.

Cybulsky, A.V., Quigg, R.J. and Salant, D.J. (1986). The membrane attack complex in complement-mediated glomerular epithelial cell injury: formation and stability of C5b-9 and C5b-7 in rat membranous nephropathy. *J. Immunol.* **137**, 1511.

Daha, M.R., Fearon, D.T. and Austen, K.F. (1976). C3 nephritic factor (C3 NeF): stabilisation of fluid phase and cell bound alternative pathway convertase. *J. Immunol.* **116**, 1.

Daha, M.R., Austen, K.F. and Fearon, D.T. (1978). Heterogeneity, polypeptide chain composition and antigenic reactivity of C3 nephritic factor. *J. Immunol.* **120**, 1389.

Daha, M.R., Hazevoet, H.M., Van Es, L.A. and Cats, A. (1980). Stabilization of the classical pathway C3 convertase C42 by a factor F42 isolated from serum of patients with systemic lupus erythematosus. *Immunology* **40**, 417.

D'Amico, G. (1987). The commonest glomerulonephritis in the world: IgA nephropathy. *Quart. J. Med.* **64**, 709.

D'Amico, G., Ferrario, F., Colosanti, G. and Bucci, A. (1984). Glomerulonephritis in essential mixed cryoglobulinaemia. *Proc. Eur. Dialysis Transplant. Assoc.* **21**, 527.

D'Amico, G., Imbasciati, E., Barbiano di Belgioioso, G. *et al.* (1985). Idiopathic IgA mesangial nephropathy: clinical and histological study of 374 patients. *Medicine* **64**, 49.

D'Apice, A.J.F., Kincaid-Smith, P., Becker, G.J., Loughhead, M.G., Freeman, J.W. and Sands, J.M. (1978). Goodpasture's syndrome in identical twins. *Ann. Intern. Med.* **88**, 61.

Date, A., Neela, P. and Shastry, J.C.M. (1983). Membranoproliferative glomerulonephritis in a tropical environment. *Ann. Trop. Med. Parasitol.* **77**, 279.

Dathan, J.R.E. and Heyworth, M.F. (1975). Glomerulonephritis associated with *Coxiella burneti* endocarditis. *Br. Med. J.* **i**, 326.

Davies, D.J., Moran, J.E., Niall, J.F. and Ryan, G.B. (1982). Segmental necrotising glomerulonephritis with anti-neutrophil antibody: possible arbovirus aetiology. *Br. Med. J.* **285**, 606.

De Heer, E., Daha, M.R., Bhakdi, S., Bazin, H. and Van Es, L.A. (1985a). Possible involvement of terminal complement complex in active Heymann nephritis. *Kidney Int.* **27**, 388.

De Heer, E., Daha, M.R. and Van Es, L.A. (1985b). The autoimmune response in active Heymann's nephritis in Lewis rats is regulated by T lymphocyte subsets. *Cell. Immunol.* **92**, 254.

Demaine, A.G., Rambausek, M. and Knight, J.F. (1988). Relation of mesangial IgA glomerulonephritis to polymorphism of immunoglobulin heavy chain switch region. *J. Clin. Invest.* **81**, 611.

De Remee, R.A., McDonald, T.J. and Welland, L.H. (1985). Wegener's granulomatosis: observations on treatment with antimicrobial agents. *Mayo Clin. Proc.* **60**, 27.

Dixon, F.J., Feldman, J.D. and Vazquez, J.J. (1961). Experimental glomerulonephritis: the pathogenesis of a laboratory model resembling the spectrum of human glomerulonephritis. *J. Exp. Med.* **113**, 899.

Donaghy, M. and Rees, A.J. (1983). Cigarette smoking and lung haemorrhage in glomerulonephritis caused by autoantibodies to glomerular basement membrane. *Lancet* **ii**, 1390.

Donker, A.J., Venuto, R.C., Vladutiu, A.O., Brentjens, J.R. and Andres, G.A. (1984). Effects of prolonged administration of D-penicillamine or captopril in various strains of rats. *Clin. Immunol. Immunopathol.* **30**, 142.

Druet, E., Sapin, C., Fournie, G., Mandet, C., Gunther, E. and Druet, P. (1982). Genetic control of susceptibility to mercury-induced immune nephritis in various strains of rat. *Clin. Immunol. Immunopathol.* **25**, 203.

Druet, P., Druet, E., Potdevin, F. and Sapin, C. (1978). Immune type glomerulonephritis induced by $HgCl_2$ in the Brown Norway rat. *Ann. Immunol. (Inst. Pasteur)* **129c**, 777.

Duncan, D.A., Drummond, K.N., Michael, A.F. and Vernier, R.L. (1965). Pulmonary hemorrhage and glomerulonephritis: report of six cases and study of the renal lesion by fluorescent antibody technique and electron microscopy. *Ann. Intern. Med.* **62**, 920.

Ebert, T.H., McCluskey, R.T., Collins, A.B. and Colvin, R.B. (1981). Modulation of autologous immune complex nephritis (AIC) by preimmunisation with autoantibodies or sensitised cells. *Kidney Int.* **19**, 181.

Edgington, T.S., Glassock, R.J. and Dixon, F.J. (1968). Autologous immune complex nephritis induced with renal tubular antigens. I. Identification and isolation of the pathogenetic antigen. *J. Exp. Med.* **127**, 555.

Egido, J., Jillian, B.A. and Wyatt, R.J. (1987). Genetic factors in primary IgA nephropathy. *Nephrol. Dial. Transplant.* **2**, 134.

Egido, K.B., Sancho, J., Rivera, F. and Hernando, L. (1984). The role of IgA and IgG immune complexes in IgA nephropathy. *Nephron* **36**, 52.

Elkon, K.B., Sutherland, D.C., Rees, A.J., Hughes, G.R.V. and Batchelor, J.R. (1983). HLA antigen frequencies in systemic vasculitis: increase in HLA-DR2 in Wegener's granulomatosis. *Arthritis Rheum.* **26**, 98.

Emancipator, S.N., Gallo, G.R. and Lamm, M.E. (1983). Experimental IgA nephropathy induced by oral immunisation. *J. Exp. Med.* **157**, 572.

Emancipator, S.N., Gallo, G.R. and Lamm, M.E. (1985). IgA nephropathy: perspective on pathogenesis and classification. *Clin. Nephrol.* **24**, 161.

Emancipator, S.N., Ovary, Z. and Lamm, M.E. (1987). The role of mesangial complement in the haematuria of experimental IgA nephropathy. *Lab. Invest.* **57**, 269.

Evans, D.J., Williams, D.G., Peters, D.K. *et al.* (1973). Glomerular deposition of properdin in Henoch Schönlein syndrome and idiopathic focal nephritis. *Br. Med. J.* **3**, 326.

Falk, R.J. and Jennette, J.C. (1988). Antineutrophil cytoplasmic antibodies with specificity for myeloperoxidase in patients with systemic vasculitis and idiopathic necrotising and crescentic glomerulonephritis. *N. Engl. J. Med.* **318**, 1651.

Falk, R.J., Dalmasso, A.P., Kim, Y. *et al.* (1983). Neoantigen of the polymerised ninth component of complement: characterisation of a monoclonal antibody and immunohistochemical localisation in renal disease. *J. Clin. Invest.* **72**, 560.

Falk, R.J., Terrell, R.S., Charles, L.A. and Jennette, J.C. (1990). Anti-neutrophil cytoplasmic autoantibodies induce neutrophils to degranulate and produce oxygen radicals *in vitro*. *Proc. Nat. Acad. Sci. (USA)* **87**, 4115.

Fauci, A.C., Hayes, B.F., Katz, P. and Wolff, S.M. (1983). Wegener's granulomatosis: prospective clinical and therapeutic experience with 85 patients for 21 years. *Ann. Intern. Med.* **98**, 76.

Feehally, J. (1988). Immune mechanisms in glomerular IgA deposition. *Nephrol. Dial. Transplant.* **3**, 361.

Feehally, J., Beattie, J.T. and Brenchley, P.E.C. (1986a). Sequential studies of the IgA system in relapsing IgA nephropathy. *Kidney Int.* **30**, 924.

Feehally, J., Samanta, A., Kinghorn, H., Barden, A.C. and Walls, J. (1986b). Red cell charge in glomerular disease. *Lancet* **ii**, 635.

Feenstra, K., Lee, R.V.D., Greben, H.A., Arends, A. and Hoedemaker, P.J. (1975). Experimental glomerulonephritis in the rat induced by antibodies directed against tubular antigens. I. The natural history: a histologic and immunohistologic study at the light microscopic and ultrastructural level. *Lab. Invest.* **32**, 235.

Feiner, H. and Gallo, G. (1977). Ultrastructure in glomerulonephritis associated with cryoglobulinaemia. *Am. J. Pathol.* **88**, 145.

Feldmann, J.D., Mardiney, M.R. and Schuler, S.E. (1966). Immunology and morphology of acute post-streptococcal glomerulonephritis. *Lab. Invest.* **15**, 283.

Felson, D.J. and Anderson, J. (1984). Evidence for the superiority of immunosuppressive drugs and prednisolone over prednisolone alone in lupus nephritis: results of a pooled analysis. *N. Engl. J. Med.* **311**, 1528.

Ferraro, G., Meroni, P.L., Tincani, A. *et al.* (1990). Anti-endothelial cell antibodies in patients with Wegener's granulomatosis and micropolyarteritis. *Clin. Exp. Immunol.* **79**, 47.

Ferri, C., Moriconi, L., Gregnai, G. *et al.* (1986). Treatment of renal involvement in mixed essential cryoglobulinaemia with prolonged plasma exchange. *Nephron* **43**, 246.

Fielder, A.H.H., Walport, M.J., Batchelor, J.R. *et al.* (1983). Family study of the major histocompatibility complex in patients with systemic lupus erythematosus: importance of null alleles of C4A and C4B in determining disease susceptibility. *Br. Med. J.* **286**, 425.

Finkelstein, A., Fraley, D.S., Stachura, I., Feldman, H.A., Gandy, D.R. and Bourke, E. (1982). Fenoprofen nephropathy: lipoid nephrosis and interstitial nephritis. A possible T lymphocyte disorder. *Am. J. Med.* **72**, 81.

Fleuren, G., Grond, J. and Hoedemaeker, P.J. (1980). *In situ* formation of subepithelial glomerular immune complexes in passive serum sickness. *Kidney Int.* **17**, 631.

Fornasieri, A., Sinico, R.A. and Madifassi, P. (1988). Food antigens: IgA immune complexes and IgA mesangial nephropathy. *Br. Med. J.* **295**, 78.

Fournie, G.J. (1988). Circulating DNA and lupus nephritis. *Kidney Int.* **33**, 487.

Frank, M.M., Hamburger, M.I., Lawley, T.J., Kimberley, R.P. and Plotz, P.H. (1979). Defective reticuloendothelial system Fc-receptor function in systemic lupus erythematosus. *N. Engl. J. Med.* **300**, 518.

Friend, P.S., Kim, Y., Michael, A.F. and Donadio, J.V. (1977). Pathogenesis of membranous nephropathy in systemic lupus erythematosus: possible role of non-precipitating DNA antibody. *Br. Med. J.* **i**, 25.

Fries, J.W.U., Mendrick, D.L. and Rennke, H.G. (1988). Determinants of immune complex-mediated glomerulonephritis. *Kidney Int.* **4**, 333.

Gallo, G.R., Caulin-Glaser, T., Emancipator, S.N. and Lamm, M.E. (1983). Nephritogenicity and differential distribution of glomerular immune complexes related to immunogen charge. *Lab. Invest.* **48**, 353.

Gallo, J.H., Russell, M.W., Hammond, D., Spotswood, M. and Mestecky, J. (1985). Environmental antigens in IgA nephropathy. *Kidney Int.* **27**, 210.

Galpin, J.E., Shinaberger, J.H., Stanley, T.M. *et al.* (1978). Acute interstitial nephritis due to methicillin. *Am. J. Med.* **65**, 756.

Gaskin, G., Savage, C.O.S., Ryan, J.J. *et al.* (1991). Anti-neutrophil cytoplasmic antibodies and disease activity during long-term follow-up of 70 patients with systemic vasculitis. *Nephrol. Dial. Transplant.* **6**, 689.

Gauthier, V.J., Mannik, M. and Stricker, G.W. (1982). Effects of cationised antibodies in preformed immune complexes on deposition and persistence in renal glomeruli. *J. Exp. Med.* **156**, 766.

Gay, S., Losman, M.J., Koopman, W.J. and Miller, E.J. (1985). Interaction of DNA with connective tissue matrix proteins reveals preferential binding to type V collagen. *J. Immunol.* **135**, 1097.

Germuth, F.G. (1953). A comparative histologic and immunologic study in rabbits of induced hypersensitivity of the serum sickness type. *J. Exp. Med.* **97**, 257.

Germuth, F.G., Senterfit, L.B. and Dressman, G.R. (1972). Immune complex disease. V. The nature of the circulating complexes associated with glomerular alterations in the chronic BSA-rabbit system. *Johns Hopkins Med. J.* **130**, 344.

Gianciacomo, J., Cleary, T.G., Cole, B.R., Hoffsten, P. and Robson, A.M. (1975). Serum immunoglobulins in the nephrotic syndrome. *N. Engl. J. Med.* **8**, 12.

Gimenez, A. and Mampaso, F. (1986). Characterisation of inflammatory cells in drug induced tubulo-interstitial nephritis. *Nephrology* **43**, 239.

Gimenez, A., Leyva-Cobian, F., Fierro, C., Rio, M., Bricio, T. and Mampaso, F. (1987). Effect of cyclosporin A on autoimmune tubulointerstitial nephritis in the Brown Norway rat. *Clin. Exp. Immunol.* **69**, 550.

Glassock, R.J. (1985). Natural history and treatment of primary proliferative glomerulonephritis: a review. *Kidney Int.* **28**, 5136.

Golbus, S.M. and Wilson, C.B. (1979). Experimental glomerulonephritis induced by *in situ* formation of immune complexes in glomerular capillary wall. *Kidney Int.* **16**, 148.

Goldman, M., Feng, H.M., Engers, H., Hochmann, A., Louis, J. and Lambert, P.H. (1983). Autoimmunity and immune complex disease after neonatal induction of tolerance in mice. *J. Immunol.* **131**, 251.

Goldschmeding, R., Van der Schoot, C.E., Ten Bokkel Huinink, D. *et al.* (1989). Wegener's granulomatosis autoantibodies identify a novel diisopropylfluorophosphate-binding protein in the lysozomes of normal human neutrophils. *J. Clin. Invest.* **84**, 1577.

Gorevic, P.D., Kassab, H.J., Levo, Y. *et al.* (1980). Mixed cryoglobulinaemia: clinical aspects and long term follow up of 40 patients. *Am. J. Med.* **69**, 287.

Gormly, A.A., Seymour, A.E., Clarkson, A.R. and Woodroffe, A.J. (1981). IgA glomerular deposits in experimental cirrhosis. *Am. J. Pathol.* **104**, 50.

Gregersen, P.K. (1989). HLA class II polymorphism: implications for genetic susceptibility to autoimmune disease. *Lab. Invest.* **61**, 5.

Gremmel, F., Druml, W., Schmidt, P. and Graninger, W. (1988). Cyclosporin in Wegener's granulomatosis. *Ann. Intern. Med.* **108**, 491.

Grishman, E., Gerber, M.A. and Churg, J. (1982). Patterns of renal injury of systemic lupus erythematosus: light and fluorescence microscopic observations. *Am. J. Kidney Dis.* **4**, 135.

Groggel, G.C., Salant, D.J., Darby, C., Rennke, H.A. and Couser, W.G. (1985). Role of terminal complement pathway in the heterologous phase of anti-glomerular basement membrane nephritis. *Kidney Int.* **27**, 643.

Gronhagen-Riska, C., Von Willebrand, E., Tikkanen, E. *et al.* (1990). The effect of cyclosporin A on interstitial mononuclear cell infiltration and the induction of Heymann's nephritis. *Clin. Exp. Immunol.* **79**, 266.

Guery, J.-C., Tournade, H., Pelletier, L., Druet, E. and Druet, P. (1990). Rat anti-glomerular basement membrane antibodies in toxin-induced autoimmunity and in chronic graft versus host reaction share recurrent idiotypes. *Eur. J. Immunol.* **20**, 101.

Guttman, R.A., Morel-Maroger Striker, L. and Striker, G.E. (1988). Glomerulonephritis with bacterial endocarditis, shunts and abdominal abscesses. In *Diseases of the Kidney*, 4th edn, ed. R. Schrier and C.W. Gottschalk, p. 1885, Little, Brown and Co., Boston.

Habib, R., Kleinknecht, C., Gubler, M.-C. and Levy, M. (1973). Idiopathic membranoproliferative glomerulonephritis in children: report of 105 cases. *Clin. Nephrol.* **1**, 194.

Habib, R., Gubler, M.-C., Loirat, C., Maiz, H.B. and Levy, M. (1975). Dense deposit disease: a variant of membranoproliferative glomerulonephritis. *Kidney Int.* **7**, 204.

Habib, R., Levy, M. and Gubler, M.-C. (1979). Clinicopathologic correlations in the nephrotic syndrome. *Pediatrician* **8**, 325.

Hahn, B.H. and Ebling, F.M. (1983). Suppression of NZB/NZW murine nephritis by administration of a syngeneic monoclonal antibody to DNA: possible role of anti-idiotypic antibodies. *J. Clin. Invest.* **71**, 1728.

Hahn, B.H. and Ebling, F.M. (1984). Suppression of murine lupus nephritis by administration of an anti-idiotypic antibody to anti-DNA. *J. Immunol.* **132**, 187.

Halbwachs, L., Leveille, M., Lesavre, P., Wattels, S. and Leibowitch, J. (1980). Nephritic factor of the classical pathway of complement: immunoglobulin G autoantibody directed against the classical pathway C3 convertase enzyme. *J. Clin. Invest.* **65**, 249.

Hale, G., McIntosh, S.L., Clarkson, A.R., Hiki, Y. and Woodroffe, A.J. (1986). Evidence for IgA specific B cell hyperactivity in patients with IgA nephropathy. *Kidney Int.* **29**, 718.

Haworth, S.J., Pusey, C.D. and Lockwood, C.M. (1985). Plasma exchange in lupus nephritis. *Proc. EDTA–ERA* **22**, 699.

Heptinstall, R.H. (1983). *Pathology of the Kidney*. Little, Brown and Co., Boston.

Heymann, W., Hackel, D.B., Harwood, S., Wilson, S.G.F. and Hunter, J.L.P. (1959). Production of nephrotic syndrome in rat by Freund's adjuvant and rat kidney suspension. *Proc. Soc. Exp. Biol. Med.* **100**, 660.

Hiki, Y., Kobayashi, T., Tateno, S., Sada, M. and Kashiwagi, N. (1982). Strong association of HLA DR4 with benign IgA nephropathy. *Nephron* **32**, 222.

Hiki, Y., Kobayashi, Y., Itoh, I. and Kashiwagi, N. (1984). Strong association of HLA-DR2 and MTI with idiopathic membranous nephropathy in Japan. *Kidney Int.* **25**, 953.

Hind, C.R.K., Paraskevakou, H., Lockwood, C.M., Evans, D.J., Peters, D.K. and Rees, A.J. (1983). Prognosis after immunosuppression of patients with crescentic nephritis requiring dialysis. *Lancet* **i**, 263.

Hinglais, N., Garcia-Torres, R. and Kleinknecht, D. (1974). Long term prognosis in acute glomerulonephritis: the predictive value of early clinical and pathological features observed in 65 patients. *Am. J. Med.* **56**, 52.

Hirsch, F., Couderc, J., Sapin, C., Fournie, G. and Druet, P. (1982). Polyclonal effect of $HgCl_2$ in the rat, its possible role in an experimental autoimmune disease. *Eur. J. Immunol.* **12**, 620.

Holdsworth, S.R., Neale, T.J. and Wilson, C.B. (1981). Abrogation of macrophage dependent injury in experimental glomerulonephritis in the rabbit. *J. Clin. Invest.* **68**, 698.

Hoyer, P.F., Knell, F. and Brodehl, J. (1986). Cyclosporin in frequently relapsing minimal change nephrotic syndrome. *Lancet* **i**, 335.

Hudson, B.G., Wieslander, J., Wisdom, B.J. and Noelken, M.E. (1989). Goodpasture's syndrome: molecular architecture and function of basement membrane antigen. *Lab. Invest.* **61**, 256.

Hyman, L.R., Colvin, R.B. and Steinberg, A.D. (1976). Immunopathogenesis of autoimmune tubulo-interstitial nephritis. I. Demonstration of different susceptibility in strain II and strain XIII guinea pigs. *J. Immunol.* **116**, 327.

Hyman, L.R., Ballow, M. and Knieser, M.R. (1978). Diphenylhydantoin interstitial nephritis: roles of cellular and humoral immunological injury. *J. Pediatr.* **92**, 915.

Iitaka, K. and West, C.D. (1979). A serum inhibitor of blastogenesis in idiopathic nephrotic syndrome transferred by lymphocytes. *Clin. Immunol. Immunopathol.* **12**, 62.

Imbasciati, E., Gusmano, R., Edefonti, A. *et al.* (1985). Controlled trial of methyl prednisolone and low dose oral prednisolone for the minimal change nephrotic syndrome. *Br. Med. J.* **291**, 1305.

Isaacs, K.L. and Miller, F. (1982). Role of antigen size and charge in immune complex glomerulonephritis. *Lab. Invest.* **47**, 198.

Izui, S., Lambert, P.H. and Miescher, P.A. (1976). *In vitro* demonstration of a particular affinity of glomerular basement membrane and collagen for DNA: a possible basis for local formation of DNA-anti-DNA complexes in systemic lupus erythematosus. *J. Exp. Med.* **144**, 428.

Jacob, L., Lety, M.A., Choquette, D. *et al.* (1987). Presence of antibodies against a cell-surface protein, cross-reactive with DNA, in systemic lupus erythematosus: a marker of the disease. *Proc. Nat. Acad. Sci. (USA)* **84**, 2956.

Jennette, J.C., Wilkman, A.S. and Falk, R.J. (1989). Anti-neutrophil cytoplasmic autoantibody associated glomerulonephritis and vasculitis. *Am. J. Pathol.* **135**, 921.

Jennings, L., Roholt, O.A., Pressman, D., Blaum, M., Andres, G.A. and Brentjens, J.R. (1981). Experimental anti-alveolar basement membrane antibody-mediated pneumonitis. I. The role of increased permeability of the alveolar capillary wall induced by oxygen. *J. Immunol.* **127**, 129.

Johnson, J.P., Moore, J., Austin, H.A., Balow, J.E., Antonovych, T.T. and Wilson, C.B. (1985). Therapy of anti-glomerular basement membrane antibody disease: analysis of prognostic significance of clinical, pathologic and treatment factors. *Medicine* **64**, 219.

Julian, B.A., Quiggins, P.A., Thompson, J.S., Woodford, S.Y., Gleason, K. and Wyatt, R.J. (1985). Familial IgA nephropathy: evidence of an inherited mechanism of disease. *N. Engl. J. Med.* **312**, 202.

Kamata, K., Baird, L.G., Erikson, M.E., Collin, A.B. and McCluskey, R.T. (1985). Characterisation of antigens and antibody specificities induced in Heyman nephritis. *J. Immunol.* **135**, 2400.

Kasahara, M., Hamada, K., Okuyama, T. *et al.* (1982). Role of HLA system in IgA nephropathy. *Clin. Immunol. Immunopathol.* **25**, 189.

Katz, A., Dyck, R.F. and Bear, R.A. (1979). Coeliac disease associated with immune complex glomerulonephritis. *Clin. Nephrol.* **11**, 39.

Katz, A., Karanicolas, S. and Falk, J.A. (1980). Family study in IgA glomerulonephritis: the possible role of HLA antigens. *Transplantation* **29**, 505.

Kazatchkine, M.D., Fearon, D.T., Appay, M.D., Mandet, C. and Bariety, J. (1982). Immunohistochemical study of the human glomerular C3b receptor in normal kidney and in seventy-five cases of renal diseases: loss of C3b receptor antigen in focal hyalinosis and in proliferative nephritis of systemic lupus erythematosus. *J. Clin. Invest.* **69**, 900.

Kelly, C.J. and Neilson, E.G. (1987). Contrasuppression in autoimmunity: abnormal contrasuppression promotes the expression of nephritogenic effector T cells and histologic interstitial nephritis in kdkd mice. *J. Exp. Med.* **165**, 107.

Kelly, C.J., Korngold, R., Mann, R., Clayman, M., Haverty, T. and Neilson, E.G. (1986). Characterisation of a tubular antigen specific H-2K restricted Lyt-2+ effector T cell that mediates destructive tubulointerstitial injury. *J. Immunol.* **136**, 526.

Kelly, C.J., Zunier, R.B., Krakauer, K.A., Blanchard, N. and Neilson, E.G. (1987). Prostaglandin E1 inhibits effector T cell induction and tissue damage in experimental murine interstitial nephritis. *J. Clin. Invest.* **79**, 782.

Kerjaschki, D. and Farquhar, M.G. (1982). The pathogenic antigen of Heymann nephritis is a membrane glycoprotein of the renal proximal tubule brush border. *Proc. Nat. Acad. Sci. (USA)* **79**, 5557.

Kerjaschki, D., Horvat, R., Binder, S. *et al.* (1987a). Identification of a 400 kD protein in the brush borders of human kidneys that is similar to gp330, the nephritogenic antigen of rat Heymann nephritis. *Am. J. Pathol.* **129**, 183.

Kerjaschki, D., Miettinen, A. and Farquhar, M.G. (1987b). Initial events in the formation of immune deposits in passive Heymann nephritis. *J. Exp. Med.* **166**, 109.

Kerjaschki, D., Schultze, M., Binder, S. *et al.* (1989). Transcellular transport and membrane insertion of the C5b-9 membrane attack complex of complement by glomerular epithelial cells in experimental membranous nephropathy. *J. Immunol.* **143**, 546.

Kim, Y., Friend, P.S., Dresner, I.G., Yunis, E.J. and Michael, A.F. (1977). Inherited deficiency of the 2nd component of complement (C2) with membranoproliferative glomerulonephritis. *Am. J. Med.* **62**, 765.

Kimberly, R.P., Lockshin, M.D., Sherman, R.L., McDougal, J.S., Inman, R.D. and Christian, C.L. (1981). High dose intravenous methylprednisolone pulse therapy in systemic lupus erythematosus. *Am. J. Med.* **70**, 817.

Klassen, J., Kano, K., Milgrom, F. *et al.* (1973). Tubular lesions produced by autoantibodies to tubular basement membrane in human renal allografts. *Int. Arch. Allergy Appl. Immunol.* **45**, 675.

Kleinknecht, D., Kanfer, A., Morel-Maroger, L. and Mery, J.P. (1978). Immunologically mediated drug-induced acute renal failure. *Contrib. Nephrol.* **10**, 42.

Kleppel, M.M., Santi, P.A., Cameron, J.D., Wieslander, J. and Michael, A.F. (1989). Human tissue distribution of novel basement membrane collagen. *Am. J. Pathol.* **134**, 813.

Klouda, P.T., Manos, J., Acheson, E.J. *et al.* (1979). Strong association between idiopathic membranous nephropathy and HLA-DRW3. *Lancet* **ii**, 770.

Knudsen, B.B., Joergensen, T. and Munch-Jensen, B. (1988). Wegener's granulomatosis in a family. *Scand. J. Rheumatol.* **17**, 225.

Kobayashi, Y., Fujii, K., Hiki, Y. and Tateno, S. (1986). Steroid therapy in IgA nephropathy: a prospective pilot study in moderate proteinuric cases. *Quart J. Med.* **61**, 985.

Koffler, D. (1974). Immunopathogenesis of systemic lupus erythematosus. *Ann. Rev. Med.* **25**, 149.

Koffler, D., Agnello, V., Thoburn, R. and Kunkel, H.G. (1971). Systemic lupus erythematosus: prototype of immune complex disease in man. *J. Exp. Med.* **134**, 169.

Komori, K., Nose, Y., Inouye, H. *et al.* (1983). Immunogenetical study in patients with chronic glomerulonephritis. *Tokai J. Exp. Clin. Med.* **8**, 135.

Kunkel, J.G., Agnello, V., Joslin, F.G., Winchester, R.J. and Capra, J.D. (1973). Cross-idiotypic specificity among monoclonal IgM proteins with anti-gammaglobulin activity. *J. Exp. Med.* **137**, 331.

Kuntel, S.L., Zanetti, M. and Sapin, C. (1982). Suppression of nephrotoxic serum nephritis in rats by prostaglandin E1. *Am. J. Pathol.* **108**, 240.

Lagrue, G., Xheneumont, S., Branellec, A. and Weil, B. (1975). Lymphokines and the nephrotic syndrome. *Lancet* **i**, 271.

Lai, K.-N., Lai, E.M. and Ho, C.P. (1986). Corticosteroid therapy in IgA nephropathy with nephrotic syndrome: a long-term controlled trial. *Clin. Nephrol.* **26**, 174.

Lai, K.-N., Chui, S.-H. and Lai, F.M. (1988). Predominant synthesis of IgA with lambda light chains in IgA nephropathy. *Kidney Int.* **33**, 584.

Lange, K., Seligson, G. and Cronin, W. (1983). Evidence for the *in situ* origin of post-streptococcal glomerulonephritis: glomerular localisation of endostreptosin and the clinical significance of the subsequent antibody response. *Clin. Nephrol.* **19**, 3.

Layrisse, Z., Rodriguez-Iturbe, B., Garcia, R., Rodriguez, A. and Tiwari, J. (1983). Family studies of the HLA system in acute post-streptococcal glomerulonephritis. *Hum. Immunol.* **7**, 177.

Leaker, B.R., Becker, G.J., Dowling, J.P. and Kincaid-Smith, P. (1986). Rapid improvement in severe lupus glomerular lesions following intensive plasma exchange associated with immunosuppression. *Clin. Nephrol.* **25**, 236.

Lehman, D.H., Lee, S., Wilson, C.B. and Dixon, F.J. (1974a). Induction of antitubular basement membrane antibodies in rats by renal transplantation. *Transplantation* **17**, 429.

Lehman, D.H., Wilson, C.B. and Dixon, F.J. (1974b). Interstitial nephritis in rats immunised with heterologous tubular basement membrane. *Kidney Int.* **5**, 187.

Lehman, D.H., Wilson, C.B. and Dixon, F.J. (1975). Extraglomerular immunoglobulin deposits in human nephritis. *Am. J. Med.* **58**, 765.

Lerner, R., Glassock, R.J. and Dixon, F.J. (1967). The role of anti-glomerular basement membrane antibody in the pathogenesis of human glomerulonephritis. *J. Exp. Med.* **126**, 989.

Levin, M., Smith, C., Walters, M.D.S., Gascoine, P. and Barratt, T.M. (1985). Steroid-responsive nephrotic syndrome: a generalised disorder of membrane charge. *Lancet* **ii**, 239.

Levy, M. and Kleinknecht, C. (1980). Membranous glomerulonephritis and hepatitis B virus infection. *Nephron* **26**, 259.

Li, P.K., Burns, A.P., So, A.K.L., Pusey, C.D., Freehally, J. and Rees, A.J. (1991). The DQw7 allele at the HLA-DQB locus is associated with susceptibility to IgA nephropathy in Caucasians. *Kidney Int.* **39**, 961.

Lianos, E.A. (1988). Synthesis of hydroxyeicosatetranoic acids and leukotrienes in rat nephrotoxic serum glomerulonephritis. *J. Clin. Invest.* **82**, 427.

Lianos, E.A., Andres, G.A. and Dunn, M.J. (1983). Glomerular prostaglandin and thromboxane synthesis in rat nephrotoxic serum nephritis: effects on renal haemodynamics. *J. Clin. Invest.* **72**, 1439.

Liebowitch, J., Leveille, M., Halbwachs, L. and Wattel, S. (1980). Glomerulonephritides and hypocomplementaemia: pathophysiology and pathogenetic implications. *Avd. Nephrol.* **9**, 295.

Linscott, W.D. and Kane, J.P. (1975). The complement system in cryoglobulinaemia. *Clin. Exp. Immunol.* **21**, 510.

Litwin, A., Bash, J.A., Adams, L.E., Donovan, R.J. and Hess, E.V. (1979). Immunoregulation of Heymann nephritis. I. Induction of suppressor cells. *J. Immunol.* **122**, 1029.

Lockwood, C.M., Worlledge, S., Nicholas, A., Cotton, C. and Peters, D.K. (1979). Reversal of impaired splenic function in patients with nephritis or vasculitis (or both) by plasma exchange. *N. Engl. J. Med.* **300**, 524.

Lomax-Smith, J.D., Zabrowarny, L.A., Howarth, G.S., Seymour,

A.E. and Woodroffe, A.J. (1983). The immunochemical characterisation of mesangial IgA deposits. *Am. J. Pathol.* **113**, 359.

Lovett, D.H. and Sterzl, R.B. (1986). Cell culture approaches to the analysis of glomerular inflammation. *Kidney Int.* **30**, 246.

Ludemann, J., Utecht, B. and Gross, W.L. (1990). Anti-neutrophil antibodies in Wegener's granulomatosis recognise an elastinolytic enzyme. *J. Exp. Med.* **357**, 362.

Lyon, M.F. and Hulse, E.V. (1971). An inherited kidney disease of mice resembling human nephronophthisis. *J. Med. Genet.* **8**, 41.

McCluskey, R.T. and Colvin, R.B. (1978). Immunological aspects of renal tubular and interstitial disease. *Ann. Rev. Med.* **29**, 191.

McKenzie, P.E., Hawke, D., Woodroffe, A.J., Thompson, A.J., Seymour, A.E. and Clarkson, A.R. (1980). Serum and tissue immune complexes in infective endocarditis. *J. Clin. Lab. Immunol.* **4**, 125.

McLean, R.H. and Hoefnagel, D. (1980). Partial lipodystrophy and familial C3 deficiency. *Hum. Hered.* **30**, 149.

MacScarraigh, E.T., Doyle, C.T., Twomey, M. and O'Sullivan, D.J. (1978). Sarcoidosis with renal involvement. *Postgrad. Med. J.* **54**, 528.

Madaio, M.P., Carlson, J., Cataldo, J., Ucci, A., Migliorini, P. and Pankewyez, O. (1987). Murine monoclonal anti-DNA antibodies bind directly to glomerular antigens and from immune deposits. *J. Immunol.* **138**, 2883.

Magil, A.B. and Wadsworth, L.D. (1982). Monocyte involvement in glomerular crescents: a histochemical and ultrastructural study. *Lab. Invest.* **47**, 160.

Mahieu, P., Lambert, P.H. and Miescher, P.A. (1974). Detection of anti-glomerular basement membrane antibodies by a radioimmunological technique: clinical application in human nephropathies. *J. Clin. Invest.* **54**, 128.

Makker, S.P. (1980). Tubular basement membrane antibody induced nephritis in systemic lupus erythematosus. *Am. J. Med.* **69**, 949.

Mampaso, F.M. and Wilson, C.B. (1983). Characterisation of inflammatory cells in autoimmune tubulointerstitial nephritis in rats. *Kidney Int.* **23**, 448.

Martini, A., Vitiello, M.A., Siena, S., Capelli, V. and Ugazio, A.G. (1981). Multiple serum inhibitors of lectin-induced lymphocyte proliferation in nephrotic syndrome. *Clin. Exp. Immunol.* **45**, 178.

Mathieson, P.W., Turner, A.N., Maidment, C.G.H., Evans, D.J. and Rees, A.J. (1988). Prednisolone and chlorambucil treatment in idiopathic membranous nephropathy with deteriorating renal function. *Lancet* **ii**, 869.

Mathieson, P.W., Cobbold, S.P., Hale, G. *et al.* (1990). Monoclonal antibody therapy in systemic vasculitis. *N. Engl. J. Med.* **323**, 250.

Matsuo, S., Fukatsu, A., Taub, M.L., Caldwell, P.R.B., Brentjens, J.R. and Andres, G. (1987). Glomerulonephritis induced in the rabbit by anti-endothelial antibodies. *J. Clin. Invest.* **79**, 1798.

Mauer, S.M., Sutherland, D.E.R., Howard, R.J., Fish, A.J., Najarian, J.S. and Michael, A.F. (1973). The glomerular mesangium. III. Acute immune mesangial injury: a new model of glomerulonephritis. *J. Exp. Med.* **137**, 553.

Melvin, T., Burke, B., Michael, A.F. and Young, K. (1983). Experimental IgA nephropathy in bile duct ligated rats. *Clin. Immunol. Immunopathol.* **27**, 369.

Mendrick, D.L. and Rennke, H.G. (1988). Epitope specific induction of proteinuria by monoclonal antibodies. *Kidney Int.* **33**, 831.

Meyrier, A., Simon, P., Perret, G. and Condamin-Meyrier, M.-C. (1986). Remission of idiopathic nephrotic syndrome after treatment with cyclosporin A. *Br. Med. J.* **292**, 789.

Michalak, T. (1978). Immune complexes of hepatitis B surface antigen in the pathogenesis of periarteritis nodosa: a study of seven necropsy cases. *Am. J. Pathol.* **90**, 619.

Mignon, F., Mery, J.-P., Mougenot, B., Ronco, P., Roland, J. and Morel-Maroger, L. (1984). Granulomatous interstitial nephritis. *Adv. Nephrol.* **13**, 219.

Miller, G.W. and Nussenzweig, V. (1975). A new complement function: solubilisation of antigen–antibody aggregates. *Proc. Nat. Acad. Sci. (USA)* **72**, 418.

Miyakawa, Y., Yamada, A., Kosaka, K., Tsuda, F., Kosugi, E. and Mayumi, M. (1981). Defective immune adherence (C3b) receptor on erythrocytes from patients with systemic lupus erythematosus. *Lancet* **ii**, 493.

Mollnes, T.E., Ng, Y.C., Peters, D.K., Lea, T., Tschapp, J. and Harboe, M. (1986). Effect of nephritic factor on C3 and on the terminal pathway of complement *in vivo* and *in vitro*. *Clin. Exp. Immunol.* **65**, 73.

Moorthy, A.V., Zimmerman, S.W. and Burtholder, P.M. (1976a). Nephrotic syndrome in Hodgkin's disease: evidence for pathogenesis alternative to immune complex deposition. *Am. J. Med.* **61**, 471.

Moorthy, A.V., Zimmerman, S.W. and Burtholder, P.M. (1976b). Inhibition of lymphocyte blastogenesis by plasma of patients with minimal change nephrotic syndrome. *Lancet* **i**, 1160.

Morimoto, C., Sano, H., Ave, T., Homma, M. and Steinberg, A.D. (1982). Correlation between clinical activity of systemic lupus erythematosus and the amounts of DNA in DNA/anti-DNA antibody immune complexes. *J. Immunol.* **129**, 1960.

Mouzon-Cambon, A., Bouisson, F., Dutau, G. *et al.* (1981). HLA-DR7 in children with idiopathic nephrotic syndrome: correlation with atopy. *Tissue Antigens* **17**, 518.

Muller, G.A., Gebhardt, M., Kompf, J., Baldwin, W.M., Ziegenhagen, D. and Bohle, A. (1984). Association between rapidly progressive glomerulonephritis and the properdin factor BfF and different HLA-D region products. *Kidney Int.* **25**, 115.

Nagy, J., Scott, H. and Brandtzaeg, P. (1988). Autoantibodies to dietary antigens in IgA nephropathy. *Clin. Exp. Immunol.* **29**, 274.

Naish, P.F., Thomson, N.M., Simpson, I.J. and Peters, D.K. (1975). Role of polymorphonuclear leucocytes in the autologous phase nephrotoxic nephritis. *Clin. Exp. Immunol.* **22**, 105.

Nakamoto, Y., Asano, Y., Dohi, D. *et al.* (1978). Primary IgA glomerulonephritis and Schönlein–Henoch purpura nephritis: clinicopathological and immuno-histological characteristics. *Quart. J. Med.* **47**, 495.

Naruse, T., Kitanura, K., Miyakawa, Y. and Shibata, S. (1983). Deposition of renal tubular epithelial antigen along the glomerular capillary walls of patients with membranous glomerulonephritis. *J. Immunol.* **110**, 1163.

Neale, T.J., Tipping, P.G., Carson, S.D. and Holdsworth, S.R. (1988). Participation of cell mediated immunity in deposition of fibrin in glomerulonephritis. *Lancet* **ii**, 421.

Neilson, E.G. and Phillips, S.M. (1982a). Suppression of interstitial nephritis by auto-anti-idiotypic immunity. *J. Exp. Med.* **155**, 179.

Neilson, E.G. and Phillips, S.M. (1982b). Murine interstitial nephritis. I. Analysis of disease susceptibility and relationship to pleomorphic gene products defining both immune-response genes and a restrictive requirement for cytotoxic T cells at H-2K. *J. Exp. Med.* **155**, 1075.

Neilson, E.G., Gasser, D.I., McCafferty, E., Zakheim, B. and Phillips, S.M. (1983). Polymorphism of genes involved in anti-tubular basement membrane disease in rats. *Immunogenetics* **17**, 55.

Neilson, E.G., McCafferty, E., Feldmann, A., Clayman, M.D., Zakheim, B. and Korngold, R. (1984a). Spontaneous interstitial nephritis in kdkd mice: an experimental model of autoimmune renal disease. *J. Immunol.* **133**, 2560.

Neilson, E.G., McCafferty, E., Phillips, S.M., Clayman, M.D. and Kelly, C.J. (1984b). Anti-idiotype immunity in interstitial nephritis. II. Rats developing anti-tubular basement membrane disease fail to make an anti-idiotype regulatory response: the modulatory role of an RT7.1+, OX8-suppressor T cell mechanism. *J. Exp. Med.* **159**, 1009.

Neilson, E.G., McCafferty, E., Mann, R., Michaud, L. and Clayman, M.D. (1985a). Murine interstitial nephritis. III. The selection of phenotypic (Lyt and L3T4) and idiotypic (RE-Id) T cell preferences by genes in Igh-I and H2-K characterises the cell mediated potential for disease expression: susceptible mice provide a unique effector T cell repertoire in response to tubular antigen. *J. Immunol.* **134**, 2375.

Neilson, E.G., McCafferty, E., Mann, R., Michaud, L. and Clayman, M.D. (1985b). Tubular antigen-derivatised cells induce a disease-protective, antigen-specific, and idiotype-specific suppressor T cell network restricted by I-J and IgH-V in mice with experimental interstitial nephritis. *J. Exp. Med.* **162**, 215.

Neilson, E.G., Sun, M.J., Emery, J. *et al.* (1989). Molecular cloning of the 3M-1 nephritogenic antigen. *Kidney Int.* **35**, 358a.

Neugarten, J. and Baldwin, D.S. (1984). Glomerulonephritis in bacterial endocarditis. *Am. J. Med.* **77**, 297.

Ng, Y.C. and Peters, D.K. (1986). C3 nephritic factor (C3NeF): dissociation of cell-bound and fluid phase stabilisation of alternative pathway C3 convertase. *Clin. Exp. Immunol.* **65**, 450.

Nochy, D., Callard, P. and Bellon, B. (1976). Association of overt glomerulonephritis and liver disease: a study of 34 patients. *Clin. Nephrol.* **6**, 422.

Nolasco, F.E., Cameron, J.S., Hartley., B., Coelho, A., Hildreth, G. and Reuben, R. (1987). Intraglomerular T cells and monocytes in nephritis: study with monoclonal antibodies. *Kidney Int.* **31**, 1160.

Nolle, B., Specks, U., Ludemann, J., Rohrbach, M.S., De Remee, R.A. and Gross, W.L. (1989). Anticytoplasmic autoantibodies: their immunodiagnostic value in Wegener's granulomatosis. *Ann. Intern. Med.* **111**, 28.

Nunex-Roldan, A., Villechenous, E., Fernandez-Andrade, C. and Martin-Govantes, J. (1982). Increased HLA-DR7 and decreased DR2 in steroid-responsive nephrotic syndrome. *N. Engl. J. Med.* **306**, 366.

Oite, T., Batsford, S.R., Mihatsch, M.J., Takamiya, H. and Vogt, A. (1982). Quantitative studies of *in situ* immune complex glomerulonephritis in the rat induced by planted, cationized antigen. *J. Exp. Med.* **155**, 460.

Ono, M., Winearls, C.G., Amos, N. *et al.* (1987). Monoclonal antibodies to restricted and cross-reactive idiotopes on monoclonal rheumatoid factors and their recognition of idiotypic positive cells. *Eur. J. Immunol.* **17**, 343.

Ooi, B.S., Orlina, A.R. and Masaitas, L. (1974). Lymphocytotoxins in primary renal disease. *Lancet* **ii**, 1348.

Papiha, S.S., Pareck, S.K., Rodger, R.S.C. *et al.* (1987). HLA-A, B, Dr and Bf allotypes in patients with idipathic membranous nephropathy. *Kidney Int.* **31**, 130.

Pardo, V., Strauss, J., Kramer, H., Ozawa, T. and McIntosh, R.M. (1975). Nephropathy associated with sickle cell anaemia: an autologous immune complex nephritis. II. Clinocopathological study of seven patients. *Am. J. Med.* **59**, 650.

Parkinson, D.T., Baker, P.J., Couser, W.G., Johnson, R.J. and Adler, S. (1985). Membrane attack complex deposition in experimental glomerular injury. *Am. J. Pathol.* **120**, 121.

Paul, L.C., Stuffers-Heiman, M., Van Es, L.A. and De Graeff, J. (1979). Antibodies directed against brush border antigens of proximal tubules in renal allograft recipients. *Clin. Immunol. Immunopathol.* **14**, 238.

Pelletier, L., Pasquier, R., Hirsch, F., Sapin, C. and Druet, P. (1986). Autoreactive T cells in mercury-induced autoimmune disease: *in vitro* demonstration. *J. Immunol.* **137**, 2548.

Pelletier, L., Pasquier, R., Rossert, J., Vial, M.-C., Mandet, C. and Druet, P. (1988). Autoreactive T cells in mercury-induced autoimmunity: ability to induce the autoimmune disease. *J. Immunol.* **140**, 750.

Peters, D.K., Rees, A.J., Lockwood, C.M. and Pusey, C.D. (1982). Treatment and prognosis in anti-GBM antibody-mediated nephritis. *Transplant. Proc.* **14**, 513.

Pickering, R.J., Michael, A.F., Herdman, R.C., Good, R.A. and Gewurz, H. (1971). The complement system in chronic glomerulonephritis: three newly associated aberrations. *J. Pediatr.* **78**, 30.

Pietromonaco, S., Kerjaschki, D., Binder, S., Ullrich, R. and Farquhar, M.G. (1990). Molecular cloning of a cDNA encoding a major pathogenic domain of the Heyman nephritis antigen gp330. *Proc. Nat. Acad. Sci. (USA)* **87**, 1811.

Pilia, P.A., Boackle, R.J., Swain, R.P. and Ainsworth, S.R. (1983). Complement independent nephrotoxic serum nephritis in Munich Wister rats. *Lab. Invest.* **48**, 585.

Pinching, A.J., Lockwood, C.M., Pussell, B.A. *et al.* (1983). Wegener's granulomatosis: observations on 18 patients with severe renal disease. *Quart. J. Med.* **52**, 435.

Ponticelli, C., Zucchelli, P., Imbasciati, E. *et al.* (1984). Controlled trial of methyl prednisolone and chlorambucil in idiopathic membranous nephropathy. *N. Engl. J. Med.* **310**, 946.

Pusey, C.D. and Lockwood, C.M. (1989). Autoimmunity in rapidly progressive glomerulonephritis. *Kidney Int.* **35**, 929.

Pusey, C.D., Bowman, C., Peters, D.K. and Lockwood, C.M. (1983a). Effect of cyclophosphamide on auto-antibody synthesis in the Brown Norway rat. *Clin. Exp. Immunol.* **54**, 697.

Pusey, C.D., Lockwood, C.M. and Peters, D.K. (1983b). Plasma exchange and immunosuppressive drugs in the treatment of glomerulonephritis due to antibodies to the glomerular basement membrane. *Int. J. Artificial Organs* **6**, 15.

Pusey, C.D., Saltissi, D., Bloodworth, L., Rainford, D.J. and Christie, J.L. (1983c). Drug associated acute interstitial nephritis: clinical and pathological features and the response to high dose steroid therapy. *Quart. J. Med.* **52**, 194.

Pusey, C.D., Dash, A., Kershaw, M.J. *et al.* (1987). A single autoantigen in Goodpasture's syndrome identified by a monoclonal antibody to human glomerular basement membrane. *Lab. Invest.* **56**, 28.

Pusey, C.D., Venning, M.C. and Peters, D.K. (1988). Immunopathology of glomerular and interstitial disease. In *Diseases of the Kidney*, 4th edn., ed. R.W. Schrier and C.W. Gottschalk, p. 1827, Little, Brown and Co., Boston.

Pusey, C.D., Bowman, C., Morgan, A., Weetman, A.P., Hartley, B. and Lockwood, C.M. (1990). Kinetics and pathogenicity of autoantibodies induced by mercuric chloride in the Brown Norway rat. *Clin. Exp. Immunol.* **81**, 76.

Pusey, C.D., Holland, M.J., Cashman, S.J. *et al.* (1991a). Experimental autoimmune glomerulonephritis induced by homologous and isologous glomerular basement membrane in Brown Norway rats. *Nephrol. Dial. Transplant.* **6**, 457.

Pusey, C.D., Rees, A.J., Evans, D.J., Peters, D.K. and Lockwood, C.M. (1991b). Plasma exchange in focal necrotizing glomerulonephritis without anti-GMB antibodies. *Kidney Int.* **40**, 757.

Pussell, B.A., Bourke, E., Nayef, M., Morris, S. and Peters, D.K. (1980). Complement deficiency and nephritis. *Lancet* **i**, 675.

Rees, A.J. (1984). The HLA complex and susceptibility to glomerulonephritis. *Plasma Ther. Transfusion Technol.* **5**, 455.

Rees, A.J., Demaine, A.G. and Welsh, K.I. (1984a). The association between immunoglobulin allotypes with autoantibodies to glomerular basement membrane and their titre. *Hum. Immunol.* **10**, 213.

Rees, A.J., Peters, D.K., Amos, N., Welsh, K.I. and Batchelor, J.R. (1984b). The influence of HLA-linked genes on the severity of anti-GBM antibody-mediated nephritis. *Kidney Int.* **26**, 444.

Reynolds, J., Cashman, S.J., Evans, D.J. and Pusey, C.D. (1991). Cyclosporin A in the prevention and treatment of experimental autoimmune glomerulonephritis in the Brown Norway rat. *Clin. Exp. Immunol.* **85**, 28.

Rich, A.R. and Gregory, J.E. (1943). The experimental demonstration that periarteritis nodosa is a manifestation of hypersensitivity. *Bull. Johns Hopkins Hosp.* **72**, 65.

Richards, W., Olson, D. and Church, J.A. (1977). Improvement of idiopathic nephrotic syndrome following allergy treatment. *Ann. Allergy* **39**, 332.

Rifai, A. and Millard, K. (1985). Glomerular deposition of immune complexes prepared with monomeric or polymeric IgA. *Clin. Exp. Immunol.* **60**, 363.

Rifai, A., Small, P.A., Teague, P.O. and Ayoube, M. (1979). Experimental IgA nephropathy. *J. Exp. Med.* **150**, 1161.

Rifai, A., Chen, A. and Imai, H. (1987). Complement activation in experimental IgA nephropathy: an antigen-mediated process. *Kidney Int.* **32**, 838.

Roberts, J.L., Wyatt, R.J., Schwartz, M.M. and Lewis, E.J. (1983). Differential characteristics of immune-bound antibodies in diffuse proliferative and membranous forms of lupus glomerulonephritis. *Clin. Immunol. Immunopathol.* **29**, 223.

Rodriguez-Iturbe, B. (1984). Epidemic post-streptococcal glomerulonephritis. *Kidney Int.* **25**, 129.

Rodriguez-Iturbe, B., Castillo, L., Valbuena, B. and Cuenca, L. (1979). Acute post-streptococcal glomerulonephritis: a review of recent developments. *Paediatrician* **8**, 307.

Rodriguez-Iturbe, B., Rubio, L. and Garcia, R. (1981). Attack rate of post-streptococcal nephritis in families. *Lancet* **i**, 401.

Rolink, A.G., Gleichmann, H. and Gleichmann, E. (1983). Diseases caused by reactions of T lymphocytes to incompatible structures of the major histocompatibility complex. VII. Immune-complex glomerulonephritis. *J. Immunol.* **130**, 209.

Roman-Franco, A.A., Turiello, M., Albini, B., Ossi, E., Milgrom, F. and Andres, G.A. (1978). Anti-basement membrane antibodies and antigen–antibody complexes in rabbits injected with mercuric chloride. *Clin. Immunol. Immunopathol.* **9**, 464.

Ronco, P., Verroust, P., Mignon, F. *et al.* (1983). Immunopathological studies of polyarteritis nodosa and Wegener's granulomatosis: a report of 43 patients with 51 renal biopsies. *Quart. J. Med.* **52**, 212.

Ronco, P., Neale, T.J., Wilson, C.B., Galceran, M. and Verroust, P. (1986). An immune pathological study of a 330kd protein defined by monoclonal antibodies and reactive with anti-RTEα5 antibodies and kidney eluates from active Heymann nephritis. *J. Immunol.* **136**, 125.

Row, P.G., Cameron, J.S., Turner, D.R. *et al.* (1975). Membranous nephropathy: long term follow-up and association with neoplasia. *Quart. J. Med.* **44**, 207.

Ruder, H., Scharer, K., Lenhard, V., Wingen, A.M. and Opelz, G. (1982). HLA phenotypes and idiopathic nephrotic syndrome in children. *Proc. Eur. Dialysis Transplant. Assoc.* **19**, 602.

Rudofsky, U.H. and Pollara, B. (1976). Studies on the pathogenesis of experimental autoimmune renal tubulointerstitial disease in guinea-pigs. II. Passive transfer of renal lesions by anti-tubular basement membrane autoantibody and non-immune bone marrow cells to leukocyte-depleted recipients. *Clin. Immunol. Immunopathol.* **6**, 107.

Rudofsky, U.H., Steblay, R.W. and Pollara, B. (1975). Inhibition of experimental autoimmune renal tubulointerstitial disease in guinea-pigs by depletion of complement with cobra venom factor. *Clin. Immunol. Immunopathol.* **3**, 396.

Rudofsky, U.H., Dilwith, R.L. and Tung, K.S.K. (1980). Susceptibility differences of inbred mice to induction of autoimmune renal tubulointerstitial lesions. *Lab. Invest.* **43**, 463.

Sabatier, J.C., Genin, C., Assenat, H., Colon, S., Drucret, F. and Berthoux, F.C. (1979). Mesangial IgA glomerulonephritis in HLA identical brothers. *Clin. Nephrol.* **11**, 35.

Sado, T., Okigaki, T., Takamiya, H. and Seno, S. (1984). Experimental autoimmune glomerulonephritis with pulmonary haemorrhage in rats: the dose–effect relationship of the nephritogenic antigen from bovine glomerular basement membrane. *J. Clin. Lab. Immunol.* **15**, 199.

Sado, T., Naito, I. and Okigati, T. (1989). Transfer of anti-glomerular basement membrane antibody-induced glomerulonephritis in inbred rats with isologous antibodies from the urine of nephritic rats. *J. Pathol.* **158**, 325.

Salant, D.J., Belok, S., Madaio, M.P. and Couser, W.G. (1980). A new role for complement in experimental membranous nephropathy in rats. *J. Clin. Invest.* **66**, 1339.

Salant, D.J., Adler, S., Darby, C. *et al.* (1985). Influence of antigen distribution on the mediation of immunological glomerular injury. *Kidney Int.* **27**, 938.

Salant, D.J., Quigg, R.J. and Cybulsky, A.V. (1989). Heymann nephritis: mechanisms of renal injury. *Kidney Int.* **35**, 976.

Sancho, J., Egido, J., Sanchez-Crespo, M. and Blasco, R. (1982).

Detection of monomeric and polymeric IgA containing immune complexes in serum and kidney from patients with alcoholic liver disease. *Clin. Exp. Immunol.* **47**, 327.

Sancho, J., Egido, J., Rivera, F. and Hernando, L. (1983). Immune complexes in IgA nephropathy: presence of antibodies against diet antigens and delayed clearance of specific polymeric IgA immune complexes. *Clin. Exp. Immunol.* **54**, 194.

Sandberg, D.H., McIntosh, R.M., Bernstein, C.W., Carr, R. and Strauss, J. (1977). Severe steroid-responsive nephrosis associated with hypersensitivity. *Lancet* **i**, 388.

Sapin, C., Druet, E. and Druet, P. (1977). Induction of anti-glomerular basement membrane antibodies in the Brown Norway rat by mercuric chloride. *Clin. Exp. Immunol.* **28**, 173.

Sato, M., Ideura, T. and Koshikawa, S. (1986). Experimental IgA nephropathy in mice. *Lab. Invest.* **54**, 377.

Saulsbury, F.T. (1987). The role of IgA rheumatoid factor in the formation of IgA-containing immune complexes in Henoch–Schönlein purpura. *J. Clin. Lab. Immunol.* **23**, 123.

Saus, J., Wieslander, J., Langeveld, J.P.M., Quinones, S. and Hudson, B.G. (1988). Identification of the Goodpasture antigen as the α3 (IV) chain of collagen IV. *J. Biol. Chem.* **263**, 13374.

Savage, C.O.S., Winearls, C.G., Evans, D.J., Rees, A.J. and Lockwood, C.M. (1985). Microscopic polyarteritis: presentation, pathology and prognosis. *Quart. J. Med.* **56**, 467.

Savage, C.O.S., Pusey, C.D., Bowman, C., Rees, A.J. and Lockwood, C.M. (1986). Anti-glomerular basement membrane antibody mediated disease in the British Isles 1980–1984. *Br. Med. J.* **292**, 301.

Savage, C.O.S., Winearls, C.G., Jones, S., Marshall, P.D. and Lockwood, C.M. (1987). Prospective study of radioimmunoassay for antibodies against neutrophil cytoplasm in diagnosis of systemic vasculitis. *Lancet* **i**, 1389.

Savage, C.O.S., Pottinger, B.E., Gaskin, G., Lockwood, C.M., Pusey, C.D. and Pearson, J.D. (1991). Vascular damage in Wegener's granulomatosis and microscopic polyarteritis: presence of anti-endothelial cell antibodies and their relation to anti-neutrophil cytoplasmic antibodies. *Clin. Exp. Immunol.* **85**, 14.

Scheer, R.L. and Grossman, M.A. (1964). Immune aspects of the glomerulonephritis associated with pulmonary hemorrhage. *Ann. Intern. Med.* **60**, 1009.

Schena, F.P., Pertosa, G., Stanziale, P., Vox, E., Pecoraro, C. and Andreucci, V.E. (1982). Biological significance of the C3 nephritic factor in membranoproliferative glomerulonephritis. *Clin. Nephrol.* **18**, 240.

Schena, F.P., Pertosa, G., Pastore, A., De-Tommasi, A., Montagna, M.T. and Bonomo, L. (1983). Circulating immune complexes in infected ventriculoatrial and ventriculoperitoneal shunts. *J. Clin. Immunol.* **3**, 173.

Schena, F.P., Mastrolitti, G. and Frasasso, A.R. (1986). Increased immunoglobulin secreting cells in the blood of patients with active idiopathic IgA nephropathy. *Clin. Nephrol.* **26**, 163.

Scher, I. (1982). CBA/N immune defective mice: evidence for the failure of a B cell subpopulation to be expressed. *Immunol. Rev.* **64**, 117.

Schifferli, J.A. and Taylor, R.P. (1989). Physiological and pathological aspects of circulating immune complexes. *Kidney Int.* **35**, 993.

Schifferli, J.A., Bartolotti, S.R. and Peters, D.K. (1980). Inhibition of immune precipitation by complement. *Clin. Exp. Immunol.* **42**, 387.

Schnaper, H.W. and Aune, T.M. (1985). Identification of the lymphokine soluble immune response suppressor in urine of nephrotic children. *J. Clin. Invest.* **76**, 341.

Schreiner, G.F., Cottran, R.S., Pando, V. and Unanue, E.R. (1978). A mononuclear cell component in experimental immunological glomerulonephritis. *J. Exp. Med.* **147**, 369.

Schulte-Wisserman, H., Lemmel, E.M., Reitz, M., Beck, J. and Straube, E. (1977). Nephrotic syndrome of childhood and disorder of T cell function. *Eur. J. Pediatr.* **124**, 121.

Scott, D.M., Amos, N., Sissons, J.G.P., Lachmann, P.J. and Peters, D.K. (1978). The immunoglobulin nature of nephritic factor (Nef). *Clin. Exp. Immunol.* **32**, 12.

Scott, D.M., Amos, N. and Bartolotti, S.R. (1981). The role of carbohydrate in the structure and function of nephritic factor. *Clin. Exp. Immunol.* **46**, 120.

Serra, A., Cameron, J.S., Turner, D.R. *et al.* (1984). Vasculitis affecting the kidney: presentation, histopathology and long-term outcome. *Quart. J. Med.* **53**, 181.

Shalhoub, R.J. (1974). Pathogenesis of lipoid nephrosis: a disorder of T cell function. *Lancet* **ii**, 556.

Sheth, K.J., Casper, J.T. and Good, T.A. (1977). Interstitial nephritis due to phenytoin hypersensitivity. *J. Pediatr.* **91**, 438.

Short, C.D., Dyer, P.A., Cairns, S.A. *et al.* (1983). A major histocompatibility system haplotype associated with poor prognosis in idiopathic membranous nephropathy. *Dis. Markers* **1**, 189.

Simpson, I.J., Amos, N., Evans, D.J., Thomson, N.M. and Peters, D.K. (1975). Guinea-pig nephrotoxic nephritis. I. The role of complement and polymorphonuclear leucocytes and effect of antibody subclass and fragments in heterologous phase. *Clin. Exp. Immunol.* **19**, 499.

Simpson, I.J., Moran, J., Evans, D.J. and Peters, D.K. (1978). Prolonged complement activation in mice. *Kidney Int.* **13**, 467.

Singer, D.R.J., Venning, M.C., Lockwood, C.M. and Pusey, C.D. (1986). Cryoglobulinaemia: clinical features and response to treatment. *Ann. Méd. Interne* **137**, 251.

Sinico, R.A., Fornasieri, A. and Oreni, M. (1986). Polymeric IgA rheumatoid factor in idiopathic IgA mesangial nephropathy (Berger's disease). *J. Immunol.* **137**, 536.

Sinniah, R. (1984). Heterogeneous IgA glomerulonephropathy in liver cirrhosis. *Histopathology* **8**, 947.

Sissons, J.G.P., West, R.J., Fallows, J. *et al.* (1976). The complement abnormalities of lipodystrophy. *N. Engl. J. Med.* **294**, 461.

Smith, H.R. and Steinberg, A.D. (1983). Autoimmunity — a perspective. *Ann. Rev. Immunol.* **1**, 175.

Specks, U., Wheatley, C.L., McDonald, T.J., Rohrbach, M.S. and De Remee, R.A. (1989). Anticytoplasmic antibodies in the diagnosis and follow-up of Wegener's granulomatosis. *Mayo Clin. Proc.* **64**, 28.

Spencer, S.J.W., Burns, A., Gaskin, G., Pusey, C.D. and Rees, A.J. (1992). HLA class II specificities in the vasculitis with antibodies to neutrophil cytoplasmic antigens. *Kidney Int.* **41**, 1059.

Spitzer, R.E., Vallota, E.H., Forristal, J. *et al.* (1969). Serum C3 lytic system in patients with glomerulonephritis. *Science* **164**, 436.

Srivastava, R.N., Agarwal, R.K., Mondgil, A. and Bhuyan, U.N. (1986). Late resistance to corticosteroids in nephrotic syndrome. *J. Pediatr.* **108**, 66.

Stachura, I., Si, L. and Whitside, T.L. (1984). Mononuclear-cell subsets in human idiopathic crescentic glomerulonephritis (ICGN): analysis in tissue sections with monoclonal antibodies. *J. Clin. Immunol.* **4**, 202.

Stanton, M.C. and Tange, J.D. (1958). Goodpasture's syndrome: pulmonary haemorrhage associated with glomerulonephritis. *Aust. Ann. Med.* **7**, 132.

Steblay, R.W. (1962). Glomerulonephritis induced in sheep by injections of heterologous glomerular basement membrane and Freund's complete adjuvant. *J. Exp. Med.* **116**, 253.

Steblay, R.W. (1963). Glomerulonephritis induced in monkeys by injections of heterologous glomerular basement membrane and Freund's adjuvant. *Nature* **197**, 1173.

Steblay, R.W. and Rudofsky, U. (1968a). *In vitro* and *in vivo* properties of autoantibodies eluted from kidneys of sheep with autoimmune glomerulonephritis. *Nature* **218**, 1269.

Steblay, R.W. and Rudofsky, U. (1968b). Autoimmune glomerulonephritis induced in sheep by injections of human lung and Freund's adjuvant. *Science* **160**, 204.

Steblay, R.W. and Rudofsky, U. (1971). Renal tubular disease and autoantibodies against tubular basement membrane induced in guinea pigs. *J. Immunol.* **107**, 589.

Steblay, R.W. and Rudofsky, U. (1973). Transfer of experimental autoimmune renal cortical tubular and interstitial disease in guinea pigs by serum. *Science* **180**, 966.

Steinman, T.I. and Silva, P. (1984). Acute interstitial nephritis and iritis: reno-ocular syndrome. *Am. J. Med.* **77**, 189.

Stenglein, B., Thoenes, G.H. and Gunther, E. (1978). Genetic control of susceptibility to autologous immune complex glomerulonephritis in inbred rat strains. *Clin. Exp. Immunol.* **33**, 88.

Stetson, C.A., Rammelkamp, C.H., Krause, R.M., Kohen, R.J. and Perry, W.D. (1955). Epidemic acute nephritis: studies on etiology, natural history and prevention. *Medicine* **34**, 431.

Strom, T.B. and Kelly, V.E. (1989). Towards more selective therapies to block undesired immune responses. *Kidney Int.* **35**, 1026.

Stuffers-Heiman, M., Gunther, E. and Van Es, L.A. (1979). Induction of autoimmunity to antigens of the glomerular basement membrane in inbred Brown Norway rats. *Immunology* **36**, 759.

Sugisaki, T., Klassen, J., Milgrom, F., Andres, G.A. and McCluskey, R.T. (1973). Immunologic study of an autoimmune tubular and interstitial renal disease in Brown Norway rats. *Lab. Invest.* **28**, 658.

Takata, Y., Tamura, N. and Fujita, T. (1984). Interaction of C3 with antigen–antibody complexes in the process of solubilization of immune precipitates. *J. Immunol.* **132**, 2531.

Tarantino, A., Anelli, A., Costantino, A., De Vecchi, A., Monti, G. and Massaro, L. (1978). Serum complement pattern in essential mixed cryoglobulinaemia. *Clin. Exp. Immunol.* **32**, 77.

Tarantino, A., De Vecchi, A., Montagnino, G. *et al.* (1981). Renal disease in essential mixed cryoglobulinaemia: long-term follow-up of 44 patients. *Quart. J. Med.* **50**, 1.

Taube, D., Chapman, S., Brown, Z. and Williams, D.G. (1981). Depression of normal lymphocyte transformation by sera of patients with minimal change nephropathy and other forms of nephrotic syndrome. *Clin. Nephrol.* **15**, 286.

Teitlebaum, D., Rauch, J., Stollar, B.D. and Schwartz, R.S. (1984). *In vivo* effects of antibodies against a high frequency idiotype of anti-DNA antibodies in MRL mice. *J. Immunol.* **132**, 1282.

Tejani, A., Nicastri, A.D., Sen, D., Chen, C.K. and Butt, K.M.H. (1983). Long term evaluation of children with nephrotic syndrome and focal segmental glomerulosclerosis. *Nephron* **35**, 225.

Tejani, A., Phadke, K., Nicastri, A. *et al.* (1985). Efficacy of cyclophosphamide in steroid sensitive nephrotic syndrome with different morphological lesions. *Nephron* **41**, 170.

Tejani, A., Butt, K., Trachtman, H., Suthanthiran, M. and Madras, P.N. (1987). Cyclosporin induced remission of relapsing nephrotic syndrome in children. *J. Pediatr.* **111**, 1056.

Theofilopoulos, A.N., Prud'homme, G.J., Fieser, T.M. and Dixon, F.J. (1983). B-cell hyperactivity in murine lupus. II. Defects in response to and production of accessory signals in lupus-prone mice. *Immunol. Today* **4**, 317.

Thomson, N.M., Naish, P.F., Simpson, I.J. and Peters, D.K. (1976). The role of C3 in the autologous phase of nephrotoxic nephritis. *Clin. Exp. Immunol.* **24**, 464.

Thomson, N.M., Holdsworth, S.R., Glasgow, E.F. and Atkins, R.C. (1979). The macrophage in the development of experimental crescentic glomerulonephritis. *Am. J. Pathol.* **94**, 223.

Tipping, P.G., Neale, T.J. and Holdsworth, S.R. (1985). T lymphocyte participation in antibody induced experimental glomerulonephritis. *Kidney Int.* **27**, 530.

Tipping, P.G., Boyce, N.W. and Holdsworth, S.R. (1989). Relative contributions of chemoattractant and terminal components of complement to anti-glomerular basement membrane (GBM) glomerulonephritis. *Clin. Exp. Immunol.* **78**, 444.

Todd, J.A., Acha-Orbea, H., Bell, J.I. *et al.* (1988). A molecular basis for MHC class II associated autoimmunity. *Science* **240**, 1003.

Tomino, Y., Endoh, M., Nomoto, Y. and Sakai, H. (1982a). Specificity of eluted antibody from renal tissues of patients with IgA nephropathy. *Am. J. Kidney Dis.* **1**, 276.

Tomino, Y., Sakai, H., Miura, M., Endoh, M. and Nomoto, Y. (1982b). Detection of polymeric IgA in glomeruli from patients with IgA nephropathy. *Clin. Exp. Immunol.* **49**, 419.

Tomizawa, S., Suzuki, S., Oguri, M. and Kuroume, T. (1979). Studies of T lymphocytes function and inhibitory factors in minimal change nephrotic syndrome. *Nephron* **24**, 179.

Tomizawa, S., Mariiyama, K., Nagasawa, N., Susuki, S. and Kuroume, T. (1985). Studies of vascular permeability factor derived from T lymphocytes and inhibitory effect of plasma on its production of minimal change nephrotic syndrome. *Nephron* **41**, 157.

Tomosugi, N.I., Cashman, S.J., Hay, H. *et al.* (1989). Modulation of antibody-mediated glomerular injury *in vivo* by bacterial lipopolysaccharide, tumour necrosis factor and IL-1. *J. Immunol.* **142**, 3083.

Tornroth, T. and Skrifvars, B. (1974). Gold nephropathy prototype of membranous glomerulonephritis. *Am. J. Pathol.* **75**, 573.

Tron, F. and Bach, J.F. (1977). Relationship between antibodies to native DNA and glomerulonephritis in systemic lupus erythematosus. *Clin. Exp. Immunol.* **28**, 426.

Tsai, C.D., Giangiacormo, J. and Zuckner, J. (1975). Dermal IgA deposits in Henoch Schönlein purpura and Berger's nephritis. *Lancet* **i**, 342.

Turner, N., Mason, P.J., Brown, R. *et al.* (1992). Molecular cloning of the human Goodpasture antigen demonstrates it to be the α3 chain of type IV collagen. *J. Clin. Invest.* **89**, 592.

Ulich, T.R. and Ni, R.-X. (1986). Inhibition of experimental autoimmune tubulointerstitial nephritis in Brown Norway rats by (155)-15-methyl prostaglandin E1. *Am. J. Pathol.* **124**, 286.

Unanue, E.R. and Dixon, F.J. (1967). Experimental glomerulonephritis: immunological events and pathogenetic mechanisms. *Adv. Immunol.* **6**, 1.

Unanue, E.R., Dixon, F.J. and Feldman, J.D. (1967). Experimental allergic glomerulonephritis induced in the rabbit with homologous renal antigens. *J. Exp. Med.* **125**, 163.

Valentijin, R.M., Radl, J., Haaijman, J.J. *et al.* (1984). Circulating and mesangial secretory component-binding IgA-1 in primary IgA nephropathy. *Kidney Int.* **26**, 760.

Van Damme, B.J.C., Fleuren, G.J., Bakker, W.W., Vernier, R.L. and Hoedemaeker, P.J. (1978). Experimental glomerulonephritis in the rat induced by antibodies directed against tubular antigens. V. Fixed glomerular antigens in the pathogenesis of heterologous immune complex glomerulonephritis. *Lab. Invest.* **38**, 502.

Van den Wall Bake, A.W., Daha, M.R., Haaijman, J.J., Radl, J., Van der Ark, A. and Van Es, L.A. (1989). Elevated production of polymeric and monomeric IgA1 by the bone marrow in IgA nephropathy. *Kidney Int.* **35**, 1400.

Van de Rijn, I., Fillit, H., Brandeis, W.E. *et al.* (1978). Serial studies on circulating immune complexes in post-streptococcal sequelae. *Clin. Exp. Immunol.* **34**, 318.

Van der Woude, F.J., Rasmussen, N., Lobatto, S. *et al.* (1985). Autoantibodies against neutrophils and monocytes: tool for diagnosis and marker of disease activity in Wegener's granulomatosis. *Lancet* **i**, 425.

Vanhaesebrouck, P., Carton, D., DeBel, C., Praet, M. and Proesmans, W. (1985). Acute tubular interstitial nephritis and uveitis syndrome (TINU Syndrome). *Nephron* **40**, 418.

Verroust, P.J., Wilson, C.B. and Dixon, F.J. (1974). Lack of nephritogenicity of systemic activation of the alternative complement pathway. *Kidney Int.* **6**, 157.

Verroust, P.J., Ronco, P.M. and Chatelet, F. (1986). Monoclonal antibodies and identification of glomerular antigens. *Kidney Int.* **30**, 649.

Vignon, J.D., Houssin, A., Soulillou, J.P., Denis, J., Guimbretiere, J. and Guenel, J. (1980). HLA antigens and Berger's disease. *Tissue Antigens* **16**, 108.

Villareal, H., Fischetti, V.A., Van der Rijn, I. and Zabriskie, J.B. (1979). The occurrence of a protein in the extracellular products of streptococci isolated from patients with acute glomerulonephritis. *J. Exp. Med.* **149**, 459.

Vogt, A., Rohrbach, R., Shimizu, F., Takamiya, H. and Batsford, S. (1982). Interaction of cationised antigen with rat glomerular basement membrane: *in situ* immune complex formation. *Kidney Int.* **22**, 27.

Vogt, A., Batsford, S., Rodriguez-Iturbe, B. and Garcia, R. (1983). Cationic antigens in poststreptococcal glomerulonephritis. *Clin. Nephrol.* **20**, 271.

Walker, R.G., Scheinkesterl, C., Becker, G.J., Owen, J.E., Dowling, J.P. and Kincaid-Smith, P. (1985). Clinical and morphological aspects of the management of crescentic anti-glomerular basement membrane (GBM) nephritis/Goodpasture's syndrome. *Quart. J. Med.* **54**, 75.

Walport, M.J., Black, C.M. and Batchelor, J.R. (1982). The immunogenesis of SLE. *Clin. Rheum. Dis.* **8**, 3.

Walport, M.J., Ross, G.D., Mackworth-Young, C., Watson, J.V., Hogg, N. and Lachmann, P.J. (1985a). Family studies of erythrocyte complement receptor type I levels: reduced levels in patients with SLE are acquired, not inherited. *Clin. Exp. Immunol.* **59**, 547.

Walport, M.J., Peters, A.M., Elkon, K.B., Pusey, C.D., Lavender, J.P. and Hughes, G.R.V. (1985b). The splenic extraction ratio of antibody coated erythrocytes and its response to plasma exchange and pulse methylprednisolone. *Clin. Exp. Immunol.* **60**, 465.

West, C.D. (1986). Childhood membranoproliferative glomerulonephritis: an approach to management. *Kidney Int.* **29**, 1077.

West, M.L., Jindal, K.K., Bear, R.A. and Goldstein, M.B. (1987). A controlled trial of cyclophosphamide in patients with membranous glomerulonephritis. *Kidney Int.* **32**, 579.

White, R.H.R. (1973). The familial nephrotic syndrome. I. A European survey. *Clin. Nephrol.* **1**, 215.

Wieslander, J., Bygren, P.G. and Heinegard, D. (1981). Anti-basement membrane antibody: immunoenzymic assay and specificity of antibodies. *Scand. J. Clin. Invest.* **41**, 763.

Wieslander, J., Bygren, P.G. and Heinegard, D. (1984). Isolation of the specific glomerular basement membrane antigen involved in Goodpasture's syndrome. *Proc. Nat. Acad. Sci. (USA)* **81**, 1544.

Wilson, C.B. (1981). Nephritogenic antibody mechanisms involving antigens within the glomerulus. *Immunol. Rev.* **55**, 257.

Wilson, C.B. and Dixon, F.J. (1970). Antigen quantitation in experimental immune complex glomerulonephritis. *J. Immunol.* **105**, 279.

Wilson, C.B. and Dixon, F.J. (1971). Quantitation of acute and chronic serum sickness in the rabbit. *J. Exp. Med.* **134**, 75.

Wilson, C.B. and Dixon, F.J. (1973). Anti-glomerular basement membrane antibody induced glomerulonephritis. *Kidney Int.* **3**, 74.

Wilson, J.G., Wong, W.W., Schur, P.H. and Fearon, D.T. (1982). Mode of inheritance of decreased C3b receptors on erythrocytes of patients with systemic lupus erythematosus. *N. Engl. J. Med.* **307**, 981.

Winfield, J.B. (1983). Cryoglobulinaemia. *Hum. Pathol.* **14**, 350.

Wittig, H.J. and Goldman, A.S. (1970). Nephrotic syndrome associated with inhaled allergens. *Lancet* **i**, 542.

Wofsy, D. and Seaman, W.E. (1986). Successful treatment of autoimmunity in NZB/NZW F1 mice with monoclonal antibody to L3T4. *J. Exp. Med.* **161**, 378.

Wofsy, D., Ledbetter, J.A., Hendlar, P.L. and Seaman, W.E. (1985). Treatment of murine lupus with monoclonal anti-T cell antibody. *J. Immunol.* **134**, 852.

Woo, K.T., Edmondson, R.P.S. and Yap, H.K. (1987). Effects of triple therapy on the progression of mesangial proliferative glomerulonephritis. *Clin. Nephrol.* **27**, 56.

Woodroffe, A.J., Gormly, A.A., McKenzie, P.E. *et al.* (1980). Immunologic studies in IgA nephropathy. *Kidney Int.* **18**, 366.

Wooley, P.H., Griffin, J., Panayi, G.S., Batchelor, J.R., Welsh, K.I. and Gibson, T.J. (1980). HLA-DR antigens and toxic reaction to sodium aurothiomalate and D-penicillamine in patients with rheumatoid arthritis. *N. Engl. J. Med.* **303**, 300.

Wraith, D.C., McDevitt, H.O., Steinman, L. and Acha-Orbea, H. (1989). T cell recognition as the target for immune intervention in autoimmune disease. *Cell* **57**, 709.

Wyatt, R.J., Valenski, W. and Stapleton, F.B. (1988). Immunoregulatory studies in patients with IgA nephropathy. *J. Clin. Lab. Immunol.* **25**, 109.

Yamamoto, T. and Wilson, C.B. (1987a). Complement dependence of antibody-induced mesangial cell injury in the rat. *J. Immunol.* **138**, 3758.

Yamamoto, T. and Wilson, C.B. (1987b). Binding of anti-basement membrane antibody to alveolar basement membrane after intratracheal gasoline instillation in rabbits. *Am. J. Pathol.* **126**, 497.

Yum, M.N., Edwards, J.L. and Kleit, S. (1975). Glomerular lesions in Hodgkin's disease. *Arch. Pathol.* **99**, 645.

Zakheim, B., McCafferty, E., Phillips, S.M., Clayman, M. and Neilson, E.G. (1984). Murine interstitial nephritis. II. The adoptive transfer of disease with immune T lymphocytes produces a phenotypically complex interstitial lesion. *J. Immunol.* **133**, 234.

Zanetti, M., Mandet, C., Duboust, A., Bedrossian, J. and Bariety, J. (1981). Demonstration of a passive Heymann nephritis-like mechanism in a human kidney transplant. *Clin. Nephrol.* **15**, 272.

Zanetti, M., Mampaso, F. and Wilson, C.B. (1983). Anti-idiotype as a probe in the analysis of autoimmune tubulointerstitial nephritis in the Brown Norway rat. *J. Immunol.* **131**, 1268.

100: Acute and Chronic Viral Hepatitis

H.C. Thomas

Many of the immunological phenomena associated with both acute and chronic liver disease are secondary to liver damage and have no primary pathogenic significance. Changes of diagnostic and possibly pathogenic significance in each disease state will be emphasized.

Hepatitis A

Hepatitis A is caused by a picornavirus that replicates within the liver, is excreted in the stool (Dienstag *et al.* 1976) and evokes a strong antibody response. A rapid rise in immunoglobulin M (IgM) antibody titre, which occurs at the onset, is of diagnostic use (Fig. 100.1). This antibody lasts for 3–6 months (Bradley *et al.* 1979). Immunoglobulin G antibodies are present in high titre from the clinical onset and remain for life, conferring protective immunity. The virus neutralizing antibody is directed to a conformational determinant, including sequences from the VP1 and 3 capsid peptides (Hughes *et al.* 1984; S. Lemon 1989, pers. comm.). The majority of the antibody is directed to a limited number of epitopes (MacGregor *et al.* 1983; Dawson *et al.* 1984). In North America and Western Europe, by middle age, 40–50% of people have immunity (Frosner *et al.* 1979). The prevalence of infection increases by 10% per decade of life (Frosner *et al.* 1979). The infection rate is greater in developing countries: in most tropical areas of Africa, more than 90% of the population will have immunity by 10 years of age (Wankya *et al.* 1979).

The virus probably replicates initially in intestinal epithelial cells and subsequently in hepatocytes. This is supported by the observation that in marmosets hepatitis A virus (HAV) antigens and ribonucleic acid (RNA) can be detected in the enterocytes of the upper jejunum as well as in the liver (Karayiannis *et al.* 1986, 1988), but replicative intermediates have not yet been identified in either tissue. There is an IgA-class antibody response within the intestinal mucosa (Karayiannis *et al.* 1988), and it is likely that this is important in conferring protective immunity against enteric challenge.

Cell-mediated immunity to the virus capsid antigens has been demonstrated (Fasel-Felley *et al.* 1986). Whether the liver damage is caused by a cytopathic effect of the virus or by cell-mediated immune responses directed to viral determinants on the infected hepatocytes has not been established.

During the acute phase of the infection, serum IgM concentrations increase (Thomas 1981), probably caused by an alteration in immunoregulatory cell function: CD4 : CD8 ratios are increased during the acute phase of the illness (Thomas 1981). Circulating immune complexes are present

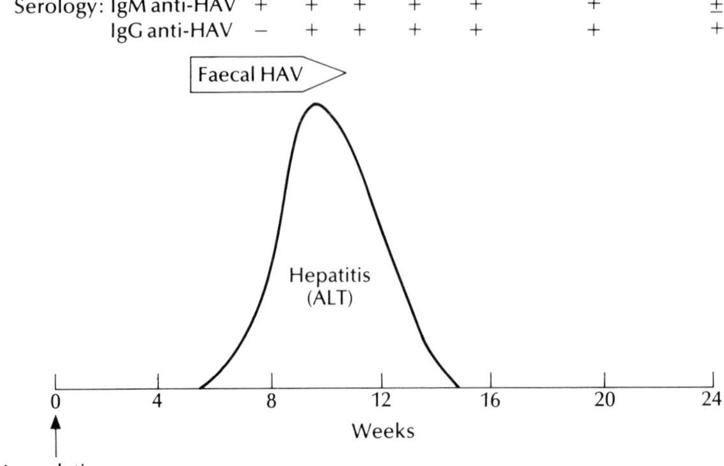

Fig. 100.1. Acute HAV infection. Immunoglobulin M class antibody is present during the acute and convalescent phases. Virus shedding in the stool precedes the onset of hepatitis.

(Thomas *et al.* 1978) but their composition is unknown. Low-titre smooth-muscle antibody is often present (Adjukiewicz *et al.* 1978). Low-titre IgM-class liver membrane antibodies (LMA) are found in most patients (Wiedmann *et al.* 1984) and may be causatively related to the piecemeal necrosis that is seen in most of these patients (Teixeira *et al.* 1982). Although protracted hepatitis has been described (Bamber *et al.* 1981; Jacobsen *et al.* 1985), chronic infection and chronic hepatitis are not seen.

Household contacts can be protected by administering immune serum globulin, 0.02 ml/kg intramuscularly (IM), within 10 days of presentation of the index case. The virus has been grown in tissue culture (Provost and Hilleman 1979) and progress has been made in developing attenuated strains. A formaldehyde-inactivated tissue culture-derived vaccine has been shown to be immunogenic in man and is now being evaluated in field trials.

Hepatitis B and D

Acute infection

Hepatitis B virus (HBV) is not cytopathic and the liver damage is caused by immune lysis of infected hepatocytes, an essential part of the recovery process. Analysis of the inflammatory infiltrate demonstrates the presence of non-specific killer (NK) and cytotoxic T (T_c) cells (Eggink *et al.* 1982; Montano *et al.* 1983). Viral antigens on the surface of the hepatocyte (Gudat *et al.* 1975) and peptides derived from these, in association with the Class I major histocompatibility complex (MHC) glycoproteins, make the cell a target for antibody-dependent or T_c cell lysis (Doherty and Zinkernagel 1975). Studies in patients with chronic HBV infection suggest that the nucleocapsid antigens hepatitis B core (HBc) and hepatitis Be (HBe) — a cleavage product of the precore/core protein — are important targets (Eddleston *et al.* 1982; Pignatelli *et al.* 1987). Hepatocytes usually express very little Class I MHC glycoprotein (Thomas *et al.* 1982a, b) but, in the early stage of acute HBV infection, following the production of interferon alpha (IFN-α), MHC expression on hepatocytes increases and simultaneously transaminases rise (Pignatelli *et al.* 1986) (Fig. 100.2). Interferon-α also activates the 2-5A oligoadenylate synthetase/endonuclease and protein kinase systems, which lead to inhibition of viral protein synthesis (Fig. 100.3(a)). This will produce an antiviral state in uninfected regenerating liver cells, preventing infection with virus shed during the lysis of infected hepatocytes.

Virus-neutralizing antibodies are directed to epitopes on the envelope of the virus. This is composed of three polypeptides, each with the same carboxyl terminus (Fig. 100.4). These are designated the large, middle and small (major) envelope proteins. The amino-terminal 119 amino acid (aa) region of the large protein, which is not present in the middle and small proteins, is designated pre-S1. This hydrophilic area is myristilated and recent data indicate that the region 12–32 aa is capable of binding to the membrane of the hepatocyte (Neurath *et al.* 1986) and is, therefore, probably involved in virus uptake. The pre-S2 region

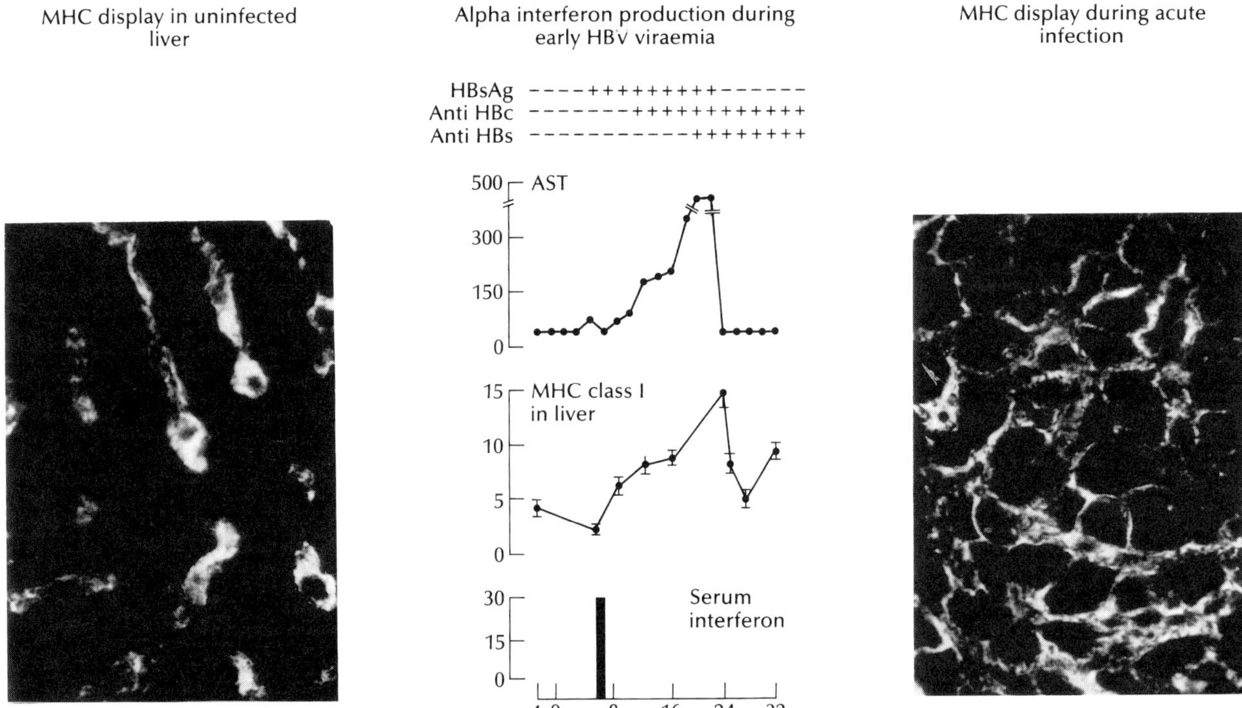

Fig. 100.2. Acute HBV infection in the chimpanzee. Markers of virus infection appear early, coinciding with a detectable pulse of circulating alpha interferon (IFN). This is followed by enhanced display of Class I MHC antigen on hepatocytes (Pignatelli *et al.* 1986). Liver damage as indicated by rising AST coincides with the first appearance of host humoral immunity to HBV (IgM anti-HBc). AST: aspartate aminotransferase (SGOT — a serum glutamic oxaloacetic transaminase).

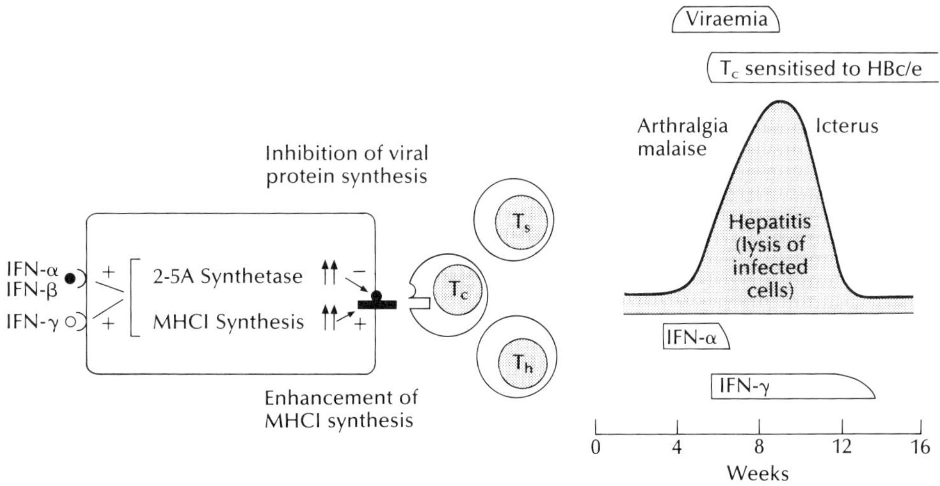

Fig. 100.3. Effect of IFNs on the virus-infected cell. Interferon-α and IFN-β acting through a common receptor and IFN-γ acting through a separate receptor activate (+) 2-5A oligoadenylate synthetase. This catalyses production of oligoadenylates, which activate an endogenous ribonuclease, leading to cleavage of viral RNA. Interferon also causes enhanced (+) expression of Class I MHC (HLA) proteins on the hepatocyte surface, facilitating recognition of virus-infected cells by the cellular immune mechanisms of the host. HBe and HBc antigens are the target of this component of the host immune response. T_c, T_s, T_h: cytotoxic, suppressor and helper T cells (+ and − denote enhancement and suppression, respectively).

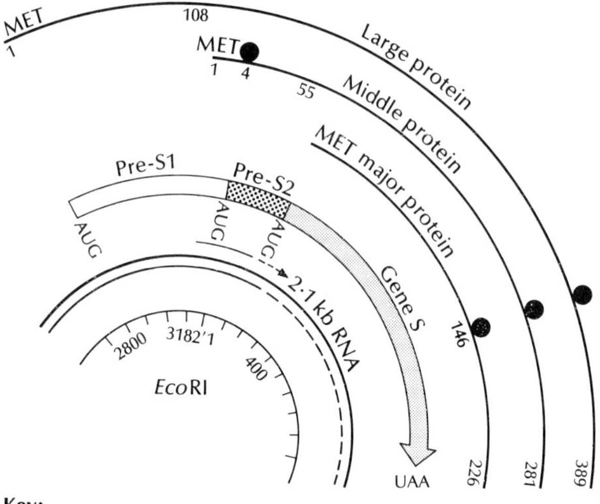

Fig. 100.4. The large, middle and small (major) proteins of the envelope of HBV have the same carboxyl terminal sequence. (MET, methionine.)

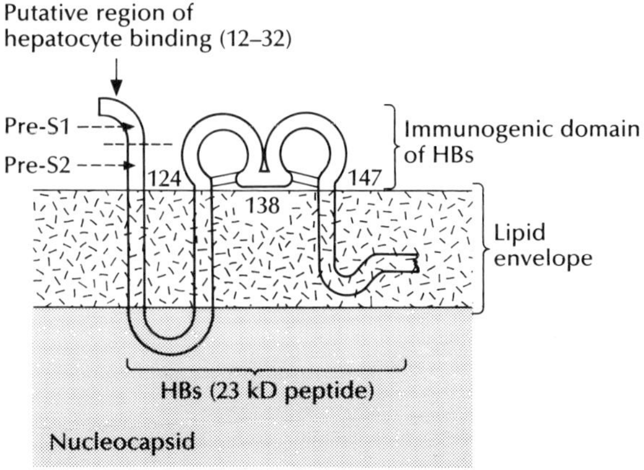

Fig. 100.5. The hydrophilic regions of the pre-S and S gene products are potential immunogenic regions. The pre-S1 amino-terminal sequence binds to the hepatocyte membrane. Antibodies to pre-S1 and the region 124–137 of HBs peptide inhibit infection.

of 55 aa, present in the large and middle proteins, binds polymerized human serum albumin (pHSA) (Machida *et al.* 1983). Because this protein also binds selectively to the hepatocytes of species that are susceptible to HBV infection and not to non-susceptible species (Trevisan *et al.* 1982), it has been proposed that pHSA acts as a bridge between the pre-S2 region of the viral envelope and the hepatocyte, facilitating uptake and infection of the cell. More recent observations showing that pHSA is not present in serum and that native albumin in physiological concentrations blocks the binding of pHSA to hepatitis B surface (HBs) antigen (Ishihara *et al.* 1987) make this hypothetical uptake system unlikely to occur *in vivo* in man.

The envelope antibodies found in convalescent serum bind predominantly to the epitopes of the HBs gene-encoded region (Brown *et al.* 1984), the carboxyl terminal region of which is present in all the envelope proteins. The hydrophilic region of this polypeptide, aa 124–147 (Fig. 100.5), forms loops because of intramolecular disulphide bridges and these are the binding regions for the majority (>80%) of the antigen-binding capacity of the convalescent sera. Using monoclonal antibodies binding to these regions (Waters *et al.* 1986), it has been possible to show that administration to chimpanzees of antibody to the region 124–136 prevents infection (Iwarson *et al.* 1985). Antibodies to this region, as well as to other epitopes on the S gene-encoded polypeptide, are present in the serum of patients convalescent from HBV infection and in normal subjects immunized with plasma-derived and recombinant deoxyribonucleic acid (DNA)-produced HBs vaccine (Thomas *et al.* 1987).

Although patients vaccinated with HBs antigen alone are protected from further infection, there has been considerable debate on whether the middle pre-S2-bearing and large pre-S1-bearing polypeptides should be added to existing vaccines. During natural infection, antibodies to pre-S1 and pre-S2 regions appear before antibodies to the HBs region (Neurath *et al.* 1985; Petit *et al.* 1986) and, if pre-S1 is the region of the envelope of the virus that binds to the hepatocyte during infection (Neurath *et al.* 1986), antibodies to this region might be virus-neutralizing and therefore inclusion of the pre-S region in a vaccine might be desirable. Furthermore, 15% of normal individuals do not respond to HBs small (major) polypeptide, and inclusion of pre-S2 facilitates, by recruiting additional helper T (T_H) cells, the development of antibody to the HBs epitopes (Milich *et al.* 1985). More recent data indicate that the inclusion of HBc antigen with HBs antigen further enhances the humoral response to HBs epitopes (Milich *et al.* 1987) (Fig. 100.6).

The recent description of the appearance of escape mutants of HBV in immunized children born to chronically infected mothers (Zanetti *et al.* 1988)

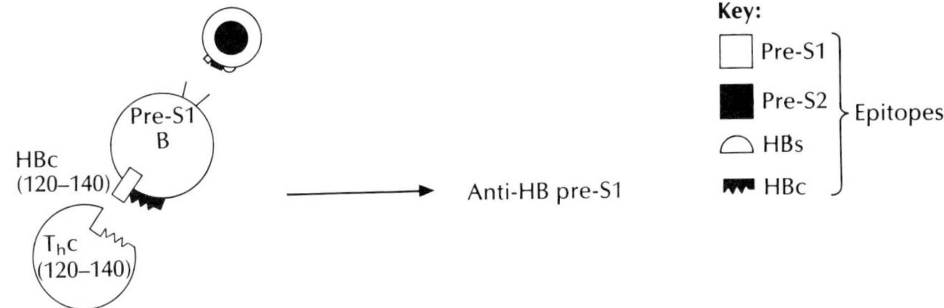

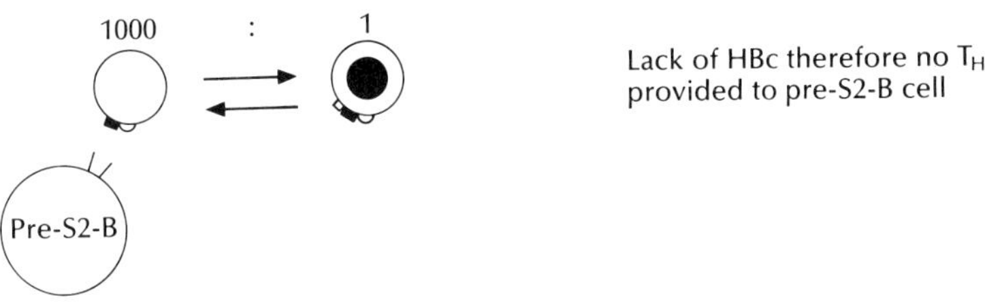

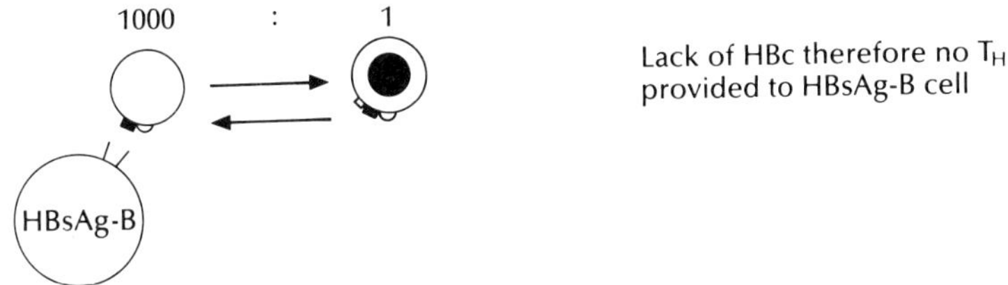

Fig. 100.6. Pre-S1 peptides are present in higher concentration in HBV particles than in non-infectious particles. Pre-S1-reactive B cells will bind and take up HBV particles more frequently than 22 nm HBs antigen particles. Hepatitis B core antigen within B cells will be processed and attract help from HBc-reactive T_h cells (Milich *et al.* 1987). Pre-S2- and S-reactive B cells will take up 22 nm particles as well as HBV and therefore will be less likely to be able to attract HBc-reactive T_h cells.

has focused attention on the adequacy of the current vaccines. One such mutant has been sequenced and shown to have undergone a glycine-to-arginine substitution at position 145 in the region of the 'a' determinant of the envelope proteins (Carman *et al.* 1990). This mutation destroys the antigenicity of the common determinants (Waters *et al.* 1992) and thus this variant is not neutralized by the anti-envelope response initiated by the HBs vaccines.

Chronic infection

It is likely that there are many different reasons why patients develop chronic infection.

CHRONIC HEPATITIS B VIRUS INFECTION FOLLOWING EXPOSURE IN NEONATAL LIFE

Ninety per cent of babies born to HBV 'e' antigen +ve mothers become infected, and over 90% of these develop a chronic carrier state (Fig. 100.7) (Beasley *et al.* 1982). These infants probably receive a large inoculum of virus from maternal blood before or during birth, and by close contact with secretions soon after birth. The reason for these infants failing to clear the virus is unknown but likely to relate to the immaturity of the neonatal immune system (Nash 1985). HBe antigen, a low-molecular-weight (15 kD) soluble protein, derived from the pre-core/core polypeptide by cleavage of both the amino- and carboxy-terminal ends, passes across the placenta and may suppress the development of the cellular immune response to the nucleocapsid proteins, which are the target during immune clearance of infected hepatocytes (Fig. 100.8) (Thomas *et al.* 1988). Support for this hypothesis has stemmed from the study of transgenic mice bearing the precore/core-encoding gene: the progeny of these mice, exposed at birth to HBe antigen, are tolerant to HBe and HBc at the T cell level but, because HBc may also function as a thymus-independent antigen, the mice develop anti-HBc (Milich *et al.* 1990).

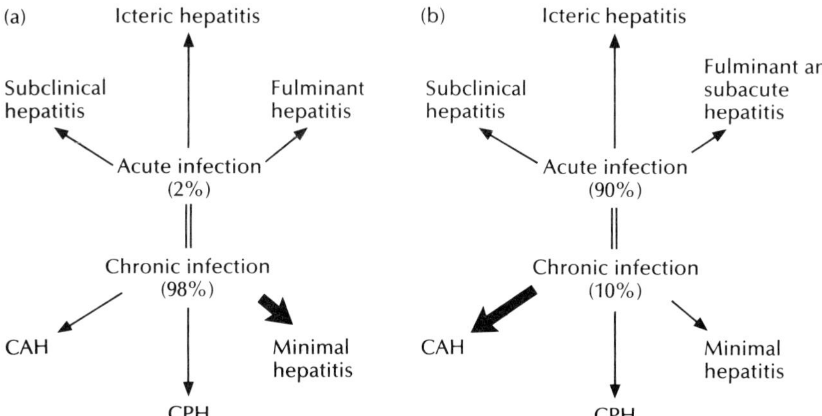

Fig. 100.7. Natural history of HBV infection after (a) neonatal or (b) adult exposure. CPH — chronic persistent hepatitis; CAH — chronic active hepatitis.

Rarely, children born to HBs antigen anti-HBe +ve mothers develop fulminant hepatitis. The mechanism is once again unknown. One hypothesis is that maternal anti-HBe and antiHBc pass across the placenta and initially modulate the lysis of infected hepatocytes by the cell-mediated immune response of the child (Pignatelli *et al.* 1987). The virus, it is argued, would spread throughout the liver and, as the maternal antibodies disappear at 3–6 months, T_c cells sensitized to HBe and HBc would then rapidly destroy the infected cells, resulting in hepatic failure. More recently it has been observed that many patients with fulminant hepatitis in adult life are infected with a variant of HBV which cannot encode the infected cell to produce HBe antigen (Carman *et al.* 1989, 1991); in the absence of the HBe antigen, clearance of infected cells is rapid and liver failure ensues. It is

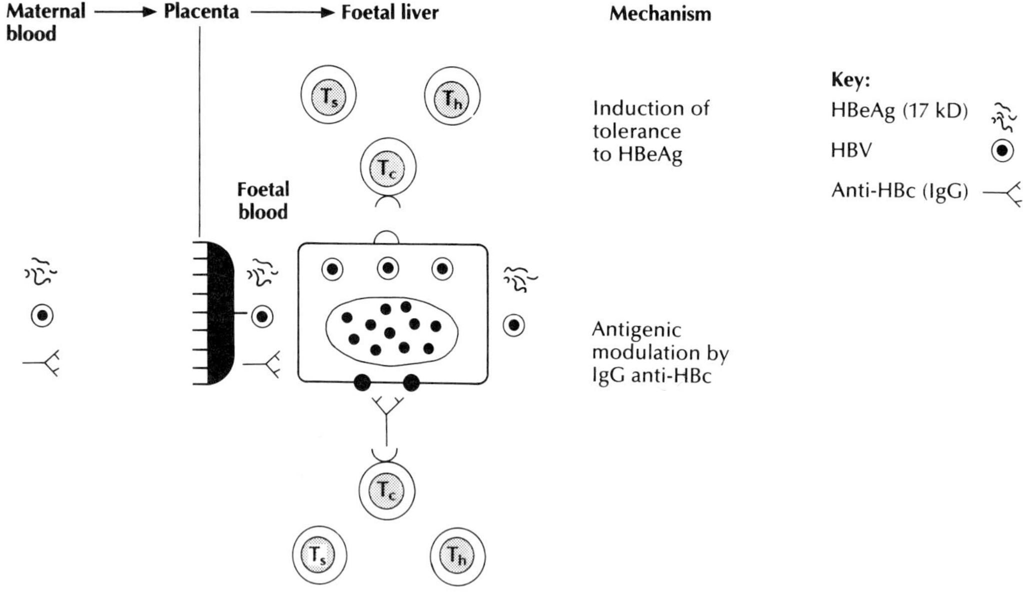

Fig. 100.8. Neonatal HBV infection: postulated mechanism of viral persistence. It is proposed that HBe antigen crosses the placenta from the maternal blood and in neonates and induces tolerance to HBe antigen, which is one of the targets of the cellular immune response. Maternal IgG anti-HBc also crosses the placenta into the neonatal circulation. Persistence of HBV-infected cells in the fetal liver is facilitated, as maternal IgG blocks recognition of virus-infected cells by cytotoxic T cells (Eddleston *et al.* 1982; Pignatelli *et al.* 1987). Early exposure to soluble virus protein (HBe) may induce a state of antigenic tolerance to the virus with specific suppressor cells inhibiting the host defence mechanism.

possible, but currently unproven, that this variant is also involved in the causation of fulminant hepatitis in the neonate.

CHRONIC HEPATITIS B VIRUS INFECTION FOLLOWING EXPOSURE AFTER THE NEONATAL PERIOD

In marked contrast to the situation at birth, after 2 years of age only 2–10% of subjects infected develop chronic infection (Fig. 100.7). There are probably several different causes for the development of chronic infection at this stage of life. One defect which has recently been documented is the production of subnormal quantities of IFN-α by peripheral blood mononuclear cells (Kato *et al.* 1982; Tolentino *et al.* 1985; Abb *et al.* 1985; Ikeda *et al.* 1986a). These individuals also have evidence of abnormal activation of their hepatocytes by IFN: levels of hepatic 2-5A synthetase (an enzyme induced by IFN) are only minimally elevated (Ikeda *et al.* 1986b), and Class I MHC glycoproteins, which are induced by IFN-α, are present in very low density on infected hepatocytes (Montano *et al.* 1982), whereas levels of 2-5A synthetase and Class I MHC display are markedly increased in peripheral blood lymphocytes of chronic HBV carriers (Poitrine *et al.* 1985). These data suggest interferon activation of peripheral blood lymphocytes but not of infected hepatocytes and raise the possibility that HBV within the hepatocyte has selectively 'switched off' the responsiveness of the hepatocyte to IFN. *In vitro* transfection of HBV genomes into cells in tissue culture makes them partially susceptible to lysis by Sindbis virus, and MHC induction by IFN does not occur (Onji *et al.* 1989). This inhibitory effect of HBV on the hepatocytes' response to IFN has now been shown to be caused by expression of the terminal protein of HBV at high levels within the hepatocyte. This protein stops the production of an IFN-inducible transcription regulating factor within the cell (Foster *et al.* 1991). Over-expression of this virally encoded protein may be a mechanism contributing to chronicity in some patients. Thus, during HBV replication, it is hypothesized that T cells cannot lyse infected cells because the virus suppresses the expression of Class I MHC glycoproteins.

IMMUNE SELECTION OF INFECTED HEPATOCYTES THAT CONTAIN INTEGRATED HEPATITIS B VIRUS SEQUENCES AND DO NOT EXPRESS NUCLEOCAPSID PROTEINS

Hepatocytes that contain integrated HBV sequences usually do not express HBV nucleocapsid proteins because the preferred site of integration within the viral genome is within the regulatory region of the gene encoding for this protein (Fowler *et al.* 1986) and thus HBc/e gene transcription is disrupted following integration (Fig. 100.9).

As the level of HBV replication within the hepatocytes falls, the suppression of MHC glycoprotein display is reduced and some cells are lysed by T_c cells. This reduction in hepatocyte mass constitutes a stimulus to the remaining hepatocytes, including those containing integrated HBV sequences, to

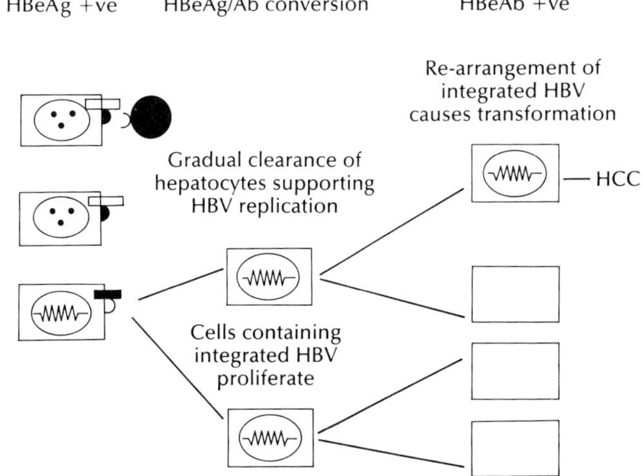

Fig. 100.9. During the HBe antigen +ve phase (left-hand column), hepatocytes containing HBV show suppression of Class I MHC antigen display and avoid T cell lysis. During the HBe antibody phase (right-hand column), hepatocytes containing integrated HBV sequences avoid T cell lysis because they do not express nucleocapsid proteins. HCC — hepatocellular carcinoma; • — HBV particles; ▲ membrane HBc antigen; ⌓ absent membrane HBc; ▮ membrane Class I MHC protein; ▯ suppressed Class I MHC protein.

divide. Ultimately, it is argued that during cell division the integrated sequences rearrange (Shafritz 1982) and cause malignant transformation of the hepatocyte. Clinically evident hepatocellular carcinoma then appears within months and the patients rapidly die.

IMMUNOLOGICAL ASPECTS OF THE TREATMENT OF CHRONIC HEPATITIS B VIRUS INFECTION

Carriers resulting from neonatal infection are resistant to all present attempts at treatment. Interferons are probably of no value in this group (Thomas and Scully 1985). Procedures to modify the immune response to the virus will be required to treat this subgroup. Preliminary data suggest that a short course of prednisolone, rapidly withdrawn, can precipitate rebound immune lysis of hepatocytes so that IFN-α given at this stage results in clearance of the virus (Perillo *et al.* 1988).

Patients who contract the infection later in life and who are actively replicating the virus (HBe antigen +ve) may be treated with either IFN-α or adenine arabinoside monophosphate (Thomas and Scully 1985; Weller *et al.* 1985). Both of these agents will reproducibly inhibit viral replication and, in cases with continuing immune competence, during the period of inhibition of viral replication, lysis of residual infected cells will occur. Lymphoblastoid IFN is effective in approximately 45% of patients, including homosexual as well as heterosexual cases (Thomas and Scully 1985). Adenine arabinoside monophosphate is effective only in the heterosexual group; the homosexual patients respond less frequently (Novick *et al.* 1985), probably because of secondary immunodeficiency (Regenstein *et al.* 1983).

Attempts at immunotherapy have largely been unsuccessful but this approach has the theoretical advantage of perhaps destroying clones of cells that contain integrated as well as replicating HBV (Thomas *et al.* 1982a).

HEPATITIS D VIRUS CO-INFECTION AND SUPERINFECTION DURING ACUTE AND CHRONIC HEPATITIS B VIRUS INFECTION

Hepatitis D virus (HDV) agent is an RNA virus that replicates only in patients with HBV infection. Both HDV and HBV may be introduced in the same inoculum (co-infection) (Fig. 100.10) and give rise to acute hepatitis with a 5–10% chance of chronicity. In other cases, HDV superinfects an established chronic HBV carrier (Fig. 100.10) and causes an acceleration of the course of the chronic hepatitis, so that the patient rapidly progresses to cirrhosis. Both co-infection and superinfection can, in the acute phase, be diagnosed by the demonstration of delta antigen or IgM anti-delta in the serum. In co-infection, but not in superinfection, high-titre IgM anti-HBc is also present. In chronic HDV infection, higher-titre IgG antibody to HDV is found and continuing IgM antibody responses are observed. Recent data demonstrate that im-

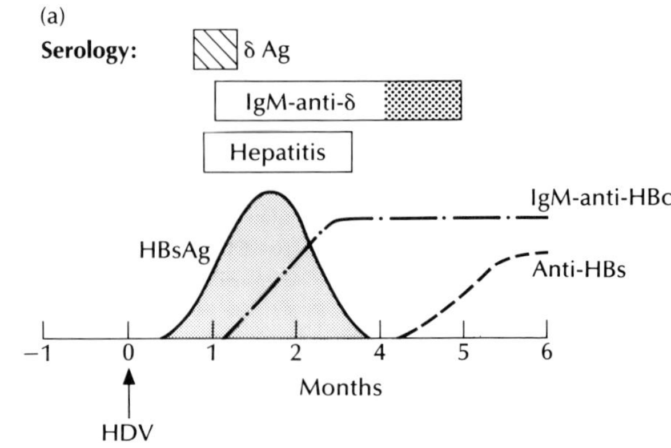

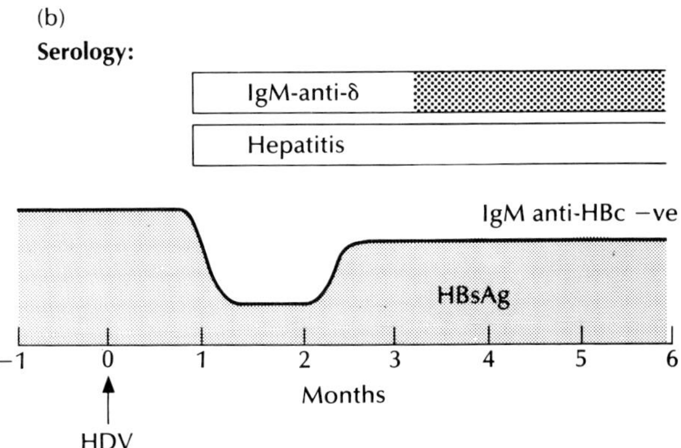

Fig. 100.10. (a) Co-infection of HBV and HDV. Immunoglobulin M-class antibodies to the nucleocapsid proteins of both viruses are present in the patients' serum. There may be one or two peaks of transaminase elevation. (b) Hepatitis D virus superinfection in a patient with established HBs antigenaemia. These patients are usually anti-HBe +ve. Immunoglobulin M-class anti-HDV is present and IgM anti-HBc absent.

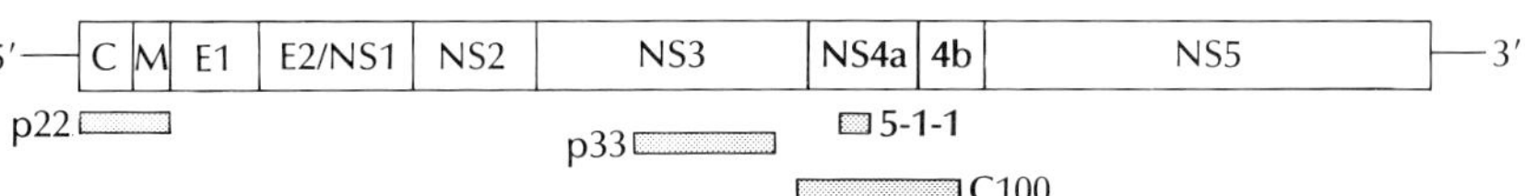

Fig. 100.11. Organization of genome of HCV. The major immunogenic regions are p22, p33 and C-100.

munization to HDV antigen results in more protracted and a higher-level viraemia (Karayiannis *et al.* 1990). Whether antibody facilitates uptake of HDV or inhibits the clearance process is unknown. Interferon alpha, given for a prolonged period, has been shown to control viraemia (Hoofnagle *et al.* 1987; Rosino *et al.* 1987; Thomas *et al.* 1987) but its clinical value remains to be determined.

Hepatitis E

An epidemic form of enterally transmitted non-A, non-B hepatitis has been described in Kashmir (Khuroo 1980) and North Africa (Belabbes *et al.* 1984). This form of the disease is similar to acute HAV infection. Whether the virus is the same as that causing sporadic non-A, non-B (Bamber *et al.* 1981) has not been established. The epidemic form is particularly severe in pregnant women. A virus particle has been identified in the stools and gallbladder bile of these patients, and a serum antibody of IgM class has been identified (Balayan *et al.* 1983; Kane *et al.* 1984). The virus genome has now been cloned and sequenced. The virus has a single positive-stranded RNA genome of approximately 10 000 bases with similarities to the caliciviruses (Reyes *et al.* 1990).

Hepatitis C

Post-transfusion (parenterally transmitted) non-A, non-B hepatitis is important in that, although the acute illness is mild, 20–80% of patients develop chronic infection, ultimately leading, in some cases, to cirrhosis. There are at least two parenterally transmitted viruses that can be differentiated by their physical characteristics (Bradley 1985).

One of the agents responsible for the majority of cases of post-transfusion hepatitis has recently been cloned and sequenced (Choo *et al.* 1989). This has been designated hepatitis C virus (HCV). The organization of the genome of HCV (Fig. 100.11) is similar to that of the pestiviridae. The structural and non-structural proteins have all been expressed and used to make antibody detection assays. The first assays detected antibody to the NS4 region (5-1-1 in figure 100.11): IgG antibody to this protein was detectable in the majority of patients with chronic post-transfusion hepatitis but, in an acute infection, did not appear until 2–6 months after infection (Kuo *et al.* 1989). More recent assays also detect antibody to the nucleocapsid (Dourakis *et al.* 1991) and additional nonstructural regions and became positive several weeks earlier in an acute infection.

The parenterally transmitted viruses are probably cytopathic. Low-titre smooth muscle antibody occurs, but hyperglobulinaemia is not evident until cirrhosis is present. A high incidence of antibodies to HCV has been reported in liver–kidney microsomal (LKM) antibody +ve (autoimmune) chronic hepatitis (type 2 autoimmune chronic hepatitis). It is hypothesized that HCV may initiate the formation of LKM antibodies and thus autoimmume liver damage. Confirmation of these results is required because of the possibility of false positivity of the antibody assay in patients with dysproteinaemia.

Treatment and prevention

Immune serum globulin may confer protection if given before blood transfusion (Knodell *et al.* 1977) or with clotting factor concentrates (Kernoff *et al.* 1985) (pre-exposure prophylaxis). Its value in preventing infection in needle-stick victims (post-exposure prophylaxis) is not proved. The dosage and use of immune serum globulin are currently under investigation: no definitive recommendations can be made at the present time.

Preliminary reports suggest that IFN-α may have some clinical value in patients with chronic non-A, non-B hepatitis. Low doses cause transaminases to return to normal but relapse rates are high (Hoofnagle *et al.* 1986; Jacyna *et al.* 1989).

References

Abb, J., Zachoval, R. and Eisenberg, J. (1985). Production of interferon alpha and interferon gamma by peripheral blood leucocytes from patients with chronic hepatitis B virus infection. *J. Med. Virol.* **16**, 171–6.

Adjukiewicz, A.B. *et al.* (1978). Immunological studies in an epidemic of infective short incubation hepatitis. *Lancet* **ii**, 380.

Balayan, M.S., Audjaparidze, A.G., Savinskaya, S.S. *et al.* (1983). Evidence for a virus in non-A, non-B hepatitis transmitted via the fecal–oral route. *Intervirology* **20**, 23–31.

Bamber, M., Murray, A., Arborgh, B.A. *et al.* (1981). Short incubation non-A, non-B hepatitis transmitted by factor VIII concentrates in patients with congenital coagulation disorders. *Gut* **22**, 854–9.

Beasley, R.P. (1982). Hepatitis B virus as the etiological agent in hepatocellular carcinoma — epidemiologic considerations. *Hepatology* **2**, 21S–26S.

Belabbes, H. *et al.* (1984). Non-A, non-B epidemic viral hepatitis in Algeria: strong evidence for its water spread. In *Viral Hepatitis and Liver Disease*, ed. G.N. Vyas, J.C. Dienstag and J.H. Hoofnagle, Grune and Stratton, New York.

Bradley, D.W. (1985). The agents of non-A non-B hepatitis. *J. Virol. Methods* **10**, 307–19.

Bradley, D.W., Fields, H.A., McCaustland, K.A. *et al.* (1979). Serodiagnosis of viral hepatitis A by a modified competitive binding radioimmunoassay for IgM anti-HAV. *J. Clin. Microbiol.* **9**, 120–7.

Brown, S.E., Howard, C.R., Zuckerman, A.J. and Steward, M.W. (1984). Affinity of antibody responses in man to hepatitis B vaccine determined with synthetic peptides. *Lancet* **ii**, 184–7.

Carman, W.F., Jacyna, M.R., Hadziyannis, S. *et al.* (1989). Mutation preventing formation of HBe antigen in patients with chronic HBV infection. *Lancet* **ii**, 588–91.

Carman, W.F., Zanetti, A.R., Karayiannis, P. *et al.* (1990). Vaccine induced escape mutants of hepatitis B virus. *Lancet* **336**, 325–9.

Carman, W.F., Fagan, E.A., Hadziyannis, S. *et al.* (1991). Association of precore genomic variants of hepatitis B virus with fulminant hepatitis. *Hepatology* **14**, 219–22.

Choo, Q.-L., Kuo, G., Weiner, A.J., Overby, L.R., Bradley, D.W. and Houghton, M. (1989). Isolation of a cDNA derived from a blood borne non-A non-B viral hepatitis genome. *Science* **244**, 259–362.

Dawson, G.J., Decker, R.H., Norton, D.K. *et al.* (1984). Monoclonal antibodies to hepatitis A virus. *J. Med. Virol.* **14**, 1–8.

Dienstag, J.L. *et al.* (1976). Hepatitis A antigen isolated from liver and stool: immunologic comparison of antigen prepared in guinea pigs. *J. Immunol.* **117**, 876–81.

Doherty, P.C. and Zinkernagel, R.M. (1975). A biological role for the major histocompatibility antigen. *Lancet* **i**, 1405–9.

Dourakis, S., Brown, J., Kumar, U. *et al.* (1991). Serological response and detection of viraemia in acute hepatitis C virus infection. *J. Hepatol.* (in press).

Eddleston, A.W.L.F., Mondelli, M., Mieli-Vergani, G. and Williams R. (1982). Lymphocyte cytotoxicity to autologous hepatocytes in chronic hepatitis B virus infection. *Hepatology* **2**, 122S–127S.

Eggink, H.F., Houthoff, H.J., Huitema, S., Gips, C.H. and Poppema, S. (1982). Cellular and humoral immune reactions in chronic active liver disease: lymphocyte subsets in liver biopsies of patients with untreated idiopathic autoimmune hepatitis, chronic active hepatitis B and primary biliary cirrhosis. *Clin. Exp. Immunol.* **50**, 17–24.

Fasel-Felley, J., Overby, L.R. and Frei, P.C. (1986). A specific immune response to purified HA antigen demonstrated by leukocyte migration inhibitors in patients recovering from viral hepatitis. *J. Hepatol.* **2**(2), 237–44.

Foster, G., Ackerill, A., Goldin, R., Kerr, I.M., Thomas, H.C. and Stark, G. (1991). Expression of the terminal protein region of HBV inhibits cellular responses to interferons alpha and gamma and double stranded RNA. *Proc. Nat. Acad. Sci. (USA)* **88**, 2888–92.

Fowler, M.J.F, Thomas, H.C. and Monjardino, J. (1986). Cloning and analysis of integrated hepatitis B virus of the adr subtype derived from a human primary liver cell carcinoma. *J. Gen. Virol.* **67**, 771–5.

Frosner, G.G., Papaevangelou, G., Butler, R. *et al.* (1979). Antibody against hepatitis A in seven European countries: comparison of prevalence data in different age groups. *Am. J. Epidemiol.* **110** (1), 63–9.

Gudat, F., Bianchi, L., Sonnabend, W. *et al.* (1975). Pattern of core and surface expression in liver tissue reflects state of immune response in hepatitis B. *J. Lab. Invest.* **32**, 1–9.

Hoofnagle, J.H., Mullen, K.D., Jones, B. *et al.* (1986). Treatment of chronic non-A, non-B hepatitis with recombinant human alpha interferon. *N. Engl. J. Med.* **315**, 1575–8.

Hoofnagle, J.H., Muller, K.D., Peters, M. *et al.* (1987). Treatment of chronic HDV with recombinant human alpha interferon. *Prog. Clin. Biol. Res.* **234**, 291–8.

Hughes, J.V., Stanton, L.W., Tomassini, J.E., Long, W.S. and Scolnick, E.M. (1984). Neutralising monoclonal antibodies to hepatitis A virus: partial localisation of a neutralising antigen site. *J. Virol.* **52**, 465–73.

Ikeda, T., Lever, A.M.L. and Thomas, H.C. (1986a). Evidence for a deficiency of IFN production in patients with chronic HBV infection acquired in adult life. *Hepatology* **6**, 962–5.

Ikeda, T., Pignatelli, M., Lever, A.M.L. and Thomas, H.C. (1986b). Relationship of HLA protein display to activation of 2-5A synthetase in HBe antigen or anti-HBe positive chronic HBV infection. *Gut* **27**, 1498–501.

Ishihara, K., Waters, J., Pignatelli, M. and Thomas, H.C. (1987). Characterisation of the polymerised and monomeric human serum albumin binding sites on hepatitis B surface antigen. *J. Med. Virol.* **21**, 89–95.

Iwarson, S., Tabor, E., Thomas, H.C. *et al.* (1985). Neutralisation of hepatitis B virus infectivity by a murine monoclonal antibody: an experimental study in the chimpanzee. *J. Med. Virol.* **16**, 89–96.

Jacobsen, I.M., Nath, B.J. and Dienstag, J.L. (1985). Relapsing viral hepatitis type A. *J. Med. Virol.* **16**, 163–9.

Jacyna, M.R., Brooks, M.G., Loke, R.H.T., Main, J., Murray-Lyon, I. and Thomas, H.C. (1989). Randomised controlled trial of interferon alpha in chronic non-A, non-B hepatitis. *Br. Med. J.* **298**, 80–2.

Kane, M.A., Bradley, D.W., Shresthna, S.M. *et al.* (1984). Epidemic non-A, non-B hepatitis in Nepal: recovery of a possible etiological agent and transmission studies in marmosets. *JAMA* **252**, 3140–5.

Karayiannis, P., Jowett, T., Enticott, M. *et al.* (1986). Studies of hepatitis A virus replication and the host immune response to HAV in relation to the pathogenesis of liver cell damage. *J. Med. Virol.* **18**, 261–76.

Karayiannis, P., McGarvey, M.J., Fry, M.A. and Thomas, H.C.

(1988). Detection of hepatitis A virus RNA in tissues and faeces of experimentally infected tamarins by cDNA-RNA hybridisation. In *Viral Hepatitis and Liver Disease*, ed. A.J. Zucherman, pp. 117–20, Alan Liss, New York.

Karayiannis, P., Saldanha, J., Monjardino, J. *et al.* (1990). Immunisation of woodchucks with recombinant hepatitis delta antigen does not protect against hepatitis delta virus infection. *Hepatology* **12**, 1125–8.

Kato, Y., Nakagawa, H. and Kobayashi, K. (1982). Interferon production by peripheral lymphocytes in HBsAg positive liver disease. *Hepatology* **2**, 789–90.

Kernoff, P.B.A., Lee, C.A., Karayiannis, P. and Thomas, H.C. (1985). High risk of non-A, non-B hepatitis after a first exposure to volunteer or commercial clotting factor concentrates: effects of prophylactic immune serum globulin. *Br. J. Haematol.* **60**, 469–79.

Khuroo, M.S. (1980). Study of an epidemic of non-A, non-B hepatitis: possibility of another human hepatitis virus distinct from post-transfusion. *Am. J. Med.* **68**, 818–24.

Knodell, R.G., Conrad, M.E. and Ishak, K.G. (1977). Development of chronic liver disease after acute non-A, non-B post-transfusion hepatitis: role of gamma-globulin prophylaxis in its prevention. *Gastroenterology* **72**, 902–9.

Kuo, G., Choo, Q.-L., Alter, H.J. *et al.* (1989). An assay for circulating antibodies to a major aetiologic virus of human non-A non-B hepatitis. *Science* **244**, 362–4.

MacGregor, A., Kornitschuk, M., Hurrell, J.G. *et al.* (1983). Monoclonal antibodies against hepatitis A virus. *J. Clin. Microbiol.* **18**, 1237–43.

Machida, A., Kishimoto, S., Ohnuma, H. *et al.* (1983). A hepatitis B surface antigen polypeptide (p31) with the receptor for polymerised human as well as chimpanzee albumin. *Gastroenterology* **85**, 268–74.

Milich, D.R., McNamara, M.K., McLachlen, A., Thornton, G.B. and Chisari, F.V. (1985). Distinct H-2 linked regulation of T-cell responses to the pre-S and S regions of the same hepatitis B surface antigen polypeptide allows circumvention of non-responsiveness to the S regions. *Proc. Nat. Acad. Sci. (USA)* **82**, 8168–72.

Milich, D.R., McLachlan, A., Thornton, G.B. and Hughes, J.L. (1987). Antibody production to the nucleocapsid and envelope of the hepatitis B virus primed by a single synthetic T-cell site. *Nature* **329**, 547–9.

Milich, D.R., Jones, J., Hughes, J., Price, J., Raney, A. and McLachlan, A. (1990). Is a function of the secreted HBe antigen to induce immunological tolerance in utero? *Proc. Nat. Acad. Sci. (USA)* **87**, 6599–603.

Montano, L., Miescher, G.C., Goodhall, A.H., Weidmann, K.H., Janossy, G. and Thomas, H.C. (1982). Hepatitis B virus and HLA display in the liver during chronic hepatitis B virus infection. *Hepatology* **2**, 557–61.

Montano, L., Aranguibel, F., Boffil, M., Goodall, A.H., Janossy, G. and Thomas, H.C. (1983). An analysis of the composition of the inflammatory infiltrate in autoimmune and hepatitis B virus induced chronic liver disease. *Hepatology* **3**, 292–5.

Nash, A.A. (1985). Tolerance and suppression in virus diseases. *Br. Med. Bull.* **41**, 41–5.

Neurath, A.R., Kent, S.B.H., Strick, N. Taylor, P. and Stevens, C.E. (1985). Hepatitis B virus contains pre-S gene encoded domains. *Nature* **315**, 154–6.

Neurath, A.R., Kent, S.B.H., Strick, N., and Parker, K. (1986). Identification and chemical synthesis of a host receptor binding site on hepatitis B virus. *Cell* **46**, 429–36.

Novick, D.M., Lok, A.S.F. and Thomas, H.C. (1985). Diminished responsiveness of homosexual men to antiviral therapy for HBsAg positive chronic liver disease. *J. Hepatol.* **1**, 29–35.

Onji, M., Lever, A. and Thomas, H.C. (1989). Hepatitis B virus reduces the sensitivity of cells to interferon. *Hepatology* **9**, 92–6.

Perrillo, R., Regenstein, F.G., Peters, M. *et al.* (1988). Prednisolone withdrawal followed by recombinant alpha interferon in treatment of chronic HBV. *Ann. Int. Med.* **109**, 95–100.

Petit, M.A., Maillard, P., Capel, F. and Pillot, J. (1986). Immunochemical structure of the hepatitis B surface antigen vaccine. II. Analysis of antibody responses in human sera against the envelope proteins. *Mol. Immunol.* **23**, 511–23.

Pignatelli, M., Waters, J., Brown, D. *et al.* (1986). HLA Class I antigens on hepatocyte membrane: increased expression during interferon therapy of chronic hepatitis B. *Hepatology* **6**, 349–53.

Pignatelli, M., Waters, J., Lever, A.M.L., Iwarson, S., Gerety, R. and Thomas, H.C. (1987). Cytotoxic T-cell responses to the nucleocapsid proteins of HBV in chronic hepatitis. *J. Hepatol.* **4**, 15–21.

Poitrine, A., Chousterman, S., Chousterman, M., Naveau, S., Thang, M.N. and Chaput, J.C. (1985). Lack of *in vivo* activation of the interferon system in HBsAg positive chronic active hepatitis. *Hepatology* **5**, 171–4.

Provost, P.J. and Hilleman, M.R. (1979). Propagation of human hepatitis A virus in cell culture *in vitro*. *Proc. Soc. Exp. Biol. Med.* **160**, 213.

Regenstein, F.G., Roodman, S.T. and Perillo, R.P. (1983). Immunoregulatory T cells subsets in chronic HBV infection — the influence of homosexuality. *Hepatology* **3**, 951–4.

Reyes, G.R., Purdy, M.A., Kim, J.P. *et al.* (1990). Isolation of a cDNA from the virus responsible for enterically transmitted non-A, non-B hepatitis. *Science* **247**, 1335–9.

Rosina, F., Saraceo, G., Lattore, V. *et al.* (1987). Alpha 2 recombinant interferon in treatment of HDV. *Prog. Clin. Biol. Res.* **234**, 299–304.

Shafritz, D.A. (1982). Hepatitis B virus DNA molecules in the liver of HBsAg carriers: mechanistic considerations in the pathogenesis of hepatocellular carcinoma. *Hepatology* **2**, 355–415.

Teixeira, M.R., Weller, I.V., Murray, A. *et al.* (1982). The pathology of hepatitis A in man. *Liver* **2**, 53–60.

Thomas, H.C. (1981). T-cell subsets in patients with acute HAV, acute and chronic HBV infection, primary cirrhosis, and alcohol-induced liver disease. *J. Immunopharmacol.* **3**, 301–5.

Thomas, H.C. (1987). The immune response to hepatitis B virus. *Postgrad. Med. J.* **63** (suppl. 2), 51–6.

Thomas, H.C. and Scully, L.J. (1985). Interferon in the management of chronic HBV infection. *Br. Med. Bull.* **41**, 374–80.

Thomas, H.C., De Villiers, D., Potter, B. *et al.* (1978). Immune complexes in acute and chronic liver disease. *Clin. Exp. Immunol.* **31**, 150–7.

Thomas, H.C., Montano, L., Goodall, A., de Koning, R., Oladapo, J. and Wiedmann, K.H. (1982a). Immunological mechanisms in chronic hepatitis B virus infection. *Hepatology* **2**, 116S–121S.

Thomas, H.C., Shipton, U. and Montano, L. (1982b). The HLA system: its relevance to the pathogenesis of liver disease. *Prog. Liver Dis.* **16**, 517–27.

Thomas, H.C., Farci, P., Sheim, R. *et al.* (1987). Inhibition of HDV replication by lymphoblastoid interferon. *Prog. Clin. Biol. Res.* **234**, 277–90.

Thomas, H.C., Jacyna, M., Waters, J. and Main, J. (1988). Virus host interaction in chronic hepatitis B virus infection. *Semin. Liver Dis.* **8**, 342–9.

Tolentino, P., Dianzani, F. and Zucea, M. (1985). Decreased interferon response by lymphocytes from children with chronic hepatitis. *J. Infect. Dis.* **132**, 459–61.

Trevisan, A., Gudat, F., Guggenheim, R. *et al.* (1982). Demonstration of albumin receptors on isolated human hepatocytes by light and scanning E.M. *Hepatology* **2**, 832–5.

Wankya, B.M., Hanson, D.P., Ngindu, A.M., Feinstone, S.F. and Purcell, R.H. (1979). Seroepidemiology of hepatitis A and B in Kenya: a rural population survey in Machakos district. *East African Med. J.* **56**, 134–8.

Waters, J.A., Pignatelli, M., Galpin, S., Ishihara, K. and Thomas, H.C. (1986). Virus neutralising antibodies to hepatitis B virus: the nature of an immunogenic epitope on the S gene peptide. *J. Gen. Virol.* **67**, 2467–73.

Waters, J.A., Kennedy, M., Vock, P., Hauser, P., Petre, J. and Thomas, H.C. (1992). Loss of the common 'a' determinant of hepatitis B surface antigen by a vaccine-induced escape mutant. *J. Clin. Invest.* (in press).

Weller, I.V.D., Lok, A.S., Mindel, A. *et al.* (1985). A randomised controlled trial of ARAMP for chronic type B hepatitis. *Gut* **26**, 745–51.

Wiedmann, K.H., Bartholomew, T.C, Brown, D.J. and Thomas, H.C. (1984). Liver membrane antibodies detected by immunoradiometric assay in acute and chronic virus-induced and autoimmune liver disease. *Hepatology* **4**, 199–204.

Wiedmann, K.H., Trejdosiewicz, L.K., Goodall, A.H. and Thomas, H.C. (1985). Analysis of the antigenic composition of liver-specific lipoprotein using murine monoclonal antibodies. *Gut* **26**, 510–17.

Zanetti, A., Tanzi, E., Manzillo, G., Waters, J., Thomas, H.C. and Zuckerman, A. (1988). Hepatitis B variants in Europe. *Lancet* **ii**, 1132–3.

Zhuang, H., Kaldor, J., Locarnini, S.A. and Gust, I.D. (1982). Serum immunoglobulin levels in acute A, B, and non-A, non-B hepatitis. *Gastroenterology* **82**, 549–53.

101: Autoimmune Liver Disease

I.G. McFarlane, J.M. Farrant and A.L.W.F. Eddleston

Aberrant autoreactivity has been implicated in a number of chronic liver disorders, of which the so-called 'autoimmune' chronic active hepatitis (AI-CAH), primary biliary cirrhosis (PBC) and primary sclerosing cholangitis (PSC) are the principal conditions. Although the precise immunopathogenesis is not yet clear, it seems likely that each of these conditions is associated with an autoimmune attack against one or more of the cellular components of the liver — principally hepatocytes in AI-CAH, and bile-duct epithelial cells in PBC and PSC. However, all are variously associated (at least at some stage) with features of chronic active hepatitis (CAH). This is defined histologically (Plate 101.1, between pages 1930 and 1931) as a dense inflammatory infiltrate of mononuclear cells (including lymphocytes, plasma cells, monocytes and fibroblasts) in the portal tracts, spilling out into the surrounding parenchyma with 'piecemeal' necrosis of periportal hepatocytes (the hallmark feature) and, in severe cases, extending along fibrous septa towards adjacent portal tracts ('bridging necrosis'). The natural history of CAH includes a tendency to progress to cirrhosis and, as one of the relatively common, and often treatable, precirrhotic conditions, it is of considerable importance in hepatology.

Autoimmune chronic active hepatitis

The first description of AI-CAH, predominantly affecting women and characterized by fluctuating jaundice, pyrexia, arthralgia and myalgia, hepatosplenomegaly, amenorrhoea, acneform rashes and hypergammaglobulinaemia (due mainly to raised immunoglobulin G (IgG) levels), is usually attributed to Waldenstrom (1950), but it seems likely that the syndrome was recognized much earlier (Cullinan 1936; Amberg 1942). The finding of lupus erythematosus (LE) cells in the blood of many patients suggested an association with systemic LE (SLE) and, initially, the condition was described as 'lupoid hepatitis' (Joske and King 1955; Mackay *et al.* 1956, 1959; Bartholomew *et al.* 1958, 1960; Aronson and Montgomery 1959; Mackay and Wood 1962). However, the recognition that only a minority (about 20%) have LE cells and that clinically significant renal involvement is extremely uncommon led to acceptance that this condition was distinct from SLE (Doniach *et al.* 1966; Whittingham *et al.* 1966a, b). Autoimmune CAH is an aggressive disorder that is exquisitely responsive to corticosteroid therapy, but has a high mortality (up to 80% at 5 years) if untreated (Willcox and Isselbacher 1961; Soloway *et al.* 1972).

Autoantibodies

Today, the disorder is subclassified into two subtypes according to the autoantibody serology: 'classical' (type 1) AI-CAH is associated with antinuclear (ANA) and/or smooth-muscle (SMA) autoantibodies, while type 2 AI-CAH is characterized by the presence of liver–kidney microsomal (LKM-1) antibodies (Homberg *et al*. 1987). Females predominate (4 : 1) in both types and, although the disease (particularly type 2) was originally described as mainly affecting younger subjects, it is now recognized that it also presents later in life and has a bimodal distribution with two peaks of onset — at 10–30 years of age and >40 years (i.e. postmenopausal in women). There is, in addition, a group of patients with idiopathic (cryptogenic) CAH who are seronegative for ANA, SMA and LKM antibodies but who, in all other respects (including responsiveness to steroids), have a condition that is indistinguishable from type 1 or type 2 AI-CAH (Czaja *et al*. 1990; Johnson *et al*. 1990). However, whether these patients constitute a third, distinct, subtype or whether they represent less aggressive forms of the other two is not yet clear.

The ANA in AI-CAH give a 'homogeneous' immunofluorescent staining pattern on rodent tissue sections similar to that seen with ANA in SLE and are usually associated with antibodies against double-stranded deoxyribonucleic acid (DNA), but they react with a different nuclear antigen from that recognized by ANA in SLE (Gurian *et al*. 1985) — although the precise target has not yet been identified. The SMA in AI-CAH were thought to be specific for the smooth-muscle protein F-actin but a recent study (Dighiero *et al*. 1990) has shown that anti-actin antibodies occur in only about 50% of SMA +ve AI-CAH patients, and it is now known that high titres of SMA with anti-actin specificity also occur in a number of other disorders not necessarily involving the liver (McFarlane 1991).

The LKM-1 autoantibody reacts with cytochrome P450 IID6 (formerly P450 db1) (Manns *et al*. 1989), the major target epitope of which is an octapeptide with the sequence –Asp–Pro–Ala–Gln–Pro–Pro–Arg–Asp–. Liver–kidney microsomal antibody 1 is distinct from similar antibodies found in tienilic acid-induced hepatitis (LKM-2) (Beaune *et al*. 1987), delta virus hepatitis (LKM-3) (Crivelli *et al*. 1983), and the liver microsomal antibodies seen in hydralazine hepatitis (Bourdi *et al*. 1990), which react with different cytochrome P450 isoenzymes — although there has been a recent report (Manns *et al*. 1990) of a case of apparently idiopathic AI-CAH with antibodies reacting with cytochrome P450 IA2, the target of the hydralazine hepatitis-associated liver microsomal antibody.

A number of other autoantibodies are reported with varying frequencies in patients with AI-CAH. These include antithyroid, reticulin, and gastric parietal cell antibodies as well as rheumatoid factor, but they seem to be of little direct relevance to the pathogenesis or classification of AI-CAH. In addition, antimitochondrial antibodies (AMA) occur in about 10% of patients and constitute part of a well-recognized clinical, histological and immunological overlap between AI-CAH and PBC (see below). An antibody (anti-SLA) that reacts with a soluble liver antigen (SLA) has been described which, it is claimed (Manns *et al*. 1987), identifies a separate subgroup of AI-CAH with cryptogenic CAH (see above), which responds to steroids, but this has not yet been confirmed.

Perhaps more relevant to the pathogenesis of AI-CAH are the anti-LSP and anti-ASGP-R autoantibodies, which are directed at other liver constituents. Anti-LSP antibodies react with the so-called 'liver-specific membrane lipoprotein' preparation (LSP) (McFarlane *et al*. 1977). This is a crude macromolecular fraction of normal liver containing fragments of hepatocellular membranes (De Kretser *et al*. 1980; Lebwohl and Gerber 1981; Jensen *et al*. 1983), and thus comprises numerous antigenic components. Some of these are liver-specific but only one, the hepatic asialoglycoprotein receptor (ASGP-R), has so far been identified (McFarlane *et al*. 1984a). 'Anti-LSP' therefore represents a group of autoantibodies that react with several different antigens in LSP, and the antigenic specificities of these antibodies may vary according to the type of liver disease.

The asialoglycoprotein receptor is involved in the binding and endocytosis of glycoproteins bearing terminal galactose residues (McFarlane 1983; Schwartz 1984; Steer and Ashwell 1986). It is specific to hepatocytes and is preferentially expressed on the surfaces of cells in the periportal areas of the liver lobules (Daniels *et al*. 1987; McFarlane *et al*. 1990), the principal sites of tissue damage in CAH. Being a membrane-bound receptor, it is not surprising that ASGP-R is also present in LSP (McFarlane *et al.* 1984a). In some liver disorders, 'anti-LSP' is therefore comprised in part of anti-ASGP-R antibodies. The contribution of anti-ASGP-R to the total 'anti-LSP' activity varies but can be as much as 70% (Wojcicka-McFarlane 1990).

Approximately 90% of patients with either type 1 or type 2 AI-CAH have high titres of anti-LSP and anti-ASGP-R antibodies at presentation (McFarlane 1984; McFarlane and Williams 1985; McFarlane *et al.* 1986; Treichel *et al.* 1990). This is true also of those patients with cryptogenic (presumed autoimmune) CAH whose disease is steroid-responsive (Johnson *et al.* 1990). Titres of both autoantibodies correlate with histologically assessed severity of disease (particularly with piecemeal necrosis) and decline rapidly and predictably with response to corticosteroid therapy (unlike ANA, SMA or LKM), with many patients becoming seronegative. The reappearance and/or rising titres of the antibodies during reduction or withdrawal of immunosuppressive therapy herald relapse — up to 3 months and more before the first rise in serum aminotransferases or clinical signs of disease exacerbation develop (McFarlane *et al.* 1984b) (Fig. 101.1).

Immunogenetics

Mackay and Morris (1972) first showed that AI-CAH is strongly associated with the histocompatibility antigens human leucocyte antigen (HLA)-A1 and B8, the antigens found at high frequency in many of the other organ-specific autoimmune diseases. Galbraith *et al.* (1974) confirmed these findings in a series of 57 patients

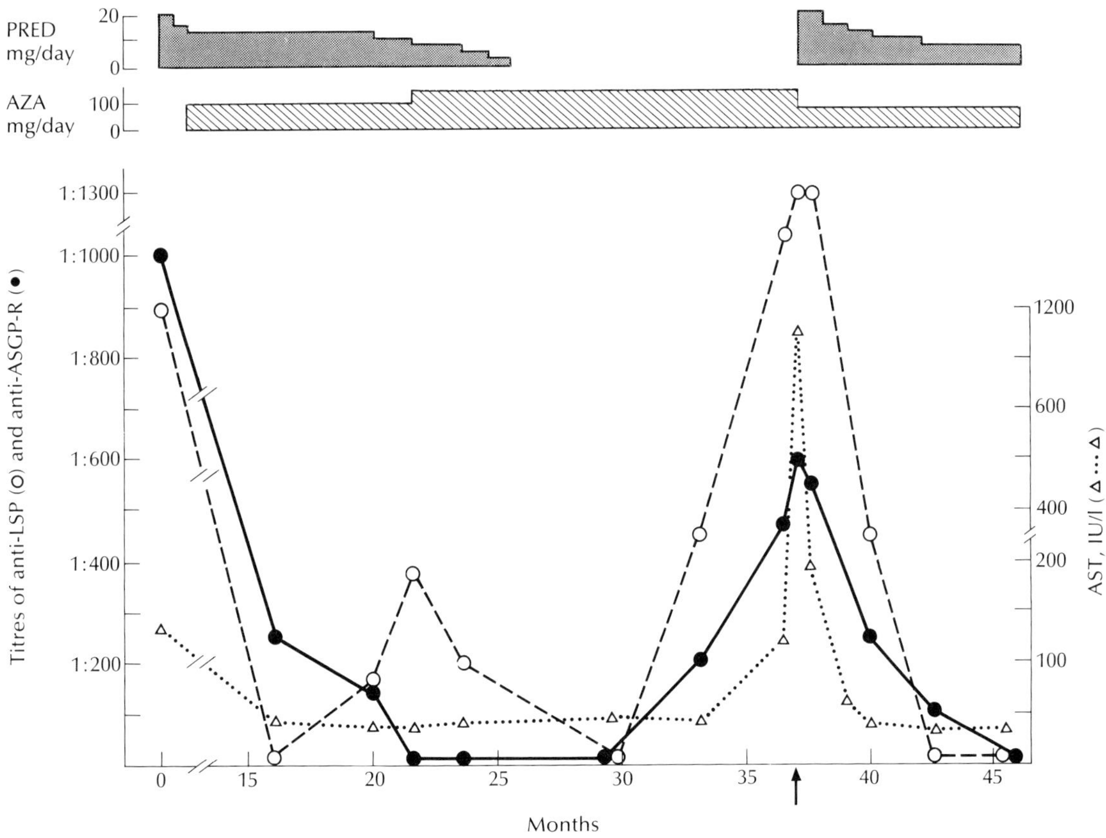

Fig. 101.1. Changes in titres of anti-LSP and anti-ASGP-R antibodies in a patient with AI-CAH during immunosuppressive therapy with prednisolone (PRED) and azathioprine (AZA). Note transient rise in anti-LSP during initial withdrawal of prednisolone, and rises in titres of both autoantibodies 3.5 months before symptomatic relapse (arrow), accompanied by increased serum aminotransferase activities (AST, normal range <40 IU/l).

with CAH and suggested that the HLA-B8 association was confined to the 'autoimmune' form of the disease, patients with CAH due to chronic hepatitis B virus (HBV) infection (HBs antigen +ve) having a different immunogenetic background. A close association with a newly discovered Class II HLA allele, Dw3, was reported by Opelz *et al.* (1977), and confirmed by Mackay and Tait (1980), who showed that in AI-CAH, as in other autoimmune diseases, B8 and DR3 are inherited together as a haplotype.

Donaldson *et al.* (1991b) have reviewed HLA associations in AI-CAH and found that the two classical presenting ages for the disease almost certainly mark out two genetically different subgroups, which may represent two major forms of the disease. The classical B8, DR3-associated type is found in the younger age-group, while the older subset, often presenting in women around the menopause, is strongly associated with DR4 (Fig. 101.2). Interestingly, in Japan, where the median age of presentation with AI-CAH is 51 years, the principal HLA association is with Bw54 and DR4, some 90% of Japanese patients having this haplotype (compared with 39% in controls) (Seki *et al.* 1990).

An association of AI-CAH with the immunoglobulin allotype Gm a +ve, x +ve was reported (Whittingham *et al.* 1981) but this has not been confirmed by later segregation and logistic regression analyses, which failed to find support for inheritance of a disease-susceptibility gene (Walsh and Cox 1984; Krawitt *et al.* 1987).

The recent visualization of the antigen-presenting groove in HLA molecules by X-ray crystallography has focused attention on the possibility that the HLA linkages described above could be associated with enhanced binding of particular autoantigenic peptides from relevant organ-specific antigens (such as ASGP-R) to Class II HLA molecules on antigen-presenting cells.

Although antigen-specific mechanisms of disease susceptibility are usually invoked to explain the HLA associations with the organ-specific auto-immune diseases, it is also possible that a generalized increase in immune reactivity could predispose to autoimmunity. The hypothesis that HLA-B8 might be associated with such a non-antigen-specific increase in immune responsiveness was originally proposed by Eddleston and Williams (1974). This concept was supported by a study by Galbraith *et al.* (1975 and 1976), who showed that titres of autoantibodies and of anti-viral antibodies were higher in B8 +ve AI-CAH patients and their first-degree relatives than in subjects without HLA-B8. Direct evidence of a link between B8 and defective non-antigen-specific suppressor cell function in relatives of patients with AI-CAH was obtained by Nouri-Aria *et al.* (1982). Further studies showed that this was due

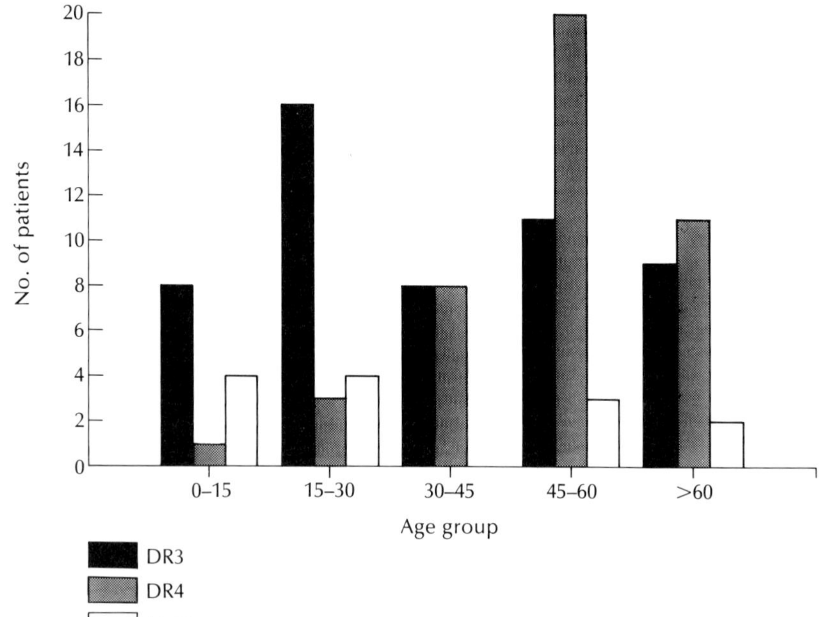

Fig. 101.2. The association between the Class II HLA antigens, DR3 and DR4, and the age of presentation with AI-CAH, showing a bimodal distribution of DR3 (but predominantly associated with the younger age-group) and an association of DR4 with the older patients.

to a T cell defect which was correctable *in vitro* by pharmacological concentrations of prednisolone in AI-CAH but not in cases of steroid-insensitive HBV-related CAH (Nouri-Aria *et al.* 1985a, b).

Mechanisms

Early studies using the leucocyte migration inhibition test with peripheral blood leucocytes (PBL) established that patients with AI-CAH have circulating lymphocytes that recognize antigens in LSP (Miller *et al.* 1972). These findings have since been confirmed using an indirect agarose microdroplet assay for T lymphocyte migratory inhibitory factor (T-LIF) production and, also using this assay, it has been shown that T cell sensitization to ASGP-R is an almost invariable finding in patients with AI-CAH but is rare in HBV-induced cases (Vento *et al.* 1984, 1986). The T cells recognizing the ASGP-R in this assay belong to the CD4 +ve helper/inducer subset (Vento *et al.* 1987). In addition, it was found that CD4 +ve T cells from normal subjects (or T cells from patients with unrelated illnesses) can suppress ASGP-R-stimulated T-LIF production by AI-CAH patients' T cells in co-culture experiments, implying that the patients have a specific defect in controlling the autoreactive response to this antigen (Vento *et al.* 1986, 1987). Family studies revealed that this antigen-specific and disease-specific functional defect in T cell suppression is inherited in an autosomal, non-major histocompatibility complex (MHC)-linked mode (O'Brien *et al.* 1986).

Although results obtained with any indirect bioassay of lymphokines, and particularly one which purports to reflect suppressor T cell (T_s) activity, are the subject of intense debate, the advent of T cell cloning has lent considerable support to these findings. Thus, clonally expanded T cells, both from peripheral blood and from liver biopsies of patients with AI-CAH: (i) recognize ASGP-R (Fig. 101.3); (ii) are almost exclusively of the CD4 +ve phenotype; and (iii) provide specific help for autologous B cell production of anti-ASGP-R antibodies in culture (Lohr *et al.* 1990; Wen *et al.* 1990).

That autoreactive cytotoxic T cells do not appear to play a major role in this condition was implied from early studies showing non-T cells, antibody-mediated cytotoxic (antibody-dependent cell-mediated cytotoxic (ADCC)) reactions *in vitro* with PBL from AI-CAH patients and, as targets, isolated rodent hepatocytes or turkey erythrocytes coated with LSP (for review see McFarlane 1984). These findings were later confirmed in studies with separated T and non-T cells and using isolated autologous hepatocytes (from the patients' liver biopsies) as targets, to satisfy the requirement for histocompatibility between effector and target cells for demonstration of T cell cytotoxic events (Zinkernagel and Doherty 1979), which showed that the cytotoxic reactions are exclusively a function of the non-T cell population (Mieli-Vergani *et al.* 1979).

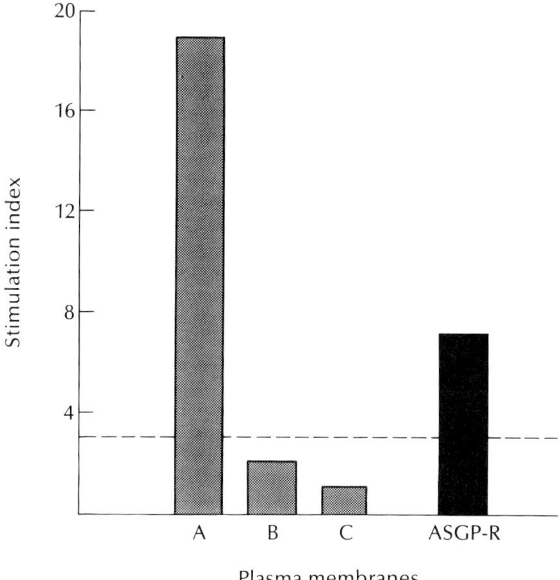

Fig. 101.3. Proliferation of T cell clones from peripheral blood of AI-CAH patients in response to 3 μg/ml of rabbit liver (A, B) or kidney (C) plasma membranes or purified asialoglycoprotein receptor (ASGP-R) with autologous (A, C, ASGP-R) or allogeneic (B) peripheral blood mononuclear cells as antigen-presenting cells. Stimulation indices >3 (dotted line) indicate significant proliferation. Adapted from Wen *et al.* (1990).

The hypothesis of Eddleston and Williams (1974) presumes that some trigger, possibly an environmental factor such as a virus, is required to initiate the disease in susceptible individuals. Certainly this seems likely, as most of the patients identified with the above-mentioned inherited defect in antigen-specific suppression (T_s) of autoreactivity to ASGP-R presented in adult life, and there is now increasing circumstantial evidence that some hepatotropic virus (e.g. hepatitis A virus (HAV) and HBV) infections are associated with liver-related autoimmune responses (for review see McFarlane 1991).

Support for viral induction of AI-CAH has come from a longitudinal study of 58 healthy first- and second-degree relatives of 13 patients with AI-CAH by Vento *et al.* (1991) in Italy. Fortuitously, three of the relatives acquired asymptomatic HAV infections with raised serum aminotransferases and seropositivity for IgM anti-HAV antibodies during the course of the study. Two were sisters whose grandmother had the disease and the third was the young nephew of a female with AI-CAH in a second family. All three developed anti-ASGP-R antibodies at onset of the acute phase and, about 4 weeks later, their lymphocytes showed *in vitro* T-LIF production in specific response to ASGP-R. One of the two sisters had an uncomplicated course and lost both anti-ASGP-R and T cells reactivity to ASGP-R by 6 weeks. In the remaining two, despite apparent resolution of the infection with normalization of aminotransferases and disappearance of IgM anti-HAV, T cell reactivity to ASGP-R and titres of anti-ASGP-R continued to increase, reaching a peak at about 18 weeks. At this point, serum aminotransferases began to rise again and both patients became seropositive for ANA and SMA, and 2 weeks later both developed classical acute-onset symptomatic AI-CAH, confirmed by liver biopsy, which subsequently responded to corticosteroid therapy. The only significant difference between the three appeared to be that the two who developed AI-CAH had inherited the antigen-specific T_s defect, whereas the one who had an uncomplicated course had not.

Animal models

The first hint at the mechanisms underlying the development of AI-CAH came from attempts by a German group to develop an animal model of the disease by immunization with various fractions of normal liver. These early studies demonstrated that rabbits immunized with LSP seemed to develop a liver lesion similar to that seen in patients (Meyer zum Buschenfelde *et al.* 1972), but attempts to convincingly reproduce this model in rabbits or mice in other laboratories met with variable success (Bartholomaeus *et al.* 1981; Feighery *et al.* 1981; Uibo *et al.* 1982; Kuriki *et al.* 1983). This may have been due to the inclusion of ethylenediamine tetra-acetic acid (EDTA) as a stabilizing agent in the buffers used to prepare LSP — which was adopted as standard practice after the German group's early studies (McFarlane *et al.* 1977) and which was later shown to inhibit induction of the lesion (Mori *et al.* 1984). In addition, the responses have been shown to be species- and strain-dependent, with C57BL/6 being the most susceptible mouse strain (Mori, Y. *et al.* 1984, 1985; Mori, T. *et al.* 1985; Lohse *et al.* 1990) and Lewis rats being resistant to development of the disease (Lohse *et al.* 1990).

These later studies have been based on immunization of mice with 100 000 g supernatants of syngeneic liver homogenates, which is the starting material for preparing LSP and presumably, therefore, also contained ASGP-R. Experiments involving passive transfer of spleen cells from immunized to unimmunized mice, leading to development of similar lesions in the recipient animals, have revealed an interplay of cellular immune events analogous to those that seemingly occur in patients with AI-CAH, (Mori, Y. *et al.* 1984, 1985; Mori, T. *et al.* 1985; Araki *et al.* 1987; Ogawa *et al.* 1988; Lohse *et al.* 1990).

Primary biliary cirrhosis

Primary biliary cirrhosis, predominantly (9:1) affecting women, is characterized by a slowly progressive destruction of intrahepatic bile-ducts leading to cirrhosis and accompanied, usually in the later stages, by periportal inflammation and piecemeal necrosis, which can resemble that seen in CAH. The initial lesion is centred on medium-sized bile-ducts, which show epithelial cell damage and are surrounded by an intense lymphocytic infiltrate sometimes with accompanying granulomata (Plate 101.2, between pages 1930 and 1931). Circulating AMA (see below) and hypergammaglobulinaemia, due mainly to markedly elevated serum IgM concentrations, are part of the diagnostic features. The disease most commonly presents around the fourth and fifth decades of life (perimenopausal in women) but has an insidious onset, and there is increasing evidence that many patients (29% in a recent series (Witt-Sullivan *et al.* 1990)) may have this condition for some time before symptoms develop.

Primary biliary cirrhosis is a multi-system disease that has been described as a 'dry gland syndrome' (Epstein *et al.* 1980). Functional impairment (often subclinical) of the pancreas, thyroid, salivary and lacrimal glands, kidney and/or other extrahepatic tissues can be demonstrated in a large proportion of patients, and features of the CREST syndrome (calcinosis, Reynaud's phenomenon, oesophageal dysmotility, sclerodactyly, telangiectasia) are not uncommon (Culp *et al.* 1982; Kaplan 1987).

Autoantibodies

The most striking serological features of PBC are AMA, which, because they are found in more than 90% of patients at presentation and are rare in other conditions, have become one of the diagnostic criteria of the disease. Indeed, the majority of asymptomatic cases are revealed by detecting AMA during investigation of patients with mildly cholestatic biochemical liver tests identified during routine health screening.

In all, nine different groups (M1 to M9) of AMA have been defined (Table 101.1), of which M2 is the one most closely related to PBC; M4 (with M2) is associated with cases of PBC that overlap with AI-CAH (Baum and Palmer 1985; Berg and Klein 1985; Gershwin *et al.* 1988), although it seems that it may not actually be specific for these cases (Berg *et al.* 1986). The target antigens of M1, M2 and M7 have been localized to the inner mitochondrial membrane and those of the remaining AMAs are thought to be located on the outer membrane.

Most of the antigenic species with which M2 AMA react have now been identified as components of the 2-oxo acid dehydrogenase complexes: pyruvate (PDC), 2-oxoglutarate (OGDC) and branched-chain 2-oxo acid (BCOADC) dehydrogenase complexes (Fussey *et al.* 1988, 1989, 1991; Van de Water *et al.* 1988; Yeaman *et al.* 1988; Surh *et al.* 1989; Fregeau *et al.* 1990; Gershwin and Mackay 1991). Each complex is loosely associated with the inner mitochondrial membrane and is comprised of three enzymes, E1, E2 and E3 (Yeaman 1989). The lipoate-containing E2 and protein X of PDC are the major M2 autoantigens (Fussey *et al.* 1988; Mutimer *et al.* 1989) but the α and β subunits of E1 of PDC are also recognized by some PBC sera (Fussey *et al.* 1989; Fregeau *et al.* 1990). The autoantibodies recognizing these antigens may be of IgM or IgG classes but, in common with other autoimmune diseases, there is a tendency for restriction to the IgG-3 isotype (Surh *et al.* 1988).

In addition to AMA, a wide range of other autoantibodies are seen in PBC. These include ANA, SMA, anti-thyroid and anti-reticulin antibodies and rheumatoid factor, which variously occur in up to about 30% of PBC patients, whether or not they have other underlying disorders (e.g. thyroid disease, rheumatoid arthritis). The ANA may give the 'homogeneous' or the 'speckled' patterns of immunofluorescent staining but anticentromere antibodies are also often found, particularly in patients with concomitant progressive

Table 101.1. Subspecificities and disease associations of antimitochondrial antibodies (AMA)

AMA type	Target antigen (location in mitochondria)	Disease associations
M1	Cardiolipin (inner membrane)	Secondary syphilis
M2	2-oxo acid dehydrogenase complex (inner membrane)	Most cases of PBC
M3	Unknown (outer membrane)	Drug-induced pseudo-lupus
M4	Unknown (outer membrane)	PBC/AI-CAH 'overlap' cases
M5	Unknown (outer membrane)	Some SLE patients
M6	Unknown (outer membrane)	Drug-induced hepatitis
M7	Unknown (inner membrane)	Various cardiomyopathies
M8	Unknown (outer membrane)	Some cases of PBC
M9	Unknown (outer membrane)	Some cases of PBC and some healthy subjects

systemic sclerosis (scleroderma) or features of the CREST syndrome (Tan 1982; Harmon 1985; Powell *et al.* 1987; Mackay and Gershwin 1989), while the SMA react with many different cytoskeletal proteins, including actin (Dighiero *et al.* 1990).

About 50% of PBC patients also have anti-LSP antibodies, mainly in the later stages of the disease, and (as in AI-CAH) titres correlate with severity of periportal inflammation and piecemeal necrosis (Tsantoulas *et al.* 1980; Bedlow *et al.* 1989). However, in contrast to AI-CAH, anti-ASGP-R is found in only about 25% of patients (McFarlane *et al.* 1986; Bedlow *et al.* 1989; Treichel *et al.* 1990). This, together with other evidence (Vento *et al.* 1986) relating to cellular immune responses to LSP discussed below, suggests that the antigens recognized by anti-LSP in PBC are different from those reacting with the anti-LSP antibodies found in AI-CAH patients.

Immunogenetics

Although there are many reports in the literature of familial occurrence of PBC (Feizi *et al.* 1972; Chohan 1973; Brown *et al.* 1975; Tong *et al.* 1976; Fagan *et al.* 1977; Jaup and Zettergen 1980; Kato *et al.* 1981; Cales *et al.* 1983; Witt-Sullivan *et al.* 1990), it is still not certain whether there is an underlying genetic basis for the disease. In particular, in contrast to AI-CAH and PSC (see below), there is no clear association of any Class I or Class II HLA antigen with PBC. Some studies have indicated linkages with DR3, DR2 and DR8 (Ercilla *et al.* 1979; Miyamori *et al.* 1983; Gores *et al.* 1987) but others have found no such associations (Mackay 1984; Bassendine *et al.* 1985; Bedlow *et al.* 1989). The only study, so far, that has investigated Class III linkages found a significant association with C4B2 (Briggs *et al.* 1987).

Nevertheless, there is evidence that inheritance of some HLA allotypes is associated (positively or negatively) with certain immunological events and with severity of disease in PBC. Thus, there is a significant positive association between inheritance of DR3 and the presence of anti-LSP and anti-ASGP-R antibodies and elevated serum IgG concentrations (Bedlow *et al.* 1989). Conversely, these parameters are negatively associated with DR2, suggesting that DR3 and DR2 are associated with one or more genes that, respectively, code for elevation or reduction of overall immune responsiveness (Bedlow *et al.* 1989). A significant negative correlation between DR2 and serum bilirubin concentrations in PBC and a non-significant increased frequency of DR2 linked to C4B2 have also been reported (Gores *et al.* 1987; Briggs *et al.* 1987). Other evidence of a possible genetic influence on the development of PBC relates to the finding of a defect in switching from an IgM to an IgG response on challenge with a foreign antigen (Thomas *et al.* 1976) and abnormalities in T_s regulation of IgM production (Nouri-Aria *et al.* 1985c; Al-Aghbar *et al.* 1986).

Mechanisms

Primary biliary cirrhosis is an immunological disease, with wide-ranging and profound abnormalities of the immune system. In addition to the circulating autoantibodies and the defects in switching from a primary to a secondary humoral immune response and in T cell regulation of IgM production, anergy to parenteral antigenic challenge (Fox *et al.* 1973), chronic activation of the classical and alternative pathways of the complement system (Potter *et al.* 1976, 1980; Wands *et al.* 1978) and high levels of circulating immune complexes (Gupta *et al.* 1978; Thomas *et al.* 1978; Wands *et al.* 1978) are demonstrable in the majority of patients.

However, these features do not establish an autoimmune pathogenesis. In particular, the antigens with which the AMA react are unlikely targets of tissue-damaging autoreactions in this condition, because: (i) they are not specific to the liver; (ii) they do not appear to be expressed on the surfaces of biliary epithelial cells; (iii) evidence as to whether they might be expressed on hepatocellular surfaces is at best conflicting (Ghadiminejad and Baum 1987; Gerken *et al.* 1988; Baum *et al.* 1990); and (iv) there is as yet no evidence that these antigens are recognized by cellular components of the immune system. Similarly, the anti-LSP, anti-ASGP-R and many of the other autoantibodies that occur in PBC are not related to the biliary tract and appear to be more a part of the background 'noise' associated with an overall heightened immune responsiveness than of primary pathogenic importance in the accompanying tissue injury (Bedlow *et al.* 1989). This impression is reinforced by the finding that, while about 50% of patients with PBC show T cell reactivity to LSP *in vitro*, they do not respond in this way to ASGP-R — suggesting that this autoreaction is directed at cryptic liver cell antigens (present in LSP) and arises as a consequence of exposure of these components to the immune system after liver damage has occurred (Vento *et al*. 1986).

More persuasive evidence of underlying autoreactive pathology that might contribute to tissue damage comes from studies of cellular immune responses to normal human-specific antigens derived from the biliary tract (Eddleston *et al*. 1973; McFarlane 1985). Two such antigens, one associated with the bile canalicular domain of the hepatocellular plasma membrane and the other with the surfaces of bile-duct epithelial cells, have been shown to be recognized by T cells from PBC patients (McFarlane *et al*. 1979; Wojcicka-McFarlane *et al*. 1981; McFarlane 1985). In addition, circulating immune complexes from PBC patients are reported to contain one or both of these antigens (Amoroso *et al*. 1980), implying the existence of corresponding autoantibodies, although these have not been directly demonstrated. The ductular epithelial antigen is specific to the bile-ducts but the canalicular antigen cross-reacts with antigens in kidney, pancreas and salivary ductules (McFarlane 1985). Interestingly, a similar pattern of cross-reactions with microbial antigens is well recognized. For example, rabbits immunized with *Schistosoma japonicum* develop anti-canalicular antibodies (Jones *et al*. 1976) and group A streptococcal antigens cross-react with antigens in the biliary tract, kidney and salivary gland (Kingston and Glynn 1971).

This raises the question of whether PBC is, after all, a primary autoimmune disorder. In addition to the lack of a definitive association with any HLA allotype, only a very modest response to one of a wide range of immunosuppressive drugs that are effective in other autoimmune conditions has been demonstrated (Christensen *et al*. 1985). In these and other respects, PBC is more reminiscent of a chronic infectious disease. Although, to date, no specific aetiological factor has been unequivocally implicated in PBC, it is worth noting that the mitochondrial antigens that are the targets of AMA (including those of the M2 antibodies) are well preserved phylogenetically and are found in a very broad range of organisms (Baum and Palmer 1985). It is possible that AMA might therefore simply be a reflection of current or previous exposure to a microbial agent and that the disease represents an unusual response to infection with what might be a common pathogen.

In support of this is a recent report of 'naturally occurring mitochondrial antibodies' (NOMA) in family members of patients with PBC (Klein and Berg 1990). These NOMA do not show immunofluorescent staining on tissue sections, but are detected either by enzyme-linked immunosorbent assay (ELISA) or by immunoblotting against antigens extracted from submitochondrial particles. They belong to the M2 and M9 groups of AMA but recognize different epitopes from those with which PBC AMA react. Thus, they occur infrequently (6%) in the patients themselves but were found in 70% of family members, including spouses of unaffected relatives. Of particular interest is the finding that 63% of unrelated laboratory technicians who regularly worked with PBC sera were also seropositive for NOMA, compared with only 17% of other technicians without such exposure and 15% of healthy blood donors (Klein and Berg 1990). The authors have suggested that these findings are indirect evidence for a contagious immunogenic agent circulating in the blood of PBC patients. They speculate that NOMA may function as a natural defence against infection, along the lines suggested by Cohen and Cooke (1986), and that PBC patients may have a defect, affecting B cell clones primed to produce NOMA, which renders them susceptible to the infection.

Animal models

There is one report of PBC occurring spontaneously in rabbits (Tison *et al*. 1982) but, strangely, no further studies seem to have been undertaken in this putative animal model. Other attempts to reproduce the disease in animals, by immunization with various biliary tract or mitochondrial antigen preparations, have not really been successful. Even immunization with 2-oxo acid dehydrogenase complex fusion proteins has yielded disappointing results (Krams *et al*. 1989a). In the latter, the animals produced AMA reacting with the same mitochondrial antigens as in PBC but did not develop biliary lesions, and studies of the fine specificities of these AMA revealed that they recognized different epitopes from those of AMA in PBC (Surh *et al*. 1990).

Somewhat more successful were experiments involving injection of PBL from PBC patients into mice with severe combined immunodeficiency (SCID). The SCID mouse lacks functional lymphocytes and can be colonized with human lymphocytes (McCune *et al.* 1988; Mosier *et al.* 1988). Injection of PBL from PBC patients led to production of AMA with similar specificity to that of the AMA in PBC, and to development of biliary lesions reminiscent of the disease (Krams *et al.* 1989b). However, caution must be exercised in attributing these findings entirely to a primary autoimmune mechanism because, if PBC is after all a chronic infectious disease (see above), the infection could presumably have been transmitted to the SCID mice during transfer of the patients' PBL. This might also account for the recurrence of PBC in the liver grafts of patients transplanted for this disease (Neuberger *et al.* 1982).

It is also interesting to note that transfer of PBL from normal healthy individuals (as a control) produced similar (albeit less severe) lesions in the SCID mice. The authors speculated that this might have been related to a type of graft-versus-host (GVH) response (Krams *et al.* 1989b). Certainly, liver lesions involving destruction of intrahepatic bile-ducts are well recognized in patients with GVH disease following bone marrow transplantation (McDonald *et al.* 1987). Indeed, an analogy has been drawn between this syndrome and PBC (Epstein *et al.* 1980), and up-regulation of Class II MHC expression on bile-duct epithelial cells has been noted in bone marrow graft recipients (Miglio *et al.* 1987), but other evidence has failed to link autoreactions to biliary tract antigens with GVH disease through cross-reacting HLA antigens (McFarlane *et al.* 1983).

Primary sclerosing cholangitis

Primary sclerosing cholangitis is a chronic liver disease of unknown aetiology, characterized by inflammation and fibrosis of the entire biliary tree (Chapman 1985). It is commoner in males than females and is associated with chronic ulcerative colitis in more than two-thirds of cases (Chapman *et al.* 1980). The disease may begin at any age from infancy onwards and the course is very variable, with some patients remaining in good health for many years, while about one-third have a rapid course and ultimately die of liver failure or require orthotopic liver transplantation (Farrant *et al.* 1991). Early in the course of the disease, the morphological abnormalities are confined to the portal tracts, with a mononuclear cell infiltrate and characteristic 'onion-skin' periductal fibrosis (stage 1) (Plate 101.3, between pages 1930 and 1931). The infiltrate is predominantly lymphocytic and in most cases the CD4/CD8 ratio is normal (Whiteside *et al.* 1985; Snook *et al.* 1989a). In later stages the inflammation is more extensive and involves the lobules periportally (stage 2), either by way of fibrosis or as 'biliary piecemeal necrosis'. Ultimately, portal–portal bridging fibrosis or necrosis (stage 3) and cirrhosis (stage 4) supervene. The diagnosis rests on the cholangiographic demonstration of widespread stricturing, dilatation and irregularity of the biliary tree in the absence of any other cause such as previous biliary surgery, choledocholithiasis or cholangiocarcinoma.

Histological features of CAH may be seen at various stages in up to two-thirds of patients with PSC (Chapman *et al.* 1980), and mild to moderate hypergammaglobulinaemia (due mainly to increased IgG) is a frequent finding. In these and other respects, especially in children (see below), the disease can be confused with AI-CAH (Lindor *et al.* 1986).

Autoantibodies

There are no definitive serological markers of PSC. In particular, it has been generally accepted that autoantibodies occur in less than one-third of adults with PSC. Certainly, AMA are exceedingly rare (Chapman *et al.* 1980; Lindor *et al.* 1986) but one study (Zauli *et al.* 1987) has reported the finding of ANA, SMA and anti-intermediate filament antibodies at titres ranging from 1 : 40 to 1 : 640 in 58–77% of patients fulfilling strict criteria for diagnosis of PSC, with ANA of the 'homogeneous' type in half. Apart from choice of substrate for immunofluorescence, the reasons for this apparent discrepancy with other studies are not clear, but the authors speculate that they might have been dealing with a selected group of patients.

Chapman *et al.* (1986) identified an autoantibody reacting with portal tracts in sera from patients with PSC, which was subsequently found to react with a component in or near the nuclei of neutrophils and to be sometimes present in very high titres (Snook *et al.* 1989b). Another group has identified an epitope shared by human skin, biliary epithelium and colon that is distinct from the neutrophil target, but this was detected using a murine monoclonal antibody and its significance in the pathogenesis of PSC in the absence of a corresponding human autoantibody is unclear (Das *et al.* 1990).

Anti-LSP and anti-ASGP-R autoantibodies occur in only about 10% of adults with PSC and their presence does not correlate with other autoantibodies or elevated serum immunoglobulins, or with any HLA allotype, or the finding of periportal inflammation and piecemeal necrosis on liver biopsy (Bedlow *et al.* 1989). In contrast, almost all children with PSC are seropositive for ANA and/or SMA and have high titres of anti-LSP at presentation but, unlike AI-CAH, these are not associated with anti-ASGP-R, only 25% being seropositive for the latter (Mieli-Vergani *et al.* 1989).

Immunogenetics

Several groups have shown that, in common with AI-CAH, type I diabetes mellitus, myasthenia gravis and coeliac disease, PSC is associated with the HLA antigens B8 (Chapman *et al.* 1983) and DR3 (Schrumpf *et al.* 1982; Shepherd *et al.* 1983), and, recently, a dual association of HLA-DR2 and DR3 with PSC has been found (Donaldson *et al.* 1991a). This latter study confirmed the linkage with the A1-B8-DR3 haplotype and also found that there is a reduction in the frequency of the antigens B44 and DR4 in PSC, resulting from the absence of the B44-DR4 haplotype — suggesting that both A1-B8-DR3 and DR2 confer susceptibility to PSC and that B44-DR4 is protective (Donaldson *et al.* 1991a). However, the closest association so far described has been with Class II MHC antigen DRw52a (Prochazka *et al.* 1990). In that study, the frequency of this antigen in a small series of patients with PSC who had been referred for liver transplantation was found to be 100%. Studies in our institute, in a larger series of less selected cases, have confirmed a strong association with DRw52a but have shown that this is by no means invariant (J.M. Farrant *et al.* 1991, submitted data). The above evidence, although circumstantial, is perhaps the strongest to date that PSC may have a genetic basis.

Mechanisms

No spontaneous or induced model of PSC in animals has been described and the mechanisms involved in the development of this condition are not at all clear. The relative infrequency of autoantibodies in adults with the disease and the generally unsatisfactory responses to immunosuppressive therapy (Lindor *et al.* 1986) suggest that autoimmunity is not a major factor. On the other hand, the prevalence of HLA-B8 and DR3 and the marked association of PSC with ulcerative colitis (Chapman *et al.* 1980; Dickson *et al.* 1984; Lindor *et al.* 1986), which is also thought to have an autoimmune basis, points to the possibility of an underlying autoreactive pathology. In addition, apart from PBC, PSC is the only condition in which a high frequency of *in vitro* T cell reactivity to normal biliary tract antigens has been demonstrated (McFarlane *et al.* 1979; McFarlane 1985).

It has been suggested that immune complexes may be involved in the pathogenesis of PSC. High circulating levels have been identified in patients' sera (Bodenheimer *et al.* 1983), and impaired clearance of immune complexes (Minuk *et al.* 1985) and IgG-tagged erythrocytes (Minuk *et al.* 1986) from the circulation has been demonstrated. Whether the elevation of circulating immune complexes is a primary or secondary phenomenon remains speculative. It is of interest that activation of complement, as measured by C3d and C4d levels, has been demonstrated in patients with PSC (Senaldi *et al.* 1989). One could speculate that immune complexes that are not cleared from the circulation at a normal rate are deposited in the portal tracts, where they might cause activation of the complement system, which in turn could lead to tissue damage.

The uncertainty as to whether PSC is an autoimmune disorder might be related to the natural history of the disease. The latter is not yet fully understood, but many adults with PSC present with a well-established biliary cirrhosis, suggesting that they must have had the disease for some time before symptoms developed. It is possible that some of the autoimmune features (particularly autoantibodies) may have disappeared by the time the condition reaches its later stages.

Some support for this suggestion comes from the contrasting findings in children with PSC of a high frequency of autoantibodies and, in many cases, of at least some response to immunosuppressive therapy (Mieli-Vergani *et al.* 1989). Such children often present with what appears to be AI-CAH and, in common with AI-CAH, their lymphocytes show (non-T) cytotoxic reactions against isolated hepatocytes *in vitro*, and they have similarly increased percentages of lymphocytes expressing the activation marker HLA-DR. However, the numbers and function of T_s cells are normal (decreased in AI-CAH), as are the percentages of T cells expressing interleukin 2 receptors (markedly increased in AI-CAH) (Mieli-Vergani *et al.* 1989). These findings, together with the relative rarity of anti-ASGP-R antibodies (see above), suggest that, if autoimmune mechanisms are involved in PSC, they are clearly different from those that obtain in AI-CAH.

A condition resembling PSC cholangiographically has been described in patients with acquired immune deficiency syndrome (AIDS). However, such patients often have frank biliary infections with cytomegalovirus and *Cryptosporidium*. The latter organisms are presumably responsible for the stricturing of the biliary tree and papillary stenosis observed and there is at present insufficient evidence to regard 'AIDS sclerosing cholangitis' and PSC as one condition.

On balance, current evidence suggests that PSC is an immunologically mediated disease and is likely to be autoimmune. The probable course of events in disease initiation is an interaction between an environmental trigger, possibly a virus, and antigen-presenting cells. The processed (viral) antigen might be presented, in conjunction with HLA Class II (possibly DRw52a), to CD4+ve T lymphocytes, which could then interact with B cells to produce an antibody directed against both the viral antigen and a cross-reacting self antigen. The latter might be soluble and deposition of immune complexes in the portal tracts might lead to tissue damage via complement activation. Alternatively, the self antigen might be located on the biliary epithelium and cell killing might be the result of ADCC.

Although the study of specific cellular immune responses to biliary epithelial cell antigens has been dormant for more than a decade, the advent of molecular biological techniques, particularly genomic libraries, and better preparations of isolated normal biliary epithelial cells will allow this avenue to be reopened, and it may be expected that this will lead to a much clearer understanding of the pathogenesis of this interesting condition.

References

Al-Aghbar, M.N.A., Alexander, G.J.M., Neuberger, J., Nouri-Aria, K.T., Eddleston, A.L.W.F. and Williams, R. (1986). The effect of prednisolone *in vitro* on immunoglobulin production in primary biliary cirrhosis. *Clin. Exp. Immunol.* **63**, 663–70.

Amberg, S. (1942). Hyperproteinaemia associated with severe liver damage. *Proc. Staff Meet. Mayo Clin.* **17**, 360–2.

Amoroso, P., Vergani, D., Wojcicka, B.M. *et al.* (1980). Identification of biliary antigens in circulating immune complexes in primary biliary cirrhosis. *Clin. Exp. Immunol.* **42**, 95–8.

Araki, K., Yamamoto, H. and Fujimoto, S. (1987). Studies on the pathogenesis of murine experimental autoimmune active hepatitis: sensitized T cell involvement in its induction. *Clin. Exp. Immunol.* **67**, 326–34.

Aronson, A.R. and Montgomery, M.M. (1959). Chronic liver disease with a 'lupus erythematosus-like syndrome'. *Arch. Intern. Med.* **104**, 544–52.

Bartholomaeus, W.N., Reed, W.D., Joske, R.A. and Shilkin, K.B. (1981). Autoantibody responses to liver-specific lipoprotein in mice. *Immunology* **43**, 219–26.

Bartholomew, L.G., Hagedorn, A.B., Cain, J.C. and Baggenstoss, A.H. (1958). Hepatitis and cirrhosis in women with positive clot tests for lupus erythematosus. *N. Engl. J. Med.* **259**, 947–56.

Bartholomew, L.G., Cain, J.C., Baggenstoss, A.H. and Hagedorn, A.B. (1960). Further observations on hepatitis in young women with positive clot tests for lupus erythematosus. *Gastroenterology* **39**, 730–6.

Bassendine, M.F., Dewar, P.J. and James, O.F.L. (1985). HLA DR antigens in primary biliary cirrhosis: lack of association. *Gut* **26**, 625–8.

Baum, H. and Palmer, C. (1985). The PBC-specific antigen. *Mol. Aspects Med.* **8**, 201–34.

Baum, H., Daffern, F., Hall, G.S. and Zilkha, K.J. (1990). M2 mitochondrial autoantigens in myelin. *Lancet* **335**, 603–4.

Beaune, P., Dansette, P.M., Mansuy, D. *et al.* (1987). Human anti-endoplasmic reticulum autoantibodies appearing in a drug-induced hepatitis are directed against a human liver cytochrome P-450 that hydroxylates the drug. *Proc. Nat. Acad. Sci. (USA)* **84**, 551–5.

Bedlow, A.J., Donaldson, P.T., McFarlane, B.M., Lombard, M., McFarlane, I.G. and Williams, R. (1989). Autoreactivity to hepatocellular antigens in primary biliary cirrhosis and primary sclerosing cholangitis. *J. Clin. Lab. Immunol.* **30**, 103–9.

Berg, P.A. and Klein, R. (1985). Clinical and prognostic relevance of different mitochondrial antibody profiles in primary biliary cirrhosis (PBC). *Mol. Aspects Med.* **8**, 235–47.

Berg, P.A., Klein, R. and Lindenborn-Fotinos, J. (1986). Antimitochondrial antibodies in primary biliary cirrhosis. *J. Hepatol.* **2**, 123–31.

Bodenheimer, H.C., LaRusso, N.F., Thayer, W.R., Charland, C., Staples, P.J. and Ludwig, J. (1983). Elevated circulating immune complexes in primary sclerosing cholangitis. *Hepatology* **3**, 150–4.

Bourdi, M., Larrey, D., Nataf, J. *et al.* (1990). Anti-liver endoplasmic reticulum autoantibodies are directed against human cytochrome P-450IA2: a specific marker for dihydralazine-induced hepatitis. *J. Clin. Invest.* **85**, 1967–73.

Briggs, D.C., Donaldson, P.T., Hayes, P., Welsh, K.I., Williams, R. and Neuberger, J.M. (1987). A major histocompatibility complex Class III allotype (C4B2) associated with primary biliary cirrhosis (PBC). *Tissue Antigens* **29**, 141–5.

Brown, R., Doniach, S. and Clark, M.L. (1975). PBC in brothers. *Postgrad. Med. J.* **51**, 110–15.

Cales, P., Calot, M., Voigt, J.J. *et al.* (1983). Pathologie auto-immune familiale compartant deux cas de cirrhose biliaire primitive. *Gastroenterol. Clin. Biol.* **7**, 777–84.

Chapman, R.W.G. (1985). Review: Primary sclerosing cholangitis. *J. Hepatol.* **1**, 179–86.

Chapman, R.W.G., Marburgh, B.A., Rhodes, R.M. *et al.* (1980). Primary sclerosing cholangitis: a review of its clinical features, cholangiography, and hepatic histology. *Gut* **21**, 870–7.

Chapman, R.W.G., Varghese, Z., Gaul, R., Patel, N., Kokinon, N. and Sherlock, S. (1983). Association of primary sclerosing cholangitis with HLA-B8. *Gut* **24**, 38–41.

Chapman, R.W.G., Cottone, M., Selby, W.S., Shepherd, H.A., Sherlock, S. and Jewell, D.P. (1986). Serum autoantibodies, ulcerative colitis and primary sclerosing cholangitis. *Gut* **27**, 86–91.

Chohan, M.R. (1973). Primary biliary cirrhosis in twin sisters. *Gut* **14**, 213–14.

Christensen, E., Neuberger, J., Crowe, J. *et al.* (1985). Beneficial effect of azathioprine and prediction of prognosis in primary biliary cirrhosis. Final results of an international trial. *Gastroenterology* **89**, 1084–91.

Cohen, I.R. and Cooke, A. (1986). Natural autoantibodies might prevent autoimmune disease. *Immunol. Today* **7**, 363–4.

Crivelli, O., Lavarini, C., Chiaberge, E. *et al.* (1983). Microsomal autoantibodies in chronic infection with the HBsAg associated delta agent. *Clin. Exp. Immunol.* **54**, 232–8.

Cullinan, E.R. (1936). Idiopathic jaundice (often recurrent) associated with subacute necrosis of the liver. *St Bartholomew's Hosp. Rep.* **69**, 55–142.

Culp, K.S., Fleming, C.R., Duffy, J., Baldus, W. and Dickson, E.R. (1982). Autoimmune associations in primary biliary cirrhosis. *Mayo Clin. Proc.* **57**, 365–70.

Czaja, A.J., Hay, J.E. and Rakela, J. (1990). Clinical features and prognostic implications of severe corticosteroid-treated cryptogenic chronic active hepatitis. *Mayo Clin. Proc.* **65**, 23–30.

Daniels, C.K., Smith, K.M. and Schmucker, D.L. (1987). Asialoorosomucoid hepatobiliary transport is unaltered by the loss of liver asialoglycoprotein receptors in aged rats. *Proc. Soc. Exp. Biol. Med.* **186**, 246–50.

Das, K.M., Vecchi, M. and Skamaki, S. (1990). A shared and unique epitope(s) on human colon, skin, and biliary epithelium detected by a monoclonal antibody. *Gastroenterology* **98**, 464–9.

De Kretser, T.A., McFarlane, I.G., Eddleston, A.L.W.F. and Williams, R. (1980). A species non-specific liver plasma membrane antigen and its involvement in chronic active hepatitis. *Biochem. J.* **186**, 679–85.

Dickson, E.R., LaRusso, N.F. and Wiesner, R.H. (1984). Primary sclerosing cholangitis. *Hepatology* **4**, 33S–35S.

Dighiero, G., Lymberi, P., Monot, C. and Abuaf, N. (1990). Sera with high levels of anti-smooth muscle and anti-mitochondrial antibodies frequently bind to cytoskeletal proteins. *Clin. Exp. Immunol.* **82**, 52–6.

Donaldson, P.T., Farrant, J.M., Wilkinson, M.L., Hayllar, K., Portmann, B.C. and Wiliams, R. (1991a). Dual association of HLA DR2 and DR3 with primary sclerosing cholangitis. *Hepatology* **13**, 129–33.

Donaldson, P.T., Doherty, D.G., Hayllar, K.M., McFarlane, I.G., Johnson, P.J. and Williams, R. (1991b). Susceptibility to autoimmune chronic active hepatitis: HLA DR4 and A1-B8-DR3 are independent risk factors. *Hepatology* **13**, 701–6.

Doniach, D., Roitt, I.M., Walker, J.G. and Sherlock, S. (1966). Tissue antibodies in primary biliary cirrhosis, active chronic (lupoid) hepatitis, cryptogenic cirrhosis and other liver diseases and their clinical implications. *Clin. Exp. Immunol.* **1**, 237–62.

Eddleston, A.L.W.F. and Williams, R. (1974). Inadequate antibody response to HBAg or suppressor T-cell defect in development of active chronic hepatitis. *Lancet* **ii**, 1543–5.

Eddleston, A.L.W.F., McFarlane, I.G., Mitchell, C.G., Reed, W.D. and Williams, R. (1973). Cell-mediated immune responses in primary biliary cirrhosis to a protein fraction from human bile. *Br. Med. J.* **4**, 340–2.

Epstein, O., Thomas, H.C. and Sherlock, S. (1980). Hypothesis: primary biliary cirrhosis is a dry gland syndrome with features of chronic graft-versus-host disease. *Lancet* **i**, 1166–8.

Ercilla, G., Pares, A., Arriaga, F. *et al.* (1979). Primary biliary cirrhosis associated with HLA-DRw3. *Tissue Antigens* **14**, 449–52.

Fagan, E., Cox, S. and Williams, R. (1977). Primary biliary cirrhosis in mother and daughter. *Br. Med. J.* **2**, 1195–7.

Farrant, J.M., Hayllar, K.M., Wilkinson, M.L. *et al.* (1991). Natural history and prognostic variables in primary sclerosing cholangitis. *Gastroenterology* **100**, 1710–17.

Feighery, C., McDonald, G.S.A., Greally, J.F. and Weir, D.G. (1981). Histological and immunological investigation of liver-specific protein (LSP) immunized rabbits compared with patients with liver disease. *Clin. Exp. Immunol.* **45**, 143–51.

Feizi, T., Naccarato, R., Sherlock, S. and Doniach, D. (1972). Mitochondrial and other tissue antibodies in relatives of patients with primary biliary cirrhosis. *Clin. Exp. Immunol.* **10**, 609–22.

Fox, R.A., Dudley, F.J. and Sherlock, S. (1973). The primary immune response to haemocyanin in patients with primary biliary cirrhosis. *Clin. Exp. Immunol.* **14**, 473–80.

Fregeau, D.R., Roche, T.E., Davis, P.A., Coppel, R. and Gershwin, M.E. (1990). Primary biliary cirrhosis: inhibition of pyruvate dehydrogenase complex activity in autoantibodies specific for E1α, a non-lipoic acid containing mitochondrial enzyme. *J. Immunol.* **144**, 1671–6.

Fussey, S.P.M., Guest, J.R., James, O.F.W., Bassendine, M.F. and Yeaman, S.J. (1988). Identification and analysis of the major M2 autoantigens in primary biliary cirrhosis. *Proc. Nat. Acad. Sci. (USA)* **85**, 8654–8.

Fussey, S.P.M., Bassendine, M.F., Fittes, D., Turner, I.B., James, O.F.W. and Yeaman, S.J. (1989). The E1 α and β subunits of the pyruvate dehydrogenase complex are M2'd' and M2'e' autoantigens in primary biliary cirrhosis. *Clin. Sci.* **77**, 365–8.

Fussey, S.P.M., West, S.M., Lindsay, J.G. *et al.* (1991). Clarification of the identity of the major M2 autoantigen in primary biliary cirrhosis. *Clin. Sci.* **80**, 451–5.

Galbraith, R.M., Smith, M.G.M., MacKenzie, R.M., Tee, D.E., Doniach, D. and Williams, R. (1974). High prevalence of seroimmunologic abnormalities in relatives of patients with chronic active hepatitis or primary biliary cirrhosis. *N. Engl. J. Med.* **290**, 63–9.

Galbraith, R.M., Eddleston, A.L.W.F., Smith, M.G.M. *et al.* (1975). Histocompatibility antigens in active chronic hepatitis and primary biliary cirrhosis. *Br. Med. J.* **4**, 77–9.

Galbraith, R.M., Eddleston, A.L.W.F., Williams, R. *et al.* (1976). Enhanced antibody responses in active chronic hepatitis: relation to HLA-B8 and HLA-B12 and portosystemic shunting. *Lancet* **i**, 930–4.

Gerken, G., Manns, M., Ramadori, G. and Meyer zum Buschenfelde, K.H. (1988). The target antigens of antimitochondrial antibodies (AMA) in primary biliary cirrhosis. *Hepatology* **8**, 705–6.

Gershwin, M.E. and Mackay, I.R. (1991). Primary biliary cirrhosis: paradigm or paradox for autoimmunity. *Gastroenterology* **100**, 822–33.

Gershwin, M.E., Coppel, R.L. and Mackay, I.R. (1988). Primary biliary cirrhosis and mitochondrial autoantigens — insights from molecular biology. *Hepatology* **8**, 147–51.

Ghadiminejad, I. and Baum, H. (1987). Evidence for the cell-surface localization of antigens cross-reacting with 'mitochondrial antibodies' of primary biliary cirrhosis. *Hepatology* **7**, 743–50.

Gores, G.J., Moore, S.B., Fisher, L.D., Powell, F.C. and Dickson, E.R. (1987). Primary biliary cirrhosis: associations with Class II major histocompatibility complex antigens. *Hepatology* **7**, 889–92.

Gupta, R.C., Dickson, E.R., McDuffie, F.C. and Bagenstoss, A.H. (1978). Circulating IgG complexes in primary biliary cirrhosis: a serial study in forty patients followed for two years. *Clin. Exp. Immunol.* **34**, 19–27.

Gurian, L.E., Rogoff, T.M., Ware, A.J., Jordan, R.E., Combes, B. and Gilliam, J.N. (1985). The immunologic diagnosis of chronic active 'autoimmune' hepatitis: distinction from systemic lupus erythematosus. *Hepatology* **5**, 397–402.

Harmon, C.E. (1985). Antinuclear antibodies in autoimmune disease. *Med. Clin. North Am.* **69**, 623–36.

Homberg, J.C., Abuaf, N., Bernard, O. *et al.* (1987). Chronic active hepatitis associated with antiliver/kidney microsome antibody type 1: a second type of 'autoimmune' hepatitis. *Hepatology* **7**, 1333–9.

Jaup, B.H. and Zettergen, L.S.W. (1980). Familial occurrence of primary biliary cirrhosis associated with hypergammaglobulinemia in descendants: a family study. *Gastroenterology* **78**, 549–55.

Jensen, D.M., Hall, C. and Majewski, T. (1983). The plasma membrane origin of liver-specific protein (LSP). *Liver* **3**, 213–19.

Johnson, P.J., McFarlane, I.G., McFarlane, B.M. and Williams, R. (1990). Autoimmune features in patients with idiopathic chronic active hepatitis who are seronegative for conventional autoantibodies. *J. Gastroenterol. Hepatol.* **5**, 244–51.

Jones, C.E., Lewert, R.M. and Ozcel, M.A. (1976). Anti-liver antibodies in rabbits infected with *Schistosoma japonicum*. *Am. J. Trop. Med. Hyg.* **25**, 613–16.

Joske, R.A. and King, W.E. (1955). The 'L.E.-cell' phenomenon in active chronic viral hepatitis. *Lancet* **ii**, 477–9.

Kaplan, M.M. (1987). Medical progress: primary biliary cirrhosis. *N. Engl. J. Med.* **316**, 521–8.

Kato, Y., Suzuki, K., Kumagai, M. *et al.* (1981). Familial PBC: immunological and genetic study. *Am. J. Gastroenterol.* **75**, 188–91.

Kingston, D. and Glynn, L.E. (1971). A cross-reaction between *Str. pyogenes* and human fibroblasts, endothelial cells and astrocytes. *Immunology* **21**, 1003–16.

Klein, R. and Berg, P.A. (1990). Demonstration of 'naturally occurring mitochondrial antibodies' in family members of patients with primary biliary cirrhosis. *Hepatology* **12**, 335–41.

Krams, S.M., Surh, C.D., Coppel, R.L. and Gershwin, M.E. (1989a). Immunization of experimental animals with dihydrolipoamide acetyltransferase, as a purified recombinant polypeptide, generates mitochondrial autoantibodies but not primary biliary cirrhosis. *Hepatology* **9**, 411–16.

Krams, S.M., Dorshkind, K. and Gershwin, M.E. (1989b). Generation of biliary lesions following transfer of human lymphocytes into SCID mice. *J. Exp. Med.* **170**, 1919–30.

Krawitt, E.L., Kilby, A.E., Albertini, R.J. *et al.* (1987). Immunogenetic studies of autoimmune chronic active hepatitis: HLA, immunoglobulin allotypes and autoantibodies. *Hepatology* **7**, 1305–10.

Kuriki, J., Murakami, H., Kakumu, S. *et al.* (1983). Experimental autoimmune hepatitis in mice after immunization with syngeneic liver proteins together with the polysaccharide of *Klebsiella pneumoniae*. *Gastroenterology* **84**, 596–603.

Lebwohl, N.A. and Gerber, M.A. (1981). Characterization and demonstration of human liver-specific protein (LSP) and apo-LSP. *Clin. Exp. Immunol.* **46**, 435–42.

Lindor, K.D., Wiesner, R.H., LaRusso, N.F. and Dickson, E.R. (1986). Chronic active hepatitis: overlap with primary biliary cirrhosis and primary sclerosing cholangitis. In *Chronic Active Hepatitis — the Mayo Clinic Experience*, ed. A.J. Czaja and E.R. Dickson, pp. 171–87, Marcel Dekker, New York.

Lohr, H., Treichel, U., Poralla, T. *et al.* (1990). The human hepatic asialoglycoprotein receptor is a target antigen for liver-infiltrating T cells in autoimmune chronic active hepatitis and primary biliary cirrhosis. *Hepatology* **12**, 1314–20.

Lohse, A.W., Manns, M., Dienes, H.P., Meyer zum Buschenfelde, K.H. and Cohen, I.R. (1990). Experimental autoimmune hepatitis: disease induction, time course and T-cell reactivity. *Hepatology* **11**, 24–30.

McCune, J.M., Namikawa, R., Kaneshima, H.S., Shultz, L.D., Lieberman, M. and Weissman, I.L. (1988). The SCID-hu mouse: murine model for the analysis of human hematolymphoid differentiation and function. *Science* **241**, 1632–9.

McDonald, G.B., Shulman, H.M., Wolford, J.L. and Spencer, G.D. (1987). Liver disease after human bone marrow transplantation. *Semin. Liver Dis.* **7**, 210–29.

McFarlane, B.M., McSorley, C.G., Vergani, D., McFarlane, I.G. and Williams, R. (1986). Serum autoantibodies reacting with the hepatic asialoglycoprotein receptor (hepatic lectin) in acute and chronic liver disorders. *J. Hepatol,* **3**, 196–205.

McFarlane, B.M., Sipos, J., Gove, C.D., McFarlane, I.G. and Williams, R. (1990). Antibodies against the hepatic asialoglycoprotein receptor perfused *in situ* preferentially bind to periportal liver cells in the rat. *Hepatology* **11**, 408–15.

McFarlane, I.G. (1983). Hepatic clearance of serum glycoproteins. *Clin. Sci.* **64**, 127–35.

McFarlane, I.G. (1984). Autoimmunity in liver disease. *Clin. Sci.* **67**, 569–78.

McFarlane, I.G. (1985). Autoreactivity against biliary tract antigens in primary biliary cirrhosis. *Mol. Aspects Med.* **8**, 249–67.

McFarlane, I.G. (1991). Autoimmunity and hepatotropic viruses. *Semin. Liver Dis.* **11**, 223–33.

McFarlane, I.G. and Williams, R. (1985). Liver membrane antibodies. *J. Hepatol.* **1**, 313–19.

McFarlane, I.G., Wojcicka, B.M., Zucker, G.M., Eddleston, A.L.W.F. and Williams, R. (1977). Purification and characterisation of human liver-specific membrane lipoprotein (LSP). *Clin. Exp. Immunol.* **27**, 381–90.

McFarlane, I.G., Wojcicka, B.M., Tsantoulas, D.C., Portmann, B., Eddleston, A.L.W.F. and Williams, R. (1979). Leukocyte migration inhibition in response to biliary antigens in primary biliary cirrhosis, sclerosing cholangitis and other chronic liver diseases. *Gastroenterology* **76**, 1333–40.

McFarlane, I.G., McFarlane, B.M., Haines, A.J., Eddleston, A.L.W.F. and Williams, R. (1983). Relationship between primary biliary cirrhosis and chronic graft-versus-host disease: investigation of histocompatibility (HLA) antigenic determinants in biliary tract antigens. *Clin. Sci.* **64**, 113–16.

McFarlane, I.G., McFarlane, B.M., Major, G.N., Tolley, P. and Williams, R. (1984a). Identification of the hepatic asialoglycoprotein receptor (hepatic lectin) as a component of liver specific membrane lipoprotein (LSP). *Clin. Exp. Immunol.* **55**, 347–54.

McFarlane, I.G., Hegarty, J.E., McSorley, C.G., McFarlane, B.M. and Williams, R. (1984b). Antibodies to liver specific protein predict outcome of treatment withdrawal in autoimmune chronic active hepatitis. *Lancet* **ii**, 954–6.

Mackay, I.R. (1984). Genetic aspects of immunologically mediated liver disease. *Semin. Liver Dis.* **4**, 26–35.

Mackay, I.R. and Gershwin, M.E. (1989). Primary biliary cirrhosis: current knowledge, perspectives, and future directions. *Semin. Liver Dis.* **9**, 149–57.

Mackay, I.R. and Morris, P.J. (1972). Association of autoimmune active chronic hepatitis with HL-A1, 8. *Lancet* **ii**, 793–5.

Mackay, I.R. and Tait, D.B. (1980). HLA associations with autoimmune type chronic active hepatitis: identification of B8-DRw3 haplotype by family studies. *Gastroenterology* **79**, 95–8.

Mackay, I.R. and Wood, I.J. (1962). Lupoid hepatitis: a comparison of 22 cases with other types of liver disease. *Quart. J. Med.* **31**, 485–507.

Mackay, I.R., Taft, L.I. and Cowling, D.C. (1956). Lupoid hepatitis. *Lancet* **ii**, 1323–6.

Mackay, I.R., Taft, L.I. and Cowling, D.C. (1959). Lupoid hepatitis and the hepatic lesions of systemic lupus erythematosus. *Lancet* **i**, 65–9.

Manns, M., Gerken, G., Kyriatsoulis, A., Staritz, M. and Meyer zum Buschenfelde, K.H. (1987). Characterisation of a new subgroup of autoimmune chronic active hepatitis by autoantibodies against a soluble liver antigen. *Lancet* **i**, 292–4.

Manns, M., Johnson, E.F., Griffin, K.J., Tan, E.M. and Sullivan, K.F. (1989). Major antigen of liver kidney microsomal autoantibodies in idiopathic autoimmune hepatitis is cytochrome P450db1. *J. Clin. Invest.* **83**, 1066–72.

Manns, M., Griffin, K.J., Quattrochi, L.C. *et al.* (1990). Identification of cytochrome P450IA2 as a human autoantigen. *Arch. Biochem. Biophys.* **280**, 229–32.

Meyer zum Buschenfelde, K.H., Kossling, F.K. and Miescher, P.A. (1972). Experimental chronic active hepatitis in rabbits following immunization with human liver proteins. *Clin. Exp. Immunol.* **11**, 99–108.

Mieli-Vergani, G., Vergani, D., Jenkins, P.J. *et al.* (1979). Lymphocyte cytotoxicity to autologous hepatocytes in HBsAg-negative chronic active hepatitis. *Clin. Exp. Immunol.* **38**, 16–21.

Mieli-Vergani, G., Lobo-Yeo, A., McFarlane, B.M., McFarlane, I.G., Mowat, A.P. and Vergani, D. (1989). Different immune mechanisms leading to autoimmunity in primary sclerosing cholangitis and autoimmune chronic active hepatitis of childhood. *Hepatology* **9**, 198–203.

Miglio, F., Pignatelli, M., Mazzeo, V. *et al.* (1987). Expression of major histocompatibility complex class II antigens on bile duct epithelium in patients with hepatic graft-versus-host-disease after bone marrow transplantation. *J. Hepatol.* **5**, 182–5.

Miller, J., Smith, M.G.M., Mitchell, C.G., Reed, W.D., Eddleston, A.L.W.F. and Williams, R. (1972). Cell-mediated immunity to human liver-specific antigen in patients with active chronic hepatitis and primary biliary cirrhosis. *Lancet* **ii**, 296–7.

Minuk, G.Y., Angus, M., Brickman, C.M. *et al.* (1985). Abnormal clearance of immune complexes from the circulation of patients with primary sclerosing cholangitis. *Gastroenterology* **88**, 166–70.

Minuk, G.Y., Hershfield, N.B., Lee, W.Y. *et al.* (1986). Reticuloendothelial system Fc receptor-mediated clearance of IgG-tagged erythrocytes from the circulation of patients with idiopathic ulcerative colitis and chronic liver disease. *Hepatology* **6**, 1–5.

Miyamori, H., Kato, Y. and Kobayashi, K. (1983). HLA antigens in Japanese patients with primary biliary cirrhosis and autoimmune hepatitis. *Digestion* **26**, 213–17.

Mori, T., Mori, Y., Yoshida, H. *et al.* (1985). Cell-mediated cytotoxicity of sensitized spleen cells against target liver cells — *in vivo* and *in vitro* study with a mouse model of experimental autoimmune hepatitis. *Hepatology* **5**, 770–7.

Mori, Y., Mori, T., Yoshida, H. *et al.* (1984). Study of cellular immunity in experimental autoimmune hepatitis in mice. *Clin. Exp. Immunol.* **57**, 85–92.

Mori, Y., Mori, T., Ueda, S. *et al.* (1985). Study of cellular immunity in experimental autoimmune hepatitis in mice: transfer of spleen cells sensitized with liver proteins. *Clin. Exp. Immunol.* **61**, 577–84.

Mosier, D.E., Galizea, R.J., Baird, S.M. and Wilson, D.B. (1988). Transfer of a functional human immune system to mice with severe combined immunodeficiency. *Nature* **355**, 256–9.

Mutimer, D.J., Fussey, S.P.M., Yeaman, S.J., Kelly, P.J., James, O.F.W. and Bassendine, M.F. (1989). Frequency of IgG and IgM autoantibodies to four specific M2 mitochondrial autoantigens in primary biliary cirrhosis. *Hepatology* **10**, 403–7.

Neuberger, J., Portmann, B., Macdougall, B.R.D., Calne, R.Y. and Williams, R. (1982). Recurrence of primary biliary cirrhosis after liver transplantation. *N. Engl. J. Med.* **306**, 1–6.

Nouri-Aria, K.T., Hegarty, J.E., Alexander, G.J.M., Eddleston,

A.L.W.F. and Williams, R. (1982). Effect of corticosteroids on suppressor-cell activity in 'autoimmune' and viral chronic active hepatitis. *N. Engl. J. Med.* **307**, 1301–4.

Nouri-Aria, K.T., Donaldson, P.T., Hegarty, J.E., Eddleston, A.L.W.F. and Williams, R. (1985a). HLA A1-B8-DR3 and suppressor cell function in first-degree relatives of patients with autoimmune chronic active hepatitis. *J. Hepatol.* **1**, 235–41.

Nouri-Aria, K.T., Hegarty, J.E., Alexander, G.J.M., Eddleston, A.L.W.F. and Williams, R. (1985b). IgG production in 'autoimmune' chronic active hepatitis: effect of prednisolone on T and B lymphocyte function. *Clin. Exp. Immunol.* **61**, 290–6.

Nouri-Aria, K.T., Hegarty, J.E., Neuberger, J., Eddleston, A.L.W.F. and Williams, R. (1985c). *In vitro* studies on the mechanism of increased serum IgM levels in primary biliary cirrhosis. *Clin. Exp. Immunol.* **61**, 297–304.

O'Brien, C.J., Vento, S., Donaldson, P.T. *et al.* (1986). Cell-mediated immunity and suppressor T-cell defects to liver-derived antigens in families of patients with autoimmune chronic active hepatitis. *Lancet* **i**, 350–3.

Ogawa, M., Mori, Y., Mori, T. *et al.* (1988). Adoptive transfer of experimental autoimmune hepatitis in mice — cellular interaction between donor and recipient mice. *Clin. Exp. Immunol.* **73**, 276–82.

Opelz, G., Vogten, A.J., Summerskill, W.H., Schalm, S.W. and Terasaki, P.I. (1977). HLA determinants in chronic active liver disease: possible relation of HLA-Dw3 to prognosis. *Tissue Antigens* **9**, 36–40.

Potter, B.J., Elias, E. and Jones, E.A. (1976). Hypercatabolism of the third component of complement in patients with primary biliary cirrhosis. *J. Lab. Clin. Med.* **88**, 427–39.

Potter, B.J., Elias, E., Thomas, H.C. and Sherlock, S. (1980). Complement catabolism in chronic liver disease: catabolism of C1q in chronic active liver disease and primary biliary cirrhosis. *Gastroenterology* **78**, 1034–40.

Powell, F.C., Scroeter, A.L. and Dickson, E.R. (1987). Primary biliary cirrhosis and the CREST syndrome: a report of 22 cases. *Quart. J. Med.* **237**, 75–82.

Prochazka, E.J., Terasaki, P.I., Park, M.S., Goldstein, L.I. and Busuttil, R.W. (1990). Association of primary sclerosing cholangitis with HLA-DRw52a. *N. Engl. J. Med.* **322**, 1842–4.

Schrumpf, E., Fausa, O., Forre, O., Dobloug, J.H., Ritland, S. and Thorsby, E. (1982). HLA antigens and immunoregulatory T cells in ulcerative colitis associated with hepatobiliary disease. *Scand. J. Gastroenterol.* **17**, 187–91.

Schwartz, A.L. (1984). The hepatic asialoglycoprotein receptor. *CRC Crit. Rev. Biochem.* **16**, 207–33.

Seki, T., Kiyosawa, K., Inoko, H. and Ota, M. (1990). Association of autoimmune hepatitis with HLA-Bw54 and DR4 in Japanese patients. *Hepatology* **12**, 1300–4.

Senaldi, G., Donaldson, P.T., Magrin, S. *et al.* (1989). Activation of the complement system in primary sclerosing cholangitis. *Gastroenterology* **97**, 1430–4.

Shepherd, H.A., Selby, W.S., Chapman, R.W.G. *et al.* (1983). Ulcerative colitis and persistent liver dysfunction. *Quart. J. Med.* **208**, 503–13.

Snook, J.A., Chapman, R.W.G., Sachdev, G.K. *et al.* (1989a). Peripheral blood and portal tract lymphocyte population in primary sclerosing cholangitis. *J. Hepatol.* **9**, 36–41.

Snook, J.A., Chapman, R.W.G., Fleming, K. and Jewell, D.P. (1989b). Anti-neutrophil nuclear antibody in ulcerative colitis, Crohn's disease and primary sclerosing cholangitis. *Clin. Exp. Immunol.* **76**, 30–3.

Soloway, R.D., Summerskill, W.H.J., Baggenstoss, A.H. *et al.* (1972). Clinical, biochemical, and histological remission of severe chronic active liver disease: a controlled study of treatments and early prognosis. *Gastroenterology* **63**, 820–33.

Steer, C.J. and Ashwell, G. (1986). Hepatic membrane receptors for glycoproteins. *Prog. Liver Dis.* **8**, 99–123.

Surh, C.D., Cooper, A.E, Coppel, R.L. *et al.* (1988). The predominance of IgG3 and IgM isotype antimitochondrial antibodies against recombinant fused mitochondrial polypeptide in patients with primary biliary cirrhosis. *Hepatology* **8**, 290–5.

Surh, C.D., Danner, D.J., Ahmed, A., Coppel, R.L., Mackay, I.R., Dickson, E.R., and Gershwin, M.E. (1989). Reactivity of primary biliary cirrhosis sera with a human fetal liver cDNA clone of branched-chain α-keto acid dehydrogenase dihydrolipoamide acyltransferase, the 52 kD mitochondrial autoantigen. *Hepatology* **9**, 63–8.

Surh, C.D., Ansari, A.A. and Gershwin, M.E. (1990). Comparative epitope mapping of murine monoclonal and human autoantibodies to human PDH-E_2, the major mitochondrial autoantigen of primary biliary cirrhosis. *J. Immunol.* **144**, 2647–52.

Tan, E.M. (1982). Autoantibodies to nuclear antigens (ANA). *Adv. Immunol.* **33**, 167–240.

Thomas, H.C., Holden, R., Verrier-Jones, J. and Peacock, D.B. (1976). Immune response to ϕX-174 in man: primary and secondary antibody production in primary biliary cirrhosis. *Gut* **17**, 844–8.

Thomas, H.C., DeVilliers, D., Potter, B.J. *et al.* (1978). Immune complexes in acute and chronic liver disease. *Clin. Exp. Immunol.* **31**, 150–7.

Tison, V., Callea, F., Morisi, C., Mancini, A.M. and Desmet, V.J. (1982). Spontaneous 'primary biliary cirrhosis' in rabbits. *Liver* **2**, 152–61.

Tong, M.J., Nies, K.M., Reynolds, T.B. and Quismorio, F.P. (1976). Immunological studies in familial primary biliary cirrhosis. *Gastroenterology* **71**, 305–7.

Treichel, U., Poralla, T., Hess, G., Manns, M. and Meyer zum Buschenfelde, K.H. (1990). Autoantibodies to human asialoglycoprotein receptor in autoimmune-type chronic hepatitis. *Hepatology* **11**, 606–12.

Tsantoulas, D., Perperas, A., Portmann, B., Eddleston, A.L.W.F. and Williams, R. (1980). Antibodies to a human liver membrane lipoprotein (LSP) in primary biliary cirrhosis. *Gut* **21**, 557–60.

Uibo, R.M., Helin, K.J. and Krohn, K.J.E. (1982). Immunological reactions to liver specific membrane lipoprotein (LSP) in experimental autoimmune liver disease in rabbits. *Clin. Exp. Immunol.* **48**, 505–12.

Van de Water, J., Fregeau, D., Davis, P. *et al.* (1988). Autoantibodies of primary biliary cirrhosis (PBC) recognize dihydrolipoamide acetyl-transferase and inhibit enzyme function. *J. Immunol.* **141**, 2321–4.

Vento, S., Hegarty, J.E., Bottazzo, G.F., Macchia, E., Williams, R. and Eddleston, A.L.W.F. (1984). Antigen-specific suppressor cell function in autoimmune chronic active hepatitis. *Lancet* **i**, 1200–4.

Vento, S., O'Brien, C.J., McFarlane, B.M., McFarlane, I.G., Eddleston, A.L.W.F. and Williams, R. (1986) T-lymphocyte sensitization to hepatocyte antigens in autoimmune chronic active hepatitis and primary biliary cirrhosis: evidence for different underlying mechanisms and different antigenic determinants as targets. *Gastroenterology* **91**, 810–17.

Vento, S., O'Brien, C.J., McFarlane, I.G., Williams, R. and Eddleston, A.L.W.F. (1987). T-cell inducers of suppressor lymphocytes control liver-directed autoreactivity. *Lancet* **i**, 886–8.

Vento, S., Garofano, T., DiPerri, G., Dolci, L., Concia, E. and Bassetti, D. (1991). Identification of hepatitis A virus as a trigger for autoimmune chronic active hepatitis type 1 in susceptible individuals. *Lancet* **337**, 1183–7.

Waldenstrom, J. (1950). Leber, Blutproteine und Nahrungseiweiss. *Deutsch Gesellschaft Z. Verdau Stoffwechselkr.* **15**, 113–19.

Walsh, L.J. and Cox, D.W. (1984). Immunoglobulin (Gm) markers and α-1 antitrypsin (pi) types in rheumatoid arthritis and early onset chronic active hepatitis. *J. Immunogenet.* **11**, 115–20.

Wands, J.R., Dienstag, J.L., Bhan, A.K., Feller, E.R. and Isselbacher, K.J. (1978). Circulating immune complexes and complement activation in primary biliary cirrhosis. *N. Engl. J. Med.* **298**, 233–7.

Wen, L., Peakman, M., Lobo-Yeo, A. *et al.* (1990). T-cell-directed hepatocyte damage in autoimmune chronic active hepatitis. *Lancet* **336**, 1527–30.

Whiteside, T.L., Lasky, S., Si, L. and Van Thiel, D.H. (1985). Immunologic analysis of mononuclear cells in liver tissues and blood of patients with primary sclerosing cholangitis. *Hepatology* **5**, 468–74.

Whittingham, S., Mackay, I.R. and Irwin, J. (1966a). Autoimmune hepatitis: immuno-fluorescence reactions with cytoplasm of smooth muscle and glomerular cells. *Lancet* **i**, 1333–5.

Whittingham, S., Irwin, J., Mackay, I.R. and Smalley, M. (1966b). Smooth muscle autoantibody in 'autoimmune' hepatitis. *Gastroenterology* **51**, 499–505.

Whittingham, S., Mathews, J.D., Scanfield, M.S., Tait, D.B. and Mackay, I.R. (1981). Interaction of HLA and Gm in autoimmune chronic active hepatitis. *Clin. Exp. Immunol.* **43**, 80–6.

Willcox, R.G. and Isselbacher, K.J. (1961). Chronic liver disease in young people: clinical features and course of thirty-three patients. *Am. J. Med.* **30**, 185–95.

Witt-Sullivan, H., Heathcote, J., Cauch, K. *et al.* (1990). The demography of primary biliary cirrhosis in Ontario, Canada. *Hepatology* **12**, 98–105.

Wojcicka-McFarlane, B.M. (1990). The asialoglycoprotein receptor as an autoantigen. PhD thesis, University of London.

Wojcicka-McFarlane, B.M., McFarlane, I.G., Amoroso, P. and Williams, R. (1981). Differential *in vitro* immune responses to biliary tract antigens in primary biliary cirrhosis and chronic active hepatitis. *Liver* **1**, 268–79.

Yeaman, S.J. (1989). The 2-oxo acid dehydrogenase complexes: recent advances. *Biochem. J.* **257**, 625–32.

Yeaman, S.J., Fussey, S.P.M., Danner, D.J., James, O.F.W., Mutimer, D.J. and Bassendine, M.F. (1988). Primary biliary cirrhosis: identification of two major M2 mitochondrial autoantigens. *Lancet* **i**, 1067–70.

Zauli, D., Schrumpf, E., Crespi, C., Cassani, F., Fausa, O. and Aadland, E. (1987). An autoantibody profile in primary sclerosing cholangitis. *J. Hepatol.* **5**, 14–18.

Zinkernagel, R.M. and Doherty, P.C. (1979). MHC-restricted cytotoxic T cells: studies on the biological role of polymorphic major transplantation antigens determining T-cell restriction-specificity, function and responsiveness. *Adv. Immunol.* **27**, 51–177.

102: Autoimmune Endocrine Disease

A.P. Weetman and A.M. McGregor

Introduction

The autoimmune endocrine diseases belong to the group of organ-specific autoimmune diseases which, in addition, include insulin-dependent diabetes mellitus, myasthenia gravis, pernicious anaemia, coeliac disease, vitiligo and alopecia. These autoimmune endocrine disorders (which are reviewed in detail elsewhere (Weetman 1991a)) encompass a range of clinical problems from the common autoimmune thyroid diseases to the rare but clinically important conditions such as adrenal failure and hypophysitis. These diseases are characterized not only by their association within the same individual or family with other organ-specific autoimmune diseases but also by a female predominance, human leucocyte antigen (HLA) associations, lymphocytic infiltration of the target organ and evidence of immune activation, particularly during the active phase of the disease, when circulating autoantibodies and activated T cells and abnormalities of cell-mediated immunity are detectable (Weetman and McGregor 1984; De Groot and Quintans 1989). The clinical manifestations of this group of diseases are outside the scope of this review but are discussed extensively elsewhere (De Groot 1989).

Graves' disease

Understanding of the biology of the normal thyroid follicular cell is crucial to the understanding of Graves' disease (Fig. 102.1). The initial demonstration in 1956 by Adams and Purves of a thyroid-stimulating activity quite distinct from thyroid-stimulating hormone (TSH) in the sera of patients with hyperthyroid Graves' disease, which they described, because of its biological activity, as a long-acting thyroid stimulator (LATS), was the key observation in the development of our understanding of the pathogenesis of the hyperthyroidism in Graves' disease. The subsequent establishment of an improved and simplified bioassay (McKenzie 1958) for LATS, using mouse thyroid gland tissue, allowed both the confirmation of the existence of LATS activity in the sera

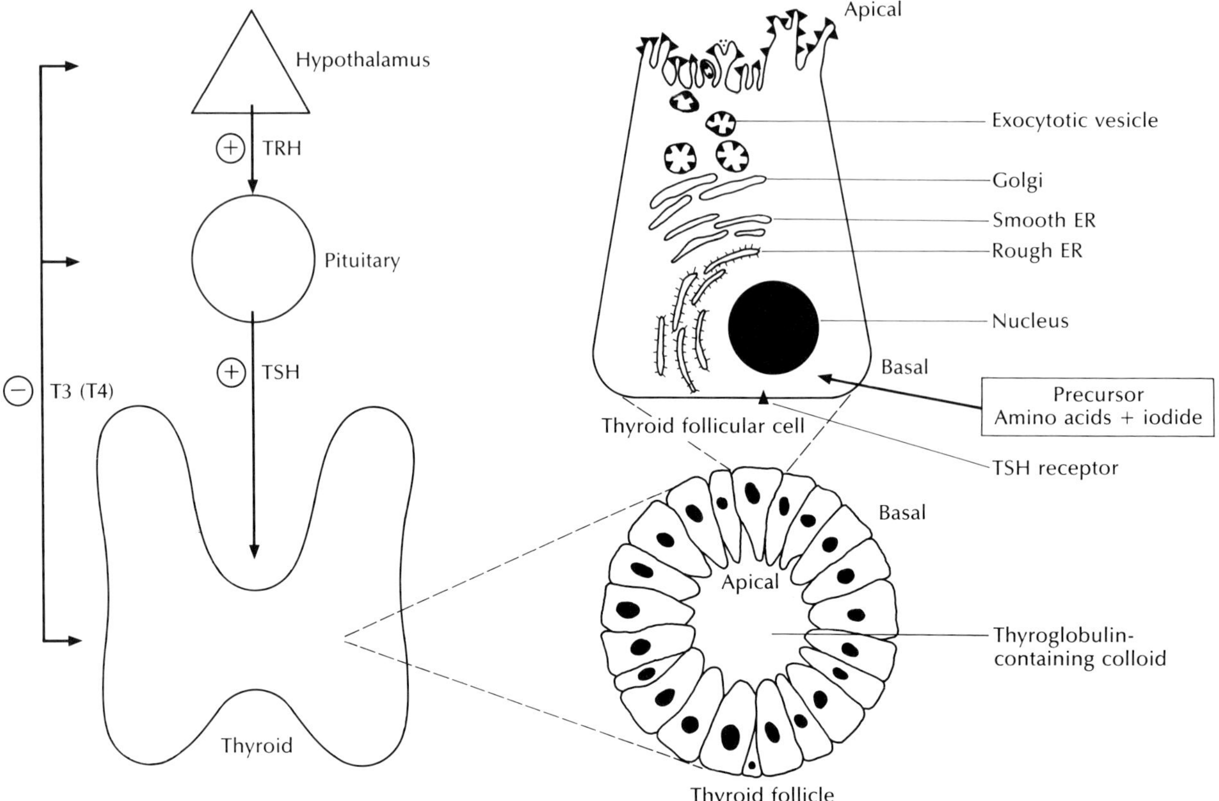

Fig. 102.1. The hypothalamic–pituitary–thyroid axis. Thyrotropin-releasing hormone (TRH), secreted by the hypothalamus, stimulates the pituitary to secrete thyrotropin (TSH), which, on binding to the thyroid follicular cell TSH receptor, stimulates the synthesis and release of thyroid hormone, which, in turn, feeds back to regulate the hypothalamic–pituitary axis.

of patients with hyperthyroid Graves' disease and further characterization of the activity. In particular, the demonstration that LATS was an immunoglobulin (Kriss *et al.* 1964) and that, when present at sufficiently high levels in the sera of pregnant women, it was likely to lead to the development of transient neonatal hyperthyroidism in their offspring, suggesting that the biologically active stimulator was crossing the placenta and inducing this transient syndrome (McKenzie 1964), led to the concept of Graves' disease being an antibody-mediated condition. Long-acting thyroid stimulator activity, however, was noted in less than 50% of patients with hyperthyroid Graves' disease, and only with the development of assay systems using human tissue (Adams and Kennedy 1967; Rapoport *et al.* 1984) did the rate of detection rise to levels more supportive of the association between the presence of antibody activity and hyperthyroidism. Infusion of Graves' immunoglobulins into man *in vivo* provided evidence of increased radio-isotope turnover in the recipients' thyroid and gave further credence to the role of the antibody in thyroid stimulation (Adams *et al.* 1974). The recognition thereafter that Graves' immunoglobulins were able to inhibit the binding of radiolabelled TSH to its receptor in thyroid membrane preparations (Mehdi *et al.* 1973; Manley *et al.* 1974; Smith and Hall 1974) and in particular the demonstration that these immunoglobulins could not bind to the receptor at the same time as radiolabelled TSH led to the concept that Graves' immunoglobulins were indeed immunoglobulins directed against the human TSH receptor (Rees Smith *et al.* 1988). Studies extending these initial observations confirmed beyond doubt that TSH and Graves' immunoglobulins could not bind simultaneously to the TSH receptor. From this early work therefore emerged the concept that Graves' disease was due to antibodies to the TSH receptor. Clinically the disease is characterized by hyperthyroidism, associated usually with diffuse enlargement of the thyroid gland, demonstrable on radio-isotope examination as a diffuse uptake of isotope in the thyroid, and with the presence or absence of Graves' ophthalmopathy, pretibial myxoedema and thyroid acropachy. The infrequency with which acropachy and pretibial myxoedema are observed has made understanding of these abnormalities difficult. In contrast, ophthalmopathy occurs more commonly, but the difficulty of access to target tissue (extraocular muscles) has again made elucidation of the association between ophthalmopathy and Graves' disease and the pathogenesis of the ophthalmopathy difficult to determine. Untreated Graves' disease is associated with considerable morbidity and mortality, but with currently available therapies, which are directed towards either inhibition of thyroid hormone synthesis or removal or destruction of thyroid gland tissue, the disease is easily controllable and relatively benign. Serendipitously, methods used to control the disease may be doing so partly by their effect on the autoimmune process (Ratanachaiyavong and McGregor 1985). The absence of an animal model of this disease has certainly delayed progress in elucidating its aetiology and pathogenesis.

Aetiology

Graves' disease occurs more commonly in women than men but when it does occur in men is a much more severe disease with a much higher relapse rate (Barnett *et al.* 1990). Remission during pregnancy tends to be followed by exacerbation of the disease so that hormonal changes clearly contribute to the natural history of the disease, but their exact role remains uncertain. No evidence has emerged to date which suggests that there is any structural abnormality in the TSH receptor present on the thyroid follicular cell surface of a Graves' thyroid as compared with that of a normal individual. The impact of stress on the induction of Graves' disease has attracted considerable interest but has always proved exceedingly difficult to assess scientifically. The few valid data available have proved conflicting (Gorman 1990; Winsa *et al.* 1991). Considerable attention has been directed to dissecting the immune response in patients with Graves' disease, and from this has grown a body of evidence, particularly associated with Volpé and his colleagues, which purports to demonstrate a defect in 'suppressor' T lymphocyte function in patients with hyperthyroid Graves' disease (Volpé 1988). The field has proved controversial because of the methodologies used, the focus on peripheral blood rather than target organ (thyroid) T lymphocyte function and, most importantly, lack of access to purified target autoantigen (TSH receptor) (Ludgate *et al.* 1985). Evidence of increased levels of activated T cells and, in particular, reduced levels of OKT8 +ve (suppressor T) cells in the peripheral blood of patients with hyperthyroid Graves' disease (Ludgate *et al.* 1984) have been used to support the concept of a suppressor T cell defect, but without justification. What seems much more likely is that Graves' disease is multifactorial in its aetiology, with the dominant contributors to its initiation being genetic and environmental factors but with the immune system having a key role to play both in the induction of hyperthyroidism through TSH receptor antibody activity and in the maintenance of the autoimmune response through a variety of mechanisms. These mechanisms include: (i) thyroid cell Ia (Class II major histocompatibility complex (MHC)) molecule expression, perhaps as a mechanism for enhancing self antigen presentation (Bottazzo *et al.* 1983); (ii) cytokine secretion, particularly by the immune infiltrate but also by thyrocytes of lymphokines such as interleukin 6, a major B lymphocyte stimulator (Weetman *et al.* 1990b); and (iii) adhesion molecule expression, again by the lymphoid infiltrate and thyroid cells (Weetman *et al.* 1990a). Whilst Graves' disease is clearly multifactorial in its origin, the key contributors to the development of this disease seem most likely to be genetic and environmental.

IMMUNOGENETICS

Three sets of genes have attracted particular attention in the attempt to dissect the genetic contribution to the development of Graves' disease (Ratanachaiyavong and McGregor 1990): genes of the HLA system, the T cell receptor and the immunoglobulin molecule. The early family studies of Graves' disease and the demonstration that just under 50% of monozygotic twins are concordant for Graves' disease, compared with less than 10% of HLA-identical siblings (Stenszky *et al.* 1985), demonstrate the undoubted hereditary contribution to the aetiology of Graves' disease.

Extensive investigation of the HLA genes in patients with Graves' disease, initially by serology and more recently by Southern blotting, restriction fragment length polymorphism analysis and oligonucleotide probing following deoxyribonucleic acid (DNA) amplification by the polymerase chain reaction, have continued to confirm the association with HLA-DR3 (Ratanachaiyavong and McGregor 1990) and have extended the association to genes in the DQ and DP regions of Class II MHC (Ratanachaiyavong *et al.* 1990), to genes in the Class III MHC region (Ratanachaiyavong *et al.* 1989) and to more recently identified new genes lying within the three HLA regions associated with the disease (Ratanachaiyavong *et al.* 1991). The search has clearly been for susceptibility genes but, unlike in insulin-dependent diabetes mellitus, has been confounded, at least in Caucasians, by problem of linkage disequilibrium in HLA-DR3 individuals. Molecular characterization of the T cell receptor (Weiss 1990) has begun to allow the examination of T cell variability in Graves' disease. Restriction fragment length polymorphism analysis of both constant and variable (V) regions of the T cell receptor has been carried out, using patients with Graves' disease, and has demonstrated associations which have proved conflicting (Demaine *et al.* 1987, 1989; Weetman *et al.* 1987a; Mangklabruks *et al.* 1991). Preliminary data examining 18 Vα gene families of intrathyroidal T cells have demonstrated restricted Vα gene family usage (Davies *et al.* 1991). Data extending this observation, and particularly its interpretation in conjunction with the Class II HLA haplotypes of patients studied, will be of importance in determining the significance of T cell receptor usage and its restriction in Graves' disease. Since Graves' disease is antibody-mediated, considerable interest has focused on the immunoglobulin genes. The frequent observation of light-chain (usually lambda) restriction of TSH receptor antibodies (Zakarija 1983; Williams *et al.* 1988), in conjunction with the observation that these antibodies are nearly always of the IgG-1 subclass (Weetman *et al.* 1990d), suggests that TSH receptor antibodies may have an oligoclonal or even monoclonal origin; sequencing of the V genes encoding the TSH receptor antibody will resolve issues such as whether these antibodies are germline-encoded, conserved in all individuals and clonally restricted.

ENVIRONMENT

Dietary iodine, a key constituent of thyroid hormones, has an important role in the modulation of the autoimmune response in autoimmune thyroid disease (McGregor *et al.* 1985). In areas of the world where iodine deficiency predominates, autoimmune thyroid disease is uncommon. With the introduction of iodine into the diet of such populations, autoantibodies to thyroid constituents and lymphocytic infiltration of the thyroid gland are more commonly observed. Across Europe the variation in the frequency with which Graves' disease is the cause of hyperthyroidism ranges from 45% in Göttingen, an area of iodine deficiency, to 87% in Athens, an area of high iodine intake. In the United Kingdom, milk provides the main source of iodine and, as a result, milk iodine levels vary through the year, with the highest levels occurring during the winter months, when cows are frequently brought indoors and, for a variety of reasons, their dietary supplements are high in iodine. The seasonal variation of Graves' disease follows that of iodine in milk, with the peak of Graves' disease following the winter peak in milk iodine content (Phillips *et al.* 1988). In genetically susceptible strains of rats and chickens, increasing iodine in the diet exacerbates their thyroid autoimmunity (Braverman 1990). It seems likely that, at least in animal models, alterations in the iodine content of thyroglobulin alter the immunogenicity of this molecule and its role in the induction of experimental thyroiditis (Sundick *et al.* 1987). Smoking has been shown to be associated with the development of both Graves' ophthalmopathy (Shine *et al.* 1990) and post-partum thyroid dysfunction (PPTD) (Fung *et al.* 1988). The mechanism for this remains unknown. Considerable evidence has accumulated supporting the possible role of infectious agents in the induction of autoimmunity in the thyroid. Elegant studies by Ingbar and his colleagues demonstrated beyond doubt that normal gut pathogens have determinants on their cell surface which are able to bind TSH, with characteristics very similar to those of the human TSH receptor on the thyroid follicular cell (Ingbar *et al.* 1987). These studies raise the concept of molecular mimicry. Studies in animal models have demonstrated a marked reduction in thyroiditis in animals maintained in a pathogen-free environment, with the normal disease incidence being restored by the transfer of intestinal microflora from animals maintained in a normal non-pathogen-free environment (Penhale and Young 1988). The concept that begins to emerge, therefore, is that the thyroid gland itself is probably normal but that, in individuals who are genetically predisposed, exposure to an environmental insult leads to immune activation. Whilst retroviruses have been shown to infect and transform rat thyroid cell lines, early claims of human immunodeficiency virus (HIV)-1 gene sequences in the thyroid cell genomic DNA obtained from patients with Graves' disease have not been substantiated (Humphrey *et al.* 1991). The possibility that other retroviruses may have a role to play cannot be excluded and indeed seems likely.

Autoantibodies

Considerable confusion has surrounded the pathogenic autoantibodies of Graves' disease. The use of different assay systems led to a profusion of terminologies and a profusion of results, which meant that, for far too long, research in the field was devoted to comparisons of antibody activity in different assay systems. Terminology has been simplified with the recognition that the autoantibodies which cause Graves' disease are antibodies to the TSH receptor, and this activity is now referred to collectively as TSH receptor autoantibodies (McGregor 1990). Bioassays for the measurement of TSH receptor antibody activity can, by and large, be divided into bioassays using human thyroid gland cells grown in monolayer (Kasagi *et al.* 1982; Rapoport *et al.* 1984) or the FRTL5 rat thyroid cell line, which offers the prospect of an immortal cell line (Vitti *et al.* 1983). The FRTL5 cell line allows the measurement of both cyclic adenosine monophosphate (AMP) production and the ability of these cells to take up radioactive iodine in response to TSH receptor antibody activity. The drift with time in culture of these cells in their responsiveness to autoantibodies and the relative insensitivity of these cells as compared with human thyroid cells in cultures make the FRTL5 cell line less attractive than at first seemed likely. In contrast to the bioassay, the establishment of a commercially available, robust, rapid, less cumbersome and easily standardized radioreceptor assay (Southgate *et al.* 1984), in which the TSH receptor antibodies inhibit the binding of ^{125}I-labelled TSH to thyroid membrane preparations, has provided a sensitive and specific marker of TSH receptor antibody activity although it is clearly not able to discriminate between binding to the receptor and actual thyroid cell stimulation. This latter concept has become exceedingly important recently as a series of studies by Konishi and his colleagues in Japan have demonstrated that patients with atrophic, as opposed to goitrous, thyroiditis have TSH receptor antibody activity in their circulation, as measured by the radioreceptor assay which, on binding to the receptor, inhibits the interaction of TSH with it and leads to hypothyroidism (Endo *et al.* 1978). The most convincing biological proof of the existence of such antibodies comes from the same group, who demonstrated initially the transient neonatal hypothyroidism occurring in babies in whom maternal antibodies crossed the placenta (Matsuura *et al.* 1980). There clearly exists, therefore, a spectrum of agonist and antagonist autoantibodies directed against the TSH receptor which, as a result of their binding to the receptor, have the capacity, on the one hand, to stimulate thyroid cell function directly and, on the other, to induce hypothyroidism by preventing the binding of TSH to its receptor.

The use of a human thyroid cell bioassay system, again by Konishi and his colleagues, has demonstrated beyond doubt that the sera of patients with atrophic thyroiditis have antibodies in them which inhibit TSH-stimulated cyclic AMP production by these cells (Konishi *et al.* 1983). The frequency of TSH receptor-blocking antibody activity in patients with atrophic thyroiditis still remains uncertain but may be present in up to 60% of patients with the disease. A further group of antibodies which demonstrate either growth-stimulating or growth-blocking activity have been described in patients with autoimmune thyroid disease, and their contribution to the pathogenesis of this group of diseases continues to be evaluated. The role of TSH receptor antibody measurement in the management of patients with autoimmune thyroid disease remains less well defined. Whilst there is little doubt that assays for the detection of this antibody activity provide vital research tools for understanding the pathogenetic mechanisms involved, the role of such measurements in routine clinical practice is limited. There is no doubt that the level of antibody activity coincides closely with the natural history of the disease, with antibody activity declining on treatment of Graves' disease and returning with recurrence (Weetman and McGregor 1984). Persistence of antibody activity following partial thyroidectomy or radioactive iodine therapy is an important indicator of subsequent disease recurrence (Weetman and McGregor 1984). The one area in which measurements of antibody activity have an undoubted role is in the situation of pregnancy in women with autoimmune thyroid disease. Whilst TSH receptor antibody activity will tend to fall during pregnancy, persistent elevation of such activity, particularly in the third trimester of pregnancy, is an important indicator of the likely development in the offspring of a transient neonatal syndrome of altered thyroid function, which may be hyper- or hypothyroidism depending on the nature of the TSH receptor antibody crossing the placenta (Munro *et al.* 1978; Zakarija *et al.* 1990).

Thyroid-stimulating hormone receptor

Considerable controversy has surrounded attempts to characterize the TSH receptor. The biochemical approaches used prior to the cloning of the receptor in 1989 (Libert *et al.* 1989a) led to a variety of claims as to the structure of the receptor. The receptor proposed by Rees Smith and his colleagues, using photoaffinity labelling of receptors cross-linked to ^{125}I-TSH, comes closest to reflecting the characteristics of the cloned human TSH receptor (Rees Smith *et al.* 1988). The major impetus to the successful cloning of the TSH receptor followed the cloning of the luteinizing hormone–human chorionic gonadotrophin (LH–HCG) receptor and its recognition as a member of the G protein-coupled group of receptors (McFarland *et al.* 1989). This group of receptors is characterized by seven transmembrane segments and, using a mixture of oligonucleotides based on these transmembrane segments as primers in a polymerase chain reaction (Libert *et al.* 1989b), with human thyroid complementary DNA (cDNA) as the template, cloning of the TSH receptor followed (Fig. 102.2) when oligonucleotides based on the second and seventh transmembrane segments of the LH–HCG receptor were used (Libert *et al.* 1989a). The 764 amino acid receptor is predicted to have a molecular weight of approximately 86 000, which is remarkably close to the molecular weight derived by Rees Smith. The successful cloning of the receptor has meant that, besides its characterization (Table 102.1), expression of the receptor in CHO cells (Perret *et al.* 1990) will allow elucidation of both the interaction between receptor autoantibodies and the receptor and discrimination in this interaction between antibodies that bind and stimulate and those that bind without stimulation of the thyroid cell. In the same way that these transfected cells offer the prospect of establishing more stable human bioassays for TSH receptor antibody activity, so the use of recombinant human TSH receptor material has allowed the development of a radioreceptor assay (Filetti *et al.* 1991) for the measurement of TSH receptor autoantibody activity. Creation of chimeric receptors will allow further characterization of the receptor antibody–receptor interaction (Nagayama *et al.* 1991).

Treatment

Patients with hyperthyroid Graves' disease have high levels of TSH receptor antibody activity prior to treatment and, with the modern assay systems available, this activity is detectable in 90–95% of such patients. In response to therapy with the antithyroid drug carbimazole, autoantibody levels fall, usually into the normal range (McGregor *et al.* 1980). Persistence of autoantibody activity following a course of antithyroid drug therapy is associated with disease recurrence, just as reappearance of antibody activity after the cessation of therapy is associated with relapse. Similarly, following partial thyroidectomy, levels of antibody tend to disappear and this is usually indicative of disease cure, whereas, interestingly, in patients treated with radio-iodine, an initial acute rise in antibody activity, peaking at about 3 months after the dose of radio-iodine and then succeeded by gradual disappearance over the next 9 months of the antibody activity, is associated with control of the disease (Weetman and McGregor 1984). Considerable effort has been expended on trying to characterize the underlying mechanisms leading to these changes in antibody activity, and *in vitro* systems (McGregor *et al.* 1980) and animal models (Rennie *et al.* 1983) have shown beyond doubt that the antithyroid drugs such as carbimazole are immunosuppressive (Ratanachaiyavong and McGregor 1985). The mechanism of this effect is

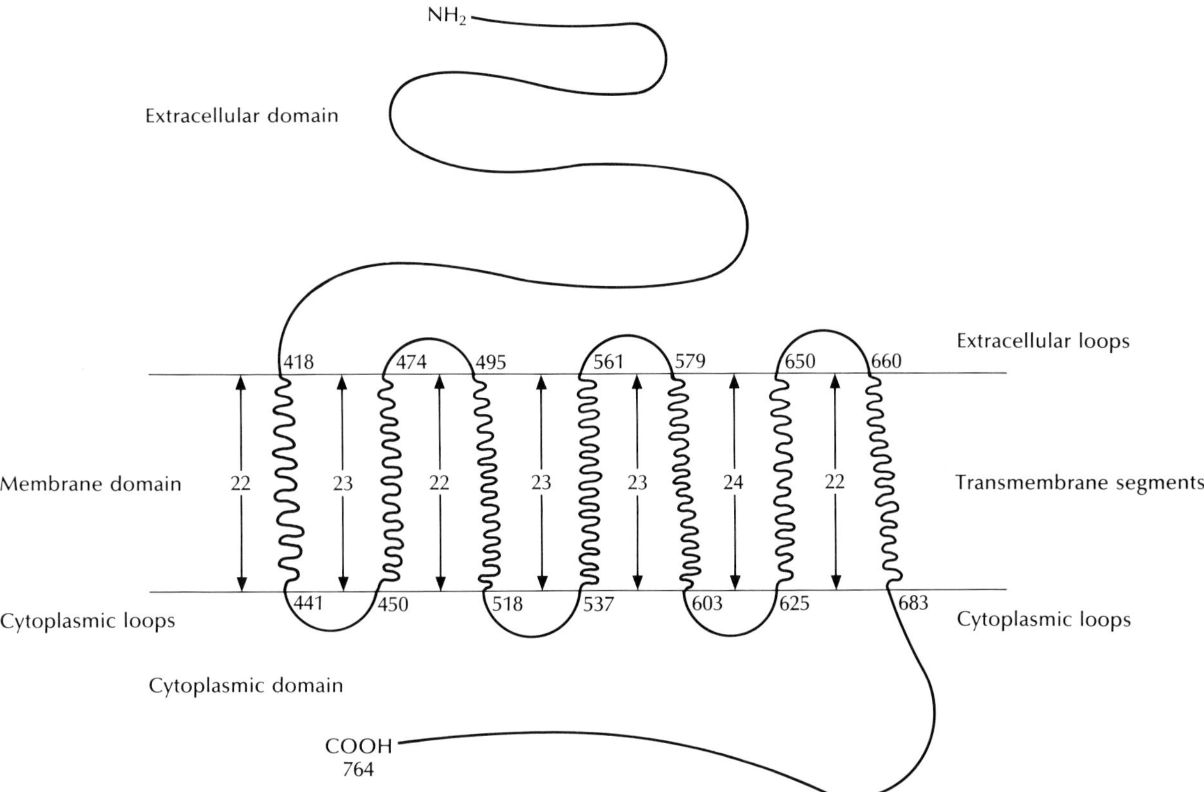

Fig. 102.2. The thyrotropin (TSH) receptor.

likely to be dependent on the uptake of these drugs by antigen-presenting cells (Weetman *et al.* 1983), and their impact on antigen presentation in these cells is via an action on oxygen radical generation (Weetman *et al.* 1984b).

Graves' ophthalmopathy

Whilst the majority of patients with ophthalmopathy have autoimmune thyroid disease, which in the majority of cases is hyperthyroid Graves' disease, the ophthalmopathy need not be associated with hyperthyroidism. Limited access to the extraocular tissues, the infrequency of severe eye disease, absence of an appropriate animal model, poor understanding of the association between the ophthalmopathy and thyroid disease and confusion as to the pathogenesis of this condition have led to it being associated with considerable controversy (Weetman 1991b). Immunogenetic studies have contributed little to our understanding of the disease although smoking (Shine *et al.* 1990) seems strongly associated with its development. A variety of assay systems have been developed for the detection of autoantibody activity against retrobulbar tissues and have relied particularly on porcine material (Atkinson *et al.* 1984). A consensus view on these antibody activities has not been reached. Alternative studies have suggested a variety of other possible autoantigens (Wall *et al.* 1991). Cross-reactivity between thyroglobulin and eye muscle acetylcholinesterase has been offered as a possible explanation for the link between the eye and the thyroid (Ludgate *et al.* 1989), although again this work has progressed no further. The recent cloning and sequencing of a 64 kD autoantigen, initially recognized by screening a human thyroid cDNA library with sera from patients with Hashimoto's thyroiditis, was followed by the recognition that the messenger ribonucleic acid (mRNA) for this protein could also be detected in eye muscle but not skeletal muscle (Dong *et al.* 1991). Studies currently under way seek to examine the possibility that autoantibodies previously described as reacting with a molecule of this size may in fact be

Table 102.1. Autoantigens in autoimmune thyroid disease

	Thyroglobulin	Thyroid peroxidase	Thyrotropin (TSH) receptor
Protein	Iodinated glycoprotein	Haemoprotein enzyme	G-binding protein-linked receptor
Glycosylated	+	+	+
Function	Biosynthetic precursor of T3 and T4	Catalyses iodination and coupling of tyrosine to yield T3 and T4	Receptor for TSH
Thyroid location	Follicular lumen Circulation	Membrane-bound Cell surface (apical) Exo/endocytotic vesicles	Membrane-bound — cell surface (basal)
Molecular weight	660 000	105 000; 110 000	86 000
Amino acids	2748	TPO-1 933; TPO-2 876; alternatively spliced products	764 (excludes 20 amino acid signal sequence)
Regions			
Extracellular	—	842 (TPO-1)	418
Transmembrane	—	29	265 (7 transmembrane domains)
Intracellular	—	62	81
Chromosome location	8	2	14
Homologies	Acetylcholinesterase	Myeloperoxidase	LH/HCG, FSH receptors

interacting with the newly described cloned autoantigen. The absence of muscle destruction has made the likelihood of immune cytotoxic mechanisms less likely. The possibility exists that cytokine release by T cells in the muscles leads to fibroblast proliferation and that this may then, through a mass effect, contribute to the changes observed clinically in the orbit (Weetman 1991b).

Autoimmune hypothyroidism

Thyroiditis has the distinction of being the first disease ascribed to autoimmune processes, a discovery based on the translation of findings in experimental animal models (Rose and Witebsky 1956) to patients with lymphadenoid (Hashimoto's) goitre (Roitt *et al.* 1956). Further studies, using several types of experimental autoimmune thyroiditis (EAT), have shown that disease severity is, in part, governed by genes within the MHC and outside it, including those controlling T cells and possibly target organ function (Rose *et al.* 1980). There is strong evidence for disordered T cell regulation as a cause of the autoimmune process in some of these models, particularly since thymectomy results in EAT in certain strains of rat and mouse, and autoantigen-responsive T cells have been identified in good responder strain animals (Weetman 1991a). Several effector mechanisms probably combine to produce the target organ damage in EAT, including antibodies, cytotoxic T cells and natural killer/killer (NK/K) cells (Wick *et al.* 1982). These experimental models have continued to provide insights into the human counterpart, and thyroiditis remains a useful paradigm generally for organ-specific autoimmune disease. However, one limitation of EAT is that thyroglobulin is the key autoantigen, whereas in the human counterpart autoimmunity against the microsomal antigen and the TSH receptor seems more related to disease pathogenesis.

The prevalence of autoimmune hypothyroidism is 2–3% in women, tenfold higher than in men (Tunbridge *et al.* 1977). A range of distinct clinical and pathological variants exist, from patients who present with a lymphocytic goitre, sometimes with fibrosis (oxyphil and fibrous Hashimoto's thyroiditis), to those with primary myxoedema, whose hypothyroidism is not accompanied by goitre but rather a shrunken, fibrotic gland remnant (Doniach *et al.* 1979). Goitre size in Hashimoto's thyroiditis may decrease over a period of years in about 50% of patients, especially with thyroxine treatment, but histological findings are usually surprisingly constant (Hayashi *et al.* 1985). Focal asymptomatic thyroiditis is even more common, being found in 6% of male and 22% of female autopsies (Williams and Doniach 1962), and is strongly associated with serum thyroid autoantibodies, even in the absence of overt clinical disease (Yoshida *et al.* 1978).

Immunogenetics

The clinicopathological heterogeneity is reflected by differences in HLA associations, but these are less clear than previously believed. Originally an association of Hashimoto's thyroiditis with HLA-DR5 and primary myxoedema with HLA-DR3 was reported in Caucasians (Weissel *et al.* 1980; Farid *et al.* 1981), but later studies, with new serological typing reagents, have shown an association of Hashimoto's thyroiditis with HLA-DR4 in Newfoundland and HLA-DR3 in Hungary and the United Kingdom (Stenszky *et al.* 1987; Tandon *et al.* 1991). Whether these differences all relate to technical factors, or are due in part to temporal and geographical heterogeneity, remains to be identified. Other D region genes, in particular DQ and DP, do not appear to contribute further susceptibility. Non-MHC genes are also associated with autoimmune hypothyroidism, including those encoding Gm allotypes (which interact with HLA-DR3 (Stenszky *et al.* 1987)) and the T cell receptor (Weetman *et al.* 1987a).

Autoantibodies

Thyroglobulin and microsomal antibodies are the hallmark of autoimmune hypothyroidism. They are undetectable in about 15% of primary myxoedema patients but are usually present in Hashimoto's thyroiditis, although recently patients have been reported in whom there was no serological evidence for biopsy-proved Hashimoto's disease (Franklyn *et al.* 1987; Baker *et al.* 1988). These antibodies are also non-specific, since about three-quarters of Graves' disease patients will have one or both antibodies (depending on assay sensitivity), as do most asymptomatic patients with focal thyroiditis. Population studies show that the development of thyroid autoantibodies and the evolution of hypothyroidism are slow, but a raised serum TSH in the presence of thyroid antibodies (Fig. 102.3) identifies those patients with asymptomatic thyroiditis at risk of progressing to overt hypothyroidism (Tunbridge *et al.* 1981). Thyroid antibodies are synthesized within the thyroid itself and in the lymph nodes draining the gland; the bone marrow may also be a major site of production (Weetman *et al.* 1984a).

THYROGLOBULIN ANTIBODIES

Thyroglobulin antibodies recognize a 660 kD glycoprotein dimer (Table 102.1) which is synthesized and secreted by thyroid epithelial cells. Thyroglobulin serves as the substrate for thyroid hormone synthesis and as a store for these hormones in the thyroid follicular colloid. Full-length copies of cDNA from thyroglobulin mRNA have been made (De Martynoff *et al.* 1980), but there are no reports of abnormal forms in pathological conditions. The only remarkable feature of the chemical composition of this protein is the high concentration of iodinated tyrosine residues (which depend on dietary iodine); these represent thyroid hormones or their precursors. Despite the molecule's large size, only two major and one minor autoantigenic epitope exist, although heterologous thyroglobulins display about 40 epitopes when used in immunization experiments (Nye *et al.* 1980). Animal studies have also shown that highly iodinated thyroglobulin is more immunogenic than that derived from animals fed on a low-iodine diet (Sundick *et al.* 1987). Antibodies binding to thyroxine are found in about 20% of patients with thyroiditis (and occasionally in other subjects); it is possible that thyroglobulin with bound hormone may act as a carrier–hapten system to trigger their formation (Premachandra and Blumenthal 1985). These antihormone antibodies are clinically important because they may interfere with thyroxine assays.

The vast majority of thyroglobulin antibodies are polyclonal (Nye *et al.* 1981) and, although public cross-reactive idiotypes are present, private

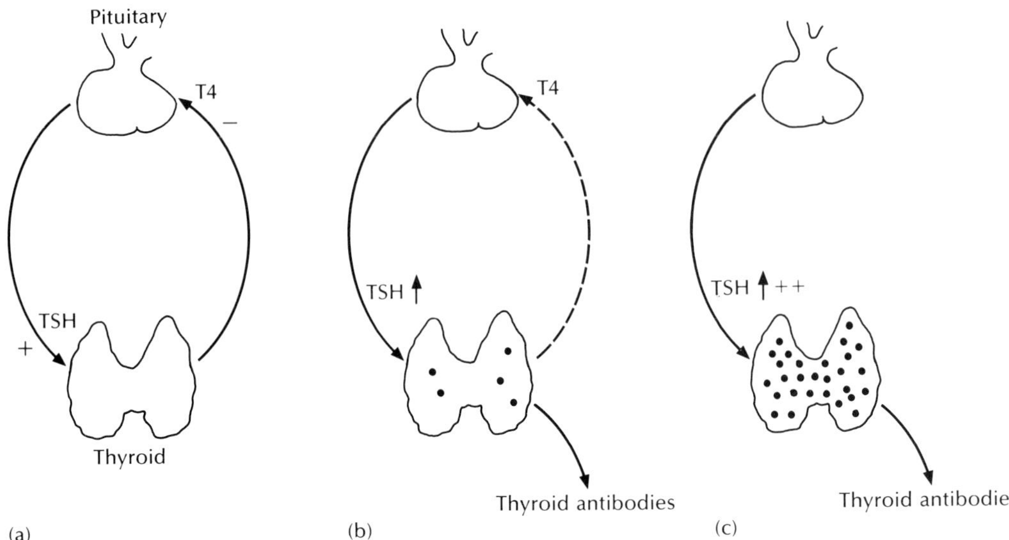

Fig. 102.3. The pituitary–thyroid axis in autoimmune hypothyroidism. (a) Pituitary thyroid-stimulating hormone (TSH) is normally under negative feedback control from circulating thyroid hormones (T4); (b) as the gland suffers autoimmune damage, reduced output of T4 leads to a raised TSH sufficient to maintain normal T4 levels by stimulating the damaged gland; many such patients will progress to (c) in which, despite very high TSH levels, the thyroid damage is too severe to sustain normal T4 production.

idiotypes are probably more important (Delves and Roitt 1984; Kojima *et al.* 1986). These antibodies are predominantly immunoglobulin G (IgG), with about 20% of sera also having IgA and 5% IgM class. The IgG subclass distribution has been controversial, probably due to technical factors (Weetman *et al.* 1989a). It now seems clear that all four subclasses are represented but with about a sixfold excess (over expected) of IgG-4 antibodies (Fig. 102.4). Such over-representation of the IgG-4 subclass is similar to that found in other situations of chronic immunization and is insufficient to explain the inability of thyroglobulin antibodies to fix complement; this is probably due to the lack of cross-linking between antibodies attached to the widely spaced epitopes (Adler *et al.* 1984). These antibodies and those against microsomal antigen are usually detected by the haemagglutination technique, using commercially available kits. It is likely that these will be supplanted eventually by newer methods such as the enzyme-linked immunosorbent assay (ELISA), which is more sensitive and easier to perform.

MICROSOMAL ANTIBODIES

Microsomal antibodies produce immunofluorescent staining of the cytoplasm and apical portion of the thyroid cell surface and react with thyroid peroxidase (TPO) (Table 102.1), a membrane-bound 105 kD haemoprotein which catalyses the iodination of thyroglobulin (Czarnocka *et al.* 1985). Cloning of the cDNA of TPO has revealed a 42% homology with myeloperoxidase, which may explain the occurrence of anti-neutrophil anti-

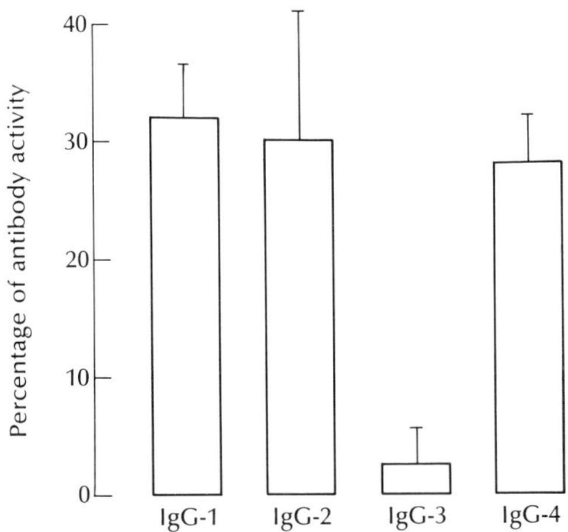

Fig. 102.4. Immunoglobulin G subclass distribution of thyroglobulin antibodies. The results are the mean (+ SD) of nine Hashimoto's sera purified, by negative-depletion affinity chromatography, into subclasses and then assayed by ELISA for thyroglobulin antibodies. Immunoglobulin G-4, which comprised 5% of total IgG, is over-represented in these antibodies.

bodies in some patients with autoimmune thyroid disease (Libert *et al.* 1987). At least six autoantigenic epitopes exist (Doble *et al.* 1988), and some microsomal antibodies may inhibit TPO activity *in vitro* (Kohno *et al.* 1986). Whether this action contributes to the development of hypothyroidism *in vivo* remains to be determined. Microsomal antibodies have a similar IgG subclass distribution to thyroglobulin antibodies but fix complement and are cytotoxic to thyroid cells *in vitro* (Khoury *et al.* 1981). Characterization of TPO at the molecular and immunological level is clarifying its role as a potential target for the aberrant autoimmune response (Banga *et al.* 1991).

OTHER ANTIBODIES

Other thyroid-specific antibodies exist but are much less well characterized; they include the second (non-iodinated) colloid antigen, detectable at present only by immunofluorescence (Balfour *et al.* 1961). Antibodies to the TSH receptor are found in a number of patients with autoimmune hypothyroidism and, as discussed earlier, may be of the 'blocking type'.

Cell-mediated immunity

T cell sensitization to thyroglobulin and the microsomal antigen has been demonstrated using assays of T cell proliferation and migration inhibition factor (MIF) production (Aoki and De Groot 1979; Okita *et al.* 1980). However, these and other similar studies have used circulating lymphocytes, which probably inadequately reflect events within the thyroid, the site of the autoimmune process. This may partly account for the inconsistent or weak responses reported (Ludgate *et al.* 1984). Similar constraints apply to the descriptions of a defect in concanavalin A-inducible T suppressor cell function, depression of CD8 +ve cells and increased numbers of Ia +ve T cells in the circulation of these patients (Aoki *et al.* 1979; Canonica *et al.* 1982; Bonnyns *et al.* 1983).

Despite these difficulties, Volpé's group have used the MIF test to assay thyroid antigen-specific T suppressor cell function (Okita *et al.* 1981). In these experiments, normal T cells were able to prevent the autoantigen-induced production of MIF by T cells from patients with Hashimoto's thyroiditis (and Graves' disease). This has been taken to show the existence of defective thyroid antigen-specific T suppressor cells in autoimmunity; conversely, normal subjects must possess activated suppressor cells in adequate numbers to prevent autoimmunity. More recently, this group have also shown that, in contrast to controls, CD8 +ve cells from patients with thyroid autoimmunity do not suppress microsomal antibody synthesis by polyclonally activated B cells (Iitaka *et al.* 1988). The hypothesis of a defect in antigen-specific suppression is certainly appealing as an explanation for the aetiology of thyroid autoimmunity (Volpé 1988), but artefactual suppressor effects in such systems (particularly those which involve mixing allogeneic cells) are difficult to exclude. These may arise, for example, as a result of limiting dilutions or non-specific lymphokine production. The implications of this hypothesis are that a large proportion of the normal T cell repertoire is continually activated, in order to suppress autoimmunity, as are, presumably, a similar number of T helper cells. This is somewhat easier to envisage for an antigen like thyroglobulin, which circulates, than for the TSH receptor; *in vitro* systems have not yet been devised to test whether active suppression is also the normal mechanism for avoiding autoimmunity to this particular antigen. Recent advances in culture techniques and the identification of cytokines which support suppressor cell growth should permit precise, clonal analysis of a possible thyroid-specific T suppressor cell defect in the near future.

Pathogenesis

In autoimmune hypothyroidism (and Graves' disease) the normally Ia antigen −ve thyroid epithelial cells express these molecules (Hanafusa *et al.* 1983), leading to the hypothesis that such aberrant Ia expression could convert thyrocytes into autoantigen-presenting cells and thereby initiate autoimmunity (Bottazzo *et al.* 1983). T cell lines and clones have been derived from the thyroid-infiltrating T cells which proliferate in response to Ia +ve thyrocytes, but the nature of the cell surface autoantigen recognized by these T cells is not clear (Londei *et al.* 1985a; Weetman *et al.* 1986). Thyroid cells seem unable to process antigen (Londei *et al.* 1985b), so it is arguable whether they could truly initiate T cell autoreactivity, unless autoantigenic peptides were available, by endogenous synthesis, to bind to Ia.

Moreover, thyroid cell Ia expression seems to depend critically on the T cell lymphokine interferon gamma (IFN-γ), although tumour necrosis factor will enhance the action of IFN-γ, and the effect of IFN-γ is increased late in the cell cycle, so that TSH and TSH receptor antibodies, which are mitogenic, could exacerbate Ia expression in Hashimoto's thyroiditis and Graves' disease respectively (Todd *et al.* 1985; Weetman *et al.* 1985, 1987b). This prime dependence on IFN-γ is reflected by the limitation of Ia antigen expression to thyroid cells adjacent to areas of lymphocytic accumulation (Aichinger *et al.* 1985), and studies in EAT have confirmed that thyroid cell Ia expression occurs only after T cell infiltration into the gland (Cohen *et al.* 1988; Hassman *et al.* 1988). Based on these observations, it seems likely that thyroid cell Ia expression may perpetuate, but does not initiate, autoimmunity (Fig. 102.5). It is also possible that aberrant Ia antigen expression could increase the susceptibility of thyroid cells to cytotoxic attack by CD4 +ve T cells.

A wider range of cytokines, including IFN-γ, tumour necrosis factor and interleukin 1, can induce thyroid cell expression of the intercellular adhesion molecule (ICAM)-1, and the thyroid cells in both Graves' disease and Hashimoto's thyroiditis are positive for ICAM-1 staining by immunohistochemistry (Weetman *et al.* 1989b). This may be of considerable importance in initiating T cell recognition of thyroid cells, and blocking thyroid cell ICAM-1 interaction with its receptor, lymphocyte function-associated antigen (LFA)-1, on T cells prevents subsequent cell-mediated cytotoxicity *in vitro* (Weetman *et al.* 1990a). Moreover, the thyroid cells themselves may release important cytokines which can modify the intrathyroidal autoimmune response. In particular, these endocrine cells secrete interleukin 6 in response to T cell-derived lymphokines and this may in turn stimulate local B and T cell activation (Weetman *et al.* 1990b).

Thyroid cell damage probably results from several effector mechanisms. Microsomal antibodies are certainly cytotoxic; both thyroglobulin and microsomal antibodies (except those of the

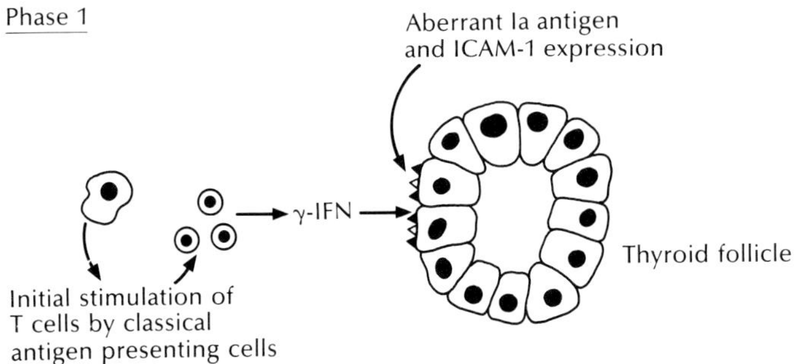

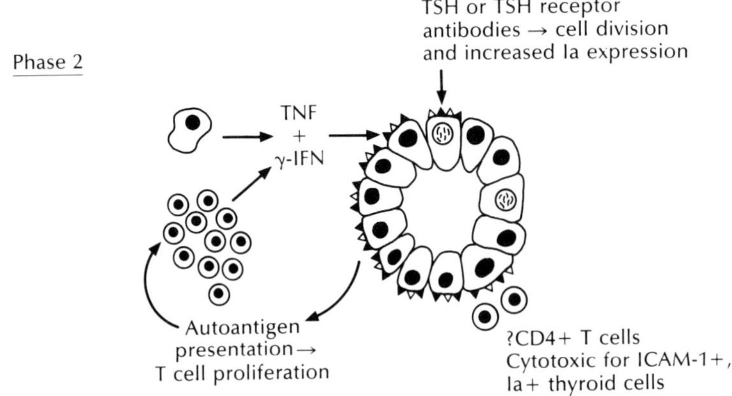

Fig. 102.5. The possible role of thyroid cell Ia and ICAM-1 expression in autoimmunity.

IgG-2 subclass) can mediate antibody-dependent cell-mediated cytotoxicity (ADCC) *in vitro* (Weetman *et al*. 1989a). Circulating levels of functioning K cells which mediate ADCC have been reported to be increased in Hashimoto's thyroiditis, but this has not been supported by other studies (Bogner *et al*. 1984; Sack *et al*. 1986). There are relatively few such cells in the thyroid infiltrate by immunohistochemical analysis; macrophages could also mediate ADCC. Cytotoxic T cells are of probable importance in producing thyroid damage, as suggested by studies in EAT (Creemers *et al*. 1983). However, while there are many CD8 +ve cells in the thyroid infiltrate (Aichinger *et al*. 1985), which are cytotoxic to a broad range of targets upon *in vitro* activation (Canonica *et al*. 1985; Del Prete *et al*. 1986), there is as yet no evidence for cytotoxicity with thyroid cell specificity, and of course it is possible that CD4 +ve could also be cytotoxic for Ia +ve thyroid cells, as mentioned above. Finally, the role of cytokines is now being explored, with some preliminary evidence that interleukin 1, in particular, can produce thyroid cell injury.

Triggering factors

A variety of factors have now been identified which are associated with the development of autoimmune thyroiditis, even though in most cases the natue of the relationship is obscure. Trisomy 21, Turner's (but not Klinefelter's) syndrome and Alzheimer's disease predispose to thyroid autoimmunity (Baxter *et al*. 1975; Doniach *et al*. 1968; Ewins *et al*. 1991). Pregnancy certainly exacerbates the autoimmune process *post partum*, as discussed below, and infection remains a possible triggering factor, although hypothyroidism only occurs after viral (de Quervain's) thyroiditis if there is preceding autoimmune or surgical thyroid damage. About 50% of patients with viral thyroiditis have transiently positive thyroid antibodies, especially against the second colloid antigen. Iodine deficiency appears to protect against thyroid autoimmunity, whereas iodine excess exacerbates it (McGregor *et al*. 1985). This has been particularly well demonstrated in EAT (Allen *et al*. 1986; Sundick *et al*. 1987) and it is possible that increasing iodine intake could be an important factor in the development of thyroiditis, not just in previously deficient areas, but in countries such as Britain where there has been a recent threefold increase in iodine intake (from milk) due to iodine supplementation of cattle foods. The adverse effect of iodine could be due to direct thyroid cell damage with autoantigen release, non-specific effects on the immune system or increased antigenicity of heavily iodinated antigens.

Post-partum thyroid dysfunction

Typically, during pregnancy autoimmune diseases are seen to improve clinically, with exacerbation of the disease following in the post-partum period. In the case of the autoimmune thyroid diseases, this pattern is characteristic. In contrast to this situation, a group of women have been identified without previous personal history of thyroid disease and often with no family history of thyroid disease who, following pregnancy, develop changes in thyroid function which are often transient but which may lead on to permanent thyroid failure (Learoyd *et al*. 1991). The condition has been referred to as post-partum thyroid dysfunction and is usually characterized initially by a period of transient thyroid over-activity and thence later by thyroid hypofunction (Fung *et al*. 1988), which may remit spontaneously or persist indefinitely. The initial description of this group of conditions (Roberton 1948) long predated the recognition of its autoimmune basis. More recent studies in Japan (Amino and Miyai 1983) and Europe (Jansson and Karlsson 1986) have contributed considerably to the characterization of this syndrome. Post-partum thyroid dysfunction is seen in about 7% of all women and, besides the evidence of altered thyroid function, is usually associated with painless enlargement of the thyroid, undetectable TSH receptor antibody activity and a low uptake of radio-iodine during the hyperthyroid phase of the disease (in contrast to the situation in Graves' disease), histological evidence of profuse lymphocytic infiltration of the thyroid gland and circulating antibody activity to the thyroid microsome. In British women the disease is associated with the HLA-A1, B8, DR3 haplotype (Kologlu *et al*. 1990) and seems to occur more commonly in women who smoke heavily during pregnancy (Fung *et al*. 1988). Whilst antibodies to the thyroid microsome are present in the majority of women developing post-partum thyroiditis, their exact role in the induction of the disease process remains uncertain. Earlier claims that there was an association between the development of the syndrome and the ability of antimicrosomal antibodies, on the basis of their immunoglobulin subclass, to fix complement have not been substantiated in more recent and extensive studies (Weetman *et al.* 1990c). A role for the functional affinity of these antibodies in the pathogenesis of the disease process has been suggested. Other mechanisms offered to explain the pathological process and the evidence of thyroid destruction observed histologically have provided conflicting evidence on the role of cell-mediated cytotoxic mechanisms (Hayslip *et al.* 1988). The changes occurring during the post-partum period in thyroid function may contribute to many of the changes noted in mood and behaviour seen in women in the post-partum period (Harris *et al.* 1989). Of particular importance, however, in the recognition of this syndrome is the observation that in a significant number of women, particularly with repeated pregnancies, the hypothyroid phase may either persist or, having recovered transiently, go on with time to permanent thyroid failure (Tachi *et al.* 1988; Othman *et al.* 1990).

Congenital and juvenile hypothyroidism

Congenital hypothyroidism affects about 1 in 4000 new-born and in most cases appears to be due to absence or maldevelopment of the thyroid. Two reports have suggested that at least some forms may be the result of transplacental passage of maternal antibodies which block (fetal) TSH-induced thyroid growth (Dussault and Bernier 1985; Van der Gaag *et al.* 1985). However, a more recent study was unable to distinguish between thyroid growth-inhibiting antibodies and TSH receptor-blocking antibodies, and found evidence for the latter in only one of 24 cases of congenital hypothyroidism (Brown *et al.* 1990). Further prospective studies are required to evaluate the importance of this mechanism and the biochemical site of maternal immunoglobulin action. Juvenile thyroiditis usually presents with a small, painless goitre and mild lymphocytic thyroiditis between the ages of 11 and 13; antibody levels are much lower than in adult thyroiditis (Doniach *et al.* 1979). This form of the disease is characterized by exacerbations and remissions.

Disease associations

Autoimmune hypothyroidism and, more commonly, the mere presence of thyroid autoantibodies are frequently associated with other auto-immune conditions. As well as the distinctive polyendocrine syndromes discussed below, there are associations with chronic active hepatitis, primary biliary cirrhosis, dermatitis herpetiformis and a variety of rheumatological conditions: Sjögren's syndrome, rheumatoid arthritis, temporal arteritis, systemic sclerosis and systemic lupus erythematosus. Another important causal relationship is with primary non-Hodgkin's lymphoma of the thyroid (usually B cell in origin). In one series, 24 of 30 such lymphomas were in glands with pre-existing Hashimoto's thyroiditis (Hamburger *et al.* 1983), a situation similar to the lymphoma risk with coeliac disease and Sjögren's syndrome.

Autoimmune hypophysitis

Lymphocytic hypophysitis is now an established entity of unknown incidence; most patients have presented with space-occupying lesions of the pituitary (which enlarges due to the mononuclear cell infiltrate) and these cases may well represent the most extreme form of the condition. Of 23 well-documented patients only two were men (Guay *et al.* 1987; Pestell *et al.* 1990) and in many of the women the onset was during pregnancy or in the year *post partum* (Mazzone *et al.* 1983). Other autoimmune diseases, including thyroiditis, adrenalitis and pernicious anaemia, have been associated with hypophysitis, and various (occasionally fatal) degrees of pituitary insufficiency may occur, together with local compressive signs from the infiltrated gland. Pituitary antibodies have been assessed by immunofluorescence in six patients and were only detected in one.

This form of pituitary autoimmunity, therefore, seems distinct from that associated with the appearance of antibodies (detectable by immunofluorescence) against discrete anterior pituitary hormone-producing cells, particularly those making prolactin or growth hormone. Such antibodies are found in 20–30% of insulin-dependent diabetics and their islet cell antibody +ve relatives (Mirakian *et al.* 1982), which is probably indicative of a widespread autoimmune phenomenon, although the sporadic occurrence of antibodies to distinct pituitary cells has been suggested as a cause of isolated hormone deficiencies (Bottazzo *et al*. 1980). It is not yet clear how common such syndromes are. About half of the patients with isolated adrenocorticotrophic hormone (ACTH) deficiency have autoantibodies against these particular pituitary cells, suggesting that this is a distinctive (but very rare) form of pituitary autoimmunity (Sauter *et al*. 1990). Idiopathic diabetes insipidus can be associated with other autoimmune diseases, especially thyroiditis, and a third of these patients have antibodies against the hypothalamic vasopressin-producing cells, suggesting that some examples of this condition may also be the result of an autoimmune process (Scherbaum and Bottazzo 1983).

Autoimmune gonadal failure

The occurrence of ovarian failure in about 25% of patients with Addison's disease is well recognized and correlates with the presence of circulating antibodies, detectable by immunofluorescence, against steroid-producing cells (Irvine and Barnes 1975). Biopsy of the ovary has revealed lymphocytic infiltration in some cases, although others show merely fibrosis. Less commonly, antibodies react with Leydig cells in the testes and, more rarely still, are associated with testicular failure. Further characterization of this family of antibodies (Table 102.2) has shown the absence of antibodies against ovary and testis in sera from 95 patients whose amenorrhoea or infertility was not associated with Addison's disease, and it also appears that at least some of these antibodies react with antigens unique to the ovary (Sotsiou *et al*. 1980). There is increasing evidence that sporadic autoimmune oöphoritis may account for a proportion of premature ovarian failure, as ovarian antibodies can be detected in almost half of these patients (Luborsky *et al*. 1990). Moreover, some sporadic cases of the gonadotrophin-resistant ovary syndrome could be the result of ovary-specific autoimmunity, possibly as the result of gonadotrophin receptor-blocking immunoglobulins (Chiauzzi *et al*. 1982).

Polyendocrine autoimmunity

The foregoing sections have alluded to the frequent close associations between autoimmune endocrine disorders; the occurrence of two or more such conditions in the same person constitutes an autoimmune polyglandular syndrome (Neufeld *et al*. 1981). There are two main types (Table 102.3). The type 1 syndrome is rare and is probably an autosomal recessive disorder which is not HLA-DR associated (Eisenbarth and Jackson 1981); siblings of a proband may have only one of the three prime features, namely mucocutaneous (never systemic) candidiasis, hypoparathyroidism and adrenal failure. Recently some tentative associations with HLA-A region genes have been reported, particularly in individuals homozygous for the type 1 polyglandular syndrome gene: HLA-A28 appears to confer susceptibility to hypoparathyroidism, HLA-A3 to ovarian failure and HLA-A2 to kerato-

Table 102.2. Immunofluorescence patterns of steroid cell autoantibodies

Organ	Reactivity	Positivity (%)[a]
Adrenal cortex	Usually all three cortical zones	100
Testis	Leydig cells	94
Ovary	Interstitial cells Hilar cells	
Graafian follicle	Theca cells	98
Corpus luteum	Paralutein cells	100
Corpus luteum	Lutein cells (three patterns)	94

a In 50 selected cases from 152 adrenal antibody +ve patients with Addison's disease (Sotsiou *et al*. 1980).

Table 102.3. Polyglandular syndromes

Type 1	Type 2
Mucocutaneous candidiasis	Graves' disease/autoimmune hypothyroidism
Hypoparathyroidism	Insulin dependent (type 1) diabetes mellitus
Primary adrenal failure (often later onset)	Primary adrenal failure ± gonadal failure
Associated with keratopathy, alopecia, vitiligo, malabsorption, chronic active hepatitis, pernicious anaemia and gonadal failure	Coeliac disease
	Myasthenia gravis
	Hypophysitis
	Associated with vitiligo, alopecia and pernicious anaemia

pathy (Ahonen *et al.* 1988). These associations are weak but they do suggest the possible location of the gene(s) responsible for the syndrome on chromosome 6. Antibodies to parathyroid and adrenal antigens are known to occur (Blizzard *et al.* 1966), but there is little recent information on T cell function (Children *et al.* 1969). In one small series a defect in non-specific T suppressor cell function was documented (Arulanantham *et al.* 1979).

The type 2 polyglandular autoimmunity syndrome is much more common than type 1 and appears to be an autosomal dominant disorder, strongly associated with the HLA-A1, B8, DR3 haplotype which acts as a permissive factor in the development of this condition (Eisenbarth and Jackson 1981). There does not seem to be anything unique about the endocrinopathies of the type 2 syndrome compared with the sporadic forms of these disorders, and separate components may occur 20 years apart in an individual, making follow-up important. Prospective screening for other disorders seems worth while in all patients with autoimmune Addison's disease and, once a polyendocrine syndrome has been identified, family members should also be examined regularly.

References

Adams, D.D. and Kennedy, T.H. (1967). Occurrence in thyrotoxicosis of a gamma globulin which protects LATS from neutralisation by an extract of thyroid gland. *J. Clin. Endocrinol. Metab.* **27**, 173–7.

Adams, D.D. and Purves, H.D. (1956). Abnormal responses in the assay of thyrotropin. *Proc. Univ. Otago Med. School* **34**, 11–12.

Adams, D.D., Kennedy, T.H. and Stewart, R.D.H. (1974). Correlation between LATS-protector levels and thyroid ^{131}I uptake in thyrotoxicosis. *Br. Med. J.* **2**, 199–201.

Adler, T.R., Beall, G.N., Curd, J.G., Heiner, D.G. and Sabharwal, U.K. (1984). Studies of complement activation and IgG subclass restriction of anti-thyroglobulin. *Clin. Exp. Immunol.* **56**, 383–9.

Ahonen, P., Koskimies, S., Lokki, M.-L., Tilitainen, A. and Perheentupa, J. (1988). The expression of autoimmune polyglandular disease type 1 appears associated with several HLA-A antigens but not with HLA-DR. *J. Clin. Endocrinol. Metab.* **66**, 1152–7.

Aichinger, G., Fill, H. and Wick, G. (1985). *In situ* immune complexes, lymphocyte subpopulations and HLA-DR positive epithelial cells in Hashimoto's thyroiditis. *Lab. Invest.* **52**, 132–40.

Allen, E.M., Appel, M.C. and Braverman, L.E. (1986). The effect of iodide ingestion on the development of spontaneous lymphocytic thyroiditis in the diabetes-prone BB/W rat. *Endocrinology* **118**, 1977–81.

Amino, N. and Miyai, K. (1983). Post-partum autoimmune endocrine syndromes. In *Autoimmune Endocrine Disease*, ed. T.F. Davies, pp. 247–72, J. Wiley and Sons, New York.

Aoki, N. and De Groot, L.J. (1979). Lymphocyte blastogenic response to human thyroglobulin in Graves' disease, Hashimoto's thyroiditis and metastatic thyroid cancer. *Clin. Exp. Immunol.* **38**, 523–30.

Aoki, N., Pinnamaneni, K.M. and De Groot, L.J. (1979). A study on suppressor cell function in thyroid disease. *J. Clin. Endocrinol. Metab.* **48**, 803–10.

Arulanantham, K., Dwyer, J.M. and Genel, M. (1979). Evidence for defective immunoregulation in the syndrome of familial candidiasis endocrinopathy. *N. Engl. J. Med.* **300**, 164–8.

Atkinson, S., Holcombe, M. and Kendall-Taylor, P. (1984). Ophthalmopathic immunoglobulin in patients with Graves' ophthalmopathy. *Lancet* **ii**, 374–6.

Baker, J.R., Saunders, N.B., Wartofsky, L., Tseng, Y.-C.L. and Burman, K.D. (1988). Seronegative Hashimoto's thyroiditis with thyroid autoantibody production localised to the thyroid. *Ann. Int. Med.* **108**, 26–30.

Balfour, B.M., Doniach, D., Roitt, I.M. and Couchman, K.G. (1961). Fluorescent antibody studies in human thyroiditis: autoantibodies to an antigen of the thyroid colloid distinct from thyroglobulin. *Br. J. Exp. Pathol.* **42**, 307–16.

Banga, J.P., Barnet, P.S. and McGregor, A.M. (1991). Immunological and molecular characteristics of the thyroid peroxidase autoantigen. *Autoimmunity* **8**, 335–43.

Barnett, P.S., Huang, G.C., Ratanachaiyavong, S. *et al.* (1990). Autoimmunity in the thyroid. In *Horizons in Medicine* 2, ed. L.K. Borysiewicz, pp. 91–101, Transmedica Europe Ltd, Tunbridge Wells.

Baxter, R.G., Larkins, R.G., Martin, F.I.R., Heyma, P., Myles, K. and Ryan, L. (1975). Downs syndrome and thyroid function in adults. *Lancet* **ii**, 794–5.

Blizzard, R.M., Chee, D. and Davis, W. (1966). The incidence of parathyroid and other antibodies in the sera of patients with idiopathic hypoparathyroidism. *Clin. Exp. Immunol.* **1**, 119–28.

Bogner, U., Schleusener, H. and Wall, J.R. (1984). Antibody-dependent cell-mediated cytotoxicity against human thyroid cells in Hashimoto's thyroiditis but not Graves' disease. *J. Clin. Endocrinol. Metab.* **59**, 734–8.

Bonnyns, M., Bentin, J., Devetter, G. and Duchateau, J. (1983). Heterogeneity of immunoregulatory T cells in human thyroid autoimmunity: influence of thyroid status. *Clin. Exp. Immunol.* **56**, 251–4.

Bottazzo, G.F., McIntosh, C., Stanford, W. and Preece, M. (1980). Growth hormone cell antibodies and partial growth hormone deficiency in a girl with Turner's syndrome. *Clin. Endocrinol.* **12**, 1–9.

Bottazzo, G.F., Pujol-Borrell, R., Hanafusa, T. and Feldmann, M. (1983). Role of aberrant HLA-DR expression and antigen presentation in induction of endocrine autoimmunity. *Lancet* **ii**, 1115–19.

Braverman, L.E. (1990). The role of iodine in the pathogenesis of lymphocytic thyroiditis in animal models. In *The Thyroid Gland, Environment and Autoimmunity*, ed. H.A. Drexhage, J.J.M. de Vijlder and W.M. Wiersinga, pp. 279–88, Elsevier Science Publishers BV, Amsterdam.

Brown, R.S., Keating, P. and Mitchell, E. (1990). Maternal thyroid-blocking immunoglobulins in congenital hypothyroidism. *J. Clin. Endocrinol. Metab.* **70**, 1341–6.

Canonica, G.W., Bagnasco, M., Corte, G., Ferrini, S., Ferrini, O. and Giordano, G. (1982). Circulating T lymphocytes in Hashimoto's thyroiditis: imbalance of subsets and presence of activated cells. *Clin. Immunol. Immunopathol.* **23**, 616–25.

Canonica, G.W., Caria, M., Bagnasco, M., Cosulich, M.E., Giordano, G. and Moretta, L. (1985). Proliferation of T9-positive cytolytic T lymphocytes in response to thyroglobulin in human autoimmune thyroiditis: analysis of cell interactions and culture requirements. *Clin. Immunol. Immunopathol.* **36**, 40–8.

Chiauzzi, V., Cigorraga, S., Escobar, M.E., Rivalrola, M.A. and Charreau, E.H. (1982). Inhibition of follicle-stimulating hormone receptor binding by circulating immunoglobulins. *J. Clin. Endocrinol. Metab.* **54**, 1221–8.

Chilgren, R.A., Meuwissen, H.J., Quie, P.G., Good, R.A. and Hong, R. (1969). The cellular immune defect in chronic mucocutaneous candidiasis. *Lancet* **i**, 1286–8.

Cohen, S.B., Dijkstra, C.D. and Weetman, A.P. (1988). Sequential analysis of experimental autoimmune thyroiditis induced by neonatal thymectomy in the Buffalo strain rat. *Cell. Immunol.* **114**, 126–36.

Creemers, P., Rose, N.R. and Kong, Y.M. (1983). Experimental autoimmune thyroiditis: *in vitro* cytotoxic effects of T lymphocytes on murine monolayers. *J. Exp. Med.* **157**, 559–71.

Czarnocka, B., Ruf, J., Ferrand, M., Carayon, P. and Lissitzky, S. (1985). Purification of human thyroid peroxidase and its identification as the microsomal antigen involved in autoimmune thyroid diseases. *FEBS Lett.* **190**, 147–51.

Davies, T.F., Martin, A., Conception, E.S., Graves, P., Cohen, L. and Ben-Nun, A. (1991). Evidence of limited variability of antigen receptors on intrathyroidal T cells in autoimmune thyroid disease. *N. Engl. J. Med.* **325**, 238–44.

De Groot, L.J. (1989). *Endocrinology*, 2nd edn, vols. I–III. W.B. Saunders Company, Philadelphia.

De Groot, L.J. and Quintans, J. (1989). The causes of autoimmune thyroid disease. *Endocrine Rev.* **10**, 537–62.

Del Prete, G.F., Vercelli, D., Tiri, A. *et al.* (1986). *In vitro* activated cytotoxic T cells in the thyroid infiltrate of patients with Hashimoto's thyroiditis. *Clin. Exp. Immunol.* **65**, 140–7.

Delves, P.J. and Roitt, I.M. (1984). Idiotypic determinants on human thyroglobulin autoantibodies derived from the serum of Hashimoto patients and EB virus transformed cell lines. *Clin. Exp. Immunol.* **57**, 33–8.

Demaine, A.G., Welsh, K.I., Hance, B.S. and Farid, N.R. (1987). Polymorphism of the T cell receptor beta-chain in Graves' disease. *J. Clin. Endocrinol. Metab.* **65**, 643–6.

Demaine, A.G., Ratanachaiyavong, S., Pope, R., Ewins, D., Millward, B.A. and McGregor, A.M. (1989). Thyroglobulin antibodies in Graves' disease are associated with T cell receptor beta-chain and major histocompatibility complex loci. *Clin. Exp. Immunol.* **77**, 21–4.

De Martynoff, G., Pays, E. and Vassart, G. (1980). Synthesis of a full length cDNA complementary to thyroglobulin 33S messenger RNA. *Biochem. Biophys. Res. Comm.* **93**, 645–61.

Doble, N.D., Banga, J.P., Pope, R., Lalor, E., Kilduff, P. and McGregor, A.M. (1988). Autoantibodies to the thyroid microsomal/thyroid peroxidase antigen are polyclonal and directed to several distinct antigenic sites. *Immunology* **64**, 23–9.

Dong, Q., Ludgate, M. and Vassart, G. (1991). Cloning and sequencing of a novel 64kDa autoantigen recognised by patients with autoimmune thyroid disease. *J. Clin. Endocrinol. Metab.* **72**, 1375–81.

Doniach, D., Roitt, I.M. and Polani, P.E. (1968). Thyroid antibodies and sex-chromosome anomalies. *Proc. Roy. Soc. Med.* **61**, 278–80.

Doniach, D., Bottazzo, G.F. and Russell, R.C.G. (1979). Goitrous autoimmune thyroiditis (Hashimoto's disease). *Clin. Endocrinol. Metab.* **8**, 63–80.

Dussault, J.H. and Bernier, D. (1985). ^{125}I uptake by $FRTL_5$ cells: a screening test to detect pregnant women at risk of giving birth to hypothyroid infants. *Lancet* **ii**, 1029–31.

Eisenbarth, G.S. and Jackson, R.A. (1981). Immunogenetics of polyglandular failure and related diseases. In *HLA in Endocrine and Metabolic Disorders*, ed. N.R. Farid, pp. 235–64, Academic Press, New York.

Endo, K., Kasagi, K., Konishi, J. *et al.* (1978). Detection and properties of TSH-binding inhibitor immunoglobulins in patients with Graves' disease and Hashimoto's thyroiditis. *J. Clin. Endocrinol. Metab.* **46**, 734–9.

Ewins, D.L., Rosser, M.N., Butler, J., Roques, P.K., Mullan, M.J. and McGregor, A.M. (1991). Association between autoimmune thyroid disease and familial Alzheimer's disease. *Clin. Endocrinol.* **35**, 93–6.

Farid, N.R., Sampson, L., Moens, H. and Barnard, J.M. (1981). The association of goitrous autoimmune thyroiditis with

HLA-DR5. *Tissue Antigens* **17**, 265–8.

Filetti, S., Foti, D., Costante, G. and Rapoport, B. (1991). Recombinant human thyrotropin (TSH) receptor in a radioreceptor assay for the measurement of TSH receptor autoantibodies. *J. Clin. Endocrinol. Metab.* **72**, 1096–101.

Franklyn, J.A., Fitzgerald, M.G., Oates, G.D. and Sheppard, M.C. (1987). Fine needle aspiration cytology in the management of euthyroid goitre. *Quart. J. Med.* **65**, 997–1003.

Fung, H.Y.M., Kologlu, M., Collison, K. *et al.* (1988). Postpartum thyroid dysfunction in mid-Glamorgan. *Br. Med. J.* **296**, 241–4.

Gorman, C.A. (1990). A critical review of the role of stress in hyperthyroidism. In *The Thyroid Gland, Environment and Autoimmunity*, ed. H.A. Drexhage, J.J.M. de Vijlder and W.M. Wiersinga, pp. 191–200, Elsevier Science Publishers, Amsterdam.

Guay, A.T., Agnello, V., Tronic, B.C., Gresham, D.G. and Friedberg, S.R. (1987). Lymphocytic hypophysitis in a man. *J. Clin. Endocrinol. Metab.* **64**, 631–4.

Hamburger, J.I., Miller, J.M. and Kini, S.R. (1983). Lymphoma of the thyroid. *Ann. Int. Med.* **99**, 685–93.

Hanafusa, T., Pujol-Borrell, R., Chiovato, L., Russell, R.C.G., Doniach, D. and Bottazzo, G.F. (1983). Aberrant expression of HLA-DR antigen on thyrocytes in Graves' disease: relevance for autoimmunity. *Lancet* **ii**, 1111–15.

Harris, B., Fung, H.Y.M., Johns, S., Kologlu, M., Bhatti, R. and McGregor, A.M. (1989). Transient post-partum thyroid dysfunction and post-natal depression. *J. Affective Disorders* **17**, 243–9.

Hassman, R., Solic, N., Jasani, B., Hall, R. and McGregor, A.M. (1988). Immunological events leading to destructive thyroiditis in the AUG rat. *Clin. Exp. Immunol.* **73**, 410–16.

Hayashi, Y., Tamai, H., Fukata, S. *et al.* (1985). A long term clinical, immunological and histological follow up study of patients with goitrous chronic lymphocytic thyroiditis. *J. Clin. Endocrinol. Metab.* **61**, 1172–8.

Hayslip, C.C., Baker, J.R., Wartofsky, L., Klein, T.A., Opsalis, M.S. and Burman, K.D. (1988). Natural killer cell activity and serum autoantibodies in women with post-partum thyroiditis. *J. Clin. Endocrinol. Metab.* **66**, 1089–93.

Humphrey, M., Mosca, J., Baker, J.R. *et al.* (1991). Absence of retroviral sequences in Graves' disease. *Lancet* **337**, 17–18.

Iitaka, M., Aguayo, J.F., Iwatani, Y., Row, V.V. and Volpé, R. (1988). Studies of the effect of suppressor T lymphocytes on the induction of antithyroid microsomal antibody-secreting cells in autoimmune thyroid disease. *J. Clin. Endocrinol. Metab.* **66**, 708–14.

Ingbar, S.H., Weiss, M., Cushing, G.W. and Kasper, D.L. (1987). A possible role for bacterial antigens in the pathogenesis of autoimmune thyroid disease. In *Thyroid Autoimmunity*, ed. A. Pinchera, S.H. Ingbar, J.M. McKenzie and G.F. Fenzi, pp. 35–44, Plenum Press, New York.

Irvine, W.J. and Barnes, E.W. (1975). Addison's disease, ovarian failure and hypoparathyroidism. *Clin. Endocrinol. Metab.* **4**, 379–434.

Jansson, R. and Karlsson, A. (1986). Autoimmune thyroid disease in pregnancy and the post-partum period. In McGregor A.M. (ed) *Immunology of Endocrine Disease*, ed. A.M. McGregor, pp. 181–96, MTP Press Ltd, Lancaster.

Kasagi, K., Konishi, J., Iida, Y. *et al.* (1982). A new *in vitro* assay for human thyroid stimulator using cultured thyroid cells: effect of sodium chloride on adenosine 3',5'-monophosphate increase. *J. Clin. Endocrinol. Metab.* **54**, 108–14.

Khoury, E.L., Hammond, L., Bottazzo, G.F. and Doniach, D. (1981). Presence of the organ-specific 'microsomal' autoantigen on the surface of human thyroid cells in culture: its involvement in complement-mediated cytotoxicity. *Clin. Exp. Immunol.* **45**, 316–28.

Kohno, Y., Hiyama, Y., Shimojo, N., Niimi, H., Nakajima, H. and Hosoya, T. (1986). Autoantibodies to thyroid peroxidase in patients with chronic thyroiditis: effect of antibody binding on enzyme activities. *Clin. Exp. Immunol.* **65**, 534.

Kojima, K., Matsuyama, T. and Tanaka, H. (1986). Suppression of *in vitro* human antithyroglobulin antibody secretion by private and cross-reactive anti-idiotypic antibodies. *Clin. Immunol. Immunopathol.* **39**, 337–43.

Kologlu, M., Fung, H., Darke, C., Richards, C.J., Hall, R. and McGregor, A.M. (1990). Post-partum thyroid dysfunction and HLA status. *Eur. J. Clin. Invest.* **20**, 56–60.

Konishi, J., Iida, Y., Endo, K. *et al.* (1983). Inhibition of thyrotropin-induced adenosine 3',5'-monophosphate increase by immunoglobulins from patients with primary myxoedema. *J. Clin. Endocrinol. Metab.* **57**, 544–9.

Kriss, J.P., Pleshakov, V. and Chien, J.R. (1964). Isolation and identification of the long-acting thyroid stimulator and its relation to hyperthyroidism and circumscribed pretibial myxoedema. *J. Clin. Endocrinol. Metab.* **24**, 1005–28.

Learoyd, D.L., Fung, H.Y.M. and McGregor, A.M. (1992). Postpartum thyroid dysfunction. *Thyroid* **2** (in press).

Libert, F., Ruel, J., Ludgate, M. *et al.* (1987). Thyroperoxidase: an autoantigen with a mosaic structure made of nuclear and mitochondrial gene modules. *EMBO J.* **6**, 4193–6.

Libert, F., Lefort, A., Gerard, C. *et al.* (1989a). Cloning, sequencing and expression of the human thyrotropin (TSH) receptor: evidence for binding of autoantibodies. *Biochem. Biophys. Res. Comm.* **165**, 1250–5.

Libert, F., Parmentier, M., Lefort, A. *et al.* (1989b). Selective amplification and cloning of four new members of the G protein-coupled receptor family. *Science* **244**, 569–72.

Londei, M., Bottazzo, G.F. and Feldmann, M. (1985a). Human T cell clones from autoimmune thyroid glands: specific recognition of autologous thyroid cells. *Science* **228**, 85–9.

Londei, M., Lamb, J.R., Bottazzo, G.F. and Feldmann, M. (1985b). Epithelial cells expressing aberrant MHC class II determinants can present antigen to clonal human T cells. *Nature* **312**, 639–41.

Luborsky, J.L., Visintin, L., Boyers, S., Asari, T., Caldwell, B. and De Cherney, A. (1990). Ovarian antibodies detected by immobilized antigen immunoassay in patients with premature ovarian failure. *J. Clin. Endocrinol. Metab.* **70**, 69–75.

Ludgate, M.E., McGregor, A., Weetman, A.P. *et al.* (1984). Analysis of T cell subsets in Graves' disease: alterations associated with carbimazole. *Br. Med. J.* **288**, 526–30.

Ludgate, M.E., Ratanachaiyavong, S., Weetman, A.P., Hall, R. and McGregor, A.M. (1985). Failure to demonstrate cell-mediated immune responses to thyroid antigen in Graves' disease using *in vitro* assays of lymphokine-mediated migration inhibition. *J. Clin. Endocrinol. Metab.* **60**, 98–102.

Ludgate, M.E., Dong, Q., Dreyfus, P.A. *et al.* (1989). Definition, at the molecular level, of a thyroglobulin-acetylcholinesterase shared epitope: study of its pathophysiological significance in patients with Graves' ophthalmopathy. *Autoimmunity* **3**, 167–76.

McFarland, K.C., Sprengel, R., Phillips, H.S. *et al.* (1989). Lutropin-choriogonadotropin receptor: an unusual member of the G protein-coupled receptor family. *Science* **245**, 494–9.

McGregor, A.M. (1990). Autoantibodies to the TSH receptor in patients with autoimmune thyroid disease. *Clin. Endocrinol.* **33**, 683–5.

McGregor, A.M., Petersen, M.M., McLachlan, S.M., Rees Smith, B. and Hall, R. (1980). Carbimazole and the autoimmune response in Graves' disease. *N. Engl. J. Med.* **303**, 302–7.

McGregor, A.M., Weetman, A.P., Ratanachaiyavong, S., Owen, G.M., Ibbertson, H.K. and Hall, R. (1985). Iodine: an influence on the development of autoimmune thyroid disease? In *Thyroid Disorders Associated with Iodine Deficiency and Excess*, ed. R. Hall and J. Kobberling, pp. 209–16, Raven Press, New York.

McKenzie, J.M. (1958). Delayed thyroid response to serum from thyrotoxic patients. *Endocrinology* **63**, 865–8.

McKenzie, J.M. (1964). Neonatal Graves' disease. *J. Clin. Endocrinol. Metab.* **24**, 660–8.

Mangklabruks, A., Cox, N. and De Groot, L.J. (1991). Genetic factors in autoimmune thyroid disease analysed by restriction fragment length polymorphisms of candidate genes. *J. Clin. Endocrinol. Metab.* **73**, 236–44.

Manley, S.W., Bourke, J.R. and Hawker, R.W. (1974). The TSH receptor in guinea-pig thyroid homogenate: interaction with the long-acting thyroid stimulator. *J. Endocrinol.* **61**, 437–45.

Matsuura, N., Yamada, Y., Nohara, Y. *et al.* (1980). Familial neonatal transient hypothyroidism due to maternal TSH-binding inhibitor immunoglobulins. *N. Engl. J. Med.* **303**, 738–41.

Mazzone, T., Kelly, W. and Ensinck, J. (1983). Lymphocytic hypophysitis associated with antiparietal cell antibodies and vitamin B_{12} deficiency. *Arch. Intern. Med.* **143**, 1794–5.

Mehdi, S.Q., Nussey, S.S., Gibbons, C.P. and El Kabir, D.J. (1973). Binding of thyroid stimulators to human thyroid membranes. *Biochem. Soc. Trans.* **1**, 1005–6.

Mirakian, R., Cudworth, A.G., Bottazzo, G.F., Richardson, C.A. and Doniach, D. (1982). Autoimmunity to anterior pituitary cells and the pathogenesis of insulin-dependent diabetes mellitus. *Lancet* **i**, 755–8.

Munro, D.S., Dirmikis, S.M., Humphries, H., Smith, T. and Broadhead, G.D. (1978). The role of thyroid stimulating immunoglobulins of Graves' disease in neonatal thyrotoxicosis. *Br. J. Obstet. Gynaecol.* **85**, 837–43.

Nagayama, Y., Wadsworth, H.L., Russo, D., Chazenbalk, G.D. and Rapoport, B. (1991) Binding domains of stimulatory and inhibitory thyrotropin (TSH) receptor autoantibodies determined with chimeric TSH-lutropin/chorionicgonadotropin receptors. *J. Clin. Invest.* **88**, 336–40.

Neufeld, M., Maclaren, N.K. and Blizzard, R.M. (1981). Two types of autoimmune Addison's disease associated with different polyglandular autoimmune (PGA) syndromes. *Medicine* **60**, 355–62.

Nye, L., De Carvalho, L.P. and Roitt, I.M. (1980). Restrictions in the response to autologous thyroglobulin in the human. *Clin. Exp. Immunol.* **41**, 252–63.

Nye, L., De Carvalho, L.P. and Roitt, I.M. (1981). An investigation of the clonality of human thyroglobulin autoantibodies and their light chains. *Clin. Exp. Immunol.* **46**, 161–70.

Okita, N., Kidd, A., Row, V.V. and Volpé, R. (1980). Sensitization of T-lymphocytes in Graves' and Hashimoto's diseases. *J. Clin. Endocrinol. Metab.* **57**, 316–20.

Okita, N., Row, V.V. and Volpé, R. (1981). Suppressor T-lymphocyte deficiency in Graves' disease and Hashimoto's thyroiditis. *J. Clin. Endocrinol. Metab.* **52**, 523–7.

Othman, S., Phillips, D.I.W., Parkes, A.B. *et al.* (1990). Long term follow-up of post-partum thyroiditis. *Clin. Endocrinol.* **32**, 559–64.

Penhale, W.J. and Young, P.R. (1988). The influence of microbial environment on susceptibility to experimental autoimmune thyroiditis. *Clin. Exp. Immunol.* **72**, 288–92.

Perret, J., Ludgate, M., Libert, F. *et al.* (1990). Stable expression of the human TSH receptor in CHO cells and characterisation of differentially expressing clones. *Biochem. Biophys. Res. Comm.* **171**, 1044–50.

Pestell, R.G., Best, J.D. and Alford, F.P. (1990). Lymphocytic hypophysitis: the clinical spectrum of the disorder and evidence for an autoimmune pathogenesis. *Clin. Endocrinol.* **33**, 457–66.

Phillips, D.I., Nelson, M., Barker, D.J., Morris, J.A. and Wood, T.J. (1988). Iodine in milk and the incidence of thyrotoxicosis in England. *Clin. Endocrinol. (Oxford)* **28**, 61–6.

Premachandra, B.N. and Blumenthal, H.J. (1985). Significance of thyroid hormone autoantibodies. In *Autoimmunity and the Thyroid*, P.G. Walfish, J.R. Wall and R. Volpé, pp. 189–208, Academic Press, London.

Rapoport, B., Greenspan, F.S., Filetti, S. and Pepitone, M. (1984). Clinical experience with a human thyroid cell bioassay for thyroid stimulating immunoglobulin. *J. Clin. Endocrinol. Metab.* **58**, 332–8.

Ratanachaiyavong, S. and McGregor, A.M. (1985). Immunosuppressive effects of antithyroid drugs. *Clin. Endocrinol. Metab.* **14**, 449–66.

Ratanachaiyavong, S. and McGregor, A.M. (1990). Immunogenetics of Graves' disease. In *The Thyroid Gland, Environment and Autoimmunity*, ed. H.A. Drexhage, pp. 167–80, Elsevier Science Publishers BV, Amsterdam.

Ratanachaiyavong, S., Lloyd, L. and McGregor, A.M. (1989). C4A gene deletion: association with Graves' disease. *J. Mol. Endocrinol.* **3**, 145–53.

Ratanachaiyavong, S., Gunn, C.A., Bidwell, E.A., Darke, C., Hall, R. and McGregor, A.M. (1990). DQA2 U allele: a genetic marker for relapse of Graves' disease. *Clin. Endocrinol.* **32**, 241–51.

Ratanachaiyavong, S., Demaine, A.G., Campbell, R.D. and McGregor, A.M. (1991). Heat shock protein 70 (HSP 70) and complement C4 genotypes in patients with hyperthyroid Graves' disease. *Clin. Exp. Immunol.* **84**, 48–52.

Rees Smith, B., McLachlan, S.M. and Furmaniak, J. (1988). Autoantibodies to the thyrotropin receptor. *Endocrinol. Rev.* **9**, 106–21.

Rennie, D.P., McGregor, A.M., Keast, D. *et al.* (1983). The influence of methimazole on thyroglobulin-induced autoimmune thyroiditis in the rat. *Endocrinology* **112**, 326–30.

Roberton, H.E.W. (1948). Lassitude coldness and hair changes following pregnancy and their response to treatment with thyroid extract. *Br. Med. J.* **2**, 93.

Roitt, I.M., Doniach, D., Campbell, P.N. and Vaughan Hudson, R. (1956) Autoantibodies in Hashimoto's disease (lymphadenoid goitre). *Lancet* **ii**, 820–1.

Rose, N.R. and Witebsky, E. (1956). Studies on organ specificity. V. Changes in the thyroid glands of rabbits following active immunization with rabbit thyroid extracts. *J. Immunol.* **76**, 417–27.

Rose, N.R., Kong, Y.M. and Sundick, R.S. (1980). The genetic lesions of autoimmunity. *Clin. Exp. Immunol.* **39**, 545–50.

Sack, J., Baker, J.R., Weetman, A.P., Wartofsky, L. and Burman, K.D. (1986). Killer cell activity and antibody-dependent cell-mediated cytotoxicity are normal in Hashimoto's disease. *J. Clin. Endocrinol. Metab.* **62**, 1059–64.

Sauter, N.P., Toni, R., McLauchlin, C.D., Dyess, E.M., Kritzman, J. and Lechan, R.M. (1990). Isolated adrenocorticotropin deficiency associated with an autoantibody to a corticotroph antigen that is not adrenocorticotropin or other proopiomelanocortin-derived peptides. *J. Clin. Endocrinol. Metab.* **70**, 1391–7.

Scherbaum, W.A. and Bottazzo, G.F. (1983). Autoantibodies to vasopressin cells in idiopathic diabetes insipidus: evidence for an autoimmune variant. *Lancet* **i**, 897–901.

Shine, B., Fells, P., Edwards, O.M. and Weetman, A.P. (1990). Association between Graves' ophthalmopathy and smoking. *Lancet* **335**, 1261–3.

Smith, B.R. and Hall, R. (1974). Thyroid stimulating immunoglobulins in Graves' disease. *Lancet* **ii**, 427–31.

Sotsiou, F., Bottazzo, G.F. and Doniach, D. (1980). Immunofluorescence studies on autoantibodies to steroid-producing cells, and to germline cells in endocrine disease and infertility. *Clin. Exp. Immunol.* **39**, 97–111.

Southgate, K., Creagh, F.M., Teece, M., Kingswood, C. and Rees Smith, B. (1984). A receptor assay for the measurement of TSH receptor antibodies in unextracted serum. *Clin. Endocrinol.* **20**, 539–48.

Stenszky, V., Kozma, L., Balazs, C. and Farid, N. (1985). The genetics of Graves' disease: HLA and disease susceptibility. *J. Clin. Endocrinol. Metab.* **61**, 735–40.

Stenszky, V., Balazs, C., Kraszits, E. *et al.* (1987). Association of goitrous autoimmune thyroiditis with HLA-DR3 in Eastern Hungary. *J. Immunogenet.* **14**, 143–8.

Sundick, R.S., Herdegen, D.M., Brown, T.R. and Bagchi, N. (1987). The incorporation of dietary iodine into thyroglobulin increases its immunogenicity. *Endocrinology* **120**, 2078–84.

Tachi, J., Amino, N., Tamaki, H., Aozasa, M., Iwatani, Y. and Miyai, K. (1988). Long term follow-up and HLA association in patient with post-partum hypothyroidism. *J. Clin. Endocrinol. Metab.* **66**, 480–4.

Tandon, N., Zhang, L. and Weetman, A.P. (1991). HLA association in Hashimoto's thyroiditis. *Clin. Endocrinol.* **34**, 383–6.

Todd, I., Pujol-Borrell, R., Hammond, L.J., Bottazzo, G.F. and Feldmann, M. (1985). Interferon-gamma induces HLA-DR expression by thyroid epithelium. *Clin. Exp. Immunol.* **61**, 265–73.

Tunbridge, W.M.G., Evered, D.C., Hall, R. *et al.* (1977). The spectrum of thyroid disease in a community: the Whickham survey. *Clin. Endocrinol.* **7**, 481–92.

Tunbridge, W.M.G., Brewis, M., French, J.M. *et al.* (1981). Natural history of autoimmune thyroiditis. *Br. Med. J.* **282**, 258–62.

Van der Gaag, R.D., Drexhage, H.A. and Dussault, J.H. (1985). Role of maternal immunoglobulins blocking TSH-induced thyroid growth in sporadic forms of congenital hypothyroidism. *Lancet* **i**, 246–50.

Vitti, P., Rotella, C.M., Valente, W.A. *et al.* (1983). Characterisation of the optimal stimulatory effects of Graves' monoclonal and serum immunoglobulin G on adenosine 3', 5'-monophosphate production in FRTL5 thyroid cells: a potential clinical assay. *J. Clin. Endocrinol. Metab.* **57**, 782–91.

Volpé, R. (1988). The immunoregulatory defect in autoimmune thyroid disease. *Autoimmunity* **2**, 55–72.

Wall, J.R., Salvi, M., Bernard, N.F., Boucher, A. and Haegert, D. (1991). Thyroid-associated ophthalmopathy — a model for the association of organ-specific autoimmune disorders. *Immunol. Today* **12**, 150–3.

Weetman, A.P. (1991a). *Autoimmune Endocrine Disease*. Cambridge University Press, Cambridge.

Weetman, A.P. (1991b). Thyroid-associated eye disease: pathophysiology. *Lancet* **338**, 25–32.

Weetman, A.P. and McGregor, A.M. (1984). Autoimmune thyroid disease: developments in our understanding. *Endocrine Rev.* **5**, 309–55.

Weetman, A.P., McGregor, A.M. and Hall, R. (1983). Methimazole inhibits thyroid autoantibody production by an action on accessory cells. *Clin. Immunol. Immunopathol.* **28**, 39–45.

Weetman, A.P., McGregor, A.M., Wheeler, M.H. and Hall, R. (1984a). Extrathyroidal sites of autoantibody synthesis in Graves' disease. *Clin. Exp. Immunol.* **56**, 330–6.

Weetman, A.P., Holt, M.E., Campbell, A.K., Hall, R. and McGregor, A.M. (1984b). Methimazole and generation of oxygen radicals by monocytes: potential role in immunosuppression. *Br. Med. J.* **288**, 518–20.

Weetman, A.P., Volkman, D.J., Burman, K.D., Gerrard, T.L. and Fauci, A.S. (1985). The *in vitro* regulation of human thyrocyte HLA-DR antigen expression. *J. Clin. Endocrinol. Metab.* **61**, 817–24.

Weetman, A.P., Volkman, D.J., Burman, K.D. *et al.* (1986). The production and characterisation of thyroid-derived T cell lines in Graves' disease and Hashimoto's thyroiditis. *Clin. Immunol. Immunopathol.* **39**, 139–50.

Weetman, A.P., So, A.K., Roe, C., Walport, M.J. and Foroni, L. (1987a). T cell receptor alpha-chain V region polymorphism linked to primary autoimmune hypothyroidism but not Graves' disease. *Hum. Immunol.* **20**, 167–73.

Weetman, A.P., Green, C. and Borysiewicz, L.K. (1987b). Regulation of major histocompatibility complex (MHC) class II antigen expression by the $FRTL_5$ rat thyroid cell line. *J. Endocrinol.* **115**, 481–7.

Weetman, A.P., Black, C.M., Cohen, S.B., Tomlinson, R., Banga, J.P. and Reimer, C.B. (1989a). Affinity purification of IgG subclasses and the distribution of thyroid autoantibody reactivity in Hashimoto's thyroiditis. *Scand. J. Immunol.* **30**, 83–9.

Weetman, A.P., Cohen, S.B., Makgoba, M.W. and Borysiewicz, L.K. (1989b). Expression of an intercellular adhesion molecule, ICAM-1, by human thyroid cells. *J. Endocrinol.* **122**, 185.

Weetman, A.P., Freeman, M., Borysiewicz, L.K. and Makgoba,

M.W. (1990a). Functional analysis of intercellular adhesion molecule-1-expressing human thyroid cells. *Eur. J. Immunol.* **20**, 271–5.

Weetman, A.P., Bright-Thomas, R. and Freeman, M. (1990b). Regulation of interleukin-6 release by human thyrocytes. *J. Endocrinol.* **127**, 357–61.

Weetman, A.P., Fung, H.Y.M., Richards, C.J. and McGregor, A.M. (1990c). IgG subclass distribution and relative functional affinity of thyroid microsomal antibodies in post-partum thyroiditis. *Eur. J. Clin. Invest.* **20**, 133–6.

Weetman, A.P., Byfield, P.G.H., Black, C. and Reimer, C.B. (1990d). IgG heavy-chain subclass restriction of thyrotropin-binding inhibitory immunoglobulins of Graves' disease. *Eur. J. Clin. Invest.* **20**, 406–10.

Weiss, A. (1990). Structure and function of the T cell antigen receptor. *J. Clin. Invest.* **8**, 1015–22.

Weissel, M., Hofer, R., Zasmeta, H. and Mayr, W.R. (1980). HLA-DR and Hashimoto's thyroiditis. *Tissue Antigens* **16**, 256–9.

Wick, G., Boyd, R., Hala, K., Thunold, S. and Kofler, H. (1982). Pathogenesis of spontaneous autoimmune thyroiditis in Obese strain (OS) chickens. *Clin. Exp. Immunol.* **47**, 1–18.

Williams, E.D. and Doniach, I. (1962). The post-mortem incidence of focal thyroiditis. *J. Pathol. Bacteriol.* **83**, 255–64.

Williams, R.C., Marshall, N.J., Kilpatrick, K. *et al.* (1988). Kappa/lambda immunoglobulin distribution of Graves' thyroid-stimulating antibodies: simultaneous analysis of C lambda gene polymorphisms. *J. Clin. Invest.* **82**, 1306–12.

Winsa, B., Adami, H.O., Bergstrom, R. and Karlson, A. (1991). Genetic predisposition and stressful life events as risk factors for Graves' disease. *Ann. Endocrinol.* **52**, 43 (abstract 70).

Yoshida, H., Amino, N., Yagawa, K. *et al.* (1978). Association of serum antithyroid antibodies with lymphocytic infiltration of the thyroid glands: studies of seventy autopsied cases. *J. Clin. Endocrinol. Metab.* **46**, 859–62.

Zakarija, M. (1983). Immunochemical characterisation of the thyroid-stimulating antibody in Graves' disease: evidence for restricted heterogeneity. *J. Clin. Lab. Immunol.* **10**, 77–85.

Zakarija, M., McKenzie, J.M. and Eidson, M.S. (1990). Transient neonatal hypothyroidism: characterisation of maternal antibodies to the thyrotropin receptor. *J. Clin. Endocrinol. Metab.* **70**, 1239–46.

103: The Aetiology, Genetics and Immunology of Type I (Insulin-dependent) Diabetes Mellitus

G.F. Bottazzo, R. Pujol-Borrell and E. Bonifacio

Type I or insulin-dependent diabetes mellitus (IDDM) has an autoimmune pathogenesis (reviewed in Eisenbarth 1986; Bottazzo *et al*. 1987). Evidence includes: autoantibodies to islet cells; cell-mediated immune (CMI) abnormalities detected in the peripheral blood (reviewed in Buschard 1985; Bach 1988); lymphocytic infiltration and other immune abnormalities in 'diabetic' islets (Foulis and Bottazzo 1988); and induced or experimental animal models of the disease (reviewed in Tarui *et al*. 1986; Mordes and Rossini 1987; Shafrin and Renold 1988). In addition to the autoimmune phenomena, environment and genetic susceptibilities (reviewed in Bottazzo *et al*. 1986) appear important.

Aetiology

It is clear that the environment plays a role in the causation of IDDM. Data supporting this are indirect and include: the 30–50% concordance for IDDM among identical twins (Barnett *et al*. 1981); the sharp increase of the disease among certain ethnic groups who have moved from countries with low incidence of IDDM to countries where there is a higher occurrence of the disease (Siemiatycki *et al*. 1988); the seasonal variations in the incidence of new cases of IDDM, with peaks in the autumn and winter (Durruty *et al*. 1979); and the coincidence of the peak ages of onset of IDDM with the ages at which children join primary and secondary schools (reviewed in Gamble 1980). These point to common viruses as potential causative factors of IDDM (reviewed in Gamble 1980; Diabetes Epidemiology Research International Group 1988). Chemical substances and food additives have also been implicated (reviewed in Bottazzo 1986). Neonatal events, including breast-feeding habits, could also be important (reviewed in Bingley and Gale 1990).

Despite these indications, there have been few advances in identifying viruses or other agents which may be the aetiological agents of IDDM. There are reports of increased titres of antibodies to Coxsackie virus in newly diagnosed IDDM patients (King *et al*. 1983), but these were not confirmed when appropriate age-, sex- and environmentally matched controls were included in the comparative analysis (Tuvemo *et al*. 1989). Furthermore, no Coxsackie virus envelope proteins are detected in the beta cells of pancreases of newly diagnosed diabetics (reviewed in Foulis 1989).

Cytomegalovirus (CMV) sequences have been found in the deoxyribonucleic acid (DNA) extracted from lymphocytes of IDDM patients (Pak *et al*. 1988) but unexpectedly the virus seems to be present in islets of type II rather than type I diabetic patients (Lohr and Oldstone 1990). Insulin-dependent diabetes mellitus occurs with increased frequency in patients with congenital rubella syndrome (reviewed in Rayfield and Ishimura 1987). This represents an interesting model of IDDM in humans, but nowadays the introduction of large-scale vaccination programmes for rubella has almost defeated the disease and, despite this, the incidence of IDDM continues to increase (reviewed in Diabetes Epidemiology Research International Group 1988).

Although IDDM manifests itself acutely, it is preceded by a long prodromal period (Gorsuch *et al*. 1981). The common viruses mentioned acutely damage beta cells *in vitro*, and hence, except for rare cases (Yoon *et al*. 1979), such viral infection probably acts to precipitate rather than initiate beta cell damage (reviewed in Bottazzo 1986). In view of this long latency, slow viruses with tropism for the beta cells have been postulated to cause IDDM. Electron-microscopy studies in the non-obese diabetic (NOD) strain of mice, which develops IDDM spontaneously, have shown an enhancement of endogenous retroviral-like particles in the beta cells and not in the glucagon (alpha), somatostatin (delta) and pancreatic polypeptide (PP) cells (Leiter 1985). In humans, it was shown that, in thyroid DNA obtained from Graves' patients, human immunodeficiency virus (HIV)-1-like sequences were identified (Ciampolillo *et al*. 1989), but these data are not easy to confirm (Humphrey *et al*. 1991). However, in patients with Graves' disease, IDDM DNA analysis of peripheral blood lymphocytes (PBLs) revealed the presence of human T cell lymphotrophic virus (HTLV)-1 homologous sequences (Lagaye *et al*. 1991). Whether a family of these slow viruses is ultimately implicated in IDDM or other autoimmune diseases remains an interesting hypothesis.

Regardless of the difficulty in identifying them, environmental factors are almost certainly involved in the aetiology of IDDM. This is further substantiated by the presence of interferon (IFN)-α, a product of virally infected cells, in human beta cells of 'diabetic' pancreases (Foulis *et al*. 1987a).

Genetic markers

The genetics of IDDM appears complex. Studies indicate that a number of genes may be involved (reviewed in Trucco and Dorman 1989). Many autoimmune diseases are associated with particular human leucocyte antigen (HLA) alleles and haplotypes (reviewed in Farid 1988). Type 1 diabetes is no exception and, like many other autoimmune endocrine disorders, is associated with HLA-DR3, but also, and more frequently, with HLA-DR4 (reviewed in Rotter *et al*. 1986). The risk of developing IDDM is greater for individuals who have HLA-DR3 or DR4 than for those with other HLA-DR types and is even greater for individuals who are heterozygous for HLA-DR3 and DR4. These findings indicate that there is more than one susceptibility gene for IDDM, and that these operate interactively. Human leucocyte antigen DR2 is rarely detected in diabetic patients and this allele, or a gene in linkage disequilibrium with it, appears to confer resistance to the disease. In addition, only some HLA-DR3 or DR4 containing haplotypes confer an increased risk (McCluskey *et al*. 1983), indicating that genes close to HLA-DR, or the combinations of several alleles within the major histocompatibility complex (MHC), are important in the pathogenesis.

In the genetics of IDDM, the excess DR3/DR4 heterozygosity remains intriguing. It is in part a result of a decreased maternal transmission of DR4-bearing haplotypes to males, compared with the father, leaving a relative excess of DR3 haplotypes derived from the mother (Rubenstein *et al*. 1990). This most likely suggests *trans* interaction between genes (Rotter *et al*. 1986). In addition to a selective haplotype transmission, there is a reduced incidence of IDDM in children from IDDM mothers (Buschard *et al*. 1989). The uncontrolled glucose metabolism in these women during pregnancy therefore may be protective for IDDM. Neonatal stimulation of beta cells by glucose in the Bio Breeding (BB) rat, the second spontaneous animal model of IDDM, markedly reduces the incidence of diabetes in these rodents (Buschard *et al.* 1990). Islet autoantigen expression increases *in vitro* under these conditions (Kampe *et al.* 1989) and this phenomenon may favour immunological tolerance to islet autoantigens in the fetal or newborn period. Indeed, an early hyperfunctional state of the beta cells may be important in protecting against IDDM in later life. The opposite is also true. A hypofunctional state induced by intensive insulin therapy in this period also prevents IDDM in these animals (Gotfredsen *et al.* 1985).

Other genes include HLA-DQ. HLA-DR4 is linked to different splits of HLA-DQ3 and IDDM is significantly associated with the DQ8 subtype (reviewed in Owerbach *et al.* 1987). Sequencing has revealed that in DQ alleles found in many of the haplotypes associated with IDDM the amino acid serine, valine or alanine is in position 57 of the DQβ chain. Those which are not associated with IDDM are more likely to possess aspartic acid in this position (Asp-57 DQβ) (reviewed in Todd *et al.* 1988). Indeed, the majority of white IDDM patients have non-Asp-57 DQβ alleles on both haplotypes (Ronningen *et al.* 1989). Despite this, IDDM does occur in individuals with Asp-57 DQβ, and a large number of non-disease individuals also possess the non-Asp-57 DQβ genotype. Nevertheless, data in whites support a potential role for the DQ genes.

The link with DQ is also found in other ethnic groups (reviewed in Hitman 1989). In the Japanese, homozygous non-Asp-57-encoding DQB genes are rare in both patients and controls (Awata *et al.* 1990). Most patients are heterozygous Asp-57/non-Asp-57, however, and thus there remains an increase in non-Asp-57 DQβ alleles in the patients. It has been speculated that the low frequency of the non-Asp-57 DQβ alleles in the Japanese may account for the rare occurrence of the disease in Japan. Variation in the distribution of the IDDM-susceptible Class II MHC alleles, in particular that of the non-Asp-57 alleles, might explain much of the geographical variations in IDDM incidence (Dorman *et al.* 1990) (Fig. 103.1).

Transethnic mapping has identified distinct HLA-DR/DQ haplotypes specific for different ethnic groups (reviewed in Todd 1990). The susceptibility to IDDM in blacks is closely linked to the DQA locus, and both DQB and DQA genes contribute to disease. In addition to the non-Asp-57-encoding DQB genes, a DQα chain bearing an arginine in position 52 is also associated with IDDM in whites (Khalil *et al.* 1990). These data suggest that disease susceptibility correlates quantitatively with the expression at the cell surface of a heterodimer composed of a DQα chain bearing an arginine at position 52 and a DQβ chain lacking aspartic acid at position 57. It has been hypothesized that the charge and the position of these two residues on the groove of the DQ heterodimer could be crucial to susceptibility via their ability to facilitate binding of antigenic peptide and subsequent autoantigen presentation to helper T cells.

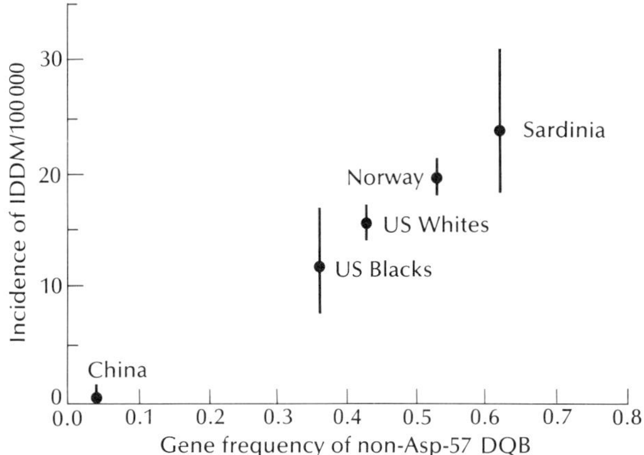

Fig. 103.1. Association between annual IDDM incidence rates and the gene frequency of non-Asp-57 DQB in different populations. Illustration courtesy of Dr M Trucco, Pittsburgh USA.

Genes in the MHC other than Class II are likely to influence susceptibility to IDDM. There are a number of genes located between HLA Class I and Class II MHC which encode mediators and amplifiers of immune responses (complement components C4, C2 and Bf, tumour necrosis factor (TNF)), together with a large number of other products of uncertain function (Spies *et al.* 1989). At least some of these genes are polymorphic. The TNF gene, for example, has polymorphisms associated with particular IDDM-susceptible haplotypes (Badenhoop *et al.* 1989).

Genes outside the MHC region have been postulated as contributing to IDDM susceptibility. These include the insulin-like growth factor (IGF)-2 gene situated on chromosome 11 (Julier *et al.* 1991), which appears to be a major susceptibility locus in HLA-DR4 +ve diabetes and, although controversial, the T cell receptor genes (Sheehy *et al.* 1989; McMillan *et al.* 1990). It is clear that IDDM is a multigenic disease, but it is also evident IDDM cannot be attributed to genetics alone.

Cell-mediated immune abnormalities

Extensive research has been carried out on the CMI processes involved in the autoimmune destruction of the beta cells. The first demonstration of CMI involvement was the leucocyte migration inhibition test (LMIT), which demonstrated that newly diagnosed IDDM patients are sensitized to pancreatic antigens (reviewed in Irvine 1980). Lymphocytes of IDDM patients can also produce cytotoxicity to various islet cell targets *in vitro* (reviewed in Bach 1988). Quantitative abnormalities of T cell phenotypes can also be demonstrated. Most commonly found are increased levels of the activated CD4 +ve population (Jackson *et al.* 1982). Although several abnormalities have been identified they are not always consistent, suggesting low precursor frequencies in the circulation.

Only by cloning can the islet-specific T lymphocytes be identified. Autoreactive CD4 +ve T cell clones have been produced from PBLs of IDDM patients (De Berardinis *et al.* 1988; Van Vliet *et al.* 1989). The reactivity against islets is HLA-DR-restricted (De Berardinis *et al.* 1988), and some of these recognize a 38 kD protein derived from insulin secretory granules (Roep *et al.* 1990). Peripheral blood lymphocytes from IDDM patients also have reactivity to this fraction (Roep *et al.* 1991). We still await the generation of an autoreactive CD8 cytotoxic T cell line from IDDM patients. The cytotoxic T cells are those most abundant in the insulitis observed at diagnosis (Bottazzo *et al.* 1985) and in the recurrent diabetes seen in diabetic identical twins transplanted with part of the pancreas of the unaffected co-twin (Sibley and Sutherland 1987).

Islet cell antibodies and other autoantibodies

Cytoplasmic islet cell antibodies

Islet cell antibodies (ICA) were first described in IDDM patients who had other coexistent autoimmune endocrine disorders (Bottazzo *et al.* 1974) and subsequently in up to 90% of newly diagnosed IDDM patients, with or without clinical endocrine manifestations (Lendrum *et al.* 1975). Islet cell antibodies tend to become undetectable in the circulation a few weeks or months after diagnosis (Lendrum *et al.* 1976).

Islet cell antibodies are demonstrated by indirect immunofluorescence (IF), and standardization programmes have defined their measurement in reference Juvenile Diabetes Foundation (JDF) units (reviewed in Gleichmann and Bottazzo 1987). They are exclusively of immunoglobulin G (IgG) class, with restriction of certain IgG subclasses (Kappler *et al.* 1987), and can fix complement (Bottazzo *et al.* 1980). Islet cell antibody +ve sera react with the cytoplasm of alpha, delta and PP cells as well as with beta cells, suggesting that the endocrine cells in the islets share a common autoantigen (reviewed in Bottazzo and Doniach 1980).

The target antigens recognized by ICA, detected by indirect IF, may be sialogangliosides, as suggested by the removal of ICA staining by certain sera upon neuraminidase treatment of pancreatic sections (reviewed in Colman and Eisenbarth 1988). Direct binding of ICA to a beta-specific sialoganglioside, however, has been difficult to demonstrate (Colman *et al.* 1988), and the identity of the autoantigen is yet to be found.

Sixty-four kilodalton/glutamic acid decarboxidase antibodies

Autoantibodies which immunoprecipitate a 64 kD protein from human and rodent islets are also detected in sera of IDDM patients (Baekkeskov *et al.* 1982). They have been reported to be as frequent and detected as early as cytoplasmic ICA (Atkinson *et al.* 1990) but, in contrast to ICA, they seem to persist longer in the circulation after the diagnosis has been established (Christie *et al.* 1990a). Their detection has involved cumbersome and expensive assays which have not allowed large population screening programmes.

The identity of the 64 kD autoantigen is reported as glutamic acid decarboxidase (GAD), the biosynthesizing enzyme of the inhibitory neurotransmitter gamma-amino butyric acid (GABA) (Baekkeskov *et al.* 1990). Antibodies to GAD were first recognized in a patient with stiff-man syndrome, a rare disorder of the nervous system (Solimena *et al.* 1988). This patient also had IDDM with associated polyendocrinopathy and high-titre ICA (Bosi *et al.* 1988). Subsequently, autoantibodies to GAD were detected in 60% of patients with the same syndrome (Solimena *et al.* 1990), and again an association with organ-specific autoimmunity, in particular ICA, was seen in patients positive for GAD antibodies.

Glutamic acid decarboxidase is in high concentration in the GABA-secreting neurone and in pancreatic beta cells (Vincent *et al.* 1983). There are at least two forms of GAD, encoded for by separate genes (Erlander *et al.* 1991; Karlsen *et al.* 1991). Homology between them is around 70% and both are found in the brain and in the islets (Giorda *et al.* 1991; Kelly *et al.* 1991).

Glutamic acid decarboxidase antibodies, measured by immunoprecipitation of GAD enzymatic activity, are found in 20–60% of IDDM sera (Martino *et al.* 1991). They are detected more frequently in patients with high levels of ICA and in female patients with thyrogastric antibodies. As in stiff-man syndrome, there seems to be an association of GAD antibodies with the polyendocrine type of patient. The relatively low prevalence of GAD antibodies detected by these assays is in contrast to the high positivity reported for anti-64 kD antibodies in newly diagnosed IDDM patients (Baekkeskov *et al.* 1987). This indicates either an inability of these assays to detect GAD antibodies or that the 64 kD autoantigen is not solely GAD.

Antibodies to 64 kD tryptic fragments

Analysis of antibody reactivity by immunoprecipitation of trypsin-digested islet homogenates results in precipitation of three major fragments of M_r 50 kD, 40 kD and 37 kD (Christie *et al.* 1990b). Patient sera can precipitate all three fragments, the 50 kD fragment alone or only the 40 kD and 37 kD fragments (Fig. 103.2). Antibodies that recognize the 50 kD fragment also bind the intact 64 kD antigen and correlate with their ability to immunoprecipitate GAD. In contrast, antibodies to the 40 kD and 37 kD fragments do not correlate with GAD antibodies and they appear to recognize cryptic determinants on the 64 kD antigen complex which are exposed by proteolytic cleavage (Christie *et al.* 1991).

Approximately 70% of diabetic patients possess antibodies to each of the tryptic fragments of the islet autoantigen and more than 90% of recent-onset IDDM patients have antibodies to at least one of the antigenic fragments (Christie *et al.* 1990b). The data suggest that 50 kD and the 40 kD/37 kD fragments may be distinct entities with different antigenic and biochemical properties (reviewed in Bottazzo *et al.* 1991).

Insulin and proinsulin autoantibodies

Spontaneous autoantibodies to insulin (IAA) were first identified in untreated, newly diagnosed IDDM patients (Palmer *et al.* 1983), using either radioimmunoassay (RIA) (Srikanta *et al.* 1986) or enzyme-linked immunosorbent assay (ELISA) (Dean *et al.* 1986b). Insulin autoantibodies are detected in 30–40% of newly diagnosed IDDM patients (reviewed in Palmer 1987). Workshops for the standardization of IAA have demonstrated

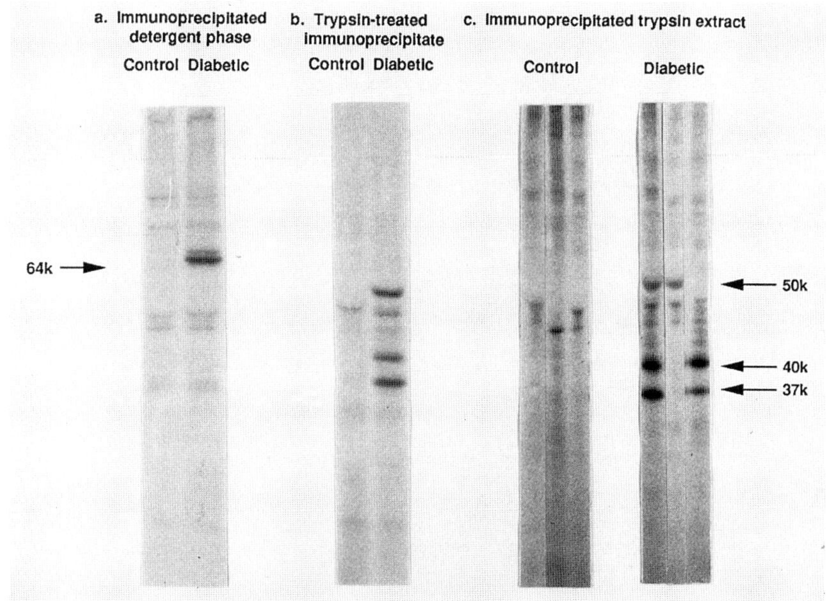

Fig. 103.2. Autoradiographs illustrating peptides immunoprecipitated from extracts of ^{35}S methionine-labelled neonatal rat islet extracts by serum antibodies from control or diabetic individuals. (a) Diabetic sera immunoprecipitate a 64 kD protein from detergent-phase purified proteins. (b) Trypsin treatment of the immunoprecipitate results in peptide fragments of 50 kD, 40 kD and 37 kD. (c) Immunoprecipitation of solubilized peptides from trypsin-digested radiolabelled islets diabetic sera can immunoprecipitate the 50, 40 and 37 kD peptides, the 50 kD peptide only, or the 40 and 37 kD peptides only. Illustration courtesy of Dr M.R. Christie.

discordance between methodologies (RIA versus ELISA) used for the detection. Radio-immunoassays produce significantly higher specific signals for the newly diagnosed diabetic sera than ELISA, and measurements from different RIA assays are more comparable to each other than those from ELISA (Kuglin *et al.* 1990a).

Autoantibodies to proinsulin have also been detected by ELISA and RIA (Kuglin *et al.* 1990b). Their frequency in IDDM is similar to that of IAA, and are sometimes found in sera which are IAA −ve.

Antibodies to heat-shock protein 65

Humoral and T lymphocyte responses to heat-shock protein (HSP)-65 of *Mycobacterium tuberculosis* have been shown in the NOD mouse model of IDDM (Elias *et al.* 1990). It was suggested that this HSP-65 antigen may also be the equivalent of the 64 kD islet antigen (Jones *et al.* 1990) but others have not confirmed these initial findings (Kampe *et al.* 1990). Heat-shock protein-65 is a ubiquitous protein and therefore unlikely to contribute to the antigen of 64 kD reactivity, but it cannot be disregarded that HSP-65 and GAD share sequence homology in their molecules (Jones and Duff 1991).

Antibodies to carboxypeptidase H

Antibodies binding to a 52 kD rat insulinoma cell protein have been found in the sera of a high proportion of NOD mice and in 30% of humans with IDDM (Karounos and Thomas 1990). Carboxypeptidase H, an enzyme involved in the conversion of proinsulin to insulin, also has a molecular weight of 52−57 kD, and it was found that 25% of diabetic sera contain antibodies to a recombinant protein which corresponds to this enzyme (Castano *et al.* 1991).

Antibodies to glucose transporter

Immunoglobulin from IDDM patients inhibits the uptake of 3-*O*-methyl-beta-D-glucose by dispersed rat islet cells. This inhibitory effect is abolished by preincubation of islet cells with membranes from hepatocytes, which contain the same glucose transporter, but not from erythrocytes, which lack it, suggesting that IDDM sera might contain antibodies to the glucose transporter (Johnson *et al.* 1990). Such antibodies could act to impair glucose-stimulated insulin secretion *in vivo*.

Islet cell surface antibodies

Islet cell surface antibodies (ICSA) are possible distinct entities of ICA. Islet cell surface antibodies were initially detected using viable cultured rodent (Lernmark *et al.* 1978) or human fetal islet cells (Pujol-Borrell *et al.* 1982), and it has been suggested that there are separate specificities for alpha, beta and PP cells (Van de Winkel *et al.* 1982). Clearly, all these data need to be confirmed using human adult islets. *In vitro*, sera of IDDM patients are cytotoxic to cultured islet cells and interfere with glucose-stimulated insulin release (Boitard *et al.* 1984).

Other autoantibodies

Not only do type I diabetic patients elicit a specific autoantibody response against islet cell components, including separate autoantibodies to alpha and delta cells (Bottazzo and Lendrum 1976), but their sera often contain a variety of other organ- and non-organ-specific autoantibodies (reviewed in Bottazzo 1984; Drell and Notkins 1987). Cytoplasmic pituitary antibodies have been demonstrated in IDDM probands and in their first-degree relatives (Mirakian *et al.* 1982), and surface antibodies to rat pituitary cells have been reported in the sera of the same patients (Vercammen *et al.* 1989). Antilymphocytic antibodies have also been demonstrated (Serjeantson *et al.* 1981). The presence of these additional autoantibodies indicate that in IDDM there is a general tendency to autoimmunity, but it remains unclear whether these other humoral specificities have any direct role in the pathogenetic process which destroys beta cells.

Predicting insulin-dependent diabetes mellitus

Measurement of ICA prospectively in first-degree relatives of IDDM patients initially established that the clinical onset of IDDM is delayed by up to several years (reviewed in Bosi *et al.* 1987). Many of the other markers found at onset of disease are also detected in the preclinical period. Hence it is possible to use the markers to predict the disease.

In order to use them for prediction, an under-

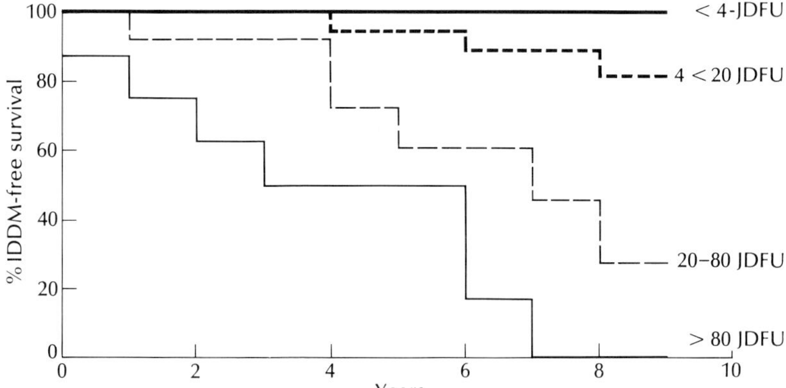

Fig. 103.3. Cumulative risk in first-degree relatives of IDDM probands for developing IDDM over 10 years. The diagram summarizes the data on 719 first-degree relatives studied in the Barts–Windsor Family Study. The risk was greatest for relatives with the highest levels of ICA.

standing of Bayes' theorem is important (reviewed in Dawkins 1985). From this theorem, the usefulness of any marker depends upon its specificity (negative in health) and sensitivity (positive in disease) and the prevalence of the disease in the population tested. Both specificity and sensitivity are dependent upon the test used to measure the marker, in particular, the threshold of positivity used. The specificity of the test will usually increase when higher positive thresholds are used.

In the case of ICA, its measurement in prospective family studies has shown that first-degree relatives with ICA titres >80 JDF units have a risk for IDDM which approaches 100% (Bonifacio *et al.* 1990; Riley *et al.* 1990) (Fig. 103.3). Using this threshold of positivity, although almost all those identified will develop IDDM, the majority of first-degree relatives who will develop IDDM have ICA <80 JDF units and therefore would not be identified (false negatives). In contrast, at a threshold of 4 JDF units, almost all of those developing IDDM will be positive for ICA but the predictive value of the test is substantially reduced, because a significant number of those who do not develop IDDM will also be positive (false positives).

The majority of individuals who develop IDDM do not have a first-degree family history of the disease. For effective prediction the tests used should be applicable to the general population. The reported frequency of ICA in the general population varies, but, in general, the prevalence of antibody is increased in countries where there is a high incidence of IDDM (Karjalainen 1990) (Fig. 103.4). In the UK, where the risk of IDDM is approximately 0.3% (Bingley and Gale 1989), around 3% of schoolchildren have detectable ICA (Bingley *et al.* 1991). Therefore, at best, the estimated predictive value of ICA at a threshold of 4 JDF units in the general population would be 10% (Fig. 103.5). At a threshold of 80 JDF units, the predictive value would increase to around 50%. Because of the very low incidence of IDDM in the general population, ICA on its own cannot provide 100% predictive value.

Several other autoantibody markers have been suggested for prediction. One of these, IAA

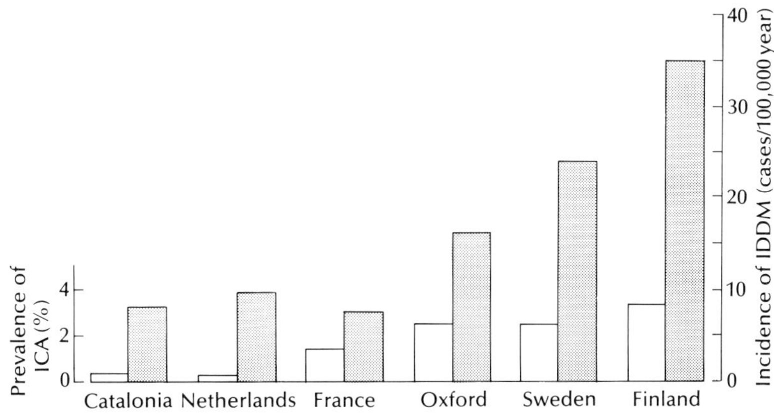

Fig. 103.4. Histogram showing the frequency of ICA (hatched bars) in a schoolchild population in several European countries. Finland, which has a high incidence of diabetes (filled bars), also has the highest prevalence of ICA. France, which has a relatively low incidence of IDDM, also has a lower frequency of ICA. Illustration courtesy of Dr P. Bingley.

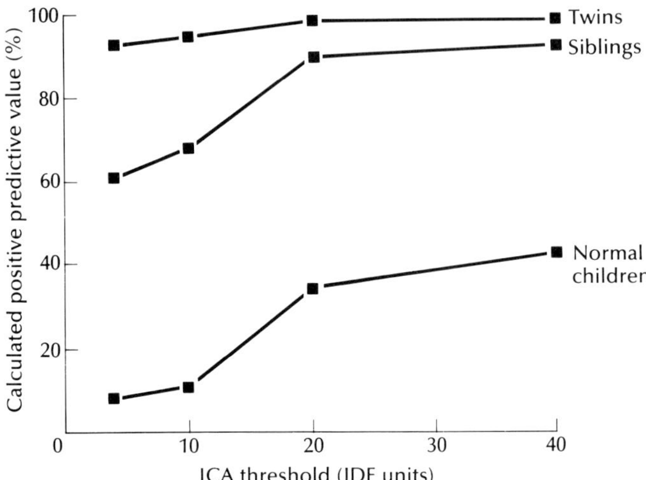

Fig. 103.5. The effect of differences in disease prevalence on the calculated positive predictive value of ICA. The positive predictive value using several thresholds of positivity for ICA is shown for discordant monozygotic twins, unaffected siblings of IDDM patients and children with no family history of IDDM. Illustration courtesy of Dr P. Bingley.

measured by RIA, appears specific for IDDM but, except in very young children, where it is detected in the majority of cases, it has a sensitivity for IDDM which is less than 50%. Nevertheless, the measurement of IAA in ICA +ve first-degree relatives, together with the use of the metabolic marker measuring first-phase insulin response to glucose, has been advocated for prediction of IDDM in first-degree relatives (reviewed in Ziegler and Eisenbarth 1990).

Another potential marker is anti-GAD antibodies, which, based on the reported frequency of 64 kD antibodies, is expected to have a sensitivity of more than 80% (Atkinson *et al.* 1990). Assays measuring GAD antibodies have been developed, but their sensitivity with respect to IDDM is too low to be used for the prediction of disease (Martino *et al.* 1991). The immunoprecipitation assay for anti-64 kD antibodies does have high sensitivity but is too cumbersome for screening. As the genes coding GAD have been cloned (Erlander *et al.* 1991; Karlsen *et al.* 1991), it is expected that other immunoassays using recombinant proteins will be developed, and that some of these may prove useful for prediction.

Antibodies to the tryptic fragments of 64 kD islet antigen may further discriminate those individuals at risk for IDDM (reviewed in Bottazzo *et al.* 1991). There is antibody heterogeneity to the fragments, and, in a study of identical twins, antibodies to 37/40 kD fragments were both specific and sensitive for IDDM (Christie *et al.* 1992). Islet cell antibodies are also heterogeneous. Patients with endocrine autoimmunity who are ICA +ve have a low risk for developing IDDM (Bosi *et al.* 1991). The majority of those who do not develop IDDM have a variant of ICA which is beta cell-selective (Genovese *et al.* 1992) (Plate 103.1, between pages 1930 and 1931). The specificity of this variant is GAD. Therefore, anti-GAD antibodies, which are found in the majority of IDDM patients are also found, even at very high titres, in the absence of diabetes. The CMI abnormalities found in IDDM can also be shown in the prediabetic period (Al-Sakkaf *et al.* 1989). In particular, the quantitative (Faustman *et al.* 1991) and functional (Schatz *et al.* 1991) abnormalities of the suppressor/inducer T cell subset (CD4 +ve/45 RA +ve) may assist prediction of IDDM.

The progression to IDDM in individuals with the autoimmune markers of IDDM is likely to be influenced factors such as age, genetic susceptibility, environmental exposure and geographical location (Leiter, 1990). The genetic markers, in particular those of the MHC, may also be useful to discriminate which ICA +ve individuals will develop IDDM. Not all ICA +ve individuals have the IDDM-susceptible MHC alleles, and selecting those with these genetic markers is likely to assist prediction of disease.

It is possible to use more than one of these markers in series. The effect of the first test is to exclude the majority of individuals who will not develop disease, effectively selecting a population with an increased incidence of IDDM to be screened by the second test. For example, selection for first-degree relatives of IDDM patients can be considered the first screen and ICA applied to this population is then an effective predictor of IDDM. The optimum is the use of tests which will result in both few false positives and few false negatives. Islet cell antibodies represent a useful first screen for IDDM. The test is relatively inexpensive and not labour-intensive, allowing large numbers of samples to be tested. International workshops have shown that precise and accurate measurement can be achieved, and, when low thresholds for positivity are used, the majority of those developing IDDM will be identified (Bonifacio *et al.* 1990).

Insulitis

One of the first clues which led to the suspicion that IDDM was an autoimmune disorder was the presence of an inflammatory infiltrate in and around the islets (reviewed in Gepts 1984). The inflammatory process is less florid than that seen in tissues affected by classic organ-specific autoimmunity.

The insulitis was seen in pancreatic specimens taken at autopsy from newly diagnosed IDDM patients. The immunohistopathology of the pancreas of newly diagnosed diabetics is complex and at least three populations of islets can be seen: (i) insulin-deficient islets which contain no beta cells but have normal or increased numbers of the other endocrine cell types, i.e. alpha cells, delta cells and PP cells; (ii) islets with 'insulitis'; and (iii) insulin-containing islets which are not inflamed. Many of these latter islets appear histological normal. Islets that are at a similar stage of destruction are anatomically grouped following the lobular structure of the pancreas (reviewed in Foulis 1989).

Studies on frozen blocks of fresh pancreases obtained at post-mortem of recently diagnosed diabetics (Bottazzo *et al.* 1985) demonstrate that the majority of the mononuclear cells in the inflammatory infiltrate are T lymphocytes of the CD8 phenotype. Other lymphocyte subsets, including natural killer/killer (NK/K) and CD4 lymphocytes, are also present. In general, macrophages are not numerous in the islet infiltrate (Foulis *et al.* 1991). A large proportion of T lymphocytes express HLA Class II MHC molecules and interleukin 2 (IL-2) receptors (Plate 103.2, between pages 1930 and 1931), indicating that they are activated, and suggesting a specific immune response directed against islet autoantigens. Many B lymphocytes are also present and this finding contrasts with that seen using classic histological techniques, which failed to observe mature plasma cells (reviewed in Gepts 1984) in the insulitis process. Immunoglobulin G and complement depositions were also detected in these islets.

Another feature of the islets in the pancreas of newly diagnosed IDDM patients is the overexpression of HLA proteins. Class I MHC molecules are markedly increased in all islet cell types and beta cells are positive for Class II (Bottazzo *et al.* 1985; Foulis and Farquharson 1986; Foulis *et al.* 1987b; Hanafusa *et al.* 1990). The 'ectopic' Class II MHC expression is specific for beta cells; alpha and delta cells do not express Class II products, consistent with the sparing of these cells in the killing process (Plate 103.3, between pages 1930 and 1931). These phenomena are present in a variety of target tissues of autoimmune disease (reviewed in Mirakian *et al.* 1990), and it has been suggested that it plays an important role in the pathogenesis of IDDM and other related disorders (Bottazzo *et al.* 1983; reviewed in Pujol-Borrell and Todd 1987).

Segmental pancreas transplantation between identical twins has generated further data. Four of these transplants were in long-standing diabetic twins who received the graft from the unaffected co-twin (Sibley and Sutherland 1987). After a few weeks, the transplanted twins became diabetic and sequential pancreatic biopsies showed intense insulitis with selective destruction of beta cells. The phenotype of the infiltrating lymphocytes was predominantly CD8. Only the beta cells in the graft were destroyed, indicating a recurrence of the IDDM caused by the 'awakening' of the same autoimmune response which originally destroyed the beta cells in the recipient, up to 20 years earlier. By contrast, in the pancreases transplanted to HLA-mismatched recipients, rejection but no disease recurrence was observed. These data support the view that the autoimmune response to the islets is HLA-restricted.

Cytokines and insulin-dependent diabetes mellitus

Cytokines are potent modulators of the immune response, and hence are likely to play a role in the pathogenesis of islet beta cell destruction in IDDM. Studies of both basal and stimulated levels of cytokines have shown inter-individual differences in IL-1 and TNF secretion by macrophages (Bendtzen *et al.* 1988; Santamaria *et al.* 1989). Some of the differences are associated with IDDM, and this association may be related to the HLA-D region-encoded genetic polymorphisms in IDDM (Santamaria *et al.* 1989).

Interferon-γ and TNF are known to be potent modulators of the expression of HLA Class I and Class II MHC molecules in certain cells (reviewed in Balkwill and Burke 1989). These cytokines have been proposed as causative factors for the observed ectopic expression of HLA molecules on 'diabetic' islets (reviewed in Bottazzo *et al.* 1988). This may be likely for the observed Class I MHC hyperexpression (Pujol-Borrell *et al.* 1986) but less so for Class II expression, since IFN-γ or TNF alone are unable to induce Class II on the same cells *in vitro*, and the combination of the two exerts the phenomenon not only on the beta cells but also on the alpha and delta cells (Pujol-Borrell *et al.* 1987), which do not express these molecules *in vivo* and are not killed.

Interleukin 1 and IFN-γ plus TNF in combination are cytotoxic to pancreatic islets (Campbell *et al.* 1988; Pukel *et al.* 1988; Mandrup-Poulsen *et al.* 1989). Again, the cytotoxic effects of these cytokines are not specific to the beta cells but also affect the alpha and delta cells (Soldevila *et al.* 1991). Furthermore, in a detailed study of Class II MHC expression and cytotoxicity induced by cytokines, it was noted that the Class II expression of the islet cells always preceded cell death or cytotoxicity (Soldevila *et al.* 1991).

As shown in NOD mice, *in vivo* these cytokines have contrasting effects to that seen *in vitro*. Tumour necrosis factor alpha suppresses insulitis and the animals do not develop diabetes (Satoh *et al.* 1989). The results correlate with a low production of TNF by these autoimmune mice. Administration of TNF-α to NOD mice also suppresses induction of IDDM after adoptive transfer of lymphocytes from diabetic mice (Jacob *et al.* 1990). Injection of a single dose of human recombinant IL-1 normalizes blood glucose in mice, indicating that, contrary to *in vitro* data, the cytokine has powerful antidiabetic properties (Del Ray and Besedovsky 1989).

The beta cell itself produces IL-6, which is upregulated by IFN-γ and/or TNF-α (Campbell 1989). Although the phenomenon is physiological, the IL-6 produced by beta cells could act as a costimulator for autoreactive T and B lymphocytes in autoimmune diabetes. No cytokines, other than IFN-α have been demonstrated in beta cells of 'diabetic' pancreases (Foulis *et al.* 1987a).

Capillary endothelial cells and adhesion molecules in insulin-dependent diabetes mellitus

In general, endothelial cells express a number of cell recognition molecules and it has been postulated that their regulation is a homing signal for immunocytes (reviewed in Stoolman 1989). Capillary endothelial cells undergo changes within 'diabetic' islets (Bottazzo *et al.* 1985; Foulis and Farquharson 1986). The cells are hypertrophied, and strongly express both Class I and Class II MHC molecules.

Physiologically, Class II MHC alone on antigen-presenting cells is not enough to activate helper T cells, and a 'second signal' is necessary. Certain cytokines can provide this, and adhesion molecules such as intercellular adhesion molecule (ICAM)-1 are known to contribute to this activation (Altmann *et al.* 1989). The cytokines which could provide the signal (e.g. IFN-γ, IL-2) have not been demonstrated in the beta cells. Whether adhesion molecules are expressed on islet cells is unclear. Intercellular adhesion molecule 1 can be induced on beta cells by cytokines *in vitro* (Vives *et al.* 1991). In thyroid autoimmunity ICAM-1 has been demonstrated on Graves' thyrocytes (Weetman *et al.* 1989; Zheng *et al.* 1990), but others have not confirmed these findings (Bagnasco *et al.* 1991).

Animal models

Three animal models of IDDM are currently studied. These are: the low-dose streptozotocin-induced diabetes model, the BB strain of Wistar rats and the NOD mice. The transgenic technology has created novel strains of diabetic mice.

Repeated injections of low-dose streptozotocin induces diabetes through a lymphocyte-mediated mechanism (Like and Rossini 1976). The use of this model is now in decline, mainly due to the availability of the two models which develop diabetes spontaneously.

In the BB rat the prevalence of diabetes at 120 days of age is about 50%. There is evidence that T lymphocytes play an important role in the pathogenesis, especially the RT6 subpopulation, which appears crucial for progression to disease (reviewed in Rossini *et al.* 1991). Natural killer cells and macrophages are also important (reviewed in Kolb-Bachofen and Kolb 1989).

In the NOD mice, insulitis commences at 4–8 weeks of age, and although there is a large variation between colonies, 70% of the females and 35% of males are overtly diabetic by 30 weeks. Islet cell surface antibodies and IAA have been detected in the sera of these mice (Tochino 1986). Lymphocyte transfer experiments have demonstrated that both CD4 and CD8 T lymphocytes are important in the pathogenesis (Bendelac *et al*. 1987).

Transgenic mice have been established in which genes encoding Class I and II MHC products or cytokines have been linked to the insulin promotor sequence, thereby causing expression of these *in vivo* (Harrison *et al*. 1989; Lipes and Eisenbarth 1990). The mice became diabetic, but without insulitis around insulin-deprived islets. The aberration of islet function is most probably due to a massive expression of the products, which interferes with insulin secretion (reviewed in Pujol-Borrell and Bottazzo 1988). In similar experiments, where the level of expression was regulated to that found on macrophages, no diabetes or insulitis developed in the mice (Bohme *et al*. 1989). Despite this, the transgenic models are a promising tool for further research in the pathogenesis of IDDM.

There are a number of similarities and dissimilarities between IDDM in humans and the diabetes seen in the animal models. For example, in the MHC region, the NOD mouse lacks the I-E genes (Hattori *et al*. 1986), while in humans the equivalent are present. Interestingly, introduction of the missing gene protects these animals from developing insulitis and diabetes (Reich *et al*. 1989). The non-aspartic acid in position 57 variant of the DQβ chain is found in both human IDDM and the NOD mice (Acha-Orhea and McDevitt 1987). The production of transgenic mice with amino acid substitutions in the DQβ chain, however, demonstrates that aspartic acid is not the sole amino acid determining susceptibility to IDDM (Lund *et al*. 1990; Miyazaki *et al*. 1990). All these data indicate that in NOD mice, and most likely in humans, IDDM is not a disease of a single amino acid substitution (Parham 1990). At least five genes (Idd 1 to 5) appear to be involved in the susceptibility of the NOD mouse, and Idd 3 and Idd 4 are located outside the MHC region (Todd *et al*. 1991). One of them has been localized on chromosome 1 and identified as the IL-1 receptor (Cornall *et al*. 1991).

The cytoplasmic ICA found in humans are not detected in BB rats and rarely seen in NOD mice (Toyota *et al*. 1982). The insulitis process is more florid in the pancreas of these animals than that seen in humans: in the NOD mice inflammatory cells extensively cap the islets (reviewed in Tarui *et al*. 1986). In the two rodents, macrophages are the predominant infiltrating cells both at the beginning of the process and at the time of acute onset of symptoms and, especially in BB rats, these cells have an important pathogenic role (reviewed in Tochino 1986). In human IDDM, macrophages, at least at the time of diagnosis, are very scarce in the islets (Foulis *et al*. 1991).

In the BB rat, very few beta cells express Class II MHC and the majority of cells which do are activated T cells and macrophages (Dean *et al*. 1986a). Expression of Class II MHC on beta cells of NOD mice is controversial (Hanafusa *et al*. 1987; Signore *et al*. 1987), but it has recently been demonstrated that such expression precedes the invasion of lymphocytes into the islets (Formby and Miller 1990). Interestingly, transgenic mice expressing IFN on their beta cells had a diffuse pancreatic inflammation and the infiltrating T cells responded to islet antigens *in vitro* (Sarvetnick *et al*. 1990).

In summary, in the two rodent models a role for both CD8 and CD4 lymphocytes (Miller *et al*. 1988; Harrison *et al*. 1989) and macrophages (Hutchings *et al*. 1990; reviewed in Tochino 1986) in the pathogenesis has been identified. It would appear that multiple mechanisms contribute to the destruction of beta cells in these animals.

Immunotherapy

The long latency period has provided a potential window for intervention where, despite the process of islet cell destruction having already commenced, there remains an adequate beta cell reserve to maintain normal endocrine function. Studies using immunosuppressive agents close to diagnosis have been performed (reviewed in Bach *et al*. 1989). It is likely that such treatments will be more effective when applied before the beta cell reserve is completely exhausted.

In the NOD mouse and BB rat animal models of IDDM a large number of therapies have proved effective in preventing IDDM. The use of immunosuppressants such as cyclosporin, the injection of autoreactive T cell clones, infection with virus, administration of cytokines such as TNF, anti-CD3, the vitamin derivative nicotinamide, change in diet, an increase in ambient temperature, and interference of macrophage function with monoclonal anti-CR3 have all led to the prevention or delay in the onset of IDDM in these animal models (Yamada *et al*. 1982; Gottlieb *et al*. 1988; Hayward and Shreiber 1989; Reich *et al.* 1989; Satoh *et al.* 1989; Scott *et al.* 1989; Hutchings *et al.* 1990; Lefkowith *et al.* 1990; Shyp *et al.* 1990; Williams *et al.* 1990). In all cases the effective treatment was applied prior to the onset of disease.

In humans the situation is more complex. Until now, strategies for immunointervention have not been applied prior to onset of disease. Cyclosporin A induces long-term remission, but continued therapy results in a loss of remissions due to increased insulin requirement of the patients, and relapse is common when cyclosporin is stopped (reviewed in Bach *et al.* 1989). Azathioprine on its own did not increase remission in children with newly diagnosed IDDM (Cook *et al.* 1989), while a combination of azathioprine and prednisolone did (Silverstein *et al.* 1988), and a number of strategies using a combination of immunosuppresive agents have been proposed. In addition to these therapies, the use of intensive insulin therapy, several monoclonal antibodies, antilymphocyte therapies and other strategies have been proposed and trials commenced (Andreani *et al.* 1989). Nicotinamide prevents or delays IDDM in NOD mice and it is reported that IDDM is alo delayed or prevented in ICA +ve individuals treated with nicotinamide (Elliott and Chase 1991).

It is possible that some patients will respond to treatment better than others. Factors which might affect this are C-peptide levels, autoantibody concentration or even MHC (Peig *et al.* 1989; Mandrup-Poulsen *et al.* 1990). Immunotherapy for the prevention of IDDM is not routine. However, a number of large trials have been or are about to commence world-wide, and there is hope that a viable therapy to prevent the disease should soon become available (reviewed in Bonifacio and Bottazzo 1991).

Acknowledgements

We are most grateful to all our colleagues whose help over the years has been instrumental in moving the subject forward. In particular, we are indebted to Professor Deborah Doniach, who launched the field of autoimmunity. Generous support has been provided by the Medical Research Council, the British Diabetic Association, the Juvenile Diabetes Foundation International (USA) and the Wellcome Trust Foundation. Lastly, we thank Ann Boswell and Valerie Verbi for patiently editing the manuscript.

References

Acha-Orhea, H. and McDevitt, H.O. (1987). *Proc. Nat. Acad. Sci. (USA)* **84**, 2435–9.

Al-Sakkaf, L., Pozzilli, P., Tarn, A.C., Schwarz, G., Gale, E.A.M. and Bottazzo, G.F. (1989). Persistent reduction of CD4/CD8 lymphocyte ratio and cell activation before the onset of type I (insulin-dependent) diabetes. *Diabetologia* **32**, 322–5.

Altmann, D.M., Hogg, N., Trowsdale, J. and Wilkinson, D. (1989). Co-transfection of ICAM-1 and HLA-DR reconstitutes human antigen-presenting cell function in mouse L cells. *Nature* **338**, 512–14.

Andreani, D., Kolb, H. and Pozzilli, P. (eds) (1989). *Immunotherapy of Type 1 Diabetes*. J. Wiley & Sons, Chichester.

Atkinson, M.A., Maclaren, N.K., Scharp, D.W., Lacy, P.E. and Riley, W.J. (1990). 64 000 Mr autoantibodies as predictors of insulin-dependent diabetes. *Lancet* **35**, 1357–60.

Awata, T., Kuzuya, T., Matsuda, A. *et al.* (1990). High frequency of aspartic acid at position 57 of HLA-DQ β-chain in Japanese IDDM patients and nondiabetic subjects. *Diabetes* **39**, 266–9.

Bach, J.F. (1988). Mechanisms of autoimmunity in insulin-dependent diabetes mellitus. *Clin. Exp. Immunol.* **72**, 1–8.

Bach, J.F., Feutren, G. and Boitard, C. (1989). Immunoprevention of insulin-dependent diabetes by cyclosporin. In *Immunotherapy of Type I Diabetes*, ed. D. Andreani, H. Kolb and P. Pozzilli, pp. 111–23, John Wiley & Sons, Chichester.

Badenhoop, K., Schwarz, G., Trowsdale, J. *et al.* (1989). TNF-α gene polymorphisms in type I (insulin-dependent) diabetes mellitus. *Diabetologia* **32**, 445–8.

Baekkeskov, S., Nielson, J.H., Marner, B., Bilde, T., Ludvigsson, J. and Lernmark, A. (1982). Autoantibodies in newly diagnosed diabetic children immunoprecipitate human pancreatic islet cell protein. *Nature* **298**, 167–9.

Baekkeskov, S., Landin, M., Kristensen, J.K. *et al.* (1987). Antibodies to a 64 000 Mr human islet cell protein precede the clinical onset of insulin-dependent diabetes. *J. Clin. Invest.* **79**, 926–34.

Baekkeskov, S., Aanstoot, H.J., Christgau, S. *et al.* (1990). Identification of the 64K autoantigen in insulin-dependent diabetes as the GABA-synthesizing enzyme glutamic acid decarboxylases. *Nature* **347**, 151–6.

Bagnasco, M., Caretto, D., Olive, D., Pedini, B., Canonica, G.W. and Betterle, C. (1991). Expression of intercellular adhesion molecule-1 on thyroid epithelial cells in Hashimoto's thyroiditis and not in Graves' disease or papillary thyroid cancer. *Clin. Exp. Immunol.* **83**, 309–13.

Balkwill, F.R. and Burke, F. (1989). The cytokine network. *Immunol. Today* **10**, 299–304.

Barnett, A.H., Eff, L., Leslie, R.D.G. and Pyke, D.A. (1981). Diabetes in identical twins: a study of 200 pairs. *Diabetologia* **20**, 87–93.

Bendelac, A., Carnaud, C., Boitard, C. and Bach, J.F. (1987). Syngeneic transfer of autoimmune diabetes from diabetic NOD mice to healthy neonates: requirement for both L3T4+ and Lyt-2+ T cells. *J. Exp. Med.* **166**, 823–32.

Bendtzen, K., Morling, N., Fomsgaard, A. *et al.* (1988). Association between HLA-DR2 and production of tumour necrosis factor a and interleukin 1 by mononuclear cells activated by lipopolysaccharide. *Scand. J. Immunol.* **28**, 599–606.

Bingley, P.J. and Gale, E.A.M. (1989). The incidence of insulin-dependent diabetes in England: a study in the Oxford region

1985–1986. *Br. Med. J.* **289**, 558–60.

Bingley, P.J. and Gale, E.A.M. (1990). The epidemiology of childhood onset diabetes; a review. *Practical Diabetes* **7** (1), 7–11.

Bingley, P.J., Bonifacio, E., Shattock, M. *et al.* (1992). Can islet cell antibodies predict insulin-dependent diabetes in the general population? *Diabetes Care* (in press).

Bohme, J., Haskins, K., Stecha, P. *et al.* (1989). Transgenic mice with I-A on islet cells are normoglycemic but immunologically intolerant. *Science* **244**, 1179–83.

Boitard, C., Sai, P., Debray-Sachs, M., Assan, R. and Hamburger, J. (1984). Anti-pancreatic immunity: *in vitro* studies of cellular and humoral immune reactions directed towards pancreatic islets. *Clin. Exp. Immunol.* **55**, 571–80.

Bonifacio, E. and Bottazzo, G.F. (1991). Immunology of IDDM (type I diabetes): entering the '90s. In *Diabetes Annual/6*, ed. K.G.M.M. Alberti and L.P. Krall, pp. 20–47, Elsevier Science Pub., Amsterdam.

Bonifacio, E., Bingley, P., Shattock, M. *et al.* (1990). Quantification of islet-cell antibodies and prediction of insulin-dependent diabetes. *Lancet* **335**, 147–9.

Bosi, E., Todd, I., Pujol-Borrell, R. and Bottazzo, G.F. (1987). Mechanisms of autoimmunity: relevance to the pathogenesis of type 1 (insulin-dependent) diabetes mellitus. *Diab./Metab. Rev.* **3**, 893–924.

Bosi, E., Vicari, A., Comi, G. *et al.* (1988). Association of stiff-man syndrome and type I diabetes with islet cell and other autoantibodies. *Arch. Neurol.* **45**, 246.

Bosi, E., Becker, F., Bonifacio, E. *et al.* (1991). Progression to type I (insulin-dependent) diabetes in autoimmune endocrine patients with islet cell antibodies. *Diabetes* **40**, 977–84.

Bottazzo, G.F. (1984). Beta-cell damage in diabetic insulitis: are we approaching the solution? *Diabetologia* **26**, 241–50.

Bottazzo, G.F. (1986). Death of a beta-cell: homicide or suicide? *Diab. Med.* **3**, 119–30.

Bottazzo, G.F. and Doniach, D. (1980). Autoimmunity in diabetes mellitus. In *Secondary Diabetes: the Spectrum of the Diabetes Syndrome*, ed. by S. Podolsky and M. Kiswanathan, pp. 391–408, Raven Press, New York.

Bottazzo, G.F. and Lendrum, R. (1976). Separate autoantibodies to human pancreatic glucagon and somatostatin cells. *Lancet* **ii**, 873–6.

Bottazzo, G.F., Florin-Christensen, A. and Doniach, D. (1974). Islet cell antibodies in diabetes mellitus with autoimmune polyendocrine deficiency. *Lancet* **ii**, 1279–83.

Bottazzo, G.F., Dean, B.M., Gorsuch, A.N., Cudworth, A.G. and Doniach, D. (1980). Complement-fixing islet-cell antibodies in type I diabetes: possible monitors of active beta-cell damage. *Lancet* **i**, 668–72.

Bottazzo, G.F., Pujol-Borrell, R., Hanafusa, T. and Feldman, M. (1983). Role of aberrant HLA-DR expression and antigen presentation in the induction of endocrine autoimmunity. *Lancet* **ii**, 1115–19.

Bottazzo, G.F., Dean, B.M., McNally, J.M., Mackay, E.H., Swift, P.G.F. and Gamble, D.R. (1985). *In situ* characterisation of autoimmune phenomena and expression of HLA molecules in the pancreas in diabetic insulitis. *N. Engl. J. Med.* **313**, 353–60.

Bottazzo, G.F., Todd, I., Mirakian, R., Belfiore, A. and Pujol-Borrell, R. (1986). Organ-specific autoimmunity: a 1986 overview. *Immunol. Rev.* **94**, 137–69.

Bottazzo, G.F., Pujol-Borrell, R. and Gale, E.A.M. (1987). Autoimmunity and type I diabetes: bringing the story up to date. In *The Diabetes Annual/3*, ed. K.G.M.M. Alberti and L.P. Krall, pp. 15–38, Elsevier Science Publ., Amsterdam.

Bottazzo, G.F., Foulis, A.K., Bosi, E., Todd, I. and Pujol-Borrell, R. (1988). Pancreatic B cell damage: in search of novel pathogenetic factors. *Diab. Care* **11** (suppl. 1), 24–8.

Bottazzo, G.F., Genovese, S., Bosi, E., Dean, B.M., Christie, M.R. and Bonifacio, E. (1991). Novel consideration on the antibody/antigen system in type I (insulin-dependent) diabetes mellitus. *Ann. Med.* **23**, 453–61.

Buschard, K. (1985). The thymus-dependent immune system in the pathogenesis of type 1 (insulin-dependent) diabetes mellitus. *Dan. Med. Bull.* **32**, 139–51.

Buschard, K., Kühl, C., Molsted-Pederson, L., Lund, E., Palmer, J. and Bottazzo, G.F. (1989). Investigations in children who were *in utero* at onset of insulin-dependent diabetes in their mothers. *Lancet* **i**, 811–14.

Buschard, K., Jorgensen, M., Aaen, K., Bock, T. and Josefsen, K. (1990). Prevention of diabetes mellitus in BB rats by neonatal stimulation of β cells. *Lancet* **335**, 134–5.

Campbell, I.L., Iscaro, A. and Harrison, L.C. (1988). IFN-gamma and tumor necrosis factor: cytotoxicity to murine islet of Langerhans. *J. Immunol.* **141**, 2325–9.

Castano, L., Russo, E., Zhou, L., Lipes, M.A. and Eisenbarth, G.S. (1991). Identification and cloning of a granule autoantigen (carboxy-peptide H) associated with type I diabetes. *J. Clin. Endocrinol. Metab.* **73**, 1197–201.

Christie, M.R., Danetian, D., Champagne, P. and Delovitch, T.L. (1990a). Persistence of serum antibodies to 64 000-Mr islet cell protein after onset of type I diabetes. *Diabetes* **39**, 653–6.

Christie, M.R., Vohra, G., Champagne, P., Daneman, D. and Delovitch, T.L. (1990b). Distinct antibody specificities to a 64-kD islet cell antigen in type 1 diabetes as revealed by trypsin treatment. *J. Exp. Med.* **172**, 789–95.

Christie, M.R., Brown, T.J. and Cassidy, D. (1992). Binding of antibodies in sera of type I (insulin-dependent) diabetes patients to glutamate decarboxylase from rat tissues: evidence for antigenic forms of the enzyme. *Diabetologia* **35**, 380–4.

Christie, M.R., Tun, R.Y.M., Lo, S.S.S. *et al.* (1992). Antibodies to glutamic acid decarboxylase and tryptic fragments of islet 64 kD antigen as distinct markers for the development of insulin-dependent diabetes: studies with identical twins. *Diabetes* (in press).

Ciampolillo, A., Marini, V., Mirakian, R. *et al.* (1989). Retrovirus-like sequences in Graves' disease: implications for human autoimmunity. *Lancet* **i**, 1096–100.

Colman, P.G. and Eisenbarth, G.S. (1988). Immunology of type I diabetes — 1987. In *The Diabetes Annual/4*, ed. K.G.M.M. Alberti and L.P. Krall, pp. 17–45, Elsevier Scientific Pub., Amsterdam.

Colman, P.G., Nayak, R.C., Campbell, I.L. and Eisenbarth, G.S. (1988). Binding of 'cytoplasmic' islet cell antibodies is blocked by human pancreatic glycolipid extracts. *Diabetes* **37**, 645–52.

Cook, J.J., Hudson, I., Harrison, L.C. *et al.* (1989). Double-blind controlled trial of azathioprine in children with newly diagnosed type I diabetes. *Diabetes* **38**, 1–7.

Cornall, R.J., Prins, J.-B., Todd, J.A. *et al.* (1991). Type 1 diabetes in mice is linked to the interleukin-1 receptor and Lsh/Ity/Bcg genes on chromosome 1. *Nature* **353**, 262–4.

Dawkins, R.L. (1985). Sensitivity and specificity of autoantibody testing. In *The Autoimmune Diseases*, ed. N.R. Rose and I.A. Mackay, pp. 669–93. Academic Press, Sydney.

Dean, B.M., Walker, R., Bone, A.J., Baird, J.D. and Cooke, A. (1986a). Pre-diabetes in the spontaneously diabetic BB/rat: lymphocytic subpopulations in the pancreatic infiltrate and expression of rat MHC Class II molecules in endocrine cells. *Diabetologia* **28**, 464–9.

Dean, B.M., Becker, F., McNally, J.M. *et al.* (1986b). Insulin autoantibodies in the pre-diabetic period: correlation with islet cell antibodies and the development of diabetes. *Diabetologia* **29**, 339–42.

De Berardinis, P., Londei, M., James, R.F.L., Lake, S.P., Wise, P.H. and Feldmann, M. (1988). Do CD4-positive cytotoxic T cells damage islet b cells in type I damage islet b cells in type I diabetes? *Lancet* **ii**, 823–4.

Del Ray, A. and Besedovsky, H. (1989). Antidiabetic effects of interleukin 1. *Proc. Nat. Acad. Sci. (USA)* **86**, 5943–7.

Diabetes Epidemiology Research International Group (1988). Geographic patterns of childhood insulin-dependent diabetes mellitus. *Diabetes* **37**, 1113–19.

Dorman, J.S., LaPorte, R.E., Stone, R.A. and Trucco, M. (1990). Worldwide differences in the incidence of type I diabetes are associated with amino acid variation at position 57 of the HLA-DQ β chain. *Proc. Nat. Acad. Sci. (USA)* **87**, 7370–4.

Drell, D.W. and Notkins, A.L. (1987). Multiple immunological abnormalities in patients with type I (insulin-dependent) diabetes mellitus. *Diabetologia* **30**, 132–43.

Durruty, P., Ruiz, F. and Garcia de los Rios, M. (1979). Age at diagnosis and seasonal variation in the onset of insulin-dependent diabetes in Chile (Southern hemisphere). *Diabetologia* **17**, 357–60.

Eisenbarth, G.S. (1986). Type 1 diabetes mellitus: a chronic autoimmune disease. *N. Engl. J. Med.* **314**, 1360–8.

Elias, D., Markovits, D., Reshef, D. *et al.* (1990). Induction and therapy of autoimmune diabetes in the non-obese diabetic (NOLDL/Lt) mouse by a 65-kDa heat shock protein. *Proc. Nat. Acad. Sci. (USA)* **87**, 1576–80.

Elliott, R.B. and Chase, H.P. (1991). Prevention or delay of type 1 (insulin-dependent) diabetes mellitus in children using nicotinamide. *Diabetologia* **34**, 362–5.

Erlander, M.G., Tillakaraine, N.J.K., Feldblum, S., Patel, N. and Tobin, A.J. (1991). Two genes encode distinct glutamate decarboxylases. *Neuron* **7**, 91–100.

Farid, N.R. (ed.) (1988). *Immunogenetics of Endocrine Disorders*. Liss, New York.

Faustman, D., Schoenfeld, D. and Ziegler, R. (1991). T lymphocyte changes linked to autoantibodies: association of insulin autoantibodies with DC4+/CD45R+ lymphocyte subpopulation in pre-diabetic subjects. *Diabetes* **40**, 590–7.

Formby, B. and Miller, N. (1990). Autologous CD4 T-cell responses to ectopic Class II major histocompatibility complex antigen-expressing single-cell islet cells: an *in vitro* insight into the pathogenesis of lymphocytic insulitis in non obese diabetic mice. *Proc. Nat. Acad. Sci. (USA)* **87**, 2438–42.

Foulis, A.K. (1989). In type I diabetes, does a non-cytopathic viral infection of insulin-secreting B-cells initiate the disease process leading to their autoimmune destruction? *Diab. Med.* **6**, 666–74.

Foulis, A.K. and Bottazzo, G.F. (1988). Insulitis in the human pancreas. In *The Pathology of the Endocrine Pancreas in Diabetes*, ed. P.J. Lefebvre and D.G. Pipeleers, pp. 41–5, Springer-Verlag, Berlin.

Foulis, A.K. and Farquharson, M.A. (1986). Aberrant expression of HLA-DR antigens in insulin containing beta cells in recent onset type I (insulin-dependent) diabetes mellitus. *Diabetes* **35**, 1215–26.

Foulis, A.K., Farquharson, M.A. and Meager, A. (1987a). Immunoreactive α-interferon in insulin-secreting β cells in type I diabetes mellitus. *Lancet* **ii**, 1423–7.

Foulis, A.K., Farquharson, M.A. and Hardman, R. (1987b). Aberrant expression of Class II major histocompatibility complex molecules by B cells and hyperexpression of Class I major histocompatibility complex molecules by insulin containing islets in type I (insulin-dependent) diabetes mellitus. *Diabetologia* **30**, 333–43.

Foulis, A.K., McGill, M. and Farquharson, M.A. (1991). Insulitis in type I (insulin-dependent) diabetes mellitus in man — macrophages, lymphocytes, and interferon-gamma containing cells. *J. Pathol.* **165**, 97–103.

Gamble, D.R. (1980). The epidemiology of insulin-dependent diabetes with particular reference to virus infection to its aetiology. *Epidemiol. Rev.* **2**, 49–70.

Genovese, S., Bonifacio, E., McNally, J.M. *et al.* (1992). Distinct cytoplasmic islet cell antibodies with different risks for type 1 (insulin-dependent diabetes mellitus. *Diabetologia* **35**, 385–8.

Gepts, W. (1984). The pathology of the pancreas in human diabetes. In *Immunology in Diabetes*, ed. D. Andreani, U. Di Mario, K.F. Federlin and L.G. Hedding, ch. 2, pp. 21–34, Kimpton, London.

Giorda, R., Pearman, M., Tan, R.C., Vergani, D. and Trucco, M. (1991). Glutamic acid decarboxylase expression in islet and brain. *Lancet* **338**, 1469–70.

Gleichmann, H. and Bottazzo, G.F. (1987). Islet-cell and insulin autoantibodies in diabetes. *Immunol. Today* **8**, 167–8.

Gorsuch, A.N., Spencer, K.M., Lister, J. *et al.* (1981). The natural history of type 1 (insulin-dependent) diabetes mellitus: evidence for a long pre-diabetic period. *Lancet* **ii**, 363–5.

Gotfredsen, C.F., Buschard, K. and Frandsen, E.K. (1985). Reduction of diabetes incidence of BB Wister rats by early prophylactic insulin treatment of diabetes-prone animals. *Diabetologia* **28**, 933–5.

Gottlieb, P.A., Rossini, A.A. and Mordes, J.P. (1988). Approaches to prevention and treatment of IDDM in animal models. *Diab. Care* **11**, 29–36.

Hanafusa, T., Fujino-Kurihara, H., Miyazaki, A. *et al.* (1987). Expression of Class II major histocompatibility complex antigens on pancreatic B cells in NOD mice. *Diabetologia* **30**, 104–8.

Hanafusa, T., Miyazaki, A., Miyagawa, J. *et al.* (1990). Examination of islets in the pancreas biopsy specimens from newly diagnosed type I (insulin-dependent) diabetic patients. *Diabetologia* **33**, 105–11.

Harrison, L.C., Campbell, I.L., Allison, J. and Miller, J.F.A.P. (1989). MHC molecules and b-cell destruction: immune and non immune mechanisms. *Diabetes* **38**, 815–18.

Hattori, M., Buse, J.B., Jackson, R.A. *et al.* (1986). The NOD mouse: recessive diabetogenic gene in the major histocompatibility complex. *Science* **231**, 733–5.

Hayward, A.R. and Shreiber, M. (1989). Neonatal injection of

CD3 antibody into non-obese diabetic mice reduces the incidence of insulitis and diabetes. *J. Immunol.* **143**, 1555–9.

Hitman, G.A. (1989). The major histocompatibility complex and insulin-dependent (type I) diabetes. *Autoimmunity* **4**, 119–30.

Humphrey, M., Mosca, J., Baker, J.R., Jr *et al.* (1991). Absence of retroviral sequences in Graves' disease. *Lancet* **337**, 17–18.

Hutchings, P., Rosen, H., O'Reilly, L., Simpson, E., Gordon, S. and Cooke, A., (1990). Transfer of diabetes in mice prevented by blockade of adhesion-promoting receptor on macrophages. *Nature* **348**, 639–42.

Irvine, W.J. (1980). Immunological aspects of diabetes mellitus: a review. In *Immunology of Diabetes*, ed. W.J. Irvine, pp. 1–53, Teviot Scient. Pub., Edinburgh.

Jackson, R.A., Morris, M.A., Haynes, B. and Eisenbarth, G.S. (1982). Increased circulating Ia-antigen bearing T cells in type I diabetes mellitus. *N. Engl. J. Med.* **306**, 785–8.

Jacob, C.O., Aiso, S., Michie, S.A., McDevitt, H.O. and Acha-Orbea, H. (1990). Prevention of diabetes in non-obese diabetic mice by tumor necrosis factor (TNF): similarities between TNF-alpha and interleukin 1. *Proc. Nat. Acad. Sci. (USA)* **87**, 968–72.

Johnson, J.H., Crider, B.P., McCorki, K., Alford, M. and Unger, R.H. (1990). Inhibition of glucose transport into rat islet cells by immunoglobulins from patients with new-onset insulin-dependent diabetes mellitus. *N. Engl. J. Med.* **322**, 653–9.

Jones, D.B. and Duff, G.W. (1991). Is there no role for heat-shock protein in diabetes? *Lancet* **337**, 115.

Jones, D.B., Hunter, R.N. and Duff, G.W. (1990). Heat-shock protein 65 kD as a β-cell antigen of insulin-dependent diabetes. *Lancet* **336**, 583–5.

Julier, C., Hyer, R.N., Davies, J. *et al.* (1991). Insulin-IGF2 region on chromosome 11p encodes a gene implicated in HLA-DR4-dependent diabetes susceptibility. *Nature* **354**, 155–8.

Kampe, O., Anderson, A., Bjork, E., Hallberg, A. and Karlsson, F.A. (1989). High-glucose stimulation of 64 000-M(r) islet cell autoantigen expression. *Diabetes* **38**, 1326–8.

Kampe, O., Velloso, L., Andersson, A. and Karlsson, F.A. (1990). No role for 65 kD heat-shock protein in diabetes. *Lancet* **336**, 1250.

Kappler, J.W., Roehm, N., Marrack, P. *et al.* (1987). T cell tolerance by clonal elimination in the thymus. *Cell* **49**, 273–80.

Karjalainen, J.K. (1990). Islet cell antibodies as predictive markers for IDDM in children with high background incidence of disease. *Diabetes* **39**, 1144–50.

Karlsen, A.E., Hagopian, W.A., Grubin, C.E. *et al.* (1991). Cloning and primary structure of a human islet isoform of glutamic acid decarboxylase from chromosome 10. *Proc. Nat. Acad. Sci. (USA)* **88**, 8337–71.

Karounos, D.G. and Thomas, J.W. (1990). Recognition of common islet antigen by autoantibodies from NOD mice and humans with IDDM. *Diabetes* **39**, 1085–90.

Kelly, C., Carter, N.D., Johnstone, A.P. and Nussey, S.S. (1991). Cloning of large isoform of human brain glutamic acid decarboxylas. *Lancet* **338**, 1468–9.

Khalil, I., d'Auriol, L., Gobet, M. *et al.* (1990). A combination of HLA-DQ Asp 57-negative and HLA-DQ Arg 52 confers susceptibility to insulin-dependent diabetes mellitus. *J. Clin. Invest.* **85**, 1315–19.

King, M.L., Shaikh, A., Bidwell, D., Voller, A. and Banatvala, J.E. (1983). Coxsackie B-virus-specific IGM responses in children with insulin-dependent diabetes mellitus. *Lancet* **i**: 1397–9.

Kolb-Bachofen, V. and Kolb, H. (1989). Hypothesis: a role for macrophage in the pathogenesis of type I diabetes. *Autoimmunity* **3**, 145–55.

Kuglin, B., Kolb, H., Greenbaum, C., Maclaren, N.K., Lernmark, A. and Palmer, J.P. (1990a). The Fourth International Workshop on standardisation of insulin autoantibody measurement. *Diabetologia* **33**, 638–9.

Kuglin, B., Rjasanowski, I., Bertrams, J., Gries, F.A., Kolb, H. and Michaelis, D. (1990b). Antibodies to pro-insulin and insulin as predictive markers of type I diabetes. *Diab. Med.* **7**, 310–14.

Lagaye, S., Vexiau, P., Morozov, V. *et al.* (1991). Detection of HTLV-1 gag related sequences in leucocyte DNA from patients with polyendocrinopathies (Basedow–Graves' disease and insulin-dependent diabetes). *C.R. Acad. Sci. (Paris) Sér. III* **312**, 309–15.

Landin-Olsson, M., Karlsson, A., Dahlquist, G., Blom, L., Lernmark, A. and Sundkvist, G. (1989). Islet cell and other organ-specific autoantibodies in all children developing type I (insulin-dependent) diabetes mellitus in Sweden during one year and in matched control children. *Diabetologia* **32**, 387–95.

Lefkowith, J., Schreiner, G., Cormier, J. *et al.* (1990). Prevention of diabetes in the BB rat by essential fatty acid deficiency: relationship between physiological and biochemical changes. *J. Exp. Med.* **171**, 729–43.

Leiter, E.H. (1985). Type C retrovirus production by pancreatic beta cells: association with accelerated pathogenesis in C3H-db (diabetic) mice. *Am. J. Pathol.* **119**, 22–32.

Leiter, E.H. (1990). The role of environmental factors in modulating insulin-dependent diabetes. In *The Role of Microorganisms in Non-infectious Disease, 14th Argenteuil Symposium, Brussels*, eds R.R.P. de Vries, I.R. Cohen and J.J. van Rood, pp. 39–54. Springer-Verlag, Berlin.

Lendrum, R., Walker, I.G. and Gamble, D.R. (1975). Islet cell antibodies in juvenile diabetes mellitus of recent onset. *Lancet* **i**, 880–2.

Lendrum, R., Walker, I.G., Cudworth, A.G. *et al.* (1976). Islet cell antibodies in diabetes mellitus. *Lancet* **ii**, 1273–6.

Lernmark, A., Freeman, Z.R., Hofman, C. *et al.* (1978). Islet cell surface antibodies in juvenile diabetes mellitus. *N. Engl. J. Med.* **299**, 375–80.

Like, A.A. and Rossini, A.A. (1976). Streptozotocin-induced pancreatic insulitis: a new model of diabetes mellitus. *Science* **193**, 415–20.

Lipes, M.A. and Eisenbarth, G.S. (1990). Transgenic mouse models of type I diabetes. *Diabetes* **39**, 879–84.

Lohr, J.M. and Oldstone, M.B.A. (1990). Detection of cytomegalovirus nucleic acid sequences in pancreas in type 2 diabetes. *Lancet* **336**, 644–8.

Lund, T., O'Reilly, L., Hutchings, P. *et al.* (1990). Prevention of insulin-dependent diabetes mellitus in non-obese diabetic mice by transgenes encoding modified I-A β-chain or normal I-E α-chain. *Nature* **345**, 727–9.

McCluskey, J., McCann, V.J., Kay, P.H. *et al.* (1983). HLA and complement allotypes in type I (insulin-dependent) diabetes. *Diabetologia* **24**, 162–5.

McMillan, S.A., Graham, C.A., Hart, P.J., Hadden, D.R. and McNeill, T.A. (1990). A T cell receptor beta chain polymorphism is associated with patients developing insulin-dependent diabetes after the age of 20 years. *Clin. Exp. Immunol.* **82**, 538–41.

Mandrup-Poulsen, T., Helquist, S., Mölvig, J., Wogensen, L.D. and Nerup, J. (1989). Cytokines as immune effector molecules in autoimmune endocrine diseases with special reference to insulin-dependent diabetes mellitus. *Autoimmunity* **4**, 191–218.

Mandrup-Poulsen, T., Molvig, J. and Andersen, H.U. (1990). Lack of predictive value of islet cell antibodies, insulin antibodies, and HLA-DR phenotype for remission in cyclosporin treated IDDM patients. *Diabetes* **39**, 204–10.

Martino, G.V., Tappaz, M., Braghi, S. *et al.* (1991). Autoantibodies to glutamic acid decarboxylase in insulin-dependent diabetes mellitus. *J. Autoimmunity* **4**, 915–23.

Miller, B.J., Appel, M.C., O'Neill, J.J. and Wicker, L.S. (1988). Both the Lyt-2+ and L3T4+ T cell subsets are required for the transfer of diabetes in nonobese diabetic mice. *J. Immunol.* **140**, 52–8.

Mirakian, R., Cudworth, A.G., Bottazzo, G.F., Richardson, C.A. and Doniach, D. (1982). Autoimmunity to anterior pituitary cells and the pathogenesis of type I (insulin-dependent) diabetes mellitus. *Lancet* **i**, 755–9.

Mirakian, R., Ciampolillo, A., Duess, U., Miyazaki, A. and Bottazzo, G.F. (1990). Inappropriate HLA molecule expression in epithelial cells: relevance for human autoimmunity. In *The Role of Microorganisms in Non-infectious Diseases*, ed. R. de Vries, I. Cohen and J. van Rood, pp. 131–54. Springer-Verlag, London.

Miyazaki, T., Uno, M., Uehira, M. *et al.* (1990). Direct evidence for the contribution of the unique I-ANOD to the development of insulitis in non-obese diabetic mice. *Nature* **345**, 722–4.

Mordes, J.P. and Rossini, A.A. (1987). Keys to understanding autoimmune diabetes mellitus: the animal models of insulin-dependent diabetes mellitus. In *Endocrine and Other Organ-orientated Autoimmune Disorders*, ed. D. Doniach and G.F. Bottazzo. *Clin. Immunol. Allergy* **1**, 29–52.

Owerbach, D., Rich, C., Carnegie, S. and Tanga, K. (1987). Molecular biology of the HLA system in insulin-dependent diabetes mellitus. *Diab./Metab. Rev.* **3**, 819–34.

Pak, C.Y., Eun, H.-M., McArthur, R.G. and Yoon, J.W. (1988). Association of cytomegalovirus infection with autoimmune type I diabetes. *Lancet* **i**, 1–4.

Palmer, J.P. (1987). Insulin autoantibodies: their role in the pathogenesis of IDDM. *Diab./Metab. Rev.* **3**, 1005–15.

Palmer, J.P., Asplin, C.M., Clemons, P. *et al.* (1983). Insulin antibodies in insulin-dependent diabetics before insulin treatment. *Science* **222**, 1337–9.

Parham, P. (1990). A diversity of diabetes. *Nature* **345**, 662–4.

Peig, M., Gomis, R., Ercilla, G., Casamitjana, R., Bottazzo, G.F. and Pujol-Borrell, R. (1989). Correlation between residual B cell function and islet cell antibodies in newly diagnosed type I diabetes. *Diabetes* **38**, 1396–401.

Pujol-Borrell, R. and Bottazzo, G.F. (1988). Puzzling diabetic transgenic mice: do they contain a lesson for human type I diabetes? *Immunol. Today* **9**, 303–6.

Pujol-Borrell, R. and Todd, I. (1987). Inappropriate HLA Class II in autoimmunity: is it the primary event? In *Endocrine and Other Organ-orientated Autoimmune Disorders*, ed. D. Doniach and G.F. Bottazzo. *Clin. Immunol. Allergy* **1**, 1–27.

Pujol-Borrell, R., Khoury, E.L. and Bottazzo, G.F. (1982). Islet cell surface antibodies in type I (insulin-dependent) diabetes mellitus: use of human fetal pancreas cultures as substrate. *Diabetologia* **22**, 89–96.

Pujol-Borrell, R., Todd, I., Doshi, M., Gray, D., Feldman, M. and Bottazzo, G.F. (1986). Differential expression and regulation of MHC products in the endocrine and exocrine cells of the human pancreas. *Clin. Exp. Immunol.* **65**, 128–39.

Pujol-Borrell, R., Todd, I., Doshi, M. *et al.* (1987). HLA Class II induction in human islet cells by interferon-gamma plus tumor necrosis factor or lymphotoxin. *Nature* **326**, 304–6.

Pukel, C., Bacquerizo, H. and Rabinovitch, A. (1988). Destruction of rat islet cell monolayer cultures by cytokines: synergistic interactions of interferon-γ, tumor necrosis factor, lymphotoxin and interleukin-1. *Diabetes* **37**, 133–6.

Rayfield, J.R. and Ishimura, K. (1987). Environmental factors and insulin-dependent diabetes mellitus. *Diab./Metab. Rev.* **3**, 925–57.

Reich, E.P., Sherwin, R.S., Kanagawa, O. and Janeway, C.A. (1989). An explanation for the protective effect of the MHC Class II I-E molecule in murine diabetes. *Nature* **341**, 326–8.

Riley, W.J., Maclaren, N.K., Krischer, J. *et al.* (1990). A prospective study of the development of diabetes in relatives of patients with insulin-dependent diabetes. *N. Engl. J. Med.* **323**, 1167–72.

Roep, B.O., Arden, S.D., de Vries, R.P. and Hutton, J.C. (1990). T-cell clones from a type-I diabetes patient respond to insulin secretory granule proteins. *Nature* **345**, 632–4.

Roep, B.O., Kallan, A.A., Hazenbos, W.L.W. *et al.* (1991). T-cell reactivity to 38kD insulin-secretory-granule protein in patients with recent-onset type I diabetes. *Lancet* **337**, 1439–41.

Ronningen, K.S., Iwe, T., Halstensen, T.S., Spurkland, A. and Thorsby, E. (1989). The amino acid at position 57 of the HLA-DQB chain and susceptibility to develop insulin-dependent diabetes mellitus. *Hum. Immunol.* **26**, 215–25.

Rossini, A.A., Handlez, E.S., Greiner, D.L. and Moroles, J.P. (1991). Insulin dependent diabetes mellitus hypothesis of autoimmunity. *Autoimmunity* **8**, 221–35.

Rotter, J.I., Vanheim, C.M., Raffel, L.J., Rimoin, D.L., Riley, W.J. and Maclaren, N.K. (1986). Genetic aetiologies of diabetes. *Pediatr. Adolesc. Endocrinol.* **15**, 1–8.

Rubenstein, P., Walker, M., Mollen, N. *et al.* (1990). No excess of DR 3/4 in Ashkenazi Jewish or Hispanic IDDM patients. *Diabetes* **39**, 1138–43.

Santamaria, P., Gehrz, R.C., Bryan, M.K. and Barbosa, J.J. (1989). Involvement of Class II MHC molecules in the LPS-induction of IL-1/TNF secretions by human monocytes: quantitative differences at the polymorphic level. *J. Immunol.* **143**, 913–92.

Sarvetnick, N., Shizuru, J., Liggit, D. *et al.* (1990). Loss of pancreatic islet tolerance induced by β cell expression of interferon-gamma. *Nature* **346**, 844–7.

Satoh, J., Seino, H., Abo, T. *et al.* (1989). Recombinant human tumor necrosis factor suppresses autoimmune diabetes in non-obese diabetic mice. *J. Clin. Invest.* **84**, 1345–8.

Schatz, D.A., Riley, W.J., Maclaren, N.K. and Barrett, D.J. (1991). Defective inducer T cell function before the onset of insulin-dependent diabetes mellitus. *J. Autoimmunity* **4** (1), 125–36.

Scott, F.W., Elliott, R.B. and Kolb, H. (1989). Diet and autoimmunity: prospects of prevention of type I diabetes. *Diab. Nutr. Metab./Clin. Exp.* **2**, 61–6.

Serjeantson, S., Theophilus, J., Zimmet, P., Court, J., Crossley, J.R. and Eliott, R.B. (1981). Lymphocytotoxic antibodies and histocompatibility antigens in juvenile-onset diabetes mellitus. *Diabetes* **30**, 26–9.

Shafrin, E., and Renold, A.E. (eds) (1988). *Frontiers in Diabetes Research: Lesson from Animal Diabetes*, vol. II. J. Libby (John) & Co., London.

Sheehy, M.J., Meske, L.M., Emler, C.A. *et al.* (1989) Allelic T-cell receptor a complexes have little or no influence on susceptibility to type I diabetes. *Hum. Immunol.* **26**, 261–71.

Shyp, S., Tishon, A. and Oldstone, M.B.A. (1990). Inhibition of diabetes in BB rats by virus infection. II. Effect of virus infection on the immune response to non-viral and viral antigens. *Immunology* **69**, 501–7.

Sibley, R.K. and Sutherland, D.E.R. (1987). Pancreas transplantation: an immunohistologic and histopathologic examination of 100 grafts. *Am. J. Pathol.* **128**, 151–70.

Siemiatycki, J., Colle, E., Campbell, S., Dewer, R., Aubert, D. and Belmonte, M.M. (1988). Incidence of IDDM in Montreal by ethnic group and by social class, and comparison with ethnic groups living elsewhere. *Diabetes* **37**, 1096–102.

Signore, A., Cooke, A., Pozzilli, P., Burcher, G., Simpson, E. and Beverley, P.C.L. (1987). Class II and Il-2 receptor positive cells in the pancreas of NOD mice. *Diabetologia* **30**, 902–5.

Silverstein, J., Maclaren, N., Riley, W., Spillar, R., Radjenovic, D. and Johnson, S. (1988). Immunosuppression with azathioprine and prednisolone in recent-onset insulin-dependent diabetes mellitus. *N. Engl. J. Med.* **319**, 599–604.

Soldevila, G., Buscema, M., Doshi, M., James, R.F.L., Bottazzo, G.F. and Pujol-Borrell, R. (1991). Cytotoxic effect of IFN-gamma plus TNF-alpha on human islet cells. *J. Autoimmunity* **4**, 291–306.

Solimena, M., Folli, F., Denis-Donini, S., Comi, G.C., Pozza, G., De Camili, P. and Vicari, A.M. (1988). Autoantibodies to glutamic acid decarboxylase in a patient with stiff-man syndrome, epilepsy and type I diabetes mellitus. *N. Engl. J. Med.* **318**, 1012–20.

Solimena, M., Folli, F., Aparisi, R., Pozza, G. and De Camilli, P. (1990). Autoantibodies to GABA-ergic neurons and pancreatic beta cells in stiff-man syndrome. *N. Engl. J. Med.* **322**, 1555–60.

Spies, T., Blanck, G., Bresnahan, M., Sands, J. and Strominger, J.L. (1989). A new cluster of genes within the human major histocompatibility complex. *Science* **243**, 214–17.

Srikanta, S., Ricker, A.T., McCulloch, D.K., Soeldner, J.S., Eisenbarth, G.S. and Palmer, S.P. (1986). Autoimmunity to insulin, beta cell dysfunction and development of insulin-dependent diabetes mellitus. *Diabetes* **39**, 139–42.

Stoolman, L.M. (1989). Adhesion molecules controlling lymphocyte migration. *Cell* **56**, 907–10.

Tarui, S., Tochino, Y. and Nonaka, K., I (eds) (1986). *Insulitis and Type 1 Diabetes: Lessons from the NOD Mouse*. Academic Press, Tokyo.

Tochino, Y. (1986). Discovery and breeding of the NOD mouse. In *Insulitis and Type I Diabetes: Lessons from the NOD Mouse*. ed. S. Tarui, Y. Tochino and K. Nonaka, pp. 3–10, Tokyo Academic Press, Tokyo.

Todd, J.A. (1990). Genetic control of autoimmunity in type I diabetes. *Immunol. Today* **11**, 122–9.

Todd, J.A., Acha-Orbea, H., Bell, J.I. *et al.* (1988). A molecular basis for MHC Class II-associated autoimmunity. *Science* **240**, 1003–9.

Todd, J.A., Aitman, T.J., Cornall, R.J. *et al.* (1991). Genetic analysis of autoimmune type I diabetes-mellitus in mice. *Nature* **351**, 542–7.

Toyota, T., Kataoka, S., Sato, J. *et al.* (1982). *Clinico-genetic Genesis of Diabetes Mellitus*. Excerpta Medica, Amsterdam.

Trucco, M. and Dorman, J.S. (1989). Immunogenetics of insulin-dependent diabetes mellitus in humans. *Crit. Rev. Immunol.* **9**, 201–45.

Tuvemo, T., Dahlquist, G., Frist, G., Blom, L. and Friman, G. (1989). The Swedish childhood diabetes study III: IgM against coxsackie B viruses in newly diagnosed type I (insulin-dependent) diabetic children: no evidence of increased antibody frequency. *Diabetologia* **32**, 745–7.

Van de Winkel, M., Smets, G., Gepts, W. and Pipeleers, D.G. (1982). Islet cell surface antibodies from insulin-dependent diabetics bind specifically to pancreatic B cells. *J. Clin. Invest.* **70**, 41–9.

Van Vliet, E., Roep, B., Meulenbrock, L., Bruining, G.J. and De Vries, R.R.P. (1989). Human T cell clones with specificities for insulinoma cell antigens. *Eur. J. Immunol.* **19**, 213–16.

Vercammen, M., Gorus, F., Foriers, A. *et al.* (1989). Cell surface antibodies in type I (insulin-dependent) diabetic patients. I. Presence of immunoglobulins M which bind to rat pituitary cells. *Diabetologia* **32**, 611–17.

Vincent, S.R., Hokfelt, T., Wu, J.Y., Elde, R.P., Morgan, L.M. and Kimmel, J.R. (1983). Immunohistochemical studies of the GABA system in the pancreas. *Neuroendocrinology* **36**, 197–204.

Vives, M., Soldevilla, G., Alcalde, L., Lorenzo, L., Somoza, N. and Pujol-Borrell, R. (1991). Expression and modulation of adhesion molecules ICAM-1 and LFA-3 in human islet cells. *Diabetes* **40**, 1382–90.

Weetman, A.P., Cohen, S., Makgoba, M.W. and Borysiewiecz, L.K. (1989). Expression of an intercellular adhesion molecule, ICAM-1, by human thyroid cells. *J. Endocrinol.* **122**, 185–91.

Williams, A.J.K., Krug, J., Lampeter, E.F. *et al.* (1990). Raised temperature reduces the incidence of diabetes in the NOD mouse. *Diabetologia* **33**, 635–7.

Yamada, K., Nonaka, K., Hanafusa, T., Miyazaki, A., Toyoshima, H. and Tarui, S. (1982). Preventive and therapeutic effects of large-dose nicotinamide injections on diabetes associated with insulitis — an observation in non obese diabetic (NOD) mice. *Diabetes* **31**, 749–53.

Yoon, J.W., Austin, M., Onodera, T. and Notkins, A.B. (1979). Virus-induced diabetes-mellitus: isolation of a virus from the pancreas of a child with diabetic ketoacidosis. *N. Engl. J. Med.* **300**, 1173–9.

Zheng, R.Q.H., Abney, E.A., Grubeck-Loebenstein, B., Dayan, C., Maini, R.N. and Feldmann, M. (1990). Expression of intercellular adhesion molecule-1 and lymphocyte function-associated antigen-3 and Hashimoto's diseases. *J. Autoimmunity* **3**, 727–36.

Ziegler, A.G. and Eisenbarth, G.S. (1990). Immunology of IDDM (type I diabetes) — 1989. In *The Diabetes Annual/5*, ed. K.G.M.M. Alberti and L.P. Krall, pp. 22–50, Elsevier Scientific Pub., Amsterdam.

104: Immunological Aspects of Oral Disease

T. Lehner

Introduction

The mouth is the site of entry for numerous microbial and food antigens which are swallowed down the alimentary canal. One of the difficulties involved in studying any infection in the mouth is the complex commensal oral flora. Although this consists of non-pathogens, probably many of these organisms, individually or in combination with others, may under appropriate conditions become pathogenic. The commensal–pathogen relationship in the mouth, as exemplified by *Streptococcus mutans*, *Candida albicans* and herpes simplex virus (HSV), can be changed by environmental factors. *Streptococcus mutans* on the tooth surface in the presence of sugars may induce dental caries; *C. albicans* may proliferate to form candidiasis in the presence of a raised concentration of salivary glucose; and HSV can be triggered off by a variety of stimuli to give rise to recurrent herpetic infections. However, the selected examples of common bacterial, fungal and viral infections may develop in subjects with lowered immune responses, which permit the commensal–pathogen relationship to be upset in favour of disease.

Before any of the oral diseases are described some relevant immunological and microbial features of the mouth will be briefly reviewed.

The establishment of micro-organisms in the mouths of infants

The mouth of the new-born is sterile and normally acquires streptococci during the 1st day of life (McCarthy *et al.* 1965). Indeed, *Streptococcus salivarius* is acquired within hours of the first feed of the new-born (Zinner and Jablon 1969; Carlsson *et al.* 1970a). Staphylococci may also appear on the 1st day, though not consistently (McCarthy *et al.* 1965). *Candida albicans* has been cultured from the mouths of about 4% of infants on the 1st day of birth and this rises to 12% by the 6th day (Anderson *et al.* 1944). Gram-positive rods, probably lactobacilli, appear on the 2nd day. Anaerobes, such as *Veillonella alcalescens*, may be detected as early as the 1st day of the infant's life but can be cultured regularly from the 7th day (Berger *et al.* 1959). Fusiform bacilli are occasionally found by the 5th day, though consistently only by the 8th month (Hurst 1957). Herpes virus is not usually isolated from the mouth before 6 months of age but the carrier rate rises to 12% by the 3rd year (Buddingh *et al.* 1953).

Although streptococci constitute on average about 98% of the cultivable bacteria on the 1st day of life, this may decrease to about 70% by the end of the 1st year, due to the appearance of 12 other groups of micro-organisms; *Nocardia*, *Neisseria*, staphylococci, *Actinomyces*, fusobacteria, *Veillonella*, *Bacteroides*, *Leptotrichia*, lactobacilli, coliforms, corynebacteria and *Candida* (McCarthy *et al.* 1965).

With the eruption of deciduous teeth there may be a shift in balance from aerobic to anaerobic forms of bacteria. *Streptococcus sanguis* becomes established in the mouth within 3 months of eruption of the deciduous teeth, that is by about 14 months of age (Carlsson *et al.* 1970b). *Streptococcus mutans* requires the tooth surface as a site for colonization (Carlsson 1967) and is found predominantly in the presence of caries.

Oral immunity

The three fluid compartments of the oral cavity

Tissues in the oral cavity may be influenced by three related fluid compartments: blood, saliva and gingival crevicular fluid. Like other epithelial tissues, the oral mucosa is maintained by a rich blood supply on its deep surface, but in addition the exposed surface of the mucosa is bathed in saliva. This dual fluid system is supplemented at the most vulnerable junction of the soft and hard tissue by gingival crevicular fluid. This minute fluid compartment is situated between the gum and the tooth, the gingival crevice, and may play an essential part in the development of gingival disease. Crevicular fluid is formed from selected components of blood, which pass into the mouth and thus contribute to the composition of mixed saliva (Fig. 104.1).

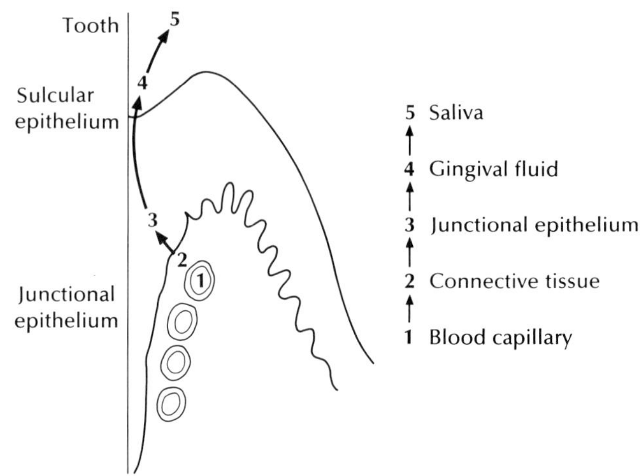

Fig. 104.1. The origin and flow of gingival crevicular fluid.

The tooth can be divided functionally into the 'salivary domain' and the 'gingival crevicular domain'. Saliva alone may exert its protective effect on the 'salivary domain' of the tooth. This includes the buccolingual surface of teeth (excluding the cervical fifth) and the pits and fissures. Whereas the incidence of caries of the buccolingual surface is very low, that of pits and fissures is rather high. It is uncertain whether the humoral and cellular components of saliva can gain access to the pits and fissures.

Crevicular fluid functions in the 'gingival domain', which includes about the cervical fifth and approximal surfaces of teeth. Caries is not very common in the cervical region, although it particularly affects the middle-aged and elderly, but approximal caries is common. The systemic mechanism of protection exerts its effects through the crevicular fluid.

SALIVA

There are two principal sources of saliva. Most of the saliva originates from the major salivary glands; a pair each of parotid, submandibular and sublingual glands. The second source is the numerous minor salivary glands scattered under the mucosa lining the oral cavity. The rate of flow varies considerably, but an average rate of resting flow is about 19 ml/hour and this may vary among different subjects from 0.5 to 111 ml/hour.

Several microbicidal components are found in saliva. Lysozyme (muramidase) is an enzyme which has bactericidal properties. Peroxidase is also an enzyme which, in the presence of thyocyanate ions and hydrogen peroxide, kills lactobacilli and may inactivate some streptococci. Lactoferrin is a heat-stable protein which has a bacteriostatic effect on a wide spectrum of microorganisms and may achieve its effect by depleting the environment of iron to a concentration which will fail to support bacterial growth.

COMPLEMENT

Sensitive techniques have failed to detect complement component 3 (C3) in parotid or submandibular saliva (Table 104.1), but small amounts, 0.05 mg/100 ml, have been found in most samples of mixed saliva (Williams *et al*. 1975). The source of C3 in the mixed saliva is almost certainly gingival crevicular fluid, which contains it in high concentrations. It is evident, therefore, that complement-dependent immune responses and damage are unlikely to take place in saliva because of lack of C3 and because immunoglobulin A (IgA) is not capable of fixing complement.

A somewhat paradoxical finding, however, is that large amounts of antibody to C3 (immunoconglutinin) are found in all samples of parotid saliva, but only low titres in about one-third of mixed salivary samples (Williams *et al*. 1975). The function of immunoconglutinins in saliva is not at all clear, but again implies that complement-dependent reactions are unlikely to operate in the salivary environment.

LEUCOCYTES

A large number of leucocytes are found in whole saliva (Calonius 1958), and it has been estimated that leucocytes migrate at a rate of about a million/minute. These leucocytes originate from blood and migrate predominantly through the gingival crevice into the oral cavity (Schiott and Löe 1970). Differential counts have established that 98–99% of salivary leucocytes are polymorphonuclear, about 1% are lymphocytes and a few monocytes and eosinophils can also be found. Cytological examination of salivary polymorphs has shown that more than 60% of them are poorly preserved, with rounded and fused lobes of nuclei resulting from degenerative changes (Raeste 1972). These changes have been ascribed to saliva being hypotonic. However, a comparative study has shown that salivary leucocytes are viable (47%), though to a lesser extent than crevicular (78%) or blood (96%) leucocytes (Scully and Lehner 1980).

Secretory immunoglobulin A in saliva

The oral mucosa, gingiva and teeth are continuously bathed in saliva. Assuming a resting flow of 19 ml of saliva/hour, and that this increases with eating and decreases with sleeping, the daily secretion is about 500 ml. As saliva contains about 19 mg/100 ml of IgA (Table 104.1), about 100 mg of IgA is secreted daily into the mouth (Brandtzaeg *et al*. 1970). By contrast only about 1.4 mg of IgG and 0.2 mg of IgM are found per 100 ml of saliva. The relative amounts of IgG and IgM in parotid saliva are much smaller (Table 104.1). The discrepancy between the immunoglobulin concentrations of whole saliva and parotid saliva can be accounted for only partly by the contribution of

Table 104.1. Concentration of immunoglobulins and C3 (in mg/100 ml) in four fluids

Fluid	IgG	IgA	IgM	IgG : IgA	C3
Serum	1250	220	80	5.7	150
Whole saliva[a]	1.4	19.4	0.2	0.07	0.05
Parotid saliva[b]	0.04	19.4	0.04	0.009	0
Gingival crevicular fluid	350[c]	110[c]	25[c]	3.2	40

a Unstimulated.
b Stimulated.
c Determined in periodontitis.
From Brandtzaeg P. *et al*. (1970). *Scand. J. Haematol.*, **12** (suppl.), 58.

submandibular, sublingual and the minor salivary glands. The contribution made by crevicular fluid is probably responsible for the increased IgG and IgM concentrations of whole saliva.

Clearly IgA is quantitatively the most important immunoglobulin secreted in saliva, and parotid saliva shows a ratio of IgA to IgG 400 times greater than the corresponding ratio in serum (Brandtzaeg *et al.* 1970). Indeed, there is a mechanism which selectively secretes IgA and this is dependent on the presence of a secretory component (SC).

There is convincing evidence to suggest that secretory IgA (sIgA) does not pass from blood to the salivary glands to be then secreted in saliva. Immunofluorescent studies have shown that IgA is produced by plasma cells locally in the salivary glands (Tomasi and Cebra 1971; Brandtzaeg 1976). These plasma cells produce not only heavy and light chains of IgA but also joining (J) chains, which are polypeptides combining with the Fc part of IgA to produce dimeric IgA. It is significant that most of the IgA plasma cells in salivary glands produce IgA dimers and not monomeric serum IgA. Only the dimeric IgA complexes with SC and the affinity of SC for IgA (and indeed IgM) may be due to the dimeric (or polymeric) conformations and not necessarily the α (or μ) chains. Secretory component appears to be synthesized by the secretory epithelial cells of salivary acini, where complexing of dimeric IgA with SC occurs. The assembled sIgA is then transported into the duct lumen and excreted into the mouth. As J chains and SC are synthesized in excess, they are found in a free state in saliva. Immunoglobulin A biosynthesis and immune responses have been reviewed by Mestecky and McGhee (1987).

The origin of predominantly IgA-secreting plasma cells in the salivary gland suggests a selective mechanism for B cells programmed to produce IgA. There are two possibilities:

1 Direct entry of antigenic material from the mouth to the salivary tissue may stimulate uncommitted B lymphocytes to form IgA-secreting plasma cells. This view is supported by the induction of sIgA antibodies on direct instillation of antigen into the salivary gland duct. Direct antigenic stimulation of sIgA antibodies in minor salivary glands was convincingly demonstrated in monkeys (Nair and Schroeder 1986). They termed the salivary gland lymphoid cell aggregation 'duct-associated lymphoid tissue' (DALT), which might be comparable to gut-associated lymphoid tissue (GALT). Direct gingivo-mucosal immunization with synthetic peptides of *S. mutans* antigen induces specific sIgA antibodies, which were most probably elicited by direct entry of the small peptides of 17–21 amino acids into the minor salivary glands (Lehner *et al.* 1989).

2 The alternative view, which has gained support, is that lymphocytes from the GALT, i.e. Peyer's patches, mostly home to salivary and other secretory glands (Cebra *et al.* 1977; Husband *et al.* 1977). Gut-associated lymphoid tissue is a major source of B lymphocytes, which can generate IgA plasma cells, whereas IgG or IgM plasma cells with only a few IgA cells are generated from lymph nodes.

Unlike systemic immune responses, which have a well-established immunological memory, there is little convincing evidence for this in the local synthesis of sIgA. Thus, repeated administration of an antigen by mouth may not induce a secondary response with a prolonged and high titre of antibodies (Mestecky *et al.* 1978; Challacombe and Lehner 1979). This apparent lack of memory on the part of secretory B cells might be a disadvantage in oral immunization, which relies on a brisk secondary immune response when a micro-organism is encountered some time after immunization. It seems that a potent, long-lasting response depends on immunization with live micro-organisms, which may give rise to a local depot of replicating antigenic material. A possible exception is cholera toxin, which generates greater IgA immunological memory in the gut lamina propria than other soluble antigens (Holmgren and Lycke 1986).

Secretory IgA has at least two functional advantages:

1 It is preferentially transferred from the gland to the mucosal surface by means of the SC on epithelial cells.

2 Secretory IgA is more resistant to proteolytic degradation by bacterial and digestive hydrolases than other immunoglobulins, so that it is particularly suited to function on mucous membranes, which either are colonized by a variety of micro-organisms or have potent digestive juices.

The function of sIgA has been aptly summarized by Macfarlane Burnett as an 'antiseptic paint' for mucosal surfaces. This may prevent absorption of the vast array of food and bacterial antigens from the gut and thereby prevent both overloading the immune system and development of undesirable allergic responses. A mechanism of action of sIgA, which may apply to all micro-organisms, is to prevent their adherence to the corresponding receptors on the mucosal surface (Williams and Gibbons 1972). This mechanism would overcome the difficulty that IgA probably does not fix complement and therefore cannot induce bacteriolysis. There is some evidence, however, that sIgA combined with complement and lysozyme may cause lysis of *Escherichia coli*. Secretory IgA antibodies have been found in saliva to a variety of bacteria, viruses and fungi, including *Streptococcus mutans*, poliovirus and *Candida* (Brandtzaeg 1972).

Gingival crevicular fluid

Components of blood can reach the tooth surface through the junctional epithelium of the gingiva and they are then referred to as crevicular fluid (Fig. 104.2). This fluid contains both the humoral and cellular elements of blood, although in lower amounts and different proportions (Table 104.1). It is likely that the flow is secondary to the bacterial plaque, which accumulates continuously, even within minutes of its removal, and causes a physiological inflammatory response in the gingiva. Crevicular flow increases greatly with the inflammatory changes of gingivitis and periodontitis. It is of some importance to appreciate that the total surface area of crevicular epithelium around 28 teeth is approximately 760 mm^2 and this can increase 10-fold with periodontal disease.

Four methods have been used for the collection of gingival crevicular fluid (Cimasoni *et al.* 1977). These employ capillary tubes, filter strips and plastic strips and are best suited for fluid collection in periodontal disease. A gingival washing method is perhaps most suitable for examination of the normal gingiva and it enables functional assessment to be made of the leucocytes and fluid components (Skapski and Lehner 1976).

The relationship between blood and crevicular fluid has been examined in the rhesus monkey (Challacombe *et al.* 1978; Scully and Challacombe 1979). Immunoglobulin G, IgA or IgM have been separated from the serum of rhesus monkeys, labelled with ^{125}I and replaced intravenously (Challacombe *et al.* 1978). Gingival crevicular fluid

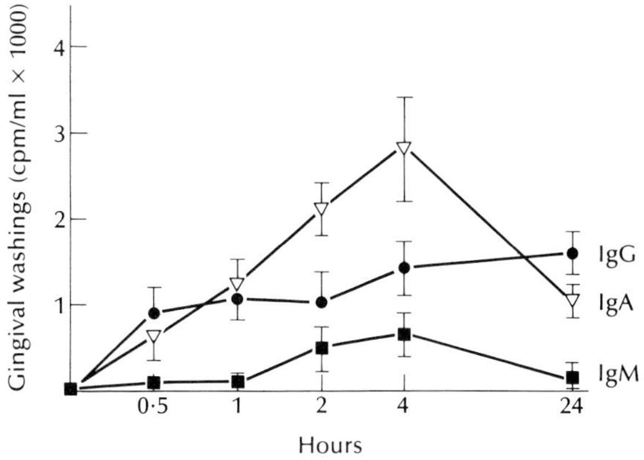

Fig. 104.2. Sequential levels of immunoglobulins in gingival washings after intravenous injection of ^{125}I-labelled immunoglobulins.

was collected at short intervals of time and this showed that the labelled IgG and IgA were detected in the fluid within 30 minutes and IgM within 2 hours of injection (Fig. 104.2). Similarly, labelled neutrophils were detectable within 20 minutes of intravenous injection (Scully and Challacombe 1979). These experiments show that humoral and cellular components from blood can reach the tooth surface. The immunological reactions of blood are therefore directly relevant to those found in crevicular fluid and they may affect the health of the tooth and gingiva. Crevicular fluid passes from the gingival crevice into the mouth, where it is mixed with saliva from the major and minor glands, and imparts to mixed saliva a number of new characteristics.

Fluid components

In addition to IgG, IgA and IgM, C3, C4, C5 and factor B have been detected in gingival crevicular fluid (Holmberg and Killander 1971; Shillitoe and Lehner 1972; Attstrom *et al.* 1975). This suggests that both the classical and the alternative complement pathways might be activated in the gingival crevice. Complement component 3 is also found in the converted form, so that complement activation may have occurred *in vivo*.

The presence of antigen and corresponding antibodies may lead to formation of immune complexes (IC), which activate the classical complement pathway. The alternative pathway of complement might also be activated, in the absence of antibody, by plaque or some of its constituents: lipopolysaccharides from Gram-negative organisms (e.g. *Veillonella*, fusobacteria) and dextran from *S. mutans* if it is sulphated. The relative importance of the two pathways, however, has not been assessed.

There are a number of other components in crevicular fluid, including albumin, transferrin, haptoglobins, glycoproteins and lipoproteins, the functions of which have not been elucidated. Perhaps, some of the most important components are enzymes released by the cells of both the host and bacteria (Cimasoni *et al*. 1977). Lysosomal enzymes released by phagocytic cells, proteases formed by bacteria, lysozyme, hyaluronidase and collagenase may all be intimately associated with maintenance of health or causing disease in the gingiva. Not only may the enzymes affect specific tissues, such as collagen, but specific proteases have been described which selectively inactivate IgA.

Cellular components

Examination of the cells found in gingival crevicular fluid has consistently shown that neutrophils constitute by far the largest number (about 92%). The remaining cells are mononuclear, consisting of macrophages and T and B lymphocytes (Wilton *et al*. 1976). These cells migrate continuously from blood through the junctional epithelium, where they may have ingested bacteria, into the gingival crevice. The increased proportion of neutrophils in crevicular fluid (92%), compared with that normally found in blood (about 70%), is consistent with the known capacity of neutrophils to migrate. This may be enhanced by the chemotactic substances formed by dental plaque, inducing neutrophils to migrate towards the tooth surface (Lindhe and Socransky 1979). Although about 40% of the crevicular neutrophils have ingested bacteria in vacuoles, over 80% are viable and functional. The cells are capable of phagocytosis of micro-organisms, although the efficacy is impaired as compared with blood neutrophils (Wilton *et al*. 1977a, b). However, crevicular neutrophils show unimpaired killing capacity.

The functions of the mononuclear cells have not been studied, although the presence of blast cells suggests that lymphocytes might be stimulated to functional activity. As viable macrophages and T and B lymphocytes are found in the crevicular domain, it is possible that some cell-mediated immune responses may take place near the surface of the tooth.

The role of local and systemic immunity

A remarkable feature of the tooth surface is that it is influenced by both local salivary and systemic immune mechanisms. The line of division between the two immune mechanisms occurs near the gingival margin, which is one of few sites of the body where an interphase can be found between the secretory and systemic immune mechanisms. A comparison of the salivary with the gingival crevicular domain suggests that, whereas the salivary domain is largely dependent on the function of sIgA, the gingival crevicular domain is controlled by most, if not all, of the immune components found in blood (Table 104.2). It is evident that the gingival crevicular domain is influenced by more versatile and diverse immune mechanisms than the salivary domain. Of course, the pulp of the tooth is supplied by the immune components of its blood circulation and, although the humoral factors may influence the dentine, it is most unlikely that they will reach the tooth surface.

The localization of the two domains also suggests that the gingival crevicular domain will affect both periodontal disease and approximal and crevicular caries, whereas the salivary domain plays a part in fissure caries and in the protection of much of the bucco-lingual surfaces of the tooth.

Periodontal disease

Dental bacterial plaque initiates gingival inflammation and, since plaque is found in almost all subjects, it follows that gingivitis affects most people. The transition from chronic gingivitis to destructive periodontitis, in most instances, appears to be related to age. Whereas bacteria trigger off the inflammatory reaction, it now appears that the host immune responses may be involved in both the chronic gingival inflammation and the progression to a destructive periodontitis. This may take many years, with breakdown of the periodontal ligament and loss of supporting bone, leading to pocket formation and loosening and eventually loss of the teeth.

Development of bacterial plaque

The causative factors responsible for periodontal disease are not entirely known but deposits of bacterial plaque are involved in the pathogenesis of this disease. There is no convincing evidence

Table 104.2. Comparison of salivary and gingival crevicular domains

Characteristic	Salivary domain	Gingival domain
Localization	Buccolingual and occlusal surfaces, excluding the cervical zone of the tooth	Cervical and approximal sites of the tooth
Source of fluid	Salivary glands	Blood
Major Ig components	Secretory IgA	IgG, IgM, IgA
Complement	Practically absent	C3, C4, C5 demonstrated
Polymorphonuclear leucocytes (PMNL)	Derived from the gingival domain and about 50% are viable	Derived from peripheral blood and over 80% are viable and capable of phagocytosis and killing
Macrophages	Not investigated	Account for about 18% of the mononuclear cells T and B lymphocytes with a ratio of 1 : 3
Antigenic stimulation	Antigens in the gut and direct oral entry of antigens	Local antigens and mitogens
Chemotaxis of PMNL and macrophages	Not studied	Both cells attracted locally by plaque-induced chemotaxis and leucocyte migration inhibition factor
Homing of lymphocytes	Circulating IgA blast cells from gut-associated lymphoid tissue	Circulating IgG (and a few IgA and IgM) blast cells from lymph nodes
Type of humoral immunity	Local secretory	Systemic, with a minor local addition of IgG and IgA
Cell-mediated immunity	Not investigated but unlikely	T cells, B cells, blast cells and macrophages present so that cellular immunity is very likely to function
Function	Inhibition of microbial adherence	Opsonization by Ig and C3b; phagocytosis and killing; complement-dependent lysis; inhibition of microbial adherence; cellular immune responses

that a single organism causes periodontal disease, but an accumulation of a large number of mixed organisms, especially Gram-negative bacteria, has been implicated (Loesche 1976; Theilade and Theilade 1976; Socransky 1977). A close relationship has been found between accumulation of bacterial plaque and gingivitis, and during this process a change occurs from a predominantly Gram-positive coccal form to a complex population of filamentous organisms, spirochaetes, vibrios and Gram-negative cocci (Löe *et al.* 1965).

Unlike the mixed non-specific bacterial flora exerting their pathogenic potential, there is some evidence that specific organisms are associated with the pathogenesis of some defined periodontal lesions (Socransky 1977). The specific microbial aetiology hypothesis has received support from the observation that *Bacteroides gingivalis* is the predominant organism isolated from both human and monkey periodontal disease (Slots and Genco 1984; Slots and Listgarten 1988). Furthermore, a specific type of juvenile and rapidly progressing adult periodontitis is associated with *Actinobacillus actinomycetem-comitants* (Newman and Socransky 1977; Socransky *et al.* 1988). The cell walls of the Gram-negative organisms contain lipopolysaccharides (LPS), which may exert toxic effects (Elin and Wolff 1976), and those of the Gram-positive organisms have lipoteichoic acids (LTA), dextrans or levans, which may contribute to a variety of immunological functions in periodontal disease (Lehner 1977a).

Correlation between local immunopathological and systemic immune responses in the four stages of periodontal disease

Quantitative analysis of the histopathological and ultrastructural changes in experimental gingivitis and periodontal disease has suggested four stages of development: initial, early, established and advanced lesions (Page and Schroeder 1976). Parallel studies of immunopathological events in the gingiva and the systemic immune responses have not been carried out during plaque-induced experimental gingivitis. Nevertheless, sequential

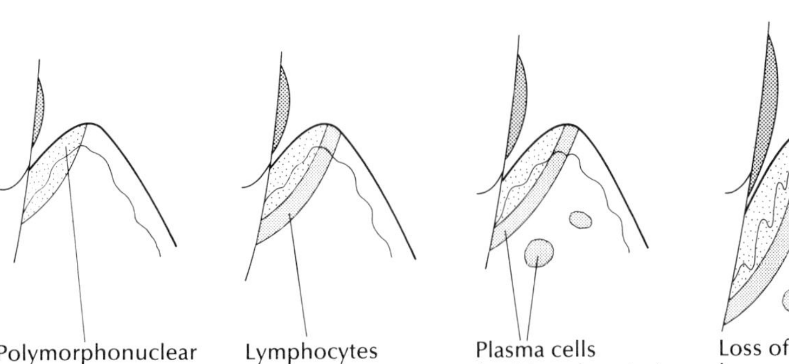

Fig. 104.3. Diagrammatic representation of the local immunopathological and systemic immune responses during the four stages of development of periodontal disease.

studies make it possible to relate the local immunopathological changes with the systemic immune responses (Fig. 104.3; Lehner *et al.* 1974a).

INITIAL LESION

As bacteria and their products are normally found on the teeth, it is difficult to distinguish between the normal and pathological tissue reactions.

Local immunopathology

There is an acute inflammatory response, which develops within 2–4 days of plaque accumulation. The lesion is localized to the gingival sulcus and the adjacent epithelium and connective tissue. The gingival blood-vessels dilate and there is exudation of fluid, with immunoglobulin (especially IgG), complement, fibrin and polymorphonuclear leucocytes (PMNL) being found in extravascular spaces. A few lymphocytes and macrophages are also found. The histological changes suggest an IC, type III hypersensitivity.

Systemic immunity

Serum antibodies to a variety of plaque bacteria are present at this stage, so that IC might well be formed with some of the plaque antigens. The IC will activate the classical complement pathway and LPS and other plaque substances may activate the alternative pathway. The biological effects of complement activation seem to be adequate to account for the initial lesion; C3a and C5a induce vascular permeability and C5a is chemotactic for PMNL, which may account for the inflammatory changes. The initial lesion may be a response to bacterial plaque, especially by activation of the complement pathways directly or by IC.

EARLY LESION

A dense lymphoid cell infiltration develops within 4–7 days of plaque accumulation at the site of the initial lesion. The early lesion is often found in the clinically normal gingiva, when plaque control is not practised efficiently.

Local immunopathology

Lymphocytes constitute 75% of the leucocytic infiltration and there are only a few plasma cells and macrophages. Most of the lymphocytes are of the T cell series, with a small number of B cells. There are some macrophages and blast cells. Fibroblasts in association with lymphocytes show degenerative changes and there is a localized loss of collagen fibres. The exudation of serum immunoglobulins, complement, fibrinogen and leucocytes is increased. The gingival crevicular fluid and leucocytes reach a maximum level 6–12 days after the onset of clinical gingivitis. The features of the early lesion are consistent with the concept that cell-mediated immunity (CMI) (type IV) plays an important part at this stage of disease.

Systemic immunity

Lymphoid cells, especially newly stimulated blast cells in the circulation, have a heightened affinity for inflamed tissue and may therefore be seeded into the gingival focus of inflammation developed in the initial lesion. Lymphocytes at this stage are capable of releasing at least some lymphokines, and these may further augment the localization of leucocytes and proliferation of lymphocytes.

ESTABLISHED LESION

The established lesion develops within 2–3 weeks

of plaque accumulation and its distinguishing feature is the predominantly plasma cell infiltration, as compared with the lymphoid infiltration in the early lesion. It is probable that some of the B lymphocytes found in the early lesion have been stimulated by plaque antigens to differentiate into plasma cells.

Local immunopathology

The lesion is still confined to a small site adjacent to the gingival sulcus but consists mostly of a plasma cell infiltration. However, clusters of plasma cells are also found among blood-vessels and collagen fibres. Most of the plasma cells produce IgG, some IgA and a few IgM. Extravascular connective tissue and the junctional epithelium contain immunoglobulin, complement and probably IC and there is loss of collagen. The gingival sulcus may deepen and the junctional epithelium may be converted into a pocket. This lesion has some features of a type IV and others of a type III hypersensitivity.

Systemic immunity

The proliferative response of lymphocytes to plaque antigen becomes evident 14–21 days after plaque accumulation. Specific plaque antigens may be involved in this process, but the polyclonal B cell mitogens found in plaque (LPS, dextran and levan) might also act as potential activators and adjuvants. As both T and B lymphocytes are stimulated by plaque antigens and newly stimulated blast cells are preferentially seeded to inflammatory foci, there is a continuous influx of these cells in the established lesion. Plasma cells are secretory cells, so that for the established lesion to be maintained for years or decades (as it often is) a continuous influx of lymphocytes is required.

ADVANCED LESION

The established lesion can persist for many years and the change into the advanced lesion marks the transition from a chronic and successful defence reaction to a destructive immunopathological mechanism. It is not certain what factors are responsible for the progression from an established to an advanced lesion but there is little doubt that this transition is crucial in the development of destructive periodontal disease.

Local immunopathology

This stage is recognized clinically as periodontitis, with pocket formation, ulceration of the pocket epithelium, destruction of the collagenous periodontal ligament and bone resorption. These changes lead to mobility and eventually loss of the tooth. The features of acute vasculitis are maintained, with the further development of chronic inflammation and reparative fibrosis. The pathological changes now extend apically and laterally, with a dense infiltration of plasma cells, lymphocytes and macrophages. There is a breakdown of the epithelial barrier between plaque and periodontal tissue and this might be associated with a significant change in the immune responses, so as to permit direct access of plaque antigens and metabolites. The essential feature of this stage of periodontal disease is that there is irreversible loss of periodontal ligament and bone, with a progressive increase in pocket formation. Gingival fluid collected at this stage contains high concentrations of IgG, IgA, IgM and complement, as well as a predominantly PMNL infiltration, with some mononuclear cells.

Systemic immunity

It is now becoming clear that the chronic destructive process may involve all the mechanisms known to contribute to the immunopathology of chronic lesions. The complexity of development of the advanced lesion of periodontal disease will become evident when it is appreciated that all four types of allergic reactions have been implicated. Whilst these reactions may contribute to the complex mechanism of bacterial elimination and the inevitable tissue destruction and tissue repair, the biological significance of any one mechanism is not known. The diverse mechanisms will be briefly described, although some aspects have been dealt with in the section on the immune responses to dental plaque.

Immunopathology and mechanism of adult periodontitis

Systematic description of the development of periodontal disease from the initial, to early, then established and finally advanced lesion is not meant to imply that this progression necessarily takes place. Indeed, the greatest difficulty is to establish the factors responsible for the transition from the reversible stage of gingivitis to the irreversible, destructive stage of periodontitis. There is no real evidence to suggest that destructive periodontitis necessarily develops from a pre-existing gingivitis.

The cellular infiltration in adult periodontitis is of particular importance, as this may help us to understand the mechanism responsible for the disease which causes the most common loss of teeth. Immunocytochemical investigation of the tissue from adult periodontitis revealed that the proportion of CD4 to CD8 T cell subsets changes from a ratio of about 2 : 1 in the circulation to about 1 : 1 in the periodontal lesion. Hence, the CD4 helper–inducer subset decreases relatively to the increased CD8 cytotoxic–suppressor subset (Taubman *et al.* 1984; Johanneson *et al.* 1987). Furthermore, both CD4 and CD8 cells appear to be activated at the site of the lesion, as some of the cells express the major histocompatibility complex (MHC) Class 2 antigen (human leucocyte antigen (HLA)-DR)). Whilst these findings are open to functional interpretation, only experimental evidence can establish whether the phenotypic expression of these cells is a true representation of their functional activities. There is, however, evidence, at least in severe adult periodontitis, that a decrease in lymphoproliferative responses to stimulation with oral micro-organisms (e.g. *Actinomyces*, *Veillonella* or *Bacteroides*) is due to the activity of CD8 suppressor T cells and their soluble products (Ivanyi 1986).

In addition to T cells there are macrophages, Langerhans cells, B cells and plasma cells. However, with repeated immunization, primed B cells may become more efficient in antigen binding through their membrane-bound antibodies, followed by the antigen binding to HLA Class II MHC and then presenting the HLA–antigen complex to T cells.

Amongst the wealth of antigenic and mitogenic stimulants found in dental plaque and its constitutive micro-organisms, polyclonal B cell activators are of particular significance (Smith *et al.* 1980; Lehner 1982a). These may elicit non-specific B cell proliferation and antibody production and may account for the large numbers of B cells and plasma cells. However, the regulatory function of T cells extends to polyclonal B cell activation. Hence, in adult periodontitis, whilst quantitatively B cell activity may predominate, the immunological changes are under T cell control. Indeed, it is possible that the lesion develops as a result of imbalance in T cell immunoregulation. The importance of T cells in the mechanism of periodontal destruction has been demonstrated by the presence of cytokines (Walsh *et al.* 1987). Interleukin 2 (IL-2) causes expansion of T and B cells, leucocyte migration inhibition factor (MIF) may immobilize passing macrophages and PMNL and lymphotoxins may damage fibroblasts. Osteoclast-activating factor, which is probably a function of IL-1, causes bone resorption (Gowen *et al.* 1983).

Macrophages are consistently found in periodontal lesions and they may have a variety of functions other than antigen processing. One of these is IL-1 production, which activates T cells to proliferate. Interleukin 1 has numerous other effects on the connective tissue, especially collagenase, production in fibroblast and bone resorption (Trechsel *et al.* 1982; Postlethwaite *et al.* 1983). A number of oral micro-organisms can induce macrophages to produce IL-1 but this is not directly related to the ability of the organism to induce periodontal disease. Macrophages release prostaglandins, which may affect immune responses. They play an important role in phagocytosis and killing bacteria and may release lysosomal enzymes, which enhance local damage.

Tissue destruction enables more plaque antigen to enter the periodontal tissue, thereby activating further immune reactions, which leads to a vicious cycle. Suppressor mechanisms an be activated, involving CD8 cells and macrophages, which release prostaglandin, and these may suppress some of the cellular or humoral immune responses.

Four types of hypersensitivity reactions

It is not clear to what extent the four different types of hypersensitivity play a part in adult periodontitis. However, it is not entirely surprising that they might all participate, if one considers the complex nature of the constituents of dental bacterial plaque and their numerous metabolic products.

TYPE I OR ANAPHYLACTIC HYPERSENSITIVITY

The observation that mast cells are found in the normal gingiva provides evidence that type I reactions could occur, but they decrease in number with inflammation. Immunoglobulin E has been found in normal gingiva and it coats some plaque bacteria (Nisengard *et al.* 1968, 1971). Antigens might induce degranulation of the gingival mast cells associated with IgE and release histamine and other vasoactive substances. It is of interest that increased levels of prostaglandins E_1 and E_2 were found in gingivitis and these may also cause increased vascular permeability (Goodson *et al.* 1974).

TYPE II OR ANTIBODY-DEPENDENT HYPERSENSITIVITY

Antibodies to periodontal tissue have not been detected, although autoimmunity has been evoked as a cause of periodontitis (Brandtzaeg and Kraus 1965). The three components of type II hypersensitivity, i.e.: (i) antibody binding to cell surface, antigens and causing phagocytosis; (ii) antibody-dependent killer cell activity; and (iii) antibody complement-dependent lysis, might, however, be involved in attempts to eliminate plaque bacteria. Although antibody and complement-mediated phagocytosis and killing may play a part in controlling Gram-positive organisms, there is no evidence that similar mechanisms are involved against the cells of periodontal tissue.

TYPE III OR IMMUNE COMPLEX-MEDIATED HYPERSENSITIVITY

Although IC have not been found directly in diseased gingiva (Clagett and Page 1978), evidence implicating their involvement in periodontitis exists (Genco *et al.* 1974). Plaque antigens (Ranney 1978) and antibodies to these (Schneider *et al.* 1966; Berglund 1979) have been reported in the gingiva. Furthermore, crevicular fluid PMNL have membrane-bound IgG, IgM and C3, and the C3b receptors are blocked in crevicular PMNL from patients with periodontal disease, consistent with the presence of IC (Wilton *et al.* 1977a, b). However, C1q-binding complexes could not be detected in sera (Mackler *et al.* 1979), although this does not exclude the possibility of complexes being found by other methods. Immune complexes might play a part in periodontal disease by activating the classical complement pathway to produce a number of biologically active mediators. This is associated with the release of lysosomal enzymes, both by PMNL and by macrophages, and will cause local damage (Page *et al.* 1973; Taichman and McArthur 1976). The macrophage is a particularly versatile cell, capable of secreting collagenase, which can degrade the collagen of the periodontal ligament (Mergenhagen *et al.* 1976). Complement activation may result in cell lysis and can also cause bone resorption, involving both the classical and the alternative pathways (Sandberg *et al.* 1977). This type of bone resorption is mediated by prostaglandins and can be inhibited by indomethacin, a prostaglandin inhibitor (Raisz *et al.* 1974). There is evidence for activation of the alternative complement pathway by plaque antigens (Allison *et al.* 1976; Wilton 1977).

TYPE IV OR CELL-MEDIATED HYPERSENSITIVITY

There is strong evidence implicating type IV reactions in periodontal disease. The activation of CMI by plaque antigens stimulates proliferation of T and B lymphocytes (Ivanyi and Lehner 1970; Horton *et al.* 1972a; Mackler *et al.* 1974). Lymphocytes maintain a supply of soluble mediators: leucocyte MIF (Ivanyi *et al.* 1972) may immobilize macrophages and PMNL, chemotactic factor may attract further leucocytes (Mackler *et al.* 1974), lymphotoxin may damage fibroblasts (Horton *et al.* 1973) and osteoclast-activating factor may cause further bone resorption (Horton *et al.* 1972b, 1974). Tissue destruction enables more plaque antigen to enter the periodontal tissues, thereby activating further immune reactions, and this leads to a vicious circle.

There are considerable individual variations in the CMI immune responses, and the pattern of cellular responses might be an indication of the patient's sensitization to plaque antigens. Attempts to correlate quantitatively the stimulation index of lymphocytes with the periodontal index of disease have been largely unsuccessful.

The existence of an immunological memory for plaque antigens has been found in experimental gingivitis (Lehner *et al.* 1974a) and the cellular immune response to some plaque antigens may persist for some time after the teeth are extracted (Baker *et al.* 1976). This might be associated with the persistence of some micro-organisms, such as *Actinomyces* or *Veillonella* in the edentulous mouth (Patters *et al.* 1976). Further evidence in favour of an immunological memory and the presence of a suppressive agent is that, in those patients with severe periodontitis whose lymphocytes are not stimulated by plaque antigens, significant lymphocyte stimulation results within 2 weeks of extraction of the diseased teeth (Baker *et al.* 1976).

The role of CMI in periodontal disease has been studied in animals. Treatment of dogs with antithymocyte serum caused a reduction of the cellular infiltrate in the gingiva but failed to influence the severity of the disease, as measured by the amount of gingival fluid and its cellular contents (Nobreus *et al.* 1974a, b). Although this result suggested that CMI was not involved in the development of periodontal disease, both the gingival fluid and the infiltrate reflect only the chemotactic capacity of plaque. Indeed, if dinitrochlorobenzene (DNCB) was applied topically to the gingiva of antithymocyte-treated dogs, the normally developed gingival disease was suppressed both clinically and histologically (Nobreus *et al.* 1974a, b). However, a damaging effect of CMI in the rat and rhesus monkey was found on the basis of histological changes and bone loss (Wilde *et al.* 1977; Crawford *et al.* 1978). Furthermore, athymic nude rats develop greater periodontal bone loss than reconstituted animals (Yoshie *et al.* 1985).

The effect of immunosuppression or immunomodulation on human periodontal disease

Immunosuppressive drugs used in renal transplantation and immunodeficiencies in man appear to be associated with reduction in periodontal inflammation (Schuller *et al.* 1973; Kardachi and Newcomb 1978; Tollefsen *et al.* 1978; Robertson *et al.* 1979; Scully *et al.* 1979).

Juvenile periodontitis (periodontosis)

This is a less common disease which affects one or several teeth of young people under the age of 21 (Baer 1971). There is rapid destruction of the periodontal membrane and the supporting bone, leading to loosening and loss of teeth. There is evidence to suggest that *Actinobacillus actinomycetemcomitans* causes juvenile periodontal disease (Newman and Socransky 1977). This organism has a cytotoxic effect on neutrophils in the periodontium, which may impair the removal of bacteria (Baehni *et al.* 1979). A remarkable defect in chemotaxis of PMNL has been described and this may be due to inhibitors directed against both the cells and the chemotactic factor (Cianciola *et al.* 1977; Lavine *et al.* 1979). The possibility that phagocytosis by PMNL might also be defective (Cianciola *et al.* 1977) has not been confirmed (Lavine *et al.* 1979). It is therefore possible that patients with juvenile periodontitis develop a rapidly advancing disease early in life, because of defects in chemotaxis. A polyclonal B cell mitogenic effect might account for the increased serum immunoglobulin concentrations. (Lehner *et al.* 1974b). A scanty inflammatory cell infiltrate in juvenile periodontitis might therefore be explained on the basis of lack of attraction or actual killing of PMNL by specific micro-organisms.

Immunology of dental caries

Dental decay (caries) is one of the most common diseases of mankind. It has reached epidemic proportions in modern times, since a fine-consistency diet, rich in refined sugars, has come to be consumed. The prevalence of caries in developed countries varies but affects 50% of 5–17-year-old and 84% of 17-year-old children (Newbrun 1989). Socioeconomic factors are important in determining the prevalence of caries. The disease has been increasing in developing countries, with the increase in popularity of highly refined sugars. The development of dental caries requires the presence of cariogenic bacteria that are capable of rapidly producing acid below the critical pH required for dissolving enamel, and the presence of a sugar in the diet that favours colonization of these bacteria and that can be metabolized by the bacteria to form acid. This process can be interfered with by the presence of an effective immune response.

Micro-organisms

There are a number of cariogenic organisms, which can be defined by their ability to colonize teeth, to reduce the pH to about 4.1 in the presence of a suitable sugar substrate and to induce caries in germ-free animals. *Streptococcus mutans*, *S. sanguis*, *Lactobacillus acidophilus* and *Actinomyces viscosus* fulfil most of these criteria (Keyes and Jordan 1964; Fitzgerald *et al.* 1966). However, *S. mutans* appears to be the most efficient cariogenic organism, as it induces caries rapidly in germ-free rodents (Fitzgerald *et al.* 1960). As most of the immunological studies in caries have been concerned with *S. mutans*, this will be described in some detail. Nevertheless, it should be remembered that the other organisms may also contribute to the development of the disease. *Streptococcus mutans* is a facultative, nonhaemolytic, acidogenic anaerobe, producing extracellular polysaccharides. The organism fulfils Koch's postulates as a cause of dental caries:

1 *Streptococcus mutans* is found in the plaque of carious teeth and cannot usually be isolated in the absence of caries.

2 The organism can be grown in pure culture.

3 Infection of germ-free rats or normal hamsters with *S. mutans* induces caries.

4 The organism can then be recovered from the carious lesion and grown in pure culture.

5 Antibodies to this organism are increased in patients with caries.

Streptococcus mutans has been separated into seven serotypes (a–g) by means of precipitation and immunofluorescence techniques (Brathall 1970; Coykendall 1974; Perch *et al.* 1974). The serotype antigen appears to be a polysaccharide residing in the cell wall of the coccus. Over 70% of *S. mutans* isolated from man appear to belong to serotype c, the next most common being serotypes d, e and g.

The structure and antigenic composition of *S. mutans* are of considerable importance in our understanding of the immune responses to this organism. It consists of a cell wall and protoplast membrane, which enclose the protoplast of the organism. A large number of cell wall antigens have been identified and these include proteins (Russell and Lehner 1978) and the enzyme glucosyl transferase, which converts sucrose into dextran or mutan (Guggenheim and Newbrun 1969). The group specificity resides in the group carbohydrate (a–g) and these are polymers of glucose, rhamnose, galactose or galactosamine. Serotype c, e and f polysaccharides share glucose and rhamnose (Hamada and Slade 1976; Linzer *et al.* 1976), whereas serotypes a, d and g share glucose and galactose (Linzer *et al.* 1975). Lipoteichoic acid is inserted in the protoplast membrane and penetrates the cell wall to function as a surface component. Lipoteichoic acid is a glycerol teichoic acid which has a phospholipid moiety (Wicken and Knox 1978). The main component of LTA is polyglycerol phosphate, which forms the backbone common to all glycerol teichoic acids and is probably responsible for most of the cross-reactions between Gram-positive bacteria.

Proteins

The constitutive enzyme glucosyltransferase (GTF) converts sucrose into glucan (dextran), which may be responsible for adhesion of *S. mutans* to the tooth surface (Guggenheim and Newbrun 1969). Four protein antigens (I, II, I/II, III) have been identified on examination of culture supernatant and cell extracts of *S. mutans* (serotype c) (Russell and Lehner 1978; Russell *et al.* 1980). Streptococcal antigens (SA) I and II appear to be two determinants usually present in a single molecule termed antigen I/II. Antigen I/II has a molecular weight of 185 000 and this is consistent with the sum of the molecular weights of antigens I (150 000) and antigen II (48 000). Antigen III has a molecular weight of about 40 000. Immunization with GTF and the protein antigens can protect against caries in experimental animals.

Polysaccharides

Extracellular dextran (glucan) is synthesized in large amounts by the action of the constitutive enzyme GTF (dextran sucrase). *Streptococcus mutans* synthesizes an $\alpha(1-3)$-linked water-insoluble dextran, termed mutan, as well as an $\alpha(1-6)$-linked water-soluble dextran (Guggenheim 1970). Glucosyltransferase from *S. sanguis*, however, synthesizes predominantly the $\alpha(1-6)$-linked water-soluble dextran. The difference in solubility of these two polysaccharides may reflect the greater efficiency in plaque and caries formation by *S. mutans*. The mutan may play an important part in the adherence mechanism of the *Streptococcus* to the tooth.

An extracellular levan (fructan) is synthesized to a limited extent by *S. mutans* (Gibbons and Nygaard 1968) but larger quantities are produced by *Actinomyces viscosus* (Howell and Jordan 1967). Although levan is found in plaque, it can be rapidly hydrolysed by plaque bacteria, so that, unlike dextran, it is not efficient in plaque formation.

An intracellular amylopectin is an iodine-staining polysaccharide found in *S. mutans* and dental plaque (Gibbons and Socransky 1962).

Amylopectin is synthesized when exogenous carbohydrate is available, and it forms an intracellular storage material. The intracellular amylopectin is metabolized to lactic acid when environmental carbohydrate becomes depleted, and this may be responsible for the prolonged acid formation inside the plaque.

The most important source of acid is glucose, which may enter plaque from the diet, but quantitatively the richest source of glucose is sucrose. Plaque bacteria and *S. mutans* contain invertase, which hydrolyses sucrose to glucose and fructose (Hartles 1965). Since streptococci do not possess a cytochrome system but contain the Embden–Meyerhof glycolytic enzymes, glucose will be converted to lactic and other organic acids. The pH inside the plaque may fall within 2–3 minutes of rinsing the mouth with glucose or sucrose from a level of about 6.5 to about 5 (Stephan 1940; Jenkins and Kleinberg 1956); the critical pH below which decalcification of enamel occurs is thought to be about 5.5. Caries is the end result of a complex sequence of microbial and biochemical processes terminating in acid formation, which attacks the tooth enamel to cause caries.

Immunology of caries in man

SALIVARY ANTIBODIES

The concentration of secretory IgA in whole saliva can be significantly less in subjects with high caries as compared with those having low caries experience (Lehner *et al.* 1967). This finding is dependent on the rate of secretion of saliva, which is difficult to standardize, and a greater proportion of the IgA may be contributed by submaxillary than parotid saliva (Zengo *et al.* 1971; Ostarvik and Brandtzaeg 1975).

Specific sIgA antibodies to *S. mutans* have been detected in saliva (Challacombe and Lehner 1976). However, contrary to expectations from the IgA concentrations, a significant increase in salivary IgA antibodies to *S. mutans* was not found in subjects with low caries experience. It appears that the salivary IgA antibodies increase with the number of carious lesions, so that they may reflect the cumulative caries experience. Salivary IgA antibodies to *S. mutans* have been induced in man by swallowing daily capsules filled with 10^{10} organisms, but the duration of the antibody titre was limited, even on secondary immunization (Mestecky *et al.* 1978).

As salivary IgA antibodies may function by preventing bacterial adherence (Williams and Gibbons 1972; Gibbons 1989), it is possible that this mechanism is efficient in preventing caries on the exposed smooth surfaces of the teeth. However, the susceptible sites (fissures, approximal and cervical sites) may not be accessible to the salivary components and a protective relationship has not been found between the antibody titres and caries index.

SERUM ANTIBODIES

Serum antibodies to cell, cell wall, GTF and SAI/II of *S. mutans* have been studied in adults and children. Both IgG and IgA classes of antibodies have been found in man (Challacombe and Lehner, 1976; Challacombe *et al.* 1984; Aaltonen *et al.* 1985; 1987), with a negative correlation between the titre and caries index in adults free of or with treated caries (i.e. fillings). The reverse, namely a positive correlation, was found in subjects with untreated caries, between the antibody titre and caries index. Sequential studies showed that the development of caries is associated with a modest but significant increase in serum IgG and IgM antibodies to *S. mutans*, as is the case with any infection (Challacombe and Lehner 1976). The somewhat modest change in the antibody level may reflect the chronic nature of caries, which may take many months to develop. It is therefore particularly significant that if the carious lesion is treated the serum antibody titre falls and salivary antibodies increase. However, recent studies have shown some inconsistencies in the results of serum antistreptococcal antibodies and the prevalence of caries.

NATURAL DEFENCES DURING THE PERINATAL PERIOD AND INFANCY

The mother can influence her baby *in utero* by transplacental transfer of the maternal IgG class of antistreptococcal antibodies (Ivanyi and Lehner 1978). However, due to the limited half-life of these passively transferred antibodies, they are cleared from the infant 3–6 months after birth (Ivanyi and Lehner 1978). Indeed, treatment for caries during pregnancy affects serum and salivary antibodies to *S. mutans* and the prevalence of caries in the offspring (Aaltonen *et al.* 1988). A surprising feature in studies of the maternal–fetal relationship was to find that, if the mother's lymphocytes are sensitized to *S. mutans*, so are the lymphocytes of the new-born. It is not clear, as yet, how long these lymphocytes remain sensitized. If, as might be assumed, sensitization has been acquired passively *in utero* by a soluble lymphocyte factor from the mother, then sensitization may be of short duration.

After birth, the mother is the most likely source of infection by *S. mutans*, due to the close contact and kissing of the baby (Kohler and Bratthal 1978; Berkowitz and Jones 1985). Exposure of the infant to the high numbers of *S. mutans* in the mother's saliva may lead to ingestion of these bacteria and production of antibodies (Aaltonen *et al.* 1985). In the young infant before eruption of teeth (0–5 months), the streptococci have no teeth to adhere to, so that oral colonization does not occur. However, salivary IgA antistreptococcal antibodies may be elicited either (i) by direct entry of antigen into the minor salivary glands scattered under the oral mucosa or (ii) indirectly by swallowing an adequate concentration of streptococci and stimulating the GALT to mount an immune response (Arnold *et al.* 1976). Furthermore, serum antistreptococcal antibodies might be more readily elicited in the new-born infant, as the intestinal epithelium is permeable to foreign proteins, before the antigen exclusion mechanism begins to function with age and this mode of entry of antigen is closed. It is therefore evident that under these conditions, a high maternal salivary content of *S. mutans* might elicit serum antibodies. The resulting immune response may prevent subsequent colonization of the erupting teeth by *S. mutans*. Salivary IgA may directly prevent streptococcal adherence, but serum IgM or IgG may also be functional, during the trauma of eruption of teeth through the gingiva or later via the gingival crevicular fluid. Whichever mechanism may operate, this type of protective relationship between mother and young child has been observed (Aaltonen *et al.* 1985, 1987). However, if, for one of many possible reasons, an effective immune response is not evoked or indeed tolerance to an important cell surface antigen is elicited, then colonization of the infant's teeth will take place by direct transmission of *S. mutans* in maternal saliva. It should be noted that, the earlier the infection of teeth by *S. mutans*, the greater the risk of development of dental caries.

A major source of antibodies and leucocytes in the mouth of the baby is breast milk. This contains sIgA, complement, PMNL and macrophages, which are capable of opsonization, phagocytosis and killing of micro-organisms. Indeed, human milk contains antibodies to *S. mutans* (Arnold *et al.* 1976), so that breast-fed babies receive an additional supply of IgA antibodies, as well as phagocytic cells, which may alter the pattern of microbial colonization of the mouth.

It is noteworthy that low serum IgG antibodies in preschool children were associated with increased caries activity (Aaltonen *et al.* 1987). In another series of children (2–5 years old), who had only deciduous teeth, the IgG (or IgM) antibody levels to *S. mutans* failed to show a relationship with dental caries (Lehner *et al.* 1978a). However, the higher the ratio of IgG to IgA antibodies, the lower the prevalence of caries, suggesting that IgA antibodies might interfere with the protective function of IgG antibodies.

OPSONIZATION, PHAGOCYTOSIS AND KILLING

Serum antibodies are capable of opsonizing *S. mutans* and this appears to be particularly a function of the IgG class of antibodies (Scully and Lehner 1979, 1980). Polymorphonuclear leucocytes then phagocytose and kill the streptococci. There is a correlation between phagocytosis of *S. mutans* and the IgG class of antibody titre to this organism. Complement is also involved in opsonization of the streptococcus. Opsonization, phagocytosis and killing by PMNL or macrophages might be one of the essential protective functions against colonization by *S. mutans*.

CELLULAR IMMUNE RESPONSES

Streptococcus mutans can induce human lymphocytes to proliferate and to release cytokines (Lehner *et al.* 1974a). Although the response of lymphocytes is modest, this can be boosted by the immunopotentiating effect of accumulation of plaque. Under these conditions a negative correlation was established between the caries index and the stimulation index of lymphocytes; this is consistent with the findings between serum antibody and the caries index. Hence, the lower the caries index, the higher the lymphoproliferative responses and antibody titres. The stimulated cells are predominantly the CD4 subset of T cells, which are involved in helping B cells to produce antibodies. Indeed, there is evidence that human T cells can be stimulated by *S. mutans* antigens to induce helper or suppressor function which may increase or decrease antibody synthesis by B cells (Lamb *et al.* 1980).

APPARENT FAILURE OF NATURAL IMMUNITY IN PROTECTION AGAINST DENTAL CARIES

As a high proportion of the population in Western countries develops caries, natural immunity is evidently inadequate. Yet the data concerning humoral and cellular immunity to *S. mutans* would suggest that these may have a protective function. This apparent contradiction can be interpreted on the basis that *S. mutans* is a poor immunogen, particularly as it preferentially colonizes enamel surfaces. Sensitization to the organism might depend on the entry of a sufficient dose of antigenic material through the junctional epithelium of the gingiva to immunologically competent cells and efficiency of this route of immunization is questionable. Indeed, natural immunization induces a low antibody titre, which is relatively higher for IgM than for IgG antibodies, and these may not be directed against an essential antigen of *S. mutans*. The T cell response to *S. mutans* also appears to be of a low order of magnitude and may need boosting for effective sensitization.

It can be assumed that *S. mutans* in saliva is swallowed and, although the organism does not colonize the gut mucosa, it may nevertheless induce an immune response in the GALT. Sensitized cells may then home to salivary glands to produce the IgA antibodies found in saliva. We have seen that the antibody titre in saliva increases with the caries index, so that salivary antibodies may be an indirect index of the frequency and possibly the magnitude of colonization by *S. mutans*.

The ability of man to produce an effective immune response to *S. mutans* may depend on the Ia gene products. This may determine the balance between helper and suppressor activity in response to streptococcal stimulation (Lamb *et al.* 1979, 1980). There is evidence to suggest that man has the potential to mount cellular and humoral immune responses to *S. mutans* but that under conditions of natural immunization these are usually inadequate (Lehner *et al.* 1976b).

PREVENTION OF DENTAL CARIES BY IMMUNIZATION

As dental decay fulfils the criteria of an infectious disease, the possibility of preventing it by vaccination has been pursued. The rationale is that immunization with *S. mutans* should induce an immune response, which might prevent the organism from colonizing the tooth surface and thereby prevent decay.

Rats and monkeys have been used in the immunization studies. The principal design in most of the experiments has been first to immunize the animals with antigens from *S. mutans* and an adjuvant, as frequently as is necessary to attain high antibody levels, followed by implantation of the same organism in the mouth and placing the animals on a high sucrose diet. Control animals are maintained under identical conditions of diet and bacterial implantation, but they are sham-immunized, that is, they are injected with saline instead of the vaccine. The teeth are then examined for the number of *S. mutans* colonized and for the number of carious lesions produced. Blood and saliva are assayed for antibody titres to *S. mutans* antigens. Some of the experiments have been designed so as to aim for salivary immunity and others for systemic immunity.

In general four routes of immunization were used with *S. mutans*: (i) oral; (ii) systemic (subcutaneous); (iii) active gingivo-salivary; and (iv) passive dental immunization (Fig. 104.4).

Oral route of immunization

Killed *S. mutans* was administered to germ-free rats in the drinking-water for 45 days before implantation of live *S. mutans*, and then throughout the experimental period (Michalek *et al.* 1976). A significant reduction in caries was related to an increased level of salivary IgA antibodies to *S. mutans*, but the serum antibody titre was minimal. Reduction in caries was also achieved by feeding GTF to rodents and this was related to salivary IgA antibodies (Smith *et al.* 1979). That IgA can be involved in the protection against

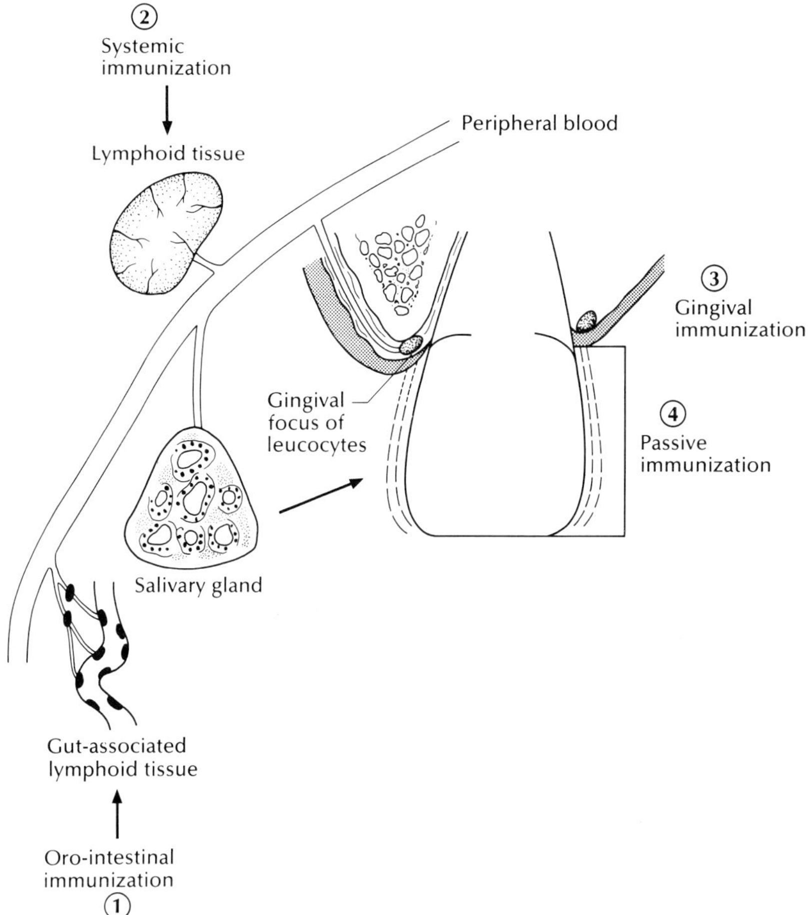

Fig. 104.4. Routes of immunization of the oral cavity.

caries has been confirmed by passive transfer of sIgA antibodies in the milk of lactating rats to their litter (Michalek and McGhee 1977). However, milk also contains IgG antibodies, which, unlike IgA antibodies, are absorbed by the gastrointestinal tract of the offspring to enter the blood and are found in both serum and saliva. Indeed, administration of cow's milk, containing mostly IgG antibodies, to gnotobiotic rats prevented oral colonization by *S. mutants* and dental caries (Michalek *et al*. 1987).

Oral immunization with *S. mutans* did not induce significant sIgA in monkeys. Daily administration of 10^{11} cells of *S. mutans* in capsules produced small increases in sIgA. Oral immunization failed to reduce caries significantly, as compared with subcutaneous immunization (Lehner *et al*. 1980; Walker 1981). The rise in secretory antibodies produced was small and of short duration, even after secondary immunization. Experiments in humans ingesting *S. mutans* in gelatine capsules resulted in an increase in sIgA antibodies in saliva, although for a limited duration (Mestecky *et al*. 1978). Immunological memory in sIgA responses is short and this may curtail the value of oral immunization. Ingestion of *S. mutans* in humans induces circulating IgA-producing cells within 7 days and these disappear by about 21 days (Czerkinsky *et al*. 1987). The central IgA-producing cells can be stimulated to release anti-*S. mutans* antibodies, which are also found peripherally in saliva and tears.

Systemic route of immunization

Subcutaneous administration of *S. mutans* was used successfully in monkeys (Bowen *et al*. 1975; Lehner *et al*. 1975a, b, 1976a, 1981) and elicited predominantly serum IgG, IgM and IgA antibodies. The antibodies find their way into the oral cavity via the gingival crevicular fluid and are protective against dental caries (Challacombe *et al.* 1978; Smith and Lehner 1981). Whole cells, cell walls and the 185 kD SA have been effective after two to four administrations.

The rhesus monkey model has been developed to induce caries and to immunize the monkeys in a way that would be acceptable in man (Lehner *et al.* 1975a, b). The significance and advantages of using this subhuman primate will be mentioned briefly. The teeth are similar to those in man in their number, morphology and eruption of deciduous and permanent teeth (Hurme and van Wagenen 1956). The pattern of approximal, cervical and fissure caries and the rate at which caries develops in the deciduous dentition are consistent with those found in man (Lehner *et al.* 1975a). The monkeys acquire *S. mutans* (serotype c) naturally, without resorting to artificial implantation of large numbers of organisms, which might alter the bacteriological balance and act as a further route of immunization (Caldwell *et al.* 1977). The monkeys are fed entirely on a human type of diet. It contains about 15% sucrose and its consistency and content are similar to those used by man. The immune responses parallel those found in man, in the IgG, IgA and IgM serum antibody classes and in the T and B lymphocyte responses (Lehner *et al.* 1976a).

Immunization reduced approximal, cervical and fissure caries by 60–80%. The reduction in caries was associated with a reduction in the number of *S. mutans* in the plaque of the immunized monkeys (Caldwell *et al.* 1977).

The immune response. A subcutaneous injection of killed cells of *S. mutans* in Freund's incomplete adjuvant elicits IgG, IgM and IgA classes of antibodies (Lehner *et al.* 1976a, 1979c). Sequential studies of these isotypes to *S. mutans* over a period of up to 3 years has shown that the IgG antibodies are maintained at a high titre, IgM antibodies progressively fall and IgA antibodies increase slowly in titre. The development of serum IgG antibodies takes place within 2 months of immunization, reaching a titre of up to 1:1280, with no change in antibodies being found in the corresponding sham-immunized monkeys. The increase in salivary IgA antibodies is very modest and not significantly different between the immunized and sham-immunized monkeys. Most of the antibody assays utilized immunofluorescence, radio-immunoassay or enzyme-linked immunosorbent assay (ELISA) to estimate antibodies to the streptococcal cells or antigen I/II in serum and crevicular fluid.

A functional opsonizing antibody assay for phagocytosis and killing of *S. mutans* by blood PMNL showed that *S. mutans* is opsonized *in vitro* by high dilution of antibodies and by complement; this leads to ingestion and killing of the organisms (Scully and Lehner 1979b). Protection against caries was associated predominantly with increased serum IgG antibodies. This is consistent with the findings that IgG, unlike IgA, antibodies are involved in opsonization of *S. mutans*.

Skin delayed hypersensitivity *in vivo* and the lymphoproliferative and leucocyte migration inhibition reactions *in vitro* are induced by immunization with *S. mutans*. The skin induration is maximal at 24–48 hours after intradermal injection of the SA and histological examination of the injected site is consistent with delayed hypersensitivity. The increased deoxyribonucleic acid (DNA) synthesis of lymphocytes from immunized monkeys stimulated with *S. mutans* is CD4-cell-dependent (Lehner 1982b). Skin delayed hypersensitivity reaction and the lymphoproliferative response to *S. mutans* have been significantly correlated with IgG and IgA but not IgM antibody titres (Lehner *et al.* 1976a). This finding is consistent with the observation that IgG and IgA antibodies are T-cell-dependent to a greater extent than IgM antibodies.

The results of systemic immunization suggest that a significant reduction in caries is associated with a reduction in the number of *S. mutans* and an increase in IgG, IgM and IgA antibody titres and T cells that are sensitized to SA (Fig. 104.5). To study directly the role of immunoregulation in T and B cell interactions, T cell helper and suppressor functions were assayed in immunized monkeys (Lehner 1982b; Lehner *et al.* 1984). Both functions were detected; however, a significantly greater amount of helper activity was found in immunized than in control monkeys. T cell helper activity is one of the essential objects of immunization, in order to elicit a prompt and effective antibody response by B cells.

Immune mechanisms in the prevention of caries

The experiments in rats and monkeys suggest

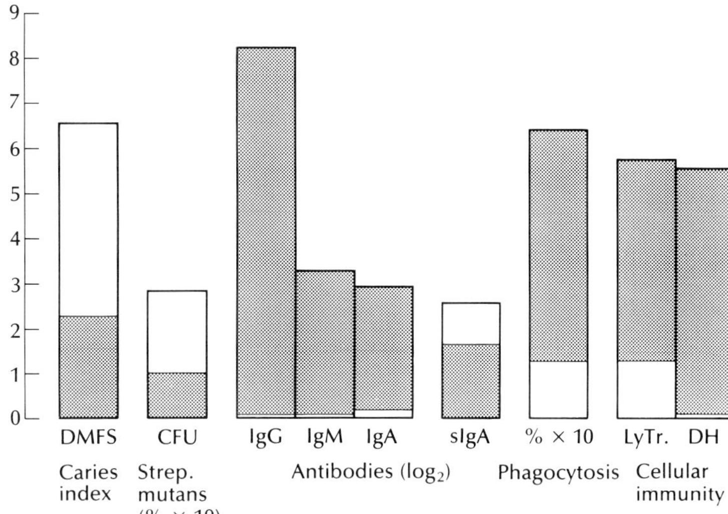

Fig. 104.5. Immunological indices, caries and the number of streptococci in immunized (shaded) and control (white) monkeys. DMFS, decayed/missing/filled surfaces; CFU, colony-forming units; LyTr, lymphocyte transformation; DH, delayed hypersensitivity.

two principal immune mechanisms of protection against caries. One involves saliva and acts on the salivary domain and the other involves gingival crevicular fluid, which affects the gingival domain. The salivary glands produce sIgA antibodies either by direct immunization of the salivary glands or, more probably by immunization of GALT, from where sensitized B cells may home to the salivary glands. Salivary IgA antibodies have, of course, direct access to the tooth surface. They may prevent *S. mutans* adhering to the enamel surface or forming dextran, by inhibiting the activity of GTF.

The gingival crevicular mechanism involves all the humoral and cellular components of the systemic immune system which may exert their functions at the tooth surface. There is now sufficient evidence to postulate what happens after subcutaneous immunization with *S. mutans*. The organism is phagocytosed and undergoes antigenic processing by macrophages. In the central lymphoid tissue T and B lymphocytes are sensitized, with formation of CD4 helper cells and CD8 cell functions. These and the related cytokines may play an essential part in modulating the formation of IgG, IgA and IgM classes of antibodies by B lymphocytes. Antibodies, complement, sensitized lymphocytes, PMNL and macrophages pass from the gingival vasculature through the junctional epithelium into crevicular fluid. Chemotactic factors for PMNL and monocytes can be generated by plaque antigens, LPS and IC, and these will activate the classical or alternative complement pathways, to generate C3a and C5a, which are chemotactic for phagocytes. Polymorphonuclear leucocytes and macrophages may be immobilized at this site by antigenic stimulation of sensitized lymphocytes, which may release macrophage and leucocyte inhibitory factors. Immunoglobulin G antibodies and complement play an essential part in opsonization which leads to binding, phagocytosis and killing by phagocytes, and this could be the principal immune mechanism against *S. mutans*. Inhibition of adherence, especially by IgA antibodies in the gingival domain, needs to be examined further. Local T and B lymphocyte responses to antigen may supplement the immune responses elicited centrally and increase the effective antibody titre and the number of phagocytes adjacent to the site of bacterial colonization.

It should not be particularly surprising that two different immune mechanisms may be involved in protection against caries. We know this to be true of other vaccines; in poliomyelitis both subcutaneous and oral immunization are effective, and yet different immune mechanisms seem to operate. It is, of course, possible that both systemic and local immunity might be necessary in the protection against caries, and we now have the immunological and bacteriological knowledge to test these concepts.

SAFETY ASPECTS OF DENTAL CARIES VACCINE

There is evidence that rabbits injected intravenously or subcutaneously with *S. mutans* in Freund's incomplete adjuvant may induce antibodies to heart muscle. (van de Rijn *et al.* 1976; Hughes *et al.* 1980; Forester *et al.* 1983; Stinson *et al.* 1983). On the other hand, rabbits are prone to develop low-affinity anti-heart antibodies spontaneously. A comprehensive series of safety tests will therefore have to be carried out before immunization trials can be started in man. However, experience with rhesus monkeys for over 10 years has not revealed any systemic side-effects or lesions at the site of injection if aluminium hydroxide or Freund's incomplete adjuvant was used as adjuvant (Bergmeier and Lehner 1983). Haematological indices were unchanged and no abnormalities were found in the heart, lungs, kidneys, liver or brain on post-mortem examination. Examination of serum for cross-reactive antibodies to heart muscle by immunofluorescence and radioimmunoassay were negative. Experience over many years in raising monoclonal antibodies to SA I/II failed to detect any anti-heart antibodies, although these were routinely screened for among thousands of antibody-forming hybridomas. Furthermore, recent evidence, using a mutant of *S. mutans* which was lacking in antigen I/II, suggests that any heart cross-reactive antigen does not reside in antigen I/II but in the cell membrane (Lee *et al.* 1989). Hence, SA I/II does not have undesirable properties and is a strong candidate for a caries vaccine.

A comprehensive review on the heart cross-reactivity with *S. mutans* was published recently (Russell and Wu 1990).

ACTIVE GINGIVO-SALIVARY IMMUNIZATION

The active gingivo-salivary immunization route has been explored in order to exclude any potential systemic side-effect and to localize the immune response to the oral cavity (Lehner *et al.* 1986b). Any objections that could be levelled against systemic immunization overloading central immunity or antigenic competition adversely affecting the immune response to other antigens is thereby overcome.

A local source of antibody synthesis in the gingival tissue has been assessed to contribute about 20% of the IgG in gingival fluid (Challacombe 1980). Investigations of the biology of the gingiva suggests that it contains a fast-migrating neutrophil population, as well as a much less mobile mononuclear cell population, i.e. monocytes, T and B lymphocytes and plasma cells. The gingiva is therefore a potential site for local immunization. Indeed, direct injection of lysozyme into rabbit gingiva elicited local antibody-forming cells to lysozyme (Brandtzaeg and Tolo 1977), and culture of mononuclear cells from the gingival tissue showed lymphoproliferative responses to mitogens and antigens (Ivanyi 1980). However, attempts at direct immunization by brushing live *S. mutans* on to the gingiva in rhesus monkeys failed to induce antibodies or prevent the development of caries (Lehner 1980).

The prerequisite for successful gingival immunization was the preparation of a smaller-molecular-weight SA (3.8 kD). A comparison of gingival applications of a high-molecular-weight (185 kD) with a low-molecular-weight (3.8 kD) SA in monkeys revealed that only the 3.8 kD peptide elicited antibodies (Lehner *et al.* 1986b). Indeed, repeated topical application of the antigen to the gingival sulcus over a period of about 1 year elicited a low but detectable increase in the IgG antistreptococcal antibody titre in the gingival fluid and IgA antibodies in the saliva. This was associated with a significant decrease in colonization of *S. mutans* and the development of caries.

The difference between the results of using the 185 kD peptide and the 3.8 kD peptide was attributed to the greater ease with which the 3.8 kD peptide can penetrate the crevicular epithelial barrier. There is evidence that the permeability through oral epithelium is related to the size of the molecule. The interesting finding in this non-invasive gingival immunization (topical applications and not injection) is that salivary IgA antibodies were also elicited. The mechanism is thought to be a retrograde entry of antigen along the ducts into the minor salivary glands.

Synthetic peptides derived from the amino acid sequences of the 3.8 kD peptide are even smaller, as they consist of 17 or 21 amino acid residues. Gingival application of these synthetic peptides again elicited a dual gingival IgG and salivary IgA antibodies to the peptide but also to the native 3.8 kD SA (Lehner *et al.* 1989). There was a significant reduction in colonization of *S. mutans* as compared with control monkeys. This rather convenient route of immunization is non-invasive, has not caused detectable side-effects and bypasses systemic immune responses and their sequelae.

PASSIVE DENTAL IMMUNIZATION

The rationale for local passive immunization was the finding that systemic passive immunization by intravenous injection of IgG antibodies to *S. mutans* protects rhesus monkeys from dental caries (Lehner *et al.* 1978). This was followed by evidence that ^{125}I-labelled serum IgG administered intravenously will pass through the gingival tissue and is detectable in gingival fluid within 30 minutes of injection (Challacombe *et al.* 1978). Furthermore, a specific IgG class of antibody to *S. mutans* was detected in the gingival fluid of animals that developed specific serum IgG antibodies after systemic immunization with *S. mutans*. These investigations led to the concept that IgG antibodies prevent colonization of *S. mutans* and the development of caries. This was then tested directly by passive immunization with an IgG class of monoclonal antibodies. Monoclonal antibodies were prepared to the streptococcal cell surface antigen I/II and applied repeatedly to the teeth of monkeys (Lehner *et al.* 1986). This resulted in decreased colonization of the teeth by *S. mutans* and prevented development of dental caries. Polyclonal antibodies in cow's milk applied directly to the teeth of rats also significantly reduced colonization of the streptococci and caries (Michalek *et al.* 1987).

Passive dental immunization with monoclonal antibodies to the cell surface SA (185 kD) has now been applied to human subjects (Ma *et al.* 1987). A purified IgG preparation of the monoclonal antibody was applied four times to the teeth and attempts were made to implant exogenous *S. mutans*. Monoclonal antibodies prevented or significantly decreased colonization of *S. mutans*, as compared with control subjects who had unrelated monoclonal antibody applied to the teeth. In subsequent experiments, recolonization with indigenous *S. mutans* was also prevented by monoclonal antibodies after this organism was reduced to undetectable levels by an antimicrobial agent (Ma *et al.* 1989). Indeed, *S. mutans* was not found for a period of over 2 years, as compared with recolonization after 2–4 weeks in control subjects. Investigations of the specificity of this human experiment revealed that only colonization of *S. mutans* and not of *S. sanguis* is prevented. Monoclonal antibody to the related *S. sobrinus* (serotypes d and g) does not prevent colonization of *S. mutans* (serotypes c, e and f). Epitope specificity of the monoclonal antibody appears to be the most important factor in preventing adherence of *S. mutans*. However, the adhesion molecule on the streptococcus might be either a carbohydrate or a protein moiety.

The $F(ab')_2$ fragment of the IgG-1 monoclonal antibody to SA I/II was as protective as the intact IgG, but the Fab fragment failed to prevent recolonization of *S. mutans* (Ma *et al.* 1990). This suggests that the two binding sites of the monoclonal antibody may be essential in preventing streptococcal colonization but that the Fc fragment-mediated phagocytosis was not essential.

The long duration of protection from colonization by *S. mutans* cannot be accounted for by functional antibody being retained on the teeth for more than a week. A four-phase hypothesis was proposed to account for the prolonged action of monoclonal antibody:

1 Monoclonal antibody adheres to the salivary glycoprotein pellicle on the tooth surface.

2 *Streptococcus mutans* cell surface determinants will be recognized by the corresponding antibody binding sites.

3 The streptococci will be opsonized by the antibodies, affecting adherence and/or proliferation of the organism and facilitate opsonization and killing by local neutrophils.

4 The ecological niche vacated by *S. mutans* is filled by another plaque organism, preventing recolonization of *S. mutans* long after the antibody function has ceased.

Immunology of oral infections

The most common infections of the oral mucosa are caused by HSV and *Candida albicans*. Oral manifestations of acquired immune deficiency syndrome (AIDS), however, are commonly found.

Herpes simplex virus infections

Clinical or subclinical primary infection by HSV type I is commonly acquired in early childhood, and in the 2nd and 3rd years of life. Primary herpetic infection in the 1st year is very rare, possibly because most mothers have neutralizing antibodies to the virus which are transferred through the placenta to the fetus. Placental transfer of cellular immunity may also take place in a small proportion of fetuses. Serum virus complement-fixing and neutralizing antibodies are found in about 50% of children at 5 years of age (Holzel *et al.* 1953; Smith *et al.* 1967).

PRIMARY HERPETIC GINGIVOSTOMATITIS

Primary herpetic infection is usually seen in the mouths of young children and less frequently in adults. The disease is recognized by an acute onset of sore mouth and often throat, fever and diffuse inflammation of the gum, followed by formation of vesicles and ulcers of the oral mucosa and regional lymphadenitis. Infants display considerable fretfulness, sleeplessness and refusal to eat. Initially there are crops of small ulcers but these coalesce to produce large, shallow, irregular ulcers with surrounding inflammation. The natural course of this infection lasts 7–14 days and healing of ulcers occurs spontaneously.

Herpetic keratitis is not often associated with herpetic stomatitis, and encephalitis is rare but may occasionally complicate the stomatitis. Herpetic infection of the nail-bed is sometimes seen in dentists who have treated patients with herpes labialis. Recurrences of herpetic lesions inside the mouth are very rare, though occasionally seen as localized crops of ulcers (Weathers and Griffin 1970). Extraoral recurrent herpetic infetion, however, commonly affects the lips.

IMMUNOPATHOLOGY OF PRIMARY HERPES VIRUS INFECTION

Herpes simplex virus is a DNA virus and there are two types: type 1 is found predominantly in the oro-facial region and type 2 in the genital region. There are three genes (α, β, γ) and the β gene codes for viral glycoproteins gB, gC, gD and gE. These viral glycoproteins have been well characterized; gB is involved in viral penetration of the cell membrane, gC constitutes the C3b receptors (binding the activated C3b) and gE is the Fc receptor for IgG. Antibodies against gD neutralize HSV and block penetration of HSV. Hence, HSV infection generates a number of significant immunological molecules in the host cell, in addition to expressing a viral antigen on the cell surface.

Herpes simplex virus gains entrance into epithelial cells of the oral mucosa. Virus replication takes place inside the nucleus and this is associated with formation of intranuclear inclusion bodies and giant cells. As more epithelial cells become infected, degenerative and oedematous changes give rise to vesicle formation, and these rupture early, resulting in ulcers. The incubation period for primary herpetic infection is 2–7 days.

Within the 1st week of onset of clinical manifestations (therefore within 2 weeks of viral infection), lymphocytes sensitized to HSV can be detected in the peripheral blood; at this time significant antibodies or macrophage MIF are not found. However, after 2 weeks, significant antibody titres and MIF appear, whilst the stimulation index of lymphocytes falls (Shillitoe *et al.* 1978). Recovery from infection coincides, therefore, with the appearance of antibody and MIF. Infection with HSV in animals is also associated with an early development of delayed skin hypersensitivity or the lymphoproliferative response, to be followed by that of antibody and MIF formation (Meyers and Pettit 1973; Rosenberg and Notkins 1974). In animals, antibody alone was not protective against dissemination of HSV and macrophages were required. Migration inhibition factor may immobilize macrophages to the site of the infection and it may also enhance their viricidal activity.

Seropositive subjects give delayed hypersensitivity reactions to HSV (Nagler 1944) and *in vitro* sensitized lymphocytes from these subjects will undergo blast cell transformation (Wilton *et al.* 1972) and produce the following lymphokines: macrophage MIF, lymphotoxin, chemotactic factor and interferon (Rasmussen *et al.* 1974; Rosenberg *et al.* 1974). In addition the lymphocytes are cytotoxic for HSV-infected target cells. There are a number of cytotoxic mechanisms and their action may depend upon the surface markers of both effector and target cells. It is a remarkable feature of HSV that within less than 6 hours of infection the infected cell surface acquires two surface markers: a virus-specific glycoprotein antigen and an Fc receptor for IgG (Watkins 1964; Westmorland and Watkins 1974). Antibodies may combine with the surface antigen and cell lysis is caused by complement activation. Antibody-dependent cellular cytotoxicity is a particularly sensitive killing mechanism and both the virus-specific surface antigen and the Fc receptor of the infected cell might be involved (Rager-Zisman and Bloom 1974; Shore *et al*. 1974). The Fc receptor of the killer cell may combine with the Fc portion of IgG antibody and the Fab portion with the HSV antigen on the cell surface (Lehner *et al*. 1975). Alternatively, IC of HSV and IgG antibodies could bind to the Fc receptors of both the target and the effector cells and result in killing the target cell.

LATENCY OF HERPES SIMPLEX VIRUS

It is now clearly recognized that, in man, HSV often remains latent after the primary infection, for years and probably throughout life. The propensity of HSV to gain entrance into the nucleus of a cell, where it may remain dormant in a non-replicating phase, has been the subject of great interest. Although oral epithelial cells and salivary glands have been considered as the reservoirs for latency of HSV (Nahmias and Roizman 1973), there is convincing evidence, in man and in animals, that the trigeminal ganglion is the principal reservoir for HSV (Stevens and Cook 1971; Waltz *et al*. 1974). The virus can be grown from trigeminal ganglia in man (Baringer and Swoveland 1973). Herpes simplex virus can also be recovered from the trigeminal ganglia in 65% of mice which have had the virus inoculated into the lips or cornea. Both clinical and subclinical infection in animals can result in latency.

The mode of entry of HSV into the trigeminal ganglion is not clear, but it appears that, during primary infection of the oral mucosa, the virus may be sequestrated to the neurones as a result of neurotropism of the virus or the inaccessibility of mononuclear killer cells to the nerves. Herpes simplex virus may enter the demyelinated nerve endings and undergo centripetal axonal migration (Paine 1964; Kristensson 1970) to the nerve cells in the trigeminal ganglion (Fig. 104.6). The mechanism of latency is unknown; it has been suggested that, as the neurone is a non-replicating cell, it may lack the specific transcriptase capable of reproducing the virus, so that both the virus and the host cell are maintained (Roizman 1974).

RECURRENT HERPES SIMPLEX VIRUS INFECTION

Recurrent HSV infection is a common condition which is usually limited to the vermilion border of the lips and the adjacent skin, and it is often referred to as a cold sore. A single vesicle or a crop of vesicles may develop a day after the prodromal phase of a tingling or burning sensation. The duration of the lesion varies usually between 3 and 10 days and the lesion recurs at various intervals for many years. A number of activating factors will precipitate recurrent HSV infection and among the most common are sunlight, cold, fever, stress, trauma, menstruation and section of the sensory root of the trigeminal ganglion. It is not clear whether there is a common mechanism for the various activating factors, but depression of HSV may lead to replication. The virus will then migrate centrifugally along the axon and will be shed at the nerve endings (Paine 1964). There is ample evidence for axonal transport of proteins and organelles (Weiss *et al*. 1962; Graftstein 1969). There is a slow and a fast axonal flow rate, and the latter, which may be greater than 40 mm/day, might

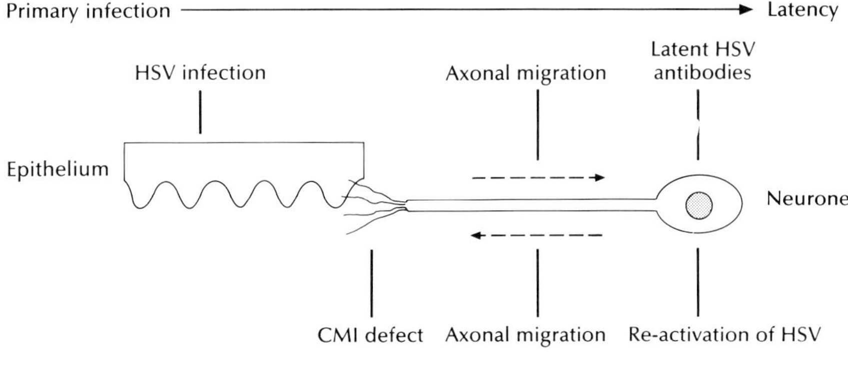

Fig. 104.6. Primary infection, latency and recurrent infection by herpes simplex virus (HSV). CMI = cell-mediated immunity.

account for recurrent HSV infection 2 days after section of the sensory root of the trigeminal ganglion. Once the virus is shed at the nerve endings a lesion may not appear if the cellular immunity is intact and the virus will be shed into the mouth, as is found in 2% of the normal population. However, in the presence of a selective cell-mediated immunodeficiency, the virus will replicate at the epithelial site of shedding and produce a recurrent lesion. The constant site for recurrences might be due to the involvement of only those neurones which innervate a restricted peripheral epithelial area.

A number of cellular defects have been recorded in patients with recurrent herpes labialis. A deficiency of MIF production and decreased cytotoxicity by CD8 cells may play a part in recurrent infection (Wilton *et al*. 1972; Shillitoe *et al*. 1977). CD4 cells produce interferon, and decreased interferon production has been correlated with an increased frequency of recurrent HSV infections (Rasmussen *et al*. 1974). Detailed sequential studies of recurrent HSV infection have shown a cyclical pattern of proliferation of lymphocytes and the release of MIF (O'Reilly *et al*. 1977; Shillitoe *et al*. 1977). Recurrent HSV infection is associated with a minimal lymphoproliferative response and MIF and interferon-γ formation. Lymphocyte stimulation is low, and increases rapidly within about 7 days. In contrast, the MIF reaction is weak or negative and takes more than 14 days to develop into a functional response. Recurrent HSV infection appears therefore to be related to a defect in lymphocyte function which consists of sluggish formation of some lymphokines. A rapid influx of macrophages and killer cells might be necessary to prevent the HSV from replicating and producing a recurrent lesion. These responses are functions of T lymphocytes, and antibody responses are intact, with perhaps slight variation in titre, during recurrent infections (Shillitoe *et al*. 1978).

In summary, therefore, recurrent HSV infection is envisaged as occurring in two stages. Herpes simplex virus in the trigeminal ganglion is released from its latent stage, permitting virus replication, axonal migration and shedding from the nerve endings near the epithelium. A selective deficiency in CMI will then enable the virus to proliferate and cause a local lesion. The importance of cellular immunity is highlighted by the intractable HSV infections found in cell-mediated immunodeficiency states (Cooper *et al*. 1968; Glasgow 1970) and in patients receiving immunosuppressive therapy.

Candidiasis

Candida is a commensal organism of the gastrointestinal tract in man. The oral carrier rate in a normal population varies between 20 and 40%. The genus *Candida* contains a number of species which are associated with disease in man. *Candida albicans* is the principal organism associated with infection, but other species such as *C. parapsilosis* and *C. kruseii* are also pathogenic for man. *Candida albicans* is a dimorphic fungus with two growth phases, the yeast form and the hyphal form.

ORAL CANDIDIASIS

There are four varieties of oral candidiasis; they are superficial infections, usually caused by *C. albicans* (Lehner 1966):

1 Acute pseudomembranous candidiasis. This disease commonly referred to as thrush, is seen in infants as well as in debilitated adults, particularly in those with diabetes, leukaemia and lymphoma. Iatrogenic agents are also important predisposing factors; systemic antibiotics, corticosteroids and immunosuppressive drugs seem to enhance *Candida* infection (Winner and Hurley 1964). Local antibiotic and corticosteroid treatment can enhance oral candidiasis. Clinical manifestations of thrush are usually symptomless white papules or cotton wool-like exudates, which can be rubbed off, leaving an erythematous mucosa.

2 Acute atrophic candidiasis. This may follow acute pseudomembranous candidiasis and is usually associated with broad-spectrum antibiotic therapy; hence it is referred to as 'antibiotic-sore tongue' (Lehner and Ward 1970). It is a type of oral candidiasis that is consistently painful, showing a smooth erythematous tongue, with angular cheilitis and, less often, inflamed lips and cheeks.

3 Chronic atrophic candidiasis. This type of *Candida* infection is better known as 'denture stomatitis', for it presents as a diffuse erythema of the palate, limited to the denture-bearing mucosa. The denture covering the palatal mucosa predisposes to proliferation of *Candida*. The lesion is usually symptomless but is often associated with angular cheilitis.

4 Chronic hyperplastic candidiasis. This is a less common type of candidiasis, which presents as a firm white patch which cannot be rubbed off and commonly affects the tongue, cheeks and lips. The lesion may persist for years; it is resistant to antimycotic treatment and has been referred to as 'candidal leucoplakia' (Cawson and Lehner 1968).

CHRONIC MUCOCUTANEOUS CANDIDIASIS

Although chronic mucocutaneous candidiasis is much less common, it has attracted a great deal of attention because of its intractable nature and the association with a variety of immunodeficiencies. The disease is characterized by persistent, superficial *Candida* infection of the mouth, nails and skin, sometimes producing granulomatous masses over the face and scalp. It can be associated with endocrine disorders, especially Addison's disease and hypoparathyroidism. Four clinical types have been described (Lehner 1964b, 1966; Hermans *et al*. 1969):

1 Chronic oral hyperplastic candidiasis. This is limited to the mouth and presents as a firm, diffuse white patch on the tongue, cheeks or lips. The lesion may persist for many years, or indeed for life, and has been differentiated from leucoplakia (Cawson and Lehner 1968).

2 Chronic localized mucocutaneous candidiasis. This condition starts in childhood as an intractable oral *Candida* infection, with involvement of nails and sometimes the adjacent skin of hands and feet. A number of other skin sites may show persistent *Candida* infection (Lehner 1966; Hermans *et al*. 1969).

3 Chronic localized mucocutaneous candidiasis with granuloma. The onset of this condition is in infancy and the clinical manifestations are similar to those in the previous type of candidiasis, with the important additional feature of granulomatous masses affecting the face and scalp. Recurrent respiratory tract infection was recorded in about a quarter of these children.

4 Chronic localized mucocutaneous candidiasis with endocrine disorder. This condition used to be found in children only, as the mortality was particularly high in the presence of Addison's disease, but nowadays the disease is also seen in young adults. A strong familial incidence is often found and candidiasis commonly precedes the endocrine abnormalities (Lehner 1966). The syndrome was named familial juvenile hypoadrenocorticism and superficial moniliasis by Whitaker *et al*. (1956). The clinical features of *Candida* infection are similar to those seen in the localized mucocutaneous variety, and the association with hypoparathyroidism illustrates the relationship between cell-mediated immunodeficiencies and autoimmune endocrine disorders.

DISSEMINATED CANDIDIASIS

In contrast to superficial candidiasis, affecting the mucous membranes and skin, *Candida* can occasionally spread to internal organs (kidneys, heart, liver, brain). This occurs, usually under the influence of iatrogenic agents, in patients suffering from other debilitating diseases (Winner and Hurley 1964).

LABORATORY DIAGNOSIS

A culture from the lesion usually yields *C. albicans*, and direct examination of scrapings shows Gram-positive hyphae and yeast cells of *Candida*. Biopsy of the lesion in chronic oral hyperplastic candidiasis and chronic mucocutaneous candidiasis is helpful, as, in addition to the superficial invasion of epithelium by *Candida* hyphae, there is parakeratosis and extensive epithelial hyperplasia. The lamina propria or dermis shows an intense mononuclear cell infiltration, with a large proportion of plasma cells. Serological tests can also be helpful when there is a rise in antibody titre. Moreover, an anti-47 kD antibody can be significant in the prognosis of systemic candidiasis.

IMMUNOLOGY OF CANDIDIASIS

There is a great deal of experimental support for the view that T cell immunity is important in preventing mucocutaneous candidiasis, whereas serum antibodies are involved in the prevention of systemic (disseminated) candidiasis.

Serum antibodies

Agglutinating antibodies to *Candida* are found in 64% of an apparently uninfected population (Winner 1955). The agglutination method assays IgG, IgM and IgA classes of antibodies (Lehner *et al*. 1972a). Precipitating antibodies, which belong mostly to the IgG class, were found more often in systemic candidiasis (Stalybrass 1964) but also in some healthy controls (Pepys *et al*. 1968; Murray *et al*. 1969) and were therefore not a reliable measure of systemic candidiasis. However, significantly increased immunoglobulin class-specific IgG and to a lesser extent IgM antibody levels were found by the immunofluorescence technique in patients with candidiasis, as compared with controls (Lehner 1966, 1970). Recent evidence suggests that serum IgG and IgM antibodies to immunodominant antigens in the range of 44–60 kD may be protective, as they are found in patients who recover from systemic candidiasis (Stockbine *et al*. 1984; Matthews *et al*. 1987). There is experimental evidence that humoral immunity is more important than CMI in preventing systemic candidiasis. Athymic mice (nude mice) are more resistant to disseminated candidiasis than normal mice after intravenous administration of *C. albicans* (Rogers and Balish 1977). Transfer of immune serum to unprotected mice conferred resistance to candidiasis, whereas transfer of immune lymphocytes had no effect, in spite of inducing skin delayed hypersensitivity reactions.

Secretory immunoglobulin A antibodies

Secretory IgA antibodies to *C. albicans* are found in saliva, and a parallel investigation of *Candida* antibodies in serum and saliva revealed a similar relationship between them, though at a much lower titre in saliva. It is, however, well recognized that the rate of secretion of saliva varies and is difficult to standardize, so that comparisons between different subjects can be misleading. In order to overcome this difficulty, Chilgren *et al*. (1967) expressed antibodies as a ratio between the salivary IgA concentration and the titre of antibody to *C. albicans*. Using this formula for expressing salivary *Candida* antibody levels, a significant differentiation into three groups was possible: non-carrier controls, *Candida* carriers and patients with chronic mucocutaneous candidiasis (Lehner *et al*. 1972b).

The relationship between salivary IgA and serum IgG, IgM and IgA antibodies to *C. albicans* runs in parallel in the control, carrier and oral candidiasis group of subjects and this suggests that antigenic stimulation, initiated in the mouth and probably in the alimentary canal, induced both local secretory and systemic antibody responses. This relationship, however, breaks down when patients with chronic mucocutaneous candidiasis are considered.

Chemotaxis, opsonization, phagocytosis and killing of Candida

Chemotactic defects in PMNL have been found in patients who are susceptible to *Candida* infections, for example new-born infants (Miller 1969) and diabetics (Clark and Kimball 1971). Chemotactic defects have also been reported for monocytes in chronic mucocutaneous candidiasis (Snyderman *et al*. 1973). Antibody and complement are necessary for optimal phagocytosis of *Candida* by PMNL or macrophages. Both opsonizing agents are found in normal serum, which can induce phagocytosis and killing of live *Candida* blastospores. The hyphal forms, however, can escape phagocytosis, particularly if they are large in size (Davies and Denning 1972).

Immune complexes of *Candida* and antibodies activate the classical complement pathway, but whole *C. albicans* or soluble extracts of the blastospores activate the alternative pathway of complement (Ray and Wuepper 1975). Indeed, depressed levels of serum complement have been recorded, and C3 and properdin have been found in biopsies of some patients with chronic mucocutaneous candidiasis (Sohnle *et al*. 1976). Phagocytic defects have been reported in some patients prone to develop candidiasis, but these patients have usually been treated with antibiotics, steroids or cytotoxic drugs (Wilton and Lehner 1979a). These agents are associated with depressed phagocytosis, and antibiotics such as tetracycline and gentamycin can inhibit C3 consumption.

Poor resistance to *Candida* infection can be found in patients with high titres of *Candida* antibodies and normal complement levels, so that other factors may be more important in the defence against *Candida*. Indeed, a *Candida* clumping factor has been found in practically all normal sera; this factor seems to be absent in mucocutaneous and systemic candidiasis and is reduced in diabetes, leukaemia and carcinoma (Louria *et al*. 1972). Furthermore, a candidacidal factor has also been found in normal human serum, and inhibiting antibodies to this factor have been detected in some patients with mucocutaneous candidiasis.

The biological role of these factors is not clear, but they are not antibodies. Complement deficiencies may also play a part in mucocutaneous candidiasis (Kirkpatrick *et al.* 1971).

Normal PMNL and monocytes can kill *C. albicans in vitro* and the principal mechanism of killing is mediated by myeloperoxidase and hydrogen peroxide (Klebanoff 1967; Lehner and Cline 1969). Some patients with leukaemia show a depression of killing of *C. albicans* by PMNL. Systemic candidiasis can also be associated with the absence of myeloperoxidase in phagocytes. The defect, however, might reside in migration of the phagocytes to the inflammatory site. Such a chemotactic defect has been found in PMNL of patients susceptible to *Candida* infections, for example diabetics (Mowat and Baum 1971), and in PMNL and monocytes of patients with chronic mucocutaneous candidiasis (Snyderman *et al.* 1973; Van Scoy *et al.* 1975). It is of interest that cell wall mannan and complement are chemotactic for PMNL.

Cell-mediated immunity

Cutaneous delayed hypersensitivity reactions and *in vitro* tests for *C. albicans* in a normal population are usually positive, although the actual incidence varies with the protein : mannan ratio of the antigen and the population tested. Positive skin induration, 24–28 hours after intradermal administration of *C. albicans* antigen, varies between 46 and 94% (Lewis *et al.* 1937; Shannon *et al.* 1966). The lymphocyte transformation and macrophage migration inhibition tests for *Candida* are also positive in a high proportion of the normal population.

Cell-mediated immunity has been studied comprehensively in chronic mucocutaneous candidiasis and a spectrum of CMI defects have been reported. Skin anergy to *C. albicans*, and often to other unrelated antigens, has been found in most patients and a deficiency of macrophage MIF was postulated by Chilgren *et al.* (1967) as the defect responsible for skin anergy in the presence of intact lymphocyte transformation. This was also reported by Valdimarsson *et al.* (1970) and Lehner *et al.* (1972b). A serum inhibitory factor which prevents lymphocyte transformation was found in one patient with mucocutaneous candidiasis by Canales *et al.* (1969).

Investigation of 15 patients with the four types of chronic mucocutaneous candidiasis revealed a heterogeneous pattern of immunodeficiencies and these have been ranked into a spectrum of increasing cell-mediated immunodeficiencies (Lehner *et al.* 1972b). The largest group of patients show a defect in skin delayed hypersensitivity, macrophage migration inhibition and the lymphoproliferative responses to *C. albicans*, and, less commonly, to unrelated antigens. It was suggested that T suppressor cells might be responsible for some of the defects in mucocutaneous candidiasis (De Sousa *et al.* 1976).

TREATMENT

All varieties of oral candidiasis except the chronic hyperplastic type respond readily to topical oral treatment with antifungal drugs; tablets of nystatin 500 000 units qds or amphotericin B 10 mg qds used for 1–2 weeks are very effective. Chronic mucocutaneous candidiasis, however, usually does not respond to topical oral treatment and necessitates intravenous administration of amphotericin B. Although almost complete eradication of the lesions can be accomplished, the disease tends to return after the drug is discontinued and the drug is highly nephrotoxic. Some of the other antifungal agents (e.g. clotrimazole) suffer from the same disadvantage — that the disease recurs if treatment is stopped. This is comprehensible on the basis of an underlying immunological defect, which, if not rectified, will lead to reinfection with *Candida*.

A number of immunotherapeutic measures have been tried with some success. Transplantation of bone marrow (Buckley *et al.* 1968), thymus (Levy *et al.* 1971) and immunocompetent allogeneic lymphocytes (Kirkpatrick *et al.* 1971) resulted in clinical improvement and restoration of some of the cell-mediated immune markers. Transfer factor has been used in the past with variable results in patients lacking MIF, cutaneous delayed hypersensitivity and/or DNA synthesis of stimulated lymphocytes (Chilgren *et al.* 1969; Rocklin *et al.* 1970; Valdimarsson *et al.* 1972; Lawrence 1974; Grob *et al.* 1975).

Oral manifestations of acquired immune deficiency syndrome

Although there is little convincing evidence that

the human immunodeficiency virus (HIV) directly infects oral tissues, lesions in the mouth are commonly found and indeed can be the presenting feature of this disease (Center for Disease Control 1986; Greenspan and Greenspan 1987). There is a wide variety of clinical manifestations of AIDS in the mouth, which will be described briefly.

FUNGAL INFECTIONS

Infection occurs with the most common species *C. albicans*, although the other candidal species can be involved. All varieties of oral candidiasis (see above) have been recorded in AIDS, but it appears that the chronic hyperplastic and atrophic varieties are more frequent than the pseudomembranous variety. Other fungal lesions may occur but are rare (e.g. histoplasmosis and cryptococcosis).

VIRAL INFECTIONS

Herpes simplex virus

Recurrent oral herpetic lesions are frequently found on the palate or gums in AIDS patients, starting as painful vesicles that ulcerate. It should be remembered that recurrent intraoral herpetic lesions are extremely uncommon in the rest of the population (unlike recurrent herpes labialis). Orofacial lesions due to herpes zoster have also been recorded but are rather rare.

Epstein–Barr virus

Hairy leucoplakia is a raised white plaque, commonly affecting the tongue, and is clinically similar to chronic hyperplastic candidiasis. There is some evidence that it might be caused by the Epstein–Barr virus found in the epithelial cells. Similar lesions have not been recorded in the general population.

Papillomavirus

Papillomavirus is the common wart virus; it causes single or multiple warts in the mouth of AIDS patient.

NEOPLASIA

Kaposi's sarcoma is a neoplasm of the vascular endothelial cells. Oral lesions present as red or purple macules or papules, often affecting the palate and frequently the tongue. Other neoplasias are less common but non-Hodgkin's lymphomas and squamous carcinomas have been recorded.

GINGIVITIS AND PERIODONTITIS

The gingiva may show changes similar to those of acute necrotizing ulcerative gingivitis, except that these may be superimposed on rapidly progressing periodontitis. The condition can be painful and can be associated with rapid loss of soft tissue and bone support, leading to loss of teeth.

OTHER LESIONS

Recurrent oral ulcers are probably more common in patients with AIDS than in the general population. Salivary gland enlargement, especially the parotid glands, might be caused by some viral infection.

NATURE OF EPITHELIAL ORIFICES IN TRANSMISSION OF HUMAN IMMUNODEFICIENCY VIRUS

There may be some special feature about rectal mucosa which makes receptive anogenital sex by far the highest risk factor, in contrast to vaginal intercourse, which carries a smaller risk, and oral mucosa in orogenital sex, with a very low risk of infection.

The presence of appropriate viral receptors, such as CD4 glycoprotein, in the epithelial lining

The very thin epithelium of the rectal mucosa differs greatly from the stratified squamous epithelium of vaginal and oral mucosa. A comparative study of CD4 glycoprotein on these mucosal surfaces showed that CD4 was not expressed on the epithelial cell surface, although CD4 cells were found under all three epithelia (Hussain *et al.* 1991).

Humoral and cellular immune defences of the orifices

Whereas the three mucosal surfaces may have in common sIgA and some aggregated lymphoid tissue, any local immunodeficiency has not been explored. Indeed, promiscuity, with multiple partners, induces a variety of infections, which may affect rectal immunity to a relatively greater extent than that of the other orifices.

SALIVARY TRANSMISSION OF HUMAN IMMUNODEFICIENCY VIRUS

The potential of salivary transmission of HIV is of immense significance to the public at large, as saliva is encountered during daily social interchanges of talking, coughing, sneezing and kissing. We must recognize that oral fluid consists of saliva and gingival fluid. Most if not all the cellular components in oral fluid (whole saliva) originate from blood, passing into gingival fluid and then mixing with saliva to result in oral fluid. Although about 90% of the gingival fluid cells are neutrophils, the rest consists of T and B cells and macrophages. Oral fluid may then contain some CD4 +ve cells, thereby creating the essential conditions for HIV transmission. Nevertheless, there is little or no evidence that salivary transmission of HIV can occur (Groopman *et al*. 1984). Comparative isolation studies of HIV from body fluids have been carried out and these suggest that, whilst HIV can be cultured from oral fluid (whole saliva), the frequency of isolation is low (1.2–9%), as compared with semen (21%) or plasma (55%) (Ho *et al*. 1985). The quantity of HIV isolated from saliva is also very low. The available evidence suggests that it is the cellular fraction of oral fluid, presumably CD4 cells and macrophages, and not the fluid fraction, originating mostly from the salivary glands, which is the potential source of HIV infection.

The special significance to the dentist of oral transmission of HIV is self-evident, as he works in a pool of saliva and often gingival bleeding. Yet no known seropositive conversions were found among about 1000 dental staff in the US and the same number tested in Germany (Klein *et al*. 1988). Only one out of 1309 dentists in another US study was seropositive and he was a man who did not wear protective gloves (Gerberding *et al*. 1987). This is almost a negligible prevalence of HIV seropositivity in a population of dentists among whom more than 90% admitted to needlestick injuries. The very low risk, if any, to dentists is both surprising and gratifying, when compared with the high risk of transmission of hepatitis B viral infection; about 20% of health workers exposed to accidental injuries with infected needles acquire the virus. This can be explained by the enormous difference in the concentration of infectious particles in the blood — up to 10^{13} viral particles per ml of blood in hepatitis B, compared with only 10^4 particles in AIDS.

IMMUNOLOGY OF HUMAN IMMUNODEFICIENCY VIRUS

The immunology of HIV is outside the scope of this section and the reader is referred to Chapter 71. There are, however, a number of features which will be discussed.

Immune responses to human immunodeficiency virus

Humoral responses. Viral neutralizing antibodies are found in AIDS and AIDS-related complex (ARC) and have been tested by replication of HIV in target cells or by inhibition of syncytium formation. However, the diagnosis of HIV infection is routinely carried out by ELISA and confirmed by the immunoblotting (Western) method (Jeffries *et al*. 1985; Redfield and Burke 1988). The time from HIV exposure to a full antibody response (seroconversion) varies when HIV is transmitted by blood (e.g. in haemophiliacs) and the latent period is 6–8 weeks. Seroconversion can, however, be delayed for years, when there is evidence of free HIV antigen in blood or HIV-specific ribonucleic acid (RNA) in the circulating mononuclear cells.

Extensive investigation for HIV antibodies has revealed low-level IgA or IgM class of antibody responses to the core antigen p24 or p17 during the earliest stages of seroconversion. All immunoglobulin classes are increased, probably due to polyclonal B cell stimulation. However, the patient usually fails to produce specific antibodies on immunization with an antigen and most patients have circulating IC.

Cellular responses. There is a marked lymphopenia and the CD4 cells are decreased to less than 400 cells/mm^2. Functional *in vitro* tests of peripheral blood lymphocytes show reduced responses to mitogens (e.g. phytohaemagglutinin (PHA)) and to antigens (e.g. *Candida*). *In vivo* tests of skin delayed hypersensitivity are impaired. There is also a reduced IL-2 production by T cells. Natural killer cell activity and specific cytotoxicity are reduced. It is noteworthy that patients with Kaposi's sarcoma also have impaired T and B cell immunity but these tend to be less severe than in patients with opportunistic infections. Phagocytic functions are normal and so are the levels of complement.

Salivary immunoglobulin A antibodies

Immunoglobulin A concentration in whole saliva of patients with AIDS is reduced as compared with controls, and the reduction was ascribed predominantly to that of the IgA-2 isotype (Jackson 1990). A detailed investigation of parotid salivary IgA confirmed the reduction of salivary IgA in patients with AIDS, as compared with asymptomatic seropositive subjects or seronegative controls (Müller *et al.* 1991). However, both IgA-1 and IgA-2 isotypes were decreased. It is noteworthy that, whilst salivary IgA was significantly decreased, serum IgA was significantly increased. Despite the decrease in salivary IgA concentration, sIgA antibodies to HIV antigens are found in parotid saliva of patients with AIDS (Archibald *et al.* 1986, 1987).

Autoallergic manifestations

Recurrent oral ulcers

Recurrent oral ulcers (ROU) are the most common lesions affecting the oral mucosa and the incidence varies between 10 and 34%. The clinical features have been well described by Sircus *et al.* (1957), Farmer (1958) and Cooke (1961). There are three varieties of ROU: minor aphthous ulcers, major aphthous ulcers and herpetiform ulcers (Lehner 1968). The differentiating clinical features of these ulcers are shown in Table 104.3. An association of any one of these three types of oral ulcers with genital, ocular, cutaneous, joint, vascular or neurological manifestations is known as Behçet's syndrome (BS) (Behçet 1937). The latter is considered here because the immunopathological features share a number of features with those found in ROU.

MINOR APHTHOUS ULCERS

The term minor aphthous ulcers was introduced by Truelove and Morris-Owen (1958) but the disease is also known by its traditional name of Mickulicz aphthae (Mickulicz and Kummel 1898). About 80% of ROU are of this type; they are extremely common, especially in the 10–40 age-group, more frequently in females than males.

A prodromal phase is recognized by most patients 1–2 days before the onset of ulceration as a burning or pricking sensation. With the breakdown of epithelium and associated inflammatory reaction, the pain increases in severity, particularly on eating. The patients are, however, usually free of general symptoms. The ulcers are round or oval, up to five in number, and enlarge in size, although they remain well under 10 mm in diameter. They have a yellow floor, with a slightly raised margin and often marked surrounding erythema and oedema. The most common sites of involvement are the mucosa of the lips and cheeks and margin of the tongue, and the ulcers last 4–14

Table 104.3. Differentiating features of three varieties of recurrent oral ulcers

	Minor aphthous ulcers	Major aphthous ulcers	Herpetiform ulcers
Sex ratio F : M	1.3 : 1	0.8 : 1	2.6 : 1
Age of onset (year) (peak incidence)	10–19	10–19	20–29
Number of ulcers	1–5	1–10	10–100
Size (mm)	<10	>10	1–2
Duration (days)	4–14	10–30	7–10
Healing by scar (%)	8	64	32
Recurrence (months)	1–4	< Monthly	< Monthly
Sites	Lips, cheeks, tongue	Lips, cheeks, tongue, pharynx, palate	Lips, cheeks, tongue, pharynx, palate, floor, gum
Total duration (year)	<5	>15	>5
Associated oral lesions	—	Erythema migrans	—
Treatment (local)	Corticosteroids	Corticosteroids	Tetracycline

days. The rate of recurrences varies from 1 to 4 months and is usually irregular. However, in some females, recurrence of ulceration is related to the menstrual period. Enlargement of lymph nodes is uncommon and the patients do not have a raised temperature.

MAJOR APHTHOUS ULCERS

Major aphthous ulcers are severe variants of minor aphthous ulcers and less than 10% of patients with ROU have this type of ulcer. The pain which develops after the prodromal symptoms can be severe and persistent, so that patients find it difficult to eat and often lose weight.

Examination may reveal 1–10 ulcers at a time and some of these may enlarge to about 30 mm in diameter. The ulcers are necrotic, with a raised margin and inflammation of the adjacent tissues, so they occasionally mimic a carcinomatous ulcer. In addition to the lips, cheeks and tongue, the soft palate and tonsillar region are commonly involved. Healing of an ulcer may take 10–40 days and recurrences are so frequent that there are periods of continuous ulceration. Multiple scars may result from the large ulcers and these may assist in the diagnosis of major aphthous ulcers. The incidence of major aphthous ulcers is probably significantly raised in ulcerative colitis (Edwards and Truelove 1964).

HERPETIFORM ULCERS

Herpetiform ulcers are recurrent crops of small ulcers, up to 100 in number, affecting any part of the mouth, including the gums, palate and dorsum of the tongue. The term herpetiform was coined by Cooke (1960) and does not imply that the ulcers are caused by herpes virus. They account for less than 10% of ROU and are much more common in females than males. Patients present with pain on eating and talking, and often with dysphagia; malaise and loss of weight can be prominent features. The lesions persist for 7–14 days and commonly new ulcers appear before the previous crop has healed, so that ulceration becomes continuous.

AETIOLOGY OF RECURRENT APHTHOUS ULCERS

Although a large variety of causes have been suggested, the aetiology of recurrent aphthous ulcers (RAU) has not been established. Trauma is unlikely to play an essential role, although it might precipitate ulceration. There is no evidence that vitamin deficiency or food allergy is involved. Whilst emotional stress may influence the pattern of the disease, it is unlikely to be the direct cause. A family history of recurrent aphthous ulceration is often present, and the highest incidence of ulcers is recorded in siblings in whom both parents have recurrent aphthous ulcers. A hormonal disturbance may play a part, as in some female patients there is a relationship between the ulcers and the menstrual period, the onset of ulceration may coincide with puberty and the ulcers often disappear during pregnancy.

About 8% of hospital out-patients with ROU may have iron, folate or vitamin B_{12} deficiency anaemias (Wray *et al.* 1975; Challacombe *et al.* 1977a). About 2% may suffer from malabsorption syndrome due to allergy to dietary gluten (Ferguson *et al.* 1976).

Streptococcus sanguis or its L form was suggested as a cause of RAU, as the L form was thought to be isolated preferentially from patients with RAU and *S. sanguis* elicited a delayed hypersensitivity reaction in most of these patients (Barile *et al.* 1963; Graykowski *et al.* 1966). The same organism, however, stimulated lymphocyte transformation to a lesser extent in patients than in controls (Francis and Oppenheim 1970), and it was commonly found in normal subjects.

The possibility has been recently raised that cross-reactivity between heat-shock proteins of bacterial origin (e.g. the 65 kD protein in mycobacteria, *S. sanguis* and others) and the homologous heat-shock proteins in oral mucosa may account for some of the autoimmune manifestations (Lehner *et al.* 1991). The HSV genome was found in lymphocytes of some patients with ROU and this might have an effect on the pahogenesis of this disease (Eglin *et al.* 1982). Many patients have some immunological abnormality, with autoimmune responses to oral mucosal antigens or some cross-reacting microbial antigen (Lehner 1964a; Dolby 1969; Donatsky 1976).

IMMUNOLOGICAL FEATURES

Histocompatibility antigens

Patients with ROU show an association with HLA-B12 (Challacombe *et al.* 1977b). Although the relative risk is low (2.9), this increases with HLA-B12 and/or DR2 to a relative risk of 5.2 (Lehner *et al.* 1982). The significance of either of these HLA antigens is not clear, although they offer an immunogenetic basis for ROU, which has a strong association among family members.

Immunoglobulin, complement and antibodies

A slight increase in serum IgA was found, especially in major aphthous ulcers (Lehner 1969b). Normal concentrations of C3 and C4 were found in ROU. An increased concentration of C9, but not of the classical acute-phase reactants, was found in ROU (Lehner and Adinolfi 1980).

Nuclear thyroid and gastric autoantibodies are not found in ROU. Early studies suggested that autoantibodies to saline homogenates of oral mucosa are found in some patients with ROU, as compared with controls (Lehner 1964a). The autoantibodies belong predominantly to the IgM and IgG classes and they are not specific to oral mucosa. As pointed out above, these autoantibodies may be accounted for by the homology between bacterial and mucosal heat-shock proteins. Indirect immunofluorescence with sera from patients with ROU have shown significant cytoplasmic fluorescence of human buccal mucosa (Donatsky and Dabelsteen 1974).

Immune complexes

Immune complexes have been found in about 40% of patients with ROU (Levinsky and Lehner 1978). Their significance is not clear, especially as IC have not been detected at the site of the lesion. Nevertheless, they may be involved in activating complement, with an effect on chemotaxis of PMNL, as well as in complement-dependent lysis of cells.

In vitro cell-mediated immunity

A significant lymphoproliferative response was induced by homogenates of oral mucosa in ROU, but not in controls (Lehner 1967). Furthermore, lymphocytes induce cytotoxicity in cultures of gingival epithelial target cells (Dolby 1969; Rogers *et al.* 1974). A correlation was found in sequential studies between the clinical features of ROU and CMI, as assessed by proliferation of lymphoand cytotoxicity. The histological and functional studies suggest that the cellular responses may play an important effector part in the recurrences of oral ulcers.

IMMUNOPATHOLOGY

An intense lymphomonocytic infiltration is found, on histological examination of the early stages of ulceration, in the lamina propria, the adjacent epithelium and around blood-vessels (Graykowski *et al.* 1966; Lehner 1969a). Later a mixed response becomes evident, with PMNL predominating and some plasma cells. The early stages are suggestive of a type IV delayed hypersensitivity reaction and this is supported by electron-microscopic findings of mononuclear cell infiltration near the basement membrane and the adjacent epithelial cells. A qualitative and quantitative immunohistological investigation of biopsies from oral ulcers of patients with ROU revealed that HLA-DR is expressed on the cell membrane of keratinocytes (Poulter and Lehner 1989). A prominent mononuclear cell infiltration consisted predominantly of T lymphocytes, and the proportion of the CD4 and CD8 subsets was about 2:1. There was a significant increase in the number of Langerhans' cells in the epithelium and macrophages in the lamina propria. The results suggest an enhanced immune response:

1 In the epithelium, keratinocytes express Class II MHC antigen (HLA-DR) and an increased number of Langerhans' cells.

2 In the lamina propria, there is a prominent infiltration of CD4, CD8 and macrophage-like cells.

The characteristic pattern of exacerbations and remissions of oral ulcers can be interpreted by the hypothesis that an initiating microbial agent may induce mononuclear cell infiltration, with the release of cytokines and the expression of Class II MHC antigen in keratinocytes, causing ulceration. This is followed by down-regulation of immunity by tolerant T cells, induced by the Class II MHC +ve keratinocytes, leading to remission of ulceration (Poulter and Lehner 1989).

TREATMENT

Topical corticosteroids are the most helpful agents in alleviating aphthous ulcers. They are most effective if application is started during the prodromal phase, before mucosal ulceration and the intensity of lymphocyte transformation has reached peak values (Lehner 1969b). If steroids are applied early, an ulcer may not appear, but application at a later stage may reduce the severity and duration of ulceration. Triamcinolone in Orabase ointment or betamethasone sodium phosphate tablets (0.5 mg) used as a mouthwash (qds) are particularly helpful. Topical tetracycline is the drug of choice in controlling herpetiform ulcers, but is also useful in controlling some major aphthous ulcers, particularly when there is an excessive amount of inflammation. Its mode of action is not clear.

Behçet's disease

Behçet's disease (BD) was first described as recurrent oral and genital ulceration with iridocyclitis (Behçet 1937, 1938). A variety of other manifestations were later added and these include cutaneous, vascular, joint, neurological and gastrointestinal manifestations (Dowling 1961; Oshima *et al.* 1963; Shimizu *et al.* 1965). The clinical manifestations of the multisystem disease have been reviewed by Chajek and Fainaru (1975) and Lehner and Barnes (1979).

Recently, international criteria for the diagnosis of BD were established (International Study Group 1990). These state that ROU must be present, with two of the following manifestations: recurrent genital ulcers, skin lesions, eye lesions and positive pathergy test (Table 104.4). The pathergy test elicits a vesicular lesion within 24–48 hours of pricking the skin with a needle (International Study Group 1990). The spectrum of clinical manifestations has led to a classification of BD (Table 104.5).

Table 104.4. International criteria for the diagnosis of Behçet's disease

Recurrent oral ulcers and two of the following:
1 Recurrent genital ulcers
2 Skin lesions (erythema nodosum, papulo-pustular or acneiform lesion)
3 Eye lesions (uveitis, retinal vasculitis or cells in vitreous)
4 Positive pathergy test

Table 104.5. Classification of Behçet's disease

Mucocutaneous type: international criteria, with genital ulcers and skin lesions
Arthritic type: international criteria and joint lesions
Neurological type: international criteria and brain lesions
Ocular type: international criteria and eye lesions

EPIDEMIOLOGY

The world literature on 907 patients has been surveyed; this included 716 patients reviewed in 1966 and eight series of 10 or more patients reported between 1966 and 1976 (Lehner 1977b). The geographical distribution is given in Fig. 104.7. Although this type of survey, at best, gives only a general trend of the prevalence of BD, nevertheless the very large number reported in Japan (more than 412 patients) is striking. A high prevalence of

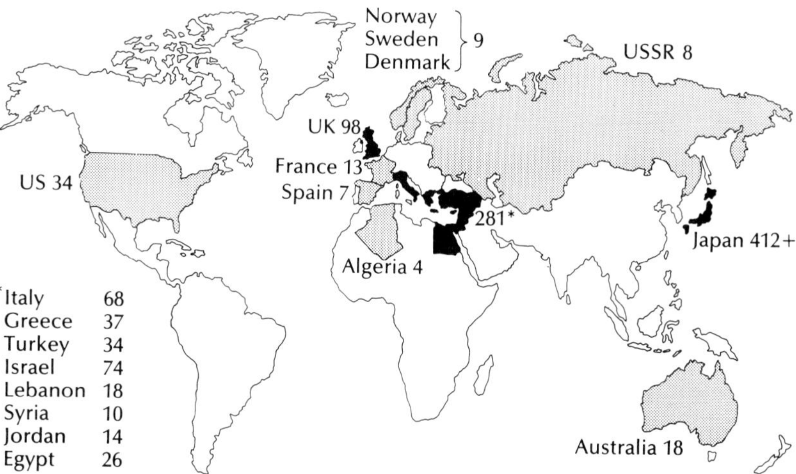

Fig. 104.7. Geographical distribution of Behcet's syndrome.

BD has now also been reported from China (Zhang 1989). The true prevalence of BD has not been determined but in an epidemiological study from the Hokkaido district a prevalence of 1 in 10 000 of the population has been recorded. This compares with 1 : 300 000 in North America (O'Duffy 1978) and about 1 : 170 000 in England (Chamberlain 1977). The prevalence is also high in countries bordering the Mediterranean (312 patients), where the disease was first reported (Turkey and Greece). Somewhat surprisingly, a relatively high prevalence has been reported from Britain (98 patients), in the list of 33 countries. It is difficult to account for the geographical distribution by some common environmental factor, viral agent or susceptibility to BD. However, the suggestion has been made that the disease follows the old silk route between latitudes 30° and 45°N in Asian and Eurasian populations (Ohno and Matsuda 1986). This covers not only Japan and the Middle East but also China, Korea and Iràn, suggesting the possibility that the disease was spread from one site, both east and west, along the migration route of the people involved in the silk route.

Although BD may develop at any age, the mean age of onset is 20–30 years. Behçet's disease may follow ROU after an interval ranging from 1 to 20 years. There is no way of predicting in any patient with ROU the development of BD, but this must be infrequent. Although most commonly oral, genital and cutaneous manifestations precede neuro-ocular or joint involvement, the sequence can be reversed. Behçet's disease develops more often in men than in women and the mean M : F ratio calculated from a review of 683 patients was 2.3 : 1. Familial association has been recorded in many patients so that genetic factors may be significant.

AETIOLOGY OF BEHÇET'S DISEASE

A viral aetiology was postulated by Behçet (1937) and a virus was isolated from the eyes of two patients by Sezer (1953) and from the eye and brain of another patient by Evans *et al.* (1957). They also showed a raised titre of neutralizing antibodies in patients but not controls. From a review of the literature, Dudgeon (1961) concluded that a viral aetiology was not proved, as there were many unsuccessful attempts at growing viruses.

The role of HSV in the aetiology of BD is not that of a direct infection causing the disease but most probably as an effect on T cell immunoregulation (Denman *et al.* 1986; Lehner 1986). The initial demonstration of part of the HSV genome in circulating mononuclear cells by *in situ* DNA–RNA hybridization (Eglin *et al.* 1982) was confirmed by the dot blot DNA–DNA hybridization method (Bonass *et al.* 1986). The polymerase chain reaction was then applied and this revealed that an EcoRI cut of HSV-1 is found in the circulating lymphocytes but not at the site of oral ulceration of patients with BD (Studd *et al.* 1991).

The possibility that *Mycoplasma pneumoniae* may be associated with the aetiology of BD was raised by finding cold agglutinins in two patients (Strom 1965). However, complement-fixing antibodies to *M. pneumoniae* were not raised in 12 sera from patients with BD (unpublished data).

Streptococcus sanguis (or the L form) was first implicated in the aetiology of oral aphthous ulcers (Barile *et al.* 1963) but the prevalence of organisms and the immune responses were difficult to differentiate between patients and healthy controls (Graykowski *et al.* 1966). Antigenic cross-reactivity between *S. sanguis* and mucosal antigens was postulated but not detected (Lehner 1972), though claimed by others (Donatsky 1976). Recently, a significant association was postulated between *S. sanguis* and BD (Mizushima 1989). This was based on finding an increased proportion of uncommon serotypes of *S. sanguis*, raised agglutinating antibody titres, more severe skin reactions and enhanced chemiluminescence of circulating leucocytes in BD, as compared with controls.

Streptococcus pyogenes was also implicated in the aetiology of BD, by finding streptococcal antigen in the plasma of patients with uveitis and a significant decrease in antibody titre, compared with controls (Namba *et al.* 1984). Furthermore, group D streptococcal antigens were found at the site of the leucocyte infiltration and in the vascular wall of oral ulcers in BD (Kaneko *et al.* 1985). In addition to β-haemolytic streptococci and *S. sanguis*, *S. salivarius* and *S. faecalis* may also be involved in BD (Mizushima 1989).

Especially significant was the finding that whole cell and cell wall preparations of four groups of streptococci elicit strong 48-hour skin reactions and provoke exacerbations in ocular symptoms, oral and genital ulcers, skin lesions or arthritis in 18% of patients with BD (Mizushima 1989). The extensive antigenic cross-reactivity between heat-shock proteins of Gram-positive bacteria (Thole *et al.* 1988) and the corresponding mammalian antigens (Jindal *et al.* 1989) led to the unified hypothesis that common epitopes within heat-shock proteins might account for the immunological responses to the diverse species of streptococci and herpes simplex virus and the autoantibodies to oral mucosal and retinal antigens (Lehner *et al.* 1991). Indeed, monoclonal antibodies to the 65 kD mycobacterial heat-shock protein revealed a band of about 65 kD with *S. sanguis* (Lehner *et al.* 1991). Furthermore, a significant increase in the IgA antibody titre to the 65 kD heat-shock protein was found in patients with BD, as compared with healthy controls. A high degree of homology was established between human and microbial heat-shock proteins (Jindal *et al.* 1989). The results suggest that at least some of the responses to the four diverse species of streptococci might be interpreted on the basis of a common epitope between the cross-reacting stress proteins. Furthermore, four monoclonal antibodies to the heat-shock protein reacted on immunoblotting with oral mucosal homogenate. The early reports with tissue homogenates (Lehner 1967; Oshima *et al.* 1963) might therefore also be accounted for by an immune response to mammalian stress proteins. Herpes simplex virus 1 failed to react on immunoblotting with anti-65 kD antibodies (Lehner *et al.* 1991) but HSV-1 does not induce the 65 kD but the 40 kD stress proteins (La Thangue and Latchman 1988).

A vascular theory was suggested by France *et al.* (1951), based on the frequent occurrence of thrombosis and microscopical findings of endothelial proliferation, leading to occlusion of the lumen of vessels. Fibrinoid necrosis has been described in BD, though not as a consistent pathological feature, but no similarity with periarteritis nodosa has been substantiated.

IMMUNOGENETIC BASIS OF BEHÇET'S DISEASE

The most significant marker of BD is HLA-B51, as described in Japan (Ohno *et al.* 1975), Turkey (Yazici *et al.* 1977), Israel (Brautbar *et al.* 1978), Tunisia (Hamza *et al.* 1979) and France (Godeau *et al.* 1976). This was apparently not found in a British series (Chamberlain 1977) or North American series (O'Duffy *et al.* 1974). However, if patients with ocular manifestations of BD were selected, their HLA-B51 was significantly increased (Lehner *et al.* 1979a). Indeed, the RR of 7.3 in the British series compares well with that found in Japan (6.7), Israel (5.2) and France (7.9).

Analysis of HLA-A, B and DR antigens according to the spectrum of tissues involved showed that HLA-B44 (B12) was significantly increased in the mucocutaneous type (RR 7.1) and to a lesser extent in the arthritic type (RR 3.2) (Lehner *et al.* 1979a). However, the RR is increased with B44 and/or DR2 in the arthritic type (RR 9.6). Human leucocyte antigen was significantly associated with the neurological (RR 7.2) and ocular (RR 8.5) types (Lehner *et al.* 1982), but surprisingly DR7 is not found in Japan. However, HLA-DRw52 shows a significant increase in Japanese patients with BD (Ohno and Matsuda 1986), as well as in the neurological and ocular types of BD in a British series (Lehner *et al.* 1982). The primary disease association is with Class I MHC gene products, as HLA-B51 is significantly increased in all ethnic groups studied. The relevance of Class II MHC antigen is uncertain, owing to the linkage disequilibrium with the Class I MHC molecules; HLA-B44 and HLA-B51 are in linkage disequilibrium with DR7 and DRw52 (Welsh and Kerr 1986).

IMMUNOGLOBULINS

Measurement of IgA, IgG and IgM by radial immunodiffusion was carried out in serum, saliva and tears (Scully *et al.* 1979). Serum IgA concentrations were significantly increased in the arthritic, neurological and ocular types of BD. However, parotid IgA concentrations were decreased in the arthritic, ocular and mucocutaneous types of BD.

COMPLEMENT

Serum C3, C4 and CH50 are generally normal in BD (Lehner *et al.* 1979b). However, C3, C4 and C2 were markedly reduced before an attack of uveitis, suggesting complement consumption by the classical pathway (Shimada *et al.* 1974). The involvement of complement in the pathogenesis of BD is supported by electron-microscopic evidence of membrane fragments, showing the appearance of complement-induced lesions, in the sera of certain patients (Lehner *et al.* 1978a).

ANTIBODIES

Nuclear, thyroid and gastric antibodies are not found in BD and the Rose–Waaler test is also negative, even with joint involvement. However, autoantibodies to saline homogenates of oral mucosa were found in patients with BD. Significant haemagglutinating antibodies were detected in patients with BD but not in a variety of controls (Oshima *et al.* 1963; Lehner 1964a). These antibodies belong predominantly to the IgM and, to a lesser extent, IgG classes; they were not specific to oral mucosa, as common antigenic determinants were shared with other epithelial saline extracts (Lehner 1969b). Direct immunofluorescent staining of predominantly IgG and IgM was found in the cytoplasm of keratinocytes in biopsies of ulcers from patients with BD (Lehner 1969a). As indirect immunofluorescent staining of normal human buccal mucosal cells with serum from patients with ROU was not detected, non-specific inflammatory binding could not be excluded. However, cytoplasmic antibodies to epithelial cells of human oesophagus were found by the indirect method in five patients with BD and in none of the 20 controls (O'Duffy *et al.* 1971). Autoantibodies to S antigen (retina-derived soluble protein) were reported in about half of the patients with the ocular type of BD (Dumonde *et al.* 1982), although a correlation was not found between these antibodies and the severity of ocular disease.

IMMUNE COMPLEXES

Circulating IC have been detected in BD and ROU by six independent methods, first by C3 haemagglutination inhibition assay of the macromolecular fraction of plasma (Williams and Lehner 1977) and then by Raji cell and C1q-binding radio-immunoassay (Gupta *et al.* 1978), the agglutination inhibition technique of IgG- or IgA-coated latex particles (Levinsky and Lehner 1978), the cold-precipitable complex technique (Lehner *et al.* 1979b) and the polyethylene glycol-precipitable method (Burton-Kee *et al.* 1979). Specific circulating IC to HSV-1 were found in BD in polyethylene glycol precipitable material (Hussain *et al.* 1986). This was more significant in the arthritic (61%) and ocular (63%) types than in the mucocutaneous (31%) or neurological (27%) type of BD. Although there is no clear evidence for a pathogenic role for IC, there is a significant association between the levels of IC and clinical indices of disease.

CHEMOTAXIS AND PHAGOCYTOSIS

An investigation of chemotaxis in BD revealed increased chemotactic activity in the serum from patients with BD (Matsumura and Mizushima 1975; Sobel *et al.* 1977). In contrast PMNL from patients with BD showed a depressed response to chemotactic stimuli (Abdulla and Lehner 1979). The paradoxical response of the serum and cells from patients with BD can be accounted for by IgA and IgG cold-precipitable IC. Immunoglobulin A complexes suppress chemotaxis of PMNL whereas IgG complexes may stimulate the release of serum chemotactic factors. It is conceivable that the IgA complexes lead to a failure of clearance of the potentially more tissue-damaging IgG complexes. Phagocytosis of PMNL was studied, using *Candida* (Wilton and Lehner 1979). The results showed that 42% of patients with BD had a depressed phagocytic capacity and the defect was more frequent in patients with the arthritic and ocular types.

CELL-MEDIATED IMMUNITY

There is no impairment of CMI in BD, as assessed by skin testing with purified protein derivative (PPD), *Candida* and streptokinase–streptodornase. The *in vitro* lymphoproliferative responses to the mitogen PHA or pokeweed or to antigens, such as PPD and *Candida*, were normal. However, a significant lymphoproliferative response was induced by homogenates of oral mucosa in BD but not in controls (Lehner 1967). Lymphocytes from patients with BD, but not from control subjects, also showed cytotoxicity against cultures of gingival epithelial cells (Rogers *et al.* 1974). These results suggest a cellular immune response to some epithelial antigen. S antigen also induces significant lymphoproliferative responses in the ocular type of BD (Nussenblatt *et al.* 1980), suggesting that lymphocytes had been sensitized to retinal antigens.

Recent investigations of circulating T cells showed a relative shift of CD8 cells from the unprimed CD45RA to the primed CD29 memory cells in BD (Fortune *et al*. 1990). A significant proportion of circulating T cells was activated, as they expressed the HLA-DR antigen. Of particular significance was the finding of CD8 cells expressing an increase in the $\gamma\delta$ T cell receptor, which might represent a response to some common microbial agent. The mucosal involvement in BD was manifested by circulating CD4 and CD8 cells with membrane-bound IgA (Fortune *et al*. 1990).

ACUTE-PHASE PROTEINS

The serum concentrations of C-reactive protein (CRP), C9, factor B, α1-acid glycoprotein (α1AG) and α1-antitrypsin (α1AT) were examined in BD (Adinolfi *et al*. 1979). The levels of C9 were significantly increased in BD as well as in ROU. Complement component 9 was a good marker of disease activity and its estimation proved to be useful in monitoring treatment. C-reactive protein was significantly increased in BD but it was of limited value as an index of disease activity. Factor B was also increased in BD, particularly in the neurological type. In contrast, α1AG was significantly increased mostly in the ocular type of BD. The clinical significance of these findings is not clear. The increased levels of acute-phase proteins (APP) could be non-specific and ascribed to tissue damage. Alternatively, APP may have some specific immunological functions (Kaplan and Volanakis 1974; Mortensen *et al*. 1975).

IMMUNOPATHOLOGY

Biopsies of oral ulcers in BD have shown an intense lympho-monocytic infiltration around blood-vessels of the lamina propria during the early stages of ulceration, but later a mixed response becomes evident, with PMNL and plasma cells (Lehner 1969a), as described in ROU. The early stages suggest a delayed hypersensitivity reaction: electron microscopy shows intracytoplasmic phagosome-like bodies of epithelial cells, adjacent to mononuclear cells, and phagocytosing macrophages, associated with prickle cells (Saito *et al*. 1971). Initially small blood-vessels, especially venules, are affected, with vascular endothelial proliferation, loss of the internal elastic lamina, fibrinoid necrosis and often obliteration of the lumen (Shikano 1966; Lehner 1969a), suggesting IC disease. The relationship between the type IV and type III reactions is not clear.

Immunofluorescence studies of biopsies from patients with ROU and BD show C3 in the absence of C1q and IgG in most biopsies, suggesting that the alternative complement pathway might be activated (Lehner 1979). In view of the finding of circulating IC in BD, it is surprising that a significant deposition of immunoglobulins was not detected in the oral lesions. This might be due to the IC not being pathogenic for oral mucosa; the latter may be the initial source of antigen and the IC might be responsible for the extraoral disease. Alternatively, IC may be deposited at a later stage of ulceration, possibly after the initial cell-mediated phase has failed. As in ROU, HLA-DR is expressed on the cell membrane of keratinocytes and there is an increase in the number of Langerhans' cells (Poulter and Lehner 1989). The lamina propria is infiltrated with CD4 and CD8 cells (with a ratio of about 2 : 1) and macrophage-like cells.

IMMUNOLOGICAL MECHANISM

A tentative mechanism is suggested to account for the reported immunological findings (Fig. 104.8). A specific microbial agent may be involved, in spite of the failure hitherto to find a causative micro-organism. Alternatively, heat-shock proteins, possibly derived from *S. sanguis* or *S. oralis*, with HSV type 1 as an associated agent, may affect the immunoregulatory mechanism in the HLA-B51 (and possibly B12, DR7 and DRw52) predisposed subjects, leading to the development of BD (Fig. 104.8). An early infiltration of T cells and macrophages in oral ulcers (Muller and Lehner 1982) and erythema nodosum in BD (Yamana *et al*. 1982), with HLA Class II MHC expression in keratinocytes (Poulter and Lehner 1989) and an increase in Langerhans' cells, might facilitate autoantigen presentation to T cells. This is followed by increased chemotaxis of neutrophils, which may account for the pathergy reaction. Local mucocutaneous immunopathology is associated with central changes in circulating lymphocytes — activated T cells, up-regulated $\gamma\delta$ T cell receptors and heat-shock protein-sensitized cells. The proportion of the IgA class of B cells is increased, as are antibodies and IC, presumably in response

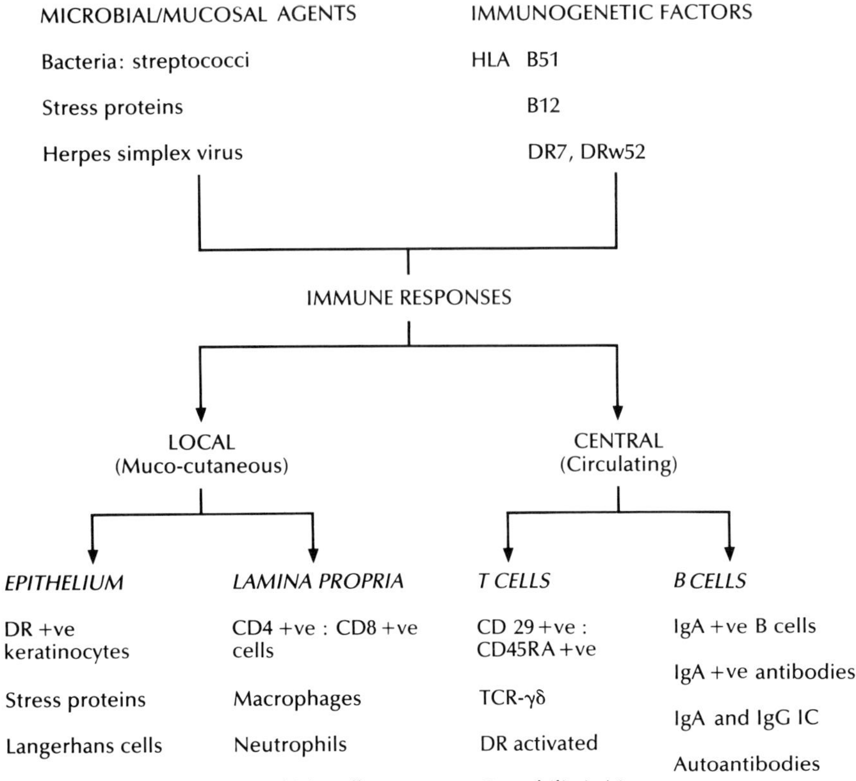

Fig. 104.8. Immunomicrobial mechanism in the development of Behçet's disease.

to mucosal immunization. The hypothesis is suggested that heat-shock proteins may affect the immune response at the mucosal surface, so as to up-regulate the IgA system and the T cells with the γδ receptors, both of which are thought to be involved in protection of the surface epithelium.

TREATMENT

The management of patients with BD can be difficult, as it requires close liaison between different specialties. Whenever possible, topical treatment of local lesions should be attempted before embarking on systemic anti-inflammatory or immunosuppressive therapy. Oral and genital ulcers often respond to topical application of steroids or tetracycline or both, as described for ROU. Uveitis is also initially treated with local steroids. However, systemic prednisolone is often administered, with a starting daily dose of 20–60 mg, which is rapidly brought down to a minimum effective maintenance dose of about 10 mg. There is usually a prompt response, although a small core of patients are resistant to steroids. Azathioprine is often used with prednisolone (2–3 mg/kg bodyweight daily). There is now evidence from a controlled trial that azathioprine has beneficial effects (Yazici *et al.* 1990); in addition, it acts as a steroid-sparing agent. Colchicine has been particularly advocated in Japan (Mizushima *et al.* 1979) for the treatment of BD and the recommended dose is 0.5 mg bd. The rationale is that the drug inhibits the motility of PMNL, which is increased in BD. There is general consensus that chlorambucil is effective in patients with unresponsive uveitis, although it has serious side-effects (O'Duffy *et al.* 1986). Recently cyclosporin has been applied successfully in the treatment of uveitis in BD (Nussenblatt *et al.* 1985) and has been evaluated in a controlled trial against colchicine (Masuda *et al.* 1989). It was found significantly more effective than colchicine in reducing the ocular attacks, oral ulcers and skin lesions, but had more side-effects, especially nephrotoxicity. Thalidomide has been found to be effective in the treatment of orogenital ulcers, cutaneous lesions, arthritis and, to a lesser extent, uveitis (Hamza 1986), but the teratogenic effect of this drug may severely restrict its use.

Oral manifestations of diseases with autoallergic features

Most diseases with autoallergic features show oral manifestations but it is outside the scope of this account to give a detailed description of these.

PEMPHIGUS VULGARIS

Pemphigus vulgaris presents in the mouth in about half the patients, but the mouth is involved at some stage of the disease in most patients. Painful vesicles or bullae may appear and burst within a few hours, resulting in shallow ulcers. These persist for weeks or months, but new lesions recur throughout the disease process. Oral manifestations of the disease may persist for many months without overt ill-health, although malaise and loss of weight may occur later.

Microscopic examination of direct scrapings from the lesion may be diagnostic, in the presence of acantholytic cells. A biopsy examination is, however, essential, for this will show intraepithelial bullae and acantholytic cells, with a diffuse leucocytic infiltration of the lamina propria.

Pemphigus vegetans is a less common and less severe variant of pemphigus vulgaris. Vegetations may be found on the oral mucosa and lips and histological examination shows intraepithelial abscesses containing numerous eosinophils.

A significant association was established with DR4 and DRw6 in patients with pemphigus. Either the DR4 or the DRw6 gene product confers disease susceptibility, and with DRw6 this has now been located to a single amino acid substitution of residue 57, from valine to aspartic acid.

The autoantibodies to the intercellular substance of epithelial cells are usually of the IgG class and are found both in the circulation and bound to keratinocytes at the site of the disease (Beutner and Jordan 1964). The serum autoantibodies are of diagnostic significance and, as they fluctuate with disease activity, they are also useful markers of disease activity. However, a biopsy is mandatory and the features of diagnostic significance are: (i) intraepithelial bullae; (ii) acantholysis; and (iii) IgG anti-intercellular substance antibodies. The target antigen for the autoantibodies has not been identified but electron-microscopic investigations have indicated that the cytoplasmic processes of keratinocytes, intercellular cementing substance or desmosomes of the epithelial cells are involved (Jones *et al*. 1984). Clearly, the antigen is a normal epithelial membrane glycoprotein. The molecular weight of a glycoprotein immunoprecipitated from human epidermal extracts was 210 kD, with a glycosylated 130 kD chain, linked to an 85 kD chain (Stanley *et al*. 1984). A smaller glycoprotein of 66 kD was also purified, using concanavalin (Peterson and Wuepper 1984). However, a 150 kD protein was identified by immunoblotting of a tongue extract and localized by electron microscopy to the area between desmosomal plates (Jones *et al*. 1984). Irrespective of these differences, it appears that, for normal expression of the antigenic structure targeted by the autoantibodies, three conditions are required: (i) newly synthesized protein; (ii) *N*-asparagine glycosylation; and (iii) calcium ions (Konohana *et al*. 1988). This high-molecular-weight, glycosylated protein chain may play an important role in epithelial morphology, cell-to-cell adhesion and stability of cell surface antigens.

There is convincing experimental evidence that the loss of interepithelial adhesion is caused by the autoantibodies binding to keratinocytes (Hashimoto *et al*. 1983). Transfer of human autoantibodies to mice can induce the clinical and histopathological features of pemphigus. The mechanism of loss of adhesion and acantholysis are unknown, but the release of proteolytic enzymes from the epithelial cells has been proposed. Indeed, epithelial cells incubated with the autoantibodies release plasminogen activators, which activate plasmin, and this may lead to acantholysis (Hashimoto *et al*. 1983). The role of complement has not been fully elucidated and does not appear to be essential in this process, although complement activation may exacerbate the response, possibly by chemotaxis of the neutrophils.

BENIGN MUCOUS MEMBRANE PEMPHIGOID

Benign mucous membrane pemphigoid (BMMP) is a mucosal lesion affecting the mouth, genitals and conjunctiva of the eyes. The disease is seen mostly in the elderly, with diffuse erosions of the mucosa, which start as blisters that readily burst. Often the patient presents with a desquamative gingivitis, which can be recognized by the diffuse erosions affecting the attached gingiva. The oral lesions usually heal without scarring, unlike those of the conjunctiva, which may leave rather troublesome cicatrization.

Biopsy examination is necessary for diagnosis and this shows a subepithelial bulla and bound IgG, IgA or IgM (with or without complement) at the basement membrane (Bean *et al.* 1979). Although circulating anti-basement membrane antibodies can be detected, these are rather variable. Benign mucous membrane pemphigoid needs to be differentiated from: (i) linear IgA disease, which is rather uncommon in the mouth and shows a linear IgA in the basement membrane; and (ii) dermatitis herpetiformis, in which papillary deposits of IgA are found (Williams *et al.* 1984). The latter may have circulating anti-gliadin antibodies, which are found both in dermatitis herpetiformis and coeliac disease (Kieffer and Barnetson 1983).

The mechanism of subepithelial bullous formation is ill-understood but it has been suggested that the autoantibodies react with the lamina lucida of the basement membrane (Sams and Gammon 1982). Complement activation (C5a) leads to chemotaxis of neutrophils and eosinophils, which release enzymes, causing destruction and blister formation.

Treatment

Treatment of pemphigus with corticosteroids has completely changed the prognosis of this disease and morbidity is minimized. Azathioprine is commonly used, with prednisolone as a steroid-sparing agent. In BMMP of the mouth, topical corticosteroids alone often suffice.

LUPUS ERYTHEMATOSUS

Oral manifestations in systemic and discoid lupus erythematosus are rarely essential features of the disease, although occasionally oral lesions may be a presenting feature. They can be recognized clinically as localized atrophic or erosive lesions, surrounded by hyperkeratotic papules or striae, and they may involve the lips, cheeks, palate or tongue. Biopsy examination shows hyperkeratosis, epithelial atrophy, liquefaction degeneration of the basal cell layer and a prominent mononuclear cell infiltration around the blood-vessels, as well as in the lamina propria. Fibrinoid degeneration may affect the connective tissue and vessel walls.

PERNICIOUS ANAEMIA

Soreness of the tongue, with burning and dryness of the mouth, are sometimes presenting symptoms of pernicious anaemia. The tongue appears smooth, due to loss of the filiform papillae, and may also be inflamed. Recurrent oral ulcers are occasionally found in pernicious anaemia. They mimic minor aphthous ulcers but they are usually shallow and two or three in number; the ulcers last only 2–4 days before they heal and a new crop develops. The oral manifestations disappear when the anaemia is treated with vitamin B_{12}.

SJÖGREN'S SYNDROME

Dryness of the mouth is a prominent feature in Sjögren's syndrome. The patient may complain of a burning sensation of the tongue, lips and cheeks, and of considerable discomfort on eating and speaking. Recurrent swelling of the parotid glands may occur. The mucosa is atrophic and devoid of saliva, and this makes movements between the tongue and mucosal surfaces rather difficult. *Candida* infection of the chronic atrophic variety commonly affects the oral mucosa and may give rise to angular cheilitis. Objective evidence of lack of saliva can be seen by giving the patient a few drops of lemon juice and observing the salivary duct openings. Usually, salivary flow cannot be seen in the established disease, but in the early stages impaired salivary flow can be established with some confidence by measuring the volume of saliva secreted over a given period of time.

The diagnosis of Sjögren's syndrome is aided by a raised erythrocyte sedimentation rate (ESR), increased concentration of immunoglobulins, positive rheumatoid factor and Rose–Waaler test and presence of antinuclear factor, antibodies to extractable nuclear antigen (Ro and La), organ-specific autoantibodies and salivary duct antibodies. An abnormal sialogram and histological evidence of sialadenitis in a lip biopsy (Chisholm and Mason 1968) may be more significant in the diagnosis of Sjögren's syndrome. Management of the oral features of Sjögren's syndrome includes clearing up any *Candida* infection by topical amphotericin B, 10 mg tablets qds, followed by application of carboxymethylcellulose (Glandosane) and frequent sips of water.

References

Aaltonen, A.S., Tenovuo, J., Lehtonen, O.P., Saksala, R. and Meurman, O. (1985). Serum antibodies against oral *Streptococcus mutans* in young children in relation to dental caries and maternal close contacts. *Arch. Oral Biol.* **30**, 331.

Aaltonen, A.S., Tenovuo, J. and Lehtonen, O.P. (1987). Increased caries activity in preschool children with low base line levels of serum IgG antibodies against the bacterial species *Streptococcus mutans*. *Arch. Oral Biol.* **32**, 55.

Aaltonen, A.S., Tenovuo, J. and Lehtonen, O.P. (1988). Antibodies to the oral bacterium *Streptococcus mutans* and the development of caries in children in relation to maternal dental treatment during pregnancy. *Arch. Oral Biol.* **33**, 33.

Abdulla, Y.H. and Lehner, T. (1979). The effect of immune complexes on chemotaxis in Behçet's syndrome and recurrent oral ulcers. In *Behçet's Syndrome: Clinical and Immunological Features*, ed. T. Lehner and C.G. Barnes, p. 53, Academic Press, London.

Adinolfi, M., Beck, S.E. and Lehner, T. (1979). Serum levels of acute phase proteins, C9, factor B and lysozyme in Behçet's syndrome and recurrent oral ulcers. In *Behçet's Syndrome: Clinical and Immunological Features*, ed. T. Lehner and C.G. Barnes, p. 107. Academic Press, London.

Allison, A.C., Schorlemmer, H.U. and Bitter-Suermann D. (1976). Activation of complement by the alternative pathway as a factor in the pathogenesis of periodontal disease. *Lancet* **ii**, 1001.

Anderson, N.A., Sage, D.N. and Spaulding, E.H. (1944). Oral moniliasis in newborn infants. *Am. J. Dis. Child.* **67**, 450.

Archibald, D.W., Zon, L., Groopman, J.E., McLane, M.F. and Essex, M. (1986). Antibodies to human T-lymphotrophic virus type III (HTLV-III) in saliva of acquired immunodeficiency syndrome (AIDS) patients and in persons at risk for AIDS. *Blood* **67**, 831.

Archibald, D.W., Barr, C.E., Torosian, J.P., McLane, M.F. and Essex, M. (1987). Secretory IgA antibodies to human immunodeficiency virus in the parotid saliva of patients with AIDS and AIDS-related complex. *J. Infect. Dis.* **155**, 793.

Arnold, R.R., Mestecky, J. and McGhee, J.R. (1976). Naturally occurring secretory immunoglobulin A antibodies to *Streptococcus mutans* in human colostrum and saliva. *Infect. Immun.* **14**, 355.

Attstrom, R., Laurell, A.B., Larsson, U. and Sjoholm, A. (1975). Complement factors in gingival crevice material from healthy and inflamed gingiva in humans. *J. Periodontal Res.* **10**, 19.

Baehni, P., Tsai, C.C., McArthur, W.P., Hammond, B.F. and Taichman, N.S. (1979). Interaction of inflammatory cells and oral microorganisms. VIII. Detection of leukotoxic activity of a plaque-derived Gram negative microorganism. *Infect. Immun.* **24**, 233.

Baer, P.N. (1971). The case for periodontosis as a clinical entity. *J. Periodontol.* **42**, 516.

Baker, J.J., Chan, S.P., Socransky, S.S., Oppenheim, J.J. and Mergenhagen, S.E. (1976). Importance of *Actinomyces* and certain Gram negative anaerobic organisms in the transformation of lymphocytes from patients with periodontal disease. *Infect. Immun.* **13**, 1363.

Barile, M.F., Graykowski, E.A., Driscoll, E.J. and Riggs, D.B. (1963). L form of bacteria isolated from recurrent aphthous stomatitis lesions. *Oral Surg.* **16**, 1395.

Baringer, J.R. and Swoveland, P. (1973). Recovery of herpes simplex virus from human trigeminal ganglions. *N. Engl. J. Med.* **288**, 648.

Bean, S.F., Rogers, R.S., Jordan, R.E., Finey, N.L. and Michel, B. (1979). Cicatricial pemphigoid. In *Immunology of the Skin*, 2nd edn., ed. E.W. Beutner, T.P. Chorzelski and S.F. Bean, p. 257, Wiley, New York.

Behçet, H. (1937). Über rezidivierende Aphthose durch ein Virus verursachte Geschwure am Mund, am Auge und an den Genitalie. *Dermatol. Wschr.* **105**, 1152.

Behçet, U. (1938). Considérations sur les lésions aphtheuses de la bouche et des parties génitales ainsi que sur les manifestations oculaires d'origine probablement parasitaire et observations concernant leur foyer d'infection. *Bull. Soc. Franc. Dermatol. Syph.* **45**, 420.

Berger, U., Kaparits, M. and Pfeifer, G. (1959). Zur Besiedlung de kindlichen Mundhohler mit anaeroben Mikroorganismen. *Z. Hyg. Infektions Krankh.* **145**, 564.

Berglund, J.E., Rizzo, A.A. and Mergenhagen, S.E. (1969). The immune response in rabbits to bacterial somatic antigen administered via the oral mucosa. *Arch. Oral Biol.* **14**, 7.

Bergmeier, L.A. and Lehner, T. (1983). Lack of antibodies to human heart tissue in sera of rhesus monkeys immunized with *Streptococcus mutans* antigens and comparative study with rabbit antisera. *Infect. Immun.* **40**, 1075.

Berkowitz, R.J. and Jones, P. (1985). Mouth-to-mouth transmission of the bacterium *Streptococcus mutans* between mother and child. *Arch. Oral Biol.* **30**, 377.

Beutner, E.H. and Jordan, R.E. (1964). Demonstration of skin antibodies in sera of pemphigus vulgaris patients by indirect immunofluorescence staining. *Nature* **208**, 353.

Bonass, W.A., Bird-Stewart, J.A., Chamberlain, M.A. and Halliburton, I.W. (1986). Molecular studies in Behçet's syndrome. In *Recent Advances in Behçet's Disease*, ed. T. Lehner and C.G. Barnes, pp. 37–41, Royal Society of Medicine Services, London.

Bowen, W.H., Cohen, B., Cole, M.F. and Colman, G. (1975). Immunisation against dental caries. *Br. Dent. J.* **139**, 45.

Brandtzaeg, P. (1972). Local formation and transport of immunoglobulins related to the oral cavity. In *Host Resistance to Commensal Bacteria*, ed. T.T. MacPhae, p. 116, Churchill Livingstone, Edinburgh.

Brandtzaeg, P. (1976). Studies on J chain and binding site for secretory component in circulating human B cells. *Clin. Exp. Immunol.* **25**, 59.

Brandtzaeg, P. and Kraus, F.W. (1965). Autoimmunity and periodontal disease. *Odontol. Tidskr.* **73**, 281.

Brandtzaeg, P. and Tolo, K. (1977). In *The Borderland between Caries and Periodontal Disease*, ed. T. Lehner, p. 145, Academic Press, London.

Brandtzaeg, P., Fjellanger, I. and Gjeruldsen, S.T. (1970). Human secretory immunoglobulins. I. Salivary secretions from individuals with normal or low levels of serum immunoglobulins. *Scand. J. Haematol.* **12** (suppl.), 58.

Brathall, D. (1970). Demonstration of five serological groups of streptococcal strains resembling *Streptococcus mutans*. *Odontol. Rev.* **21**, 143.

Brautbar, C., Chajek, T., Ben-Tuvia, S., Lamm, L. and Cohen, T. (1978). A genetic study of Behçet's disease in Israel. *Tissue*

Antigens **11**, 113–20.

Buckley, R.H., Lucas, Z.J., Hattler, B.G., Jr, Zmijewski, C.M. and Amos, D.B. (1968). Defective cellular immunity associated with chronic mucocutaneous moniliasis and recurrent staphylococcal botryomycosis: immunological reconstitution by allogeneic bone marrow. *Clin. Exp. Immunol.* **3**, 153.

Buddingh, G.J., Schrum, D.I., Lanier, J.C. and Guidry, G.J. (1953). Studies on the natural history of herpes simplex infections. *Pediatrics (Springfield)* **11**, 595.

Burton-Kee, E.J., Lehner, T. and Mowbray, J.F. (1979). In *Behçet's Syndrome: Clinical and Immunological Features*, ed. T. Lehner and C.G. Barnes, p. 45, Academic Press, London.

Caldwell, J., Challacombe, S.J. and Lehner, T. (1977). A sequential bacteriological and serological investigation of rhesus monkeys immunised against dental caries with *Streptococcus mutans*. *J. Med. Microbiol.* **10**, 213.

Calonius, P.E.B. (1958). The leukocyte count in saliva. *Oral Surg.* **11**, 43.

Canby, C.P. and Bernier, J.L. (1942). Bacteriologic and immunologic studies in dental caries: preliminary report. *J. Am. Dent. Assoc.* **29**, 606.

Carlsson, J. (1967). Presence of various types of non-haemolytic streptococci in dental plaque and in other sites of the oral cavity in man. *Odontol. Rev.* **18**, 55.

Carlsson, J., Grahnen, H., Jonsson, G. and Winker, S. (1970a). Early establishment of *Streptococcus salivarius* in the mouth of infants. *J. Dent. Res.* **49**, 415.

Carlsson, J., Grahnen, H., Jonsson, G. and Wikner, S. (1970b). Establishment of *Streptococcus sanguis* in the mouth of infants. *Arch. Oral Biol.* **15**, 1143.

Cawson, R.A. and Lehner, T. (1968). Chronic hyperplastic candidiasis candidal leukoplakia. *Br. J. Dermatol.* **80**, 9.

Cebra, J.J., Kamat, R., Gearhart, P., Robertson, S.M. and Tzeng, J. (1977). The secretory IgA system of the gut. In *Immunology of the Gut*, p. 5, Excerpta Medica, Elsevier, North-Holland, Amsterdam.

Center for Disease Control (1986). Classification system for human T-lymphotrophic virus type III/lymphadenopathy associated virus infections. *Morb. Mort. Weekly Rep.* **35**, 334.

Chajek, T. and Fainaru, M. (1975). Behçet's disease: report of 41 cases and a review of the literature. *Medicine* **54**, 179.

Challacombe, S.J.C. (1980). Passage of serum immunoglobulins into the oral cavity. In *The Borderland between Caries and Periodontal Disease*, ed. T. Lehner and G. Cimasoni, Vol. II, p. 51, Academic Press, London.

Challacombe, S.J. and Lehner, T. (1976). Serum and salivary antibodies to cariogenic bacteria in man. *J. Dent. Res.* **55**, C139.

Challacombe, S.J. and Lehner, T. (1979). Salivary antibodies in rhesus monkeys immunised with *Streptococcus mutans* by the oral submucosal or subcutaneous routes. *Arch. Oral Biol.* **24**, 917.

Challacombe, S.J., Barkhan, P. and Lehner, T. (1977a). Haematological features and differentiation of recurrent oral ulceration. *Br. J. Oral Surg.* **15**, 37.

Challacombe, S.J., Batchelor, J.R., Kennedy, L. and Lehner, T. (1977b). HLA-antigens in patients with recurrent oral ulceration. *Arch. Dermatol.* **113**, 1717.

Challacombe, S.J., Russell, M.W., Hawkes, J.E., Bergmeier, L.A. and Lehner, T. (1978). Passage of immunoglobulins from plasma to the oral cavity in rhesus monkeys. *Immunology* **35**, 923.

Challacombe, S.J., Bergmeier, L. and Rees, A. (1984). Natural antibodies in man to a protein antigen from the bacterium *Streptococcus mutans* related to dental caries experience. *Arch. Oral Biol.* **29**, 179.

Chamberlain, M.A. (1977). Behçet's syndrome in 32 patients in Yorkshire. *Ann. Rheum. Dis.* **36**, 491.

Chilgren, R.A., Quie, P.G., Meuwissen, H.J. and Hong, R. (1967). Chronic muco-cutaneous candidiasis, deficiency of delayed hypersensitivity and selective local antibody defect. *Lancet* **ii**, 688.

Chilgren, R.A., Quie, P.G., Meuwissen, H.J., Good, R.A. and Hong, R. (1969). The cellular immune defect in chronic mucocutaneous candidiasis. *Lancet* **i**, 1286.

Chisholm, D.M. and Mason, D.K. (1968). Labial salivary gland biopsy in Sjögren's syndrome. *J. Clin. Pathol.* **21**, 656.

Chorzelski, T.P. and Beutner, E.H. (1969). Factors contributing to occasional failures in demonstration of pemphigus antibodies by the immunofluorescence test. *J. Invest. Dermatol.* **53**, 188.

Cianciola, L.J., Genco, R.J., Patters, M.T., McKenna, J. and Van Oss, C.J. (1977). Defective polymorphonuclear leukocyte function in a human periodontal disease. *Nature* **265**, 445.

Cimasoni, G., Ishikawa, I. and Jaccard, F. (1977). Enzyme activity in the gingival crevice. In *The Borderland between Caries and Periodontal Disease*, ed. T. Lehner, p. 13, Academic Press, London.

Clagett, J.A. and Page, R.C. (1978). Insoluble immune complexes and chronic periodontal diseases in man and the dog. *Arch. Oral Biol.* **23**, 153.

Clark, R.A. and Kimball, H.R. (1971). Defective granulocyte chemotaxis in the Chediak–Hingashi syndrome. *J. Clin. Invest.* **50**, 2645.

Cochrane, C.G., Weigle, W.O. and Dixon, F.J. (1959). The role of polymorphonuclear leukocytes in the initiation and cessation of the Arthus vasculitis. *J. Exp. Med.* **110**, 481.

Cole, K.L., Seymour, G.J. and Powell, R.N. (1987). Phenotypic and functional analysis of T-cells extracted from chronically inflamed human periodontal tissues. *J. Periodontol.* **58**, 569.

Cooke, B.E.D. (1960). The diagnosis of bullous lesions affecting the oral mucosa. *Br. Dent. J.* **109**, 83.

Cooke, B.E.D. (1961). Recurrent Mikulicz's aphthae. *Dent. Practitioner* **12**, 119.

Cooper, M.D., Chase, H.P., Lowman, J.T., Krivit, W. and Good, R.A. (1968). Wiskott–Aldrich syndrome: an immunologic deficiency disease involving the afferent limb of immunity. *Am. J. Med.* **44**, 449.

Coykendall, A.L. (1974). Four types of *Streptococcus mutans* based on their genetic, antigenic and biochemical characteristics. *J. Gen. Microbiol.* **82**, 327.

Crawford, J.M., Taubman, M.A. and Smith, D.J. (1978). The effects of immunisation with periodontopathic microorganisms on periodontal bone loss in gnotobiotic rats. *J. Periodontal Res.* **13**, 445.

Czerkinsky, C., Prince, S.J., Michalek, S.M. *et al.* (1987). IgA antibody-producing cells in peripheral blood after antigen ingestion: evidence for a common mucosal immune system in humans. *Proc. Nat. Acad. Sci. (USA)* **84**, 2449.

Davies, R.R. and Denning, T.J.V. (1972). Growth and form in

Candida albicans. *Sabouraudia* **10**, 180.

Denman, A.M., Hylton, W., Pelton, B.K., Palmer, R.G., Topper, R. and Smith-Burchenell, C. (1986). The viral aetiology of Behçet's syndrome. In *Recent Advances in Behçet's Disease*, ed T. Lehner and C.G. Barnes, pp. 23–30, Royal Society of Medicine Services, London.

De Sousa, M., Cochran, R., MacKie, R., Parratt, D. and Arala-Chaves, M. (1976). Chronic mucocutaneous candidiasis treated with transfer factor. *Br. J. Dermatol.* **94**, 79.

Dolby, A.E. (1969). Recurrent aphthous ulceration; effect of sera and peripheral blood upon epithelial tissue culture cells. *Immunology* **17**, 709.

Donatsky, O. (1976). Comparison of cellular and humoral immunity against streptococcal and adult human oral mucosa antigens in relation to exacerbation of recurrent apthous stomatitis. *Acta Pathol. Microbiol. Scand. Sec. C* **84**, 270.

Donatsky, O. and Dabelsteen, E. (1974). An immunofluorescence study on the humoral immunity to adult human oral mucosa in recurrent aphthous stomatitis. *Acta Allergol.* **29**, 308.

Dowling, G.B. (1961). Behçet's disease. *Proc. Roy. Soc. Med.* **54**, 101.

Dudgeon, J.A. (1961). Virological aspects of Behçet's disease. *Proc. Roy. Soc. Med.* **54**, 104.

Dumonde, D.C., Kasp-Grochowska, E., Graham, E. *et al.* (1982). Anti-retinal autoimmunity and circulating immune complexes in patients with retinal vasculitis. *Lancet* **ii**, 787.

Edwards, F.C. and Truelove, S.C. (1964). The course and prognosis of ulcerative colitis. III. Complications. *Gut* **5**, 1.

Eglin, R.P., Lehner, T. and Subak-Sharpe, J.H. (1982). Detection of RNA complementary to herpes simplex virus in mononuclear cells from patients with Behçet's syndrome and recurrent oral ulcers. *Lancet* **ii**, 1356.

Elin, R.J. and Wolff, S.M. (1976). Biology of endotoxin. *Ann. Rev. Med.* 127.

Evans, A.D., Pallis, C.A. and Spillane, J.D. (1957). Involvement of the nervous system in Behçet's syndrome: report of three cases and isolation of virus. *Lancet* **ii**, 349.

Farmer, E.D. (1958). Recurrent aphthous ulcers. *Dent. Practitioner* **8**, 177.

Ferguson, R., Basu, M.K., Asquith, P. and Cooke, W.T. (1976). Jejunal mucosal abnormalities in patients with recurrent aphthous ulceration. *Br. Med. J.* **1**, 11.

Fitzgerald, R.J., Jordan, H.V. and Stanley, H.R. (1960). Experimental caries and gingival pathologic changes in the gnotobiotic rat. *J. Dent. Res.* **39**, 923.

Fitzgerald, R.J., Jordan, H.V. and Archard, H.O. (1966). Dental caries in gnotobiotic rats infected with a variety of lactobacillus acidophilus. *Arch. Oral Biol.* **11**, 473.

Forester, H., Hunter, N. and Knox, K.W. (1983). Characteristics of a high molecular weight protein of *Streptococcus mutans*. *J. Gen. Microbiol.* **129**, 2779.

Fortune, F., Kingston, J., Barnes, C.S. and Lehner, T. (1990). Identification and characterization of IgA and *Vicia villosa*-binding T cell subsets in rheumatoid arthritis. *Clin. Exp. Immunol.* **79**, 202.

France, R., Buchanan, R.N., Wilson, M.W. and Sheldon, M.D. (1951). Relapsing iritis with recurrent ulcers of the mouth and genitalia (Behçet's syndrome): Review with report of an additional case. *Medicine (Baltimore)* **30**, 335.

Francis, T.C. and Oppenheim, J.J. (1970). Impaired lymphocyte stimulation by some streptococcal antigens in patients with recurrent aphthous stomatitis and rheumatic heart disease. *Clin. Exp. Immunol.* **6**, 573.

Genco, R.J., Mashimo, P.A., Krygier, C. and Ellison, S.A. (1974). Antibody mediated effects on the periodontium. *J. Periodontol.* **45**, 330.

Gerberding, J.L., Bryant-LeBlanc, C.E., Nelson, K. *et al.* (1987). Risk of transmitting the human immunodeficiency virus, cytomegalovirus, and hepatitis B virus to health care workers exposed to patients with AIDS and AIDS-related conditions. *J. Infect. Dis.* **156**, 1.

Gibbons, R.J. (1989). Bacterial adhesion to oral tissue: a model for infectious diseases. *J. Dent. Res.* **68** (5), 750.

Gibbons, R.J. and Nygaard, M. (1968). Synthesis of insoluble dextran and its significance in the formation of gelatinous deposits by plaque-forming streptococci. *Arch. Oral Biol.* **13**, 1249.

Gibbons, R.J. and Socransky, S.S. (1962). Intracellular polysaccharide storage by organisms in dental plaque; its relations to dental caries and microbial ecology of oral cavity. *Arch. Oral Biol.* **7**, 73.

Glasgow, L.A. (1970). Cellular immunity in host resistance to viral infections. *Arch. Intern. Med.* **126**, 125.

Godeau, P., Terre, D., Campinchi, R. *et al.* (1976). HLA B-5 and Behçet's disease. In *HLA and Disease 101*, vol. 58, abstract No 117–7. Editions INSERM, Paris.

Goodson, J.M., Dewhirst, F.E. and Brunetti, A. (1974). Prostaglandin E2 levels and human periodontal disease. *Prostaglandins* **6**, 81.

Gowen, M., Wood, D.D., Ihrie, E.J., McGuire, M.K.B. and Russell, R.G.G. (1983). An interleukin 1 like factor stimulates bone resorption *in vitro*. *Nature* **306**, 378.

Graftstein, B. (1969). Axonal transport: communications between soma and synapse. *Adv. Biochem. Psychopharmacol.* **1**, 11.

Graykowski, E.A., Barile, M.F., Lee, W.B. and Stanley, H.R. (1966). Recurrent aphthous stomatitis: clinical, therapeutic, histopathologic and hypersensitivity aspects. *JAMA* **196**, 637.

Greenspan, D. and Greenspan, J.S. (1987). Oral mucosal manifestations of AIDS. *Dermatol. Clin.* **5** (4), 733.

Grob, P.J., Franke, C., Reymond, J.F. and Frei-Wetenstein, M. (1975). Therapeutic use of transfer factor. *Eur. J. Clin. Invest.* **5**, 33.

Groopman, J.E., Salahuddin, S.Z., Serngadharan, M.D. *et al.* (1984). HTLV-III in saliva of people with AIDS related complex and healthy homosexual men at risk for AIDS. *Science* **266**, 447.

Guggenheim, B. (1970). Enzymatic hydrolysis and structure of water insoluble glucan produced by glucosyltransferases from a strain of *Streptococcus mutans*. *Helv. Odontol. Acta* **14** (suppl. 5), 89.

Guggenheim, B. and Newbrun, E. (1969). Extracellular glucosyltransferase activity of an HS strain of *Streptococcus mutans*. *Helv. Odontol. Acta* **13**, 84.

Gupta, R.C., O'Duffy, J.D., McDuffie, F.C., Meurer, M. and Jordon, R.E. (1978). Circulating immune complexes in the blood of patients with Behçet's syndrome. *Clin. Exp. Immunol.* **34**, 213.

Hamada, S. and Slade, H.D. (1976). The adherence of serotype e

Streptococcus mutans and the inhibitory effect of Lancefield group E and *Strep. mutans* type e antiserum. *J. Dent. Res.* **55**, C65.

Hamza, M. (1986). Treatment of Behçet's disease with thalidomide. In *Recent Advances in Behçet's Disease*, ed. T. Lehner and C.G. Barnes, p. 359, Royal Society of Medicine Services, London.

Hamza, M., Sohier, R., Betuel, H. and Ben Ayed, B. (1979). HLA-B5 and Behçet's disease. In *Behçet's Disease*, ed. N. Dilsen, M. Konice and C. Ovul, p. 265, Excerpta Medica, International Congress Series, Amsterdam.

Hartles, R.L. (1965). Dietary and environmental factors influencing caries resistance. In *Caries Resistant Teeth*, ed. G.E.W. Wolstenholme and M. O'Connor, p. 289, Ciba Foundation Symposium, Little, Brown & Co., Boston, Mass.

Hashimoto, K., Shafran, K.M., Webber, P.S., Lazarus, G.S. and Singer, K.H. (1983). Anti-cell surface pemphigus autoantibody stimulates plasminogen activator activity of human epidermal cells. *J. Exp. Med.* **157**, 259.

Hermans, P.E., Ulrich, J.A. and Morkowitz, H. (1969). Chronic muco-cutaneous candidiasis as a surface expression of deep-seated abnormalities. *Am. J. Med.* **47**, 503.

Ho, D.D., Byinton, R.E., Schooley, R.T., Flynn, T., Rota, T.R. and Hirsch, M.S. (1985). Infrequency of isolation of HTLV-III virus from saliva in AIDS. *N. Engl. J. Med.* **313**, 1606.

Holmberg, K. and Killander, J. (1971). Quantitative determination of immunoglobulins (IgG, IgA and IgM) and identification of IgA-type in the gingival fluid. *J. Periodontal Res.* **6**, 1.

Holmgren, J. and Lycke, J. (1986). Immune mechanisms in enteric infections. In *Development of Vaccines and Drugs against Diarrhea. Nobel Conference 11*, ed. A. Lindburg and R. Mollby, p. 9, Studentlitteratur Lund/Chartwell-Bratt, Bromley, England.

Holzel, A., Feldman, G.V., Tobin, J.O'H. and Harper, J. (1953). Herpes simplex: a study of complement-fixing antibodies at different ages. *Acta Paediatr. (Stockholm)* **42**, 206.

Horton, J.E., Leiken, S. and Oppenheim, J.J. (1972a). Human lymphoproliferative reaction to saliva and dental plaque deposits: an *in vitro* correlation with periodontal disease. *J. Periodontol.* **43**, 522.

Horton, J.E., Raisz, L.G., Simmons, H.A., Oppenheim, J.J. and Mergenhagen, S.E. (1972b). Bone resorbing activity in supernatant fluid from cultured human peripheral blood leukocytes. *Science* **177**, 793.

Horton, J.E., Oppenheim, J.H. and Mergenhagen, S.E. (1973). Elaboration of lymphotoxin by cultured human peripheral blood leukocytes stimulated with dental plaque deposits. *Clin. Exp. Immunol.* **13**, 383.

Horton, J.E., Oppenheim, J.J., Mergenhagen, S.E. and Raisz, L.G. (1974). Macrophage–lymphocyte synergy in the production of osteoclast-activating factor. *J. Immunol.* **113**, 1278.

Howell, A. and Jordan, H.V. (1967). Production of an extracellular levan by *Odontomyces viscosus*. *Arch. Oral Biol.* **12**, 571.

Hughes, M., Machardy, S.M., Sheppard, A.J. and Woods, N.C. (1980). Evidence for an immunological relationship between *Streptococcus mutans* and human cardiac tissue. *Infect. Immun.* **27**, 276.

Hurme, V.O. and Van Wagenen, G. (1956). Emergence of permanent first molars in the monkey (*Macaca mulatta*): association with other growth phenomena. *Yale J. Biol. Med.* **28**, 538.

Hurst, V. (1957). *Staphylococcus aureus* in the infant upper respiratory tract. I. Observations on hospital born babies. *J. Hyg. (Cambridge)* **55**, 299.

Husband, A.J., Monie, H.J. and Gowans, J.L. (1977). The natural history of the cells producing IgA in the gut. In *Immunology of the Gut*, p. 29, Excerpta Medica, Elsevier, North-Holland, Amsterdam.

Hussain, L., Ward, R.G., Barnes, C.G. and Lehner, T. (1986). Antibodies to herpes simplex virus in polyethylene glycol precipitable complexes and in sera from patients with Behçet's syndrome. In *Recent Advances in Behçet's Disease*, ed. T. Lehner and C.G. Barnes, pp. 73–7, Royal Society of Medicine Services, London.

Hussain, L., Kelly, C., Hecht, E.M., Fellower, R., Jourdan, M. and Lehner, T. (1991). The expression of Fc receptors for IgG in human rectal epithelium demonstrated by immunohistology and PCR amplification of gene transcripts. *AIDS* **5**, 1089.

International Study Group for Behçet's Disease (1990). Criteria for diagnosis of Behçet's disease. *Lancet* **335**, 1078.

Ishikawa, I. and Cimasoni, G. (1978). Partial purification of a neutral protease from human polymorphonuclear leucocytes and its proteolytic effect on immunoglobulin G. *Arch. Oral Biol.* **23**, 933.

Ivanyi, L. (1980). Stimulation of gingival lymphocytes by antigens from oral bacteria. In *The Borderland between Caries and Periodontal Disease*, ed. T. Lehner and G. Cimasoni, vol. II, p. 125.

Ivanyi, L. (1986). Immunosuppression in severe periodontitis. In *Borderland between Caries and Periodontal Disease*, ed. T. Lehner and G. Cimasoni, p. 223, Médecine et Hygiène, Geneva.

Ivanyi, L. and Lehner, T. (1970). Stimulation of lymphocyte transformation by bacterial antigens in patients with periodontal disease. *Arch. Oral Biol.* **15**, 1089.

Ivanyi, L. and Lehner, T. (1978). The relationship between caries index and stimulation of lymphocytes by *Streptococcus mutans* in mothers and their neonates. *Arch. Oral Biol.* **23**, 851.

Ivanyi, L., Wilton, J.M.A. and Lehner, T. (1972). Cell-mediated immunity in periodontal disease: cytotoxicity, migration inhibition and lymphocyte transformation studies. *Immunology* **22**, 141.

Jackson, S. (1990). Secretory and serum IgA are inversely altered in AIDS patients. In *Advances in Mucosal Immunology*, ed. T.T. MacDonald, S.J. Challacombe, P.W. Bland, C.R. Stokes, R.V. Heatly and A.McI. Mowat, p. 665, Kluwer Academic Publishers, Lancaster.

Jeffries, E., Willoughby, B., Boyko, W.J. *et al.* (1985). The Vancouver lymphadenopathy — AIDS study II: seroepidemiology of HTLV-III antibody. *Can. Med. Assoc. J.* **132**, 1373.

Jenkins, G.N. and Kleinberg, I. (1956). Studies on the pH of plaque in interproximal areas after eating sweets and starchy foods. *J. Dent. Res.* **35**, 964 (abstract no. 24).

Jindal, S., Dudani, A.K., Singh, B., Harley, C.B. and Gupta, R.S. (1989). Primary structure of a human mitochondrial protein homologous to the bacterial and plant chaperonins and to the 65-kilodalton mycobacterial antigen. *J. Immunol.* **9**, 2279–83.

Johannessen, A.C., Nilsen, R., Knudsen, G.E. and Kristoffersen, T. (1987). *In situ* characterization of mononuclear cells in human chronic marginal periodontitis using monoclonal antibodies. *J. Periodontal Res.* **21**, 113.

Jones, J.C.R., Arnn, J., Straehelin, L.A. and Golman, R.D. (1984). Human autoantibodies against desmosomes: possible causative factors in pemphigus. *Proc. Nat. Acad. Sci. (USA)* **81**, 2781.

Kaneko, F., Takahashi, T., Muramatsu, Y. and Miura, Y. (1985). Immunological studies on aphthous ulcer and erythema nodosum-like eruptions in Behçet's disease. *Br. J. Dermatol.* **113**, 303–12.

Kaplan, M.H. and Volanakis, J.E. (1974). Interaction of C reactive protein complexes with the complement system. *J. Immunol.* **112**, 2135.

Kardachi, B.J.R. and Newcomb, G.M. (1978). A clinical study of gingival inflammation in renal transplant recipients taking immunosuppressive drugs. *J. Periodontol.* **49**, 307.

Keyes, P.H. and Jordan, H.V. (1964). Periodontal lesions in the Syrian hamster. III. Findings related to an infectious and transmissible component. *Arch. Oral Biol.* **9**, 377.

Kieffer, M. and Barnetson, R. St C. (1983). Increased gliadin antibodies in dermatitis herpetiformis and pemphigoid. *Br. J. Dermatol.* **108**, 673.

Kirkpatrick, C.H., Rich, R.R. and Bennett, J.E. (1971). Chronic mucocutaneous candidiasis: model-building in cellular immunity. *Ann. Intern. Med.* **74**, 955.

Klebanoff, S.J. (1967). Iodination of bacteria: a bactericidal mechanism. *J. Exp. Med.* **126**, 1063.

Klein, R.S., Phelan, J.A., Freeman, K. *et al.* (1988). Low occupational risk of human immunodeficiency virus infection among dental professionals. *N. Engl. J. Med.* **318**, 86.

Köhler, B. and Bratthall, D. (1978). Intrafamilial levels of *Streptococcus mutans* and some aspects of bacterial transmission. *Scand. J. Dent. Res.* **86**, 35.

Konohana, I., Konohana, A., Xia, P., Jordon, R.E., Geoghegan, W.D. and Duvic, M. (1988). Expression of pemphigus vulgaris antigen in cultured human keratinocytes: effect of inhibitors, tunicamycin and lectins. *J. Invest. Dermatol.* **90** (5), 708.

Kristensson, K. (1970). Morphological studies of the neural spread of herpes simplex virus to the central nervous system. *Acta Neuropathol. (Berlin)* **16**, 54.

Lamb, J., Kontiannen, S. and Lehner, T. (1979). Generation of specific T cell suppressor function induced by *Streptococcus mutans* in monkeys and mice. *Infect. Immun.* **26**, 903.

Lamb, J., Kontiannen, S. and Lehner, T. (1980). A comparative investigation of the generation of specific T cell helper function by *Streptococcus mutans* in monkeys and mice. *J. Immunol.* **124**, 2384.

La Thangue N. and Latchmann, D. (1988). A cellular protein related to heat-shock protein 90 accumulates during herpes simplex virus infection and is overexpressed in transformed cells. *Exp. Cell. Res.* **178**, 169–79.

Lavine, W.S., Maderazo, E.G., Stolman, J. *et al.* (1979). Impaired neutrophil chemotaxis in patients with juvenile and rapidly progressing periodontitis. *J. Periodontal Res.* **14**, 10.

Lawrence, H.S. (1974). Selective immunotherapy with transfer factor. *Adv. Clin. Immunol.* **4**, 115.

Lee, S.F., Progulske-Fox, A., Erdos, G.W. *et al.* (1989). Construction and characterization of isogenic mutants of *Streptococcus mutans* deficient in the major surface protein antigen P1 (I/II). *Infect. Immun.* **57**, 3306.

Lehner, T. (1964a). Recurrent aphthous ulceration and autoimmunity. *Lancet* **ii**, 1154.

Lehner, T. (1964b). Chronic candidiasis. *Dermatol. Trans.* **50**, 8.

Lehner, T. (1966). Classification and clinico-pathological features of *Candida* infections in the mouth. In *Symposium on Candida Infections*, ed. H.I. Winner and R.E. Hurley, p. 119, E. & S. Livingstone Ltd, London.

Lehner, T. (1967). Stimulation of lymphocyte transformation by tissue homogenates in recurrent oral ulceration. *Immunology* **13**, 159.

Lehner, T. (1968). Autoimmunity in oral disease, with special reference to recurrent oral ulceration. *Proc. Roy. Soc. Med.* **61**, 515.

Lehner, T. (1969a). Pathology of recurrent oral ulceration and oral ulceration in Behçet's syndrome: light, electron and fluorescence microscopy. *J. Pathol. Bacteriol.* **97**, 481.

Lehner, T. (1969b). Characterization of mucosal antibodies in recurrent aphthous ulceration and Behçet's syndrome. *Arch. Oral Biol.* **14**, 843.

Lehner, T. (1970). Serum fluorescent antibody and immunoglobulin estimations in candidosis. *J. Med. Microbiol.* **3**, 475.

Lehner, T. (1986). The role of a disorder in immunoregulation, associated with herpes simplex virus type 1 in Behçet's disease. In *Recent Advances in Behçet's Disease*, ed. T. Lehner and C.G. Barnes, pp. 31–6, Royal Society of Medicine Services, London.

Lehner, T. (1977a). Immunological responses to bacterial plaque in the mouth. In *Immunology of the Gut*, p. 135, Excerpta Medica, Elsevier, North-Holland, Amsterdam.

Lehner, T. (1977b). Progress report: oral ulceration and Behçet's syndrome. *Gut* **18**, 491.

Lehner, T. (1979). Immunopathology of Behçet's syndrome. In *Behçet's Syndrome: Clinical and Immunological Features*, p. 127, Academic Press, London.

Lehner, T. (1980). The role of serum and salivary antibodies in protection against dental caries. In *The Borderland between Caries and Periodontal Disease*, ed. T. Lehner and G. Cimasoni, vol. II, p. 193.

Lehner, T. (1982a). Cellular immunity in periodontal disease: an overview. In *Host–Parasite Interactions in Periodontal Diseases*, ed. R.J. Genco and S.E. Mergenhagen, pp. 202–16, American Society for Microbiology, Washington, DC.

Lehner, T. (1982b). The relationship between human helper and suppressor factors to a streptococcal protein antigen. *J. Immunol.* **129**, 1936.

Lehner, T. and Adinolfi, M. (1980). Acute phase proteins, C9, factor B, and lysozyme in recurrent oral ulceration and Behçet's syndrome. *J. Clin. Pathol.* **33**, 269.

Lehner, T. and Barnes, C.G. (1979). Criteria for diagnosis and classification of Behçet's syndrome. In *Behçet's Syndrome: Clinical and Immunological Approach*, ed. T. Lehner and C.G. Barnes, p. 4, Academic Press, London.

Lehner, T. and Ward, R.G. (1970). Iatrogenic candidosis. *Br. J. Dermatol.* **83**, 161.

Lehner, T. and Wilton, J.M.A. (1979). *In vivo* and *in vitro* effect of levamisole on lymphocytes from patients with Behçet's syndrome and recurrent oral ulceration. In *Drugs and Immune Responsiveness*, ed. J.L. Turk and D. Parker, p. 119, Macmillan Press Ltd., London and Basingstoke.

Lehner, T., Cardwell, J.E. and Clarry, E.D. (1967). Immunoglobulins in saliva and serum in dental caries. *Lancet* **i**, 1294.

Lehner, T., Buckley, H.E. and Murray, I.G. (1972a). The relationship between fluorescent, agglutinating and precipitating antibodies to *Candida albicans* and their immunoglobulin classes. *J. Clin. Pathol.* **25**, 344.

Lehner, T., Wilton, J.M.A. and Ivanyi, L. (1972b). Immunodeficiencies in chronic muco-cutaneous candidosis. *Immunology* **22**, 775.

Lehner, T., Wilton, J.M.A., Challacombe, S.J. and Ivanyi, L. (1974a). Sequential cell-mediated immune responses in experimental gingivitis in man. *Clin. Exp. Immunol.* **16**, 481.

Lehner, T., Wilton, J.M.A., Ivanyi, L. and Manson, J.D. (1974b). Immunological aspects of juvenile periodontitis (periodontosis). *J. Periodontol.* **45**, 261.

Lehner, T., Challacombe, S.J. and Caldwell, J. (1975a). An experimental model for immunological studies of dental caries in the rhesus monkey. *Arch. Oral Biol.* **20**, 299.

Lehner, T., Challacombe, S.J. and Caldwell, J. (1975b). An immunological investigation into the prevention of caries in deciduous teeth of rhesus monkeys. *Arch. Oral Biol.* **20**, 305.

Lehner, T., Challacombe, S.J., Wilton, J.M.A. and Caldwell, J. (1976a). Cellular and humoral immune responses in vaccination against dental caries. *Nature* **264**, 69.

Lehner, T., Challacombe, S.J., Wilton, J.M.A. and Ivanyi, L. (1976b). Immunopotentiation by dental microbial plaque and its relationship to oral disease in man. *Arch. Oral Biol.* **21**, 749.

Lehner, T., Russell, M.W., Challacombe, S.J., Scully, C.M. and Hawkes, J.E. (1978). Passive immunisation with serum and immunoglobulins against dental caries in rhesus monkeys. *Lancet* **i**, 693.

Lehner, T., Murray, J., Winter, G. and Caldwell, J. (1978b). Antibodies to *Streptococcus mutans* and immunoglobulin levels in children with dental caries. *Arch. Oral Biol.* **23**, 1061.

Lehner, T., Batchelor, J.R., Challacombe, S.J. and Kennedy, L. (1979a). An immunogenetic basis for the tissue involvement in Behcet's syndrome. *Immunology* **37**, 895.

Lehner, T., Losito, A. and Gwyn Williams, D. (1979b). Cryoglobulins in Behçet's syndrome and recurrent oral ulcerations. *Clin. Exp. Immunol.* **38**, 436.

Lehner, T., Russell, M.W., Scully, C.M., Challacombe, S.J. and Caldwell, J. (1979c). The role of IgG, IgA and IgM classes of antibodies to *Streptococcus mutans* in protection against caries in rhesus monkeys. In *Pathogenic Streptococci*, ed. M.T. Parker, p. 215. Reedbooks, Chertsey.

Lehner, T, Lavery, E., Smith, R., van der Zee, Mizushima, Y. and Shinnick, T. (1991). Association between the 65-kilodalton heat shock protein, *Streptococcus sanguis*, and the corresponding antibodies in Behçet's syndrome. *Infect. Immun.* **59**, 1434.

Lehner, T., Challacombe, S.J. and Cardwell, J. (1980). Oral immunisation with *Streptococcus mutans* in rhesus monkeys and the development of immune responses and dental caries. *Immunology* **41**, 857.

Lehner, T., Russell, M.W., Caldwell, J. and Smith, R. (1981). Immunization with purified protein antigens from *Streptococcus mutans* against dental caries in rhesus monkeys. *Infect. Immun.* **34**, 407.

Lehner, T., Welsh, K.L. and Batchelor, J.R. (1982). The relationship of HLA-B and DR phenotypes to Behçet's syndrome, recurrent oral ulceration and the class of immune complexes. *Immunology* **47**, 581.

Lehner, T., Caldwell, J. and Avery, J. (1984). Sequential development of helper and suppressor function, antibody titres and functional avidities to a streptococcal antigen in rhesus monkeys. *Eur. J. Immunol.* **14**, 814.

Lehner, T., Caldwell, J. and Smith, R. (1986a). Local passive immunization by monoclonal antibodies against streptococcal antigen I/II in the prevention of dental caries. *Infect. Immun.* **50**, 796.

Lehner, T., Mehlert, A. and Caldwell, J. (1986b). Local active gingival immunization by a 3,800-molecular-weight streptococcal antigen in protection against dental caries. *Infect. Immun.* **52**, 682.

Lehner, T., Haron, J., Bergmeier, L.A. *et al.* (1989). Local oral immunization with synthetic peptides induces a dual mucosal IgG and salivary IgA antibody response and prevents colonization of *Streptococcus mutans*. *Immunology* **67**, 419.

Lehrer, R.I. and Cline, M.J. (1969). Leukocyte myeloperoxidase deficiency and disseminated candidiasis: the role of myeloperoxidase in resistance to *Candida* infection. *J. Clin. Invest.* **48**, 1478.

Levinsky, R.J. and Lehner, T. (1978). Circulating soluble immune complexes in recurrent oral ulceration and Behçet's syndrome. *Clin. Exp. Immunol.* **32**, 193.

Levy, R.L., Bach, M.L., Huang, S.W. *et al.* (1971). Thymic transplantation in a case of chronic mucocutaneous candidiasis. *Lancet* **ii**, 898.

Lewis, G.M., Hopper, M.E. and Montgomery, R.A. (1937). Infections of skin due to *Monilia albicans*. 1. Diagnostic value of intradermal testing with commercial extract of *Monilia albicans*. *NY State J. Med.* **37**, 878.

Lindhe, J. and Socransky, S.J. (1979). Chemotaxis and vascular permeability produced by human periodontopathic bacteria. *J. Periodontal Res.* **14**, 138.

Linzer, R., Mukasa, H. and Slade, H.D. (1975). Serological purification of polysaccharide antigens from *Streptococcus mutans* serotypes a and d: characterization of multiple antigenic determinants. *Infect. Immun.* **12**, 791.

Linzer, R., Gill, K. and Slade, H.D. (1976). Chemical composition of *Streptococcus mutans* type c antigen: comparison to type a, b and d antigens. *J. Dent. Res.* **55**, A109.

Löe, H., Theilade, E. and Jensen, S.B. (1965). Experimental gingivitis in man. *J. Periodontol.* **36**, 177.

Loesche, W.J. (1976). Chemotherapy of dental plaque infection. *Oral Sci. Rev. (Copenhagen)* **9**, 65.

Louria, D.B., Smith, J.K., Brayton, R.G. and Buse, M. (1972). Anti-*Candida* factors in serum and their inhibition. I. Clinical and laboratory observations. *J. Infect. Dis.* **125**, 102.

Ma, J.K.-C., Smith, R. and Lehner, T. (1987). Use of monoclonal antibodies in local passive immunization to prevent colonization of human teeth by *Streptococcus mutans*. *Infect. Immun.* **55**, 1274.

Ma, J.K.-C., Hunjan, M., Smith, R. and Lehner, T. (1989). Specificity of monoclonal antibodies in local passive immunization against *Streptococcus mutans*. *Clin. Exp. Immunol.* **77**, 331.

Ma, J.K.-C., Hunjan, M., Smith, R., Kelly, C. and Lehner, T. (1990). An investigation into the mechanism of protection by local passive immunization with monoclonal antibodies against *Streptococcus mutans*. *Infect. Immun.* **58**, 3406.

McCarthy, C., Snyder, M.L. and Parker (1965). The indigenous oral flora of man. I. The newborn to the 1 year old infant. *Arch. Oral Biol.* **10**, 61.

Mackler, B.F, Altman, L.C., Wahl, S., Rosenstreich, D.L., Oppenheim, J.J. and Mergenhagen, S.E. (1974). Blastogenesis and lymphokine synthesis by T and B lymphocytes from patients with periodontal disease. *Infect. Immun.* **10**, 844.

Mackler, B.F., Schur, P., Waldrop, T., Coker, E. and Rossen, R. (1979). IgG subclasses in human periodontal disease. III. Serum concentrations of IgG subclass immunoglobulins and circulating immune complexes. *J. Dent. Res.* **58**, 1701.

Masuda, K., Nakajima, A., Urayama, A., Nakae, K., Kogure, M. and Inaba, G. (1989). Double-masked trial of cyclosporin versus colchicine and long-term open study of cyclosporin in Behçets disease. *Lancet* **i**, 1093.

Matsumura, N. and Mizushima, Y. (1975). Leucocyte movement and colchicine treatment in Behçet's disease. *Lancet* **ii**, 813.

Matthews, R.C., Burnie, J.P. and Tabaqchali, S. (1987). Isolation of immunodominant antigens from sera of patients with systemic candidiasis and characterization of serological response to *Candida albicans*. *J. Clin. Microbiol.* **25**, 230.

Mergenhagen, S.E., Rosenstreich, D.L., Wilton, J.M.A., Wahl, S.M. and Wahl, L.K. (1976). Interaction of endotoxin with lymphocytes and macrophages. In *The Role of Immunological Factors in Infections, Allergic and Autoimmune Processes*, ed. R.F. Beers and E.G. Bassett, p. 170, Johns Hopkins University Press, Baltimore.

Mestecky, J. and McGhee, J.R. (1987). Immunoglobulin (IgA): molecular and cellular interactions involved in IgA biosynthesis and immune responses. *Adv. Immunol.* **40**, 153.

Mestecky, J., McGhee, J.R., Arnold, R.R., Michalek, S.M., Prince, S.J. and Babb, J.L. (1978). Selective induction of an immune response in human external secretions by ingestion of bacterial antigen. *J. Clin. Invest.* **61**, 731.

Meyers, R.L. and Pettit, T.H. (1973). Corneal immune response to herpes simplex virus antigens. *J. Immunol.* **110**, 1575.

Michalek, S.M. and McGhee, J.R. (1977). Effective immunity to dental caries: passive transfer to rats of antibodies to *Streptococcus mutans* elicits protection. *Infect. Immun.* **17**, 644.

Michalek, S.M., McGhee, J.R., Mestecky, J., Arnold, R.R. and Bozzo, L. (1976). Ingestion of *Streptococcus mutans* induces secretory immunoglobulin A and caries immunity. *Science* **192**, 1238.

Michalek, S.M., Gregory, R.L., Harmon, C.C. *et al.* (1987). Protection of gnotobiotic rats against dental caries by passive immunization with bovine antibodies to *Streptococcus mutans*. *Infect. Immun.* **55**, 2341.

Mikulicz, J. von and Kummel, W. (1898). *Die Krankheiten des Mudes*. Gunter Fischer, Jena.

Miller, M.E. (1969). Deficiency of chemotactic function in the human neonate: a previously unrecognised defect of the inflammatory response. *Abstr. Paediatr. Res.* **3**, 497.

Mizushima, Y., Matsumura, N., Mori, M. and Matsumura, Y. (1979). Colchicine in the treatment of Behçet's disease. In *Behçet's Disease: Proceedings of an International Symposium on Behçet's Disease, Istanbul*, ed. N. Dilsen, M. Konice and C. Ovul, p. 286, Excerpta Medica, Elsevier, North-Holland, Amsterdam.

Mizushima, Y. (1989). Skin hypersensitivity to streptococcal antigens and the induction of systemic symptoms by the antigens in Behçet's disease — a multicenter study. *J. Rheumatol.* **16**(4), 506–11.

Mortensen, R.F., Osmand, A.P. and Gewurz, H. (1975). Effects of C reactive protein on the lymphoid system. *J. Exp. Med.* **141**, 821.

Mowat, A.F. and Baum, J. (1971). Chemotaxis of polymorphonuclear leukocytes from patients with diabetes mellitus. *N. Engl. J. Med.* **284**, 621.

Müller, F., Froland, S.S., Hvatum, M., Radl, J. and Brandtzaeg, P. (1991). Both IgA subclasses are reduced in parotid saliva from patients with AIDS. *Clin. Exp. Immunol.* **83**, 203.

Muller, W. and Lehner, T. (1982). Quantitative electron microscopical analysis of leukocyte infiltration in oral ulcers of Behçet's syndrome. *Br. J. Dermatol.* **106**, 535.

Murray, I.G., Buckley, H.R. and Turner, G.C. (1969). Serological evidence of *Candida* infection after open-heart surgery. *J. Med. Microbiol.* **2**, 463.

Nagler, F.P.O. (1944). Specific cutaneous reaction in persons infected with virus of herpes simplex. *J. Immunol.* **48**, 213.

Nahmias, A.J. and Roizman, B. (1973). Infection with herpes simplex virus 1 and 2. *N. Engl. J. Med.* **289**, 667.

Nair, P.N.R. and Schroeder, H.E. (1986). Duct associated lymphoid tissue (DALT) of minor salivary glands and mucosal immunity. *Immunology* **57**, 171.

Namba, K., Ueno, T., Matsumi, F., Okita, M. *et al.* (1984). Behçet's disease and streptococcus infection: time course of streptococcus antigen titre and comparison with other uveitis. Behçet's Disease Research Committee of Japan. In *Studies on Etiology Treatment and Prevention of Behçet's Disease*, pp. 367–72, Ministry of Welfare, Japan.

Newbrun, E. (1989). Guest editorial: Uses and abuses of the news release/press conference. *J. Dent. Res.* **67**, 1442.

Newman, M.G. and Socransky S.S. (1977). Predominant cultivable microbiota in periodontosis. *J. Periodontal Res.* **12**, 120.

Nisengard, R.J., Beutner, E.H. and Hazen S.P. (1968). Immunologic studies of periodontal disease. IV. Bacterial hypersensitivity and periodontal disease. *J. Periodontol.* **39**, 329.

Nisengard, R.J., Beutner, E.H. and Gauto, M. (1971). Immunofluorescence studies of IgF in periodontal disease. *Ann. NY Acad. Sci.* **177**, 39.

Nobreus, N., Attstrom, R. and Egelberg, J. (1974a). Effect of anti-thymocyte serum on development of gingivitis in dogs. *J. Periodontal Res.* **9**, 227.

Nobreus, N., Attstrom, R. and Egelberg, J. (1974b). Effect of anti-thymocyte antiserum on chronic gingival inflammation in dogs. *J. Periodontal Res.* **9**, 236.

Nussenblatt, R.B., Grey, I., Ballintine, E.J. and Wacker, W.B. (1980). Cellular immune response of uveitis patients to retinal S-antigen. *Am. J. Ophthalmol.* **89**, 173.

Nussenblatt, R.B., Palestine, A.G., Chan, C.C., Mochizuki, M. and Yancey, K. (1985). Effectiveness of cyclosporin therapy for Behçet's disease. *Arthritis. Rheum.* **28**, 671.

O'Duffy, J.D. (1978). Summary of International Symposium on

Behçet's Disease. *J. Rheumatol.* **5**, 229.

O'Duffy, J.D., Carney, J.A. and Deodhar, S. (1971). Behçet's disease: report of 10 cases, 3 with new manifestations. *Ann. Intern. Med.* **75**, 561.

O'Duffy, J.D., Bowles, C.A. and O'Fallon, W.M. (1986). The immunosuppressive treatment of Behçet's disease with emphasis on chlorambucil. In *Recent Advances in Behçet's Disease*, ed. T. Lehner and C.G. Barnes, p. 301, International Congress and Symposium Series no. 103, Royal Society of Medicine Services, London.

Ohno, S. (1986). Behçet's disease in the world. In *Recent Advances in Behçet's Disease*, ed. T. Lehner and C.G. Barnes, p. 181, International Congress and Symposium Series no. 103, Royal Society of Medicine Services, London.

Ohno, S. and Matsuda, H. (1986). Studies of HLA antigens in Behçet's disease in Japan. In *Recent Advances in Behçet's Disease*, ed. T. Lehner and C.G. Barnes, pp. 11–15, Royal Society of Medicine Services, London.

Ohno, S., Nakayama, E., Sugiura, S., Itakura, K., Aoki, K. and Aizawa, M. (1975). Specific histocompatibility antigens associated with Behçet's disease. *Am. J. Ophthalmol.* **80**, 636.

O'Reilly, R.J., Chibbaro, A., Anger, E. and Lopez, C. (1977). Cell-mediated immune responses in patients with recurring herpes simplex infections. II. Infection associated deficiency of lymphokine production in patients with recurrent herpes progenitalis. *J. Immunol.* **118**, 1095.

Oshima, Y., Shimizu, T, Yokohari, R. *et al.* (1963). Clinical studies on Behçet's syndrome. *Ann. Rheum. Dis.* **22**, 36.

Ostarvik, J. and Brandtzaeg, P. (1975). Secretion of parotid IgA in relation to gingival inflammation and dental caries experience in man. *Arch. Oral Biol.* **20**, 701.

Page, R.C. and Schroeder, H.E. (1976). Pathogenesis of inflammatory periodontal disease: a summary of current work. *Lab. Invest.* **33**, 235.

Page, R.C, Davies, P. and Allison, A.C. (1973). Effects of dental plaque on the production and release of lysosomal hydrolases by macrophages in culture. *Arch. Oral Biol.* **18**, 1481.

Paine, T.F., Jr (1964). Latent herpes simplex infection in man. *Bacteriol. Rev.* **28**, 472.

Patters, M.R., Genco, R.J., Reed, M.J. and Mashimo, P.A. (1976). Blastogenic response of human lymphocytes to oral bacterial antigens: comparison of individuals with periodontal disease to normal and edentulous subjects. *Infect. Immun.* **14**, 1213.

Pepys, J., Faux, J.A., McCarthy, D.S. and Hargreave, F.E. (1968). *Candida albicans* precipitins in respiratory disease in man. *J. Allergy* **41**, 305.

Perch, B., Kjems, E. and Ravn, T. (1974). Biochemical and serological properties of *Streptococcus mutans* from various human and animal sources. *Acta Pathol. Microbiol. Scand. Sec. B* **28**, 357.

Peterson, L.L. and Wuepper, K.D. (1984). Isolation and purification of a pemphigus vulgaris antigen from human epidermis. *J. Clin. Invest.* **73**, 1113.

Postlethwaite, A.E., Lachman, L.B., Minardi, C.L. and Kang, A.H. (1983). Interleukin 1 stimulation of collagenase: production by cultured fibroblasts. *J. Exp. Med.* **157**, 801.

Poulter, L.W. and Lehner, T. (1989). Immunohistology of oral lesions from patients with recurrent oral ulcers and Behçet's syndrome. *Clin. Exp. Immunol.* **78**, 189.

Raeste, A.M. (1972). The differential count of oral leukocytes. *Scand. J. Dent. Res.* **80**, 63.

Rager-Zisman, B. and Bloom, B.R. (1974). Immunological destruction of herpes simplex virus 1 infected cells. *Nature* **251**, 542.

Raisz, L., Sandberg, A., Goodson, J., Simmons, H. and Mergenhagen, S. (1974). Complement-dependent stimulation of prostaglandin synthesis and bone resorption. *Science* **185**, 789.

Ranney, R.R. (1978). Immunofluorescent localisation of soluble dental plaque components in human gingiva affected by periodontitis. *J. Periodontal Res.* **13**, 99.

Rasmussen, L.E., Jordan, G.W., Stevens, D.A. and Merigan, T.C. (1974). Lymphocyte interferon production and transformation after herpes simplex infections in humans. *J. Immunol.* **112**, 728.

Ray, T.C. and Wuepper, K.D. (1975). Experimental cutaneous *Candida albicans* infections in rodents; role of complement. *Clin. Res.* **23**, 2304.

Redfield, R.R. and Burke, D.S. (1988). HIV infection: the clinical picture. *Sci. Am.* **259** (4), 70.

Rocklin, R.E., Chilgren, R.A., Hong, R. and David, J.R. (1970). Transfer of cellular hypersensitivity in chronic mucocutaneous candidiasis monitored *in vivo* and *in vitro*. *Cell. Immunol.* **1**, 290.

Rogers, R.S., Sams, W.M. and Shorter, R.G. (1974). Lymphocytotoxicity in recurrent aphthous stomatitis. *Arch. Dermatol.* **109**, 361.

Rogers, T.J. and Balish, E. (1977). The role of activated macrophages in resistance to experimental renal candidiasis. *J. Reticuloendothelial Soc.* **22**, 309.

Roizman, B. (1974). Herpes virus, latency and cancer: a biochemical approach. *J. Reticuloendoth. Soc.* **15**, 312.

Rosenberg, G.L. and Notkins, A.L. (1974). Induction of cellular immunity to herpes simplex virus: relationship to the humoral immune response. *J. Immunol.* **112**, 1019.

Rosenberg, G.L., Snyderman, R. and Notkins, A.L. (1974). Production of chemotactic factor and lymphotoxin by human leukocytes stimulated with herpes simplex virus. *Infect. Immun.* **10**, 111.

Russell, M.W. and Lehner, T. (1978). Characterisation of antigens extracted from cells and culture fluids of *Streptococcus mutans* serotype c. *Arch. Oral Biol.* **23**, 7.

Russell, M.W. and Wu, H. (1990). *Streptococcus mutans* and the problem of heart cross-reactivity. *Oral Biol. Med.* **1**, 191.

Russell, M.W., Bergmeier, L.A., Zanders, E.D. and Lehner, T. (1980). Protein antigens of *Streptococcus mutans*: purification and properties of a double antigen and its protease-resistant component. *Infect. Immun.* **28**, 486.

Saito, T., Honma, T., Sato, T. and Fujioka, Y. (1971). Autoimmune mechanisms as a probable aetiology of Behçet's syndrome, an electron microscopic study of the oral mucosa. *Virchows Archiv A Pathologische Anatomie* **353**, 261.

Sams, W.M. and Gammon, W.R. (1982). Mechanism of lesion production in pemphigus and pemphigoid. *J. Am. Acad. Dermatol.* **6**, 431.

Sandberg, A.L., Raisz, L.G., Goodson, J.M., Simmons, H.A. and Mergenhagen, S.E. (1977). Initiation of bone resorption by the classical and alternative complement pathways and its mediation by prostaglandins. *J. Immunol.* **119**, 1378.

Sanders, M.D. (1979). Ophthalmic features of Behçet's disease.

In *Behçet's Syndrome: Clinical and Immunological Approach*, ed. T. Lehner and C.G. Barnes, p. 183, Academic Press, London.

Schiott, C.R. and Löe, H. (1970). The origin and variation in number of leukocytes in the human saliva. *J. Periodontol. Res.* **5**, 36.

Schneider, T.F., Toto, P.D., Garguilo, A.W. and Pollock, R.J. (1966). Specific bacterial antibodies in the inflamed human gingiva. *Periodontics* **4**, 53.

Schuller, P.D., Freedman, H.L. and Levins, D.W. (1973). Periodontal status of renal transplant patients receiving immunosuppressive therapy. *J. Periodontol.* **44**, 167.

Scully, C.M. and Challacombe, S.J. (1979). The migration of ^{111}Indium radiolabelled polymorphonuclear leucocytes into the oral cavity in the rhesus monkey. *J. Periodontal Res.* **14**, 475.

Scully, C.M. and Lehner, T. (1979). Bacterial and strain specificities in opsonisation, phagocytosis and killing of *Streptococcus mutans*. *Clin. Exp. Immunol.* **35**, 128.

Scully C.M. and Lehner, T. (1980). Comparative opsonic activity for *Streptococcus mutans* in oral fluids and phagocytic activity of blood, crevicular and polymorphonuclear leukocytes in rhesus monkeys. *Immunology* **39**, 101.

Scully, C.M., Lehner, T. and Harfitt, R. (1979). Serum, salivary and lacrimal immunoglobulins in Behçet's syndrome and recurrent oral ulceration. In *Behçet's Syndrome: Clinical and Immunological Features*, ed. T. Lehner and C.G. Barnes, p. 77, Academic Press, London.

Sezer, F.N. (1953). The isolation of a virus as the cause of Behçet's disease. *Am. J. Ophthalmol.* **36**, 301.

Shannon, D.C., Johnson, G., Rosen, F.S. and Austen, K.F. (1966). Cellular reactivity to *Candida albicans* antigen. *N. Engl. J. Med.* **275**, 690.

Shikano, S. (1966). Ocular pathology of Behçet's syndrome. In *International Symposium on Behçet's Disease*, ed. M. Monacelli and P. Nazzaro, p. 111, Karger, Basle.

Shillitoe, E.J. and Lehner, T. (1972). Immunoglobulins and complement in crevicular fluid, serum and saliva in man. *Arch. Oral Biol.* **17**, 241.

Shillitoe, E.J., Wilton, J.M.A. and Lehner, T. (1977). Sequential changes in cell-mediated immune responses to herpes simplex virus following recurrent herpetic infection in man. *Infect. Immunol.* **18**, 130.

Shillitoe, E.J., Wilton, J.M.A. and Lehner, T. (1978). Sequential changes in T and B lymphocyte responses to herpes simplex virus in man. *Scand. J. Immunol.* **7**, 357.

Shimada, K., Kogure, M., Kawashima, T. and Nishioka, K. (1974). Reduction of complement in Behçet's disease and drug allergy. *Med. Biol.* **52**, 234.

Shimizu, T., Kagami, T., Matsumoto, T. and Matsumura, N. (1965). Clinical studies of Behçet's syndrome: analysis of epidemiology and attack-inducing factor of the disease. *Medicine (Japan)* **12**, 526.

Shore, S.L., Nahmias, A.J., Starr, S.E., Wood, P.A. and McFarlin, D.E. (1974). Detection of cell-dependent cytotoxic antibody to cells infected with herpes simplex virus. *Nature* **251**, 350.

Sircus, W., Church, R. and Kelleher, J. (1957). Recurrent aphthous ulceration of the mouth: a study of the natural history, aetiology and treatment. *Quart. J. Med.* **26**, 235.

Skapski, H. and Lehner, T. (1976). A crevicular washing method for investigating immune components of crevicular fluid in man. *J. Periodontal Res.* **11**, 19.

Slots, J. and Genco, R.J. (1984). Black pigmented *Bacteroides* species, *Capnocytophaga* species and *Actinobacillus actinomycetemcomitans* in human periodontal disease. *J. Dent. Res.* **63**, 412.

Slots, J. and Listgarten, M.A. (1988). *Bacteroides gingivalis, Bacteroides intermedius* and *Actinobacillus actinomycetemcomitans* in human periodontal diseases. *J. Clin. Periodontol.* **15**, 85.

Smith, R. and Lehner, T. (1981). A radioimmunoassay for serum and gingival crevicular fluid antibodies to a purified protein of *Streptococcus mutans*. *Clin. Exp. Immunol.* **43**, 417–24.

Smith, D.J., Taubman, M.A. and Ebersole, J.L. (1979). Effect of oral administration of glucosyltransferase antigens on experimental caries. *Infect. Immun.* **26**, 82.

Smith, I.W., Peutherer, J.F. and McCallum, F.O. (1967). The incidence of herpesvirus hominis antibody in the population. *J. Hyg. (Cambridge)* **65**, 395.

Smith, S., Bick, P.H., Miller, G.A. *et al.* (1980). Polyclonal B-cell activation: severe periodontal disease in young adults. *Clin. Immunol.* **16**, 354.

Snyderman, R., Altman, L.C., Franlel, A. and Blaese, R.M. (1973). Defective mononuclear chemotaxis: a previously unrecognised immune dysfunction. Studies in a patient with chronic mucocutaneous candidiasis. *Ann. Intern. Med.* **78**, 509.

Sobel, J.D., Haim, S.M., Obedeanu, M., Meshulam, T. and Merzbach, D. (1977). Polymorphonuclear leucocyte function in Behçet's disease. *J. Clin. Pathol.* **30**, 250.

Socransky, S.S. (1977). Microbiology of periodontal disease — present status and future considerations. *J. Periodontol.* **48**, 497.

Socransky, S.S., Haffajee, A.D., Dzink, J.L. and Hillman, J.D. (1988). Associations between microbial species in subgingival plaque samples. *Oral Microbiol. Immunol.* **3**, 1.

Sohnle, P.G., Frank, M.M. and Kirkpatrick, C.H. (1976). Deposition of complement components in the cutaneous lesion of chronic mucocutaneous candidiasis. *Clin. Immunol. Immunopathol.* **5**, 340.

Stalybrass, F.C. (1964). *Candida* precipitins. *J. Pathol. Bacteriol.* **87**, 89.

Stanley, J.R., Koulu, L. and Thivolet, C. (1984). Distinction between epidermal antigens binding pemphigus vulgaris and pemphigus foliaceus autoantibodies. *J. Clin. Invest.* **74**, 313.

Stephan, R.M. (1940). Changes in hydrogen-ion concentration on tooth surfaces and in carious lesions. *J. Am. Dent. Assoc.* **27**, 718.

Stevens, J.G. and Cook, M.L. (1971). Restriction of herpes simplex virus by macrophages: an analysis of the cell–virus interaction. *J. Exp. Med.* **133**, 19.

Stinson, M.W., Nisengard, R.J., Neiders, M.E. and Albini, B. (1983). Serology and tissue lesions in rabbits immunized with *Streptococcus mutans*. *J. Immunol.* **131**, 3021.

Stockbine, N.A., Largen, M.T., Zweibel, S.M. and Buckley, H.R. (1984). Indentification and molecular weight characterization of antigens from *Candida albicans* that are recognized by human sera. *Infect. Immun.* **43**, 715.

Strom, J. (1965). Ectodermosis erosiva pluriorificalis, Stevens–

Johnson's syndrome in cold-agglutination-positive infections. *Lancet* **i**, 457.

Studd, M., McCance, J. and Lehner, T. (1991). Detection of HSV-1 DNA in patients with Behçet's syndrome and in patients with recurrent oral ulcers by the polymerase chain reaction. *J. Med. Microbiol.* **34**, 39–43.

Taichman, N.S. and McArthur, W.P. (1976). Interaction of inflammatory cells and oral bacteria: release of lysosomal hydrolases from rabbit polymorphonuclear leukocytes exposed to Gram-positive plaque bacteria. *Arch. Oral Biol.* **21**, 257.

Taubman, M.A. and Smith, D.J. (1977). Effects of local immunisation with glucosyltransferase fractions from *Streptococcus mutans* on dental caries in rats and hamsters. *J. Immunol.* **118**, 710.

Taubman, M.A., Stoufi, E.D., Ebersole, J.L. and Smith, D.J. (1984). Phenotypic studies of cells from periodontal disease tissues. *J. Periodontal Res.* **19**, 587.

Theilade, E. and Theilade, J. (1976). Role of plaque in the etiology of periodontal disease and caries. *Oral Sci. Rev. (Copenhagen)*, 23.

Thole, J.E.R., Keulen, W.J., Kolk, A.H.J. *et al.* (1987). Characterization, sequence determination, and immunogenicity of a 64-kilodalton protein of *Mycobacterium bovis* BCG expressed in *Escherichia coli* K-12. *Infect. Immun.* **55**, 1466–75.

Tollefsen, T., Saltvedt, E. and Koppang, H.S. (1978). The effect of immunosuppressive agents on periodontal disease in man. *J. Periodontal Res.* **13**, 240.

Tomasi, T.B. and Cebra, J.J. (1971). Secretory immunoglobulins. In *Progress in Immunology*, p. 1481, Academic Press, New York.

Trechsel, U., Dew, G., Murphy, G. and Reynolds, J.J. (1982). Effects of products from macrophages, blood mononuclear cells and of retinol on collagenase secretion and collagen synthesis in chondrocyte culture. *Biochem. Biophys. Acta* **720**, 364.

Truelove, S.C. and Morris-Owen, R.M. (1958). Treatment of aphthous ulceration of the mouth. *Br. Med. J.* **1**, 603.

Valdimarsson, H., Holt, L., Riches, R.C. and Hobbs, J.R. (1970). Lymphocyte transformation abnormality in chronic mucocutaneous candidosis. *Lancet* **i**, 1259.

Valdimarsson, H., Wood, C.B.S., Hobbs, J.R. and Holt, P.J.L. (1972). Immunological features in a case of chronic granulomatous candidiasis and its treatment with transfer factor. *Clin. Exp. Immunol.* **11**, 151.

van de Rijn, I., Bleiweis, A.S. and Zabriskie, J.B. (1976). Antigens in *Streptococcus mutans* cross reactive with human heart muscle. *J. Dent. Res.* **55**, C59.

Van Scoy, R.E., Hill, H.R., Ritts, R.E. and Quie, P.G. (1975). Familial neutrophil chemotaxis defect, recurrent bacterial infections, mucocutaneous candidiasis and hyperimmunoglobulinaemia E. *Ann. Intern. Med.* **82**, 766.

Walker, J. *et al.* (1981). Antibody responses of monkeys to oral and local immunisation with *Streptococcus mutans*. *Infect. Immun.* **31**, 61.

Walsh, L.J., Lander, P.E., Seymour, G.J. and Powell, R.N. (1987). Isolation and purification of ILS, an interleukin 1 inhibitor produced by human gingival epithelial cells. *Clin. Exp. Immun.* **68**, 366.

Waltz, M.A., Price, R.W. and Notkins, A.L. (1974). Latent ganglionic infection with herpes simplex virus types 1 and 2: viral reactivation *in vivo* after neurectomy. *Science* **184**, 1185.

Watkins, J.F. (1964). Adsorption of sensitized sheep erythrocytes to HeLa cells infected with herpes simplex virus. *Nature* **202**, 1364.

Weathers, D.R. and Griffin, J.W. (1970). Intraoral ulcerations of recurrent herpes simplex and recurrent aphthae: two distinct clinical entities. *J. Am. Dent. Assoc.* **81**, 81.

Weiss, P., Taylor, A.C. and Pillai, P.A. (1962). The nerve fiber as a system in continuous flow: microcinematographic and electronmicroscopic demonstrations. *Science* **136**, 330.

Welsh, K.I. and Kerr, L.A. (1986). The immunogenetics of Behçet's disease – do they give an indication to the likely mechanism of the disease? In *Recent Advances in Behçet's Disease*. In ed. T. Lehner and C.G. Barnes, pp. 3–9, Royal Society of Medicine Services, London.

Westmorland, D. and Watkins, J.F. (1974). The IgG receptor induced by herpes simplex virus studies using radiodinated IgG. *J. Gen. Virol.* **24**, 167.

Whitaker, J., Landing, B.H., Esselborn, W.H. and Williams, R.R. (1956). The syndrome of familial juvenile hypoadrenocorticism, hypoparathyroidism and superficial moniliasis. *J. Clin. Endocrinol. Metab.* **16**, 1374.

Wicken, A.J. and Knox, K.W. (1978). Studies on the group F antigen of lactobacilli: isolation of a teichoic acid lipid complex from *Lactobacillus fermenti*, NCTC 6991. *J. Gen. Microbiol.* **60**, 293.

Wilde, G., Cooper, M. and Page, R.C. (1977). Host tissue response in chronic periodontal disease. VI. The role of cell-mediated hypersensitivity. *J. Periodontal Res.* **12**, 179.

Williams, B.D. and Lehner, T. (1977). Immune complexes in Behçet's syndrome and recurrent oral ulceration. *Br. Med. J.* **1**, 1387.

Williams, B.D., Challacombe, S.J., Slandy, J.M., Lachmann, P.J. and Lehner, T. (1975). Immunoconglutinins and C3 in human saliva. *Clin. Exp. Immunol.* **19**, 423.

Williams, D.M., Leonard, J.N., Wright, P. *et al.* (1984). Benign mucous membrane (cicatricial) pemphigoid revisited: a clinical and immunological reappraisal. *Br. Dent. J.* **157**, 313.

Williams, R.C. and Gibbons, R.J. (1972). Inhibition of bacterial adherence by secretory immunoglobulin A: a mechanism of antigen disposal. *Science* **177**, 697.

Wilton, J.M.A. (1977). The function of complement in crevicular fluid. In *The Borderland between Caries and Periodontal Disease*, ed. T. Lehner, p. 223, Academic Press, London.

Wilton, J.M.A. (1978). Suppression by IgA of IgG-mediated phagocytosis by human polymorphonuclear leucocytes. *Clin. Exp. Immunol.* **34**, 423.

Wilton, J.M.A. and Lehner, T. (1979). Detective polymorphonuclear leukocyte phagocytosis in patients with Behçet's syndrome and recurrent oral ulceration. In *Behçet's Syndrome: Clinical and Immunological Features*, ed. T. Lehner and C.G. Barnes, p. 67, Academic Press, London.

Wilton, J.M.A., Ivanyi, L. and Lehner, T. (1972). Cell mediated immunity in herpesvirus hominis infections. *Brit. Med. J.* **1**, 723.

Wilton, J.M.A., Renggli, H.H. and Lehner, T. (1976). The isolation and identification of mononuclear cells from the gingival crevice in man. *J. Periodontal. Res.* **11**, 262.

Wilton, J.M.A., Renggli, H.H. and Lehner, T. (1977a). A functional comparison of blood and gingival inflammatory polymorphonuclear leucocytes in man. *Clin. Exp. Immunol.* **27**, 152.

Wilton, J.M.A., Renggli, H.H. and Lehner, T. (1977b). The role of Fc and C3 receptors in phagocytosis by inflammatory polymorphonuclear leucocytes in man. *Immunology* **32**, 955.

Winner, H.I. (1955). A study of *Candida albicans* in human sera. *J. Hyg. (Cambridge)* **53**, 509.

Winner, H.I. and Hurley, R. (1964). *Candida albicans*, p. 62. Churchill, London.

Wray, D., Ferguson, M.M., Mason, D.K., Hutcheon, A.W. and Dagg, J.H. (1975). Recurrent aphthae: treatment with vitamin B_{12}, folic acid and iron. *Br. Med. J.* **2**, 490.

Yamana, S., Aoi, K., Yamamoto, M. and Ofuji, T. (1982). Studies on the pathogenesis of Behçet's disease: is Behçet's disease mediated by mononuclear cells? In *Behçet's Disease: Pathogenetic Mechanism and Clinical Features*, ed. G. Inaba, p. 454, Japan Medical Research Foundation Publication no. 18, University of Tokyo Press, Tokyo.

Yazici, H., Akokan, G., Yalcin, B. and Muftuogla, A. (1977). The high prevalence of HLA B-5 in Behçet's disease. *Clin. Exp. Immunol.* **30**, 259–61.

Yazici, H., Pazarli, H., Barnes, C.G. *et al.* (1990). A controlled trial of azathioprine in Behçet's syndrome. *N. Engl. J. Med.* **322**, 281.

Yoshie, H., Taubman, M.A., Ebersole, J.L., Smith, D.J. and Olson, C.L. (1985). Periodontal bone loss and immune characteristics of congenitally athymic and thymic cell-reconstruction athymic rats. *Infect. Immun.* **50**, 403.

Zengo, A.N., Mandel, I.D., Goldman, R. and Khurana, H.S. (1971). Salivary studies in human caries resistance. *Arch. Oral Biol.* **16**, 557.

Zhang, X.-Q. (1989). (In Chinese.) *Chin. J. Intern. Med.* **19**, 15.

Zinner, D.D. and Jablon, J.M. (1969). Cariogenic streptococci in infants. *Arch. Oral Biol.* **14**, 1429.

105: Immunology of the Gut

W.F. Doe

Introduction

The mucosa of the gut represents a massive surface area exposed to the external environment. There is constant challenge from micro-organisms and ingested foreign antigens, including the products of food digestion and drugs. In common with other exposed surfaces, the gut has developed an immune system that is specially adapted to the mucosal environment, as outlined in Chapter 5. In considering immunological aspects of the gut, it is not surprising that primary antibody immunodeficiency and deficiency of cellular immunity, as in human immunodeficiency virus (HIV) infection, commonly result in gastrointestinal diseases due to infection or, in some cases, to tumour development. The gut diseases arising from primary immune deficiency states and from HIV infection are discussed in Chapters 66 and 72.

This chapter is concerned principally with chronic diseases of the gastrointestinal tract in which the immune system is implicated in the pathogenesis of the disease. The involvement of the immune system may vary from possible molecular mimicry in coeliac disease, to autoimmunity in gastritis and to mediation of tissue injury in secondary immune responses, as has been proposed for inflammatory bowel disease (IBD).

Coeliac disease

Coeliac disease (gluten-sensitive enteropathy) results from exposure of a genetically susceptible population to a defined fraction of cereal proteins found in wheat, rye, oats and barley grain. Two characteristics define the disease: (i) there is a malabsorption of many nutrients due to a diffuse abnormality of the small intestine, which extends distally in continuity from the duodenum for varying lengths of the small intestine; (ii) clinical recovery and improvement in the morphology of the jejunal mucosa occur after treatment with a gluten-free diet.

Several hypotheses have been advanced to explain the pathogenesis of coeliac disease. An inherited mucosal peptidase deficiency resulting in failure to digest a putative toxic gliadin peptide and, more recently, an intrinsic permeability defect in the small-intestinal mucosa have been suggested (Bjarnson and Peters 1984), but evidence is lacking. The strong association between coeliac disease and gene products of the human leucocyte antigen (HLA)-D region and the essential role of dietary gluten and, possibly, an adenovirus, together with the similarities of the lesion to graft-versus-host disease in mice, point to immune mechanisms being responsible for the mucosal tissue injury.

Genetic factors

Family studies reveal a prevalence rate of 10–15% for either symptomatic or asymptomatic coeliac disease in first-degree relatives (Mylotte *et al.* 1973) and disease susceptibility maps to the HLA-D region of the Class II major histocompatibility complex (MHC) of the sixth chromosome. The HLA-DR3 and DQw2 serological markers are found in over 80% of Caucasian coeliac patients, compared with 20% of the normal population. In Italians and Spaniards, the HLA-DR7 and DQw2 serotypes are associated with coeliac disease. Recent molecular analysis has revealed heterogeneity of the DR and DQ serotypes. Using restriction fragment length polymorphism (RFLP) analysis, genomic fragments which distinguish DR3 +ve, DQw2 +ve coeliac disease patients from serologically identical, normal controls were identified on the HLA-DP β chain. Using a deoxyribonucleic acid (DNA)-based method for HLA-DP typing to investigate the distribution of DP β-chain alleles, either DPB4.2 or DPB3 was found in 78% of the Italian coeliac population compared with 21% of identically matched controls (relative risk 13.5). Moreover, the polymorphic residues at position 69 and at 56 and 57 on the DP β chain that appear to be critical in conferring disease susceptibility do not appear to be linked to the serological markers DR3 and DR7 (Bugawan *et al.* 1989). A related but different pattern of DP β associations was reported in a group of American coeliac patients, who displayed an increase in the DPB1 allele frequency, as well as that of DPB3 and a slight increase in DPB4.2 (Kagnoff *et al.* 1989).

Because the DR3 and DR7 serotypes each have the DQB2 allele at the DQB locus which encodes the DQw2 specificity, the DQ antigen appears to be another major determinant of susceptibility. The DQ heterodimer (DQB2 and DQA4) in combination with DPB4.2 (or DPB3) allele confers high risk for coeliac disease. This extended haplotype of different Class II MHC molecules may be implicated in coeliac disease at the level of peptide binding and presentation to T lymphocytes or at the level of the T cell repertoire (Bugawan *et al.* 1989). Differences in concordance rates for coeliac disease between monozygotic twins (around 75%) and between siblings thought to be HLA-identical (around 40%), however, indicate that genes located outside the HLA region also confer susceptibility to coeliac disease, and this is supported by the observation that coeliac disease occurs more frequently among family members sharing the HLA susceptibility haplotypes than in non-family members that have the same haplotype. One possible example is the association between immunoglobulin allotype markers and coeliac disease, which is restricted to the minority of coeliac patients who lack the DR3 and DQw2 specificities. It has been proposed that immunoglobulin genes may increase susceptibility to coeliac disease by regulating the nature of the antibody response to gliadin.

Environmental factors

A fraction of gluten called alpha-gluten has been shown to contain the toxic peptide, which remains to be precisely characterized. The discordance for coeliac disease in monozygotic twins suggested that additional environmental factors may be implicated in the pathogenesis of coeliac disease. Kagnoff (1984) showed that alpha-gluten and the E1B protein of adenovirus 12 (Ad12) shared a region of homology. Increased titres of Ad12-neutralizing antibodies, a recognized cause of enteric infection in infants, were found in 89% of untreated coeliac patients, compared with 17% of disease controls (Kagnoff 1989). By contrast, no serological response to the E1B protein was evident in a study of 23 coeliac patients (seven untreated) and only one showed antibodies to the synthetic gliadin peptide homologous to the E1B protein (Howdle *et al.* 1989). This intriguing hypothesis, suggesting that peptides shared by alpha-gluten and the E1B protein of Ad12 may cross-react at the level of T cell recognition, remains to be proved.

Immunopathology

The evolving mucosal lesion of coeliac disease is initiated by infiltration of the villous and crypt epithelium of normal villi by small lymphocytes. Crypt hypertrophy occurs and then loss of villous height, the effacement of villous structure and large mitotic intraepithelial lymphocytes appear (Marsh 1989). This sequence of events closely parallels that reported for intestinal cell-mediated reactions reported in graft-versus-host reactions (Mowat and Ferguson 1982). Both treated and untreated coeliac mucosa show a striking increase in the T cell receptor (TCR)-associated lymphocytes (CD3 +ve) which belong to the γ/δ subset (median 20%; range 11–53%), compared with normal controls (median 2%; range 0–39%), and the TCR γ/δ cells were concentrated within the epithelium, where they were CD8 −ve. Studies of the intraepithelial lymphocyte component in coeliac disease confirm the increase in the T cell subset characterized as CD7 +ve, CD3 +ve, CD4 −ve, CD8 −ve, which is not found in non-coeliac enteropathy. In the enteropathy associated with T cell lymphomas, the T cell subset distribution is identical to that of coeliac disease, strongly suggesting that T cell lymphoma of the intestine is a complication of coeliac disease (Spencer *et al.* 1989).

The correlation between high titres of serum and intestinal antibodies to proved toxic fractions of gluten and the severity of the coeliac mucosal damage has provoked suggestions that the immunopathology of coeliac disease involves an antibody-dependent mechanism. This view strengthened with the finding of circulating immune complexes that bound complement (Doe *et al.* 1972). The antibody specificities in serum and intestinal fluid to a range of toxic gluten-derived peptides, however, were the same in untreated coeliacs as in normal controls and no significant binding was found to alpha-gluten-derived peptides or to the 12 amino acid A-gliadin peptide (Devery *et al.* 1989). Coeliac anti-gliadin antibodies, therefore, are not specific for the gluten peptides toxic to coeliac patients. Taken together, the present evidence favours a cell-mediated immune pathogenesis in coeliac disease, in which the strong association between several HLA-D region proteins and disease susceptibility may involve the binding of peptides derived from the processing of gliadin and the interaction of this Class II MHC–peptide complex with T cells.

Eosinophilic gastroenteritis

Eosinophilic gastroenteritis is an uncommon entity characterized by diffuse eosinophilic infiltrations and oedema of the gastrointestinal tract, peripheral blood eosinophilia, iron-deficiency anaemia, protein-losing enteropathy and, occasionally, malabsorption. There is dense eosinophilic infiltration of the mucosa, muscularis mucosa or serosa, which principally affects the stomach and, to a lesser extent, the small intestine, where the lesion is more patchy in distribution (Katz *et al.* 1977). The gastric infiltrate is associated with necrosis of epithelial cells, and the infiltrated small intestine shows villous shortening and crypt hyperplasia, apparently due to the toxic effects of eosinophil granule proteins, particularly major basic protein. Although the presence of high serum immunoglobulin E (IgE) levels and the associations of food allergy and intestinal helminthiasis (Croese 1988) implicate reaginic mechanisms, the pathogenesis of the condition remains a mystery.

Gastritis

Gastritis is defined as the inflammatory response of the gastric mucosa to injury. Despite its worldwide prevalence, the causes of the lesion have been difficult to identify. The presence of organ-specific antibodies directed against gastric antigens, the ease of access to the stomach provided by fibre optic endoscopy, the recent discovery of a bacterium, *Helicobacter pylori*, in association with the gastritis lesion and the development of an animal model have helped elucidate the pathogenesis of inflammatory disorders of the stomach. A new classification of gastritis, the Sydney System, incorporates these recent developments into a framework that integrates aetiology with the histological and endoscopic findings (Misiewicz *et al.* 1990). The discussion here will be confined to autoimmune chronic gastritis and to *Helicobacter*-associated gastritis (Table 105.1).

Gastric autoantibodies

Autoantibodies against two separate components of the gastric parietal cell have been identified in

Table 105.1. Chronic gastritis

	Autoimmune	*Helicobacter* +ve
Histology	Chronic gastritis Neutrophil infiltration absent	Chronic gastritis with neutrophil infiltration
Topography	Diffuse involvement of gastric body but antral-sparing	Predominantly antral involvement; variable focal involvement of the gastric body, which can extend to pangastritis
Serum gastritis	High to very high	Low
Parietal cell antibody	Positive >90%	Negative
Intrinsic factor antibody	Positive >75%	Negative

serum and gastric juice. Parietal cell antibodies (PCA) are organ- and cell-specific antibodies which are directed against a 94 kD antigen identified as the H^+,K^+-adenosine triphosphatase (ATPase), the parietal cell acid pump and pepsinogen (41 kD) located in the chief cells (Mardh and Song 1989). A surface-reactive PCA may be directed against the gastrin receptor. Although PCA are not species-specific, they are most sensitively detected using unfixed cryostat sections of human gastric fundus mucosa.

Intrinsic factor antibodies (IFA) are directed against the 60 000 kD glycoprotein which is a secretory product of the gastric parietal cell in man. Intrinsic factor binds dietary vitamin B_{12} to form a stable complex during its transit to the terminal ileum, where vitamin B_{12} is absorbed via specific receptors on the surface of the ileal epithelial cells. Two distinct IFA have been shown to interfere with intrinsic factor function. Almost all sera containing IFA show an antibody specificity for the vitamin B_{12}-binding site on the intrinsic factor molecule (blocking antibody) which prevents attachment of vitamin B_{12}. Some 60% of IFA-containing sera also have an antibody against the vitamin B_{12}–intrinsic factor complex which is specific for a site on intrinsic factor distant from its vitamin B_{12}-binding site and has been named binding antibody. While the presence of IFA in the serum may have little influence on the uptake of vitamin B_{12}, gastric juice IFA clearly diminish absorption of this vitamin (Rose and Chanarin 1971). Detection of gastric juice IFA, however, may be rendered more difficult by their presence as antigen–antibody complexes, which need to be dissociated before IFA can be identified (Rose and Chanarin 1969). Gastric juice PCA and IFA are synthesized and secreted by plasma cells of the gastric mucosa and may be IgG or secretory IgA antibody. In pernicious anaemia (PA), gastric juice yields a higher frequency of IFA antibodies than is found in serum (Strickland *et al.* 1971).

Serum PCA are rarely found in the presence of a healthy gastric mucosa, and their frequency, like that of chronic atrophic gastritis, increases with advancing age. Chronic atrophic gastritis was found in 90% of subjects whose serum was positive for PCA. In PA, serum PCA are detected in about 90% of patients and gastric juice PCA in about 75%. Parietal cell antibodies are absent in most patients whose gastritis is associated with *Helicobacter*. Intrinsic factor antibodies are a very rare finding in chronic atrophic gastritis patients when their vitamin B_{12} absorption is normal. By contrast, in PA, IFA are found in about 75% of PA patients' serum and in a slightly higher percentage of patients' gastric juice.

Autoimmune gastritis

Parietal cell antibody +ve gastritis is a progressive autoimmune condition that evolves slowly towards full PA, which is characterized by antral sparing, hypergastrinaemia and chronic atrophic gastritis, affecting predominantly the body of the stomach. Autoimmune gastritis (AIG) is usually a histological diagnosis that is clinically silent, and only in severe advanced disease are there abnormalities visible at endoscopy. Unlike the chronic gastritis associated with *Helicobacter* infection, AIG is not associated with polymorph infiltration (Misiewicz *et al.* 1990).

Recent models of AIG have been developed in mice that have been thymectomized on day 3 of life, which appears to prevent the generation of a T cell population that suppresses autoreactive T cells (Fukuma *et al*. 1988). A development of AIG in mice can be prevented by transfer of normal adult T cells, suggesting that T cell regulation of self-reactivity may be the fundamental lesion in AIG (Elson 1990).

As the prevalence of PCA is only 2–4% in Western adults, rising to 10% in the elderly, AIG is an uncommon cause of gastritis and only 15–20% of AIG patients will progress to PA. Autoimmune gastritis is associated with a number of complications. Carcinoid tumours may develop from the strong trophic drive to enterochromaffin-like cells due to prolonged hypergastrinaemia. There is also an increased risk of epithelial cell dysplasia and of hyperplastic polyps and a threefold increase in gastric cancer risk.

Helicobacter gastritis

The commonest form of chronic gastritis is that associated with *H. pylori* infection, which excites a gastric infiltrate with lymphocytes, plasma cells and granulocytes. Long-standing *H. pylori* infection is a pangastritis that is predominantly antral and evolves to an atrophy affecting either the antrum on the body of the stomach or both (Paull and Yardley 1989). The condition is common, affecting 50% of the population in developed countries after the fifth decade of life. Although gastric function, including acid and intrinsic factor secretion, may be severely impaired, PA is rare in *Helicobacter*-associated chronic gastritis, but there is an increased risk of gastric carcinoid tumours, polyps and carcinoma of the intestinal type (three to four times) and a tenfold enhanced susceptibility to peptic ulcer disease, especially duodenal ulceration.

Class II MHC proteins are strongly expressed on epithelial cells from *H. pylori*-infected gastric mucosa but not on control normal gastric epithelial cells, and an increase in intraepithelial CD8 +ve lymphocytes has been reported (Engstrand *et al*. 1989). The question as to whether this induced Class II MHC protein expression may lead to aberrant or enhanced local immune responses is unresolved, but Class II MHC protein expression in the gastric epithelium may merely represent the production of interferon gamma by the intraepithelial lymphocyte population.

Immunoproliferative small-intestinal disease and alpha-chain disease

Immunoproliferative small-intestinal disease (IPSID) is characterized by diffuse, primary intestinal lymphoid infiltration of the small intestine and mesenteric nodes, associated with a chronic malabsorption syndrome that affects young patients, predominantly in developing countries. In over 70% of cases, the condition involves a monoclonal expansion of IgA B lymphocytes, which proliferate in the intestinal lamina propria and synthesize and secrete an abnormal IgA fragment comprising α heavy chains free of light chains. Clinical studies suggest the evolution of IPSID from a benign plasma cell infiltration confined to the lamina propria to a frank lymphoma comprising more primitive immunoblasts. It is now recognized that 'Mediterranean lymphoma', a diffuse primary intestinal lymphoma with clinical and pathological features which clearly distinguish it from intestinal lymphomas found in Western countries, represents the malignant development of IPSID (reviewed in Doe 1985).

Pathology

The small-intestinal villi are shortened and broadened, resulting in partial or total effacement of villous architecture (Fig. 105.1). There is a diffuse, dense mononuclear cell infiltrate of the lamina propria, causing wide separation of the crypts and loss of villous structure without significant impairment of the surface epithelium. The cellular infiltrate consists mainly of plasma cells of varying degrees of maturity (Fig. 105.2). Topographically, the infiltrate usually begins in the jejunum and extends distally to involve most of the small intestine. In early cases, the cellular infiltrate is confined to the lamina propria and appears benign — a finding consistent with the clinical evidence for a premalignant stage of the disease. The infiltrate may invade the submucosa, destroy the architecture of the mesenteric lymph nodes, and spread to other parts of the intestine and the bone marrow.

There is evidence that the lymphoma that supervenes in IPSID results from malignant transformation of the same clone of proliferating plasma

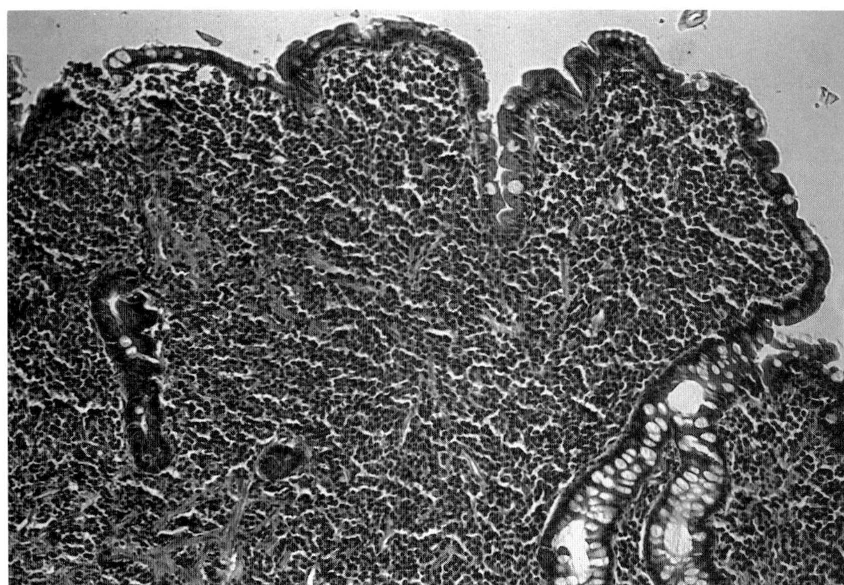

Fig. 105.1. Jejunal biopsy from an IPSID patient, showing flat deformed villi, sparse crypts, preservation of luminal epithelium and a very dense cellular infiltrate (haematoxylin and eosin (HE × 49)).

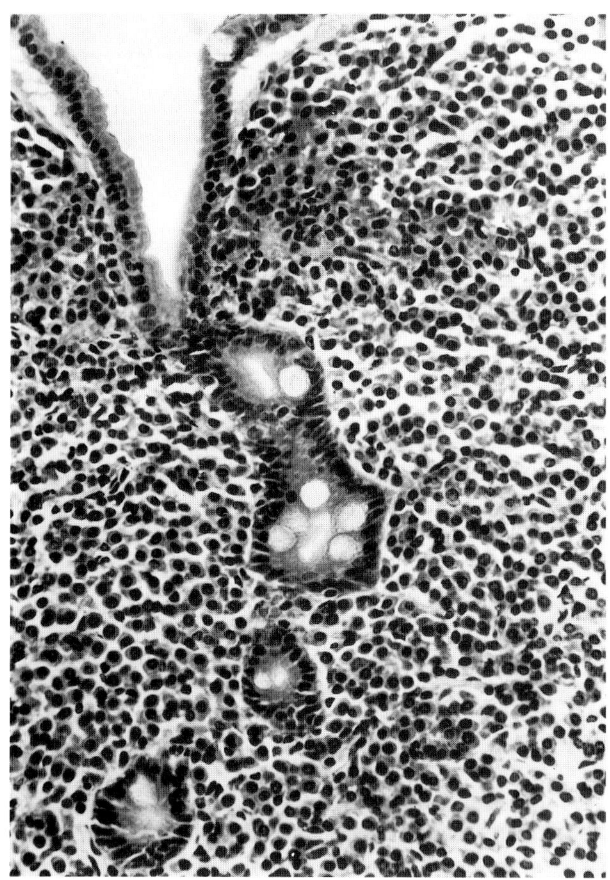

Fig. 105.2. Detail from an IPSID jejunal biopsy showing the relatively normal surface epithelium and the dense cellular infiltrate, which is composed largely of immature plasma cells (HE × 230).

cells that constituted the premalignant phase. Biosynthetic studies of cells from an IPSID lymphoma showed that both the lymphoma cells and the apparently benign plasma cells of the premalignant infiltrate synthesized the alpha-chain disease (ACD) α-chain peptide, suggesting that the immunoblastic lymphoma cells arose from dedifferentiation of the same defective clone (Preud'homme *et al.* 1979).

Protein studies

The characteristic immunoglobulin fragment of ACD is usually found in the serum, urine and intestinal fluid. The fragment comprises α1 heavy chains devoid of light chains. The monomeric ACD polypeptide varies from 20 000 to 34 000 kD. The missing portion of the α heavy chain is located in the Fd fragment and involves both the heavy-chain variable (V_H) and heavy-chain constant (C_H)1 domains (Seligmann 1975). Failure of light-chain synthesis has been confirmed by biosynthetic studies of nascent immunoglobulin subunits (Buxbaum and Preud'homme 1972).

The mechanisms underlying the synthesis of the abnormal ACD protein fragment are unknown. Detailed study of ACD fragments from one patient showed short α1 chains lacking the V_H and C_H1 domains. The ACD messenger ribonucleic acid (mRNA) was shortened and the corresponding complementary DNA (cDNA) had a leader sequence and 84 base pair sequence of unknown origin and the C_H2 and C_H3 exons of the α1 gene (Tsapis *et al*. 1989).

The most sensitive technique for immunodiagnosis of ACD involves an immunoselection technique. Test serum is electrophoresed into agarose containing an antiserum which recognizes the conformational specificities of the Fab fragment of normal IgA, which are absent from ACD polypeptide. This step results in the precipitation of the normal IgA close to the origin and allows the ACD fragment to migrate and be detected by monospecific antiserum for IgA (Doe *et al*. 1979). The immunoselection technique can also be used with anti-light-chain antisera, but occasional false positives may occur because some myeloma proteins fail to precipitate with anti-light-chain antisera (Fig. 105.3).

Clinical variants

In about 30% of IPSID patients, ACD polypeptide is not detectable in the serum. This group is heterogeneous and in the majority of cases no evidence of associated gammopathy is present (Tabbane *et al*. 1988). The rare variants include a non-secretory ACD, in which the mucosal plasma cell infiltrate contained a shortened mRNA for α1 that lacked the coding sequences for the C_H1 exon. The pathological findings and clinical causes were similar to those of secretory ACD (Matuchansky *et al*. 1989). Immunoproliferative small-intestinal disease has also been associated with a monoclonal IgA gammopathy, and γ heavy-chain protein has been demonstrated in a further IPSID patient (Seligmann 1975). Colonic (Savilahti *et al*. 1980) and pulmonary presentations of ACD have been reported. An IPSID-like clinicopathological picture without evidence of ACD has been found in two untravelled Frenchwomen who have a predominantly lymphocytic mucosal infiltrate (Matuchansky *et al*. 1988).

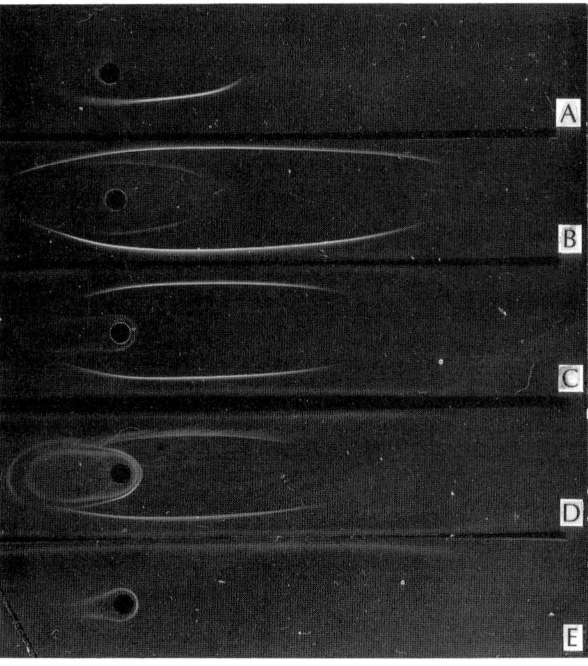

Fig. 105.3. Immunoselection plates for detecting α CD polypeptide, showing the appearances seen in normal control serum (A) and the positive findings in an IPSID serum (B), jejunal fluid (C) and concentrated urine (D). No α CD polypeptide is seen in the patient's saliva (E).

Inflammatory bowel disease

Although no specific aetiological agents have been identified for IBD, considerable progress has been made in understanding the pathogenesis of the chronic inflammatory lesion and in elucidating the pathways of tissue injury. The predominant localization of IBD to the terminal ileum and colon closely corresponds to the distribution of the commensal bacteria in the lumen of the intestine. Many different insults may cause acute damage to the intestinal epithelium, and the persistence of mucosal inflammation may be less related to the nature of the initial insult than to the massive exposure of the lamina propria to luminal contents, including intestinal microflora and their bioactive constituents, such as endotoxin. The pathology of the mucosal lesions in both ulcerative colitis (UC) and Crohn's disease (CD), therefore, is highly complex and probably involves the activation of inflammatory cells and their mediators directly and as part of the immune response.

Familial clustering

Although most cases of IBD arise sporadically, there is an increased susceptibility in IBD relatives, which varies from 10 to 35%. The age-corrected empiric risk estimates in Ashkenazi Jews in Los Angeles are 8.9% in offspring, 8.8% in siblings and 3.5% in parents in a sample of 188 IBD patients, of whom 23.4% had a positive family history (Roth *et al.* 1989). Although the observed familial aggregation does not discriminate between genetic and environmental aetiological factors, other evidence suggests a genetic contribution to susceptibility. There is a high concordance in monozygotic twins, a higher risk of IBD in children when both parents suffer from IBD and no increased frequency of IBD in spouses of IBD patients. Moreover, the onset of IBD amongst different members of the same family may be separated by many years. Evidence for a firm association with the HLA system is lacking in Caucasians but a marked segregation to HLA-DR2 has been reported in Japanese UC patients (Asakura *et al.* 1982). Inflammatory bowel disease is associated with several genetically determined disorders, including Hermansky–Pudlak syndrome, ankylosing spondylitis and Turner's syndrome. In addition, many studies have reported the occurrence of CD and UC in the same family, suggesting that they may both be associated with the same genetic predisposition or that they share one or more such genes in common.

Reports of defects in intestinal permeability in patients with CD and their relatives (Hollander *et al.* 1986) and evidence of immune reactivity against a restricted set of epithelial cell macromolecules in 62–73% of IBD patients and 54–57% of healthy first-degree relatives (Fiocchi *et al.* 1989) suggest that one or more genetically determined defects may determine susceptibility to IBD.

Environmental factors

An infectious aetiology has been suggested for CD but convincing evidence remains to be established. Lymphocytotoxic antibodies reactive with synthetic double-stranded RNA have been reported in IBD patients and their family and household contacts, suggesting the possibility of viral infection in IBD (Korsmeyer *et al.* 1975), but little further supporting evidence has emerged. Because of similarities in the histopathology between CD, intestinal tuberculosis and Johne's disease, CD tissue specimens were studied for *Myobacterium paratuberculosis* infection. A slow-growing *M. paratuberculosis* has been isolated from a small proportion of CD tissue specimens by several laboratories, and oral inoculation of neonatal goats has produced a granulomatous non-caseating ileitis within 3–5 months from which mycobacteria were reisolated (van Kruiningen *et al.* 1986). However, detection and precise identification of mycobacteria in mucosal tissue, using cloned DNA probes and RFLP analysis, have not supported a role for mycobacteria in the pathogenesis of CD (Butcher *et al.* 1988).

Immunopathology

Immunohistological studies of the involved ileum and colon in IBD reveal increased staining for Class II MHC proteins by epithelial cells in the small intestine and *de novo* expression on the colonic epithelium (Hirata *et al.* 1986). Because helper T cells recognize processed antigen in association with Class II MHC gene products, these findings raise the question of whether Class II MHC antigen expression on the surface of epithelial cells in IBD enables them to present antigen and to induce abnormal immune responses that contribute to the inflammation and tissue injury in IBD. There is evidence that intestinal epithelial cells can process and present antigen *in vitro* (Mayer and Shlien 1987), but whether the induction of Class II MHC expression on IBD epithelial cells results in abnormal immune responses or whether it merely reflects increased levels of interferon gamma in the inflammatory lesion is unknown. In active CD, mucosal T lymphocyte numbers appear reduced but the subset distribution is normal (Hirata *et al.* 1986). While the subepithelial population of mature macrophages (HLA-DR +ve, 25F9 +ve, CD4 +ve, CD11b −ve) is preserved in active CD, there is also a marked monocyte infiltration (CD11b +ve, HLA-DR −ve, CD4 −ve). The giant cells and epithelioid cells in granulomas stain heavily with OKM1 and, in some microgranulomas, with the mature macrophage marker 25F9. In active CD, mesenteric nodes show extensive infiltration of T-dependent areas with 25F9 +ve macrophages (Hume *et al.* 1987). The inflammatory infiltrate can also be studied *in vivo* in a more dynamic way, using autologous radiolabelled leucocytes and scanning. Selective labelling of neutrophils and monocytes (Pullman *et al.* 1988b) provides an objective measure of inflammatory cell turnover which correlates closely with clinical and histological indices of disease activity.

Mucosal T cells and macrophages produce colony-stimulating factors (CSF) and some interleukins (IL) which induce differentiation, maturation and activation of granulocytes and macrophages. In addition, granulocyte–monocyte (GM)-CSF and granulocyte (G)-CSF produced in the mucosa contribute to the circulating CSF pool, which induces the proliferation of bone marrow stem cells into the myeloid series. In IBD, mucosal CSF production is greatly increased, especially G-CSF, which more than doubles on a per cell basis. Similarly, IL-1 production by mucosal macrophages is greatly increased, particularly in CD (Pullman *et al.* 1992a). Exposure to foreign antigen and bacterial lipopolysaccharide is a major factor in the induction of mucosal CSF production. The enhanced production of CSF in the mucosal lesion of IBD is suppressed by hydrocortisone and 5-aminosalicylic acid. Similarly, mucosal IL-2 production is suppressed by cyclosporin, suggesting that mucosal T cells and macrophages are central to the pathogenesis of inflammation and tissue injury in IBD (Pullman *et al.* 1992b).

CYTOTOXIC CELLS

Extensive study of peripheral blood cells in IBD has yielded a plethora of observations, which have mostly proved to be non-specific findings related to the duration, severity and type of IBD, the nutritional state of the patient or the nature of therapy (reviewed by MacDermott and Stenson 1988). The presence of lymphocytotoxic antibodies (Korsmeyer *et al.* 1975) directed against lymphocyte subpopulations, however, may be relevant to the altered immunity observed in some IBD patients. Some antibodies are directed towards the precursors of suppressor T cells, while in other patients there is lymphocytotoxic activity against B cells, which may alter antibody synthesis and secretion. Both cold and warm anti-lymphocyte antibodies against B cells and macrophages have been reported with broad DRw specificities, implying sensitization to DR antigens. The induction of DR determinants on intestinal epithelial cells associated with active IBD may result in both anti-lymphocyte and anti-colon epithelial antibodies, which could react with DR antigens on B cells, macrophages and dendritic cells, thereby modulating immune function (MacDermott and Stenson 1988).

Although peripheral blood mononuclear cells (PBMC) from ulcerative colitis have been reported to lyse fetal human colon cells (Perlmann and Broberger 1963) and adult human autologous colon epithelial cells in the absence of complement (Shorter *et al.* 1984), these studies lacked disease controls. The validity of these cytotoxicity assays has been questioned by Gibson *et al.* (1986), who used a freshly isolated radiolabelled population of normal epithelial cells of proved viability as targets and showed similar levels of cytotoxicity in PBMC from normal subjects and UC and CD patients. Mucosal mononuclear cell populations from normal and actively inflamed IBD colon failed to lyse normal colon epithelial cell targets (Gibson *et al.* 1986), despite evidence for marked lymphokine-activated killer (LAK) cell activity against freshly isolated colon carcinoma cells and normal mucosal fibroblasts (Hogan *et al.* 1990). Moreover, the levels of IL-2 found in supernatants of IBD lamina propria mononuclear cells (LPMC) are decreased compared with normal (Fiocchi *et al.* 1984). These results indicate that cell-mediated cytotoxicity by either natural killer (NK) or LAK cells is unlikely to play a significant role in the generation of colonic epithelial cell injury in IBD. There is evidence, however, for the presence of specific mucosal cytotoxic T cells which can lyse chicken red blood cells coated with antigens isolated from colonic epithelial cells (Roche *et al.* 1985), but whether these findings indicate a pathogenic mechanism is unclear.

ANTIBODY SECRETION

There is a greatly expanded IgG-containing plasma cell population in both active UC and CD mucosa by a factor of 30 compared with controls, while IgA- and IgM-containing cells are only slightly increased (Brandtzaeg *et al.* 1974). T cell subsets show normal numbers and distribution in IBD mucosa (Selby *et al.* 1984), mucosal T cell subsets from CD display normal helper function and there is no evidence of suppression of IgA synthesis (James *et al.* 1985), suggesting that T cell regulation of antibody synthesis in the active lesion of IBD is normal. Intestinal LPMC from IBD patients, however, show decreased unstimulated IgA secretion but increased IgG secretion, especially in UC patients, whose LPMC secrete markedly increased quantities of IgG-1, while, in CD, IgG-2 secretion is increased (Scott *et al.* 1986). The differences in IgG subclass emphasis between UC and CD have led to speculation about the nature of antigenic signals exciting IgG-1 responses in UC (proteins and T-cell-dependent antigens) and IgG-2 responses in CD (carbohydrates and bacterial antigens) (MacDermott and Stenson 1988). Reports of an IgG antibody eluted from a colon resected for UC that binds to a 40 kD protein on epithelial cells from IBD patients and normal controls raise the possibility of a disease-specific antibody that has yet to be confirmed (Takahashi and Das 1985).

MEDIATORS OF INFLAMMATION

Soluble mediators of inflammation appear to be largely responsible for the clinical and histological findings in IBD. Agents used in the treatment of IBD, including corticosteroids and 5-aminosalicylic acid, block the synthesis of many of the soluble mediators, including prostaglandins and leukotrienes (MacDermott and Stenson 1988). Prostaglandin levels, especially PGE_2, are increased in stool, rectal mucosa and venous blood in IBD (Sharon *et al.* 1978). Yet clinical trials of non-steroidal anti-inflammatory drugs (NSAIDs) show no improvement in UC, despite causing a decrease in prostaglandin production (Campieri *et al.* 1980), indicating that prostaglandins are unlikely to be significant mediators of inflammation in IBD.

The lipoxygenase pathway, which appears confined to myeloid cells, including mast cells, neutrophils and macrophages, generates 5-hydroxy-eicosatetraenoic acid (5-HETE) and, especially, leukotriene B-4 (LTB-4), which is a powerful chemoattractant for neutrophils. Leukotriene B-4 is present in high concentration in IBD mucosa and in IBD rectal dialysates (Lauritsen *et al.* 1985), but not in normal mucosa. Incubation of IBD mucosa with radio-labelled arachidonic acid results in the synthesis of large amounts of LTB-4 and 5-HETE and lesser amounts of PGE_2 and thromboxane B_2 (Sharon and Stenson 1984), and the patterns of arachidonate metabolites are similar for UC and CD. As LTB-4 may represent 60–90% of the chemotactic activity of the whole mucosa, a therapeutic attack aimed at blocking LTB-4 synthesis or impairing neutrophil responsiveness may represent a useful advance in treatment.

Whipple's disease

Whipple's disease is a rare systemic illness characterized by fever, weight loss, malabsorption, arthritis, lymphadenopathy and central nervous system involvement. The pathognomonic histology of the involved organs comprises aggregations of 'foamy' macrophages which stain positively with the periodic acid–Schiff reagent and contain large numbers of bacteria. No single pathogen has been consistently isolated from affected tissue. While alterations of both humoral and cellular immunity have been reported, there is no consistent evidence of specific immune defect in patients in complete remission. Longitudinal studies in one patient showed that, although phagocytosis was normal, there was impairment of intracellular degradation of phagocytosed zymosan particles and bacteria, accompanied by a reduced blood T lymphocyte count which persisted over 4 years' observation during full clinical remission, suggesting a primary defect of monocyte function (Bjerknes *et al.* 1988).

References

Asakura, H., Tsuchiya, M., Aiso, S. *et al.* (1982). Association of the human lymphocyte-DR2 antigen with Japanese ulcerative colitis. *Gastroenterology* **82**, 413–18.

Bjarnson, I. and Peters, T.J. (1984). *In vitro* determination of small intestinal permeability: demonstration of a persistent defect in patients with celiac disease. *Gut* **25**, 145–50.

Bjerknes, R., Ødegaard, S., Bjerkvig, R., Børkje, B. and Lærum, O.D. (1988). Whipple's disease: demonstration of a persisting monocyte and macrophage dysfunction. *Scand. J. Gastroenterol.* **23**, 611–19.

Brandtzaeg, P., Baklien, K., Fausa, O. and Hoel, P.S. (1974). Immunohistochemical characterization of local immunoglobulin formation in ulcerative colitis. *Gastroenterology* **66**, 1123–36.

Bugawan, T.L., Angelini, G., Larrick, J., Auricchio, S., Ferrara, G. and Erlich, H.A. (1989). A combination of a particular HLA-DP β allele and an HLA-DQ heterodimer confers susceptibility to coeliac disease. *Nature* **339**, 470–3.

Butcher, P.D., McFadden, J.J. and Hermon-Taylor, J. (1988). Investigation of mycobacteria in Crohn's disease tissue by Southern blotting and DNA hybridisation with cloned mycobacterial genomic DNA probes from a Crohn's disease isolated mycobacteria. *Gut* **29**, 1222–8.

Buxbaum, J.N. and Preud'homme, J.L. (1972). Alpha and gamma heavy chain diseases in man: intracellular origin of the aberrant polypeptides. *J. Immunol.* **109**, 1131–7.

Campieri, M., Lanfranchi, G.A., Bazzochi, G. *et al.* (1980). Prostaglandins, indomethacin, and ulcerative colitis. *Gastroenterology* **78**, 193.

Croese, T.J. (1988). Eosinophilic enteritis — a recent North Queensland experience. *Aust. NZ J. Med.* **18**, 848–53.

Devery, J.M., La Brooy, J.T., Krillis, S., Davidson, G. and Skerritt, J.H. (1989). Anti-gliadin antibody specificity for gluten-derived peptides toxic to coeliac patients. *Clin. Exp. Immunol.* **76**, 384–90.

Doe, W.F. (1985). Lymphoma and alpha-chain disease. In *Disorders of the Small Intestine*, ed. A. Booth and G. Neale, pp. 179–94, Blackwell Scientific Publications, Oxford.

Doe, W.F., Henry, K. and Booth, C.C. (1972). Complement in coeliac disease. In *Coeliac Disease: Proceedings of the Second International Coeliac Symposium*, ed. W.T.J.M. Hekkens and A.S. Pena, pp. 189–94, Stenford Kroese, Leiden.

Doe, W.F., Danon, F. and Seligmann, M. (1979). Immunodiagnosis of alpha-chain disease. *Clin. Exp. Immunol.* **36**, 189–97.

Elson, C.O. (1990). Do organ-specific suppressor T cells prevent autoimmune gastritis? *Gastroenterology* **98**, 226–9.

Engstrand, L., Scheynius, A., Påhlson, C., Grimelius, L, Schwan, A. and Gustavsson, S. (1989). Association of *Campylobacter pylori* with induced expression of class II transplantation antigens on gastric epithelial cells. *Infect. Immunity* **57**, 827–32.

Fiocchi, C., Hilfiker, M.L., Youngman, K.R., Doerder, N.C. and Finke, J.H. (1984). Interleukin 2 activity of human intestinal mucosa mononuclear cells: decreased levels in inflammatory bowel disease. *Gastroenterology* **86**, 734–42.

Fiocchi, C., Roche, J.K. and Michener, W.M. (1989). High prevalence of antibodies to intestinal epithelial antigens in patients with inflammatory bowel disease and their relatives. *Ann. Intern. Med.* **110**, 786–94.

Fukuma, K., Sakaguchi, S., Chen, W.-L. *et al.* (1988). Immunological and clinical studies on murine experimental autoimmune gastritis induced by neonatal thymectomy. *Gastroenterology* **94**, 274–83.

Gibson, P.R., Van der Pol, E., Pullman, W. and Doe, W.F. (1986). Lysis of colonic epithelial cells by allogeneic mononuclear and lymphokine activated killer cells derived from peripheral blood and intestinal mucosa: evidence against pathogenic role in inflammatory bowel disease. *Gut* **29**, 1076–84.

Hirata, I., Berrebi, G., Austin, L.L., Keren, D.F. and Dobbins, W.O. (1986). Immunohistological characterisation of intraepithelial and lamina propria lymphocytes in control ileum and colon and in inflammatory bowel disease. *Dig. Dis. Sci.* **31**, 593–603.

Hogan, P.G., Gibson, P.R., Hapel, A.J. and Doe, W.F. (1991). Intestinal lymphokine-activated killer cells in inflammatory bowel disease. *J. Gastroenterol. Hepatol.* **6**, 455–60.

Hollander, D., Vadheim, C.M., Brettholz, E., Petersen, G.M., Delahunty, T. and Rotter, J.I. (1986). Increased intestinal permeability in patients with Crohn's disease and their relatives: a possible etiologic factor. *Ann. Intern. Med.* **105**, 883–5.

Howdle, P.D., Blair Zajdel, M.E., Smart, C.J., Trejdosiewicz, L.K., Blair, G.E. and Losowsky, M.S. (1989). Lack of a serologic response to an E1B protein of adenovirus 12 in coeliac disease. *Scand. J. Gastroenterol.* **24**, 282–6.

Hume, D.A., Allan, W., Hogan, P.G. and Doe, W.F. (1987). Immunohistochemical characterisation of macrophages in human liver and gastrointestinal tract: expression of CD4, HLA-DR, OKM1 and the mature macrophage marker 25F9 in normal and diseased tissue. *J. Leucocyte Biol.* **42**, 474–84.

James, S.P., Fiocchi, C., Graeff, A.S. and Strober, W. (1985). Immunoregulatory function of lamina propria T cells in Crohn's disease. *Gastroenterology* **88**, 1143–50.

Kagnoff, M.F. (1984). Possible role for a human adenovirus in the pathogenesis of celiac disease. *J. Exp. Med.* **160**, 1544–57.

Kagnoff, M.F. (1989). Celiac disease: adenovirus and alpha gliadin. *Curr. Topics Microbiol. Immunol.* **145**, 67–78.

Kagnoff, M.F., Harwood, J.I., Bugawan, T.L. and Erlich, H.A. (1989). Structural analysis of the HLA-DR, -DQ, and -DP alleles on the celiac disease-associated HLA-DR3 (DRw17) haplotype. *Proc. Nat. Acad. Sci. (USA)* **86**, 6274–8.

Katz, A.J., Goldman, H. and Grand, R.J. (1977). Gastric mucosal biopsy in eosinophilic (allergic) gastroenteritis. *Gastroenterology* **73**, 705–9.

Korsmeyer, S.J., Williams, R.C., Wilson, I.D. and Strickland, R.G. (1975). Lymphocytotoxic antibody in inflammatory bowel disease: a family study. *N. Engl. J. Med.* **293**, 1117–20.

Lauritsen, K., Laursen, L.S., Bukhave, K. and Rask-Madsen, J. (1985). Effects of systemic prednisolone on arachidonic acid metabolites determined by equilibrium *in vivo* dialysis of rectum in severe relapsing ulcerative colitis. *Gastroenterology* **88**, A 1466.

MacDermott, R.P. and Stenson, W.R. (1988). Alterations of the immune system in ulcerative colitis and Crohn's disease. *Adv. Immunol.* **42**, 285–328.

Mardh, S. and Song, Y.-H. (1989). Characterization of antigenic structures in autoimmune atrophic gastritis with pernicious anaemia: the parietal cell H,K-ATPase and the chief cell pepsinogen are the two major antigens. *Acta Physiol. Scand.* **136**, 581–7.

Marsh, M.N. (1989). Studies of intestinal lymphoid tissue. XIII. Immunopathology of the evolving celiac sprue lesion. *Pathol. Res. Pract.* **185**, 774–7.

Matuchansky, C., Touchard, G., Babin, P., Lemaire, M., Cogne, M. and Preud'homme, J.L. (1988). Diffuse small intestinal lymphoid infiltration in nonimmunodeficient adults from Western Europe. *Gastroenterology* **95**, 470–7.

Matuchansky, C., Cogne, M., Lemaire, M. *et al.* (1989). Nonsecretory alpha-chain disease with immunoproliferative small intestinal disease. *N. Engl. J. Med.* **320**, 1534–9.

Mayer, L. and Shlien, R. (1987). Evidence for function of Ia molecules on gut epithelial cells in man. *J. Exp. Med.* **166**, 1471–83.

Misiewicz, J.J., Tytgat, G.N.J., Goodwin, C.S. *et al.* (1990). The Sydney system: a new classification of gastritis. *J. Gastroenterol. Hepatol.* **144**, 53–7.

Mowat, A.M. and Ferguson, A. (1982). Intra-epithelial lymphocyte count and crypt hyperplasia measure the mucosal component of the graft-versus-host reaction in mouse small intestine. *Gastroenterology* **83**, 417–23.

Mylotte, M.J., Egon-Mitchell, B., Fottrell, P.I., McNicholl, B. and McCarthy, C.F. (1973). Incidence of coeliac disease in the West of Ireland. *Br. Med. J.* **1**, 703–5.

Paull, G. and Yardley, J.M. (1989). Pathology of *C. pylori* associated gastric and esophageal lesions. In Campylobacter pylori *in Gastritis and Peptic Ulcer Disease*, ed. M.J. Blaser, Igaku-Shoin, New York.

Perlmann, P. and Broberger, O. (1963). *In vitro* studies of ulcerative colitis. II. Cytotoxic action of white blood cells from patients on human fetal colon cells. *J. Exp. Med.* **117**, 717–33.

Preud'homme, J.L., Brouet, J.C. and Seligmann, M. (1979). Cellular immunoglobulins in human γ- and α-heavy chain diseases. *Clin. Exper. Immunol.* **37**, 283–91.

Pullman, W.E., Hapel, A.J. and Doe, W.F. (1988a). Colony stimulating factor production by intestinal lamina propria cells is increased in inflammatory bowel disease (IBD). *Gastroenterology* **94**, A361.

Pullman, W.E., Sullivan, P.J., Barratt, P.J., Lising, J., Booth, J.A. and Doe, W.F. (1988b). Assessment of inflammatory bowel disease activity by 99m technetium phagocyte scanning. *Gastroenterology* **95**, 989–96.

Roche, J.K., Fiocchi, C. and Youngman, K. (1985). Sensitization to epithelial antigens in chronic mucosal inflammatory disease: characterization of human intestinal mucosa-derived mononuclear cells reactive with purified epithelial cell-associated components *in vitro*. *J. Clin. Invest.* **75**, 522–30.

Rose, M.S. and Chanarin, I. (1969). Dissociation of intrinsic factor from its antibody application to study of pernicious anaemia gastric juice specimens. *Br. Med. J.* **1**, 468–70.

Rose, M.S. and Chanarin, I. (1971). Intrinsic factor antibody and absorption of vitamin B_{12} in pernicious anaemia. *Br. Med. J.* **1**, 25–6.

Roth, M.P., Petersen, G.M., McElree, C., Vadheim, C.M., Panish, J.F. and Rotter, J.I. (1989). Familial empiric risk estimates of inflammatory bowel disease in Ashkenazi Jews. *Gastroenterology* **96**, 1016–20.

Savilahti, E., Brandtzaeg, P. and Kuitenen, P. (1980). Atypical intestinal alpha-chain disease evolving into selective immunoglobulin A deficiency in a Finnish boy. *Gastroenterology* **79**, 1303–10.

Scott, M.G., Nahm, M.H., Macke, K., Nash, G.S., Bertovich, M.J. and MacDermott, R.P. (1986). Spontaneous secretion of IgG subclasses by intestinal mononuclear cells: differences between ulcerative colitis, Crohn's disease, and controls. *Clin. Exp. Immunol.* **66**, 209–15.

Selby, W.S., Janossy, G., Bofill, M. and Jewell, D.P. (1984). Intestinal lymphocyte subpopulations in inflammatory bowel disease: an analysis by immunohistological and cell isolation techniques. *Gut* **25**, 32–40.

Seligmann, M. (1975). Alpha-chain disease. *J. Clin. Pathol.* **29** (suppl. 6), 72–6.

Sharon, P. and Stenson, W.F. (1984). Enhanced synthesis of leukotriene B4 by colonic mucosa in inflammatory bowel disease. *Gastroenterology* **86**, 453–60.

Sharon, P., Ligumsky, M., Rachmilewitz, D. and Zoir, U. (1978). Role of prostaglandins in ulcerative colitis: enhanced production during active disease and inhibition by sulfasalazine. *Gastroenterology* **75**, 638–40.

Shorter, R.G., McGill, D.B. and Bahn, R.C. (1984). Cytotoxicity of mononuclear cells for autologous colonic epithelial cells in colonic diseases. *Gastroenterology* **86**, 13–22.

Spencer, J., MacDonald, T.T., Diss, T.C., Walker-Smith, J.A., Ciclitira, P.J. and Isaacson, P.G. (1989). Changes in intraepithelial lymphocyte subpopulations in coeliac disease and enteropathy associated T cell lymphoma (malignant histiocytosis of the intestine). *Gut* **30**, 339–46.

Strickland, R.G., Baur, S., Ashworth, L.A.E. and Taylor, K.B. (1971). A correlative study of immunological phenomena in pernicious anaemia. *Clin. Exp. Immunol.* **8**, 25–36.

Tabbane, F., Mourali, N., Cammoun, M. and Najjar, T. (1988). Results of laparotomy in immunoproliferative small intestinal disease. *Cancer* **61**, 1699–706.

Takahashi, F. and Das, K.M. (1985). Isolation and characterization of a colonic autoantigen specifically recognised by colon tissue-bond IgG from idiopathic ulcerative colitis. *J. Clin. Invest.* **76**, 311–18.

Tsapis, A., Bentaboulet, M., Pellet, P. *et al.* (1989). The productive gene for alpha-H chain disease protein MAL is highly modified by insertion-deletion processes. *J. Immunol.* **143**, 3821–7.

van Kruiningen, H.J., Chiodini, R.J., Thayer, W.R., Coutu, J.A., Merkal, R.S. and Runnels, P.L. (1986). Experimental disease in infant goats induced by a mycobacterium isolated from a patient with Crohn's disease. *Dig. Dis. Sci.* **31**, 1351–60.

106: Autoimmune Disorders of the Neuromuscular Junction

J. Newsom-Davis, A.C. Vincent and H.N.A. Willcox

The neuromuscular junction is the site of two antibody-mediated autoimmune disorders, myasthenia gravis (MG) and the Lambert–Eaton myasthenic syndrome (LEMS), and may be especially vulnerable because it lacks the protection of the blood–brain barrier. Both disorders can be associated with neoplasms, epithelial thymoma in about 10% of MG cases and small-cell lung cancer (SCLC) in around 60% of LEMS patients. In MG, immunoglobulin G (IgG) autoantibodies to the postsynaptic nicotinic acetylcholine receptor (AChR) lead to AChR loss and consequent fatiguable muscle weakness (Fig. 106.1). The antibodies can cross the placenta, and cause transient myasthenic weakness in the new-born 'neonatal MG'. In a small proportion of otherwise typical MG patients, no serum anti-AChR antibodies are detectable by the standard radio-immunoassay (RIA) ('seronegative' MG), but their plasma nevertheless appears to contain factor(s) that interfere with neuromuscular transmission.

In LEMS, the defects are presynaptic; IgG autoantibodies to voltage-gated calcium channels (VGCCs) at the nerve terminal lead to an impairment of nerve impulse-evoked release of ACh (Fig. 106.1). The association with SCLC found by Lambert *et al.* (1956) led to the early recognition of LEMS as a paraneoplastic neurological disorder, and it was the first of these (apart from MG) in which an autoantibody-mediated mechanism was shown to be causative. Autoimmune mechanisms are now proving to be important in other paraneoplastic disorders.

The idea that MG is an autoimmune disorder is not new. Simpson (1960) and Nastuk, Strauss and their colleagues (Nastuk *et al.* 1959, 1960) all reported evidence supporting an autoimmune basis for the defect in neuromuscular transmission. However, it was not until the 1970s that the use of snake neurotoxins, notably α-bungarotoxin (α-BuTx), to purify and quantify the nicotinic AChR made it possible to detect a loss of end-plate AChRs in muscle biopsies from MG patients (Fambrough *et al.* 1973), and to show that rabbits immunized with purified AChR developed an MG-like weakness that responded, as MG does, to anti-acetylcholinesterase medication (Patrick and Lindstrom 1973). Moreover, a clinically useful immunoprecipitation test based on extracted human AChR was developed (Lindstrom *et al.* 1976).

Experimental autoimmune MG (EAMG) has been induced in many animals by immunization with purified nicotinic AChR derived from many species (for review see Lindstrom *et al.* 1988). In LEMS there is not yet a validated animal model, but the role of antibodies to VGCCs has been

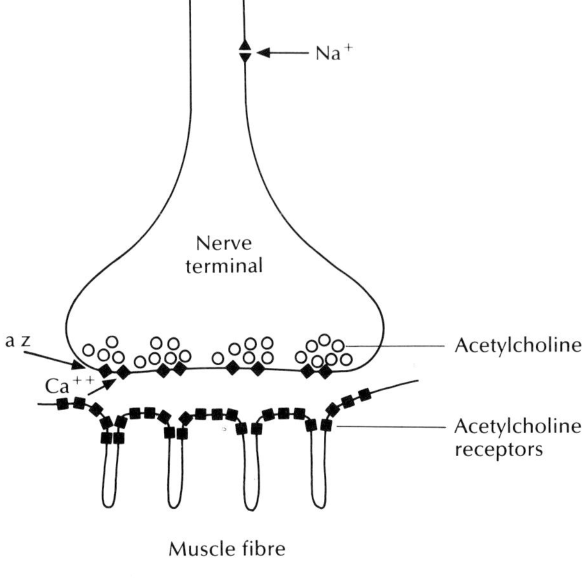

Fig. 106.1. Outline of neuromuscular transmission. When an Na^+-dependent action potential arrives at the nerve ending it opens voltage-gated calcium channels (VGCCs, ◆), which are located at 'active zones' (az), specialized regions of the nerve terminal opposite the secondary postsynaptic clefts. Influx of Ca^{2+} ions results in fusion of the ACh-containing synaptic vesicles with the nerve terminal membrane and release of around 50 of these 'quanta' of ACh into the synaptic cleft. The ACh diffuses across the synaptic cleft and binds to acetylcholine receptors (AChRs ■), which are present at very high density on the crests of the postsynaptic folds. Binding of two ACh molecules to each AChR causes transient opening of the ion channel, which allows entry of cations, principally Na^+, into the muscle fibre. This depolarizes the membrane and results in activation of voltage-gated Na^+ channels, which conduct the action potential along the muscle and activate excitation–contraction coupling. In the Lambert–Eaton Syndrome (LEMS), antibodies modulate the number and distribution of VGCCs and reduce the number of quanta released per nerve impulse. In myasthenia gravis (MG), antibodies cause loss of AChRs and decrease the response to released ACh. In both cases the defect results in weakness, but the clinical expression of the diseases differs.

extensively documented and an immunoprecipitation assay has recently been described (see Vincent *et al.* 1989).

An introduction to basic and clinical aspects of neuromuscular transmission can be found in Vincent and Wray (1990). Myasthenia gravis and LEMS should be distinguished from hereditary (congenital or familial) myasthenias, a heterogeneous group of non-immunological disorders (reviewed by Engel 1990). Much of the earlier work in MG has been reviewed extensively (e.g. Lindstrom 1979; Vincent 1980; Newsom-Davis and Vincent 1982) and is not included in this chapter; more recent developments are covered in Drachman (1987), Lindstrom *et al.* (1988) and Willcox and Vincent (1988).

Myasthenia gravis

Clinical features

The clinical features of MG are fully described in Oosterhuis (1984). The characteristic symptom is muscle weakness increasing with repeated usage. Any striated muscle can be affected; the eye muscles are commonly the first to be involved. Symptoms are often first noticed after an infection, at a time of physiological or psychological stress, or during recovery from anaesthesia.

The age at onset ranges from the first year of life to extreme old age, and helps to divide Caucasian patients into subgroups (Table 106.1). The first peak is in the second and third decades (when females predominate) and the second in the 60s, when there is a slight excess of males. In the 10% of cases with an associated thymoma, the age at onset ranges from 15 to 90, with a mode in the fifth decade and no sex bias; the same applies to the patients with persistently pure ocular symptoms, many of whom are 'seronegative'. Cases presenting below the age of 10 years are rare and are often seronegative.

DIAGNOSIS

Response to intravenous edrophonium or to intramuscular neostigmine, increased decrement in the compound muscle action potential on repetitive nerve stimulation, or increased jitter in single-fibre electromyographic studies indicate a disorder of neuromuscular transmission, but they do not distinguish between seronegative MG, hereditary myasthenia or LEMS (Newsom-Davis 1992). Serum anti-AChR antibodies are normally measured in a highly sensitive RIA using ^{125}I-α-BuTx-labelled human AChR. Their presence (>0.5 nmol/l) in about 88% of patients with generalized MG, and in 60% of those with restricted ocular weakness, establishes the diagnosis. They may sometimes only become detectable after a few months, perhaps because initially they are bound to muscle AChR. Thymic abnormalities can

Table 106.1 Clinical heterogeneity

	'Early onset' (55%)	'Thymoma' (10%)	'Late onset' (20%)	'Seronegative' (15%)
Thymus	Hyperplasia	Thymoma	Atrophy	↑ T cell areas?
Age at onset	<40 years	Any	>40 years	Any
Sex incidence	F ≫ M	F = M	M ≥ F	M > F
Anti-AChR (titre)	High	Intermediate	Low	Absent
Anti-striated muscle (incidence)	Low	Very high	Intermediate	Absent
Weakness	Generalized	Generalized	Generalized/ocular	Generalized/ocular
HLA (Caucasians)	B8, DR3	None detected (n = 62)	B7, DR2	None detected (n = 17)

sometimes be detected in MG patients by anterior mediastinal tomography (Moore 1989).

NATURAL HISTORY

In a long-term follow-up study of 73 seropositive patients living in Amsterdam between 1926 and 1965 (treated mostly with anti-cholinesterase medication only), maximum severity occurred during the first 7 years after onset in 87% of cases (Oosterhuis 1989). Thymoma was present in almost half of the 29% who had died. However, 22% were in complete remission at the end of the study, and 34% had improved. Spontaneous remissions were more common in restricted ocular cases, and appeared to occur at the rate of about 2% per year in this group and at about 1% per year in the remainder of non-thymoma cases.

ASSOCIATED DISEASES AND AUTOANTIBODIES

Occasional associations have been observed with many other autoimmune disorders, especially thyroid disease, type 1 diabetes mellitus and rheumatoid arthritis, and there is an even higher frequency of the corresponding autoantibodies. The strongest association of all is between anti-striated muscle antibody and thymoma, which is detectable in >90% of thymoma cases (Aarli *et al.* 1981) but also in a proportion of non-thymoma cases (Table 106.1).

GENETICS OF MYASTHENIA GRAVIS

Familial cases of MG are rare. A recent paper describes MG in monozygotic twins and reviews the literature (Murphy and Murphy 1986). By 1986, MG had been reported in 26 sets of twins; six of 14 sets of validated monozygotic twins were discordant for MG, to which we can add four further sets, of whom only one asymptomatic twin had serum anti-AChR antibodies. This gives a total of 18 sets of monozygotic twins, of whom seven were concordant (for seropositivity). By contrast, none of 13 sets of dizygotic twins or twins of undetermined zygosity were concordant. These findings suggest that genetically susceptible subjects only make an autoimmune response to AChR either by chance or after exposure to some unidentified environmental factor(s).

IMMUNOGENETICS

Associations with particular human leucocyte antigen (HLA) Class I and Class II major histocompatibility complex (MHC) alleles have long been recognized. As shown in Table 106.1, in Caucasian MG, young-onset cases show a strong association with HLA-B8-DR3, and late-onset cases a weaker one with HLA-B7-DR2 (Compston *et al.* 1980; Carlsson *et al.* 1990). In Chinese and Japanese patients, the associations are with Bw46 and DRw9 (Chiu *et al.* 1987). Restricted ocular MG occurring early in life is common in China and Japan, and may be a genetically controlled variant of MG, since the HLA-DRw9 association is strongest in these very young cases (Matsuki *et al.* 1990); it often coincides with ocular Graves' disease. No clear immunogenetic association has been identified in thymoma or ocular MG in Caucasians.

This evidence for disease heterogeneity is further supported by recent studies of associations with Ig heavy chain genes. Strong Gm associations have previously been reported in Japanese MG patients, especially in those with thymoma (Nakao *et al.* 1980), though not in Caucasians. More recently, however, a restriction fragment marker nearer the heavy chain, variable region genes has revealed a highly significant association in late-onset Caucasian MG (and LEMS), but not in the other subgroups (Demaine *et al.* 1991).

EPIDEMIOLOGY AND POSSIBLE PROVOKING FACTORS

Myasthenia gravis appears to occur world-wide with no major differences in prevalence, which varies only moderately in different series. In a recent survey in Norway it was $52/10^6$ for males, 127 for females and 90 overall (Storm-Mathiesen 1984), somewhat higher figures than the $30-60/10^6$ collated from earlier surveys by Kurtzke (1978). The annual incidence for the Norwegian population was 2.6 (males), 5.3 (females) and 4 overall. The relatively high frequency of very early-onset (typically <5 years), seropositive MG in HLA-DRw9 +ve subjects in China and Japan is an intriguing clue that requires further study.

The only known provoking agents in MG are thymomata (see below), and D(−)penicillamine (Dawkins *et al.* 1981), which may lead to ocular or generalized myasthenic symptoms in about 1% of treated rheumatoid arthritis patients, especially with HLA-DR1, and in Wilson's disease. Anti-AChR antibody is present in the majority of cases and shows similar properties to that in idiopathic MG of recent onset (Vincent and Newsom-Davis 1982b). After stopping treatment, most patients recover and the titre falls. Attempts to mimic D(−) penicillamine-induced MG by long-term treatment of animals have not so far been very convincing.

Provoking factors for the other main patient subgroups, with their distinct immunogenetics, are completely unknown. Molecular mimicry by viral and bacterial antigens has often been invoked, but two detailed seroepidemiological studies for the former have proved negative (Aoki *et al.* 1985; Klavinskis *et al.* 1985). The development of MG in the recipient of a bone marrow transplant (Smith *et al.* 1983) and the apparent donor origin of the AChR specific B cells are an intriguing observation. Clinical evidence of MG was lacking in the donor (although there were minimal electrophysiological abnormalities), implying a dysregulation of the donor's immune cells in their new environment.

POSSIBLE CENTRAL NERVOUS SYSTEM INVOLVEMENT

Anti-AChR antibody has been demonstrated in the cerebrospinal fluid (CSF) of MG patients but appeared to gain access by passive leakage rather than local synthesis. However, two recent studies on central cholinergic effects in MG have given conflicting results. Tucker *et al.* (1988) found memory dysfunction in a group of MG patients compared with healthy and disease control groups, which improved in one case after plasma exchange. By contrast, Lewis *et al.* (1989) were unable to demonstrate a deficit in five MG patients in an auditory vigilance test of ability to direct and sustain attention (a function that is thought to be cholinergic) in comparison with that in a control group or with the subjects' own performance after a course of plasma exchange.

MYASTHENIA GRAVIS VARIANTS

Neonatal myasthenia

Neonatal myasthenia occurs in 10−15% of babies born to myasthenic mothers. It is due to placental transfer of maternal anti-AChR antibody, which can be detected in the infant at birth, usually at a similar titre to that in the mother (Donaldson *et al.* 1981). Antibody then declines, with a half-time of about 8 days, and full recovery usually occurs by the age of 3 weeks. Occasional cases show a marked prolongation of symptoms. A higher titre or pathogenicity of the anti-AChR antibodies in some mothers, or greater neonatal complement activity, may explain why particular babies are affected. Transfer of specific antibody through breast milk is a possibility.

Seronegative myasthenia gravis

As indicated above, 10−15% of patients with generalized MG (and about 40% of those with ocular MG) have no detectable serum anti-AChR antibodies measured by the standard RIA. By other criteria, they appear to have typical MG (Soliven *et al.* 1988), although bulbar and respiratory muscle weakness, as well as ocular symptoms, may be over-represented (Mossman *et al.* 1986), and a thymoma is never found. Clinical improvement after plasmaphaeresis and immunosuppressive drug treatment strongly suggest the presence of a pathogenic humoral factor (Mossman *et al.* 1986; Soliven *et al.* 1988), as does the report of neonatal myasthenia in a baby born to a seronegative myasthenic patient (Mier and Havard 1985). Moreover, a similar defect in neuromuscular transmission could be transferred to mice with patients' Ig while not inducing appreciable AChR loss (Mossman *et al.* 1986). Seronegative plasma can inhibit carbachol-evoked $^{22}Na^+$ flux through the AChR ion channel in cultured cells, perhaps via IgM antibodies (Yamamoto *et al.* 1991). Finally, complement is detectable at end-plates in these patients (Tsujihata *et al.* 1989), again implying that their weakness is antibody-mediated.

Autoantibodies and pathophysiology

THE ACETYLCHOLINE RECEPTOR

A model of the AChR based on work with electric fish AChR is shown in Fig. 106.2; several recent reviews cover the main properties (e.g. Claudio 1989). The AChR is an integral membrane protein which consists of α_2, β, γ and δ (fetal/extrajunctional) or α_2, β, δ and ε (adult/end-plate) subunits arranged around a central cation channel. The subunits are evolutionarily related, the α being the most conserved (75% identity in man and *Torpedo*). It is represented twice and uniquely contains the ACh binding site close to Cys^{192}–Cys^{193}. Alpha-BuTx competes with ACh and binds to amino acid (aa) 179–196 on the α-subunit. Although the presence of four hydrophobic transmembrane domains in each subunit (Fig. 106.2) suggests a model for the tertiary structure (for alternative models, see Claudio 1989), very little is known about the conformation of the extracellular region. However, the ACh/α-BuTx binding site and the *N*-glycosylation site, Asn^{141}, clearly must be exposed on the surface of the molecule, as must the 'main immunogenic region' (MIR), to which a large proportion of experimentally induced antibodies bind (Tzartos and Lindstrom 1980).

ANTI-ACETYLCHOLINESTERASE RECEPTOR ANTIBODIES IN MYASTHENIA GRAVIS

Specific antibodies binding to AChRs are detected by immunoprecipitation of human muscle AChR extracted in detergent and radioactively tagged by incubation with ^{125}I-α-BuTx. Only a small minority of antibodies inhibit toxin binding. Anti-AChR

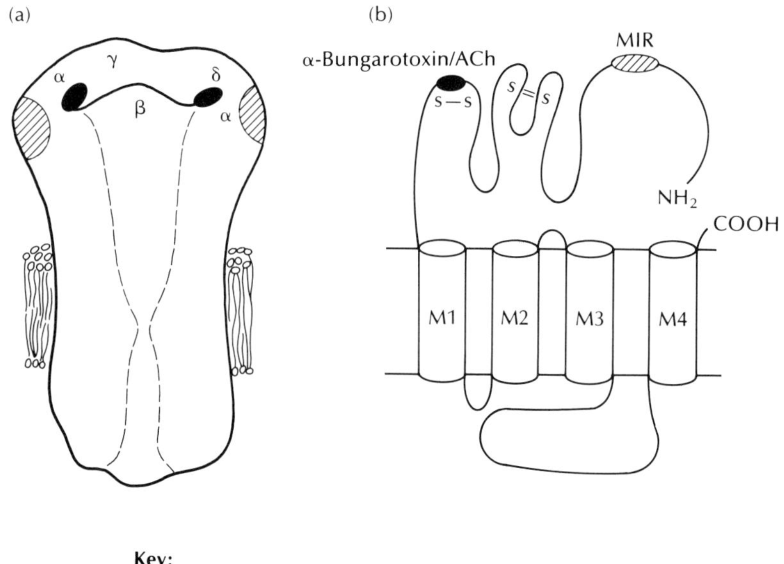

Fig. 106.2. The acetylcholine receptor. (a) The AChR is an oligomeric membrane protein consisting of five subunits, each of which projects from the muscle membrane into the extracellular space. The subunits are arranged around a central ion channel. (b) Each polypeptide chain is thought to traverse the membrane four times (M1, 2, 3, 4). The conformation of the first 200 or so amino acids, which are extracellular, is unknown, but ACh and α-BuTx bind to α 179–196, and antibodies to the main immunogenic region (MIR) bind to α 67–76. However, other sequences may also be important in contributing to the binding sites on the intact molecule.

antibodies are present in 85–90% of MG patients and are undetectable in healthy controls (Lindstrom *et al.* 1976; Vincent and Newsom-Davis 1985). However, low titres have occasionally been detected without symptoms in several groups at increased risk of MG who may be pre-myasthenic, notably those with D(−)penicillamine-treated rheumatoid arthritis, thymoma or primary biliary cirrhosis and in a few first-degree relatives. Antibodies were also detected in aged Japanese but not in aged Caucasians (see Vincent and Newsom-Davis 1985). Positive titres were found in some patients with polymyositis (Pestronk and Drachman 1985).

In many series, the absolute level of antibody has not correlated well with the clinical severity in different patients, although those with ocular MG tend to have very low or negative titres. Nevertheless, passive transfer of MG Ig clearly reduced both the miniature end-plate potential (mepp) amplitude and the binding of ^{125}I-α-BuTx in the recipient mice (Toyka *et al.* 1977). Moreover, there is a broad correlation between antibody levels and clinical state within an individual, particularly during and after plasma exchange. Thymectomy often, but by no means always, reduces the titre (Oosterhuis *et al.* 1985), and corticosteroid therapy markedly decreases it over several months in most cases (Tindall 1980; Oosterhuis *et al.* 1983). Thus it is generally accepted that the anti-AChR antibodies are responsible for the myasthenic weakness.

HETEROGENEITY OF ANTI-ACETYLCHOLINE RECEPTOR ANTIBODIES

Anti-acetylcholine receptor antibodies are almost exclusively IgGs, with all four subclasses and both κ and λ light chains represented (Vincent and Newsom-Davis 1982a). They are very heterogeneous by other criteria too; for example, they bind variably to muscle AChR from other species (Garlepp *et al.* 1981) but not to central nervous system (CNS) AChRs (Whiting *et al.* 1987). A variable but generally small proportion of the antibodies inhibits α-BuTx binding and some MG sera discriminate between end-plate and extrajunctional AChR of several species (e.g. Vincent and Newsom-Davis 1982a). To be detected in the RIA, the avidity of MG antibodies for human AChR is necessarily in the 10^{-11} M range, at least two orders of magnitude higher than that of most monoclonal antibodies (Vincent and Newsom-Davis 1982a).

FINE SPECIFICITY OF AUTOANTIBODIES IN MYASTHENIA GRAVIS

Knowledge of the aa sequences of each subunit should make it possible to map the binding sites of antibodies. However, as human sera bind nonspecifically to isolated AChR subunits in Western blots or to peptides in enzyme-linked immunosorbent assays (ELISA), a better strategy is to map human antibodies indirectly, using monoclonal anti-AChR antibodies. Some monoclonal antibodies against the MIR (see Fig. 106.2) bind in solid-phase assays to recombinant fragments or synthetic peptides containing α 67–76, and another monoclonal antibody raised against human AChR has been mapped to α 125–143 (see Tzartos *et al.* 1991). Many of these monoclonal anti-AChR antibodies can inhibit the binding of MG sera to AChR, implying overlapping specificities. Interestingly, although about 60% of polyclonal rat antibodies compete with rat monoclonal anti-MIR antibodies, mouse monoclonal antibodies appear to be more diverse. Moreover, anti-AChR antibodies from individual MG patients do not necessarily bind to MIR (Tzartos *et al.* 1982; Heidenreich *et al.* 1988a; Lennon and Griesmann 1989).

In spite of the heterogeneity of anti-AChR antibodies within and between patients, the spectrum of specificities within an individual usually remains remarkably constant with time, even when the total levels change (e.g. Tzartos *et al.* 1982; Heidenreich *et al.* 1988b).

MECHANISMS OF END-PLATE ACETYLCHOLINE RECEPTOR LOSS

The three principal modes of action of the anti-AChR antibodies are complement-mediated AChR loss, pharmacological blockade and accelerated degradation of receptors. The decrement during 3 Hz stimulation and the 'jitter' on single-fibre electromyography both reflect a defect in neuromuscular transmission at the end-plates of MG muscle, resulting from antibody-mediated loss of functional AChRs. With intracellular recording, mepps, the small postsynaptic depolarizations re-

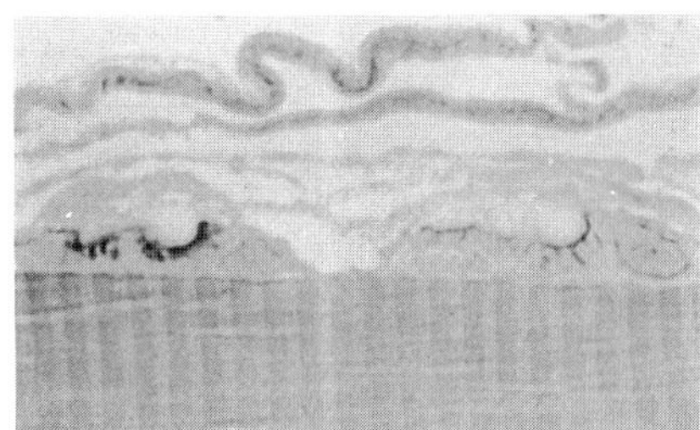

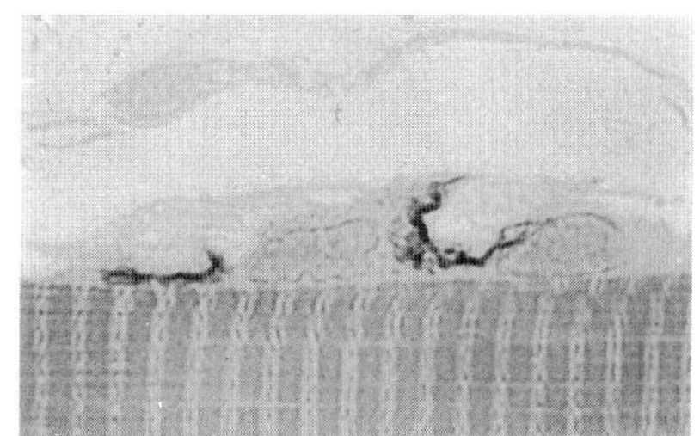

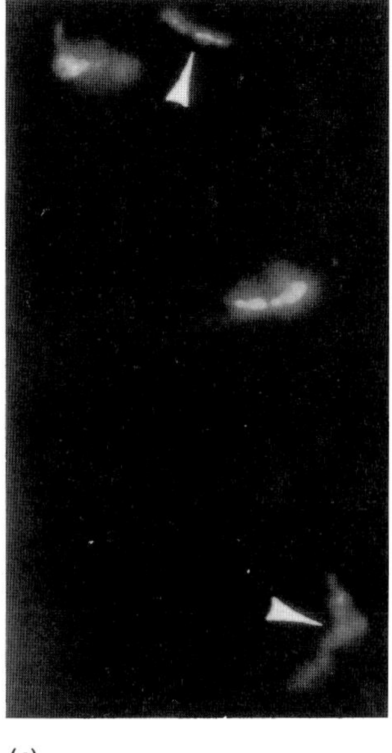

(c)

(d)

Fig. 106.3. Immunopathology of MG demonstrated by immunolabelling. Semi-thin sections show that IgG (a) and complement C3 (b) are localized at the neuromuscular junction. Involvement of complement in the loss of AChRs is shown by binding of fluorescein-labelled antibodies to the membrane attack complex (MAC) (c) and rhodamine-labelled α-BuTx (d). End-plates in MG muscle show a strong reaction with anti-MAC and reduced or absent binding of α-BuTx. Arrows in (c) indicate end-plates at which α-BuTx binding is not detected (d). End-plates in normal muscle (not shown) label with rhodamine-α-BuTx but do not show any MAC. Taken with permission from Engel *et al.* (1977) ((a) and (b)) and Engel and Arahata (1987) ((c) and (d)) (× 403).

sulting from the action of each quantum of ACh (see Fig. 106.1), are markedly reduced in amplitude (Elmqvist *et al.* 1964). Autoradiograms and gamma counting of ^{125}I-α-BuTx-labelled MG muscle show that AChR numbers are reduced at the somewhat enlarged and fragmented end-plates (Fambrough *et al.* 1973). A large study has shown generalized AChR loss, even in patients with limited or focal weakness, although a reduction is also sometimes found in some patients with polymyositis (Pestronk and Drachman 1985; Pestronk *et al.* 1985).

Morphological changes involving the postsynaptic membrane are frequently seen at MG end-plates by electron microscopy. Typically, the nerve terminal is normal but the postsynaptic folds are shallow and simplified. Immunoperoxidase or ^{125}I-α-BuTx labelling confirms a substantial reduction in both the density and the extent of AChRs along the postsynaptic membrane. There is coincident labelling for IgG and C3, and both the postsynaptic membrane and the debris in the synaptic cleft stain for complement (for a review see Engel 1984). Recent localization of the membrane attack complex (MAC) has unequivocally demonstrated complement activation on the postsynaptic membrane (Engel and Arahata 1987). Moreover, whereas IgG and C3 tend to co-localize with AChRs, C9 and the MAC are seen at the end-plates with the fewest remaining AChRs, supporting the causal relationship between complement damage and AChR loss (Fig. 106.3).

In some patients, on the other hand, a direct block of AChR function may contribute to the defect in transmission. Myasthenia gravis sera only occasionally reduce mepp amplitude or nerve-evoked muscle twitch in nerve/muscle preparations *in vitro* (e.g. Burges *et al.* 1990), but the AChRs of the cultured muscle cell line TE 671 are more accessible, and many MG sera directly block carbachol-induced Na^+ influx into them (Lang *et al.* 1988). Moreover, monoclonal antibodies specific for the α-BuTx binding site can cause acute experimental MG in passive transfer experiments (e.g. Gomez and Richman 1985).

The rate of AChR degradation is less than 5% per day at normal mouse diaphragm end-plates, but increases to around 12.5% after injection of MG sera (Stanley and Drachman 1978). Fab fragments of human MG IgG can protect mouse end-plates from this effect (Toyka *et al.* 1980), which thus depends critically on divalent antibody binding. However, at normal junctions a compensatory increase in AChR synthesis may occur (Wilson *et al.* 1983).

While none of the three mechanisms described above fully accounts for the defect in neuromuscular transmission or the clinical weakness in MG, Drachman *et al.* (1982) reported an improved correlation with clinical state when they used a combined index of degradation and pharmacological blockade. Nevertheless, a poor correlation between AChR loss, AChR with antibody bound and transmission defects was found in another study using passive transfer (Mossman *et al.* 1988), implying that other factors might be contributing to the defect.

IDIOTYPES AND ANTI-IDIOTYPES

There is, perhaps not unexpectedly, no extensive sharing of idiotypes between MG patients. One study showed cross-reactivity of two rabbit polyclonal anti-idiotypes with anti-AChR from 8 and 37% of MG patients (Lefvert 1981) but, in another only 1/3 anti-idiotype sera cross-inhibited anti-AChR in 2/19 heterologous MG samples (Lang *et al.* 1985).

A possible role for the idiotype network in the initiation of MG has been proposed. Dwyer and colleagues (1983) reported anti-idiotypic binding of MG sera to a mouse monoclonal anti-AChR antibody. Subsequently they described a network of interactions between monoclonal anti-AChR antibodies and antibodies specific for α 1:4 dextrans (bacterial polysaccharides), and found anti-dextran antibodies in about 38% of MG patients (Dwyer *et al.* 1986). The interactions were mainly demonstrated by ELISA assays in which the idiotypic specificity was not confirmed, and attempts to use other monoclonal antibodies to detect anti-idiotype antibodies in MG sera, and to confirm their presence by additional inhibition experiments in solution (Vincent 1988), have not generally been successful. Nevertheless, idiotypes and anti-idiotypic activity in serum and culture supernatants from MG patients and evidence for anti-idiotypes predating the idiotype during the course of the disease have been reported (Lefvert *et al.* 1987). Such studies would be greatly facilitated by the ready availability of panels of monoclonal anti-AChR antibodies generated from patients, but, despite much effort, very few have been obtained (e.g. Blair *et al.* 1986).

THE IMMUNOGEN IN MYASTHENIA GRAVIS

In theory, autoimmune responses could arise via a number of mechanisms (see Chapter 38) — for instance: (i) cross-reactions with extraneous antigens; (ii) via an internal image anti-idiotype; (iii) through a more complex idiotypic network (see above; Dwyer *et al.* 1986); (iv) as a result of dysregulation of normal immune responses; or (v) through *de novo* autosensitization to a normally sequestered autoantigen. Observations favouring some of these mechanisms operating in MG have been reported. For instance, Schwimmbeck *et al.* (1989) showed a cross-reaction between the AChR sequence α 160–167 and herpes simplex virus glycoprotein D (see (i) above). An example of the 'internal image' concept (see (ii) above) is the demonstration by Wassermann *et al.* (1982) that antibodies generated against the particularly rigid cholinergic agonist 'Bis Q' had ligand-binding preferences very similar to those of AChR. From a mouse immunized with Bis Q, they could generate not only receptor-mimicking monoclonal antibodies of this type, but also some anti-idiotype monoclonal antibodies that bound AChR (Cleveland *et al.* 1983). While the idiotype network can evidently operate in inbred mice (see (ii) and (iii) above; Dwyer *et al.* 1986), the relevance of these findings to human MG is questionable. For example, one would expect the initial antibodies to be directed to only one region of the AChR (e.g. the ligand-binding site) and to have a low affinity for it. In fact, as discussed above, anti-AChR antibodies are heterogeneous and of high affinity. Moreover, the high specificity for the native antigen and low reactivity with recombinant or peptide sequences implicate a native form of AChR (rather than a cross-reactive antigen or ligand) in stimulating the immune response. Such a form is present not only at the end-plate but also on myoid cells in the thymus (see below). Nevertheless, it is possible that the initiating antibodies in MG are low-affinity, perhaps derived by one of the mechanisms considered above, and cause complement-dependent release of immune complexes from end-plates or myoid cells; the high-affinity antibodies found in the patients might represent a secondary response to these complexes after their exposure to a non-tolerant immune system (e.g. in germinal centres).

The AChR is a remarkably immunogenic molecule; successive nanogram doses, injected into mice without adjuvant, can evoke antibody levels comparable with those in patients (Jermy *et al.* 1989). Thus there seems to be no natural state of unresponsiveness to AChR, possibly (see (v) above) because of its sequestration at the neuromuscular junction; possibly its multiple transmembrane regions help to target it to efficient antigen-presenting cells.

The cellular immunology of myasthenia gravis

The anti-AChR antibodies in MG are heterogeneous, high-affinity and IgG (see above), and thus seem highly mutated. They are T-cell-dependent in laboratory animals (Lennon *et al.* 1976) and probably in man too, and most workers believe that the initial activation of these helper T cells, possibly by over-enthusiastic antigen-presenting cells, is a crucial step in the induction of this response. If these T cells prove to be less heterogeneous, they might offer one of the best potential targets for selective immunotherapy.

THYMOMA IN MYASTHENIA GRAVIS

Thymoma, a tumour of epithelial cells (Rosai and Levine 1976), is apparently derived from outer thymic cortical epithelium, which often expresses unusual combinations of markers and shows a disorganized and fragmented morphology (Fig. 106.4; Willcox *et al.* 1987). It retains the normal function of generating cortical (and probably maturing) thymocytes, but often in such vast and disorganized excess (Willcox 1989) that aberrations in the positive selection processes (Chapter 36) and in self-tolerance induction (Chilosi *et al.* 1986) seem likely to occur. This might account for the 30–40% incidence of autoimmune diseases in thymoma cases (bone marrow aplasias in about 5% and MG in around 30% (Souadjian *et al.* 1974; Namba *et al.* 1978)), but their narrow spectrum demands additional explanations.

It seems more than coincidence that thymomatous MG cases have autoantibodies both to AChR and to striational (or other) muscle antigens (Aarli *et al.* 1981). Further, some of the latter cross-react with components of the thymoma epithelial cells (Gilhus *et al.* 1984). Moreover, one cytoplasmic AChR α subunit epitope (expressed on a 153 kD polypeptide chain) has recently been found in them too (Kirchner *et al.* 1988a; Marx *et al.* 1990) — more frequently than in the otherwise similar thymomata from non-MG cases. These findings suggest that the neoplastic epithelial cells actively sensitize developing T cells against these autoantigens. If so, these T cells probably initiate autoantibody responses only after export to the periphery, where they may subsequently encounter degrading autoantigen, since B cells are extremely rare in these tumours, and the MG may begin only months or even years after removal of the thymoma (Namba *et al.* 1978). In support of these suggestions, proliferative responses to *Torpedo* AChR are frequently stronger with T cells from the thymoma than from autologous blood (Sommer *et al.* 1990); identifying the epitopes these T cells recognize may help to define the putative autosensitizing molecule(s) in the thymomas.

THYMIC HYPERPLASIA IN YOUNG-ONSET MYASTHENIA GRAVIS

At first sight, the abnormalities here seem completely different. The cortex is largely normal, although prior corticosteroid treatment may deplete it drastically (Willcox *et al.* 1989). However, in the medulla there is usually infiltration by lymph node-type T cell areas and germinal centres, which are both entirely typical in appearance (Fig. 106.5). These often compress the residual true thymic medulla into bands and arches whose laminin +ve boundaries may break down close to the densest regions of the infiltrate (Bofill *et al.* 1985). The consequent dilution of maturing medullary T cells by peripheral-type T cells, B cells, blasts and antigen-presenting cells accounts for the altered cell populations so often reported in MG (e.g. Abdou *et al.* 1974). Similar infiltrates may occur in normal adult humans (e.g. Middleton 1967), and perhaps

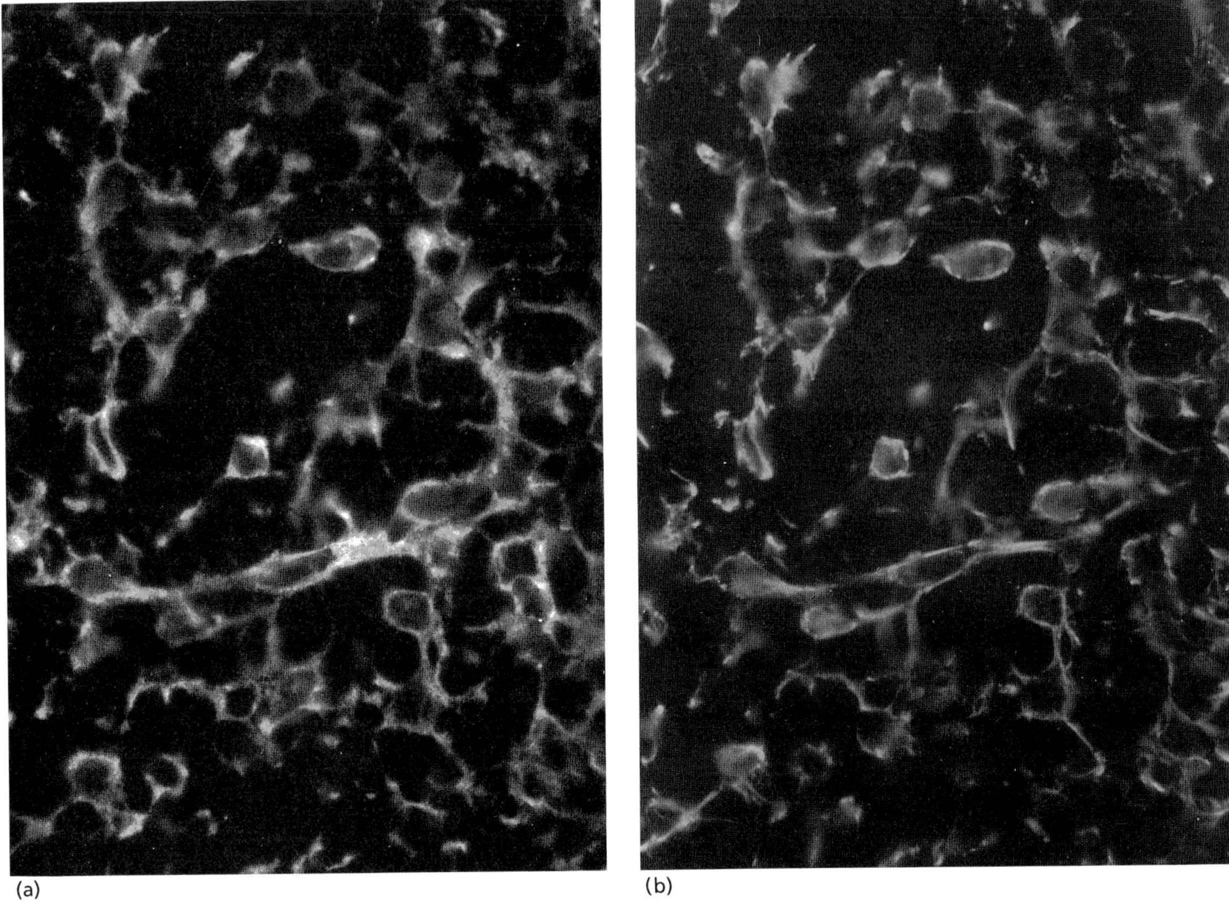

Fig. 106.4. Section of an MG thymoma showing that most of the epithelial cells express both the cortical epithelial marker MR6 ((a) fluorescein isothiocyanate (FITC)) and the subcapsular/medullary antigen detected by antibody MR19 ((b) tetramethyl rhodamine isothiocyanate (TRITC)). In the normal and hyperplastic MG thymus, there is much less double labelling (Schluep *et al.* 1988) (× 427). The donor was a 32-year-old female. Reproduced from Willcox *et al.* (1987) with permission.

in ageing animals, but are usually much less striking (although they may be even more so in other autoimmune diseases).

When suspensions of hyperplastic MG thymus are cultured, they spontaneously synthesize anti-AChR antibodies. They do so at rates that correlate strongly with the donors' serum anti-AChR titres (Scadding *et al.* 1981), and at much higher specific activity (i.e. relative to total IgG) than in autologous lymph node or bone marrow cell cultures or in serum (e.g. Fujii *et al.* 1986). While many other B cells are often present — specific for influenza virus or tetanus toxoid, for example — these only produce antibody on stimulation (e.g. with pokeweed mitogen). At the same time, total IgG synthesis increases greatly, and it correlates well with germinal centre frequencies. The AChR-specific B cells are evidently preferentially activated in hyperplastic thymus, often to generate terminal plasma cells (reviewed in Willcox and Vincent 1988). These are located mainly in the T cell areas, which seem to be the more MG-specific element (Schluep *et al.* 1988), and are also evident in seronegative MG (Willcox *et al.* 1991). Furthermore, there is also a preferential localization of AChR-specific T cells in the MG thymus relative to autologous blood, whereas purified protein derivative (PPD)-reactive cells may be present but only as a random sample of those in the circulation (Sommer *et al.* 1990). Finally, in all these histological and functional respects, the uninvolved thymus adjacent to a thymoma usually behaves exactly like the hyperplastic MG thymus (Willcox *et al.* 1987; Sommer *et al.* 1990).

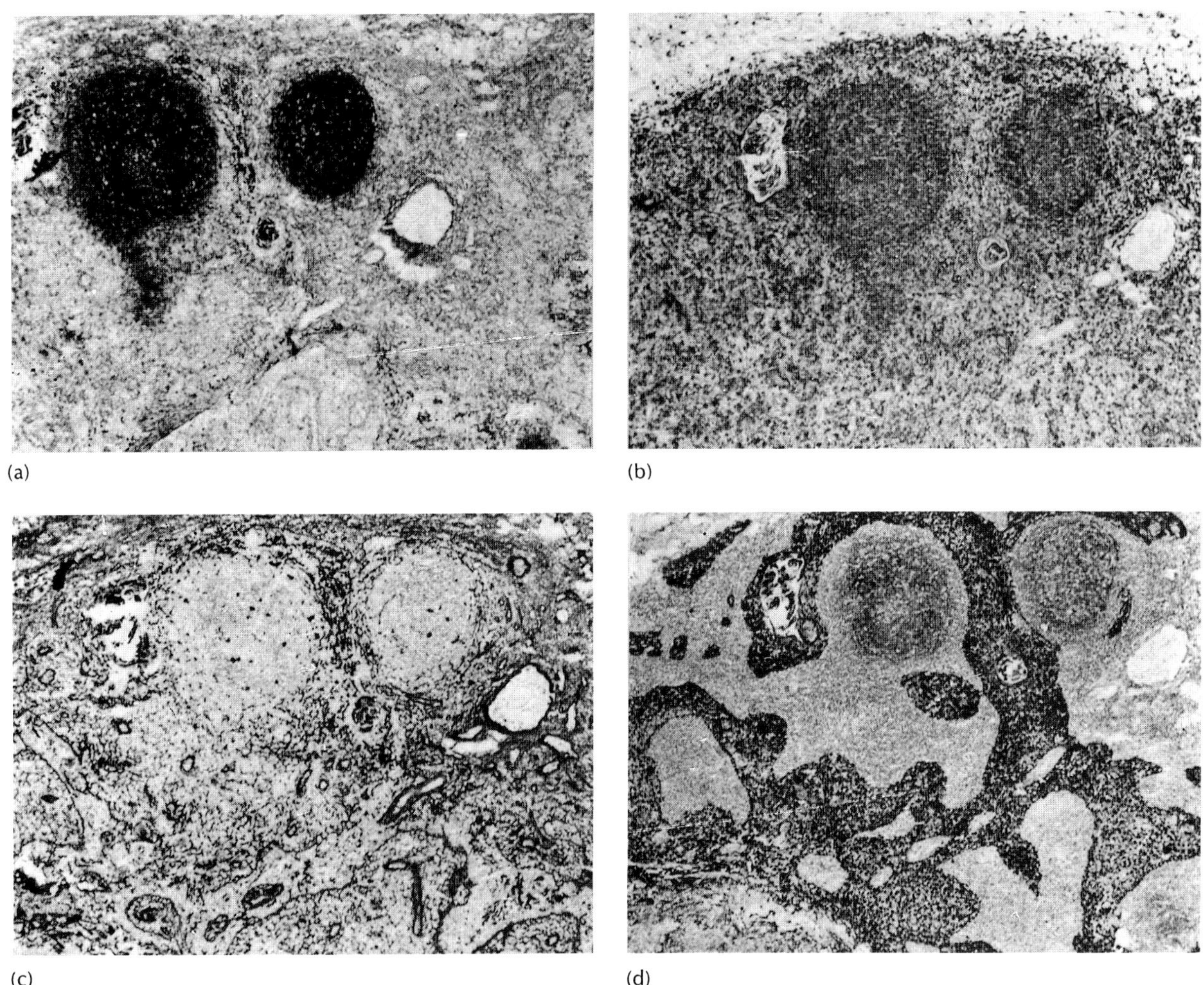

Fig. 106.5. Serial sections showing medullary hyperplasia in the thymus of an 18-year-old MG patient; residual cortex was relatively normal (not shown, but mainly situated above these photographs). Strongly labelled for B cells ((a) with RFB4) are two germinal centres; they are located in the midst of the T cell areas, which contain further HLA-DR +ve B cells and interdigitating ('dendritic') cells (b), and a fine fibronectin +ve network, including small blood-vessels and high endothelial venules (c). These T/B cell infiltrates are compressing the residual thymic medullary epithelial tissue into characteristic bands and arches ((d) MR19). (×362). Reproduced with permission from Willcox (1989).

It is an attractive suggestion — originally from Wekerle and Ketelsen (1977) and Kao and Drachman (1977) — that initial autosensitization to AChR might occur in the hyperplastic as it may in the neoplastic MG thymus. It could be caused either by the cytoplasmic epitope mentioned above, which is also present in some normal medullary epithelial cells, or (as originally proposed) by the rare muscle-like myoid cells in the normal medulla. These express complete AChR molecules, in addition to contractile proteins, and do so both in culture (Wekerle and Ketelsen 1977) and *in situ* (Plate 106.1, between pages 1930 and 1931; Schluep *et al.* 1987). They appeared to be foci of immunological attack by T cells and antigen-presenting cells in one study (Kirchner *et al.* 1988b), though not in another (Plate 106.1; Schluep *et al.* 1987). However, it is equally possible that all these hyperplastic changes are secondary, and that cells initially sensitized in the periphery are subsequently attracted into the thymus by the autoantigens expressed there. This alternative explanation seems to us to fit all the findings better — especially the similarity of the uninvolved thymus adjacent to a thymoma.

RESPONSES OF T CELLS TO ACETYLCHOLINE RECEPTOR ANTIGENS

Several groups have begun to generate T lymphocyte lines and clones from blood and thymus, initially using *Torpedo* AChR plus antigen-presenting cells and subsequent interleukin 2 (IL-2) for stimulation (Hohlfeld *et al.* 1984), and later using recombinant mouse (Melms *et al.* 1989) or human (Fig. 106.6; Newsom-Davis *et al.* 1989; Ong *et al.* 1991) AChR α subunit — apparently the main focus of T and B cell responses (Hohlfeld *et al.* 1987) — or synthetic peptides (Protti *et al.* 1990). Detection of initial responses and selection of CD4 +ve lines have both proved surprisingly easy in healthy controls as well as in MG (e.g. Sommer *et al.* 1991), and it is premature to claim disease specificity for these T cells at present. Other provisional conclusions are that: (i) responses to mammalian sequences are more frequent and stronger than to their *Torpedo* equivalents, with little T cell cross-reactivity between the two; (ii) no dominant T cell epitope or HLA Class II MHC restriction element has emerged; in DR3 +ve patients, the alternative DR allele is often involved, and sometimes even the other Class II MHC isotypes, DQ or DP; and (iii) heterogeneity of these T cells is thus considerable between patients and may be significant even within one donor (Newsom-Davis *et al.* 1989). If these T cells are disease-relevant, this heterogeneity already raises doubts about the potential of selective therapy directed either at specific T cell clones (Acha-Orbea *et al.* 1988) or at particular Class II MHC molecules (Waldor *et al.* 1983), although it remains possible that the key pathogenic T cells are more restricted. Much effort is being devoted to exploring these possibilities at present.

Management

The first line in therapy is anti-cholinesterase drug treatment, which often suffices to control mild or remitting symptoms. It is also used as an adjunct to immunosuppressive treatment in severe cases.

THYMECTOMY

The effects of thymectomy on myasthenic weak-

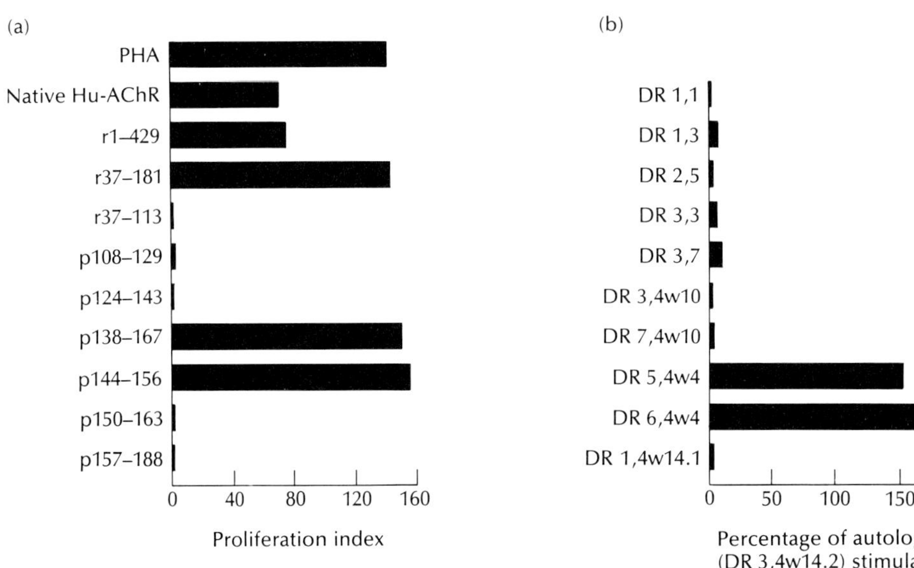

Fig. 106.6. Proliferative responses of a T cell line raised from thymic cells of a 15-year-old MG patient by stimulation with almost full-length recombinant (r) AChR α subunit. Panel (a) shows that this T cell line responds very well to picomolar concentrations of solubilized human AChR. Mapping of its epitope to the 114–180 region (deduced from responses to smaller recombinant products) was confirmed with synthetic peptides (p). There was no response to *Torpedo* AChR α subunit or the equivalent synthetic peptide. (b) Such T cells absolutely require HLA Class II MHC +ve antigen-presenting cells, which, in this case, must express the correct subtype of HLA-DR4 (i.e. Dw14.2, or the very similar Dw4). Strikingly, the totally inactive Dw14.1 differs only by a valine-for-glycine substitution at position 86 of its β chain. Modified from Ong *et al.* (1991).

ness depend on the thymic pathology. There is general agreement that early-onset patients showing medullary hyperplasia often benefit, the pooled results from several series indicating that 25–30% of patients will experience a remission (developing over 1–3 years postoperatively), and that a further 40–45% will improve. The effects of surgery on the remainder appear to be neutral. While there has been no controlled prospective trial of thymectomy, a retrospective computer-matched study clearly demonstrated a better outcome in surgically treated cases compared with those receiving anti-cholinesterase medication alone (Buckingham *et al.* 1976). Improvement is also seen in some children undergoing thymectomy (Rodriguez *et al.* 1983). In late-onset patients, in those with restricted ocular disease and in seronegative MG, the case for thymectomy is currently much weaker.

Thymoma should be sought by regular follow-up of non-thymectomized generalized seropositive patients in whom striated muscle antibodies have been detected. When a thymoma is present, surgical removal is normally undertaken to reduce the risk of local spread, which is common and can lead to premature death, although distant metastases are rare (Verley & Hollmann 1985). Paradoxically, improvement in myasthenic weakness attributable to surgery is seldom evident, and symptoms may increase or even begin after complete excision of the thymoma (Namba *et al.* 1978).

IMMUNOSUPPRESSIVE DRUG TREATMENT

The value of corticosteroids and of azathioprine is widely accepted although not assessed in prospective trials. Alternate-day dosage may reduce the risk of exacerbation of symptoms that can occur during initiation of treatment, and incrementing from an initially low dose may similarly be preferable in severe or 'bulbar' cases. When remission develops, a slow rate of dose reduction is advisable to define the effective minimal dose. Clinical improvement is accompanied by a decline in specific antibody in most cases. Patients with ocular MG appear to respond particularly well to corticosteroid treatment.

Cyclosporin A was assessed in a prospective controlled trial as the sole treatment in 20 MG patients (Tindall *et al.* 1987). Although it gave a significant improvement relative to a placebo, side-effects were frequent and the drug does not appear to offer any advantages over the use of prednisolone and azathioprine, but could be used in those intolerant of them. The use of cyclophosphamide has been reported in an uncontrolled study, but its relative toxicity limits its application in this disease.

OTHER IMMUNOLOGICAL TREATMENTS

Plasma exchange was first used in MG in 1976, and is usually given as a course of four or five daily exchanges, the size of each exchange relating to the patient's plasma volume (Pinching *et al.* 1976; Newsom-Davis *et al.* 1978). It is of particular value in the management of a myasthenic crisis (acute relapse) and as regular initial treatment in chronic severe MG. Improvement typically begins within 2–3 days and last 3–4 weeks, but sometimes less in acute severe cases. In both these situations, plasma exchange is usually used in conjunction with immunosuppressive drugs; however, there is no evidence that they are synergistic. Plasma exchange can also be used to prepare patients for thymectomy, and in the post-operative period while potential improvement is awaited.

Intravenous gamma globulin has been used in MG in similar circumstances to plasma exchange, and improvement has been reported. Results of controlled trials with both these therapies are lacking. In occasional patients resistant to, or intolerant of, immunosuppressive drugs, lymphoid irradiation has been found to be an effective treatment.

SPECIFIC IMMUNOTHERAPY

A long-term therapeutic goal in autoimmune disease is selectively to control the abnormal immune response without interfering with the function of the remainder of the immune system. Myasthenia gravis should be well suited to such an approach since the primary sequence of the target antigen is known allowing, at least in theory, the identification of critical T cell epitopes, their receptor gene usage and Class II MHC restriction, although the T cell heterogeneity already observed (see below) may seem discouraging. Prospects for specific immunotherapy in MG have recently been reviewed by Steinman and Mantegazza (1990).

Lambert–Eaton myasthenic syndrome

Clinical features

CANCER ASSOCIATION

Although LEMS was first recognized in association with bronchial carcinoma (Lambert *et al.* 1956), it can also occur independently of cancer. In our personal series of 50 cases, thoracic cancer was present in 24, being histologically proved to be of the small-cell type (SCLC) in 21 cases (O'Neill *et al.* 1988). Two other miscellaneous malignancies were probably coincidental. The neurological syndrome typically preceded the detection of the SCLC. The longest interval we have encountered between LEMS and the appearance of the cancer has been 5 years. The association with SCLC is of special interest in the immunological context, since this cancer may be of neural crest origin and might therefore share antigenic determinants with the nervous system.

EPIDEMIOLOGY

Judged by referral to a myasthenic clinic, LEMS (both forms) is at least 10 times less frequent than MG (i.e. <1 per 100 000), although it is probably often overlooked, especially when cancer-associated. A prospective survey of 150 SCLC cases and analysis of earlier studies suggest that 3% of SCLC cases have LEMS, implying an annual incidence in the United Kingdom of 250 LEMS cases (Elrington *et al.* 1991). The sex incidence is approximately equal in the non-cancer cases. In the remainder, males exceed females, which may simply reflect their commoner smoking habit.

SYMPTOMS AND SIGNS

The Lambert–Eaton myasthenic syndrome is characterized by proximal muscle weakness, augmentation of strength during sustained effort ('post-tetanic potentiation'), depressed tendon reflexes and autonomic disturbances, including dry mouth, constipation and impotence. Onset is usually subacute and the autonomic disorder can precede muscular symptoms by many months. Respiratory involvement can occur in severe cases.

AUTOIMMUNE AND IMMUNOGENETIC ASSOCIATIONS

Other autoimmune diseases and autoantibodies occur at increased frequency in LEMS (Lennon *et al.* 1982). Thyroid disease and vitiligo appear to be particularly often associated. The Lambert–Eaton myasthenic syndrome has occasionally been found to coexist with MG (Newsom-Davis *et al.* 1991). There is a weak association with HLA-B8 and DR3 in cases with or without SCLC, and a stronger one with Ig heavy chain markers (Willcox *et al.* 1985).

DIAGNOSIS

The diagnosis of LEMS can be confidently made in most cases by clinical electrophysiology. A reduced resting compound muscle action potential (CMAP) with an amplitude incrementing by >100% following 15 seconds of maximum voluntary contraction of the muscle is firm evidence of LEMS. There are often other disorders of neuromuscular transmission also, including abnormal decrement in the CMAP amplitude on repetitive nerve stimulation and increased jitter on single-fibre electromyography. Anti-calcium channel antibodies, detected by an RIA using ^{125}I-labelled ω-conotoxin (CgTx), are present at raised titre in 45–65% of cases (Lennon and Lambert 1989; Sher *et al.* 1989; Leys *et al.* 1991).

Neuromuscular pathology and pathophysiology

The defect in LEMS is presynaptic. The quantal release of ACh (see Fig. 106.1) is characteristically reduced to below 20 quanta per impulse (Lambert and Elmqvist 1971). This reduction is apparently due to a decrease in the number of functional VGCCs. Freeze-fracture electron microscopy shows a decrease and disorganization of active-zone particles at the nerve terminal, normally arrayed as a double parallel row, which are thought to represent VGCCs (Fukunaga *et al.* 1982). Evidence that anti-VGCC antibodies cause this reduction is discussed in the next section.

HUMORAL FACTORS

The first clinical clue to an autoimmune aetiology

came from the observed association of LEMS with other autoimmune diseases. It was later shown that the clinical and electrophysiologial abnormalities in LEMS improved after plasma exchange, whether the patients had an associated SCLC or not (Lang *et al.* 1981). Moreover, improvement could be maintained by long-term immunosuppressive drug treatment.

Direct evidence for an antibody-mediated process was provided by passive transfer studies (Lang *et al.* 1981; for a review see Vincent *et al.* 1989). Immunoglobulin G purified from the plasma of LEMS patients and injected intraperitoneally into mice transferred the principal physiological and morphological abnormalities. Plasma was no more effective than IgG in inducing the physiological changes, indicating that the IgG was the active factor. These changes closely followed the level of human IgG in the recipient mouse serum. *In vitro* experiments failed to show any effect of LEMS IgG on VGCC function over a period of 4 hours, arguing against direct block of the ion channel itself. The mechanism of action of LEMS IgG did not appear to involve complement in that C5-deficient animals were as susceptible as controls. Further analysis of the electrophysiological changes in the injected mice indicated that LEMS IgG antibodies act by reducing the number of functional VGCCs.

The nerve terminals in these mice revealed a significant reduction in the number of active zones, and of active-zone particles representing VGCCs (Fukunaga *et al.* 1983). Subsequent studies (see Engel *et al.* 1989 for a review) showed that the earliest change was a slight reduction in the distance separating adjacent particles in the outside pairs of rows, which are sufficiently close to be spanned by divalent antibody (Fukuoka *et al.* 1987a). Later they became more disorganized, with clustering and reduction in the number of active zones and particles as in the human disorder (Fig. 106.7(b)). Both the physiological and morphological effects apparently depended on antibody divalency. Thus LEMS IgG appears to reduce the

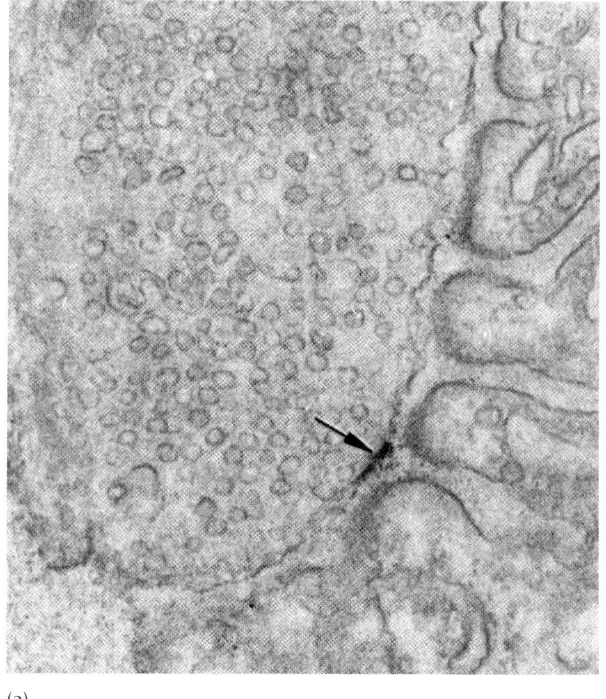

(a)

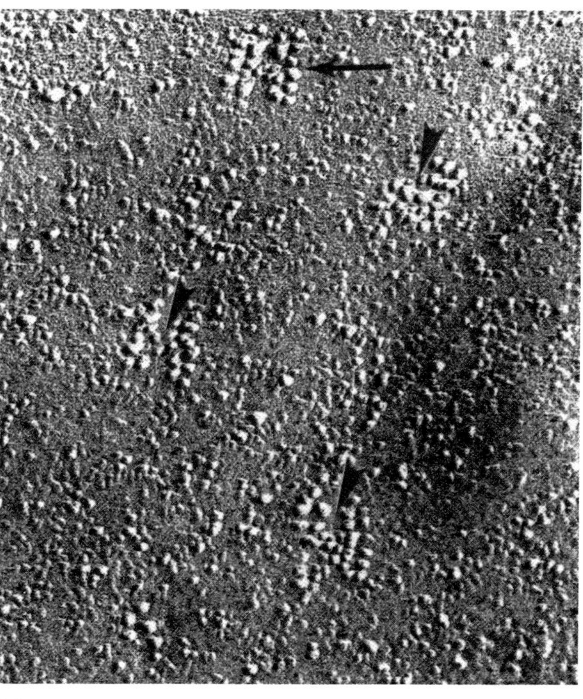

(b)

Fig. 106.7. Early morphological effects of LEMS IgG on presynaptic membrane active zones. (a) Immunoperoxidase localization of human IgG at the active-zone region in mice treated with a single 10 mg dose of LEMS IgG (×515 000). (b) Changes in distribution of active-zone particles visualized by freeze-fracture electron microscopy of the presynaptic membrane in muscle from mice treated for 2 days with LEMS IgG. One normal-appearing active zone (arrow) and several abnormal active zones (arrow heads) can be seen (×1 205 100). Reproduced with permission from Fukuoka *et al.* (1987a, b).

number of VGCCs by cross-linking, perhaps resulting in an increased rate of VGCC internalization. Immuno-electron microscopy localized the LEMS IgG in injected mice to the active zones of the presynaptic membrane (Fig. 106.7(a); Fukuoka *et al.* 1987b).

Aetiology and the role of small-cell lung cancer

Several lines of evidence indicate that the cancer cells play a critical role in triggering the autoantibody response in SCLC–LEMS. As mentioned above, SCLC is thought to be a tumour of neuroectodermal origin and thus might be expected to share some antigenic determinants with nervous system components, including VGCCs. In support of this, electrophysiological studies have shown that SCLC cells, either in organ culture or as a cell line, are capable of voltage-gated Ca^{2+} flux. This was confirmed by measuring Ca^{2+} influx following brief exposure to a high external K^{+} concentration, which induces depolarization (Roberts *et al.* 1985). $^{45}Calcium^{2+}$ flux was significantly inhibited when the SCLC cells were maintained in LEMS rather than in control IgG. The effect was observed at physiological IgG concentrations, and was dose-dependent. The time course was slow, the maximum effect being observed at 5–7 days. These results are consistent with modulation of VGCCs secondary to cross-linking of adjacent channels by LEMS IgGs. Interestingly, IgG from LEMS patients without SCLC inhibited $^{45}Ca^{2+}$ flux was effectively as IgG from those with SCLC. By contrast, IgG from an SCLC patient without LEMS had no effect.

These findings suggested that tumour VGCC determinants were triggering the autoimmune response. One might, therefore, expect disease severity (assessed by electromyography (EMG)) to correlate with these functional effects of the patient's IgG on Ca^{2+} flux; in fact this correlation proved to be highly significant (r = 0.8; Lang *et al.* 1989). The apparently specific association with SCLC but not with other lung cancers suggested that the latter may not express VGCCs, and this has proved to be the case in the lines so far examined. A rodent hybrid and a human neuroblastoma line, however, both expressed VGCCs, the latter being used as the source of antigen for the RIA to detect anti-VGCC antibodies (see above).

If tumour VGCC determinants are triggering and sustaining the autoantibody response, treatment of the tumour should influence the neurological disorder. Seven of 11 SCLC-associated LEMS cases surviving for more than 2 months following specific tumour therapy showed clinical improvement, their EMG index of disease severity returning to normal values within 6 months to 1 year (Chalk *et al.* 1990). This suggests that the autoantibody response must be provoked by remarkably small tumours in the extreme cases where LEMS onset precedes radiological evidence of the tumour by up to 5 years. This would imply that these patients are very high responders and/ or that the tumours are extremely immunogenic. The former is supported by the immune response gene associations.

In its cancer-associated form, LEMS thus provides the best current evidence that autoimmune mechanisms may underlie some paraneoplastic neurological diseases. By contrast, the autoimmune stimulus in the non-cancer-associated disorder is unknown. An occult SCLC can be excluded in view of the long history present in some cases. The phenotypic and immunological similarities between the two forms of the disease underline the observation that a single autoimmune disease may have more than one triggering factor.

Management

The compound 3,4-diaminopyridine (not yet generally available) increases ACh release from the nerve terminal and produces symptomatic improvement (McEvoy *et al.* 1989). In SCLC–LEMS, treatment of the tumour by surgery, radio- or chemotherapy may result in neurological improvement or remission (see above). In non-SCLC LEMS, treatment with prednisolone, either alone or combined with azathioprine, often results in improvement and sometimes in complete remission (Newsom-Davis and Murray 1984). The response is slow, typically taking 6 months or more to develop.

References

Aarli, J.A., Lefvert, A.-K. and Tonder, O. (1981). Thymoma-specific antibodies in sera from patients with myasthenia gravis demonstrated by indirect haemagglutination. *J. Neuroimmunol.* **1**, 421–7.

Abdou, N.I., Lisak, R.P., Zweiman, B., Abrahamsohn, I. and Penn, A.S. (1974). The thymus in myasthenia gravis: evidence for altered cell populations. *N. Engl. J. Med.* **291**, 1271–5.

Acha-Orbea, H., Mitchell, D.J., Timmermann, L. *et al.* (1988). Limited heterogeneity of T cell receptors from lymphocytes mediating autoimmune encephalomyelitis allows specific immune intervention *Cell* **54**, 263–73.

Aoki, T., Drachman, D.B, Asher, D.M., Gibbs, C.J., Bahmanyar, S. and Wolinsky, J.S. (1985). Attempts to implicate viruses in myasthenia gravis. *Neurology* **35**, 185–92.

Blair, D.A., Richman, D.P., Taves, C.J. and Koethe, S. (1986). Monoclonal antibodies to acetylcholine receptor secreted by human × human hybridomas derived from lymphocytes of a patient with myasthenia gravis. *Immunol. Invest.* **15**, 351–64.

Bofill, M., Janossy, G., Willcox, N., Chilosi, M., Trejdosiewicz, L.K. and Newsom-Davis, J. (1985). Microenvironments in the normal thymus and the thymus in myasthenia gravis. *Am. J. Pathol.* **119**, 462–73.

Buckingham, J.M., Howard, F.M., Bernatz, P.E. *et al.* (1976). The value of thymectomy in myasthenia gravis: a computer-matched study. *Ann. Surg.* **184**, 453–8.

Burges, J., Wray, D.W., Pizzighella, S., Hall, Z. and Vincent, A. (1990). A myasthenia gravis plasma immunoglobulin reduces miniature endplate potentials at human endplates *in vitro*. *Muscle Nerve* **13**, 407–13.

Carlsson, B., Wallin, J., Pirskanen, R., Matell, G. and Smith, C.I.E. (1990). Different HLA DR-DQ associations in subgroups of idiopathic myasthenia gravis. *Immunogenetics* **31**, 285–90.

Chalk, C.H., Murray, N.M.F., Newsom-Davis, J., O'Neill, J.H. and Spiro, S.G. (1990). Response of the Lambert–Eaton myasthenic syndrome to treatment of associated small-cell lung carcinoma. *Neurology* **40**, 1552–6.

Chilosi, M., Ianucci, A., Fiore-Donati, L. *et al.* (1986). Myasthenia gravis: immunohistological heterogeneity in microenvironmental organisation of hyperplastic and neoplastic thymuses suggesting different mechanisms of tolerance breakdown. *J. Neuroimmunol.* **11**, 191–204.

Chiu, H.C., Hsieh, R.P., Hsieh, K.H. and Hung, T.P. (1987). Association of HLA-DRw9 with myasthenia gravis in Chinese. *J. Immunogenet.* **14**, 203–7.

Claudio, T. (1989). Molecular genetics of acetylcholine receptor-channels. In *Frontiers in Molecular Neurobiology*, ed. D.M. Glover and B.D. Hames, pp. 63–142. IRL Press, Oxford.

Cleveland, W.L., Wassermann, N.H., Sarangarajan, R., Penn, A.S. and Erlanger, B.F. (1983). Monoclonal antibodies to the acetylcholine receptor by a normally functioning auto-anti-idiotypic mechanism. *Nature* **305**, 56–7.

Compston, D.A.S., Vincent, A., Newsom-Davis, J. and Batchelor, J.R. (1980). Clinical, pathological, HLA antigen and immunological evidence for disease heterogeneity in myasthenia gravis. *Brain* **103**, 579–601.

Dawkins, R.L., Zilko, P.J., Carrano, J., Garlepp, M.J. and McDonald, B.L. (1981). Immunobiology of D-penicillamine. *J. Rheumatol.* **8** (suppl. 7), 56–61.

Demaine, A., Willcox, N., Janer, M., Welsh, K. and Newsom-Davis, J. (1992). Immunoglobulin heavy chain gene associations in myasthenia gravis: new evidence for disease heterogeneity. *J. Neurol.* **239**, 53–6.

Donaldson, J.O., Penn, A.S., Lisak, R.P., Abramsky, O., Brenner, T. and Schotland, D.L. (1981). Anti-acetylcholine receptor antibody in neonatal myasthenia gravis. *Am. J. Dis. Child.* **135**, 222–6.

Drachman, D.B. (ed.) (1987). Myasthenia gravis: biology and treatment. *Ann. NY Acad. Sci.* **505**, 1–914.

Drachman, D.B., Adams, R.N., Josifek, L.F. and Self, S.G. (1982). Functional activities of autoantibodies to acetylcholine receptors and the clinical severity of myasthenia gravis. *N. Engl. J. Med.* **307**, 769–75.

Dwyer, D.S., Bradley, R.J., Urquhart, C.K. and Kearney, J.F. (1983). Naturally occurring anti-idiotypic antibodies in myasthenia gravis patients. *Nature* **301**, 611–14.

Dwyer, D.S., Vakil, M. and Kearney, J.F. (1986). Idiotypic network connectivity and a possible cause of myasthenia gravis. *J. Exp. Med.* **164**, 1310–18.

Elmqvist, D., Hofmann, W.W., Kugelberg, J. and Quastel, D.M.J. (1964). An electrophysiological investigation of neuromuscular transmission in myasthenia gravis. *J. Physiol.* **174**, 417–34.

Elrington, G.M., Murray, N.M.F., Spiro, S.G. and Newsom-Davis, J. (1991). Neurological paraneoplastic syndromes in patients with small cell lung cancer: a prospective survey of 150 patients. *J. Neurol. Neurosurg. Psychiatry* **54**, 764–7.

Engel, A.G. (1984). Myasthenia gravis and myasthenic syndromes. *Ann. Neurol.* **16**, 519–34.

Engel, A.G. (1990). Congenital myasthenic syndromes. In *Neuromuscular Transmission: Basic and Applied Aspects*, ed. A. Vincent and D. Wray, pp. 200–25, Manchester University Press, Manchester.

Engel, A.G. and Arahata, K. (1987). The membrane attack complex of complement at the endplate in myasthenia gravis. *Ann. NY Acad. Sci.* **505**, 326–32.

Engel, A.G., Lambert, E.H. and Howard, F.M. (1977). Immune complexes (IgG and C3) at the motor endplate in myasthenia gravis: ultrastructural and light microscopic localization and electrophysiologic correlations. *Mayo Clin. Proc.* **52**, 267–80.

Engel, A.G., Nagel, A., Fukuoka, T. *et al.* (1989). Motor nerve terminal calcium channels in Lambert–Eaton myasthenic syndrome: morphologic evidence for depletion and that the depletion is mediated by autoantibodies. *Ann. NY Acad. Sci.* **560**, 278–90.

Fambrough, D.M., Drachman, D.B. and Satyamurti, S. (1973). Neuromuscular junction in myasthenia gravis: decreased acetylcholine receptors. *Science* **182**, 293–5.

Fujii, Y., Hashimoto, J., Monden, Y., Ito, T., Nakahara, K. and Kawashima, Y. (1986). Specific activation of lymphocytes against acetylcholine receptor in the thymus in myasthenia gravis. *J. Immunol.* **136**, 887–91.

Fukunaga, H., Engel, A.G., Osame, M. and Lambert, E.H. (1982). Paucity and disorganisation of presynaptic membrane active zones in the Lambert–Eaton myasthenic syndrome. *Muscle Nerve* **5**, 686–97.

Fukunaga, H., Engel, A.G., Lang, B., Newsom-Davis, J. and Vincent, A. (1983). Passive transfer of Lambert–Eaton myasthenic syndrome with IgG from man to mouse depletes the presynaptic membrane active zones. *Proc. Nat. Acad. Sci. (USA)* **80**, 7636–40.

Fukuoka, T., Engel, A.G., Lang, B., Newsom-Davis, J., Prior, C. and Wray, D.W. (1987a). Lambert–Eaton myasthenic syndrome. I. Early morphologic effects of IgG on the presynaptic membrane active zones. *Ann. Neurol.* **22**, 193–9.

Fukuoka, T., Engel, A.G., Lang, B., Newsom-Davis, J. and Vincent, A. (1987b). Lambert–Eaton myasthenic syndrome. II. Immunoelectron microscopy localisation of IgG at the mouse motor endplate. *Ann. Neurol.* **22**, 200–11.

Garlepp, M.J.H., Kay, P.H., Dawkins, R.L., Bucknall, R.C. and Kemp, A. (1981). Cross-reactivity of anti-acetylcholine receptor autoantibodies. *Muscle Nerve* **4**, 282–8.

Gilhus, N.-E., Aarli, J.A., Christensson, B. and Matre, R. (1984). Rabbit antiserum to a citric acid extract of human skeletal muscle staining thymomas from myasthenia gravis patients. *J. Neuroimmunol.* **7**, 55–64.

Gomez, C.M. and Richman, D.P. (1985). Monoclonal anti-acetylcholine receptor antibodies with differing capacities to induce experimental autoimmune myasthenia gravis. *J. Immunol.* **135**, 235–41.

Heidenreich, F., Vincent, A., Roberts, A. and Newsom-Davis, J. (1988a). Epitopes on human acetylcholine receptor defined by monoclonal antibodies and myasthenia gravis sera. *Autoimmunity* **1**, 285–97.

Heidenreich, F., Vincent, A., Willcox, N. and Newsom-Davis, J. (1988b). Anti-acetylcholine receptor antibody specificities in serum and in thymic culture supernatants from myasthenia gravis patients. *Neurology* **38**, 1784–8.

Hohlfeld, R., Toyka, K.V., Heininger, K., Gross-Wilde, H. and Kalies, I. (1984). Autoimmune human T lymphocytes specific for acetylcholine receptor. *Nature* **310**, 244–6.

Hohlfeld, R., Toyka, K.V., Tzartos, S.J., Carson, W. and Conti-Tronconi, B.M. (1987). Human T-helper lymphocytes in myasthenia gravis recognize the nicotinic receptor alpha subunit. *Proc. Nat. Acad. Sci. (USA)* **84**, 5379–83.

Jermy, A.C., Fisher, C.A., Vincent, A.C., Willcox, N.A. and Newsom-Davis, J. (1989). Experimental autoimmune myasthenia gravis induced in mice without adjuvant: genetic susceptibility and adoptive transfer of weakness. *J. Autoimmunity* **2**, 675–88.

Kao, I. and Drachman, D.B. (1977). Thymic muscle cells bear acetylcholine receptors: possible relation to myasthenia gravis. *Science* **195**, 74–5.

Kirchner, T., Tzartos, S., Hoppe, F., Schalke, B., Wekerle, H. and Muller-Hermelink, H.K. (1988a). Pathogenesis of myasthenia gravis: acetylcholine receptor-related antigenic determinants in tumour-free thymuses and thymic epithelial tumours. *Am. J. Pathol.* **130**, 268–80.

Kirchner, T., Hoppe, F., Schalke, B. and Muller-Hermelink, H.K. (1988b). Microenvironment of thymic myoid cells in myasthenia gravis. *Virchows Arch. B Cell. Pathol.* **54**, 295–302.

Klavinskis, L.S., Willcox, N., Oxford, J. and Newsom-Davis, J. (1985). Anti-virus antibodies in myasthenia gravis. *Neurology* **35**, 1381–4.

Kurtzke, J.F. (1978). Epidemiology of myasthenia gravis. *Adv. Neurol.* **19**, 545–64.

Lambert, E.H. and Elmqvist, D. (1971). Quantal components of end-plate potentials in the myasthenic syndrome. *Ann. NY Acad. Sci.* **183**, 183–99.

Lambert, E.H., Eaton, L.M. and Rooke, E.D. (1956). Defect of neuromuscular conduction associated with malignant neoplasms. *Am. J. Physiol.* **187**, 612–13.

Lang, B., Newsom-Davis, J., Wray, D., Vincent, A. and Murray, N.M.F. (1981). Autoimmune aetiology for myasthenic (Eaton–Lambert) syndrome. *Lancet* **ii**, 224–6.

Lang, B., Roberts, A.J., Vincent, A. and Newsom-Davis, J. (1985). Anti-acetylcholine receptor idiotypes in myasthenia gravis analysed by rabbit anti-sera. *Clin. Exp. Immunol.* **60**, 637–44.

Lang, B., Richardson, G., Rees, J., Vincent, A. and Newsom-Davis, J. (1988). Plasma from myasthenia gravis patients reduces acetylcholine receptor agonist-induced Na^+ flux into TE671 cell line. *J. Neuroimmunol.* **19**, 141–8.

Lang, B., Vincent, A., Murray, N.M.F. and Newsom-Davis, J. (1989). Lambert–Eaton myasthenic syndrome: immunoglobulin G inhibition of Ca^{2+} flux in tumor cells correlates with disease severity. *Ann. Neurol.* **25**, 265–71.

Lefvert, A.-K. (1981). Anti-idiotypic antibodies against the receptor antibodies in myasthenia gravis. *Scand. J. Immunol.* **13**, 493–7.

Lefvert, A.-K., Holm, G. and Pirskanen, R. (1987). Autoanti-idiotypic antibodies in myasthenia gravis. *Ann. NY Acad. Sci.* **505**, 133–54.

Lennon, V.A. and Griesmann, G.E. (1989). Evidence against acetylcholine receptor having a main immunogenic region as target for autoantibodies in myasthenia gravis. *Neurology* **39**, 1069–76.

Lennon, V.A. and Lambert, E.H. (1989). Autoantibodies bind solubilised calcium channel–omega-conotoxin complexes from small cell lung carcinoma: a diagnostic aid for Lambert–Eaton myasthenic syndrome. *Mayo Clin. Proc.* **64**, 1498–504.

Lennon, V.A., Lindstrom, J.M. and Seybold, M.E. (1976). Experimental autoimmune myasthenia gravis: cellular and humoral immune responses. *Ann. NY Acad. Sci.* **274**, 283–99.

Lennon, V.A., Lambert, E.H., Whittingham, S. and Fairbanks, V. (1982). Autoimmunity in the Lambert-Eaton myasthenic syndrome. *Muscle Nerve* **5**, S21–S25.

Lewis, S.W., Ron, M. and Newsom-Davis, J. (1989). Absence of central functional cholinergic deficits in myasthenia gravis. *J. Neurol. Neurosurg. Psychiatry* **52**, 258–61.

Leys, K., Lang, B., Johnston, I. and Newsom-Davis, J. (1991). Calcium channel autoantibodies in the Lambert–Eaton myasthenic syndrome. *Ann. Neurol.* **29**, 307–14.

Lindstrom, J.M. (1979). Autoimmune response to acetylcholine receptors in myasthenia gravis and its animal model. *Adv. Immunol.* **27**, 1–50.

Lindstrom, J.M., Seybold, M.E., Lennon, V.A., Whittingham, S. and Duane, D.D. (1976). Antibody to acetylcholine receptor in myasthenia gravis: prevalence, clinical correlates and diagnostic value. *Neurology* **26**, 1054–9.

Lindstrom, J.M., Shelton, D. and Fujii, Y. (1988). Myasthenia gravis. *Adv. Immunol.* **42**, 233–284.

McEvoy, K.M., Windebank, A.J., Daube, J.R. and Low, P.A. (1989). 3,4-Diaminopyridine in the treatment of Lambert–Eaton myasthenic syndrome. *N. Engl. J. Med.* **321**, 1567–71.

Marx, A., O'Connor, R., Geuder, K.I. *et al.* (1990). Characterization of a protein with an acetylcholine receptor epitope from myasthenia gravis-associated thymomas. *Lab. Invest.* **62**, 279–87.

Matsuki, K., Juji, T., Tokunaga, K. *et al.* (1990). HLA antigens in Japanese patients with myasthenia gravis. *J. Clin. Invest.* **86**, 392–9.

Melms, A., Chrestel, S., Schalke, B.C.G. *et al.* (1989). Autoimmune T lymphocytes in myasthenia gravis: determination of target epitopes using T lines and recombinant products of the mouse nicotinic acetylcholine receptor gene. *J. Clin. Invest.* **83**, 785–90.

Middleton, G. (1967). The incidence of follicular structures in the human thymus at autopsy. *Aust. J. Exp. Biol. Med. Sci.* **45**, 189–99.

Mier, A.K. and Havard, C.W.H. (1985). Diaphragmatic myasthenia in mother and child. *Postgrad. Med. J.* **61**, 725–7.

Moore, N.R. (1989). Imaging in myasthenia gravis. *Clin. Radiol.* **40**, 115–16.

Mossman, S., Vincent, A. and Newsom-Davis, J. (1986). Myasthenia gravis without acetylcholine receptor antibody: a distinct disease entity. *Lancet* **i**, 116–19.

Mossman, S., Vincent, A. and Newsom-Davis, J. (1988). Passive transfer of myasthenia gravis by immunoglobulins: lack of correlation between AChR with antibody bound, acetylcholine receptor loss and transmission defect. *J. Neurol. Sci.* **84**, 15–28.

Murphy, J. and Murphy, S.F. (1986). Myasthenia gravis in identical twins. *Neurology* **36**, 78–80.

Nakao, Y., Matsumoto, H., Miyazaki, T. *et al.* (1980). IgG heavy chain allotypes (Gm) in autoimmune diseases. *Clin. Exp. Immunol.* **42**, 20–6.

Namba, T., Brunner, N.G. and Grob, D. (1978). Myasthenia gravis in patients with thymoma, with particular reference to onset after thymectomy. *Medicine (Baltimore)* **57**, 411–33.

Nastuk, W.L., Strauss, A.J.L. and Osserman, K.E. (1959). Search for a neuromuscular blocking agent in the blood of patients with myasthenia gravis. *Am. J. Med.* **26**, 394–409.

Nastuk, W.L., Plescia, O. and Osserman, K.E. (1960). Changes in serum complement activity in patients with myasthenia gravis. *Proc. Soc. Exp. Biol. Med.* **105**, 177–84.

Newsom-Davis, J. (1992) Diseases of the neuromuscular junction. In *Diseases of the Nervous System*, 2nd edn, eds A.K. Asbury, G.M. McKhann and W.I. McDonald, pp. 197–212, W.B. Saunders, Philadelphia.

Newsom-Davis, J. and Murray, N.M.F. (1984). Plasma exchange and immunosuppressive drug treatment in the Lambert–Eaton myasthenic syndrome. *Neurology* **34**, 480–5.

Newsom-Davis, J. and Vincent, A. (1982). Myasthenia gravis. In *Clinical Aspects of Immunology*, ed. P.J. Lachmann and D.K. Peters, pp. 1011–68, Blackwell Scientific Publications, Oxford/London.

Newsom-Davis, J., Pinching, A.J., Vincent, A. and Wilson, S.G. (1978). Function of circulating antibody to acetylcholine receptor in myasthenia gravis: investigation by plasma exchange. *Neurology* **28**, 266–72.

Newsom-Davis, J., Harcourt, G., Sommer, N., Beeson, D., Willcox, N. and Rothbard, J.B. (1989). T-cell reactivity in myasthenia gravis. *J. Autoimmunity* **2** (suppl.), 101–8.

Newsom-Davis, J., Leys, K., Vincent, A., Ferguson, I., Modi, G. and Mills, K. (1991). Immunological evidence for the coexistence of the Lambert–Eaton myasthenic syndrome and myasthenia gravis in two patients. *J. Neurol. Neurosurg. Psychiatry* **54**, 452–3.

O'Neill, J.H., Murray, N.M.F. and Newsom-Davis, J. (1988). The Lambert–Eaton myasthenic syndrome: a review of 50 cases. *Brain* **111**, 577–96.

Ong, B., Willcox, N., Wordsworth, P. *et al.* (1991). Critical role for the Val/Gly^{86} HLA-DR beta dimorphism in autoantigen presentation to human T cells. *Proc. Nat. Acad. Sci. (USA)* **88**, 7343–7.

Oosterhuis, H.J.G.H. (1984). Myasthenia gravis. In *Clinical Neurology and Neurosurgery Monographs*, vol. 5, Churchill Livingstone, Edinburgh.

Oosterhuis, H.J.G.H. (1989). The natural course of myasthenia gravis: a long term follow-up study. *J. Neurol. Neurosurg. Psychiatry* **52**, 1121–7.

Oosterhuis, H.J.G.H., Limburg, P.C., Hummel-Tappel, E. and The, T.H. (1983). Anti-acetylcholine receptor antibody in myasthenia gravis. II. Clinical and serological follow-up of individual patients. *J. Neurol. Sci.* **58**, 371–85.

Oosterhuis, H.J.G.H., Limburg, P.C., Hummel-Tappel, E., Van den Berg, W. and The, T.H. (1985). Anti-acetylcholine receptor antibody in myasthenia gravis. III. The effect of thymectomy. *J. Neurol. Sci.* **69**, 335–45.

Patrick, J. and Lindstrom, J. (1973). Autoimmune response to acetylcholine receptor. *Science* **180**, 871–2.

Pestronk, A. and Drachman, D.B. (1985). Polymyositis: reduction of acetylcholine receptors in skeletal muscle. *Muscle Nerve* **8**, 233–9.

Pestronk, A., Drachman, D.B. and Self, S.B. (1985). Measurement of junctional acetylcholine receptors in myasthenia gravis: clinical correlates. *Muscle Nerve* **8**, 245–51.

Pinching, A.J., Peters, D.K. and Newsom-Davis, J. (1976). Remission of myasthenia gravis following plasma exchange. *Lancet* **ii**, 1373–6.

Protti, M.P., Manfredi, A.A., Straub, C., Wu, X., Howard, J.F. and Conti-Tronconi, B.M. (1990). Use of synthetic peptides to establish anti-human acetylcholine receptor CD4+ cell lines from myasthenia gravis patients. *J. Immunol.* **144**, 1711–20.

Roberts, A., Perera, S., Lang, B., Vincent, A. and Newsom-Davis, J. (1985). Paraneoplastic myasthenic syndrome IgG inhibits $^{45}Ca^{2+}$ flux in a human small cell carcinoma line. *Nature* **317**, 737–9.

Rodriguez, M., Gomez, M.R., Howard, F.M. and Taylor, W.F. (1983). Myasthenia gravis in children: long term follow-up. *Ann. Neurol.* **13**, 504–10.

Rosai, J. and Levine, G.D. (1976). Tumours of the thymus. In *Atlas of Tumour Pathology*, 2nd series: fascicle 13, US Armed Forces Institute of Pathology, Washington, DC.

Scadding, G.K., Vincent, A., Newsom-Davis, J. and Henry, K. (1981). Acetylcholine receptor antibody synthesis by thymic lymphocytes;: correlation with thymic histology. *Neurology* **31**, 935–43.

Schluep, M., Willcox, N., Vincent, A., Dhoot, G.K. and Newsom-Davis, J. (1987). Acetylcholine receptors in human thymic myoid cells in situ: an immunohistological study. *Ann. Neurol* **22**, 212–22.

Schluep, M., Willcox, N., Ritter, M.A., Newsom-Davis, J., Larche, M. and Brown, A.N. (1988). Myasthenia gravis thymus: clinical, histological and culture correlations. *J. Autoimmunity* **1**, 445–67.

Schwimmbeck, P.L., Dyrberg, T., Drachman, D.B. and Oldstone, M.B.A. (1989). Molecular mimicry and myasthenia gravis. *J. Clin. Invest.* **84**, 1174–80.

Sher, E., Canal, N., Piccolo, G., Gotti, C. *et al.* (1989). Specificity of calcium channel autoantibodies in Lambert–Eaton myasthenic syndrome. *Lancet* **ii**, 640–3.

Simpson, J.A. (1960). Myasthenia gravis: a new hypothesis. *Scottish Med. J.* **5**, 419–39.

Smith, C.I.E., Aarli, J.A., Biberfeld, P. *et al*. (1983). Myasthenia gravis after bone-marrow transplantation: evidence for a donor origin. *N. Engl. J. Med.* **309**, 1565–8.

Soliven, B.C., Lange, D.J., Penn, A.S. *et al*. (1988). Seronegative myasthenia gravis. *Neurology* **38**, 514–17.

Sommer, N., Willcox, N., Harcourt, G.C. and Newsom-Davis, J. (1990). Myasthenic thymus and thymoma are selectively enriched in acetylcholine receptor-reactive T cells. *Ann. Neurol.* **28**, 312–19.

Sommer, N., Harcourt, G.C., Willcox, N., Beeson, D. and Newsom-Davis, J. (1991). Acetylcholine receptor-reactive T lymphocytes from healthy subjects and myasthenia gravis patients. *Neurology* **41**, 1270–6.

Souadjian, J.V., Enriquez, P., Silverstein, M.N. and Pepin, J.-M. (1974). The spectrum of diseases associated with thymoma. *Arch. Intern. Med.* **134**, 374–9.

Stanley, E.F. and Drachman, D.B. (1978). Effect of myasthenic immunoglobulin on acetylcholine receptors of intact mammalian neuromuscular junctions. *Science* **200**, 1285–7.

Steinman, L. and Mantegazza, R. (1990). Prospects for specific immunotherapy in myasthenia gravis. *FASEB J.* **4**, 2726–31.

Storm-Mathiesen, A. (1984). Epidemiology of myasthenia gravis in Norway. *Acta Neurol. Scand.* **70**, 274–84.

Tindall, R.S.A. (1980). Humoral immunity in myasthenia gravis: effect of steroids and thymectomy. *Neurology* **30**, 554–7.

Tindall, R.S.A., Rollins, J.A., Phillips, J.T., Greenlee, R.G., Wells, L. and Belendiuk, G. (1987). Preliminary results of a double-blind, randomized, placebo-controlled trial of cyclosporine in myasthenia gravis. *N. Engl. J. Med.* **316**, 719–24.

Toyka, K.V., Drachman, D.B., Griffin, D.E. *et al*. (1977). Myasthenia gravis: study of humoral immune mechanisms by passive transfer to mice. *N. Engl. J. Med.* **296**, 125–31.

Toyka, K.V., Lowenadler, B., Heininger, K. *et al*. (1980). Passively transferred myasthenia gravis: protection of mouse endplates by Fab fragments from human myasthenic IgG. *J. Neurol. Neurosurg. Psychiatry* **43**, 836–40.

Tsujihata, M., Yoshimura, T., Satoh, A. *et al*. (1989). Diagnostic significance of IgG, C3 and C9 at the limb muscle motor endplate in minimal myasthenia gravis. *Neurology* **39**, 1359–63.

Tucker, D.M., Roeltgen, D.P., Wann, P.D. and Wertheimer, R.I. (1988). Memory dysfunction in myasthenia gravis: evidence for central cholinergic effects. *Neurology* **38**, 1173–7.

Tzartos, S.J. and Lindstrom, J.M. (1980). Monoclonal antibodies used to probe acetylcholine receptor structure: localization of the main immunogenic region and detection of similarities between subunits. *Proc. Nat. Acad. Sci. (USA)* **77**, 755–9.

Tzartos, S.J., Seybold, M.E. and Lindstrom, J.M. (1982). Specificities of antibodies to acetylcholine receptors in sera from myasthenia gravis patients measured by monoclonal antibodies. *Proc. Nat. Acad. Sci. (USA)* **79**, 188–92.

Tzartos, S.J., Barkas, T., Cung, M.T. *et al*. (1991). The main immunogenic region of the acetylcholine receptor: structure and role in myasthenia gravis: *Autoimmunity* **8**, 259–70.

Verley, J.M. and Hollmann, K.H. (1985). Thymoma: a comparative study of clinical stages, histologic features, and survival in 200 cases. *Cancer* **55**, 1074–86.

Vincent, A. (1980). Immunology of acetylcholine receptors in relation to myasthenia gravis. *Physiol. Rev.* **60**, 756–824.

Vincent, A. (1988). Are spontaneous anti-idiotypic antibodies against anti-acetylcholine receptor antibodies present in myasthenia gravis? *J. Autoimmunity* **1**, 131–42.

Vincent, A. and Newsom-Davis, J. (1982a). Acetylcholine receptor antibody characteristics in myasthenia gravis. I. Patients with generalised myasthenia or disease restricted to ocular muscles. *Clin. Exp. Immunol.* **49**, 257–65.

Vincent, A. and Newsom-Davis, J. (1982b). Acetylcholine receptor antibody characteristics in myasthenia gravis. II. Patients with penicillamine-induced myasthenia or idiopathic myasthenia of recent onset. *Clin. Exp. Immunol.* **49**, 266–72.

Vincent, A. and Newsom-Davis, J. (1985). Acetylcholine receptor antibody as a diagnostic test for myasthenia gravis: results in 153 validated cases and 2967 diagnostic assays. *J. Neurol. Neurosurg. Psychiatry* **48**, 1246–52.

Vincent, A. and Wray, D. (eds.) (1990). *Neuromuscular Transmission: Basic and Applied Aspects*. Manchester University Press, Manchester.

Vincent, A., Lang, B. and Newsom-Davis, J. (1989). Autoimmunity to the voltage-gated calcium channel underlies the Lambert–Eaton myasthenic syndrome, a paraneoplastic disorder. *Trends Neurosci.* **12**, 496–502.

Waldor, M.K., Sriram, S., McDevitt, H.O. and Steinman, L. (1983). *In vivo* therapy with monoclonal anti-I-A antibody suppresses immune responses to acetylcholine receptor. *Proc. Nat. Acad. Sci. (USA)* **80**, 2713–17.

Wassermann, N.H., Penn, A.S., Freimuth, P.I. *et al*. (1982). Anti-idiotypic route to anti-acetylcholine receptor antibodies and experimental myasthenia gravis. *Proc. Nat. Acad. Sci. (USA)* **79**, 4810–14.

Wekerle, H. and Ketelsen, U.-P. (1977). Intrathymic pathogenesis and dual genetic control of myasthenia gravis. *Lancet* **i**, 678–80.

Whiting, P.J., Cooper, J. and Lindstrom, J.M. (1987). Antibodies in sera from patients with myasthenia gravis do not bind to nicotinic acetylcholine receptors from human brain. *J. Neuroimmunol.* **16**, 205–13.

Willcox, N. (1989). The thymus in myasthenia gravis patients and the *in vivo* effects of corticosteroids on its cellularity, histology and functions. *Thymus Update* **2**, 105–24.

Willcox, N. and Vincent, A. (1988). Myasthenia gravis as an example of organ-specific autoimmune disease. In *B Lymphocytes in Human Disease*, ed. G. Bird and J.E. Calvert, pp. 469–506, Oxford University Press, Oxford.

Willcox, N., Demaine, A.G., Newsom-Davis, J., Welsh, K.I., Robb, S.A. and Spiro, A.G. (1985). Increased frequency of IgG heavy chain marker (Glm(2)) and of HLA-B8 in Lambert-Eaton myasthenic syndrome with and without associated lung carcinoma. *Hum. Immunol.* **14**, 29–36.

Willcox, H.N.A., Schluep, M., Ritter, M.A., Schuurman, H.J., Newsom-Davis, J. and Christensson, B. (1987). Myasthenic and non-myasthenic thymoma: an expansion of a minor cortical epithelial cell subset? *Am. J. Pathol.* **127**, 447–60.

Willcox, N., Schluep, M., Sommer, N. *et al*. (1989). Variable corticosteroid sensitivity of thymic cortex and medullary peripheral-type lymphoid tissue in myasthenia gravis patients: structural and functional effects. *Quart. J. Med.* **73**, 1071–87.

Willcox, N., Schluep, M., Ritter, M.A. and Newsom-Davis, J. (1991). The thymus in seronegative myasthenia gravis patients. *J. Neurol.* **238**, 256–61.

Wilson, S., Vincent, A. and Newsom-Davis, J. (1983). Acetylcholine receptor turnover in mice with passively transferred myasthenia gravis. II. Receptor synthesis. *J. Neurol. Neurosurg. Psychiatry* **46**, 383–7.

Yamamoto, T., Vincent, A., Ciulla, T., Lang, B., Johnston, I. and Newsom-Davis, J. (1991). Seronegative myasthenia gravis: a plasma factor inhibiting agonist-induced acetylcholine receptor function co-purifies with IgM. *Ann. Neurol.* **30**, 550–7.

107: Immunological Mechanisms in the Eye

P.A.R. Meyer

The eye is an exquisitely delicate optical instrument, which depends for normal function upon constant geometry and the perfect clarity of its media. These features give the ophthalmologist an unrivalled opportunity to witness the events of the immune response. However, they also impose particular demands upon the immune system. Image formation requires the absence of all blood and lymphatic vessels from tissues in the optical axis. Even antigen-presenting cells are scanty or absent from the cornea and ocular interior. This chapter describes the mechanisms that allow the immune system to function within such constraints and considers the consequences of their failure.

The structure of the eye is illustrated in Fig. 112.1, but an immunologist need not dwell on the intricacies of image formation, photoelectric transduction and image processing. He can consider a different organization of the eye — into three communicating immunological compartments, the surface, the cornea and the interior, each of which has its own route for antigen presentation and facilities for mounting an immune response.

At the *surface* of the eye, tears wash antigen away from the central cornea, over the conjunctival epithelium and into the nasolachrymal ducts and gastrointestinal tract. Sensitization of the mucosa-associated lymphoid system is followed by the secretion of specific immunoglobulin A (IgA) in tears.

The healthy *cornea* lacks antigen-presenting cells, but they lie poised to migrate inwards from the corneoscleral limbus, and can then transport antigen to the regional lymph nodes and spleen. Sensitized lymphocytes and antibody can be delivered from the limbal vascular arcades. The monolayer of 'endothelial' cells (which lines the inner surface of the cornea and dehydrates the stroma by pumping water into the anterior chamber) is best considered to be part of the ocular interior.

The *interior* of the globe is continually irrigated by aqueous, a clear fluid analogous to cerebrospinal fluid. It is secreted behind the iris by a ring of vascular tufts (the ciliary apparatus), flows

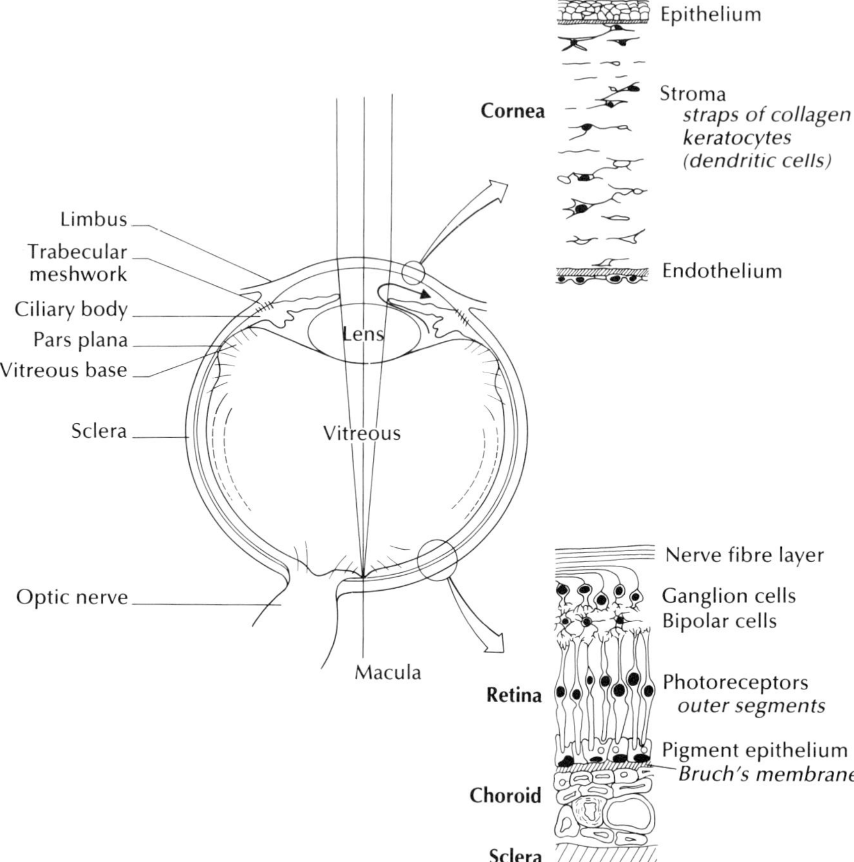

Fig. 107.1. The structure of the eye. Arrow indicates aqueous flow.

through the pupil, and is discharged directly into venous blood through a circular collagenous lattice lying at the angle between cornea and peripheral iris (the trabecular meshwork) (Fig. 107.1). Available evidence suggests that haematogenous lymphocytes and antibody are mainly distributed to this compartment from the ciliary body.

Immunological compartments

The surface (Fig. 107.2) (reviews: Robin *et al.* 1986; Friedman 1990)

The eyelids and tear film provide between them a complete immune system for the ocular surface, and tears are rich in secretory IgA and complement (Bluestone *et al.* 1975). Topical antigens can induce humoral immunity, but their principal effect is a vigorous secretory immune response, during which copious secretory IgA, and some IgG, is spread over the entire cornea and conjunctiva (Mondino *et al.* 1987).

The flow of tears carries foreign material to the peripheral corneal or conjunctival epithelium, which contain Langerhans' cells, but most is washed into the nasolachrymal ducts. It has been speculated that antigen passes into the gastrointestinal tract, where it sensitizes lymphoid tissue in the Peyer's patches (Mondino *et al.* 1987). Antigens also wash over subepithelial conjunctival lymphoid follicles, which contain immature B lymphocytes, largely committed to IgA secretion. In the rabbit, these are covered by an epithelium that lacks goblet cells, and may be capable of pinocytosis and antigen presentation (Franklin and Remus 1984). However, no such specialized epithelial dome can be found in man (Friedman 1990).

The conjunctival lymphoid follicles, gastrointestinal Peyer's patches and lymphoid follicles on other mucosal surfaces all form part of a network of mucosa-associated lymphoid tissue (MALT). It is not yet known whether conjunctival lymphoid follicles can sensitize this system, but antigen presentation in the gut is followed by the distribution

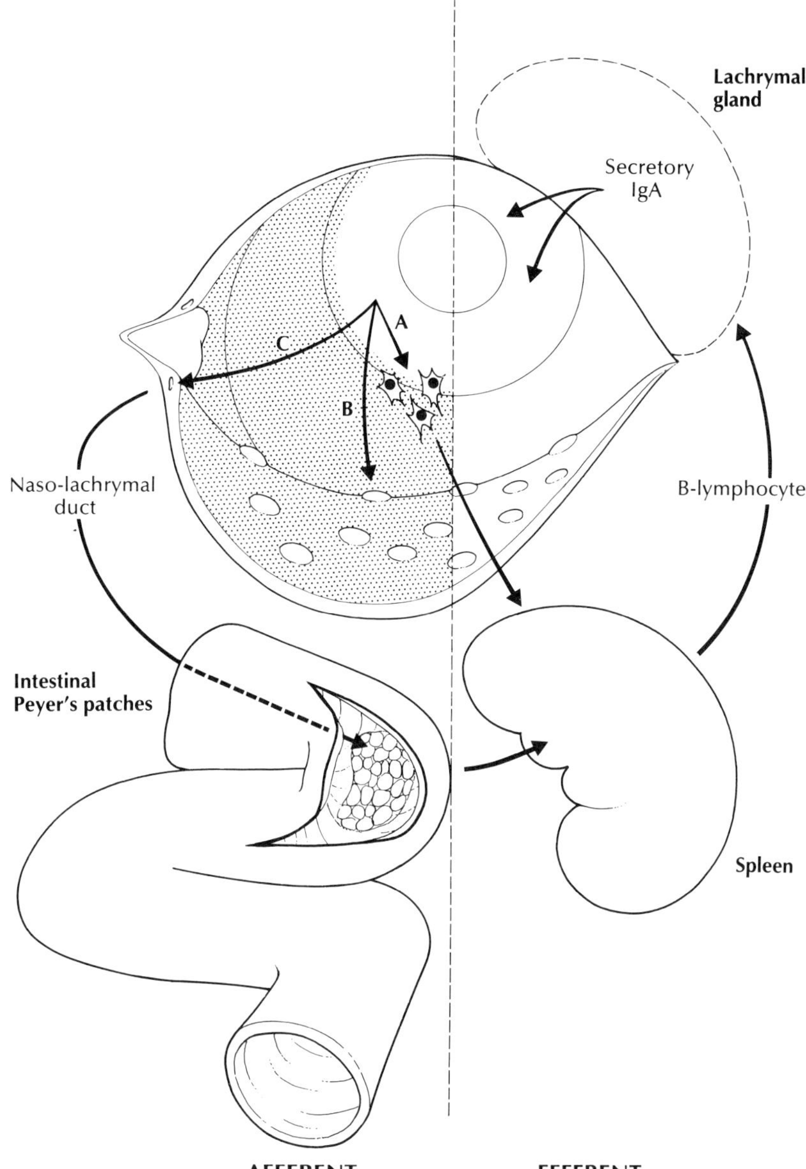

Fig. 107.2. The surface. *Afferent*: (A) Langerhans cells (*distribution shown by shading*) → cervical/pre-auricular nodes → spleen. (B)* Conjunctival lymphoid follicles (Franklin and Remus 1984). (C)* Naso-lachrymal duct → intestinal Peyer's patches (Mondino *et al*. 1987). *Efferent*: Sensitized lymphocytes → lachrymal glands: selection of those committed to IgA: secretory IgA in tears. (**Denotes unconfirmed pathways*.)

of antigen-specific B lymphocytes to other exocrine glands (Weisz-Carrington *et al*. 1979).

Antibody-producing cells of all isotypes except IgM pass through the lachrymal glands (Allansmith *et al*. 1976), but those that remain and proliferate are predominantly committed to IgA production. It seems that this selection is exacted by the lachrymal gland itself. When mixed lachrymal gland cells are co-cultured with splenic lymphocytes, they enhance the replication of IgA-committed B cells and suppress lymphocytes producing other classes of antibody, possibly by stimulating appropriate helper T lymphocytes (Franklin *et al*. 1985).

The cornea (Fig. 107.3)

Antigen-presenting cells of the monocyte/macrophage lineage are in constant transit between most tissues of the body, their regional lymph nodes and the spleen (Katz *et al*. 1979; Streilein and Bergstresser 1980). They are called Langerhans' cells in the skin and corneal epithelium, and dendritic cells in the corneal stroma, but for this discussion the distinction is largely academic. Although they form an immunological collecting network over the body's entire surface, they are scanty (Rodrigues *et al*. 1981; Gillette *et al*.

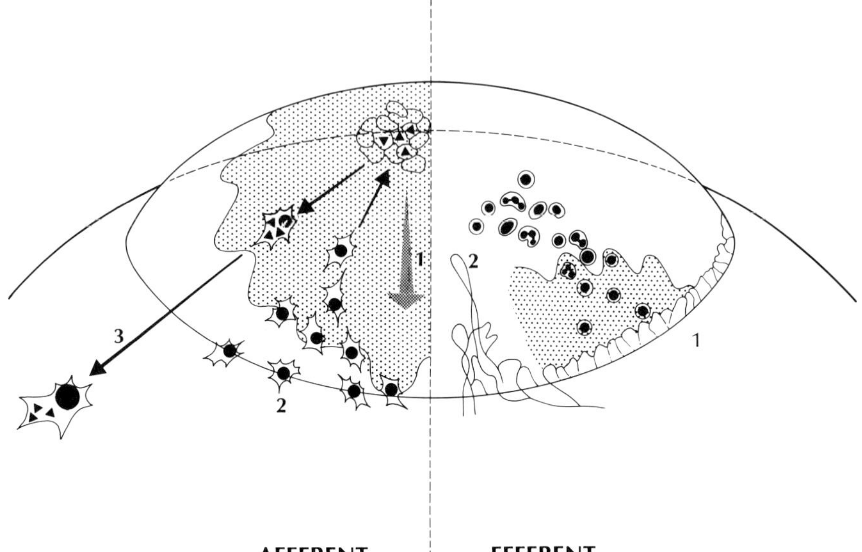

Fig. 107.3 The cornea. *Afferent*: (1) Epithelial cells phagocytose antigen and release CETAF (Grabner *et al.* 1983), which may be IL-1 (Niederkorn *et al.* 1989). (*Shading indicates diffusion of CETAF/IL-1*). (2) Langerhans' cells migrate inwards from the limbus. (3) Langerhans' cells carry antigen to lymph nodes and spleen. *Efferent*: (1) Antibody and inflammatory cells enter the cornea from the limbal circulation or tears. (*Shading indicates diffusion of antibody*). (2) Mediators from T-lymphocytes induce growth of new limbal vessels towards antigen (Epstein and Hughes 1981).

1982) or absent (Bergstresser *et al.* 1980; Peeler *et al.* 1985; Pepose *et al.* 1985) in the central corneal epithelium and stroma. Instead, they lie in wait in a ring at the limbus and can be attracted towards the centre by stimuli as varied as cautery (Williamson *et al.* 1987), topical irritants (Rubsamen *et al.* 1984), latex beads (Peeler and Niederkorn 1986; Niederkorn *et al.* 1989), bacteria (Niederkorn *et al.* 1989) and endotoxin (Gillette *et al.* 1982).

The inward migration of Langerhans' cells is thought to be initiated by corneal epithelial cells. These phagocytose particulate antigens that they encounter and then secrete a diffusible chemoattractant (named corneal epithelial thymocyte-activating factor (CETAF) from the bioassay used to detect it) (Grabner *et al.* 1983; Niederkorn *et al.* 1989). Corneal epithelial thymocyte-activating factor may be interleukin 1 (IL-1) itself, since their mitogenic effects on T cells are similar and intracorneal injections of IL-1 also attract Langerhans' cells into the central cornea (Niederkorn *et al.* 1989). Niederkorn and colleagues (Niederkorn *et al.* 1989; Niederkorn 1990) have speculated that epithelial cells may even undertake some antigen processing, passing predigested fragments to the Langerhans' cells, which can carry them to the preauricular and cervical lymph nodes (Smolin *et al.* 1973) or spleen.

Immunoglobulin enters the corneal stroma from the limbal capillaries (Breebaart and James-Witte 1959) and diffuses slowly through the dehydrated collagen matrix (Allansmith *et al.* 1979). When the epithelium is breached, it can also enter directly from the tear film (McDonnell *et al.* 1988). Components of the classical and alternative pathways of complement (C1q, C3, C4, C5, properdin and factor B) are all present in normal cornea, but direct immunofluorescence shows a decline in C1q from the limbus towards the centre, perhaps implying a similar gradient in the potential for classical pathway activation (Mondino *et al.* 1980).

During the early stages of an immune response, inflammatory cells are obliged to enter cornea from the limbus (Movat *et al.* 1963; Mohos and Wagner 1969). However, once within the stroma, activated T lymphocytes release angiogenic mediators (Epstein and Hughes 1981) which excite neovascularization from the limbal arcades — a process that is facilitated by granulocytes (Fromer and Klintworth 1976; Epstein and Hughes 1981), but not dependent upon them (Eliason 1978; Sholley *et al.* 1978). This brings the effector arm of the immune system closer to the antigenic focus.

The ocular interior (Fig. 112.4)

The ocular interior also lacks lymphatics, but aqueous flow swiftly removes any substance that is introduced into the anterior chamber and much enters venous blood unaltered. Nevertheless, there is little doubt that intraocular antigens are presented to the immune system in some form before they leave the eye, and the consequent disruption

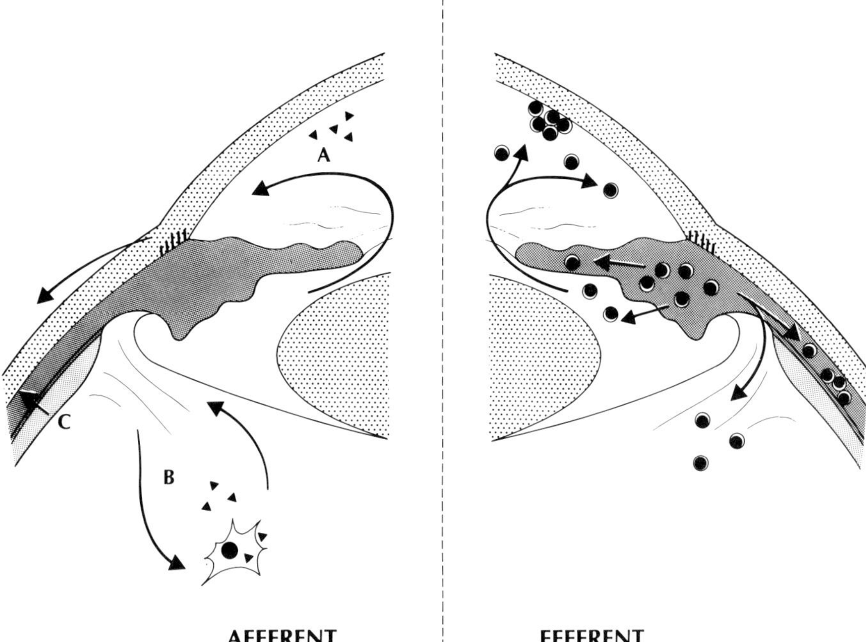

Fig. 107.4 The ocular interior. *Afferent*: (A) Anterior chamber: Arrow shows aqueous flow and drainage by trabecular meshwork. Signal initiating ACAID is uncertain: it may be *soluble (Ferguson *et al.* 1989) or *cellular (Wilbanks and Streilein 1991). (B) Vitreous: Soluble antigens diffuse into anterior chamber. Particulate antigens are scavenged by macrophages. (C) Retina: *Antigen presentation by retinal pigment epithelial cells (Percopo *et al.* 1990). *Efferent*: Haematogenous lymphocytes are distributed from ciliary body to aqueous, iris, choroid and retina. They enter the vitreous base from the pars plana. (**Denotes unconfirmed pathways.*)

of systemic immunity is a fascinating problem that will be considered later (see section on Immune privilege).

Aqueous discharges directly into venous blood, but it must first percolate through the trabecular meshwork, which is studded with cells that express Class II major histocompatibility complex (MHC) antigens (Lynch *et al.* 1987). They are strategically placed for antigen processing (Ferguson *et al.* 1989; Niederkorn 1990), but it is not yet clear whether this is their role. Other workers have described a population of leucocytes, residing in the iris and ciliary body, which carry markers common to mature macrophages but lack Ia (Williamson *et al.* 1989). These appear to be able to process soluble antigens and transport them from the eye to the spleen (Wilbanks and Streilein 1991).

In contrast, the collagenous vitreous gel, which occupies the posterior segment of the eye, allows little circulation and acts as a sump for antigens. If soluble, they may leave by diffusion (Fernando 1960); if particulate, they await phagocytosis by occasional itinerant macrophages that enter the gel through its ring of attachment to the anterior retina, known as the vitreous base (Fig. 112.1) (Spencer 1985).

The retina is separated from the choroidal circulation by the retinal pigment epithelium (RPE) (a sheet of neuroectoderm) and its basement membrane (Bruch's membrane). Retinal pigment epithelial cells normally phagocytose the outer segments of retinal photoreceptors (Young and Bok 1969), but can be induced by interferon gamma to express Ia and present either retinal or foreign antigens (S-antigen, IRBP or PPD) to suitably primed helper T lymphocytes (Percopo *et al.* 1990). Whether they can transfer antigen to choroidal macrophages, thereby initiating the afferent limb of an immune response, is still unknown.

Antibody may doubtless enter the eye from the ciliary circulation, but there is ample evidence that it is also synthesized within the globe: indeed, patients with ocular toxoplasmosis may have higher antibody concentrations in aqueous than in serum (Witmer 1978). During the immune response to intravitreal antigen, sensitized lymphocytes are delivered from the spleen to the uvea (Smith *et al.* 1969), and 10% of all uveal lymphocytes may become dedicated to the secretion of a single specific antibody (Shimada and Silverstein 1975).

In rats with experimental allergic uveitis induced by S-antigen, T cells initially accumulate in the ciliary body, then migrate to the iris and finally to the choroid and retina (Brown *et al.* 1989). The retina offers a barrier against the migration of inflammatory cells from the choroid (Aronson *et al.* 1963c) and they must usually traverse the vitreous base if they are to enter the gel.

In human inflammatory eye disease, T lymphocytes pour from damaged ciliary capillaries, giving similar helper/suppressor ratios in aqueous and blood (Deschenes *et al.* 1986). However, the lymphocytic infiltrate within the vitreous does differ from that in peripheral blood (Deschenes *et al.* 1986), indicating that lymphocytes either are selected or replicate within the eye.

Humoral immunity

For the greater part of this century, humoral immunity has been invoked to explain most of the events surrounding ocular immunity. The fund of experimental data is colossal, but much of the work antedates our awareness of anti-idiotypic antibodies and of B cell/T cell interactions. Nevertheless, some of the models of human disease are remarkably convincing, particularly those of recurrent uveitis, and they deserve consideration in any account of ocular immunological mechanisms.

Arthus response (review: Silverstein 1974)

THE CORNEA

When a foreign protein is injected into the central corneal stroma, a short-lived haziness develops as it diffuses towards the limbus. However, 10–14 days later, upon the appearance of circulating antibody, one or more well-defined, concentric rings appear in the stroma. They last for up to a week, then become granular and subside (Breebaart and James-Witte 1959). A tissue antigen depot has excited systemic antibody formation and extravascular immune complex deposition — an active Arthus response. Antibodies enter the cornea from the limbus, and the precipitation of insoluble immune complexes at antigen/antibody equivalence is demonstrated in corneal stroma as it would be in an agarose plate. Injection of antigen into the cornea of a sensitized animal produces within 24 hours a ring that is smaller and more intense (Breebaart and James-Witte 1959; Germuth *et al.* 1962).

Intracorneal immune complexes are phagocytosed by polymorphonuclear neutrophils, which migrate into the cornea (Germuth *et al.* 1962; Movat *et al.* 1963; Mohos and Wagner 1969), presumably in response to complement-derived chemotactic factors, since complement is abundantly available (Allansmith *et al.* 1973; Mondino *et al.* 1980). Whether the invading polymorphs also degranulate, fragmenting and engulfing the stromal collagen (Mohos and Wagner 1969), has been a matter of controversy (Movat *et al.* 1963), and this is not a convincing model for 'melting' of the cornea in corneoscleral inflammatory disease.

THE SCLERA

There is also insufficient evidence to implicate the Arthus response in scleral inflammatory disease. The injection of ovalbumin into the corneoscleral limbus of sensitized rabbits has been observed to cause scleral thinning at a distance from the injection site (Hembry *et al.* 1979), but this experiment could not be repeated (Watson 1982). Disordered cell-mediated immunity is responsible for the scleritis that complicates a systemic autoimmune disease in mice of the MRL/Mp-lpr/lpr strain (Jabs and Prendergast 1991a, b).

THE VITREOUS

Intravitreal antigen in a naïve animal

A single injection of foreign protein into the vitreous of a rabbit or guinea-pig causes a minor inflammatory response that quickly subsides (Zimmerman and Silverstein 1959). It remains in abeyance for the next 7–10 days as the antigen depot gradually declines (Fernando 1960), but an intense uveitis accompanies the appearance of circulating antibodies (Foss 1949; Silverstein and Zimmerman 1959; Silverstein *et al.* 1961; Gamble *et al.* 1970b) and persists until the antigen has been cleared from the gel (Silverstein *et al.* 1961). Macrophages migrate into the vitreous while polymorphs and erythrocytes extravasate from ciliary vessels (Zimmerman and Silverstein 1959 [*active Arthus*]; Waksman and Bullington 1956 [*passive Arthus*]).

Immunological memory is both central and local

Staggered injections of antigen into the two eyes cause simultaneous, bilateral uveitis (Silverstein *et al.* 1961): expected confirmation of a central immune response. However, closer examination of this model shows that each eye responds to soluble antigens with a remarkable degree of independence. When uniocular inoculation is followed by systemic exposure to the same antigen, uveitis is rekindled in the immunized eye only (Seegal and Seegal 1930a, 1931a). This occurs whether the antigen is introduced intravenously (Seegal and Seegal 1930a, b, 1931a; Foss 1949), intraperitonneally (Gamble *et al.* 1970a) or even into the gastrointestinal tract (Seegal and Seegal 1930b, 1931b).

The localization of recurrent uveitis to one eye is not simply the result of vascular damage sustained during the earlier Arthus response. When a different antigen is injected into the vitreous of each eye, uveitis can later be rekindled on either side by systemic administration of the antigen to which that particular eye was exposed (Shimada and Silverstein 1975). Therefore, the eye appears to retain local immunological memory of an antigen.

Uninvolved antigens can trigger uveitis

During an active Arthus reaction, only a proportion of the plasma cells in the eye appear to produce antibody to the antigen that has been inoculated. Lymphocytes bearing memory of other antigens are also non-specifically stimulated to proliferate within the eye, particularly those involved in a recent or current systemic immune response, which will be present in greatest numbers (Shimada and Silverstein 1975). Later intravenous (IV) challenge with the same systemic antigen can rekindle uniocular uveitis, and this discovery prompted Silverstein (1974) to propose that each successive wave of proliferating lymphocytes may contribute to a local ocular library of memory T cells. This notion has not been explored further.

Viruses as antigen

In this plausible model for recurrent uveitis, Silverstein (1974) cast viruses in the role of ocular antigens. If mouse lymphocytic choriomeningitis virus is injected into the anterior chamber of a mouse's eye, it proliferates within uveal tissue for a week, causing no immediate disease. However, the violent immune response that follows is far more damaging than any cytopathic effect: it is indistinguishable from that induced by intravitreal ovalbumin and is preventable by immunosuppression with cyclophosphamide (Ticho *et al.* 1974a). Cell-mediated immunity clearly plays an important part in this model: the uveitis can be reactivated in immunosuppressed animals by transfer of lymphocytes from immune, syngeneic animals (Ticho *et al.* 1974a), but only if they include T cells (Ticho *et al.* 1974b).

Circulating immune complexes

Circulating immune complexes increase the permeability of uveal vessels in the rabbit (Howes and McKay 1975) and repeated intravascular immune complex formation induces inflammatory foci in the ciliary body, pars plana and choroid, with an outpouring of cells and protein into aqueous (Wong *et al.* 1971). Protein leakage may be enhanced by mechanical vascular damage (Wong *et al.* 1971) or intravitreal bacterial endotoxin (Gamble *et al.* 1970a, b).

Interaction with blood rheology

When immune complexes form in the circulation of a living rabbit, they recruit circulating platelets and leucocytes, and the resulting aggregates localize in limbal capillaries (Meyer 1987). A single such shower of immune complexes excites little clinical inflammation (Meyer 1987); however, repeated IV injections of large doses of antigen into immunized rabbits do produce microscopic limbal inflammatory foci (Wong *et al.* 1971). The human limbal circulation is characterized by arterial segments in which blood flow periodically ceases (Meyer 1988); a phenomenon that could repeatedly accumulate such aggregates, then discharge them into selected lobules of the microcirculation, causing a local increase in their dose and amplification of their effects.

Endotoxin

Bacterial endotoxins can cause uveitis when introduced either locally (Howes and McKay 1975) or systemically (Ajo 1941; Howes *et al.* 1971; Rosenbaum *et al.* 1980). For 24 hours after a systemic injection, rabbits develop bilateral conjunctivitis and anterior uveitis (Ajo 1941; Howes *et al.* 1971), characterized by an enormous increase in the permeability of the ciliary vessels (Howes *et al.* 1971). Although this usually occurs in the context of a generalized Schwartzmann reaction, rats may exhibit no systemic features, making it a plausible model for recurrent anterior uveitis (Rosenbaum *et al.* 1980). However, repeated injections of bacterial lipopolysaccharide (LPS) become progressively less uveitogenic (Howes and Rosenbaum 1985).

Bacterial LPS appears to trigger the secretion of a chain of cytokines, which may begin with the production of tumour necrosis factor (TNF) and IL-1 by macrophages (Beutler *et al.* 1985). Intravitreal injections of TNF (Kulkarni and Srinivasan 1988) or IL-1 (Rosenbaum *et al.* 1987) produce pathological effects in the eyes of rabbits that closely mirror those of systemic endotoxin. Interleukin 6 (IL-6) is known to be secreted by lymphocytes in response to TNF, and can be found in the serum and aqueous of rats with endotoxin-induced uveitis. The titre in aqueous exceeds that in serum, and the responses follow a different time course, indicating intraocular synthesis (Hoekzema *et al.* 1991). A similar situation pertains in patients with anterior uveitis, in whom IL-6 can be demonstrated in aqueous but not in serum (Murray *et al.* 1990). All these effects appear to bypass the complement system (Bhattacherjee *et al.* 1983; Howes *et al.* 1985).

These inflammatory pathways, excited by LPS, interact with other immunological responses. Bacterial endotoxins within the vitreous enhance the deposition of circulating immune complexes (Gamble *et al.* 1970a, b). Conversely, 'tolerance' to systemic endotoxin is accompanied by reduced exudation of serum into the vitreous during the direct passive Arthus response (Howes and Rosenbaum 1985).

In experiments to explain the particular susceptibility of the uveal tract to systemic endotoxin, antisera from rabbits immunized with *Klebsiella* antigens were found to cross-react with a crude preparation of bovine vitreous (Avakian *et al.* 1981); conversely, the binding of rabbit anti-vitreous antibodies to bovine vitreous could be inhibited by a *Klebsiella* ultrasonicate (Welsh *et al.* 1981).

The notion that Gram-negative bacteria can trigger HLA-B27-related anterior uveitis (Ebringer *et al.* 1979; White *et al.* 1984) made models such as these particularly attractive. This is now in doubt (see section on HLA and ocular inflammation), and survivable doses of systemic endotoxin have recently been shown to have no effect upon the permeability of the blood/aqueous barrier in man (Herman *et al.* 1991). Nevertheless, this does not detract from the capacity of LPS to induce or enhance uveal inflammation.

Cell-mediated immunity

Corneal graft rejection (reviews: Niederkorn and Peeler 1988; Coster 1989; Niederkorn 1990; Katami 1991)

Clinical incidence and appearance

The rejection of clinical corneal allografts is rare (5% of uncomplicated cases) and can usually be controlled with topical steroid therapy (Coster 1989). Even the matching of MHC antigens appears to be unnecessary. This astonishing success rate stems from two characteristics that are unique to the cornea: its avascularity and its low content of antigen-presenting cells. These profoundly affect its behaviour, both as a graft and as a recipient bed.

When rejection does occur, an inflammatory infiltrate sweeps across the donor button, followed by a line of dying donor cells. This has been studied separately for each layer of rabbit cornea by carrying epithelium or endothelium from donor to recipient on buttons of recipient stoma. Host cells immediately repopulated the epithelium and stroma, but endothelium took up to 6 months to regenerate (Khodadoust and Silverstein 1969) (human corneal endothelial cells are not thought to divide *in vivo*). The inflammatory cells that effected endothelial rejection took the form of adherent lymphocytic precipitates and, by analogy with later experiments (Khodadoust and Silverstein 1975), must have been delivered from the anterior chamber.

Rejection is mediated by T lymphocytes

The role of T lymphocytes in corneal graft rejection is not in question, and nowhere else in the body can their adherence to, and destruction of, a target be observed with such directness (Khodadoust and Silverstein 1969, 1975, 1976). When transferred from a sensitized animal into the anterior chamber of a graft recipient, lymphocytes alone are sufficient to induce graft rejection (Khodadoust and Silverstein 1976 [*rabbit*]). Although humoral immunity to corneal grafts can be demonstrated experimentally (Treseler and Sanfilippo 1985 [*rat*]), its contribution to clinical rejection remains to be established.

Delayed hypersensitivity is suppressed, but cytotoxicity preserved, when antigen-presenting cells are scarce

A remarkable characteristic of corneal allografts is their failure to excite delayed hypersensitivity, despite inducing a brisk cytotoxic immune response, even after heterotopic transplantation (Peeler *et al.* 1985). This has been related to a dearth of antigen-presenting cells in the central cornea (Peeler *et al.* 1985; Peeler and Niederkorn 1986). The further depletion of antigen-presenting cells reduces the rate with which heterotopic murine corneal grafts are rejected (Ray-Keil and Chandler 1985). Conversely, their attraction into the central cornea by topical dinitrofluorobenzene (Rubsamen *et al.* 1984) or subepithelial latex beads (Peeler and Niederkorn 1986; Peeler *et al.* 1988) prior to heterotopic grafting invites rejection by delayed hypersensitivity.

The cornea is not the only site in which a lack of antigen-presenting cells confers protection from cell-mediated immunity. A similar mechanism operates within the anterior chamber (anterior chamber-associated immune deviation (ACAID): see below), and the destruction of Langerhans' cells in skin by ultraviolet light can prevent delayed hypersensitivity to a topically applied hapten (Toews *et al.* 1980).

Which antigens are responsible for graft rejection?

It is not surprising to learn, from experimental heterotopic corneal allografts, that MHC antigens are the usual targets of the lymphocytotoxic response (Peeler *et al.* 1985 [*mouse*]; Treseler *et al.* 1985 [*rat*]), although minor histocompatibility antigens may also be implicated (Peeler *et al.* 1988 [*mouse*]).

Where are major histocompatibility complex antigens expressed?

Not all workers have been equally successful at demonstrating MHC antigens on corneal cells. Class I antigens are probably expressed on all cells of epithelium, stroma and endothelium (Treseler *et al.* 1984 [*human*]; Whitsett and Stulting 1984 [*human*]; Treseler and Sanfilippo 1986 [*rat*]), although some researchers have found them to be restricted to epithelium (Williams *et al.* 1985 [*human*]). The migratory antigen-presenting cells (called Langerhans' cells in epithelium and dendritic cells in stroma) display Class II antigens (Treseler *et al.* 1984 [*human*]; Williams *et al.* 1985 [*human*]; Treseler and Sanfilippo 1986 [*rat*]). Their capacity to migrate out of a graft, and presumably to exhibit donor MHC antigens to host antigen-presenting cells, makes them powerful initiators of an immune response. Their low numbers in the central cornea (Rodrigues *et al.* 1981), and the consequent lack of Class II expression, have been used to explain the low incidence of corneal graft rejection (Streilein *et al.* 1979).

In an attempt to identify which anatomical layer of transplanted rat cornea excited a host immune response, Treseler and colleagues (1986) separated epithelium, stroma and endothelium by microdissection and transplanted each layer heterotopically on to the chest walls of separate recipients that differed from the donor at Class I MHC loci. Only the animals that received stroma and corneal endothelium developed cell-mediated immunity to the implant. The rat corneal epithelium does express Class I MHC antigens, and this experiment conflicts with clinical evidence that removal of epithelium reduces the frequency with which human corneal transplants are rejected (Tuberville *et al.* 1983).

Induction of Class II major histocompatibility complex expression

An explanation for the inconsistencies of some of these experiments may lie in the ability of local inflammation (Donelly *et al.* 1985), possibly through the medium of interferon gamma (Donelly *et al.* 1985; Young *et al.* 1985; Kusuda *et al.* 1989; Foets *et al.* 1991), to induce the expression of Class II MHC antigens in most ocular tissues, particularly the corneal endothelium (Donelly *et al.* 1985 [*rabbit*]; Young *et al.* 1985 [*human*]; Foets *et al.* 1991 [*human*]). At the time of transplantation, a graft may express little or no Class II MHC, and the response to endothelial Class I antigens may be depressed as a result of ACAID (see below). However, local or systemic inflammation may, at any subsequent moment, induce Class II expression on the graft and hence a rejection episode.

Immune privilege (reviews: Niederkorn 1990; Streilein 1990)

Intraocular antigens depress cell-mediated immunity

For more than a century the anterior chamber of the eye has been regarded as an immunologically privileged site, in which heterogeneic grafts could flourish remote from immune recognition (Greene 1947, 1949). It took an insightful study by Raju and Grogan (1969), in which the implantation of skin into the anterior chamber accelerated the rejection of subsequent orthotopic grafts, to demonstrate that antigens within the eye affect the immune system profoundly. Paradoxically, their result was exceptional. It is now apparent that inoculation via the anterior chamber depresses the cell-mediated immune response during any subsequent exposure, and this phenomenon has been called anterior chamber-associated immune deviation (ACAID).

Skin, grafted from an F1 hybrid rat to one of its parents, presents foreign MHC antigens and is rejected. Prior injection of F1 hybrid lymphocytes into the parent's subconjunctival space (Kaplan and Streilein 1974) or footpad (Kaplan and Streilein 1977) makes rejection even more rapid and vigorous — the 'second set response'. However, transfer of lymphocytes from an F1 hybrid rat to the anterior chamber of one of its parents enables subsequent skin grafts to survive (Kaplan and Streilein 1974, 1977), despite the appearance of circulating antibodies (Kaplan and Streilein 1977).

Similarly, when tumours are transplanted between mouse strains that differ only at minor histocompatibility loci, graft survival can be prolonged by prior implantation into the anterior chamber (Streilein *et al*. 1980; Niederkorn *et al*. 1981). Virus-infected cells (Whittum *et al*. 1984), soluble antigens (Mizuno *et al*. 1989; Wilbanks and Streilein 1990) and haptens (Wetzig *et al*. 1982; Waldrep and Kaplan 1983) can also induce ACAID.

Delayed hypersensitivity is suppressed in favour of lymphocytotoxicity

All these models of ACAID show depressed delayed hypersensitivity, but there is evidence that the lymphocytotoxic arm of the immune response is preserved. In mice that harbour growing MHC-incompatible intraocular tumours, subcutaneous tumour implants and metastases fail to become established (Niederkorn and Streilein 1983), even though the survival of skin grafts expressing the same MHC antigens is prolonged (Streilein and Niederkorn 1981).

The influence of ambient light

A fascinating aspect of this story, which raises new questions about the overall control of ACAID, has been the discovery that it is dependent upon ambient illumination (Ferguson *et al*. 1988). The introduction of hapten-treated lymphocytes into the anterior chamber induces ACAID if mice are exposed to visible light, but this can be prevented by just 18 hours of darkness following the injection. Twenty-four hours of light is sufficient to establish ACAID in dark-reared animals. The phenomenon is local, and unaffected by section of the optic nerve.

The mechanism of anterior chamber-associated immune deviation

Current evidence indicates that macrophages of a subset that do not display Class II MHC antigens are in some way modified as they traverse the anterior segment of the eye. Having phagocytosed and digested foreign antigens, they circulate in the blood to the spleen. There they induce suppressor T lymphocytes that prevent the generation of the specific helper T cells that would normally mediate delayed hypersensitivity.

The signal from eye to spleen

The induction of ACAID requires a functioning spleen (Kaplan and Streilein 1974; Streilein and Niederkorn 1981; Waldrep and Kaplan 1983) and an intact eye (Niederkorn and Streilein 1982) for some days after antigen has been introduced into the anterior chamber. It seems likely that a signal is elaborated in the eye, then passed to the spleen, and its nature has been the subject of intense research.

If splenic T cells are soaked in hapten and then implanted into the anterior chambers of splenectomized mice, a soluble ACAID-inducing factor appears in the serum: when injected into naïve animals with intact spleens, such serum induces the proliferation of hapten-specific splenic suppressor T cells (Ferguson *et al.* 1989). This experiment shows that a soluble factor can induce ACAID, but the message is elaborated by the implanted splenic T lymphocytes and can be likened to 'transfer factor'.

The trabecular meshwork, through which any antigen must leave the eye, itself contains cells that express HLA Class II antigens (Lynch *et al.* 1987) and it has been suggested that these may normally process antigens and secrete similar signalling proteins (Wetzig *et al.* 1982; Niederkorn 1990).

The idea of a soluble signalling factor has, however, seemed less convincing since some recent experiments by Wilbanks and Streilein. They have shown that, shortly after the injection of bovine serum albumin into the anterior chambers of splenectomized mice, certain circulating mononuclear cells (which express F4/80, but not Class II MHC) carry an ACAID-inducing signal: they can transmit ACAID to naïve animals with intact spleens (Wilbanks and Streilein 1991). Macrophages of this subset are found in some profusion in the anterior segment of the eye (Williamson *et al.* 1989).

After exposure to antigen in tissue culture, F4/80 +ve, Ia −ve cells can also transmit ACAID to naïve animals, but only when they are inoculated into the anterior chamber of the eye (Wilbanks *et al.* 1991). Therefore the anterior segment of the eye itself imparts to F4/80 +ve, Ia −ve macrophages the ability to transmit ACAID. No such transformation accompanies the passage of Ia +ve antigen-presenting cells through the anterior chamber: they prevent ACAID when introduced intracamerally (Williamson and Streilein 1989), or even into the central cornea (Williamson *et al.* 1987).

Splenic suppression

A number of elegant experiments, in which ACAID was transferred between animals using splenic T lymphocytes (Wetzig *et al.* 1982; Niederkorn and Streilein 1983; Waldrep and Kaplan 1983; Whittum *et al.* 1984), have shown that intracameral (IC) antigen triggers the replication of antigen-specific suppressor T cells (Wetzig *et al.* 1982; Whittum *et al.* 1984), which may interfere with either the afferent (Whittum *et al.* 1984), the efferent (Waldrep and Kaplan 1983) or both (Wetzig *et al.* 1982) limbs of the immune response.

Aware that the introduction of antigen into a vein also induces antigen-specific depression of immunity, early workers in this field concluded that the IC route represented an elaborate means of IV injection (Kaplan and Streilein 1974). However, the two methods of antigen administration stimulate different populations of splenic suppressor T cells, each with a characteristic effect upon the immune response. Inoculation by either route depresses cell-mediated immunity, but only IV injections affect the humoral immune response (Niederkorn and Streilein 1982). Both routes cause afferent suppression, but only IC injections suppress the efferent limb. Interestingly, afferent suppression is mediated by CD8 +ve cells after IV antigen, but by a CD4 +ve suppressor subset after IC antigen (Wilbanks and Streilein 1990).

A caution

The unfolding story of ACAID relies heavily on very few experimental techniques, and will not be secure until much of the work has been repeated, and some revised. Swelling of an ear after the local application of antigen has been used in many of the experiments to assay delayed hypersensitivity. The changes in thickness, which are measured by an engineer's micrometer, are only in the order of 10 μm (Waldrep and Kaplan 1983), and it is remarkable that statistically significant results can be achieved.

When splenic lymphocytes are exposed to dilute solutions of hapten and then injected into the anterior chamber, they must undergo many changes for which no experimental control can be devised. This technique has been used to demonstrate ACAID to haptens (Wetzig *et al.* 1982; Waldrep and Kaplan 1983), to detect a soluble signal from eye to spleen (Ferguson *et al.* 1989) and to investigate the effects of ambient light (Ferguson *et al.* 1988).

The interpretation of other experiments has been based upon reasonable assumptions, which nevertheless require confirmation (e.g. it has been assumed that antigens are expressed at the surface of the macrophages that transport them between the eye and spleen (Wilbanks and Streilein 1991) and that the timing of afferent immune suppression is identical after IV and IC inoculations of antigen (Wilbanks and Streilein 1990)).

What is the benefit of anterior chamber-associated immune deviation?

The benefit of ACAID becomes apparent when it is considered as a means of inhibiting delayed hypersensitivity, which is immensely destructive to surrounding structures (Knisely *et al.* 1987), in favour of the more discriminating lymphocytotoxic or humoral immune responses (Niederkorn and Streilein 1982; Niederkorn 1990). The discovery of ACAID to soluble antigens has placed this in a new and interesting context. The eye contains powerful corneal, lens and retinal antigens (see section on Autoimmunity below) and it has been suggested that small quantities of these may be continually released into the anterior chamber, ensuring that delayed hypersensitivity is depressed should injury occur (Mizuno *et al.* 1989; Niederkorn 1990).

Ocular immune deviation?

The suppression of delayed hypersensitivity in favour of lymphocytotoxicity is not confined to immune responses within the anterior chamber, but also characterizes the rejection of corneal grafts (see above). The central migration of corneal Langerhans' cells not only restores corneal delayed hypersensitivity (Peeler and Niederkorn 1986; Peeler *et al.* 1988), it also abrogates ACAID (Williamson *et al.* 1987). The purely anatomical boundary between the corneal and intraocular compartments appears to be of less consequence than the harmony which exists among all immune responses in the optical axis.

Autoimmunity (reviews: Duke-Elder and Perkins 1966 [*historical*]; Faure 1980)

The awareness that a penetrating injury to one eye may be followed by inflammation of its fellow appears in the literature around AD 1000 (Duke-Elder and Perkins 1966). We now call this disease sympathetic ophthalmia, and the characteristic granulomatous uveitis can be replicated experimentally by enucleating and incising a rabbit's eye, then implanting it into the peritoneal cavity of the same animal (Vannas *et al.* 1960). With an understanding of immunology arose the notion that ocular injury may reveal autoantigens, but the search for them is still gathering pace. They have now been found in the cornea, lens and retina, and all are truly organ-specific: in every case material extracted from one mammalian species can excite an autoimmune response of varying intensity in many others.

Experimental models of autoimmune eye disease bear close resemblance to some clinical syndromes. Further interest has been generated by the discovery of humoral and cell-mediated immunity to autoantigens among patients with inflammatory eye disease; however, a pathogenic role for autoimmunity in clinical ophthalmology still remains to be established.

Corneal antigens

A single 54 kD protein contributes approximately 30% of the soluble protein fraction of mammalian corneal epithelium (Alexander *et al.* 1981; Silverman *et al.* 1981). It has been purified, is not glycosylated (Alexander *et al.* 1981), and antibodies raised against it cross-react with determinants in the lens capsule, retina, retinal pigment epithelium and choroid (Silverman *et al.* 1981; Kruit *et al.* 1986).

The clinical relevance of this strikingly bland information was transformed by the discovery of humoral immunity to corneal epithelium after corneal grafting, during inflammatory corneal melting (Kruit *et al.* 1986) and in anterior uveitis (Kruit *et al.* 1985; van der Gaag *et al.* 1989). Among patients with anterior uveitis, cell-mediated immunity to corneal epithelium has also been demonstrated (van der Gaag *et al.* 1989). The incidence of antibodies to corneal epithelium approaches 90% in Fuch's heterochromic cyclitis (La Hey *et al.* 1988), a disease in which large aggregates of lymphocytes (keratic precipitates) adhere to the corneal endothelium. These plaques are indistinguishable from those which follow the injection into the anterior chamber of lymphocytes sensitized to autologous cornea (graft-versus-host disease) (Khodadoust and Silverstein 1975).

In all these circumstances the 54 kD protein has been implicated as the antigen (Kruit *et al.* 1986; van der Gaag *et al.* 1989). Although it is tempting to infer that some types of anterior ocular inflammatory disease represent a failure of tolerance to this autoantigen, the immune response to the 54 kD protein may equally be a consequence of long-standing corneal damage.

Lens antigens

After the assertion by Otto Schirmer in 1898 that lens material could induce ocular inflammation, and the subsequent description of 'phacoanaphylactic' uveitis by Verhoeff and Lemoine in 1922 (Duke-Elder and Perkins 1966), accidental rupture of the lens capsule became a feared complication of cataract surgery (Wirostko and Spalter 1967). Since the lens loses its blood supply at an early stage of embryological development, it was reasoned that its proteins must fail to invoke immunological tolerance (Rahi *et al.* 1977). But fashions in cataract surgery change and, although the capsule is now routinely ruptured early in the procedure, the incidence of postoperative uveitis is no greater. If lens matter is antigenic, then some mechanism must operate to suppress a harmful immune response.

The lens does indeed contain endogenous protein autoantigens (crystallins), of which α-crystallin appears to be the most powerful (Sandberg and Closs 1979a; Goldschmidt *et al.* 1982), and damage to its capsule can induce an intense humoral immune response (Wirostko and Spalter 1967 [*human*]; Misra *et al.* 1977 [*rabbit*]; Gery *et al.* 1981 [*rabbit*]; Goldschmidt *et al.* 1982 [*mouse*]). However, the notion that such antigens are normally sequestered from the immune system is a myth. Lens crystallins can be detected in the aqueous of normal subjects, their titre rising in those with cataract (Sandberg and Closs 1979b), and up to 50% of the population have circulating antibodies to them (Hackett and Thompson 1964; Perkins and Wood 1964; Luntz 1968; Sandberg and Closs 1979a; Angunawela 1987). It is doubtful whether they could ever be pathogenic, and the recent suggestion that they may be implicated in the formation of cataracts (Angunawela 1987) seems most unlikely.

There are minor variations between the crystallins of different species, which underlie the diverse immune responses to heterologous and autologous material. Heterologous crystallin arouses a normal cell-mediated immune response (Rahi *et al.* 1977; Goldschmidt *et al.* 1982), but immunization with autologous lens antigens is met by a complete failure of delayed hypersensitivity, despite the appearance of circulating antibodies (Gery *et al.* 1981 [*rabbit*]; Goldschmidt *et al.* 1982 [*mouse*]).

It is significant that lens antigens are continually shed into the anterior chamber, which they leave through the trabecular meshwork (Sandberg and Closs 1979b). Niederkorn (1990) has proposed that this induces ACAID, and their excitation of humoral immunity but depression of delayed hypersensitivity supports his contention. It is further reinforced by the confirmation that ACAID can arise in response to soluble antigens (Mizuno *et al.* 1989; Wilbanks and Streilein 1990).

Uveal antigens

In some of the earliest attempts to identify autoantigens responsible for ocular inflammation, guinea-pigs (Aronson *et al.* 1963a; Aronson 1965) or primates (Collins 1949) were repeatedly inoculated with homologous uveal homogenates. This produced a disease in which plasma cells and lymphocytes pervaded the ciliary apparatus and then spread to involve the iris, anterior vitreous and anterior choroid. Although lymphocytes occasionally spread directly into the sclera, the retina effectively prevented their passage from choroid to vitreous (Aronson *et al.* 1963c). This pathology bore a striking resemblance to human 'pars planitis', but it never became chronic (Aronson *et al.* 1963b).

The affected animals produced antibodies to species-specific uveal antigens (Wacker *et al.* 1964) in Bruch's membrane (Kalsow and Wacker 1975). Cell-mediated immunity was also implicated by the discovery that the disease could be transferred to normal animals with cells from the lymph nodes and spleen, but not with serum (Aronson and McMaster 1971). Unfortunately, this was a rather untidy model which used impure antigen (Aronson 1965; Wacker 1972). During the preparation of uveal tissue, retina was 'teased' away after death (Aronson *et al.* 1963a), possibly leaving photoreceptor outer segments behind (Wacker 1972).

Retinal antigens

The various retinal proteins that have been identified as autoantigens are all involved in photoelectric transduction.

S-ANTIGEN

In 1965 Wacker and Lipton produced uveitis by repeatedly injecting an emulsion of autologous retinal extract in Freund's adjuvant into the footpads of guinea-pigs. A soluble extract (S-antigen), which could be distinguished from uveal antigens by immunofluorescence (Kalsow and Wacker 1975), was found to be the most potent inducer of autoimmune uveitis (Wacker 1973). Guinea-pig (Wacker 1973), bovine (Wacker *et al.* 1977) and human (Beneski *et al.* 1984) S-antigens have all been purified, and contain epitopes which cross-react (Beneski *et al.* 1984; Doekes *et al.* 1989). The antigenicity of various fragments has been investigated (Gregerson and Putterman 1984; Kamada *et al.* 1985; Banga *et al.* 1987; Gregerson *et al.* 1989), and synthetic peptides can induce the disease (Singh *et al.* 1989).

Bovine S-antigen is a 50 kD lipoprotein and the primary structure of its 48 kD protein component is known (Shinohara *et al.* 1987). Physiologists know it as 'arrestin', a rod outer-segment protein that is responsible for modulating the biochemical cascade by which a photon absorbed by rhodopsin is translated into a nervous impulse (Wilden *et al.* 1986; Kuhn 1987; Palczewski *et al.* 1989). As its function indicates, it is confined to the outer retina (Kalsow and Wacker 1975; Wacker *et al.* 1977), where it is mainly associated with the disc membranes of rod outer segments (Uusitalo *et al.* 1985; McKechnie *et al.* 1986; Rodrigues *et al.* 1987).

Systemic immunization with bovine (Wacker *et al.* 1977) or human (Beneski *et al.* 1984) S-antigen causes ocular inflammation that culminates in the destruction of the retinal photoreceptors (Wacker and Lipton 1965, Wacker *et al.* 1977, Beneski *et al.* 1984, Forrester *et al.* 1985 [*guinea-pig*]; Nussenblatt *et al.* 1981b [*primate*]; Mochizuki *et al.* 1985, Broekhuyse *et al.* 1986, Brown *et al.* 1989 [*rat*]; Iwase *et al.* 1990 [*mouse*]). A lymphocytic infiltrate also sweeps through the pineal gland (Kalsow and Wacker 1978 [*guinea-pig*]).

In the rat, the first evidence of ocular inflammation is seen in the anterior segment. Lymphocytes swell the ciliary body, then migrate into the iris (Brown *et al.* 1989). The anterior chamber may fill with inflammatory cells (hypopyon) and the cornea becomes oedematous (Mochizuki *et al.* 1985). The multifocal choroidal and retinal inflammation that follows varies in intensity, but an outpouring of neutrophil polymorphs into the subretinal space may cause serous retinal detachment (Mochizuki *et al.* 1985).

The character of the ocular disease varies according to the dose of antigen and this has been studied in guinea-pigs (Wacker 1973; Rao *et al.* 1979). After low doses, lymphocytes, plasma cells and macrophages enter the choroid and multifocal granulomas form between the RPE cells and Bruch's membrane — an appearance indistinguishable from the Dalen–Fuchs nodules of human sympathetic ophthalmia. Purulent panophthalmitis with serous retinal detachment follows higher doses (Rao *et al.* 1979).

All available evidence implicates helper/inducer T cells in the pathogenesis of this disease. CD4 +ve cells predominate in the early stages (Brown *et al.* 1989) and uveitis can be transferred from affected to naïve, syngeneic rats by intraperitoneal injections of helper/inducer (but not suppressor/cytotoxic) T lymphocytes from the lymph nodes or spleen (Mochizuki *et al.* 1985). Cultured helper/inducer T cell lines, obtained from affected animals, can also induce the disease in syngeneic hosts (Gregerson *et al.* 1986). Such cells only proliferate in response to S-antigen if it is presented by syngeneic antigen-presenting cells (Gregerson *et al.* 1986) and the dependence upon MHC (Ia) antigens (genetic restriction) must apply *in vivo*, since S-antigen uveitis in rats can be prevented with anti-Ia antibodies (Wetzig *et al.* 1988; Rao *et al.* 1989). Delayed hypersensitivity to S-antigen closely reflects the intensity of the disease (Atkinson *et al.* 1989).

The crucial role of T cells is confirmed by the effect of cyclosporin A. Its administration to rats from the moment of immunization causes a reduction in the helper/inducer T cell fraction in lymph nodes draining the immunization site (Nussenblatt and Scher 1985) and uveitis is suppressed (Nussenblatt *et al.* 1981a, 1982a; Broekhuyse *et al.* 1986; Atkinson *et al.* 1989), although many animals develop the disease later if the drug is withdrawn (Atkinson *et al.* 1989). When given 7 days after immunization, cyclosporin A modulates the disease from a florid, purulent pan-uveitis to a granulomatous choroiditis (Nussenblatt *et al.* 1982a).

INTERPHOTORECEPTOR RETINOID-BINDING PROTEIN

Interphotoreceptor retinoid-binding protein (IRBP) is a 133 kD extracellular glycoprotein (Adler and Klucznik 1982; Adler and Evans 1985) that transports retinol between the RPE cells and photoreceptors (Chader and Wiggert 1984; Adler and Evans 1985). Immunoelectron microscopic localization indicates that it is secreted only by rod inner segments and pinealocytes (Rodrigues *et al.* 1986, 1987). Parenteral administration with adjuvant is followed by a disease of the retina and pineal gland that bears histological similarity to S-antigen-induced uveitis, but is said to be less severe (Broekhuyse *et al.* 1986 [*rat*]; Gery *et al.* 1986, Vistica *et al.* 1986 [*guinea-pig*]). In rabbits (Eisenfeld *et al.* 1987) and primates (Hirose *et al.* 1986) the choroid is more intensely involved and there is disruption of Bruch's membrane.

As with S-antigen uveitis, T lymphocytes are implicated in the pathogenesis of this disease. It can be aborted by cyclosporin A (Broekhuyse *et al.* 1986) and may be transferred to naïve, syngeneic animals by T cells (Fox *et al.* 1986; McAllister *et al.* 1986).

Opsin (Broekhuyse *et al.* 1986 [*rat*]) and rhodopsin (Schalken *et al.* 1989 [*primate*]) are also autoantigenic.

OCULAR AUTOANTIGENS AND INFLAMMATORY EYE DISEASE

In primates, retinal autoantigens can generate pathology that closely resembles human ocular inflammatory diseases. While immunization with S-antigen is said to produce a retinal vasculitis (Nussenblatt *et al.* 1981b), IRBP causes a disease that bears a striking similarity to sympathetic ophthalmia. In addition to lymphocytic sheathing of retinal veins, and multifocal infiltration of the retina and RPE with lymphocytes and histiocytes, choroidal epithelioid granulomas appear which are indistinguishable from Dalen–Fuchs nodules (Hirose *et al.* 1986). (Hirose *et al.* 1986). Immunization with rhodopsin causes an intermediate uveitis, with lymphocytic infiltration of the ciliary body and pars plana, then choroiditis, retinitis and retinal vasculitis (Schalken *et al.* 1989).

Lymphocytes from many patients with uveitis and retinal vasculitis can be transformed by S-antigen (Nussenblatt *et al.* 1980, 1982b), and circulating antibodies to retinal antigens have been found in others (Dumonde *et al.* 1982; Chan *et al.* 1985). There is also circumstantial evidence that idiotype/anti-idiotype immune complexes may protect against the deleterious effects of antiretinal autoantibodies (Dumonde *et al.* 1982). This has fired the imagination of some ophthalmic immunologists, and S-antigen has been implicated in the initiation or perpetuation of uveitis (Nussenblatt *et al.* 1980, 1982b) and even retinitis pigmentosa (Brinkman *et al.* 1980; Heredia Garcia and Carcia-Calderon 1989). However, antibodies to retinal antigens are common in people without eye disease (Forrester *et al.* 1989 [*S-antigen*]; van der Lelij *et al.* 1990a [*S-antigen, IRBP, opsin*]) and may even play a protective role (Forrester *et al.* 1989). Many normal subjects also show cell-mediated immunity to S-antigen and IRBP (van der Lelij *et al.* 1990b).

The prevailing evidence suggests that ocular autoantigens are continually exposed to the immune system, but the response to them is attenuated — presumably by ACAID. If this is true, the first stage of autoimmune uveitis must be the abrogation of ACAID. The extraocular introduction of a retinal autoantigen with adjuvant may achieve this during experimental allergic uveitis, a situation that is paralleled when injury and infection of an eye result in sympathetic ophthalmia. Should the extraocular release of autoantigens complicate uveitis of a different aetiology, autoimmune uveitis would perpetuate the disease.

Molecular mimicry offers an alternative mechanism for the induction of retinal autoimmunity. A peptide from the yeast histone (H3), which has a five amino acid sequence of homology with the uveitogenic peptide M from S-antigen, can induce uveitis in rats (Singh *et al.* 1989) and precipitates a bizarre autoimmune uveitis in monkeys (Eto *et al.* 1991). Synthetic peptides, representing fragments of viral and food proteins with even shorter sequences of homology with peptide M, have also been shown to induce uveitis and to stimulate lymph node cells from animals with peptide M-induced disease (Singh *et al.* 1990).

Human leucocyte antigen and ocular inflammation (reviews: Rahi 1979; Meyer 1986; Feltkamp 1990)

The eye is implicated in a number of systemic disorders that are linked to HLA antigens, including ankylosing spondylitis, Reiter's syndrome and reactive arthritis [HLA-B27], rheumatoid arthritis [HLA-DR4] and Behçet's syndrome [HLA-B5 (Ohno *et al.* 1975), now localized to its HLA-Bw51 subtype (Ohno *et al.* 1978)]. However, most of the early, enthusiastic reports of HLA associations with purely ocular diseases were based on the inappropriate application of statistics (Svejgaard *et al.* 1974; Meyer 1986) and the only two to survive are anterior uveitis and birdshot choroidopathy.

Anterior uveitis

Human leucocyte antigen B27 is associated with anterior uveitis

Anterior uveitis complicates ankylosing spondylitis and reactive arthropathy, both of which are strongly associated with HLA-B27 (Laitinen *et al.* 1977; Yu *et al.* 1989). This prompted Brewerton and colleagues (1973) to investigate the HLA-B27 status of patients presenting with anterior uveitis. The incidence of approximately 50% that he observed has been repeatedly confirmed (Mapstone and Woodrow 1975; Wakefield and Penny 1983; Rothova *et al.* 1987; Wakefield *et al.* 1990). Among patients with HLA-B27-associated diseases, those who do have the antigen are at additional risk of developing anterior uveitis. For example, only half the patients who acquire an arthropathy after *Yersinia* infection are HLA-B27 +ve, but all those who develop anterior uveitis belong to this group (Laitinen *et al.* 1977; Saari *et al.* 1980).

Do additional genetic factors operate?

Thirteen per cent of the first-degree relatives of patients with HLA-B27-associated acute anterior uveitis themselves claim a history of the disease, compared with 1% in the normal HLA-B27 +ve population (Derhaag *et al.* 1988a). Although this indicates that genetic factors other than HLA-B27 must determine susceptibility to anterior uveitis, the particular factor that is responsible has not been identified. There is no association between anterior uveitis and any HLA-B27 subtype (Derhaag *et al.* 1988b), and homozygosity for HLA-B27 does not increase its incidence (Derhaag *et al.* 1989). Nor does the frequency of other Class I antigens in patients with anterior uveitis differ from that in an HLA-B27 +ve healthy control population (Derhaag *et al.* 1989).

Are infections trigger factors in uveitis?

Human leucocyte antigen B27 increases the risk of a remote bacterial infection triggering an organ-specific immune response in the form of a reactive arthropathy, and several research groups, considering that anterior uveitis may be analogous, have sought evidence of bacterial infections in these patients.

Antibodies to *Yersinia* have been detected in patients with anterior uveitis but without reactive arthritis (Mattilla *et al.* 1982; Wakefield *et al.* 1990), and a recent Australian study suggests that their incidence may be higher in HLA-B27 +ve subjects (Wakefield *et al.* 1990). Cell-mediated immunity to *Chlamydia trachomatis* has also been recorded in two-thirds of unselected HLA-B27 +ve patients with anterior uveitis, but not in HLA-B27 −ve controls (Wakefield and Penny 1983).

However, it has been the notion that *Klebsiella* infection could precipitate acute anterior uveitis that has aroused most interest. It began with the observation that the carriage of *Klebsiella* in the stool increases during attacks of anterior uveitis in patients with (Ebringer *et al.* 1979) and without (White *et al.* 1984) ankylosing spondylitis, although this has been disputed (Warren and Brewerton 1979). The incidence of *Klebsiella* was thought to be highest in patients with HLA-B27, or HLA-B7 antigens that cross-react with B27 (B7, Bw22, Bw40 and Bw42) (White *et al.* 1984).

Other workers have found that, whatever their HLA-B27, status, patients with uveitis have no greater incidence of *Klebsiella* infection (Willshaw 1981; Beckingsale *et al.* 1984) and no higher antibody titres to *Klebsiella* (Kijlstra *et al.* 1986) than a control population. Cell-mediated immunity to *Klebsiella* has not been associated with uveitis (Holland *et al.* 1982).

The development of animal models of endotoxin-induced ocular inflammation lent credence to the notion that Gram-negative infections could precipitate or intensify anterior uveitis.

However, the declining effects of repeated injections have been disappointing (see above) and the failure of intravenous LPS to increase the permeability of the blood/aqueous barrier has been a further blow (Herman *et al.* 1991). The evidence that endotoxin is responsible for uveitis is at best inconsistent, at worst spurious. If an association does exist, any explanation will have to account for its presence both in HLA-B27 +ve and −ve patients (cf. reactive arthropathy: Yu *et al.* 1989; Benjamin and Perham 1990).

Does human leucocyte antigen B27 affect the character of uveitis?

There are no specific clinical features of anterior uveitis that implicate the HLA-B27 antigen, although the keratic precipitates (plaques of inflammatory cells adherent to corneal endothelium) are smaller than in granulomatous disease (Mapstone and Woodrow 1975). Nevertheless, anterior uveitis in patients with HLA-B27 is a distinct clinical entity, whether or not it is associated with arthritis. It arises at a lower age, has a high male/female ratio (Mapstone and Woodrow 1975; Rothova *et al.* 1987) and recurrences tend to be uniocular, affecting either eye (Rothova *et al.* 1987). Although the attacks are less frequent than in patients without HLA-B27, they are more severe, there is often fibrin in the anterior chamber and the incidence of complications is higher (Rothova *et al.* 1987).

Therefore, although the management of anterior uveitis must be guided by clinical findings, the identification of HLA-B27 in patients with anterior uveitis can be helpful (Feltkamp 1990). It identifies subjects who may be at risk of complications without energetic and protracted therapy, but in whom the prognosis is otherwise excellent. The expectation of relapses allows patients to make preparations for the prompt application of topical steroids and mydriatics, thereby reducing the risk of complications.

Birdshot choroidopathy

In 1980 Ryan and Maumenee described a form of relentlessly progressive, bilateral uveitis that was largely confined to the posterior segment. The vitreous contained many cells and much debris, but no snowball opacities, and there was no exudate at the pars plana. Multifocal cream-coloured plaques were scattered throughout the retinal pigment epithelium and the retinal circulation was incompetent, with disc and cystoid macular oedema and venous sheathing. Peripheral lymphocytes from these patients could be transformed by bovine retinal S-antigen (Nussenblatt *et al.* 1982b), but this was probably a secondary phenomenon.

Birdshot choroidopathy is associated with HLA-A29 in about 95% of cases. The relative risk (RR) is between 50 (Nussenblatt *et al.* 1982b) and 244 (Priem *et al.* 1988), one of the highest associations between HLA and disease reported. Subtypes of HLA-A29 exist and the possibility remains that one of these is invariably associated. The apparent association with HLA-B12 (RR = 7) is explained by linkage disequilibrium with HLA-A29 (Priem *et al.* 1988).

The very high incidence of HLA-A29 in birdshot choroidopathy suggests that this antigen may be directly implicated in its pathogenesis.

Summary

The ocular immunological compartments have distinct pathways for antigen presentation, but great similarity in the character of the immune responses that they mount. Antigens that are presented within the eye suppress delayed hypersensitivity in favour of humoral immunity and cytotoxicity (ACAID), and the immune response to corneal antigens is similar. This is linked to a dearth of antigen-presenting cells expressing Class II MHC, but the signals between eye and spleen are still incompletely characterized.

The available evidence suggests that ocular immune deviation has permitted the evolution of an organ that fails to present its unique proteins to the developing immune system, and it is ocular immune deviation that protects the resulting powerful autoantigens throughout life. This tolerance can be induced to fail experimentally, but the extent to which such failure can cause or perpetuate clinical inflammatory eye disease is still unknown.

Other challenges for the future will be to clarify the role that is played by immune complexes and bacterial endotoxins in the induction of inflammatory eye disease and explore the way in which other factors, such as blood flow and even photoelectric transduction, interact with the ocular immune response.

References

Adler, A.J. and Evans, C.D. (1985). Some functional characteristics of purified bovine interphotoreceptor retinol-binding protein. *Invest. Ophthalmol. Vis. Sci.* **26**, 273–82.

Adler, A.J. and Klucznik, K.M. (1982). Proteins and glycoproteins of the bovine interphotoreceptor matrix: composition and fractionation. *Exp. Eye Res.* **34**, 423–34.

Ajo, C. (1941). New observation on a primary ocular reaction to Schwartzman toxins. *Proc. Soc. Exp. Biol. Med.* **47**, 500–1.

Allansmith, M.R., Whitney, C.R., McClellan, B.H. and Newman, L.P. (1973). Immunoglobulin in the human eye. *Arch Ophthalmol* **89**, 36–45.

Allansmith, M.R., Kajiyama, G., Abelson, M.B. and Simon, M.A. (1976). Plasma cell content of main and accessory lacrimal glands and conjunctiva. *Am. J. Ophthalmol.* **82**, 819–26.

Allansmith, M.R., de Ramus, A. and Maurice, D. (1979). The dynamics of IgG in the cornea. *Invest. Ophthalmol. Vis. Sci.* **18**, 947–55.

Alexander, R.J., Silverman, B. and Henley, W.L. (1981). Isolation and characterization of BCP 54, the major soluble protein of bovine cornea. *Exp. Eye Res.* **32**, 205–16.

Angunawela, I.I. (1987). The role of autoimmune phenomena in the pathogenesis of cataract. *Immunology* **61**, 363–8.

Aronson, S.B. (1965). The homoimmune uveitises in the guinea pig. *Ann. NY Acad. Sci.* **124**, 365–76.

Aronson, S.B. and McMaster, P.R.B. (1971). Passive transfer of experimental allergic uveitis. *Arch. Ophthalmol* **86**, 557–63.

Aronson, S.B., Hogan, M.J. and Zweigart, P. (1963a). Homoimmune uveitis in the guinea pig. I. General concepts of auto- and homoimmunity, methods, and manifestations. *Arch. Ophthalmol* **69**, 105–9.

Aronson, S.B., Hogan, M.J. and Zweigart, P. (1963b). Homoimmune uveitis in the guinea pig. II. Clinical manifestations. *Arch. Ophthalmol.* **69**, 203–7.

Aronson, S.B., Hogan, M.J. and Zweigart, P. (1963c). Homoimmune uveitis in the guinea pig. III. Histopathologic manifestations of the disease. *Arch. Ophthalmol.* **69**, 208–19.

Atkinson, E.G., Dinning, W.J., Kasp, E., Graham, E.M. and Dumonde, D.C. (1989). Precipitation of experimental autoallergic uveoretinitis by cyclosporin A withdrawal: an experimental model of uveitis relapse. *Clin. Exp. Immunol.* **78**, 108–14.

Avakian, H., Abuknesha, R., Welsh, J. and Ebringer, A. (1981). Uveitis, vitreous humour, and *Klebsiella*. I. Binding studies with rabbit antisera. *Br. J. Ophthalmol.* **65**, 315–22.

Banga, J.P., Kasp, E., Ellis, B.A., Brown, E., Suleyman, S. and Dumonde, D.C. (1987). Antigenicity and uveitogenicity of partially purified peptides of a retinal autoantigen, S-antigen. *Immunology* **61**, 357–62.

Beckingsale, A.B., Williams, D., Gibson, J.M. and Rosenthal, A.R. (1984). *Klebsiella* and acute anterior uveitis. *Br. J. Ophthalmol.* **68**, 866–8.

Beneski, D.A., Donoso, L.A., Edelberg, K.E., Magargal, L.E., Folberg, R. and Merryman, C. (1984). Human retinal S-antigen. *Invest. Ophthalmol. Vis. Sci.* **25**, 686–90.

Benjamin, R. and Perham, P. (1990). Guilt by association: HLA-B27 and ankylosing spondylitis. *Immunol. Today* **11**, 137–42.

Bergstresser, P.R., Fletcher, C.R. and Streilein, J.W. (1980). Surface densities of Langerhans cells in relation to rodent epidermal sites with special immunologic properties. *J. Invest. Dermatol.* **74**, 77–80.

Beutler, B.A., Milsark, I.W. and Cerami, A. (1985). Cachectin/tumor necrosis factor: production, distribution, and metabolic fate *in vivo*. *J. Immunol.* **135**, 3972–7.

Bhattacherjee, P., Williams, R.N. and Eakins, K.E. (1983). An evaluation of ocular inflammation following the injection of bacterial endotoxin into the rat foot pad. *Invest. Ophthalmol. Vis. Sci.* **24**, 196–202.

Bluestone, R., Easty, D.L., Goldberg, L.S., Jones, B.R. and Petit, T.H. (1975). Lacrimal immunoglobulins and complement quantified by counter-immunoelectrophoresis. *Br. J. Ophthalmol.* **59**, 279–81.

Breebaart, A.C. and James-Witte, J. (1959). Studies on experimental corneal allergy. *Am. J. Ophthalmol.* **48**, 37–47.

Brewerton, D.A., Caffrey, M., Nicholls, A., Walters, D. and James, D.C.O. (1973). Acute anterior uveitis and HL-A27. *Lancet* **ii**, 994–6.

Brinkman, C.J.J., Pinkers, A.J.L.G. and Broekhuyse, R.M. (1980). Immune reactivity to different retinal antigens in patients suffering from retinitis pigmentosa. *Invest. Ophthalmol. Vis. Sci.* **19**, 743–50.

Broekhuyse, R.M., Winkens, H.J. and Kuhlmann, E.D. (1986). Induction of experimental autoimmune uveoretinitis and pinealitis by IRBP-comparison to uveoretinitis induced by S-antigen and opsin. *Curr. Eye Res.* **5**, 231–40.

Brown, E.C., Kasp, E. and Dumonde, D.C. (1989). Morphometric analysis of T lymphocyte compartmentation in experimental autoimmune uveoretinitis. *Clin. Exp. Immunol.* **77**, 422–7.

Chader, G.J. and Wiggert, B. (1984). Interphotoreceptor retinoid-binding protein: characteristics in bovine and monkey retina. *Vis. Res.* **24**, 1605–14.

Chan, C., Palestine, A.G., Nussenblatt, R.B., Roberge, F.G. and Benezra, D. (1985). Anti-retinal auto-antibodies in Vogt–Koyanagi–Harada syndrome, Behçet's disease, and sympathetic ophthalmia. *Ophthalmology* **92**, 1025–8.

Collins, R.C. (1949). Experimental studies on sympathetic ophthalmia. *Am. J. Ophthalmol.* **32**, 1687–99.

Coster, D.J. (1989). Mechanisms of corneal graft failure: the erosion of corneal privilege. *Eye* **2**, 251–62.

Derhaag, P.J.F.M., Linssen, A., Broekema, N., de Waal, L.P. and Feltkamp, T.E.W. (1988a). A familial study of the inheritance of HLA-B27-positive acute anterior uveitis. *Am. J. Ophthalmol.* **105**, 603–6.

Derhaag, P.J.F.M., de Waal, L.P., Linssen, A. and Feltkamp, T.E.W. (1988b). Acute anterior uveitis and HLA-B27 subtypes. *Invest. Ophthalmol. Vis. Sci.* **29**, 1137–40.

Derhaag, P.J.F.M., van der Horst, A.R., de Waal, L.P. and Feltkamp, T.E.W. (1989). HLA-B27 + acute anterior uveitis and other antigens of the major histocompatibility complex. *Invest. Ophthalmol. Vis. Sci.* **30**, 2160–4.

Deschenes, J., Freeman, W.R., Char, D.H. and Garovoy, M.R. (1986). Lymphocyte subpopulations in uveitis. *Arch. Ophthalmol.* **104**, 233–6.

Doekes, G., Gerritsen, M.J. and Kijlstra, A. (1989). Immunoreactivity and cross-reactivity of human and bovine retinal S-antigen. *Invest. Ophthalmol. Vis. Sci.* **30**, 1169–73.

Donelly, J.J., Li, W., Rockey, J.M. and Prendergast, R.A. (1985). Induction of Class II (Ia) alloantigen expression on corneal endothelium *in vivo* and *in vitro*. *Invest. Ophthalmol. Vis. Sci.* **26**, 575–80.

Duke-Elder Sir, S., Perkins, E.S. (1966). *System of Ophthalmology* vol. IX, *Diseases of the Uveal Tract*. Henry Kimpton, London, pp. 500–12, 560–1.

Dumonde, D.C., Kasp-Grochowska, E., Graham, E. *et al.* (1982). Anti-retinal autoimmunity and circulating immune complexes in patients with retinal vasculitis. *Lancet* **ii**, 787–92.

Ebringer, R., Cawdell, D. and Ebringer, A. (1979). *Klebsiella pneumoniae* and acute anterior uveitis in ankylosing spondylitis. *Br. Med. J.* **i**, 383.

Eisenfeld, A.J., Bunt-Milam, A.H. and Saari, J.C. (1987). Uveoretinitis in rabbits following immunization with interphotoreceptor retinoid-binding protein. *Exp. Eye Res.* **44**, 425–38.

Eliason, J.A. (1978). Leucocytes and experimental corneal vascularisation. *Invest. Ophthalmol. Vis. Sci.* **17**, 1087–95.

Epstein, R.J. and Hughes, W.F. (1981). Lymphocyte-induced corneal neovascularisation: a morphologic assessment. *Invest. Ophthalmol. Vis. Sci.* **21**, 87–94.

Eto, K., Singh, V.K., Usukura, J., Sunil, S. and Shinohara, T. (1991). Molecular mimicry: yeast histone H3 induced autoimmune uveitis in primates. *Invest. Ophthalmol. Vis. Sci.* **32** (suppl.), 933.

Faure, J.P. (1980). Autoimmunity and the retina. *Curr. Topics Eye Res.* **2**, 215–302.

Feltkamp, T.E.W. (1990). Ophthalmological significance of HLA associated uveitis. *Eye* **4**, 839–44.

Ferguson, T.A., Hayashi, J.D. and Kaplan, H.J. (1988). Regulation of the systemic immune response by visible light and the eye. *FASEB J.* **2**, 3017–21.

Ferguson, T.A., Hayashi, J.D. and Kaplan, H.J. (1989). The immune response and the eye III. Anterior chamber-associated immune deviation can be adoptively transferred by serum. *J. Immunol.* **143**, 821–6.

Fernando, A.N. (1960). Immunological studies with I^{131} labeled antigen in experimental uveitis. *Arch Ophthalmol.* **63**, 515–39.

Foets, B.J.J., van den Oord, J.J., Billiau, A., van Damme, J. and Missotten, L. (1991). Heterogeneous induction of major histocompatibility complex Class II antigens on corneal endothelium by interferon-gamma. *Invest. Ophthalmol. Vis. Sci.* **32**, 341–5.

Forrester, J.V., Borthwick, G.M. and McMenamin, P.G. (1985). Ultrastructural pathology of S-antigen uveoretinitis. *Invest. Ophthalmol. Vis. Sci.* **26**, 1281–92.

Forrester, J.V., Stott, D.I. and Hercus, K.M. (1989). Naturally occurring antibodies to bovine and human retinal S antigen: comparison between uveitis patients and healthy volunteers. *Br. J. Ophthalmol.* **73**, 155–9.

Foss, B. (1949). Experimental anaphylactic iridocyclitis. *Acta Pathol. Microbiol. Scand.* suppl. 81.

Fox, M., Hirose, S., Vistica, B.P. *et al.* (1986). A dissociation between lymphocyte proliferation responses and induction of disease in interphotoreceptor retinoid binding protein (IRBP) induced autoimmune uveitis (EAU). *Invest. Ophthalmol. Vis. Sci.* **27** (suppl.), 11.

Franklin, R.M. and Remus, L.E. (1984). Conjunctival-associated lymphoid tissue: evidence for a role in the secretory immune system. *Invest. Ophthalmol. Vis. Sci.* **25**, 181–7.

Franklin, R.M., McGee, D.W. and Shepard, K.F. (1985). Lacrimal gland-directed B cell responses. *J. Immunol.* **135**, 95–9.

Friedman, M.G. (1990). Antibodies in human tears during and after infection. *Surv. Ophthalmol.* **35**, 151–7.

Fromer, C.H. and Klintworth, G.K. (1976). An evaluation of the leukocytes in the pathogenesis of experimentally induced corneal vascularisation III: studies related to the vasoproliferative capability of polymorphonuclear leukocytes and lymphocytes. *Am. J. Pathol.* **82**, 157–67.

Gamble, C.N., Aronson, S.B. and Brescia, F.B. (1970a). Experimental uveitis. I. The production of recurrent immunologic (Auer) uveitis and its relationship to increased uveal vascular permeability. *Arch. Ophthalmol.* **84**, 321–30.

Gamble, C.N., Aronson, S.B. and Brescia, F.B. (1970b). Experimental uveitis. II. The pathogenesis of recurrent immunologic (Auer) uveitis. *Arch. Ophthalmol.* **84**, 331–41.

Germuth, F.G., Maumenee, A.E., Senterfit, L.B. and Pollack, A.D. (1962). Immunohistologic studies on antigen-antibody reactions in the avascular cornea. *J. Exp. Med.* **115**, 919–28.

Gery, I., Nussenblatt, R.B., Ben Ezra, D. (1981). Dissociation between humoral and cellular immune responses to lens antigens. *Invest. Ophthalmol. Vis. Sci.* **20**, 32–9.

Gery, I., Wiggert, B., Redmond, T.M. *et al.* (1986). Uveoretinitis and pinealitis induced by immunization with interphotoreceptor retinoid-binding protein. *Invest. Ophthalmol. Vis. Sci.* **27**, 1296–300.

Gillette, T.E., Chandler, J.W. and Greiner, J.V. (1982). Langerhans cells of the ocular surface. *Ophthalmology* **89**, 700–10.

Goldschmidt, L., Goldbaum, M., Walker, S.M. and Weigle, W.O. (1982). The immune response to homologous lens crystallin. *J. Immunol.* **129**, 1652–7.

Grabner, G., Luger, T.A., Luger, B.M., Smolin, G. and Oh, J.O. (1983). Biologic properties of the thymocyte-activating factor (CETAF) produced by a rabbit corneal cell line (SIRC). *Invest. Ophthalmol. Vis. Sci.* **24**, 589–95.

Greene, H.S.N. (1947). The use of the mouse eye in transplantation experiments. *Cancer Res.* **7**, 491–501.

Greene, H.S.N. (1949). Heterologous transplantation of the Brown–Pearce tumor. *Cancer Res.* **9**, 728–35.

Gregerson, D.S. and Putterman, G.J. (1984). Preparation, isolation, and immunochemical studies of the cyanogen bromide peptides from a retinal photoreceptor cell autoantigen, S-antigen. *J. Immunol.* **133**, 843–8.

Gregerson, D.S., Obritsch, W.F., Fling, S.P. and Cameron, J.D. (1986). S-antigen-specific rat T cell lines recognize peptide fragments of S-antigen and mediate experimental autoimmune uveoretinitis and pinealitis. *J. Immunol.* **136**, 2875–82.

Gregerson, D.S., Fling, S.P., Obritsch, W.F., Merryman, C.F. and Donoso, L.A. (1989). Identification of T cell recognition sites in S-antigen: dissociation of proliferation and pathogenic sites. *Cell. Immunol.* **123**, 427–40.

Hackett, E. and Thompson, A. (1964). Anti-lens antibody in human sera. *Lancet* **ii**, 663–6.

Hembry, R.M., Playfair, J., Watson, P.G. and Dingle, J.T. (1979). Experimental model for scleritis. *Arch. Ophthalmol* **97**, 1337–40.

Heredia Garcia, C.D. and Carcia Calderon, P.A. (1989). Evolution time and longitudinal studies of the anti-S-antigen antibody titers in retinitis pigmentosa. *Retina* **9**, 237–41.

Herman, D.C., Suffredini, A.F., Parrillo, J.E. and Palestine, A.G. (1991). Ocular permeability after systemic administration of endotoxin in humans. *Curr. Eye Res.* **10**, 121–6.

Hirose, S., Kuwabara, T., Nussenblatt, R.B., Wiggert, B., Redmond, T.M. and Gery, I. (1986). Uveitis induced in primates by interphotoreceptor retinoid-binding protein. *Arch. Ophthalmol.* **104**, 1698–702.

Hoekzema, R., Murray, P.I., van Haren, M.A.C., Helle, M. and Kijlstra, A. (1991). Analysis of interleukin-6 in endotoxin-induced uveitis. *Invest. Ophthalmol. Vis. Sci.* **32**, 88–95.

Holland, E.J., Loren, A.B., O'Donnell, M.J., Spence, D.J., Tessler, H.H. and Yokoyama, M.M. (1982). HLA-B27, *Klebsiella pneumoniae*, and the relation to acute anterior uveitis. *Invest. Ophthalmol. Vis. Sci.* **22**, 213–19.

Howes, E.L. and McKay, D.G. (1975). Circulating immune complexes: effects on ocular vascular permeability in the rabbit. *Arch. Ophthalmol.* **93**, 365–70.

Howes, E.L. and Rosenbaum, J.T. (1985). Lipopolysaccharide tolerance inhibits eye inflammation. II. Preliminary studies on the mechanism. *Arch. Ophthalmol.* **103**, 261–5.

Howes, E.L., McKay, D.G. and Aronson, S.B. (1971). An ultrastructural study of the ciliary process in the rabbit following systemic administration of bacterial endotoxin. *Lab. Invest.* **24**, 217–28.

Howes, E.L., Wong, K.L., Hartiala, K.T., Webster, R.O. and Rosenbaum, J.T. (1985). Complement and polymorphonuclear leukocytes do not determine the vascular permeability induced by intraocular LPS. *Am. J. Pathol.* **118**, 35–42.

Iwase, K., Fujii, Y., Nakashima, I., Kato, N., Fujino, Y. and Kawashima, H. (1990). A new method for induction of experimental autoimmune uveoretinitis (EAU) in mice. *Curr. Eye Res.* **9**, 207–16.

Jabs, D.A. and Prendergast, R.A. (1991a). Ocular inflammation in MRL/Mp-lpr/lpr mice. *Invest. Ophthalmol. Vis. Sci.* **32**, 1944–7.

Jabs, D.A. and Prendergast, R.A. (1991b). Autoimmune ocular disease in MRL/Mp-lpr/lpr mice is suppressed by anti-CD4 antibody. *Invest. Ophthalmol. Vis. Sci.* **32**, 2718–22.

Kalsow, C.M. and Wacker, W.B. (1975). Use of immunofluorescent localization in the normal guinea pig eye to differentiate three autoantisera. *Int. Arch. Allergy Appl. Immunol.* **48**, 287–93.

Kalsow, C.M. and Wacker, W.B. (1978). Pineal gland involvement in retina-induced experimental allergic uveitis. *Invest. Ophthalmol. Vis. Sci.* **17**, 774–83.

Kamada, Y., Yamada, M., Das, N.D., Samuelson, D., Leverenz, V.R. and Shichi, H. (1985). Preparation of a uveitogenic peptide by chymotryptic digestion of bovine S-antigen. *Invest. Ophthalmol. Vis. Sci.* **26**, 1274–80.

Kaplan, H.J. and Streilein, J.W. (1974). Do immunologically privileged sites require a functioning spleen? *Nature* **251**, 553–54.

Kaplan, H.J. and Streilein, J.W. (1977). Immune response to immunization via the anterior chamber of the eye. I. F1 lymphocyte-induced immune deviation. *J. Immunol.* **118**, 809–13.

Katami, M. (1991). Corneal transplantation-immunologically privileged status. *Eye* **5**, 528–48.

Katz, S.I., Tamaki, K. and Sachs, D.H. (1979). Epidermal Langerhans cells are derived from cells originating in bone marrow. *Nature* **282**, 324–6.

Khodadoust, A.A. and Silverstein, A.M. (1969). Transplantation and rejection of individual cell layers of the cornea. *Invest. Ophthalmol.* **8**, 180–95.

Khodadoust, A.A. and Silverstein, A.M. (1975). Local graft versus host reactions within the anterior chamber of the eye: the formation of corneal endothelial pocks. *Invest. Ophthalmol.* **14**, 640–7.

Khodadoust, A.A. and Silverstein, A.M. (1976). Induction of corneal graft rejection by passive cell transfer. *Invest. Ophthalmol. Vis. Sci.* **15**, 89–95.

Kijlstra, A., Luyendijk, L., van der Gaag, R., van Kregten, E., Linssen, A. and Willers, J.M.N. (1986). IgG and IgA immune response against *Klebsiella* in HLA-B27 associated anterior uveitis. *Br. J. Ophthalmol.* **70**, 85–8.

Knisely, T.L., Luckenbach, M.W., Fischer, B.J. and Niederkorn, J.Y. (1987). Destructive and nondestructive patterns of immune rejection of syngeneic intraocular tumors. *J. Immunol.* **138**, 4515–23.

Kruit, P.J., van der Gaag, R., Broersma, L. and Kijlstra, A. (1985). Circulating antibodies to corneal epithelium in patients with uveitis. *Br. J. Ophthalmol.* **69**, 446–8.

Kruit, P.J., van der Gaag, R., Broersma, L. and Kijlstra, A. (1986). Autoimmunity against corneal antigens. I. Isolation of a soluble 54 Kd corneal epithelium antigen. *Curr. Eye Res.* **5**, 313–20.

Kuhn, H. (1987). Light-regulated binding of rhodopsin kinase and other proteins to cattle photoreceptor membranes. *Biochemistry* **17**, 4389–95.

Kulkarni, R.S. and Srinivasan, B.D. (1988). Cachectin: a novel polypeptide induces uveitis in the rabbit eye. *Exp. Eye Res.* **46**, 631–3 (letter).

Kusuda, M., Gaspari, A.A., Chan, C.C., Gery, I. and Kats, S.I. (1989). Expression of Ia antigen by ocular tissues of mice treated with interferon gamma. *Invest. Ophthalmol. Vis. Sci.* **30**, 764–8.

La Hey, E., Baarsma, G.S., Rothova, A., Broersma, L., van der Gaag, R. and Kijlstra, A. (1988). High incidence of corneal epithelium antibodies in Fuchs' heterochromic cyclitis. *Br. J. Ophthalmol.* **72**, 921–5.

Laitinen, O., Leirisalo, M. and Skylv, G. (1977). Relation between HLA-B27 and clinical features in patients with *Yersinia* arthritis. *Arthritis Rheum.* **20**, 1121–4.

Luntz, M.H. (1968). Anti-uveal and anti-lens antibodies in uveitis and their significance. *Exp. Eye Res.* **7**, 561–9.

Lynch, M.G., Peeler, J.S., Brown, R.H. and Niederkorn, J.Y. (1987). Expression of HLA Class I and II antigens on cells of the human trabecular meshwork. *Ophthalmology* **94**, 851–7.

McAllister, C.G., Wiggert, B., Redmond, T.M., Kuwabara, T., Chader, G.J. and Gery, I. (1986). Uveitogenicity of lymphocytes activated by interphotoreceptor retinoid binding protein (IRBP). *Invest. Ophthalmol. Vis. Sci.* **27** (suppl.), 113.

McDonnell, P.J., Schanzlin, D.J. and Rao, N.A. (1988). Immunoglobulin deposition in the cornea after application of autologous serum. *Arch. Ophthalmol.* **106**, 1423–5.

McKechnie, N.M., Al-Mahdawi, S., Dutton, G. and Forrester, J.V. (1986). Ultrastructural localization of retinal S-antigen in the human retina. *Exp. Eye Res.* **42**, 479–87.

Mapstone, R. and Woodrow, J.C. (1975). HL-A27 and acute anterior uveitis. *Br. J. Ophthalmol.* **59**, 270–5.

Mattila, L., Granfors, K. and Toivanen, A. (1982). Acute anterior uveitis after *Yersinia* infection. *Br. J. Ophthalmol.* **66**, 209–12.

Meyer, P.A.R. (1986). Glaucoma, HLA and the immune system. In *Glaucoma*, ed. J.E. Cairns, vol. I, pp. 395–406, Grune and Stratton, London.

Meyer, P.A.R. (1987). The observation of immune complex formation and deposition in the eyes of living rabbits. *Clin. Exp. Immunol.* **69**, 166–78.

Meyer, P.A.R. (1988). Patterns of blood flow in episcleral vessels studied by low-dose fluorescein videoangiography. *Eye* **2**, 533–46.

Misra, R.N., Rahi, A.H.S. and Morgan, G. (1977). Immunopathology of the lens II. Humoral and cellular immune responses to homologous lens antigens and their roles in ocular inflammation. *Br. J. Ophthalmol.* **61**, 285–96.

Mizuno, K., Clark, A.F. and Streilein, J.W. (1989). Anterior chamber-associated immune deviation induced by soluble antigens. *Invest. Ophthalmol. Vis. Sci.* **30**, 1112–19.

Mochizuki, M., Kuwabara, T., McAllister, C., Nussenblatt, R.B. and Gery, I. (1985). Adoptive transfer of experimental autoimmune uveoretinitis in rats. *Invest. Ophthalmol. Vis. Sci.* **26**, 1–9.

Mohos, S.C. and Wagner, B.M. (1969). Damage to collagen in corneal immune injury. *Arch. Pathol.* **88**, 3–20.

Mondino, B.J., Ratajczak, H.V., Goldberg, D.B., Schanzlin, D.J. and Brown, S.I. (1980). Alternate and classical pathway components of complement in the normal cornea. *Arch. Ophthalmol.* **98**, 346–9.

Mondino, B.J., Laheji, A.K. and Adamu, S.A. (1987). Ocular immunity to *Staphylococcus aureus*. *Invest. Ophthalmol. Vis. Sci.* **28**, 560–4.

Movat, H.Z., Fernando, N.V.P., Uriuhara, T., Weiser, W.J. (1963). Allergic inflammation III. The fine structure of collagen fibrils at sites of antigen–antibody interaction in Arthus-type lesions. *J. Exp. Med.* **118**, 557–64.

Murray, P.I., Hoekzema, R., van Haren, M.A.C., deHon, F.D. and Kijlstra, A. (1990). Aqueous humor interleukin-6 levels in uveitis. *Invest. Ophthalmol. Vis. Sci.* **31**, 917–20.

Niederkorn, J.Y. (1990). Immune privilege and immune regulation in the eye. *Adv. Immunol.* **48**, 191–226.

Niederkorn, J.Y. and Peeler, J.S. (1988). Regional differences in immune regulation: the immunogenic privilege of corneal allografts. *Immunol. Res.* **7**, 247–55.

Niederkorn, J.Y. and Streilein, J.W. (1982). Analysis of antibody production induced by allogeneic tumor cells inoculated into the anterior chamber of the eye. *Transplantation* **33**, 573–7.

Niederkorn, J.Y. and Streilein, J.W. (1983). Intracamerally induced concomitant immunity: mice harboring progressively growing intraocular tumors are immune to spontaneous metastases and secondary tumor challenge. *J. Immunol.* **131**, 2587–94.

Niederkorn, J.Y., Streilein, J.W. and Shadduck, J.A. (1981). Deviant immune responses to allogeneic tumors injected intracamerally and subcutaneously in mice. *Invest. Ophthalmol. Vis. Sci.* **20**, 355–63.

Niederkorn, J.Y., Peeler, J.S. and Mellon, J. (1989). Phagocytosis of particulate antigens by corneal epithelial cells stimulates interleukin-1 secretion and migration of Langerhans cells into the central cornea. *Reg. Immunol.* **2**, 83–90.

Nussenblatt, R.B. and Scher, I. (1985). Effects of cyclosporine on T-cell subsets in experimental autoimmune uveitis. *Invest. Ophthalmol. Vis. Sci.* **26**, 10–14.

Nussenblatt, R.B., Gery, I., Ballintine, E.J. and Wacker, W.B. (1980). Cellular immune responsiveness of uveitis patients to retinal S-antigen. *Am. J. Ophthalmol.* **89**, 173–9.

Nussenblatt, R.B., Rodrigues, M.M., Wacker, W.B., Cevario, S.J., Salinas-Carmona, M.C. and Gery, I. (1981a). Cyclosporin A: inhibition of experimental autoimmune uveitis in Lewis rats. *J. Clin. Invest.* **67**, 1228–31.

Nussenblatt, R.B., Kuwabara, T., de Monasterio, F.M. and Wacker, W.B. (1981b). S-antigen uveitis in primates. *Arch. Ophthalmol.* **99**, 1090–2.

Nussenblatt, R.B., Rodrigues, M.M., Salinas-Carmona, M.C., Gery, I., Cevario, S. and Wacker, W.B. (1982a). Modulation of experimental autoimmune uveitis with cyclosporin A. *Arch. Ophthalmol.* **100**, 1146–9.

Nussenblatt, R.B., Mittal, K.K., Ryan, S., Green, W.R. and Maumenee, A.E. (1982b). Birdshot retinochoroidopathy associated with HLA-A29 antigen and immune responsiveness to retinal S-antigen. *Am. J. Ophthalmol.* **94**, 147–58.

Ohno, S., Nakayama, E., Sugiura, S., Itakura, K., Aoki, K. and Aizawa, M. (1975). Specific histocompatibility antigens associated with Behçet's disease. *Am. J. Ophthalmol* **80**, 636–41.

Ohno, S., Asanuma, T., Sugiura, S., Wakisaka, A., Aizawa, M. and Itakura, K. (1978). HLA-Bw51 and Behçet's disease. *JAMA* **240**, 529 (letter).

Palczewski, K., McDowell, J.H., Jakes, S., Ingebritsen, T.S. and Hargrave, P.A. (1989). Regulation of rhodopsin dephosphorylation by arrestin. *J. Biol. Chem.* **264**, 15770–3.

Peeler, J.S. and Niederkorn, J.Y. (1986). Antigen presentation by Langerhans cells *in vivo*: donor-derived Ia+ Langerhans cells are required for induction of delayed-type hypersensitivity but not for cytotoxic T lymphocyte responses to alloantigens. *J. Immunol.* **136**, 4362–71.

Peeler, J.S., Niederkorn, J.Y. and Matoba, A, (1985). Corneal allografts induce cytotoxic T cell but not delayed hypersensitivity responses in mice. *Invest. Ophthalmol. Vis. Sci.* **26**, 1516–23.

Peeler, J.S., Callanan, D.G., Luckenbach, M.W. and Niederkorn, J.Y. (1988). Presentation of the H-Y antigen on Langerhans' cell-negative corneal grafts downregulates the cytotoxic T cell response and converts responder strain mice into phenotypic nonresponders. *J. Exp. Med.* **168**, 1749–66.

Pepose, J.S., Gardner, K.M., Nestor, M.S., Foos, R.Y. and Pettit, T.H. (1985). Detection of HLA class I and II antigens in rejected human corneal allografts. *Ophthalmology* **92**, 1480–4.

Percopo, C.M., Hooks, J.J., Shinohara, T., Caspi, R. and Detrick B. (1990). Cytokine-mediated activation of a neuronal retinal resident cell provokes antigen presentation. *J. Immunol.* **145**, 4101–7.

Perkins, E.S. and Wood, R.M. (1964). Auto-immunity in uveitis. *Br. J. Ophthalmol.* **48**, 61–9.

Priem, H.A., Kijlstra, A., Nones, L., Baarsma, G.S., DeLaey, J.J. and Oosterhuis, J.A. (1988). HLA typing in birdshot chorioretinopathy. *Am. J. Ophthalmol.* **105**, 182–5.

Rahi, A.H.S. (1979). HLA and eye disease. *Br. J. Ophthalmol.* **63**, 283–92.

Rahi, A.H.S., Misra, R.N. and Morgan, G. (1977). Immunopathology of the lens. I. Humoral and cellular immune responses to heterologous lens antigens and their roles in ocular inflammation. *Br. J. Ophthalmol.* **61**, 164–76.

Raju, S. and Grogan, J.B. (1969). Allograft implants in the anterior chamber of the eye of the rabbit. *Transplantation* **7**, 475–83.

Rao, N.A., Wacker, W.B. and Marak, G.E. (1979). Clinicopathologic features associated with varying doses of S antigen. *Arch. Ophthalmol.* **97**, 1954–8.

Rao, N.A., Atalla, L., Linker-Israeli, M. *et al.* (1989). Suppression of experimental uveitis in rats by anti-I-A antibodies. *Invest. Ophthalmol. Vis. Sci.* **30**, 2348–55.

Ray-Keil, L. and Chandler, J.W. (1985). Rejection of murine heterotopic corneal transplants. *Transplantation* **39**, 473–7.

Robin, J.B., Schanzlin, D.J., Verity, S.M. *et al.* (1986). Peripheral corneal disorders. *Surv. Ophthalmol.* **31**, 1–36.

Rodrigues, M.M., Rowden, G., Hackett, J., and Bakos, I. (1981). Langerhans cells in the normal conjunctiva and peripheral cornea of selected species. *Invest. Ophthalmol. Vis. Sci.* **21**, 759–65.

Rodrigues, M.M., Hackett, J., Gaskins, R. *et al.* (1986). Interphotoreceptor retinoid-binding protein in retinal rod cells and pineal gland. *Invest. Ophthalmol. Vis. Sci.* **27**, 844–50.

Rodrigues, M.M., Hackett, J., Wiggert, B. *et al.* (1987). Immunoelectron microscopic localization of photoreceptor-specific markers in the monkey retina. *Curr. Eye Res.* **6**, 369–80.

Rosenbaum, J.T., McDevitt, H.O., Guss, R.B. and Egbert, P.R. (1980). Endotoxin-induced uveitis in rats as a model for human disease. *Nature* **286**, 611–13.

Rosenbaum, J.T., Samples, J.R., Hefeneider, S.H. and Howes, E.L. (1987). Ocular inflammatory effects of intravitreal interleukin 1. *Arch. Ophthalmol.* **105**, 1117–20.

Rothova, A., Van Veenendaal, W.G., Linssen, A., Glasius, E., Kijlstra, A. and de Jong, P.T.V.M. (1987). Clinical features of acute anterior uveitis. *Am. J. Ophthalmol.* **103**, 137–45.

Rubsamen, P.E., McCulley, J., Bergstresser, P.R. and Streilein, W. (1984). On the Ia immunogenicity of mouse corneal allografts infiltrated with Langerhans cells. *Invest. Ophthalmol. Vis. Sci.* **25**, 513–18.

Ryan, S.J. and Maumenee, A.E. (1980). Birdshot retinochoroidopathy. *Am. J. Ophthalmol.* **89**, 31–45.

Saari, K.M., Laitinen, O., Leirisalo, M. and Saari, R. (1980). Ocular inflammation associated with *Yersinia* infection. *Am. J. Ophthalmol.* **89**, 84–95.

Sandberg, H.O. and Closs, O. (1979a). The humoral immune response to alpha, beta and gamma crystallins of the human lens. *Scand. J. Immunol.* **10**, 549–54.

Sandberg, H.O. and Closs, O. (1979b). The alpha and gamma crystallin content in aqueous humor of eyes with clear lenses and with cataracts. *Exp. Eye Res.* **28**, 601–10.

Schalken, J.J., Winkens, H.J., van Vugt, A.H.M., de Grip, W.J. and Broekhuyse, R.M. (1989). Rhodopsin-induced experimental autoimmune uveoretinitis in monkeys. *Br. J. Ophthalmol.* **73**, 168–72.

Seegal, D. and Seegal, B.C. (1930a). Local organ hypersensitiveness. I. Experimental production in the rabbit eye. *Proc. Soc. Exp. Biol. Med.* **27**, 390–3.

Seegal, D. and Seegal, B.C. (1930b). Local organ hypersensitiveness. II. Repeated response in the rabbit eye. *Proc. Soc. Exp. Biol. Med.* **27**, 393–5.

Seegal, D. and Seegal, B.C. (1931a). Local organ hypersensitiveness. III. Further observations on its experimental production in the rabbit eye. *J. Exp. Med.* **54**, 249–63.

Seegal, D. and Seegal, B.C. (1931b). Local organ hypersensitiveness. IV. Inflammation produced in the actively sensitized rabbit eye by the introduction of homologous antigen into the gastrointestinal tract. *J. Exp. Med.* **54**, 265–9.

Shimada, K. and Silverstein, A.M. (1975). Local antibody formation within the eye: a study of immunoglobulin class and antibody specificity. *Invest. Ophthalmol.* **14**, 573–83.

Shinohara, T., Dietzschold, B., Craft, C.M. *et al.* (1987). Primary and secondary structure of bovine retinal S antigen (48-kDa protein). *Proc. Nat. Acad. Sci. (USA)* **84**, 6975–9.

Sholley, M.M., Gimbrone, M.A. and Cotran, R.S. (1978). The effects of leucocyte depletion on corneal neovascularisation. *Lab. Invest.* **38**, 32–40.

Silverman, B., Alexander, R.J. and Henley, W.L. (1981). Tissue and species specificity of BCP 54, the major soluble protein of bovine cornea. *Exp. Eye. Res.* **33**, 19–29.

Silverstein, A.M. (1974). Immunogenic uveitis. *Trans. Ophthal. Soc. (UK)* **94**, 496–517.

Silverstein, A.M. and Zimmerman, L.E. (1959). Immunogenic endophthalmitis produced in the guinea pig by different pathogenetic mechanisms. *Am. J. Ophthalmol.* **48**, 435–46.

Silverstein, A.M., Welter, S. and Zimmerman, L.E. (1961). A progressive immunization reaction in the actively sensitized rabbit eye. *J. Immunol.* **86**, 312–23.

Singh, V.K., Yamaki, K., Donoso, L.A. and Shinohara, T. (1989). Molecular mimicry: yeast histone H3-induced experimental autoimmune uveitis. *J. Immunol.* **142**, 1512–17.

Singh, V.K., Kalra, H.K., Yamaki, K., Abe, T., Donoso, L.A. and Shinohara, T. (1990). Molecular mimicry between a uveitopathogenic site of S-antigen and viral peptides. *J. Immunol.* **144**, 1282–7.

Smith, R.E., Jensen, A.D. and Silverstein, A.M. (1969). Antibody formation by single cells during experimental immunogenic uveitis. *Invest. Ophthalmol.* **8**, 373–80.

Smolin, G., Hall, J. and Cignetti, F. (1973). The afferent arc of the corneal immunologic reaction: migration inhibitory factor. *Invest. Ophthalmol.* **12**, 152–4.

Spencer, W.H. (1985). Vitreous. In *Ophthalmic Pathology*, ed. W.H. Spencer, pp. 548–88, W.B. Saunders, Co., Philadelphia.

Streilein, J.W. (1990). Anterior chamber associated immune deviation: the privilege of immunity in the eye. *Surv. Ophthalmol.* **35**, 67–73.

Streilein, J.W. and Bergstresser, P.R. (1980). Ia antigens and epidermal Langerhans cells. *Transplantation* **30**, 319–23.

Streilein, J.W. and Niederkorn, J.Y. (1981). Induction of anterior chamber-associated immune deviation requires an intact, functional spleen. *J. Exp. Med.* **153**, 1058–67.

Streilein, J.W., Toews, G.B. and Bergstresser, P.R. (1979). Corneal allografts fail to express Ia antigens. *Nature* **282**, 326–7.

Streilein, J.W., Niederkorn, J.Y. and Shadduck, J.A. (1980). Systemic immune unresponsiveness induced in adult mice by anterior chamber presentation of minor histocompatibility antigens. *J. Exp. Med.* **152**, 1121–5.

Svejgaard, A., Jersild, C., Staub-Nielsen, L. and Bodmer, W.F. (1974). HLA antigens and disease: statistical and genetical considerations. *Tissue Antigens* **4**, 95–105.

Ticho, U., Cole, G.A. and Silverstein, A.M. (1974a). Immunopathologic uveitis in the mouse due to lymphocytic choriomeningitis virus. *Invest. Ophthalmol.* **13**, 33–8.

Ticho, U., Silverstein, A.M. and Cole, G.A. (1974b) Immunopathogenesis of LCM virus-induced uveitis: the role of T lymphocytes. *Invest. Ophthalmol.* **13**, 229–31.

Toews, G.B., Bergstresser, P.R., Streilein, J.W. and Sullivan, S. (1980). Epidermal Langerhans cell density determines whether contact hypersensitivity or unresponsiveness follows skin painting with DNFB. *J. Immunol.* **124**, 445–53.

Treseler, P.A. and Sanfilippo, F. (1985). Humoral immunity to heterotopic corneal allografts in the rat. *Transplantation* **39**, 193–6.

Treseler, P.A. and Sanfilippo, F. (1986). The expression of major histocompatibility complex and leukocyte antigens by cells in the rat cornea. *Transplantation* **41**, 248–52.

Treseler, P.A., Foulks, G.N. and Sanfilippo, F. (1984). The expression of HLA antigens by cells in the human cornea. *Am. J. Ophthalmol.* **98**, 763–72.

Treseler, P.A., Treseler, C.B., Foulks, G.N. and Sanfilippo, F. (1985). Cellular immunity to heterotopic corneal allografts in the rat. *Transplantation* **39**, 196–201.

Treseler, P.A., Foulks, G.N. and Sanfilippo, F. (1986). The relative immunogenicity of corneal epithelium, stroma, and endothelium: the role of major histocompatibility complex antigens. *Transplantation* **41**, 229–34.

Tuberville, A.W., Foster, C.S. and Wood, T.O. (1983). The effect of donor cornea epithelium removal on the incidence of allograft rejection reactions. *Ophthalmology* **90**, 1351–6.

Uusitalo, H., Lehtosalo, J.I., Gregerson, D.S., Uusitalo, R. and Palkama, A. (1985). Ultrastructural localization of retinal S-antigen in the rat. *Graefe's Arch. Clin. Exp. Ophthalmol.* **222**, 118–22.

van der Gaag, R., Broersma, L., Rothova, A., Baarsma, S. and Kijlstra, A. (1989). Immunity to a corneal antigen in Fuchs' heterochromic cyclitis patients. *Invest. Ophthalmol. Vis. Sci.* **30**, 443–8.

van der Lelij, A., Doekes, G., Hwan, B.S. *et al.* (1990a). Humoral autoimmune response against S-antigen and IRBP in ocular onchocerciasis. *Invest. Ophthalmol. Vis. Sci.* **31**, 1374–80.

van der Lelij, A., Rothova, A., Stilma, J.S., Hoekzema, R. and Kijlstra, A. (1990b). Cell-mediated immunity against human retinal extract, S-antigen, and interphotoreceptor retinoid binding protein in onchocercal chorioretinopathy. *Invest. Ophthalmol. Vis. Sci.* **31**, 2031–6.

Vannas, S., Nordman, E. and Teir, H. (1960). Uveitis resembling sympathetic ophthalmia. *Acta Ophthalmol. (Kbh)* **38**, 618–34.

Vistica, P., Usui, M., Kuwabara, T. *et al.* (1986). Interphotoreceptor retinoid binding protein (IRBP) is poorly uveitogenic in guinea pigs and is identical to A-antigen. *Invest. Ophthalmol. Vis. Sci.* **27** (suppl.), 112.

Wacker, W.B. (1972). Autoimmune uveitis (choroiditis) in the guinea pig sensitized with homologous uvea and its differentiation from that following sensitization with homologous retina. *Int. Arch. Allergy* **43**, 39–52.

Wacker, W.B. (1973). Experimental allergic uveitis: studies on characterization of the pathogenic retina antigen. *Int. Arch. Allergy* **45**, 639–56.

Wacker, W.B. and Lipton, M.M. (1965). Experimental allergic uveitis: homologous retina as uveitiogenic antigen. *Nature* **206**, 253–4.

Wacker, W.B., Lipton, M.M. and Ongchua, F.E. (1964). Antibody production in the guinea pig to homologous uvea. *Proc. Soc. Exp. Biol. Med.* **117**, 150–4.

Wacker, W.B., Donoso, L.A., Kalsow, C.M., Yankeelov, J.A. and Organisciak, D.T. (1977). Experimental allergic uveitis: isolation, characterization, and localization of a soluble uveitiopathogenic antigen from bovine retina. *J. Immunol.* **119**, 1949–58.

Wakefield, D. and Penny, R. (1983). Cell-mediated immune response to *chlamydia* in anterior uveitis: role of HLA B27. *Clin. Exp. Immunol.* **51**, 191–6.

Wakefield, D., Stahlberg, T.H., Toivanen, A., Granfors, K. and Tennant, C. (1990). Serologic evidence of *Yersinia* infection in patients with anterior uveitis. *Arch. Ophthalmol.* **108**, 219–21.

Waksman, B.H. and Bullington, S.J. (1956). A quantitative study of the passive Arthus reaction in the rabbit eye. *J. Immunol.* **76**, 441–53.

Waldrep, J.C. and Kaplan, H.J. (1983). Anterior chamber associated immune deviation induced by TNP-splenocytes (TNP-ACAID). *Invest. Ophthalmol. Vis. Sci.* **24**, 1086–92.

Warren, R.E. and Brewerton, D. (1979). *Klebsiella*, spondylitis, and uveitis. *Br. Med. J.* **i**, 889 (letter).

Watson, P.G. (1982). The nature and the treatment of scleral inflammation. *Trans. Ophthal. Soc. (UK)* **102**, 257–81.

Weisz-Carrington, P., Roux, M.E., McWilliams, M., Phillips-Quagliata, J.M. and Lamm, M.E. (1979). Organ and isotype distribution of plasma cells producing specific antibody after oral immunization: evidence for a generalized secretory immune system. *J. Immunol.* **123**, 1705–8.

Welsh, J., Avakian, H. and Ebringer, A. (1981). Uveitis, vitreous humour, and *Klebsiella*. II. Cross-reactivity studies with radioimmunoassay. *Br. J. Ophthalmol.* **65**, 323–8.

Wetzig, R.P., Foster, S. and Greene, M.I. (1982). Ocular immune responses. I. Priming of A/J mice in the anterior chamber with azobenzenearsonate-derivatised cells induces second-order-like suppressor T cells. *J. Immunol.* **128**, 1753–7.

Wetzig, R.P., Hooks, J.J., Percopo, C.M., Nussenblatt, R., Chan, C. and Detrick, B. (1988). Anti-Ia antibody diminishes ocular inflammation in experimental autoimmune uveitis. *Curr. Eye Res.* **7**, 809–18.

White, L., McCoy, R., Tait, B. and Ebringer, R. (1984). A search for Gram-negative enteric micro-organisms in acute anterior uveitis: association of *Klebsiella* with recent onset of disease, HLA-B27, and B27 CREG. *Br. J. Ophthalmol.* **68**, 750–5.

Whitsett, C.F. and Stulting, R.D. (1984). The distribution of HLA antigens on human corneal tissue. *Invest. Ophthalmol. Vis. Sci.* **25**, 519–24.

Whittum, J.A., Niederkorn, J.Y., McCulley, J.P. and Streilein, J.W. (1984). Role of suppressor T cells in herpes simplex virus-induced immune deviation. *J. Virol.* **51**, 556–8.

Wilbanks, G.A. and Streilein, J.W. (1990). Characterization of suppressor cells in anterior chamber-associated immune deviation (ACAID) induced by soluble antigen: evidence of two functionally and phenotypically distinct T-suppressor cell populations. *Immunology* **71**, 383–9.

Wilbanks, G.A. and Streilein, J.W. (1991). Studies on the induction of anterior chamber-associated immune deviation (ACAID). I. Evidence that an antigen-specific, ACAID-inducing, cell-associated signal exists in the peripheral blood.

J. Immunol. **146**, 2610–17.

Wilbanks, G.A., Mammolenti, M. and Streilein, J.W. (1991). Studies on the induction of anterior chamber-associated immune deviation (ACAID). II. Eye-derived cells participate in generating blood-borne signals that induce ACAID. *J. Immunol.* **146**, 3018–24.

Wilden, U., Hall, S.W. and Kuhn, H. (1986). Phosphodiesterase activation by photoexcited rhodopsin is quenched when rhodopsin is phosphorylated and binds the intrinsic 48-kDa protein of rod outer segments. *Proc. Nat. Acad. Sci. (USA)* **83**, 1174–8.

Williams, K.A., Ash, J.K. and Coster, D.J. (1985). Histocompatibility antigen and passenger cell content of normal and diseased human cornea. *Transplantation* **39**, 265–9.

Williamson, J.S.P. and Streilein, J.W. (1989). Induction of delayed hypersensitivity to alloantigens coinjected with Langerhans cells into the anterior chamber of the eye: abrogation of anterior chamber-associated immune deviation. *Transplantation* **47**, 519–24.

Williamson, J.S.P., DiMarco, S. and Streilein, J.W. (1987). Immunobiology of Langerhans cells on the ocular surface. I. Langerhans cells within the central cornea interfere with induction of anterior chamber associated immune deviation. *Invest. Ophthalmol. Vis. Sci.* **28**, 1527–32.

Williamson, J.S.P., Bradley, D., Streilein, J.W. (1989). Immunoregulatory properties of bone marrow-derived cells in the iris and ciliary body. *Immunology* **67**, 96–102.

Willshaw, H.E. (1981). Acute anterior uveitis and *Klebsiella aerogenes*: a causal relationship? *Br. J. Ophthalmol.* **65**, 796–7.

Wirostko, E. and Spalter, H.F. (1967). Lens-induced uveitis. *Arch. Ophthalmol.* **78**, 1–7.

Witmer, R. (1978). Clinical implications of aqueous humor studies in uveitis. *Am. J. Ophthalmol.* **86**, 39–45.

Wong, V.G., Angerson, R.R. and McMaster, P.R.B. (1971). Endogenous immune uveitis. *Arch. Ophthalmol.* **85**, 93–102.

Young, E., Stark, W.J. and Prendergast, R.A. (1985). Immunology of corneal allograft rejection: HLA-DR antigens on human corneal cells. *Invest. Ophthalmol. Vis. Sci.* **26**, 571–4.

Young, R.W. and Bok, D. (1969). Participation of the retinal pigment epithelium in the rod outer segment renewal process. *J. Cell Biol.* **42**, 392–403.

Yu, D.T.Y., Choo, S.Y. and Schaack, T. (1989). Molecular mimicry in HLA-B27 related arthritis. *Ann. Intern. Med.* **111**, 581–91.

Zimmerman, L.E. and Silverstein, A.M. (1959). Experimental ocular hypersensitivity: histopathologic changes observed in rabbits receiving a single injection of antigen into the vitreous. *Am. J. Ophthalmol.* **48**, 447–63.

108: Reproductive Immunopathology

P.M. Johnson

Introduction

The natural model posed by pregnancy is a fascinating, yet not fully explored, research area within the wider spectrum of immunology. Attention has long been drawn to the uniqueness of the conceptus as an allograft and to identification of immunobiological mechanisms normally employed by the pregnant mother to tolerate and nourish a haplo-non-identical fetus *in utero* (see Chapter 40). Our understanding of the immunological adaptations which take place in pregnancy is now leading to a range of significant implications regarding both maternal disease and fetal well-being. It is the aim of this chapter to summarize the immunopathological basis of relevant clinical events and recent medical applications. The rapid pace of current advances in reproductive biotechnology, directed towards improved fecundity, prenatal diagnosis of genetic disorders and reproductive models as bizarre as interspecies chimeras, will undoubtedly result in yet further practical insight into reproductive immunopathology.

Infertility

Anti-sperm antibodies can arise in both men and women, but the interpretation of some of the laboratory assays and correlation with clinical infertility have raised some concerns in the past (Bronson *et al*. 1984; Hjort *et al*. 1985; Haas 1987). Infertility secondary to anti-sperm antibody may occur in up to 20% of couples with unexplained infertility, although this is more clinically significant in the male than in the female (Hjort *et al*. 1985). The presence of antibodies in the local genital tract, which are locally produced in cervicovaginal tissue and secreted into the mucus in the female, or bound to sperm or in seminal plasma in the male, is more significant than their detection only in serum (Jones 1987). Men with sperm autoimmunity are more likely to have female partners who also demonstrate immunity to sperm. Sperm antibody titres may be higher when autologous sperm (for autoantibodies in the male) or partner's sperm (for isoantibodies in the female) is used and compared with unrelated donor sperm, although most male and female anti-sperm antibodies are not individual-specific (Jones 1987). It is also a general observation that anti-sperm antibodies are mostly tissue-specific and unrelated to any systemic immunological or general medical disorder.

Anti-sperm antibodies may potentially influence fertility in many separate ways: disruption of spermiogenesis, impairing sperm transport, autoagglutination or cytotoxic immobilization of ejaculated sperm, antibody-mediated phagocytosis, prevention of cervical mucus penetration, interference with sperm capacitation or the acrosome reaction, blockage of functional molecules (e.g. sperm enzymes or sperm–ovum interaction sites), or disruption of the preimplantation embryo since sperm antigens may be incorporated into the early zygote. There is a correspondingly large number of methods for assay of anti-sperm antibodies, based on agglutination, immobilization and immunoglobulin-specific binding techniques, which may be applied to serum, liquefied cervical mucus or seminal plasma (Haas 1987; Jones 1987). Titres obtained in assays employing viable sperm (e.g. the tray agglutination test or immunobead binding test) have a much better correlation with clinical infertility than those using dead sperm or solubilized sperm fractions (e.g. enzyme-linked immunosorbent assay (ELISA) or immunofluorescence on fixed material), presumably in part because of their focus towards cell surface structures (Hjort *et al.* 1985). Antibodies of the immunoglobulin A (IgA) isotype appear to be the main mediators of clinical infertility and the location of binding to sperm (i.e. head and/or tail) may also be important, although there are no absolute guidelines as to the precise location or number of bound anti-sperm antibodies necessary to have a detrimental effect on reproduction (Bronson *et al.* 1984; Haas 1987). The immunobead binding test allows both isotyping and identification of the site of binding of anti-sperm antibodies (Clarke 1987). Agglutination assays are susceptible to false positive results due to agglutination by factors other than antibodies.

Overt systemic cell-mediated immunity to sperm is very uncommon and of much less clinical significance than humoral immunity, although certain cytokines, notably tumour necrosis factor alpha (TNF-α) and interferon-gamma (IFN-γ), have been shown to impair both human sperm motility and fertilization ability (Hill and Anderson 1988). Hence, local immune cellular disturbances in cytokine production in both the male and female reproductive tract tissues (e.g. during infection) could also be relevant in some cases of infertility. Although lymphocytic infiltration has been described in a small number of testicular biopsies from infertile men, the precise cellular immunological phenomena in the testis or elsewhere in male tissues that may lead to the onset of autoimmunity remain obscure (Lehmann and Emmons 1989). Nevertheless, clinical clues regarding previous infection, trauma or anatomical abnormalities can sometimes be identified that may assist in the appropriate selection of infertile couples for evaluation of antibody-mediated infertility (Haas 1987). Behavioural practices can also be relevant, and both prostitutes and homosexual men are at increased risk of developing anti-sperm antibodies (Haas 1987).

Other serum antibodies directed against zona pellucida, ovarian, endometrial or embryo/trophoblast antigens have all been implicated in the pathogenesis of reproductive failure, although none have been either reproducibly identified or shown to express a clear correlation with clinical infertility (Hjort *et al.* 1985; Hill and Anderson 1988).

Endometriosis

Endometriosis is the occurrence of endometrial tissue at ectopic (extrauterine) locations; this occurs most frequently at peritoneal sites and occasionally at sites remote from the pelvis. It accounts for a significant proportion of major gynaecological surgery and is the most common female reason for reproductive failure. The anatomical distortions that occur in moderate or severe stages of this condition will contribute a physical aspect to reduced fertility but, in mild disease, the mechanisms and level of interaction between endometriosis and infertility have been difficult to determine (Olive and Haney 1986). Causative factors for endometriosis are still not clearly established. Retrograde menstruation, a common phenomenon in women of reproductive age, has been implicated, but this does not explain its occurrence at pelvically remote sites and the correlation is by no means absolute. Dissemination by vascular and lymphatic routes, as well as surgical interventions, may be contributory and it has been proposed that an altered immune responsiveness could render some women more predisposed to develop endometriosis (Demowski *et al.* 1981; Steele *et al.* 1984).

Circulating autoantibodies to endometrial gland epithelial cells and ovarian antigens, as well as anti-phospholipid autoantibodies (APA) and other autoantibodies, have been reported in endometriosis (Mathur *et al.* 1982; Wild and Shivers 1985; Gleicher *et al.* 1987; Taylor *et al.* 1991), although these have not been confirmed in all studies (Switchenko *et al.* 1991). Studies in infertile women with endometriosis have indicated a relative reduction in CD3 +ve T cell-mediated cytotoxicity (Steele *et al.* 1984), and an apparent reduction in major histocompatibility complex (MHC)-non-restricted natural killer (NK) activity against autologous endometrium has been reported in endometriosis (Oosterlynck *et al.* 1991). It is not clear whether these findings are incidental or indicate a true association: indeed, autoimmunity or impaired cellular immunity could be consequent to endometriosis rather than causative (Hill 1992). Although there is a genetic association, in that 7% of first-degree relatives of endometriosis cases are also affected, unlike many autoimmune diseases no linkage with any human leucocyte antigen (HLA) allele has yet been established (Simpson *et al.* 1984).

Whilst studies on peripheral blood leucocytes have produced little useful information, investigation of leucocytes taken from peritoneal fluid samples or uterine endometrial tissue may prove more illuminating. Indeed, there is strong evidence for increased numbers of leucocyte populations in the peritoneal fluid of infertile women with endometriosis, most particularly macrophages (Halme *et al.* 1982; Hill *et al.* 1988). An increase in peritoneal macrophages has also been noted in subfertile compared with fertile women, even in the absence of endometriosis (Olive *et al.* 1985; Hill *et al.* 1988), and it has been suggested that this is more strongly associated with the infertility than the endometriosis (Olive *et al.* 1991). Peritoneal macrophages in endometriotic patients are highly activated compared with those from normal women, and there has been varied unresolved speculation about mechanisms by which they could contribute to infertility (Halme *et al.* 1987; Zeller *et al.* 1987). Peritoneal T lymphocytes (mostly CD4 +ve T helper cells) and NK cells are also more abundant in endometriosis, but B lymphocytes and plasma cells are rarely, if ever, found (Hill *et al.* 1988).

The possible local involvement of cytokines and growth factors in influencing the progression of endometriosis and associated infertility is also becoming the subject of increasing research interest. For example, the colony-stimulating factors (CSFs), interleukin 6 (IL-6) and TNF-α are produced extensively in endometrial tissue, and elevated levels of IL-1, IL-2, TNF-α and IFN-γ have been noted in the peritoneal fluid of sub-fertile women with endometriosis compared with fertile women without endometriosis (Halme *et al.* 1988; Hill 1992).

Maternofetal blood cell incompatibilities

Maternal isoimmunization to paternally inherited blood cell surface antigens expressed in the fetus can occur in pregnancy and results from leakage of fetal cells into maternal circulation, mostly at parturition (Jones and Need 1988). Selective transplacental transfer of IgG from maternal blood to bestow passive immunity to the fetus occurs from about the 20th week of gestation, and hence any maternal IgG antibody to fetal blood cell surface antigens will often pose a potential threat to the health of the offspring. Blood group incompatibility is clinically the most significant occurrence, although pregnancy-induced isoimmunization to platelets and leucocytes may also occur. However, maternal IgG anti-leucocyte antibodies are generally benign and do not prejudice perinatal wellbeing because of placental sequestration (Jazwinska *et al.* 1987; Jones and Need 1988; see also Chapter 40). Maternal IgG anti-neutrophil antibodies have been described, which may cause transient neonatal neutropenia, but these are extremely rare.

Maternal pregnancy-induced IgG anti-erythrocyte antibody may cross into the fetus in a subsequent pregnancy and provoke haemolysis by complement-dependent lysis and possibly by antibody-dependent cell-mediated cytotoxicity (ADCC), as well as opsonization which facilitates phagocytosis and intracellular lysis of fetal erythrocytes, and can result in severe anaemia, jaundice, hydrops and fetal death. The most common serious example involves rhesus (Rh) antigens, and the clinicopathological manifestations and management of haemolytic disease of the fetus and new-born have been described in great detail (Jones and Need 1988). Treatment for severe disease can involve intrauterine transfusion, plasmaphaeresis, pharmaceutical immunosuppression or, possibly, high-dose intravenous immunoglobulin (Jones and Need 1988). The widespread prophylactic use of Rh(D)-immune IgG fractions to prevent sensitization (Clarke 1982) has, however, significantly reduced the incidence of Rh haemolytic disease; this approach demonstrates successful specific antibody-mediated immune suppression, probably by accelerating removal of fetal Rh(D) +ve erythrocytes in the spleen before maternal sensitization occurs. Along the road of development of the topic of reproductive immunology, prophylactic immunization against Rh haemolytic disease represents one of the few major therapeutic advances in all of medicine that is not based on surgical or pharmacological intervention.

Although antibodies in the ABO blood group system are predominantly of the IgM isotype and hence cannot cross prenatally into the fetal compartment, occasional ABO blood group incompatibilities can cause mild neonatal haemolysis, notably in group O mothers (Jones and Need 1988). However, severe haemolytic disease may be produced by other blood group incompatibilities, particularly of the Kell (K) and Duffy (Fy) antigen systems (Beal 1979). Maternal antibodies to Lewis (Le) and other blood group antigens can also develop in pregnancy, although these do not generally cause haemolytic disease since fetal erythrocytes do not express surface antigens at sufficient density (Beal 1979).

Neonatal thrombocytopenia due to placental transfer of maternal IgG antibody, resulting from isoimmunization by fetal platelets, is rarer than disease caused by maternal IgG anti-platelet autoantibodies. Testing of maternal and neonatal platelets will determine whether the maternal antibody is reactive with both (due to autoimmunity) or only the neonatal platelets (due to isoimmunization). Iso(allo)immune thrombocytopenia of the neonate can be severe and fatal following intracranial haemorrhage but, if treated adequately with maternal platelets, is benign and transient for a length of time in keeping with the half-life of the offending maternal IgG antibody in fetal circulation following parturition (Jones and Need 1988).

Autoimmune disease

The hormonal and immunological perturbations that occur in pregnancy can have various effects on the progression of autoimmune disorders such as systemic lupus erythematosus (SLE), as well as vice versa — i.e. maternal autoimmune disorders can have adverse effects on the well-being of pregnancy (Gatenby 1989; Scott and Bird 1990). However, there is often conflict about the impact of pregnancy-related events on the course of maternal autoimmune disease. Thus, several autoimmune diseases, perhaps most notably rheumatoid arthritis, are known to remit during pregnancy but symptoms may rebound soon after pregnancy, whereas SLE may be exacerbated during and immediately after pregnancy and often requires careful clinical management (Scott 1984; Scott and Bird 1990). In the context of clinical immunology, nevertheless, some correlations are emerging between fetal and neonatal effects and particular types of maternal autoantibody.

Anti-phospholipid autoantibody

Anti-phospholipid autoantibodies (APA) are autoantibodies of pathogenic significance that are directed against negatively charged phospholipids. They can be detected by the prolongation of phospholipid-dependent coagulation times *in vitro*, even after plasma is mixed with an equal quantity of normal plasma (misnamed the lupus anticoagulant test), by either ELISA or radioimmunoassay (RIA) against cardiolipin or separated negatively charged phospholipid fractions, or by the biologically false positive Venereal Disease Reference Laboratory flocculation test (Scott 1984; Taylor 1988; Triplett 1989). There is overlap between these assays, but they are by no means concordant and hence detect an overlapping family of APA. They can occur as IgM or IgG or both, and are present in 15–20% of SLE patients as well as in various myeloproliferative disorders and in acute infectious and other connective tissue diseases. Antiphospholipid autoantibodies, and paradoxically the related lupus anticoagulant, promote thrombosis *in vivo* through numerous complex prothrombotic mechanisms and interference with platelet-endothelial cell interactions (Taylor 1988; Mackworth-Young 1990). Thrombotic episodes are thus the most striking clinical manifestation, although APA are associated with a syndrome also involving thrombocytopenia and intrauterine fetal death, as well as additional features such as neurological complaints, livedo reticularis and other obstetric complications including pre-eclampsia and intrauterine growth retardation (Branch *et al*. 1985; Mackworth-Young 1990).

A proportion (up to 10%) of recurrent miscarriage (RM) patients will have significant serum APA levels, although they need not necessarily have clinical evidence of connective tissue disease at the time of investigation (Scott 1984; Johnson and Ramsden 1988; Taylor *et al*. 1990; Out *et al*. 1991). Low or transient levels can occur in many asymptomatic women, although screening in early pregnancy is also advised for APA −ve women with a history of thrombosis or fetal loss. There is a correlation between maternal APA and recurrent intrauterine death in all three trimesters of pregnancy, presumably following spiral artery vasculopathy and intervillous thrombosis leading to placental infarction, although a direct effect of maternal serum APA on fetal placental trophoblast cannot yet be excluded (Lockshin *et al*. 1985; Scott *et al*. 1987). However, APA have also been detected in the normal obstetric population and it is clear that therapy is not always required for acceptable outcomes in patients without other risk factors (Lockwood *et al*. 1989; Triplett 1989). Treatment has been carried out largely on an empirical basis although, without treatment, fetal prognosis is poor in a pregnancy with a history of repeated fetal loss. Therapeutic doses of heparin anticoagulation, prednisone with low-dose aspirin or high-dose intravenous immunoglobulin have been reported to correct the serological detection of APA, with subsequent successful delivery of healthy off-spring (Scott *et al*. 1987; Johnson and Ramsden 1988; Triplett 1989). However, comparative randomized therapeutic trials have not been completed, and treatment may not always alleviate the underlying pathophysiological situation. In addition, complications have been described involving pre-eclampsia, intrauterine growth retardation and a severe maternal post-partum syndrome of cardipulmonary disease and fever (Kochenour *et al*. 1987; Scott *et al*. 1987).

Other maternal autoantibodies and neonatal autoimmune disease

Systemic lupus erythematosus sera contain multiple autoantibodies directed against nucleic acid, nucleoproteins, cell surface antigens and phospholipids. The detection of a particular serum autoantibody, however, does not necessarily imply a pathological process. One particular IgG autoantibody to a soluble ribonucleoprotein, anti-Ro (SS-A), is found in approximately 25% of SLE patients and 50% of patients with Sjögren's syndrome (Scott 1984). This autoantibody is associated with photosensitive cutaneous lesions and renal damage, usually in mild SLE, but has also been reported in asymptomatic antinuclear autoantibody −ve women. Similar neonatal lupus-like skin lesions may occur in offspring of SLE mothers due to passively acquired maternal autoantibody, and the clinical course of this neonatal lupus erythematosus (NLE) parallels the disappearance of maternal anti-Ro (SS-A) from fetal circulation (Scott 1984; Scott and Bird 1990). Most attention has focused on the potential role of anti-Ro (SS-A) antibodies, but there are data to suggest anti-La (SS-B) ribonuclear protein can also have a part to play (Provost *et al*. 1987; Taylor 1988).

There can also be haemolytic anaemia and thrombocytopenia in NLE, although the most dramatic association of anti-Ro (SS-A) autoantibodies is with congenital complete heart block (CCHB) (Scott *et al*. 1983). Anti-Ro (SS-A) and anti-La (SS-B) autoantibodies have been identified in all mothers of babies with CCHB and in 100% of affected neonates. This lesion of CCHB is permanent, whilst other neonatal symptoms resulting from passive transfer of maternal IgG autoantibody are short-lived. Although strongly associated with the transplacental passage of maternal autoantibody, the pathogenesis is not clear; indeed, postulated mechanisms have to account for why there is no evidence of a related pathological effect in the mother herself.

It is well established that various other maternal IgG autoantibodies will cross the placenta and can cause passively acquired fetal or neonatal autoimmune disease, such as myasthenia gravis, haemolytic anaemia, thyroid disease and autoimmune thrombocytopenic purpura; the mechanistic and clinical descriptions of these specific conditions have been covered in depth elsewhere (Johnson 1988; Taylor 1988; Scott and Bird 1990; see also Chapter 95).

Pemphigoid gestationis

Pemphigoid gestationis (PG) is a bullous skin disorder induced only by pregnancy, including molar pregnancy with no fetus or fetal circulation. Although very uncommon, it is particularly fascinating since pregnancy itself may cause the autoimmune disorder. The diagnosis of PG (previously termed herpes gestationis) centres on immunohistological demonstration of C3 complement deposition at the basement membrane zone of skin. A serum complement-binding IgG autoantibody which binds to this site can also be found in PG sera. The clinical and immunological similarities between PG and bullous pemphigoid suggest that the IgG autoantibody may be provoked by an immune response to a placental antigen that is cross-reactive with the skin basement membrane zone. Ortonne *et al.* (1987) have emphasized antigenic similarities also between amniotic and skin basement membrane zones, although the former is not normally exposed to the maternal immune system. There is a strong association of PG with HLA-DR3 and DR4, as well as with the HLA-A1, B8, DR3 haplotype, reflecting an immunogenetic susceptibility to autoimmune reactions. Increased numbers of Class II MHC +ve leucocytes have been identified in the chorionic villous stroma of the placentas of PG cases compared with normal pregnancy (Borthwick *et al.* 1985). The paternal genetic component is important since PG usually recurs with subsequent pregnancies unless there has been a change of sexual partner or the possibility of complete HLA-DR compatibility between mother and fetus (Holmes *et al.* 1983). The identity of the provoking placental antigen is still unknown.

Recurrent miscarriage

Much recent attention has been directed towards elucidating possible immunological mechanisms, in addition to autoimmunity (see previous section), in women suffering repeated early fetal loss. Recurrent miscarriage is usually defined in the UK by the occurrence of three or more consecutive spontaneous abortions with no more than one live birth or pregnancy exceeding 28 weeks' gestation. The prevalence of RM is around 1% of the gravida III or more female population (Johnson and Ramsden 1988). Causative or contributory factors may be identified in a proportion of these women, e.g. parental chromosomal abnormalities, cervicouterine structural malformations, corpus luteum deficiencies, prostacyclin deficiency, thrombocythaemia or preexisting maternal thyroid or other endocrine disorders (Ramsden and Johnson 1992). In at least 50% of cases, however, no predisposing mechanism can be identified (Stirrat 1990; Coulam 1991; Ramsden and Johnson 1992). These women fall into an, as yet, unexplained group of RM patients essentially by exclusion of other causes, and it is unjustified to assume a single mechanism for all these cases.

Several lines of investigation and proposals for treatment have been based on the hypothesis that certain cases of unexplained RM may be allied to some aspect of failure in early pregnancy of maternal immune adaptation to the genetically dissimilar fetal allograft, in a manner somewhat analogous to organ transplant rejection. This could involve intrinsic maternal hyporesponsiveness (which would not be specific to one partner) or a lack of maternal recognition due to repeated maternal–fetal identity of a relevant genetically polymorphic alloantigen (which would be specific to one partner).

Immunological and immunogenetic studies

Marked polymorphism within the MHC contributes substantially to fetomaternal genetic disparity. Since HLA antigens encoded within the MHC region are the focus of mechanisms of T cell restriction and allograft rejection, they may play a central role in the immunogenetic enigma of reproduction (Johnson and Ramsden 1988). Additional molecules with relevant immunobiological activities are also encoded within the MHC region, e.g. the closely linked genes for TNF-α and β as well as the tandem genes for the fourth component of complement (C4A and C4B). Significant HLA segregation distortion does not occur in man, but it is attractive to propose a connection between parental HLA haplotypes and risk of pregnancy miscarriage (Gill 1987).

Initial investigations suggested increased parental HLA sharing in RM, although inconsistent as to which Class I and II MHC loci were involved (McIntyre *et al.* 1986; Coulam *et al.* 1987; Reznikoff-Etievant *et al.* 1988). There have also been difficulties related to inconsistencies in patient referral patterns and local patient selection policy, low study numbers, the choice of an appropriate control group and data handling for HLA 'blanks'. Other investigations have shown parental HLA sharing to be of uncertain statistical significance and, more importantly, of neither diagnostic or prognostic value (Johnson *et al.* 1988; Christiansen *et al.* 1989). Indeed, HLA-identical fetomaternal combinations can be found among normal term pregnancies (Jazwinska *et al.* 1987) just as, conversely, completely HLA-haplo-non-identical combinations can be found in donor oocyte pregnancies. Additional studies have shown no consistent differences in HLA antigen or C4 allotype frequencies, although an increased prevalence of both HLA-B and C4A homozygosity in RM women has been reported (Johnson *et al.* 1988; Risk and Johnson 1992). Analysis of the genomic MHC region by restriction fragment length polymorphism (RFLP), using HLA-B, C, E, F, G, DQA1, TNF-α and C4 locus-specific gene probes, disclosed no consistent differences in banding patterns for RM women compared with controls (Risk and Johnson 1992). Thus, although tissue-typing data may suggest possible involvement of MHC genes in at least some cases of RM, genetic differences within the MHC region cannot be identified by RFLP analysis. Nevertheless, studies of MHC haplotype inheritance and fetal loss in sisters of RM women have indeed indicated that RM can be associated with a gene segregating on chromosome 6 (Christiansen *et al.* 1990).

There are no consistent differences in mean absolute numbers or relative percentages of the major peripheral blood T lymphocyte subpopulations in RM women compared with controls (Chia and Johnson 1987). Other studies have suggested decreased intrinsic maternal cellular responsiveness to paternal stimulator cells in the mixed lymphocyte culture reaction (MLR) for RM couples compared with controls (McIntyre *et al.* 1986), although this may not be a consistent phenomenon and could result from the marginally increased maternal–paternal HLA sharing (Johnson and Ramsden 1988). The production of so-called 'blocking antibodies', which inhibit a wide variety of *in vitro* lymphocyte proliferation or function assays, most notably the MLR, is a common feature in normal pregnancy (Johnson and Ramsden 1988; see also Chapter 40); these may be absent from RM women either during or after unsuccessful pregnancies (Beer *et al.* 1985), although consistent results in MLR inhibition may require up to 29% serum concentration (Takakuwa *et al.* 1990). Doubt remains about these observations since: (i) other pregnancy-related serum components, notably steroidal hormones, may be influential at such high concentrations; (ii) blocking antibody may be a consequence rather than a cause of successful pregnancy; and (iii) the interpretation of results may vary according to the equation used to calculate the inhibitory effect (Johnson and Ramsden 1988; Sargent *et al.* 1988; Park *et al.* 1990).

There is no evidence for overt maternal cell-mediated reactivity to paternal antigens being a common factor in pregnancy (Sargent *et al.* 1988), although up to 15% of women may develop serum antipaternal lymphocytotoxic antibody (LCA) after their first pregnancy. Lymphocytotoxic antibodies have been detected in only approximately 10% of all multigravid unexplained RM women (Johnson *et al.* 1988). This was interpreted initially as reflecting immunological hyporesponsiveness to fetal antigens in RM; a more pertinent comparison is with women who have had three or more elective first-trimester pregnancy terminations, who demonstrate a similar prevalence of serum LCA to that in RM (Biddle *et al.* 1987). Thus, sensitization for LCA responses is infrequent in first-trimester pregnancy.

There have been no consistent immunopathological reports of immune-mediated attack in the placentas of spontaneously aborted fetuses, although there can be difficulties in obtaining such fresh tissues and possible confusion with post-abortion inflammatory cellular changes (Bulmer 1988). Khong *et al.* (1987) have suggested that defective trophoblastic vascular invasion may be a cause of recurrent abortion, although this has also been described in pre-eclampsia and small-for-gestational-age infants. Decidual leucocyte populations, notably the characteristic CD3 −ve CD56 +ve granulated leucocyte population

(Bulmer *et al.* 1991), may deserve further study, since endometrial leucocytes with smaller cytoplasmic granules than usual have been associated with incipient abortion (Michel *et al.* 1989). Indeed, rodent models of spontaneous fetal resorption in pregnancy may operate via mechanisms involving NK cell attack against the fetoplacental unit (Gendron and Baines 1988). There are several rodent immunogenetic breeding combinations that are particularly susceptible to recurrent early fetal loss, although many of these examples may reflect endogenous genetic factors together with exogenous pathogens, endotoxins or environmental stimuli (Johnson and Ramsden 1988).

Immunotherapy

The earlier investigational studies formed the original basis for deliberate immunization with paternal or third-party unmatched leucocytes in RM in order to prime for immunoregulatory alloresponses other than by pregnancy (Beer *et al.* 1981; Taylor and Faulk 1981). The broad hypothesis that a proportion of hitherto unexplained RM cases can be ascribed to failure of normal active maternal immune adaptation to early pregnancy has provoked extensive debate of controversial concepts (Scott *et al.* 1987; Johnson and Ramsden 1988; Hill 1990).

The dose, route(s) and frequency of leucocyte immunization have varied significantly between centres, as have patient selection criteria and follow-up rates. Reports of 50–90% successful pregnancy outcome following immunization have accumulated steadily, although the vast majority of leucocyte immunization programmes have been uncontrolled open studies (McIntyre *et al.* 1986; Unander and Lindholm 1986; Reznikoff-Etievant *et al.* 1988; Gatenby *et al.* 1989; Cowchock *et al.* 1990; Takakuwa *et al.* 1990). One randomized controlled trial showed a 78% pregnancy success following immunization with paternal leucocytes, compared with 37% following administration of control autologous leucocytes (Mowbray *et al.* 1985). However, two more recent reports of randomized controlled studies, one using a similar method of paired sequential analysis, have shown no statistically significant benefit of paternal leucocyte immunization in RM and the control groups achieved pregnancy success outcome figures of the order of 70% (Cauchi *et al.* 1991; Ho *et al.* 1991). There may also be some inherent risks in administering viable leucocytes to healthy women, such as sensitization to HLA or other leucocyte antigens, or to platelet or blood group antigens; the latter could compromise a pregnancy following paternal cell immunization. Other transfusion-related risks are also potentially increased, notably following third-party immunization, such as cytomegalovirus or human immunodeficiency virus (HIV) transmission by viable leucocytes (Johnson 1988).

An alternative, but conceptually similar, approach has been assessed using an intravenous infusion of isolated sterile syncytiotrophoblast microvillous plasma membrane vesicle preparations. This mimics the fetal cell contact with maternal blood that occurs normally in pregnancy, and has an advantage in that it uses purified nonviable material that will not provoke sensitization to HLA, blood group or platelet antigens (Johnson and Ramsden 1988). However, a randomized double-blind placebo-controlled trial, as well as comparative open studies, with strict clinically defined groups of RM women, has shown no significant difference in subsequent pregnancy outcome whether immunotherapy, placebo or no immunotherapy was used (Johnson *et al.* 1991; Ramsden and Johnson 1992). The successful pregnancy outcome figures of around 60–65% in all subsequent pregnancies are comparable with results from recent retrospective and prospective epidemiological studies (Vlaanderen and Treffers 1987; Parazzini *et al.* 1988; Houwert-de Jong *et al.* 1989; Regan *et al.* 1989).

'Placebo effects' are undoubtedly strong in these immunotherapeutic studies in RM and current opinion is leaning towards, at best, only a small proportion that may be helped by such intervention. However, there is now little of a conceptual framework for this approach to be effective at a systemic level since extensive laboratory investigations have provided many leads but, as yet, no consistent results applicable to clinical use in the counselling or management of unexplained RM patients. As active immunization is not an insignificant procedure, further developments in laboratory investigation are required to improve patient selection and to avoid offering false hope. In the meantime, unexplained RM patients should be investigated fully before pregnancy and in early pregnancies for other possible aetiologies, including subclinical autoimmunity, and should receive immunotherapy only in a research context at specialist centres within the confines of further tightly controlled, randomized, clinical efficacy studies.

Pre-eclamptic toxaemia

Numerous concepts, including immunological causes, have been put forward to account for the aetiopathogenesis of pre-eclamptic toxaemia (PET), which is the main cause of maternal mortality in pregnancy. Pre-eclamptic toxaemia is a pregnancy-specific disorder, which may be characterized by maternal hypertension, proteinuria, oedema, abnormal activation of the coagulation system and fetal compromise due to disturbed placental function (Jenkins 1988). The disease can be asymptomatic until it is far advanced and eclampsia, the convulsive phase, is imminent. Clinical presentation is heterogeneous, and hence the aetiology may be multifactorial. Pre-eclamptic toxaemia is a disorder of the second half of pregnancy, more common in primigravidae, and either previous pregnancy or blood transfusions, as well as possibly more frequent preconceptual exposure to sperm or seminal plasma antigens, may be protective (Redman 1980; Need *et al.* 1983).

These observations have led to the hypothesis that PET may result from an inadequate maternal immune adaptation to pregnancy, notably in primigravidae or a first pregnancy with a new partner, and hence is a disorder of maternofetal incompatibility. However, specific immunological evidence is tenuous and gives only inconclusive support. A lower prevalence of pregnancy-induced antibodies to paternal HLA may occur in PET than in uncomplicated pregnancy, as well as an abnormal MLR between parents (Jenkins *et al.* 1977; Sargent *et al.* 1982). Other studies, in contrast, have shown no difference in antigen- or mitogen-induced lympho-proliferative responses between PET and normal pregnancy (Alanen and Lassila 1982) and hence there is little concordance of information on cell-mediated immunity. Furthermore, any relationship of immune changes to the intravascular coagulation or decreased fibrinolysis observed in PET, or to changes in the renin–angiotensin system, remain undefined (Jenkins 1988).

The placenta is of central importance, since PET can occur in complete hydatidiform molar pregnancy in the absence of fetal tissue or circulation and always regresses immediately on placental removal. Histopathological studies have shown that endovascular cytotrophoblast invasion into the spiral arteries in the placental bed is decreased in PET, resulting in inadequate physiological changes and failure of conversion into utero-placental arteries; similar events have been noted in RM pregnancies and those with small-for-gestational-age infants (Bulmer 1988). Inadequate placentation may be the central causative factor in gestational hypertension. Hypoxia due to these spiral artery changes could lead to the characteristic placental changes in PET, notably cytotrophoblast proliferation, syncytial budding, thickening of the trophoblastic basement membrane and placental infarction (Fox 1978; Redman 1991).

These histopathological changes neither show evidence of cellular immune attack on trophoblast nor appear to involve the unusual decidual CD3 −ve CD56 +ve granulated leucocyte population (Fox 1978; Khong 1987). Other investigation has indicated that the uterine spiral arteries leading into the placental bed may show changes similar to acute atherosis and are characterized by fibrinoid necrosis as well as lipid-loaded macrophage and perivascular mononuclear cell infiltration (Bulmer 1988; Redman 1991). An immunological pathogenesis for the inadequate maternal vascular response to placentation has been supported by detection of complement, IgG and fibrin deposits in placental bed vessels in PET (Kitzmiller and Benirschke 1973), although this could be the result of occluded blood flow rather than the cause. Complement deposition may also be increased in placental chorionic villous tissue in PET (Sinha *et al.* 1984), although similar necrotic foci have been identified in placentae from insulin-dependent diabetic and indeed healthy mothers. Serum APA may be found in a proportion of cases with particularly severe early-onset PET without symptomatic autoimmune disease (Branch *et al.* 1989); this could reflect an immunopathological relationship with functional endothelial cell changes.

Pre-eclamptic toxaemia runs in families and may be a single recessive gene disorder (Chesley and Cooper 1986). It is not associated with any particular HLA allele or blood group antigen, although a weak association with maternal HLA homozygosity has been claimed (Redman 1980). Nevertheless, the main maternally expressed genes affecting susceptibility to PET are not in the HLA region (Wilton *et al.* 1990). Pre-eclamptic toxaemia can be partner-specific and the relevance of a male genetic factor merits further attention since it is now recognized that inherited paternal, rather than maternal, genomic imprinting is necessary for normal development of trophoblast and extra-embryonic tissues (Reik *et al.* 1987). Pre-eclamptic toxaemia also occurs more frequently in situations with increased placental mass, including multiple pregnancy, molar pregnancy and triploidy, notably trisomy 13 (Redman 1980; Boyd *et al.* 1987; Jenkins 1988). Hence, an as yet undefined maternal–fetal genetic interaction may underlie this disorder.

Graft-versus-host disease of the fetus

There have been observations from animal models to indicate that maternal cells presensitized to paternal alloantigens may occasionally engraft the fetus, causing fetal graft-versus-host (GVH) disease and runting (Beer and Billingham 1973). In humans, intrauterine and exchange transfusions for haemolytic disease of the new-born have occasionally been followed by development of neonatal GVH disease (Parkman *et al.* 1974). Spontaneous cases have been documented most commonly in association with fetal immunodeficiency, although it is not clear whether the GVH is the result or cause of the fetal immunodeficiency (Seemayer *et al.* 1983). An increased incidence of HLA compatibility between mother and child is associated with severe combined immunodeficiency and fetal engraftment by maternal T cells in some cases (Pollack *et al.* 1982).

Gestational trophoblastic disease

Complete hydatidiform moles lack any identifiable fetal tissue, other than extraembryonic tissue, and have a diploid genome that is entirely of paternal (androgenetic) origin. Hence, they do not have any haplo-identity, and are fully allogeneic, with the maternal host (Kajii and Ohama 1977). Partial hydatidiform moles are associated with identifiable fetal tissues or vasculature and are usually triploid, the extra haploid component being paternal (Lawler and Fisher 1987a). Recently, however, rare cases have been identified that blur the apparent distinction between the two types of hydatidiform mole based on morphological and cytogenetic criteria (Fox 1991). Experimental studies of genetic imprinting of parental chromosomes in mice, using diandric and digynic diploid concepti, have identified the inherited paternal genome as playing the predominant role in placental development, whereas the maternal genome is more important in embryonic development (Kauffman and Lee 1989); this is in close agreement with clinical molar cytogenetics. Choriocarcinoma may follow normal term pregnancy, molar pregnancy or non-molar abortion, and this trophoblastic malignancy represents the only natural example of allogeneic tumours which grow and metastasize in histocompatible hosts. Trophoblastic neoplasia can often be associated with a pronounced local mononuclear cell response involving macrophages and CD3 +ve T cells (Fox 1978; Bulmer 1988).

Fetal trophoblast antigen expression in both molar pregnancy and choriocarcinoma obeys the same general rules as for normal pregnancy (see Chapter 40), according to trophoblast morphology and location (Bulmer 1988; Bulmer *et al.* 1988). The phenotypic heterogeneity of antigen expression in choriocarcinoma reflects the extensive differentiation into cellular subgroups that occurs for malignant trophoblast. The unusual maternal CD3 −ve CD56 +ve granulated leucocyte cells observed characteristically in normal pregnancy decidua (Bulmer *et al.* 1991) are also found in molar pregnancy but not in uterine tissue in choriocarcinoma, suggesting that their presence is associated with decidualization events rather than the presence of fetal trophoblast.

Unusually high serum levels of antipaternal HLA alloantibodies are formed in gestational trophoblastic disease (Shaw *et al.* 1979). Trophoblast lacks expression of HLA-A or B alloantigens and, in the case of a complete mole lacking a fetus or fetal blood cells, the immunogenic source must be stromal cells of the placental chorionic villi (Lawler and Fisher 1987b).

Choriocarcinoma may be associated with a small increase in HLA compatibility between patient and spouse, but there is a higher risk depending on the blood group antigen system. Thus, there is an increased prevalence in group A women, particularly with a group O partner, and women with ABO-compatible partners appear relatively protected from development of choriocarcinoma following evacuation of a mole (Bagshawe *et al.* 1971; Lawler and Fisher 1987b). Trophoblast does not express ABO blood group antigens, and direct immunological sensitization is clearly not involved; rather, postmolar trophoblastic proliferation may possibly be influenced instead by the action of a separate gene linked to the ABO system.

Host resistance in pregnancy

It is often suggested that maternal tolerance to the antigenically foreign fetoplacental unit during pregnancy may be associated with a reduced maternal immune response that extends to other aspects of the immune system. If this were so, manifestations such as an increased incidence of spread of infection and altered responses to vaccination, malignant tumours and transplantation might be expected. One difficulty in assessing the incidence and extent of infection in pregnancy is often the paucity of comparable available data on non-pregnant women of childbearing age. However, there is no evidence that extrauterine immune competence is significantly prejudiced in pregnancy and hence pregnant women are not generally at greater risk of acquiring or suffering more severe infections than non-pregnant women, including local recurrence of latent infection or a primary infection, other than in certain specific situations; these have been detailed elsewhere (Hart 1988). There is some indication that pregnant women may be more susceptible to malaria (Bruce-Chwatt 1983).

Vaccine administration appears to give equal and adequate protection to pregnant compared with non-pregnant individuals and host defence to malignant tumours is also not significantly altered in pregnancy although, again, differences in patient selection and methods of treatment can make data comparison difficult (Hart 1988). Organ transplantation during pregnancy is extremely rare, and hence it is not possible to assess the direct interaction between pregnancy-induced immunological changes and transplantation. Although confounded by variable concomittant immunosuppressive therapy, pregnancy is not greatly affected in individuals who have received a clinical tissue allograft, apart from some possible increased incidence of PET and premature delivery (Rudolph *et al.* 1979; Penn *et al.* 1980). In the same studies, it was apparent that pregnancy does not significantly lower host resistance to allow improved allograft survival since rejection episodes can occur. However, a reduced incidence of alloantibody production to non-inherited maternal HLA antigens compared with non-inherited paternal HLA antigens has been reported, indicating the possibility that a form of active tolerance to maternal alloantigens may be acquired by the fetus *in utero* that persists into adult life (Claas *et al.* 1988).

Immunological approaches to prenatal diagnosis

A monoclonal antibody recognizing a cell surface antigenic epitope entirely specific for fetal cells, in concert with a fluorescence-activated cell sorter, could potentially provide a means for isolating some of the small numbers of fetal cells that may gain access to maternal peripheral blood via the uterine vein (Adinolfi 1988; Mueller *et al.* 1990). This would provide a minimally invasive route for prenatal diagnosis of fetal chromosomal abnormalities and selected genetic diseases, especially since the sensitivity of polymerase chain reaction (PCR) amplification of specific deoxyribonucleic acid (DNA) sequences now enables precise genetic analysis of extremely small numbers of cells (Lo *et al.* 1989). Three types of fetal nucleated cells may theoretically be identified and isolated from maternal blood by exploiting fetomaternal antigenic differences: syncytiotrophoblast cellular elements, lymphocytes and erythroblasts (Adinolfi 1991).

With the exception of fetal HLA, the identification of fetal cell-specific antigen expression using monoclonal antibodies has been elusive (Anderson *et al.* 1987; Adinolfi 1991; Johnson 1991). Fetal blood cell traffic into maternal blood is very limited, particularly in the case of leucocytes, and may not occur independently of transplacental haemorrhage. The use of antibodies against fetal HLA determinants inherited from the father and absent from the mother for the isolation of fetal nucleated cells is hampered significantly by: (i) the difficulty of predicting the fetal phenotype; and (ii) the fact that the maternal immune system will rapidly remove incompatible leucocytes (Adinolfi 1991). In contrast, extensive numbers of syncytial sprouts can become detached from placental syncytiotrophoblast from early in the first trimester of pregnancy and have been repeatedly observed in uterine venous blood samples. However, although very promising, this approach has yet to be fully exploited because: (i) the number of nucleated fetal trophoblastic cells that cross the lung barrier into peripheral blood appears to be very small (Ganshirt-Ahlert *et al*. 1990); and (ii) there can be significant intravascular uptake of trophoblastic cell membrane fragments by maternal blood cells, which then contaminate the subsequent separation of fetal cells, using antigen identification techniques (Covone *et al*. 1988).

Birth control vaccines

Much research effort is now coming to fruition in the exciting possibility of the development of fertility-regulating birth control vaccines of limited effective duration without further reimmunization. Large numbers of women, particularly in developing countries, avoid currently available methods of contraception for cultural or practical reasons. There are over 300 million couples of reproductive age in developing countries, 80% of whom do not use adequate means of birth control (Basten 1988). Vaccination may prove to be an acceptable, affordable and dependable approach to relieve the dramatic population escalation and its associated socio-economic problems, as well as providing a novel alternative choice for contraception which avoids endocrinological, mechanical or surgical intervention.

Current strategies are directed towards the identification of immunogenic epitopes that may be engineered to form the basis for development of a vaccine capable of stimulating an active immune response that will interfere with fertilization or immediate implantation events. Thus, those potential vaccine candidates which have been and are being identified are associated with the gametes, notably acrosome-reacted sperm and the zona pellucida, as well as the preimplantation blastocyst (Basten 1988; Alexander *et al*. 1990; Johnson 1991). The expression of such target antigens or epitopes should ideally be restricted only to gametes and/or early products following fertilization, be accessible to immune (antibody) effectors, and be present transiently and in relatively low amounts compared with the predicted immune response (Griffin 1991).

Protein hormone-based vaccines have been of particular interest, notably involving the β chain of human chorionic gonadotrophin (HCG) which is a pregnancy-specific soluble secreted product of the blastocyst. Specific antibodies to HCG will neutralize its systemic action in signalling the corpus luteum, resulting in inadequate progesterone support to maintain viable pregnancy at an extremely early stage (Basten 1988). A World Health Organization (WHO)-sponsored development programme has incorporated a synthetic 37 amino acid C-terminal peptide of β-HCG conjugated to diphtheria toxoid into a vaccine administered with a muramyl dipeptide derivative adjuvant (Griffin 1991). This immunogen does not contain T cell epitopes and promotes no immune memory to HCG, and hence provokes transient anti-HCG immunity; boosting with the vaccine, but not native HCG, will regenerate the antibody response. This strategy has achieved a repeatable contragestational effect of limited time span in baboons (Stevens 1986), and a clinical trial in sterilized women has been completed which elicited antibody responses in excess of those thought to be required to neutralize HCG in maternal circulation (Jones *et al*. 1988). Phase II clinical trials for efficacy in fertile women are about to commence. Alternative HCG-based vaccines, using the whole β chain of HCG conjugated to other protein carriers (tetanus toxoid and/or cholera toxin B chain), and also with different adjuvant and delivery vehicle systems, have been developed and are currently being evaluated in other clinical trials (Singh *et al*. 1989).

References

Adinolfi, M. (1988). Immunological approaches to prenatal diagnosis. *Baillière's Clin. Immunol. Allergy* **2**, 775–90.

Adinolfi, M. (1991). On a non-invasive approach to prenatal diagnosis based on the detection of fetal nucleated cells in maternal blood samples. *Prenat. Diagn.* **11**, 799–804.

Alanen, A. and Lassila, O. (1982). Cell-mediated immunity in normal pregnancy and pre-eclampsia. *J. Reprod. Immunol.* **4**, 349–54.

Alexander, N.J., Griffin, P.D., Spieler, J.M. and Waites, G.M.H. (eds) (1990). *Gamete Interaction: Prospects for Immunocontraception*. Wiley-Liss, New York.

Anderson, D.J., Johnson, P.M., Alexander, N.J., Jones, W.R. and Griffin, P.D. (1987). Monoclonal antibodies to human trophoblast and sperm antigens: report of two WHO-sponsored workshops. *J. Reprod. Immunol.* **10**, 231–57.

Bagshawe, K.D., Rawlins, G., Pike, M. and Lawler S.D. (1971). ABO blood groups in trophoblastic neoplasia. *Lancet* **i**, 553–7.

Basten, A. (1988). Birth control vaccines. *Baillière's Clin. Immunol. Allergy* **2**, 759–74.

Beal, R.W. (1979). Non-rhesus (D) blood group isoimmunisation in obstetrics. *Clin. Obstet. Gynecol.* **6**, 493–508.

Beer, A.E. and Billingham, R.E. (1973). Procurement of runt disease of maternal origin. *Transplant. Proc.* **5**, 887–91.

Beer, A.E., Quebbeman, J.F., Ayers, J.W.T. and Haines, R.F. (1981). Major histocompatibility complex antigens, maternal and paternal immune responses, and chronic habitual abortions in humans. *Am. J. Obstet. Gynecol.* **141**, 987–99.

Beer, A.E., Semprini, A.E., Xiaoyn, Z. and Quebbeman, J.F. (1985). Pregnancy outcome in human couples with recurrent spontaneous abortion: HLA antigen profiles, HLA antigen sharing, female serum MLR blocking factors and paternal leucocyte immunization. *Exp. Clin. Immunogenet.* **2**, 137–53.

Biddle, P.K., Friedman, C.I. and Johnson, P.M. (1987). Lymphocyte-reactive antibodies and recurrent early pregnant failure. *Am. J. Obstet. Gynecol.* **157**, 785–6.

Borthwick, G., Lawlor, F., Holmes, R.C., Black, M.M. and Stirrat, G.M. (1985). Evidence for an immunological attack on the placenta in pemphigoid gestationis. *Br. J. Dermatol.* **113** (suppl. 29), 41–2.

Boyd, P.A., Lindenbaum, R.H. and Redman, C.W.G. (1987). Pre-eclampsia and trisomy 13: a possible association. *Lancet* **ii**, 425–7.

Branch, D.W., Scott, J.R., Kochenour, N.K. and Hershgold, E. (1985). Obstetric complications associated with the lupus anticoagulant. *N. Engl. J. Med.* **313**, 1322–6.

Branch, D.W., Andres, R., Digre, K.B., Rote, N.S. and Scott, J.R. (1989). The association of antiphospholipid antibodies with severe pre-eclampsia. *Obstet. Gynecol.* **73**, 541–5.

Bronson, R., Cooper, G. and Rosenfeld, G. (1984). Sperm antibodies: their role in infertility. *Fertil. Steril.* **42**, 171–83.

Bruce-Chwatt, L.J. (1983). Malaria and pregnancy. *Br. Med. J.* **286**, 1457–8.

Bulmer, J.N. (1988). Immunopathology of pregnancy. *Baillière's Clin. Immunol. Allergy* **2**, 697–734.

Bulmer, J.N., Johnson, P.M., Sasagawa, M. and Takeuchi, S. (1988). Immunohistochemical studies of fetal trophoblast and maternal decidua in hydatiform mole and choriocarcinoma. *Placenta* **9**, 183–200.

Bulmer, J.N., Morrison, L., Longfellow, M., Ritson, A. and Pace, D. (1991). Granulated lymphocytes in human endometrium: histochemical and immunohistochemical studies. *Hum. Reprod.* **6**, 791–8.

Cauchi, M.N., Lim, D., Young, D.E., Kloss, M. and Pepperell, R.J. (1991). Treatment of recurrent aborters by immunization with paternal cells — controlled trial. *Am. J. Reprod. Immunol.* **25**, 16–17.

Chesley, L.C. and Cooper, D.W. (1986). Genetics of hypertension in pregnancy: possible single gene control of pre-eclampsia and eclampsia in the descendants of eclamptic women. *Br. J. Obstet. Gynaecol.* **93**, 898–908.

Chia, K.V. and Johnson, P.M. (1987). T-lymphocyte subsets in unexplained recurrent spontaneous abortion. *Fertil. Steril.* **48**, 685–7.

Christiansen, O.B., Riisom, K., Lauritsen, J.G. and Grunnet, N. (1989). No increased histocompatibility antigen-sharing in couples with idiopathic habitual abortions. *Hum. Reprod.* **4**, 160–2.

Christiansen, O.B., Mathieson, O., Riisom, K., Lauritsen, J.G., Grunnet, N. and Jersild, C. (1990). HLA or HLA-linked genes reduce birthweight in families affected by idiopathic recurrent abortion. *Tissue Antigens* **36**, 156–63.

Claas, F.H.J., Gijbels, Y., van der Velden-de Munck, J. and Van Rood, J.J. (1988). Induction of B cell unresponsiveness to noninherited maternal HLA antigens during fetal life. *Science* **241**, 1815–17.

Clarke, C.A. (1982). Historical annotation: rhesus haemolytic disease of the newborn and its prevention. *Br. J. Haematol.* **52**, 525–36.

Clarke, G.N. (1987). An improved immunobead test procedure for detecting sperm antibodies in serum. *Am. J. Reprod. Immunol. Microbiol.* **13**, 1–3.

Coulam, C.B. (1991). Epidemiology of recurrent spontaneous abortion. *Am. J. Reprod. Immunol.* **26**, 23–7.

Coulam, C.B., Moore, S.B. and O'Fallon, W.M. (1987). Association between major histocompatibility antigen and reproductive performance. *Am. J. Reprod. Immunol. Microbiol.* **14**, 54–8.

Covone, A., Kozma, R., Johnson, P.M., Latt, S.A. and Adinolfi, M. (1988). Analysis of peripheral maternal blood samples for the presence of placenta-derived cells using Y-specific probes and McAb H315. *Prenat. Diagn.* **8**, 591–607.

Cowchock, F.S., Smith, J.B., David, S., Scher, J., Batzer, F. and Corson, S. (1990). Paternal mononuclear cell immunization therapy for repeated miscarriage: predictive variables for pregnancy success. *Am. J. Reprod. Immunol.* **22**, 12–17.

Demowski, W.P., Steele, R.W. and Baker, G.F. (1981). Deficient cellular immunity in endometriosis. *Am. J. Obstet. Gynecol.* **141**, 377–83.

Fox, H. (1978). *Pathology of the Placenta*. W.B. Saunders & Co., London.

Fox, H. (1991). Current topic: trophoblastic pathology. *Placenta* **12**, 479–86.

Ganshirt-Ahlert, D., Pohlschmidt, M., Gal, A., Miny, P., Hurst, J. and Holzgreve, W. (1990). Ratio of fetal to maternal DNA is less than 1 in 5000 at different gestational ages in maternal blood. *Clin. Genet.* **38**, 36–41.

Gatenby, P.A. (1989). Systemic lupus erythematosus and pregnancy. *Aust. NZ. J. Med.* **19**, 261–78.

Gatenby, P.A., Moore, H., Cameron, K., Doran, T.J. and Adelstein, S. (1989). Treatment of recurrent spontaneous abortion by immunization with paternal lymphocytes: correlates with outcome. *Am. J. Reprod. Immunol.* **19**, 21–7.

Gendron, R.L. and Baines, M.G. (1988). Infiltrating decidual killer cells are associated with spontaneous abortion in mice. *Cell. Immunol.* **113**, 261–7.

Gill, T.J., III (1987). Genetic factors in fetal loss. *Am. J. Reprod. Immunol. Microbiol.* **15**, 133–7.

Gleicher, N., El-Roiey, A., Confine, E. and Friberg, J. (1987). Is endometriosis an autoimmune disease? *Obstet. Gynecol.* **70**, 115–25.

Griffin, P.D. (1991). The WHO Task Force on Vaccines for Fertility Regulation: its formation, objectives and research activities. *Hum. Reprod.* **6**, 166–72.

Haas, G.G. (1987). How should sperm antibody tests be used clinically? *Am. J. Reprod. Immunol. Microbiol.* **15**, 106–11.

Halme, J., Becker, S., Hammond, M.G. and Raj, S. (1982). Pelvic macrophages in normal and infertile women: the role of patent tubes. *Am. J. Obstet. Gynecol.* **142**, 890–5.

Halme, J., Becker, S. and Haskill, S. (1987). Altered motivation and function of peritoneal macrophages: possible role in pathogenesis of endometriosis. *Am. J. Obstet. Gynecol.* **156**, 783–91.

Halme, J., White, C., Kamma, S., Ester, J. and Haskill, S. (1988). Peritoneal macrophages from patients with endometriosis release growth factor activity *in vitro*. *J. Clin. Endocrinol. Metab.* **66**, 1044–50.

Hart, C.A. (1988). Pregnancy and host resistance. *Baillière's Clin. Immunol. Allergy* **2**, 735–8.

Hill, J.A. (1990). Immunological mechanisms of pregnancy maintenance and failure: a critique of theories and therapy. *Am. J. Reprod. Immunol.* **22**, 33–7.

Hill, J.A. (1992). Immunological factors in endometriosis and endometriosis-associated reproductive failure. In *Infertility and Reproductive Medicine Clinics in North America* (in press).

Hill, J.A. and Anderson, D.J. (1988). Immunological mechanisms of female infertility. *Baillière's Clin. Immunol. Allergy* **2**, 551–76.

Hill, J.A., Faris, H.M.P., Schiff, I. and Anderson, D.J. (1988). Characterization of leukocyte subpopulations in the peritoneal fluid of women with endometriosis. *Fertil. Steril.* **50**, 216–23.

Hjort, T., Johnson, P.M. and Mori, T. (1985). An overview of the WHO international multi-centre studies on antibodies to reproductive tract antigens in clinically defined sera. *J. Reprod. Immunol.* **8**, 359–62.

Ho, H.-N., Gill, T.J., III, Hsieh, H.-J., Jiang, J.-J., Lee, T.-Y. and Hsieh, C.-Y. (1991). Immunotherapy for recurrent spontaneous abortions in a Chinese population. *Am. J. Reprod. Immunol.* **25**, 10–15.

Holmes, R.C., Black, M.M., Jurecka, W. *et al.* (1983). Clues to the aetiology and pathogenesis of herpes gestationis. *Br. J. Dermatol.* **109**, 131–9.

Houwert-de Jong, M.H., Termijtelen, A., Eskes, T.K.A.B., Mantingh, A. and Bruinse, H.W. (1989). The natural course of habitual abortion. *Eur. J. Obstet. Gynecol. Reprod. Biol.* **33**, 221–8.

Jazwinska, E.C., Kilpatrick, D.C., Smart, G.E. and Liston, W.A. (1987). Feto-maternal HLA compatibility does not have a major influence on human pregnancy except for lymphocytotoxin production. *Clin. Exp. Immunol.* **68**, 116–22.

Jenkins, D.M. (1988). Pre-eclamptic toxaemia. *Baillière's Clin. Immunol. Allergy* **2**, 625–42.

Jenkins, D.M., Need, J.A. and Rajah, S.M. (1977). Deficiency of specific HLA antibodies in severe pregnancy pre-eclampsia/eclampsia. *Clin. Exp. Immunol.* **27**, 485–6.

Johnson, P.M. (1988). Immunology of pregnancy. In *Obstetrics*, ed. A.C. Turnbull and G.V.P. Chamberlain, pp. 173–87, Churchill Livingstone, Edinburgh.

Johnson, P.M. (1991). Trophoblast membrane antigens for contragestational vaccine development. In *Female Contraception and Male Fertility Regulation*, ed. B. Runnebaum, T. Rabe and L. Kiesel, pp. 115–22. Parthenon Press, Carnforth.

Johnson, P.M. and Ramsden, G.H. (1988). Recurrent miscarriage. *Baillière's Clin. Immunol. Allergy* **2**, 607–24.

Johnson, P.M., Chia, K.V., Risk, J.M., Barnes, R.M.R. and Woodrow, J.C. (1988). Immunological and immunogenetic investigation of recurrent spontaneous abortion. *Dis. Markers* **6**, 163–71.

Johnson, P.M., Ramsden, G.H., Chia, K.V., Hart, C.A., Farquharson, R.G. and Francis, W.J.A. (1991). A combined randomised double-blind and open study of trophoblast membrane infusion (TMI) in unexplained recurrent miscarriage. *Colloque INSERM* **212**, 277–84.

Jones, W.R. (1987). Immunological factors in infertility. In *The Infertile Couple*, ed. R. Pepperell, B. Hudson and C. Wood, pp. 158–160, Churchill Livingstone, Melbourne.

Jones, W.R. and Need, J.A. (1988). Maternal–fetal cell surface antigen incompatibilities. *Baillière's Clin. Immunol. Allergy* **2**, 577–606.

Jones, W.R., Bradley, J., Judd, S.J. *et al.* (1988). Phase I clinical trials of a World Health Organization birth control vaccine. *Lancet* **i**, 1295–8.

Kajii, T. and Ohama, K. (1977). Androgenetic origin of hydatidiform mole. *Nature* **268**, 633–4.

Kauffman, M.P.H. and Lee, K.P.H. (1989). Influence of diandric and digynic triploid genotypes in early mouse embryogenesis. *Development* **105**, 137–45.

Khong, T.Y. (1987). Immunohistologic study of the leukocytic infiltrate in maternal uterine tissues in normal and pre-eclamptic pregnancies at term. *Am. J. Reprod. Immunol. Microbiol.* **15**, 1–8.

Khong, T.Y., Liddell, H.S. and Robertson, W.B. (1987). Defective haemochorial placentation as a cause of miscarriage: a preliminary study. *Br. J. Obstet. Gynaecol.* **94**, 649–55.

Kitzmiller, J.L. and Benirschke, K. (1973). Immunofluorescent study of placental bed vessels in pre-eclampsia of pregnancy. *Am. J. Obstet. Gynecol.* **115**, 248–51.

Kochenour, N.K., Branch, D.W., Rote, N.S. and Scott, J.R. (1987). A new postpartum syndrome associated with antiphospholipid antibodies. *Obstet. Gynecol.* **69**, 460–8.

Lawler, S.D. and Fisher, R.A. (1987a). Genetic studies in hydatidiform mole with clinical correlations. *Placenta* **8**, 77–88.

Lawler, S.D. and Fisher, R.A. (1987b). Immunogenicity of hydatidiform mole. *Placenta* **8**, 185–99.

Lehmann, D. and Emmons, L.R. (1989). Immunological phenomena observed in the testis and their possible role in infertility. *Am. J. Reprod. Immunol.* **19**, 43–52.

Lo, Y.-M.D., Patel, P., Wainscoat, J.S., Sampietro, M., Gillmer, M.D.G. and Fleming, K.A. (1989). Prenatal sex determination by DNA amplification from maternal peripheral blood. *Lancet* **ii**, 1363–5.

Lockshin, M.D., Druzin, M.L., Goei, S. *et al.* (1985). Antibody to cardiolipin as a predictor of fetal distress or death in pregnant patients with systemic lupus erythematosus. *N. Engl. J. Med.* **313**, 152–6.

Lockwood, C.J., Romero, R., Feinberg, R.F., Clyne, L.P., Coster, B. and Hobbins, J.C. (1989). The prevalence and biologic significance of lupus anticoagulant and anticardiolipin antibodies in a general obstetric population. *Am. J. Obstet. Gynecol.* **161**, 369–73.

McIntyre, J.A., Faulk, W.P., Nichols-Johnson, V.R. and Taylor, C.G. (1986). Immunological testing and immunotherapy in recurrent spontaneous abortion. *Obstet. Gynecol.* **67**, 169–75.

Mackworth-Young, C. (1990). Antiphospholipid antibodies; more than just a disease marker? *Immunol. Today* **11**, 60–5.

Mathur, S., Perress, M.R., Williamson, H.O. *et al.* (1982). Autoimmunity to endometrium and ovary in endometriosis. *Clin. Exp. Immunol.* **50**, 259–67.

Michel, M., Underwood, J., Clark, D.A., Mowbray, J.F. and Beard, R.W. (1989). Histologic and immunologic study of uterine biopsy tissue of women with incipient abortion. *Am.*

J. Obstet. Gynecol. **161**, 409–14.

Mowbray, J.F., Gibbings, C., Liddell, H., Reginald, P.W., Underwood, J.L. and Beard, R.W. (1985). Controlled trial of treatment of recurrent spontaneous abortion by immunisation with paternal cells. *Lancet* **i**, 941–3.

Mueller, U.W., Hawes, C.S., Wright, A.E. *et al.* (1990). Isolation of fetal trophoblast cells from peripheral blood of pregnant women. *Lancet* **336**, 197–200.

Need, J.A., Bell, B., Meffin, E. and Jones, W.R. (1983). Pre-eclampsia in pregnancies from donor inseminations. *J. Reprod. Immunol.* **5**, 329–38.

Olive, D.L. and Haney, A.F. (1986). Endometriosis. In *Reproductive Failure*, ed. P. Dechaney, pp. 153–74, Churchill Livingstone, New York.

Olive, D.L., Weinberg, J.B. and Haney, A.F. (1985). Peritoneal macrophages and infertility: the association between cell number and pelvic pathology. *Fertil. Steril.* **44**, 772–80.

Olive, D.L., Montoya, I., Riehl, R.M. and Schenken, R.S. (1991). Macrophage conditioned media enhance endometrial stromal cell proliferation *in vitro*. *Am. J. Obstet. Gynecol.* **164**, 953–9.

Oosterlynck, D.J., Cornillie, F.J., Waer, M., Vandeputte, M. and Koninckx, P.R. (1991). Women with endometriosis show a defect in natural killer activity resulting in a decreased cytotoxicity to autologous endometrium. *Fertil. Steril.* **56**, 45–51.

Ortonne, J.-P., Hsi, B.-L., Verrando, P. *et al.* (1987). Herpes gestationis factor reacts with the amniotic epithelial basement membrane. *Br. J. Dermatol.* **117**, 147–54.

Out, H.J., Bruinse, H.W., Christiaens, G.C. *et al.* (1991). Prevalence of antiphospholipid antibodies in patients with fetal loss. *Ann. Rheum. Dis.* **50**, 553–7.

Parazzini, F., Acaia, B., Ricciardiello, O., Fedele, L., Liati, P. and Candiani, G.B. (1988). Short-term reproductive prognosis when no cause can be found for recurrent miscarriage. *Br. J. Obstet. Gynaecol.* **95**, 654–8.

Park, M.I., Edwin, S.S., Scott, J.R. and Branch, D.W. (1990). Interpretation of blocking activity in maternal serum depends on the equation used for calculation of mixed lymphocyte culture results. *Clin. Exp. Immunol.* **82**, 363–8.

Parkman, R., Mosier, D., Umansky, I., Cochrane, W., Carpenter, C.B. and Rosen, F.S. (1974). Graft-versus-host disease after intrauterine and exchange transfusion for haemolytic disease of the newborn. *N. Engl. J. Med.* **290**, 359–63.

Penn, I., Makowski, E.L. and Harris, P. (1980). Parenthood following renal and hepatic transplantation. *Transplantation* **30**, 397–400.

Pollack, M.S., Kirkpatrick, D., Kapoor, N., Dupont, B. and O'Reilly, R.J. (1982). Identification by HLA typing of intrauterine-derived maternal T cells in four patients with severe combined immunodeficiency. *N. Engl. J. Med.* **307**, 662–6.

Provost, T.T., Watson, W.L., Gaither, K.K. and Harley, J.B. (1987). The neonatal lupus erythematosus syndrome. *J. Rheumatol.* **14**, 199–205.

Ramsden, G.H. and Johnson, P.M. (1992). Unexplained recurrent miscarriage and the role of immunotherapy. *Contemp. Rev. Obstet. Gynaecol.* **4**, 29–35.

Redman, C.W.G. (1980). Immunological aspects of eclampsia and pre-eclampsia. In *Immunological Aspects of Reproduction and Fertility Control*, ed. J.P. Hearn, pp. 83–103, MTP Press, Lancaster.

Redman, C.W.G. (1991). Current topic: pre-eclampsia and the placenta. *Placenta* **12**, 301–8.

Regan, L., Braude, P.R. and Trembath, P.L. (1989). Influence of past reproductive performance on risk of spontaneous abortion. *Br. Med. J.* **299**, 541–5.

Reik, W., Collick, A., Norris, M.L., Barton, S.C. and Surani, M.A. (1987). Genomic imprinting determines methylation of parental alleles in transgenic mice. *Nature* **328**, 248–51.

Reznikoff-Etievant, M.F., Durieux, I., Huchet, J., Slamon, C. and Netter, A. (1988). Human MHC antigens and paternal leucocyte injections in recurrent spontaneous abortions. In *Early Pregnancy Loss, Mechanisms and Treatment*, ed. R.W. Beard and F. Sharp, pp. 375–84, Peacock Press, Ashton-under-Lyme.

Risk, J.M. and Johnson, P.M. (1992). Immunogenetic studies in unexplained recurrent miscarriage of pregnancy. In *HLA 1991*, vol. 2, ed. K. Sasazuki, Oxford University Press, Oxford (in press).

Rudolph, J.E., Schweitzer, R.T. and Bartus, S.A. (1979). Pregnancy in renal transplant recipients. *Transplantation* **27**, 26–9.

Sargent, I.L., Redman, C.W.G. and Stirrat, G.M. (1982). Maternal cell-mediated immunity in normal and pre-eclamptic pregnancy. *Clin. Exp. Immunol.* **50**, 601–9.

Sargent, I.L., Wilkins, T. and Redman, C.W.G. (1988). Maternal immune responses to the fetus in early pregnancy and recurrent miscarriage. *Lancet* **ii**, 1099–104.

Scott, J.R. (1984). Connective tissue disease antibodies and pregnancy. *Am. J. Reprod. Immunol.* **6**, 19–24.

Scott, J.R., Rote, N.S. and Branch, D.W. (1987). Immunologic aspects of recurrent abortion and fetal death. *Obstet. Gynecol.* **70**, 645–56.

Scott, J.S. and Bird, H.A. (eds) (1990). *Pregnancy Autoimmunity and Connective Tissue Disorders.* Oxford University Press, Oxford.

Scott, J.S., Maddison, P.J., Taylor, P.V., Esscher, E., Scott, O. and Skinner, R.P. (1983). Connective tissue disease, antibodies to ribonucleoprotein, and congenital heart block. *N. Engl. J. Med.* **309**, 209–12.

Seemayer, T.A., Bolande, R.P. and Lapp, W.S. (1983). Graft vs host disease and severe combined immunodeficiency. *N. Engl. J. Med.* **308**, 160–2.

Shaw, A.R.E., Dasgupta, M.K., Kovithavongs, T. *et al.* (1979). Humoral and cellular immunity to paternal antigens in trophoblastic neoplasia. *Int. J. Cancer* **24**, 586–93.

Simpson, J.L., Malinak, R., Elias, S., Carson, S.A. and Raduary, R.A. (1984). HLA associations in endometriosis. *Am. J. Obstet. Gynecol.* **148**, 395–401.

Singh, O., Rao, L.V., Gaur, A., Sharma, N.C., Alam, A. and Talwar, G.P. (1989). Antibody response and characteristics of antibodies in women immunized with three contraceptive vaccines inducing antibodies against human chorionic gonadotrophin. *Fertil. Steril.* **52**, 739–44.

Sinha, D., Wells, M. and Faulk, W.P. (1984). Immunological studies of human placentae: complement components in pre-eclamptic chorionic villi. *Clin. Exp. Immunol.* **56**, 175–84.

Steele, R.W., Damowski, W.P. and Marmer, D.J. (1984). Immunologic aspects of human endometriosis. *Am. J. Reprod. Immunol.* **6**, 33–7.

Stevens, V.C. (1986). Current status of anti-fertility vaccines using gonadotrophin immunogens. *Immunol. Today* **7**,

369–74.

Stirrat, G.M. (1990). Recurrent miscarriage. I. Definition and epidemiology. *Lancet* **336**, 673–5.

Switchenko, A.C., Kauffman, R.S. and Becker, M. (1991). Are there antiendometrial antibodies in sera of women with endometriosis? *Fertil. Steril.* **56**, 235–41.

Takakuwa, K., Goto, S., Hasegawa, I. *et al.* (1990). Result of immunotherapy on patients with unexplained recurrent abortion: a beneficial treatment for patients with negative blocking antibodies. *Am. J. Reprod. Immunol.* **23**, 37–41.

Taylor, C.G. and Faulk, W.P. (1981). Prevention of recurrent abortion with leucocyte transfusions. *Lancet* **ii**, 68–70.

Taylor, M., Cauchi, M.N. and Buchanan, R.R.C. (1990). The lupus anticoagulant, anticardiolipin antibodies and recurrent miscarriage. *Am. J. Reprod. Immunol.* **23**, 33–6.

Taylor, P.V. (1988). Autoimmunity and pregnancy. *Baillière's Clin. Immunol. Allergy* **2**, 665–96.

Taylor, P.V., Maloney, M.D., Campbell, J.M. *et al.* (1991). Autoreactivity in women with endometriosis. *Br. J. Obstet. Gynaecol.* **98**, 680–4.

Triplett, D.A. (1989). Antiphospholipid antibodies and recurrent pregnancy loss. *Am. J. Reprod. Immunol.* **20**, 52–67.

Unander, A.M. and Lindholm, A. (1986). Transfusions of leukocyte-rich erythrocyte concentrates: a successful treatment in selected cases of habitual abortion. *Am. J. Obstet. Gynecol.* **4**, 171–8.

Vlaanderen, W. and Treffers, P.E. (1987). Prognosis of subsequent pregnancies after recurrent abortion in the first trimester. *Br. Med. J.* **295**, 92–3.

Wild, R.A. and Shivers, C.A. (1985). Antiendometrial antibodies in patients with endometriosis. *Am. J. Reprod. Immunol.* **8**, 84–9.

Wilton, A.N., Cooper, D.W., Brennecke, S.P., Bishop, S.M. and Marshall, P. (1990). Absence of close linkage between maternal genes for susceptibility to pre-eclampsia/eclampsia and HLA-DRβ. *Lancet* **336**, 653–7.

Zeller, J.M., Henig, I., Radwanska, E. and Smowski, P. (1987). Enhancement of human monocyte and peritoneal macrophage chemiluminescence activities in women with endometriosis. *Am. J. Reprod. Immunol.* **13**, 78–87.

109: Multiple Sclerosis

B.H. Waksman

Introduction

Multiple sclerosis (MS) is the commonest crippling neurological disorder of young adults in countries with a predominantly Caucasian population. For a clinical description of MS, see Hallpike *et al.* (1983) and Matthews *et al.* (1985). For research aspects, see McFarlin and McFarland (1982), Waksman (1984, 1988a), Whitaker and Snyder (1984), Koetsier (1985), Confavreux *et al.* (1988) and Raine (1988). For work with animal models, see McFarlin and Waksman (1982) and Waksman (1988b).

Clinical onset of MS is most frequently associated with weakness or visual disturbances (Table 109.1). In advanced disease, the clinical picture may be dominated by spastic paralysis, accompanied by pain, or by wild, uncontrollable intention tremor, urinary and/or bowel incontinence, or varying degrees of dementia. Fatigue may be overwhelming in many cases, and depression is frequent.

Most cases of MS start between 10 and 60 years of age. The highest age-specific incidence, in a careful population-based survey, was at the age of 22 (Fig. 109.1). However, the median age of onset is 30. Women outnumber men by a factor which varies from 1.5 : 1 to 7 : 1 in different series. At onset, most MS patients experience exacerbations (bouts, attacks, relapses) and remissions; most of these go on eventually to develop a slowly progressive course and may become completely disabled. About one-third of patients have no clear-cut exacerbations, but experience a slowly progressive disease from the start.

Traditionally, the diagnosis of MS has been based on clinical and historical evidence for 'dissemination of the disease in space and time', i.e. evidence for the presence of multiple discrete lesions in the central nervous system (CNS) white matter and the occurrence either of repeated disease episodes or of continuous disease progression (Table 109.2). The identification of clinically silent lesions by magnetic resonance imaging (MRI), the use of evoked potentials or the more recently introduced technique of magnetic cortical stimulation (Mills and Murray 1985) may be used to support a diagnosis of MS, but only if clinical evidence of at least one lesion is already present. Typical MS lesions are found at autopsy in neurologically normal people with a frequency at least comparable to that of clinically manifest disease (Gilbert and Sadler 1983). In MRI studies, such silent lesions have been found in family members of patients

Table 109.1. Multiple sclerosis as disease

Impairment of function	Onset (%)	Later (%)
Visual	36	66
Strength	40	80
Sensation	21	73
Co-ordination	10	77
Bladder, bowel, sex	9	56
Cerebral	3	>60
Clinical course		
Age at onset 10–60 years (half before 30)		
Female : male 1.75 : 1		
Relapsing–remitting, chronic progressive, stabilized		
Number of cases in North America		
Average prevalence (per 100 000)	58 (<10–130)	
Annual incidence of new cases (per 100 000)	4.2	

Table 109.2. The Poser Committee diagnostic criteria for multiple sclerosis

1 Clinically definite multiple sclerosis:
(a) Two attacks and clinical evidence of two separate lesions.
(b) Two attacks, clinical evidence of one and paraclinical evidence of another separate lesion.
2 Laboratory-supported definite multiple sclerosis:
(a) Two attacks, either clinical or paraclinical evidence of one lesion and cerebrospinal fluid oligoclonal bands.
(b) One attack, clinical evidence of two separate lesions and cerebrospinal fluid oligoclonal bands.
(c) One attack, clinical evidence of one lesion and cerebrospinal fluid oligoclonal bands.
3 Clinically probable multiple sclerosis:
(a) Two attacks and clinical evidence of one lesion.
(b) One attack and clinical evidence of two separate lesions.
(c) One attack, clinical evidence of one lesion and paraclinical evidence of another, separate lesion.
4 Laboratory-supported probable multiple sclerosis:
(a) Two attacks and CSF oligoclonal bands.

Note An 'attack' is the occurrence of a symptom or symptoms of neurological dysfunction which lasts for more than 24 hours.

From Poser *et al*. 1983.

with MS and especially in asymptomatic identical twins of MS patients (McFarland *et al*. 1985).

Using clinical criteria, MS prevalence rates in North America, Western Europe, Australia and New Zealand are found to vary significantly with latitude (Kurtzke 1985). In southern cities of the US, MS prevalence is below 10 per 100 000, while in such Canadian provinces as Saskatchewan and British Columbia the figure may exceed 130 per 100 000. In northern Scotland and the Orkney Islands, figures up to 300 per 100 000 are reported. Most epidemiologists agree that there is a true latitude effect, independent of ethnic differences in susceptibility to the disease.

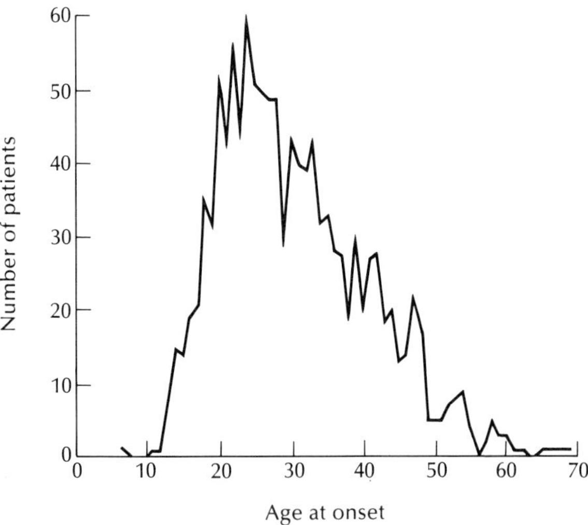

Fig. 109.1. Age of onset of multiple sclerosis in population-based survey of 1200 Canadian patients. From Ebers *et al*. (1986).

The use of MRI bids fair to change our concepts of MS substantially. Patients with minimal disease, experiencing less than one clinical attack annually, are found, with frequently repeated scans, to have as many as 20 (average about six) showers of new lesions a year (Koopmans *et al*. 1989). Exacerbating–remitting and progressive disease are found to differ only in lesion extent and the frequency with which new lesions appear. Disease activity continues, apparently unabated, in periods of clinical remission, and this is confirmed by, for example, cerebrospinal fluid (CSF) studies. Prevalence figures, of course, reflect clinical findings only; the true figures are clearly much higher if asymptomatic lesions are taken into account. Of cases diagnosed as optic (retrobulbar) neuritis or chronic progressive myelopathy, half to two-thirds are found to have brain lesions typical of MS by MRI. In the myelopathy case, the diagnosis now becomes MS. In the case of optic neuritis, this is not current practice, although from the research standpoint many of these patients are cases of MS and many progress to become clinically manifest MS over a few months or years. It should be noted, in passing, that many 'asymptomatic' brain lesions are in fact expressed clinically in disturbances of cognitive function and could be detected by proper psychological testing (Rao 1986).

Multiple sclerosis-like disease of 'specific' aetiology is increasingly capturing public attention (Table 109.3). Rabies vaccination, in a famous series of Japanese cases, was followed by chronic disease indistinguishable from MS, presumably autoimmune in character. Tropical spastic paraparesis or human T cell lymphotrophic virus (HTLV)-1-associated myelopathy (HAM), resulting from persistent HTLV-1 infection of the CNS accompanied by an immune response to the virus, is seen as progressive spinal cord disease clinically indistinguishable from MS and not infrequently with brain lesions which can be visualized by MRI (Gessain *et al.* 1985; Osame *et al.* 1986; Johnson and McArthur 1987; Bhagavati *et al.* 1988). Similarly, tertiary Lyme disease, with persistent *Borrelia burgdorferi* infection of the CNS, may give a clinical picture resembling MS (Pachner and Steere 1986). The lesions, however, are significantly more inflammatory in character (perivascular inflammation, meningitis) than those of MS.

Multiple sclerosis is a chronic 'demyelinative' disease of the CNS. The term refers to the characteristic destruction (primary) of myelin with relative sparing of axons seen in the lesions, in contrast to Wallerian (secondary) myelin breakdown after damage of the neuron. Myelin itself (or the oligodendrocyte, which makes and maintains myelin) thus appears to be the target of the disease process. The larger group of demyelinative diseases includes a condition similar to MS affecting the peripheral nerve system (PNS), chronic relapsing inflammatory polyneuropathy. Some MS cases, perhaps as many as 5–10%, have clinical and histological evidence of PNS as well as CNS lesions. The group of demyelinative diseases also includes acute monophasic disease of the CNS — post-infectious or post-rabies-vaccination encephalomyelitis (and acute disseminated encephalomyelitis without an obvious triggering event — or of the PNS — the Guillain–Barré syndrome, also occurring after viral infection or rabies vaccination (or without a visible triggering event). The evidence is compelling that the acute monophasic diseases result from viral induction of autoimmune responses to myelin basic protein (MBP) (CNS) or P2 (PNS) (see, for example, Johnson *et al.* 1984; Geczy *et al.* 1985), perhaps by molecular mimicry between short peptide sequences in certain antigens of measles virus, rubella virus or Epstein–Barr virus (EBV) and immunogenic sequences of the proteins in question (Fujinami and Oldstone 1985). This relationship tends to strengthen the implication that MS and chronic demyelinative disease of the PNS may also be autoimmune.

Table 109.3. Chronic demyelinating diseases of the central nervous system

Disease	Mode of immunization
Post-rabies vaccination encephalomyelitis	Myelin
Multiple sclerosis	Common viruses (?)
HTLV-1-associated myelopathy	HTLV-1, persisting in CNS
Tertiary Lyme disease	*Borrelia burgdorferi*, persisting in CNS

Genetic factors in multiple sclerosis

Multiple sclerosis occurs only in Caucasians with a genetically determined predisposition to this disease. African blacks, American mongoloids (Inuit, Indian), some unmixed Asian mongoloids (Yakuts) and one well-studied Caucasian group, the Hutterites of Canada, are virtually free of MS (Dean 1988). In racially mixed groups such as the Chinese, Japanese and American blacks, MS occurs at a much reduced frequency (Kuroiwa and Kurland 1982). Multiple sclerosis in Asians (Chinese, Japanese, Filipinos) also differs from MS in Caucasians in lesion distribution, with relatively greater involvement of optic nerve and spinal cord and less of brain; in intensity, with lesions often proceeding beyond demyelination to frank necrosis; and in clinical course, with relatively more acute and often rapidly fatal disease (Kuroiwa and Kurland 1982; Kuroiwa 1985).

The genetic control of MS susceptibility is underlined by family and twin studies (Table 109.4), as is the polygenic nature of this control (Ebers *et al.* 1986; McFarlin 1988). There appears to be no single susceptibility gene for MS (Compston 1986; McFarlin 1988). Instead, as in many other 'autoimmune' diseases, susceptibility has been related

Table 109.4. Occurrence of multiple sclerosis in family members

Relationship to person with MS	Probability of getting MS (%)
General population	0.1
Spouse	0.1
Identical twin	40 (70)[a]
Parent, uncle, aunt	5
Sibling	2
Fraternal twin	2 (12)[b]
Child	1

a The higher figure includes asymptomatic cases found to have lesions by MRI, evoked potential or CSF studies.
b The higher figure was obtained in a survey with a higher average age among those studied.

to genes determining T cell recognition, notably Class II major histocompatibility complex (MHC) genes encoded on chromosome 6 and genes for the T cell receptor (TCR) α and β chains encoded on chromosomes 14 and 7, respectively (Table 109.5). In some Western European studies, benign exacerbating–remitting MS of early onset, predominating in females, was associated with human leucocyte antigen (HLA)-A3B7DR2 and more severe, progressive MS of later onset, more common in males, with A1B8DR3 (Madigand *et al.* 1982; Lambalgen *et al.* 1986). However this distinction could not be found in other studies, in particular in the US.

Table 109.5. Genetic factors which may play role in multiple sclerosis

Factor	Chromosome
HLA-A3B7DR2 (DQw1), C4-A4B2, BfS A1B8DR3	6
T cell receptor	
Alpha chain	14
Beta chain	7
Gm-1 17; 21	14
α1-antitrypsin (M3 allele)	14
C3F	19
GC-IF	4
(?) Chromosomal translocation frequency (T cell rearranging gene)	7
(?) Vasoamine sensitivity (histamine)	6
(?) Myelin basic protein (three forms)	18
(?) Proteolipid protein	X
(?) Myelin-associated glycoprotein	19

Additional genes on chromosome 14 found to be associated with MS (Pandey *et al.* 1981; Propert *et al.* 1982) may be in linkage disequilibrium with the gene for the TCR α chain. Alternatively, these have been regarded as population markers for the population (of Scandinavian origin) most at risk for MS (Ebers and Bulman 1986). Associations between MS and genes on chromosomes 19 and 4 require confirmation. Still other possible associations, indicated with (?) in Table 109.5, await investigation, in particular genes governing the reported increase in sister chromatid exchange (spontaneous or induced) in MS (Gipps and Kidson 1984). Genetically controlled vasoamine sensitivity plays an important role in determining sensitivity to autoimmune demyelinative disease in animal models (Linthicum and Frelinger 1982) and may do so in MS. The question of possible abnormalities in one or another of the structural antigens of myelin has never been laid to rest. Finally, the sex difference in MS susceptibility may represent an as yet unknown chromosome-linked control (see McFarlin 1988).

Many lines of evidence suggest that MS may be initiated by a primarily T-cell-mediated process. Accordingly, a much closer disease association has been found with DW2, a 'lymphocyte-defined' HLA-D region allele, than with the 'serologically defined' DR2 (Compston 1986; McFarlin 1988). These immunological definitions can now be put aside in favour of the more precise definitions of base sequences within the various alleles of DP, DQ and DR and the TCR α- and β-chain genes and amino acid sequences in the corresponding gene products, as revealed by restriction fragment length polymorphism (RFLP) analysis and gene sequencing (Cohen and Dausset 1983). In a recent Norwegian series (Vartdal *et al.* 1989), virtually all (59/61) MS patients studied carried HLA-DR2, 4 or 6 in association with a DQW1 β-chain allele showing identical amino acid sequences at positions 23–31 (see also Cohen *et al.* 1984). In insulin-dependent diabetes mellitus (IDDM), another 'autoimmune' disease, this question has been pursued one step further and susceptibility has been found to be strongly correlated with the presence of alanine, valine or serine at residue 57 of the DQ3.2 β-chain allele linked with DR3 or DR4 (Todd *et al.* 1988). Conversely, aspartic acid at this position is strongly related to disease resistance. This single amino acid, through its steric configuration and polarity, presumably determines the ability of the HLA-DQ molecule to present the significant viral or autologous antigen to T cells and thus initiate the pathological response. Something comparable appears to be the case in MS.

The TCR presents the obverse relationship, in that it must provide a configuration capable of recognizing and binding the antigenic epitope attached to the Class II MHC molecule, in this case DQw1. Accordingly, a weak association is found between MS and the TCR β-chain haplotype (Beall *et al.* 1989), and characteristic RFLPs showing an association with MS are found in both α and β chains (Martell *et al.* 1987; Ciulla *et al.* 1988).

Factors initiating the disease process

Multiple sclerosis lesions are found in no more that 70% of monozygotic twins of affected probands with MS (McFarland *et al.* 1985). Thus exogenous factors are required to initiate the disease process. The bulk of existing epidemiological evidence (Table 109.6) favours common exanthematic and respiratory virus infections as the triggering agents (see Johnson 1982, 1985; Kurtzke 1985; Matthews *et al.* 1985; Waksman and Reingold 1986). There is a strong suggestion of a 'window of vulnerability' in adolescence, presumably related to the maturation of as yet unknown immunoregulatory processes. Data from a National Institutes of Health twin study showing this relationship and a British study of relative MS risk in relation to age of infection with measles, rubella and mumps are presented in Figs 109.2 and 109.3 as illustrations. Kurtzke, in a detailed study of the epidemic of MS among Faeroese Islanders, occurring after the arrival of British troops in World War II (Kurtzke and Hyllested 1986), also observed this 'window of vulnerability' and calculated an average latency of 6 years between the time of the triggering infection and the onset of clinical MS. Similarly, immune demyelinating disease in genetically predisposed guinea-pigs and mice is readily produced by immunization with myelin components at weaning, corresponding approximately to puberty in man, and much less readily by immunization earlier or later (Raine 1984). Widespread vaccination against measles, mumps and rubella, i.e. infection before the 'window' opens, has not lowered MS incidence rates but has perhaps not yet had time to produce its expected effect (Alvord *et al.* 1988).

Table 109.6. Infection with common viruses probably initiates both the primary multiple sclerosis process and most exacerbations

Primary MS process
MS in migrant populations can be related to environmental influences before age 15
MS occurs in epidemic form in island populations. The suggested 'window' of susceptibility is age 13–26, and suggested latency 6 years
In sibling pairs with MS starting after age 4, disease onset in sibling is related in time to onset in the first sibling rather than to age
MS in susceptible monozygotic twin pairs is related to frequency and severity of viral infection in late childhood, adolescence or early adult life
Common virus infections (measles, rubella, mumps, EBV) occur at older age in those who get MS than in matched controls
MS prevalence is increased with latitude among Caucasians
MS prevalence is increased in higher socio-economic groups
Exacerbations
A high proportion of MS exacerbations are triggered by upper respiratory, especially adenovirus, infections
Exacerbation rates are increased immediately after childbirth
It is possible that some relapses may be triggered by stress

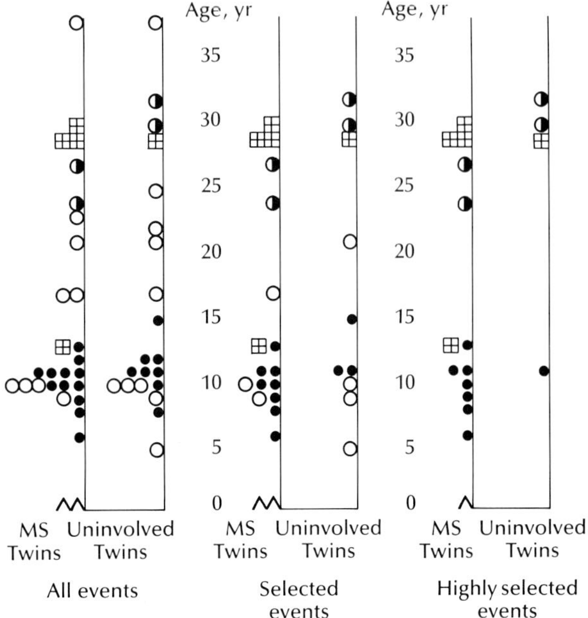

Fig. 109.2. Possible triggering events in six monozygotic long-interval twin pairs, discordant for MS. From Currier and Eldridge (1982).

The relation of MS to viral infections in adolescence may account in part for increase prevalence of the disease in higher socio-economic groups (e.g. Lauer and Firnhaber 1988) and in temperate, as compared with tropical and subtropical, latitudes (Dean 1988) (Table 109.6). As in the case of poliomyelitis, which tends to induce neurological disease only with infection at or after puberty, smaller families, larger houses and better personal and family hygiene tend to result in viral transmission at later ages and thus increased production of disease (Poskanzer *et al.* 1963).

Some confounding of genetic and environmental influences is inevitable, as in studies of MS among US veterans (see Kurtzke 1985). The clear-cut latitude effect seen in these studies may have resulted in part from the relatively greater number of people derived from Scandinavian stock in the northern tier of states (Ebers and Bulman 1986). Geographical 'clusters' of MS cases are well recognized, for example in Finland, Switzerland and Yugoslavia, but the problem of distinguishing genetic and environmental effects in these clusters has hitherto proved insoluble. Where the number of new cases has increased markedly, as in the cluster found in Møre and Romsdal counties of western Norway, with an almost threefold increase in incidence and a four- to five-fold increase in prevalence (Midgard *et al.* 1988), it is possible to suspect an introduced infection, comparable to that responsible for MS in the Faeroes. A different mechanism may be at work in the cluster of MS cases found related to a zinc factory in Rochester, NY (Stein *et al.* 1987). There is a large literature to show that zinc levels may modulate the function of immunoregulatory T cell subsets. Perhaps zinc exposure influences the 'thermostat setting' which determines which MS susceptibles will actually develop disease when stimulated by virus infection. Autoimmune encephalomyelitis is substantially increased in incidence and intensity in mice by a dietary supplement of zinc (Schiffer *et al.* 1988).

Attempts to relate MS to a single specific virus have failed, in spite of 13 different reports of isolation of one or another 'causative' agent since the late 1940s (see Johnson 1985). The epidemiological data cited above do not point at any one virus as the common trigger, although epidemics in isolated communities such as the Faeroe Islands may well result from dissemination of a single infectious agent (Kurtzke and Hyllested 1986). It appears that a variety of common viruses can trigger MS. None of these has been isolated from the CNS of MS patients, in numerous attempts by competent laboratories, and it is concluded by most workers in the field that MS is autoimmune.

An autoimmune theory is made credible by two kinds of evidence: the existence of a convincing autoimmune animal model of MS, chronic relapsing experimental allergic encephalomyelitis (EAE), induced in animals of appropriate genetic background by immunization with such myelin antigens as MBP and proteolipid protein (PLP) (McFarlin and McFarland 1982; Lassmann 1983; Raine 1984; Yoshimura *et al.* 1985; Waksman 1985; and the repeated demonstration, in both animals and man, that viral infection can immunize against MBP and result in neurological disease (Table 109.7). Experimental allergic encephalomyelitis is mediated by T cells and can be transferred between syngeneic animals by cloned MBP or PLP-specific cells of helper phenotype. However, a full-blown demyelinative lesion, like that

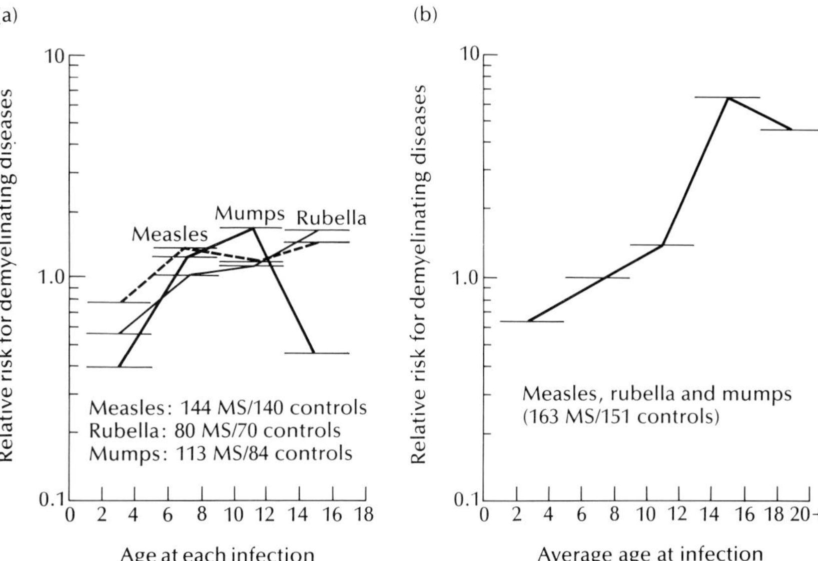

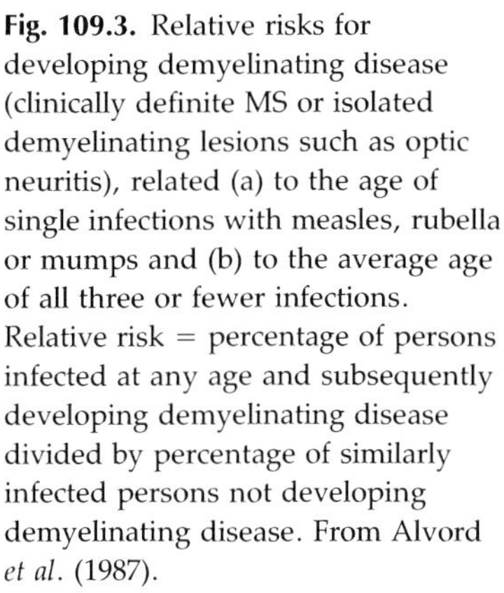

Fig. 109.3. Relative risks for developing demyelinating disease (clinically definite MS or isolated demyelinating lesions such as optic neuritis), related (a) to the age of single infections with measles, rubella or mumps and (b) to the average age of all three or fewer infections. Relative risk = percentage of persons infected at any age and subsequently developing demyelinating disease divided by percentage of similarly infected persons not developing demyelinating disease. From Alvord *et al.* (1987).

described in MS, requires the synergistic action of antibody against other myelin antigens, such as galactocerebroside (GC) or myelin–oligodendrocyte glycoprotein (MOG), apparently mediating an antibody-dependent macrophage-mediated myelinolysis (Fierz *et al.* 1988).

Viral induction of autoimmunity to CNS myelin antigens is seen with a wide variety of viruses and may depend in the majority of instances on sequence homologies between short peptides (≤10 amino acids) in certain viral antigens and in encephalitogenic regions of MBP, PLP or MOG (Stoner 1984; Fujinami and Oldstone 1985; Jahnke *et al.* 1985). However, other mechanisms may also play a role, such as myelin incorporation in the viral envelope of myxo-, paramyxo-, pox or herpes viruses (Steck *et al.* 1979) or an anti-idiotypic immune response against antiviral antibody, resulting in T cells or antibody reactive with the viral receptor on oligodendrocytes or myelin (Nepom *et al.* 1982). The majority of experiments in this area have concerned MBP, the most recent being a measles model, with triggering of MBP-specific EAE-like disease in rats (Liebert *et al.* 1988).

The most important evidence needed to support an autoimmune theory of MS, the demonstration of MBP- or PLP-specific T cells in the CNS lesions or in the blood or CSF, was first accomplished in the late 1970s (Lisak and Zweiman 1977). Several laboratories, using state-of-the-art molecular biologic techniques, have by now demonstrated the presence in blood and CSF of CD4+ve T cells reactive with specific peptides of both myelin antigens (Martin *et al.* 1990; Ota *et al.* 1990; Pette *et al.* 1990) and, more important, of *activated* T cells with similar reactivity (Allegretta *et al.* 1990). There is disagreement on the diversity of T cell receptor peptides used by these MBP-reactive cells (Pette *et al.* 1990; Wucherpfennig *et al.* 1990). While sampling of the lesions themselves to obtain living cells is logistically difficult (Hafler *et al.* 1987), it has been possible, with the polymerase chain reaction to learn that T cells in the lesions are limited in clonality (Oksenberg *et al.* 1990).

An exciting new finding is the absence in the majority of MS patients of a circulating specific CD4+ve subset of T cells identified as cytotoxic T cell precursors recognizing measles antigens in

Table 109.7. Viral immunization to myelin basic protein

Cross-immunization observed	
In man:	Measles, rubella, varicella
	Rubella (T cell clones)
In animals:	Measles, canine distemper, virus, vaccinia,
	JHM (mouse hepatitis virus)
Peptide sequence homology	
Measles, influenza, HBV, EBV, CDV, RSV, adenoviruses, SV40, JC and BK virus	

For references, see Waksman (1988a).
HBV, hepatitis B virus; RSV, respiratory syncytial virus; SV40, simian virus type 40.

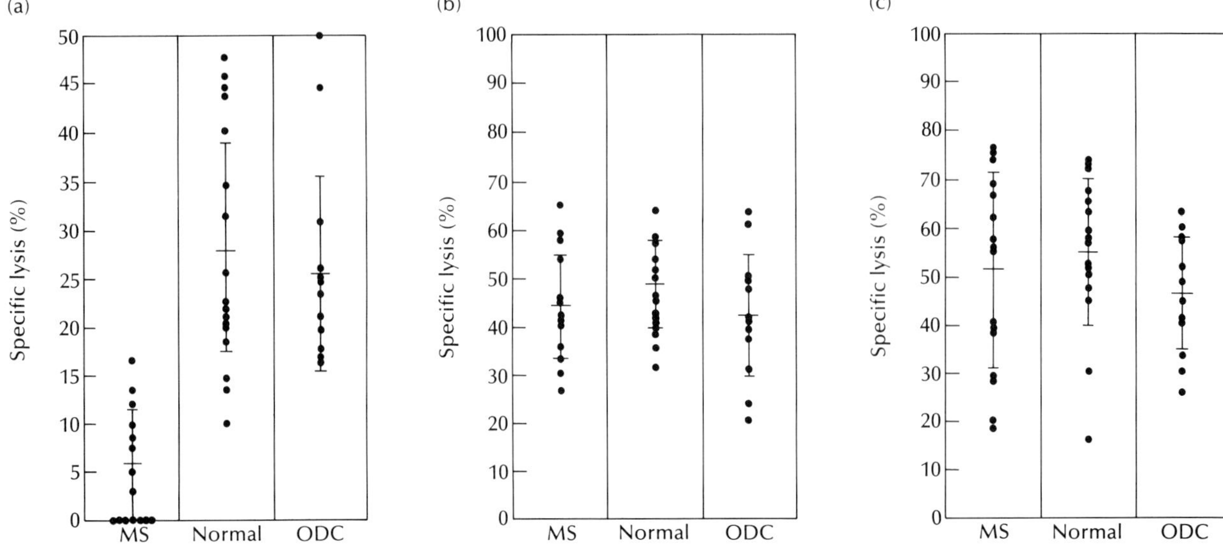

Fig. 109.4. Five-hour ^{51}Cr release assay of cytolytic activity expressed by peripheral blood lymphocytes, immunized by culture for 7 days with (a) measles virus (Edmonston) or (b) influenza A (Bankok/1/79), acting at a 40 : 1 ratio on target cells prepared by infecting EBV-transformed autologous B cell lines with the corresponding virus. Natural killer activity (c) was measured by the cytolytic activity of measles-primed lymphocytes on the NK-sensitive target K-562. Values are expressed as means of triplicate cultures. Bars indicate means ± SD. Measles virus-stimulated cells from MS patients produced significantly higher lysis of both infected and uninfected target cells than other members of this group. From Jacobson *et al.* (1985).

the context of Class II MHC (Fig. 109.4) (Jacobson *et al.* 1985). There is no comparable absence of influenza- or mumps-specific T cells. These measles-specific cells have not been shown to cross-react with myelin antigens, and the meaning of their absence from the blood remains obscure, the more so as no single antigen of measles seems to be involved (McFarland and Dhib-Jalbut 1988).

Antibodies to MBP, on the other hand, are present in MS patients' CSF (Paterson *et al.* 1981; Warren and Catz 1986; Cruz *et al.* 1988) and may vary in avidity with the clinical stage of the disease. There is reported to be a significant correlation of antibody level, measured by a sensitive radio-immunoassay (RIA), with disease activity (Fig. 109.5). This antibody is free during exacerbations of MS and bound to specific antigen in immune complexes in progressive phases of disease (Warren and Catz 1986). Antibody to glycolipid and glycoprotein antigens is also present, in immune complex form (e.g. Endo *et al.* 1984; Thuillier *et al.* 1988). It is not clear whether such antibodies should be regarded as playing a primary role in the disease or as secondary to tissue breakdown.

Increasing awareness of the viral aetiology of many cases of chronic myelopathy (Johnson and McArthur 1987; Bhagavati *et al.* 1988), together with the failure to establish an autoimmune basis for MS, have fuelled continued attempts to identify a retrovirus like HTLV-1 persisting in the CNS, as the cause of this disease (Koprowski *et al.* 1985). The reported demonstration of viral genome in CSF T cells has been vitiated by artefact (Hauser *et al.* 1986), and the antiviral antibody demonstrable by supersensitive techniques in the blood and CSF has also been found in normals or other disease controls at a lower titre. Many common antiviral antibodies, however, are also present in MS patients at a higher titre than in controls (Forghani *et al.* 1978); therefore such evidence is not convincing proof of a specific aetiological relationship.

Factors triggering exacerbation in multiple sclerosis

The process of exacerbation is played out over a period of days or weeks, in contrast to the period of several years which intervenes between the initial stimulation of MS by viral infection and the onset of clinical disease (Table 109.6). In a recent American series, over one-quarter of exacerbations could be related to upper respiratory infections

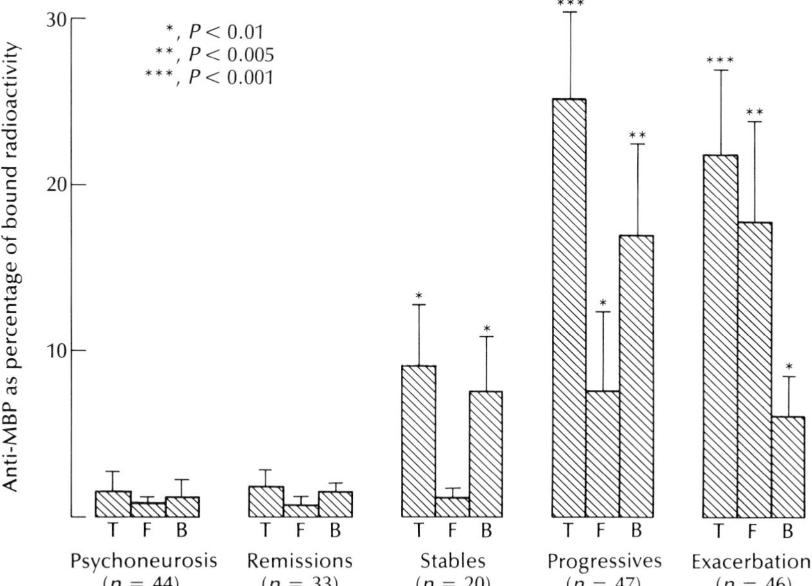

Fig. 109.5. Total (T), free (F) and bound (B) anti-MBP in control patients with psychoneurosis and in patients with multiple sclerosis. Numbers of patients in parentheses. From Warren and Catz (1986).

becoming manifest between 2 weeks before and 5 weeks after the onset of exacerbation (Sibley *et al.* 1985). The known frequency of inapparent viral infections suggests the possibility that a much higher proportion of exacerbations is so triggered. The basic finding has been confirmed in a Scandinavian study, with the addition of serological evidence that the responsible agent is frequently an adenovirus (Lygner *et al.* 1988). A British report relating exacerbation to chronic sinusitis (Gay *et al.* 1986) has not thus far been confirmed.

Two different mechanisms may play a role in virus-triggered exacerbation. There may be a renewal of the process leading to the original disease, either primary immunization with a new viral antigen or secondary (booster) stimulation of the pre-existing immune response. New specific immunocompetent cells would enter the circulation and generate new lesions in the CNS. A different process is implied by the observation, during a recent pilot study of interferon-γ in mild MS, that half the patients receiving this agent developed an exacerbation within a few days (Panitch *et al.* 1987). Exacerbation was correlated with enhanced expression of Class II MHC on circulating monocytes. A parallel increase of MHC on cerebral vascular endothelium (Pober *et al.* 1983) and astrocytes (Fontana *et al.* 1984) may be inferred. In fact, systemic infection has been shown to be associated with increased systemic release of lymphokines and with increased Class II MHC throughout the CNS (Traugott and Lebon 1988b). The exacerbations were limited to a reappearance of clinical signs experienced earlier by the same patients and seemed to represent a rekindling of pre-existing lesions, perhaps by T cells persisting at the lesion sites. These two mechanisms correspond to the finding in the MRI studies cited earlier that, even in the mildest MS cases, both frequent showers of new lesions and reactivation of old lesions occur as concomitant and seemingly independent events.

Experiments with the animal model EAE confirm the ready induction of exacerbation by manoeuvres that up-regulate MHC throughout the body, e.g. infection or systemic graft-versus-host (GVH) disease (Willenborg *et al.* 1985; Traugott and Lebon 1988b). However, other agents which eliminate suppressor T cells selectively, e.g. low-dose cyclophosphamide (Arnon 1981) and antithymocyte serum (Sobel *et al.* 1983), also induce exacerbation. Experimentally, MBP-specific suppressor T cells have been found to be present in the spleens of MBP-immunized guinea-pigs during periods of disease remission and to disappear during spontaneous exacerbation (Lyman *et al.* 1985). Corresponding observations have not been made in MS patients.

The frequency of exacerbation diminishes during pregnancy and is markedly augmented immediately *post partum* (Millar 1961) (Fig. 109.6).

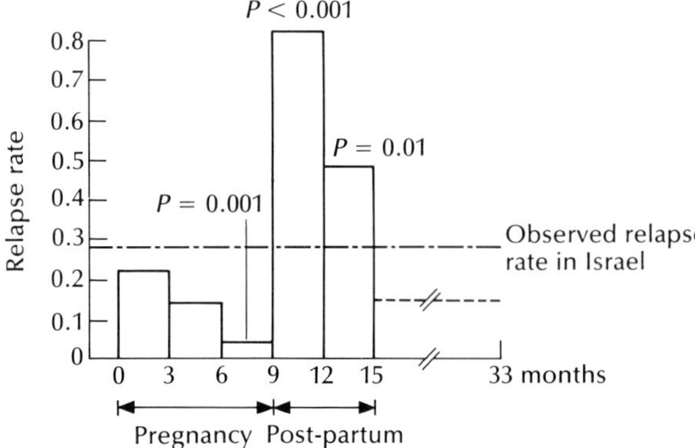

Fig. 109.6. Relapse rate in pregnancy and *post partum*, as compared with the observed relapse rate of multiple sclerosis patients in Israel. From Korn-Lubetzki *et al.* (1984).

A simple interpretation would be that pregnancy is accompanied by steroid-mediated immunosuppression or immunosuppression by α-fetoprotein and release from suppression after delivery (Korn-Lubetzki *et al.* 1984). A more complex mechanism involving α-fetoprotein and suppressor T cells may be envisaged. In the broader sense, the 'thermostat' of immune regulation appears to be reset, first in one direction, then the other.

Most physicians believe that stress plays a role in some MS exacerbations. However, in Sibley's study, analysis of 10 'stress factors', such as loss of spouse, loss of job, etc., failed to establish a statistically significant relationship between any such factor and relapse (Sibley 1988). The quality of stressful life events (desirability, controllability) rather than the quantity (number) of events may be related to the occurrence of exacerbation (Franklin *et al.* 1988). It has also been reported that quality of life influences the initiation of the MS process (Warren *et al.* 1982). It is difficult, however, to sort out true stress events from infection rates and the initiation of MS as such from the exacerbation process.

The multiple sclerosis lesion

Morphologists agree (Lassmann 1983; Raine 1984; Prineas 1985) on the following essential features of MS lesions, all of which are duplicated in acute and chronic EAE (Table 109.8, Figs 109.7–109.10): an inflammatory reaction, beginning around venules and small veins and consisting predominantly of mononuclear cells (lymphocytes, macrophages and some plasma cells); breakdown of the blood–tissue barrier and oedema, especially in acute lesions; demyelination, which is primarily segmental and is seen only in relation to, and probably secondary to, the presence of macrophages; and a loss of oligodendrocytes. There is some axonal damage, but rarely damage of neurons. Meningeal inflammation is present in many cases. Later changes include remyelination, leading to formation of 'shadow plaques', and gliosis (activation and proliferation of astrocytes), which results in scarring, i.e. the laying down of glial fibrillary acidic protein (GFAP) fibres.

Larger plaques form by coalescence and by peripheral extension of early lesions. They maintain a topographical relationship to areas of venous drainage, especially near the ventricles. They are largely limited to the CNS white matter, but there may be small wedge-shaped lesions in the cortex. A few patients show PNS lesions as well.

The details vary strikingly with the age of the lesions studied and perhaps with the underlying immunological mechanism. Prineas (1985) has stressed the role of the cell infiltrate, and of macro-

Table 109.8. Essential features of the multiple sclerosis lesion

Perivenous inflammation: T4 +ve and T8 +ve lymphocytes, many macrophages, some plasma cells
Blood–tissue barrier breakdown, oedema
Demyelination: stripping and phagocytosis, vesicular breakdown (macrophages in lesions are filled with IgG; macrophage IgG shows capping at site of myelin breakdown)
Myelin and oligodendrocytes both destroyed early
Remyelination and renewed demyelination (shadow plaques, concentric lesions)
Astrocytic gliosis, scarring
Coalescence and peripheral extension of lesions

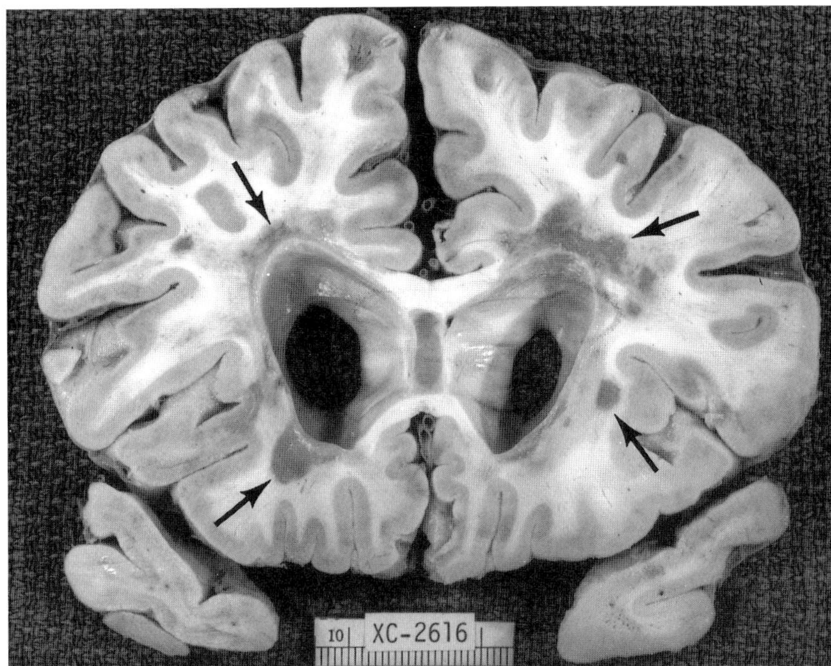

Fig. 109.7. Typical gross appearance of chronic MS plaques (arrows) in periventricular white matter. Plaques are glassy in appearance and grey, due to the loss of myelin and scarring. Courtesy of Dr C.S. Raine.

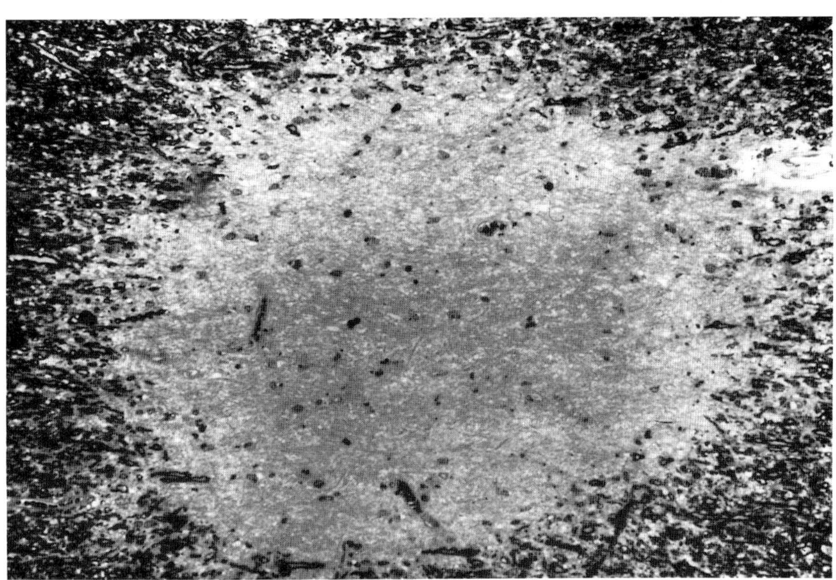

Fig. 109.8. Small MS plaque, from the brain illustrated in Fig. 114.7, stained for myelin (black) and photographed at intermediate power (×100). There is complete destruction of myelin within the plaque and an abrupt margin between the plaque and the adjacent white matter.

phages in particular, in the destruction of myelin, while Lassmann (1983) has called attention to lesions which are largely acellular. These differences are like those seen in model experiments with rats to which varying proportions of cloned MBP-immune T cells and anti-MOG antibody have been transferred (Fierz *et al.* 1988). Both CD4 +ve cells and CD8 +ve cells are found in the active zones of MS plaques. The former (Traugott *et al.* 1983) are mostly 4B4 +ve, i.e. helper–inducer in phenotype, and 2B4 +ve suppressor–inducer cells are rare (Sobel *et al.* 1988). The predominant cells in the lesions are typical CD3, 8, 11 +ve cytotoxic T cells (Boos *et al.* 1983) lacking the HNK-1 natural killer (NK) cell marker and also lacking the activation antigens TAC (interleukin 2 (IL-2) receptor), Ta1 and T11–3 (Hayashi *et al.* 1988). Thus, although regulation within the lesion is minimal, few activated effector cells appear to be present. γ/δ T cells are frequent in older lesions (Aquino and Selmaj

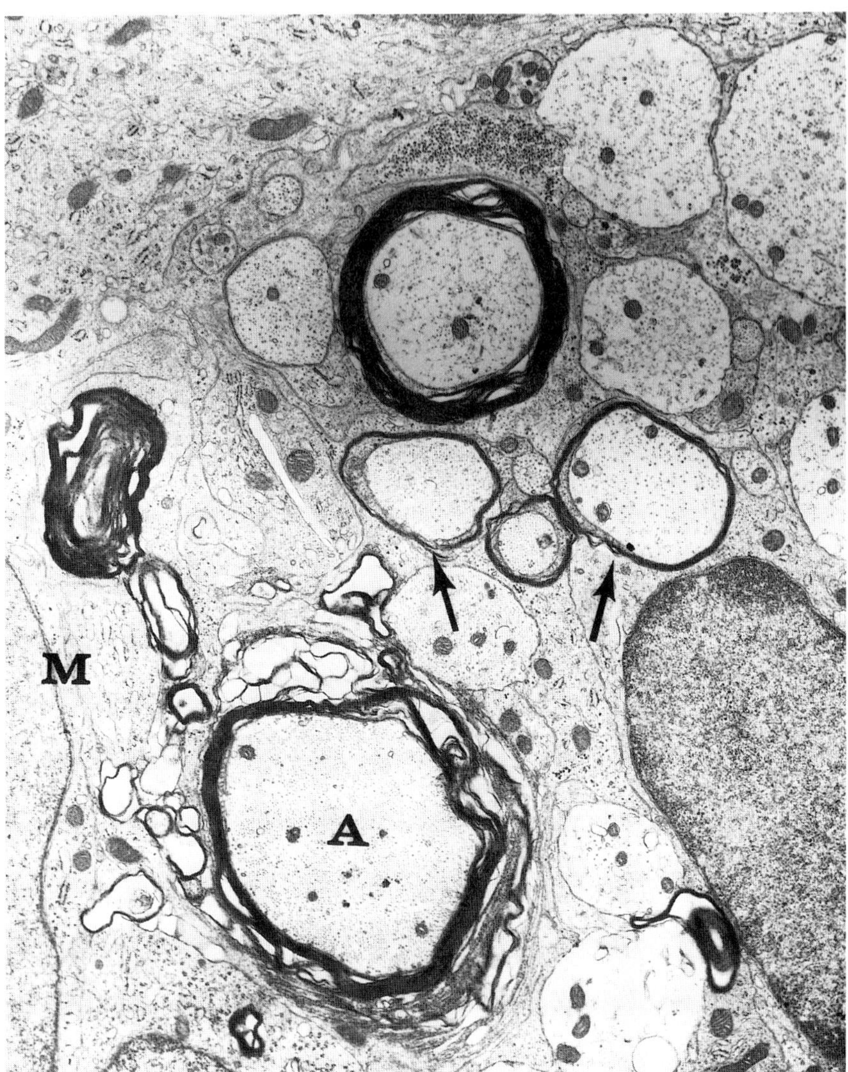

Fig. 109.9. Electron microscopic view (×8500) of chronic relapsing EAE plaque in guinea-pig spinal cord, illustrating important features of both the disease process and repair. The myelin sheath around the axon (A) shows active breakdown under the influence of the macrophage (M). There are also naked axons, which have been demyelinated. Remyelination is demonstrated by thin layers of myelin (arrows) around several axons. Courtesy of Dr C.S. Raine.

1992), but their role is completely unknown. In addition, structures resembling organized lymphoid tissue are often present in the perivascular spaces of older MS plaques (Prineas 1985). These may provide the principal sites of ongoing immune responses to tissue antigens.

Vascular damage and oedema formation in fresh lesions (Troiano *et al.* 1984) bring all the conventional plasma constituents into the tissue, including any circulating antibody and the full array of complement components. Myelin itself, in the absence of antibody, can trigger complement-mediated lysis by the classical pathway (Vanguri *et al.* 1982) and this may be one of the more important elements of early tissue damage. The procoagulant activity of macrophages, activated by T cell lymphokines, and the possible role of fibrin deposition in oedematous lesions of MS have also been stressed (Geczy 1983).

Myelin breakdown, the key element in MS lesions, takes several forms. Macrophages strip and ingest intact myelin by ligand-mediated endocytosis, with formation of typical 'coated pits' (Prineas 1985). The ligand appears to be antibody and there is immunoglobulin G (IgG) capping on the surface of the demyelinating macrophages. There is also vesiculation and dissolution of myelin in the immediate vicinity of the infiltrating cells, possibly due to release of proteases and/or phospholipases, with secondary activation of comple-

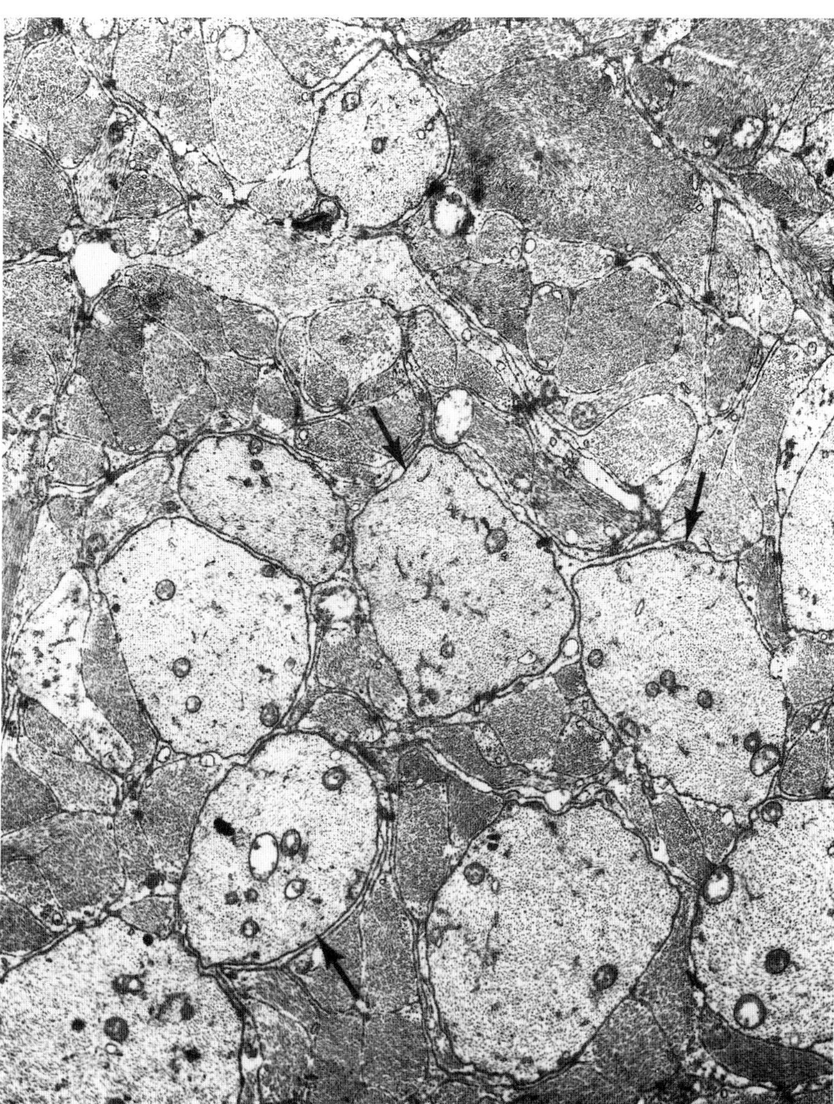

Fig. 109.10. Electron micrograph (×12 400) of chronic demyelinated MS plaque, showing naked axons (arrows) embedded in fibrous glial scar. Courtesy of Dr C.S. Raine.

ment or of endogenous proteases of the myelin itself (Sato *et al*. 1982). Free oxygen radicals, generated by activated macrophages may also play a role in myelin breakdown (Hartung *et al*. 1988). Oedema, of course, especially intramyelin oedema, increases the accessibility of the myelin lamellae to all of these damaging factors.

Analysis with modern tools, such as *in situ* hybridization with nucleic acid probes, permitting analysis of gene expression in individual cells, and the use of monoclonal antibodies to identify gene products, either immunohistochemically in the lesions or by sensitive assays like RIA in tissue extracts or CSF, has added a new dimension to current studies of MS lesions. Table 109.9 lists the classes of molecules recently studied or under investigation at the present time. Of course Class II MHC requires special comment because of its importance in recognition by most or all CD4 +ve T cells. Class II MHC is not found normally on any tissue element of the CNS but is expressed on vascular endothelium in and near MS plaques, on astrocytes in the periphery of such plaques and the adjacent normal tissue, and of course on microglia and activated macrophages infiltrating the tissue (Traugott *et al*. 1985). The up-regulating of Class II MHC by interferon-γ (Wong *et al*. 1985; Panitch *et al*. 1987), e.g. in association with systemic infection, and its down-regulation by such endogenous neurotransmitters as norepine-

Table 109.9. Important molecules in lesion formation

Antigens MBP, PLP, MOG, GC, etc. *Serum derivatives* Antibody, complement, clotting factors *T cell receptor peptides* Ti-alpha, beta or gamma, delta CD3-gamma, delta, epsilon, zeta, eta *Other T and B cell markers* CD4, CD8, mIg 2H4, 4B4, Tal, T11–3, etc. *Class II MHC* DR-alpha, beta DQ-alpha, beta	*T cell factors* IL-2–12 IFN-gamma Lymphotoxin *Macrophage factors* IL-1 and TNF Proteolytic, lipolytic enzymes O_2 radicals, NO_2^- Prostaglandins, leukotrienes Complement components *Astrocyte factors* Several of above *Other neural factors* Adhesion molecules Growth factors Neuropeptides Neurotransmitters *Receptors* For all of above

IL, interleukin; IFN, interferon; MBP, PLP, MOG, GC, myelin antigens; MHC, major histocompatibility complex; TNF, tumour necrosis factor.

phrine (Frohman *et al.* 1988) or exogenously administered interferon-β (Joseph *et al.* 1988) are crucial elements in the biology of the MS process. Class I MHC is expressed on a variety of neural cells, may be up-regulated by such macrophage products as tumour necrosis factor (TNF) (Lavi *et al.* 1988) and may also play a role in stimulating T cells. Several lymphokines are also found in MS CSF, interferon-γ being perhaps the most important (Hirsch *et al.* 1985; Traugott and Lebon 1988a).

Many potential mutagenic influences are present in the MS lesion. These include: spontaneous chromatid exchange, possible retrovirus infection (HTLV-1-related), MHC autoreactivity, IL-1 and IL-2 and the interferons, and reactive oxygen species. In cloning studies of cells from the MS lesions themselves or from CSF (Birnbaum *et al.* 1984; Hafler *et al.* 1987), continuously proliferating clones were easily isolated. These, however, have had no special attention, and their relation either to mutagenic events or to the pathogenesis of the lesions remains conjectural. On the other hand, MHC autoreactive cells have been found in the CSF (Birnbaum *et al.* 1984), and this justifies the speculation that a mixed lymphocyte reaction (MLR) or GVH-like reaction may be an important component of the established lesion (Waksman 1985, 1988a, b).

The oligodendrocytes, which produce and maintain myelin, are destroyed in early MS lesions, but new cells appear rapidly and lay down new myelin repeatedly as the lesion ages (Prineas 1985). Many questions remain unanswered here: the source of the new cells (existing oligodendrocytes reactivated by loss of their myelin burden, previously undifferentiated oligodendrocyte precursors, Schwann cells); whether the process destroying oligodendrocytes is immunological and is targeted to myelin components in the oligodendrocyte surface membrane or components of the oligodendrocyte itself; or whether it may instead result from the action of TNF or lymphotoxin-like molecules or oxygen radicals released by the infiltrating cells. Evidence exists to support all these possibilities.

Functional loss, i.e. the failure of conduction, is produced in early lesions by elements other than loss of myelin. Oedema may be the most important, since vascular leakage, demonstrable originally by the use of radio-opaque dye and computed tomography scanning and more recently with the use of gadolinium-DPTA and MRI (Grossman *et al.* 1986), often parallels symptomatology. Both are diminished in parallel after a high dose of intravenous steroids (Troiano *et al.* 1984) or intravenous mannitol (Stefoski *et al.* 1985). T cell lymphokines are reported to arrest conduction directly or indirectly (Yarom *et al.* 1983; Brosnan *et al.* 1988), as are fragments of MBP (Gähwiler and Honegger 1979). Finally, a circulating 'neuroelectric blocking factor', shown to be IgG antibody against an unknown presynaptic nerve terminal component (Schauf and Davis 1978), may play a role.

Cellular responses in the cerebrospinal fluid and blood

T cells (Table 109.10) are the main cellular constituent of the CSF in MS (Brooks *et al.* 1983). Most are continuously cycling cells of helper–inducer phenotype (Noronha *et al.* 1980; Brooks *et al.* 1983) and half carry markers characteristic of long-term, IL-2-dependent T cell lines (Hafler *et al.* 1985). Occasional reports of positive reactivity to MBP (Lisak and Zweiman 1977) or other myelin antigens (Offner *et al.* 1981) have remained unconfirmed. Most investigators regard the CSF T cells as oligo-

Table 109.10. Characteristics of cerebrospinal fluid T cells in multiple sclerosis

Continuously cycling blasts are present during both clinical activity and 'remission'
Phenotype suggests cells in late stage of activation (like cells after prolonged culture)
Cells show limited polyclonality; express limited number of T cell receptor gene rearrangements; are reactive to many viruses
Relative absence of cells reactive to myelin antigens
Predominance of MHC autoreactive cells (many with identical pattern of heteroclitic alloreactivity)

Table 109.11. Cerebrospinal fluid B cells and plasma cells in multiple sclerosis

Continuously productive cells are present during both clinical activity and 'remission'
These range from typical B cells to mature plasma cells and produce antibody of all major isotypes
Cells show limited polyclonality; produce antibody to multiple viruses and myelin antigens
Preferential synthesis of certain allotypes in heterozygotes (example: Glm(1) versus Glm(3) of IgG1)
Over-production of free monomeric and dimeric light chains similar to Bence-Jones protein
Immune complexes with viral and myelin protein and glycolipid antigens and complement fixation: C2 and C9

or polyclonal; indeed, cells reactive with a variety of viruses are often found in one and the same patient (Reunanen *et al.* 1983). However, the absence of a CD4 +ve, Class II MHC-restricted T cell subset specific for measles virus from the circulation (Utermohlen and Zabriskie 1973; Jacobson *et al.* 1985; McFarland and Dhib-Jalbut 1988) may represent a specific change; investigation of the involved measles antigen(s) and MHC locus are in progress.

Cloning studies have mainly re-emphasized the polyclonality of the CSF T cells. Restriction fragment length polymorphism analysis of T cell receptor variable (V)-region gene rearrangements in a series of clones has led to the finding in one laboratory of oligoclonality (Hafler *et al.* 1988) and in another of polyclonality (Rotteveel *et al.* 1988). A unique finding is the presence in virtually all MS patients' CSF of MHC autoreactive T cells, the majority heteroclitic, i.e. more reactive with allogeneic than syngeneic MHC (Birnbaum *et al.* 1984). Such autoreactive clones, presumably generated in response to exogenous antigenic stimuli, have the potential of contributing to the pathogenesis of chronic lesions (Waksman 1985). T cell clones reactive with MBP are readily obtained from peripheral blood (Burns *et al.* 1983). These are reactive with as many as 10 distinct MBP epitopes (Richert *et al.* 1988; Tournier-Lasserve *et al.* 1988). For recent studies of this problem, see above under 'Factors initiating the disease process'.

Plasma cells and B cell blasts are present in the lesions of MS, particularly in the perivascular inflammatory cuffs, and some are present in the CSF (Table 109.11). Elevated Ig of all isotypes produced by these cells are found in the CNS and CSF (Brooks *et al.* 1983; Tourtellotte 1985). The predominant isotype is IgG; it shows a disturbed $\kappa:\lambda$ ratio, preferential synthesis of the IgG-1 subclass and a striking allotype restriction. There is also an overproduction of monomeric and dimeric Ig light chains reminiscent of Bence-Jones proteins (Rudick *et al.* 1986). The factors determining these restrictions remain conjectural. In spite of its well-known oligoclonality, CSF IgG, even from a single patient, may contain multiple antiviral and antibacterial antibodies (Forghani *et al.* 1978; Norrby 1978), as well as antibodies to MBP (Paterson *et al.* 1981; Warren and Catz 1986; Cruz *et al.* 1988) and other CNS constituents, such as GFAP and S-100 (Melse *et al.* 1983). Immune complexes, found in both CSF and peripheral blood, contain Ig of all the isotypes, bound to a variety of common viral antigens and both MBP and myelin glycolipids (Paterson *et al.* 1981; Endo *et al.* 1984; Coyle and Procyk-Doughtery 1984; Warren and Catz 1986; Thuillier *et al.* 1988). Not expectedly, C2 and C9 levels in the CSF are low. Attempts to find unique, reproducible Ig idiotypes which would identify important antigens have been disappointing (Coyle and Procyk-Doughtery 1984; Gerhard *et al.* 1985). Thus the bulk of the CSF Ig is MS cannot be identified as antibody to any one antigen. It has been inferred that B cells move non-specifically from the blood into new plaques and persist as antibody-forming cells, perhaps continuously stimulated by the ongoing T cell and macrophage reactions in their vicinity. The polyclonality found in studies of CSF Ig is underscored by increasingly refined *in vitro* studies of CSF B cells, cultured with or without mitogenic stimulation (Link *et al.* 1988).

One is left with a picture of semi-autonomous proliferative and reactive foci of both T and B cells, scattered throughout the CNS and CSF compartments, resembling metastases of proliferating T lymphoma cells or the cells of a so-called plasma cell dyscrasia.

In the blood, the dominant finding in MS is a deficiency in mechanisms of down-regulation (Reder and Arnason 1985). A decrease in non-antigen-specific suppressor–inducer T cells and autologous MLR suppressors (CD4 +ve, 2H4 +ve) (Fig. 109.11) is clearly related to disease activity (Morimoto *et al.* 1987; Crisp and Greenstein, submitted), and there is a related deficiency in non-specific T suppressor activity, as shown by a variety of assays (see Reder and Arnason 1985). The responsible CD8 +ve T cells appear to undergo modulation, with loss of both phenotypic markers and suppressor activity, under the influence of MS serum, rather than disappearing (Reder *et al.* 1984). This effect is variously attributed to decreased

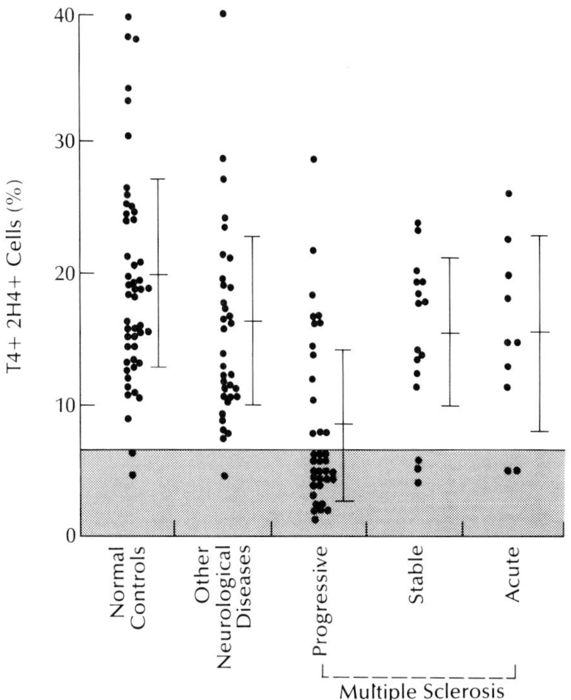

Fig. 109.11. Percentage of CD4 +ve, 2H4 +ve T cells in the peripheral blood of MS patients and controls. The shaded area indicates the lower limit of normal 2 SD below the mean percentage of CD4 +ve, 2H4 +ve cells in the peripheral blood of the healthy controls (6%). From Morimoto *et al.* (1987).

suppressor–inducer influence, to lymphocytotoxic antibodies and to prostaglandins released by other cells. Natural killer cells are also modulated, with loss of markers, killer activity and the ability to generate interferon-α/β. An increase in β-adrenergic receptors on the altered CD8 +ve cells and altered sympathetic function similar to that seen in sympathectomized animals (Arnason *et al.* 1988; Nordenbo 1988) imply an altered responsiveness of immune regulatory mechanisms to psychoneural influences in MS.

In striking contrast to this immunoregulatory deficiency is the activation of all other cells in the circulation, including cells not considered to have any relation to the MS process (see Reder and Arnason 1985; Waksman 1988a). Circulating lymphocytes express activation markers, monocytes and granulocytes express increased lysosomal enzyme activity and increased production of E-series prostaglandins and leukotrienes, and platelets, as well as the other cell types, express altered adherence properties. The cause of all this activity is unknown; it may lie among lymphokines and monokines coming from the CNS lesions. The monocytic prostaglandins play a role in modulating circulating CD8 +ve NK cells (Merrill *et al.* 1983), and their enzymes seem to account for much of the so-called myelinotoxic property of MS serum (Grundke-Iqbal and Bornstein 1979).

Non-cellular changes in cerebrospinal fluid and other body fluids

Of the known non-cellular changes in MS body fluids (Table 109.12), the most striking is the appearance of myelin breakdown products, notably MBP and its fragments, in CSF, blood and even urine (Whitaker and Snyder 1984; Tourtellotte 1985), and galactosyl ceramide in blood (Thuillier *et al.* 1988). The qualitative difference between peptides resulting from digestion of MBP by T-lymphokine-activated macrophages and those from digestion by conventional reactive macrophages, in such conditions as stroke, can be exploited by the use of appropriate (but unfortunately rare) monoclonal antibodies to give a highly specific measure of MS disease activity as expressed in the rate of myelin breakdown (Fig. 109.12).

Antibody to MBP in the CSF (Paterson *et al.*

Table 109.12. Non-cellular abnormalities in cerebrospinal fluid and other body fluids

Myelin basic protein fragments
Other CNS myelin and non-myelin breakdown products
Antibodies reactive with the above
Antibodies to pituitary (neural lobe) peptides
Antibodies to vascular endothelium
Elevated antiviral (especially anti-measles) antibodies
Elevated immunoglobulins, oligoclonal bands, free Ig light chains
Immune complexes, terminal complement complexes (C5b–9)
Decreased complement components (C2, C9)
Myelinotoxic, neuroelectric blocking and lymphocytotoxic factors
Elevated ACTH, prolactin, β-endorphin, substance P, vasopressin, cholecystokinin
Interferon-γ, other lymphokines, IL-2 receptor, prostaglandin E_2
Decreased essential fatty acids
Abnormal levels of zinc, selenium (cells and/or plasma)

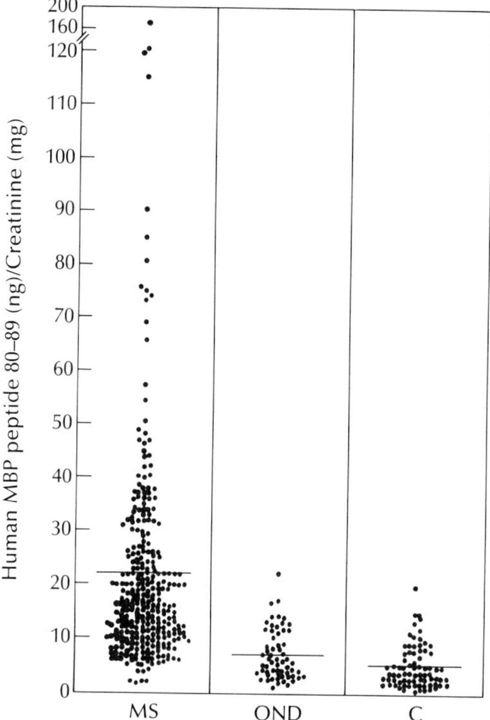

Fig. 109.12. Urinary MBP-like material measured in unconcentrated urine in a double-antibody radio-immunoassay against a standard of human MBP peptide 80–89 and expressed in relation to urinary creatinine level in patients with MS, other neurological diseases (OND) and normal control subjects (C). From Whitaker (1987).

1981; Cruz *et al.* 1988) shows a significant relation to disease activity (Warren and Catz 1986), as do immune complexes in the CSF and blood (Coyle and Procyk-Doughtery 1984). Circulating antibody titres to a variety of viruses exceed the comparable titres in other disease controls (Forghani *et al.* 1978; Norrby 1978), apparently as part of the general 'activation' of immune and other cells, combined with the faulty immune regulation characteristic of MS. This simple fact has led to successive waves of enthusiasm for measles virus, then EBV and currently HTLV-1 (Koprowski *et al.* 1985; Ohta *et al.* 1988) as the 'cause' of MS.

The hypothalamus and pituitary may have a special role in MS, as suggested by frequent rather striking alterations in the blood levels of pituitary peptides (Allen *et al.* 1980) and by cases of pituitary-related failure of sexual function (Bourdette *et al.* 1988). The dexamethasone suppression response, which depends on normal pituitary function, is also abnormal in as many as half of MS patients (Reder *et al.* 1987). While some patients may have actual MS plaques in the hypothalamic region, autoantibodies to pituitary peptides (Hansen *et al.* 1983; Heltberg *et al.* 1988) may play a significant role here, as may IL-1 and TNF, which are released by activated macrophages and astrocytes and which bind to cells in both hypothalamic nuclei and the pituitary (Breder *et al.* 1988). Some of the elevated blood adrenocorticotrophic hormone (ACTH) and endorphin may be produced directly by activated lymphocytes (Reder *et al.* 1988).

For references to studies of fatty acids and of zinc and selenium in MS, the reader is referred to Utermohlen *et al.* (1981), Neu (1983) and Waksman (1985).

Clinical management of multiple sclerosis

Diagnosis of MS today depends on the clinical neurological examination, complemented, as discussed earlier, by MRI, evoked potential, magnetic cortical stimulation and CSF studies (Table 109.2). There is no specific test for MS, but one or more of the laboratory findings under study, notably MBP

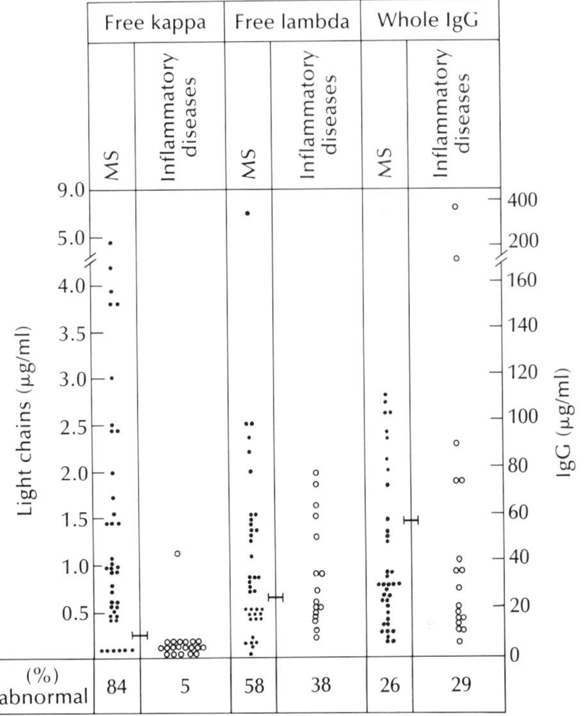

Fig. 109.13. Free light chains and whole IgG in MS and inflammatory disease controls. Bars represent upper limit of normal, as derived from non-inflammatory disease controls. The difference between MS and controls in the kappa assay was highly significant ($p < 0.0001$). From Rudick *et al.* (1986).

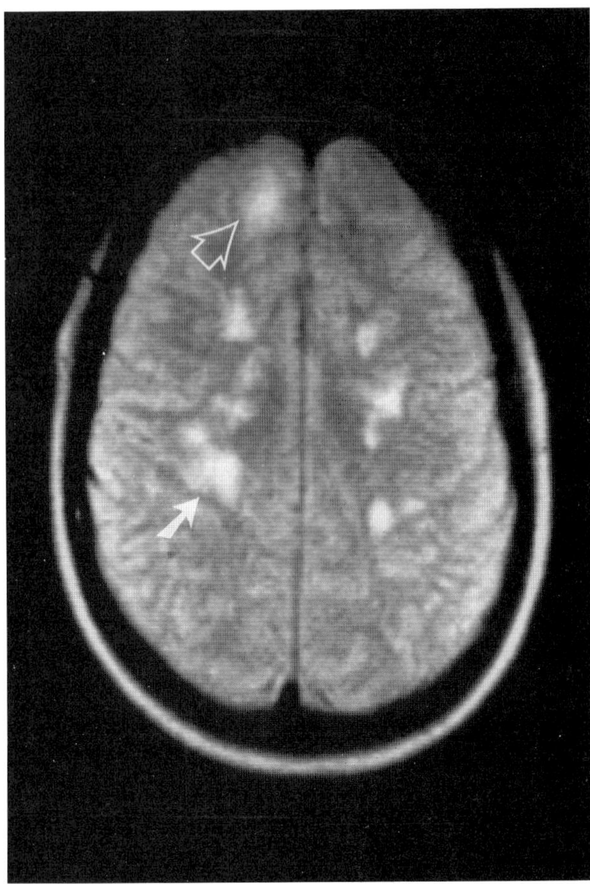

Fig. 109.14. Characteristic appearance of MS plaques in MRI scan, showing largely periventricular localization. The two arrows point to lesions that subsequently disappeared. This image was the first in a series of 13 images on this particular patient. The two lesions did not reappear during the entire study while the other lesions (white areas) remained stable. Figure kindly provided by Dr David K.B. Li, Director of MRI Research, Department of Diagnostic Radiology, University of British Columbia.

fragments in urine, GC in blood, MBP antibody in CSF and free κ chains in CSF, may ultimately provide an almost foolproof test for the disease (Fig. 109.13). Magnetic resonance imaging is the single most important laboratory test today (Fig. 109.14).

Therapies in current use or under investigation (Table 109.13) are directed either at preventing the presumed viral triggering event, preventing autoimmunization against myelin, suppressing the pathological immune response, modifying immune regulation (enhancing suppression), reducing inflammation at the lesion site or restoring conduction in demyelinated nerve fibres (Sibley *et al.* 1988). The reported efficacy of interferon-β and of copolymer-1 in reducing the frequency of exacerbations requires confirmation by more extensive trials, as does the reported efficacy of such lymphopenic agents as cyclophosphamide and total lymphoid irradiation in arresting progression. There is general agreement that ACTH or high-dose steroids stop oedema formation promptly and ameliorate acute attacks of MS, without, however, affecting the course of the disease. Agents like 4-aminopyridine can restore neurological function transiently, but have not as yet found their place in current practice.

Imaginative new approaches to therapy (Table 109.14) are for the most part extensions of the above list but depend on identification of the antigen(s) actually responsible for MS or on isolation of the specifically reactive cells (see recent review of Miller *et al.* 1991). Identification of the key DQW1 β-chain peptide (see Vartdal *et al.* 1989) and synthesis of molecules that can block this site, as has been proposed for IDDM (Todd *et al.* 1988), may provide the most practical approach to preventing or treating MS. Approaches via non-

Table 109.13. Multiple sclerosis 'treatments' in current use or under investigation

Antiviral agents: interferons, amantadine, cytarabine, acyclovir, isoprinosine
Specific immunological 'tolerance' to myelin antigens: myelin basic protein, copolymer-1, oral myelin
Non-specific immunosuppression: azathioprine, cyclophosphamide, cyclosporin, plasmaphaeresis, lymphocytophaeresis, total lymphoid irradiation
Immunomodulation: various monoclonal antibodies, interferons, interferon inducers, levamisole, thymus hormones, thymectomy, alpha-fetoprotein, transfer factor, heparin, 'immunoactive' peptides
Suppression of inflammation: ACTH, corticosteroids, colchicine, desferrioxamine, EACA, gold compounds, prazosin, calcium chelators
Restoration of conduction: 4-aminopyridine, amantadine, 3,4-diaminopyridine

Table 109.14. Specific 'immunotherapies' which may soon be tested in multiple sclerosis

Inject or feed synthetic analogues of MBP or PLP, to induce antigen-specific tolerance
Inject inactivated MBP- or PLP-specific effector T cells, cloned from CSF, to induce idiotype tolerance
Inject T cell receptor peptides from MBP- or PLP-specific effector T cells
PUVA (oral psoralen and extracorporeal UV irradiation of blood) to induce idiotype tolerance
Inject MBP- or PLP-specific suppressor T lymphocytes, cloned from blood or CSF, to maintain antigen or idiotype tolerance
Inject monoclonal antibody against T cell receptor idiotypes or antibody against non-polymorphic recognition molecules (DR2, IFN-γ (or its receptor), IL-2 receptor, Fc receptor), to block reaction or induce long-term suppression
Inject monoclonal antibody or specific peptides designed to block key sites in the DQw1 β-chain involved in antigen presentation

polymorphic molecules remain non-specific and have all the drawbacks that accompany the cruder non-specific anti-inflammatory, immunosuppressive and immunomodulatory agents in current use.

References

Allegretta, M., Nicklas, J.A., Sriram, S. and Albertini, R.J. (1990). T cells responsive to myelin basic protein in patients with multiple sclerosis. *Science* **247**, 718.

Allen, J., Powers, C., Kepic, T., Talereco, J., Garwacki, D. and Swank, R. (1980). Plasma peptide concentrations in patients with multiple sclerosis. *Clin. Res.* **28**, 255A (abstract).

Alvord, E.C., Jr, Jahnke, V., Fischer, E.H., Kies, M.W., Driscoll, B.F. and Compston, D.A.S. (1987). The multiple causes of multiple sclerosis: the importance of age of infections in childhood. *J. Child Neurol.* **2**, 313–21.

Alvord, E.C., Jr, Compston, D.A.S. and Kies, M.W. (1988). Is multiple sclerosis already being prevented? In *Trends in European Multiple Sclerosis Research*, ed. C. Confavreux, G. Aimard and M. Devic, p. 61, Excerpta Medica, Amsterdam.

Aquino, D.A. and Selmaj, K. (1992). Heat-shock proteins and gamma-delta cell responses in the central nervous system. *Chem. Immunol.* **53**, 86.

Arnason, B.G.W., Brown, M., Maselli, R., Karaszewski, J. and Reder, A. (1989). Blood lymphocyte β-adrenergic receptors in multiple sclerosis. *Ann. NY Acad. Sci.* **540**, 585–8.

Arnon, R. (1981). Experimental allergic encephalomyelitis susceptibility and suppression. *Immunol. Res.* **55**, 5–30.

Beall, S.S., Concannon, P., Charmley, P. *et al.* (1988). The germline repertoire of T-cell receptor β-chain genes in patients with chronic progressive multiple sclerosis. *J. Neuroimmunol.* **21**, 59.

Bhagavati, S., Ehrlich, G., Kula, R.W. *et al.* (1988). Detection of human T-cell lymphoma/leukemia virus type I DNA and antigen in spinal fluid and blood of patients with chronic progressive myelopathy. *N. Engl. J. Med.* **318**, 1141–7.

Birnbaum, G., Kotilinek, L., Sternad, M. and Schwartz, M. (1984). Spinal fluid lymphocytes responsive to autologous and allogeneic cells in multiple sclerosis and control individuals. *J. Clin. Invest.* **74**, 1307–17.

Boos, J., Esiri, M.M., Tourtellotte, W.W. and Mason, D.Y. (1983). Immunohistological analysis of T lymphocyte subsets in the central nervous system in chronic progressive multiple sclerosis. *J. Neurol. Sci.* **62**, 219–32.

Bourdette, D., McClung, M., Whitham, R. and Hatch, T. (1988). Hypothalamic hypogonadism may cause sexual dysfunction in some males with multiple sclerosis. *Neurology* **38** (suppl. 1), 253.

Breder, C.D., Dinarello, C.A. and Saper, C.B. (1988). Interleukin-1 immunoreactive innervation of the human hypothalamus. *Science* **240**, 321–4.

Brooks, B.R., Hirsch, R.L. and Coyle, P.K. (1983). Cellular and humoral immune responses in lumbar cerebrospinal fluid. In *Neurobiology of Cerebrospinal Fluid*, ed. J.H. Wood, vol. II, p. 263, Plenum Press, New York.

Brosnan, C.F., Selmaj, K., Schroeder, C.C., Litwak, M., Raine, C.S. and Arezzo, J.C. (1988). Recombinant human lymphokines induce changes in visual evoked potentials (VEPs) in the rabbit. *Ann. NY Acad. Sci.* **540**, 571–2.

Burns, J., Rosenzweig, A., Zweiman, B. and Lisak, R.P. (1983). Isolation of myelin basic protein-reactive T-cell lines from normal human blood. *Cell. Immunol.* **81**, 435–40.

Ciulla, T.A., Robinson, M.A., Doolittle, T. *et al.* (1988). Molecular genotyping of the T-cell receptor beta chain in families of multiple sclerosis patients. *Ann. NY Acad. Sci.* **540**, 271–6.

Cohen, D. and Dausset, J. (1983). New definition of polymorphism of HLA genes by restriction endonuclease analysis. In *Progress in Immunology*, ed. Y. Yamamura and T. Tada, vol. V, p. 1.

Cohen, D., Cohen, O. and Marcadet, A. (1984). Class II HLA-CD β-chain DNA restriction fragments differentiate among HLA-DR2 individuals in insulin-dependent diabetes and multiple sclerosis. *Proc. Nat. Acad. Sci. (USA)* **81**, 1774–8.

Compston, A. (1986). Genetic factors in the etiology of multiple sclerosis. In *Multiple Sclerosis*, ed. W.I. McDonald and D.H. Silberberg, p. 56, Butterworths, London.

Confavreux, C., Aimard, G. and Devic, M. (eds.) (1988). *Trends in European Multiple Sclerosis Research*. Excerpta Medica, Amsterdam.

Coyle, P.K. and Procyk-Doughtery, Z. (1984). Multiple sclerosis immune complexes: an analysis of component antigens and antibodies. *Ann. Neurol.* **16**, 660–7.

Crisp, D.T., Maldonado, N. and Greenstein, J.I. Regulation of the autologous mixed lymphocyte reaction in multiple sclerosis. *J. Clin. Immunol.* (submitted).

Cruz, M., Olsson, T., Ernerudh, J., Höjeberg, B. and Link, H. (1988). Oligoclonal anti-myelin basic protein IgG antibodies in cerebrospinal fluid in multiple sclerosis detected by immunoblot. In *Trends in European Multiple Sclerosis Research*, ed. C. Confavreux, G. Aimard and M. Devic, p. 217, Excerpta Medica, Amsterdam.

Currier, R.D. and Eldridge, R. (1982). Possible risk factors in multiple sclerosis, as found in a national twin study. *Arch. Neurol.* **39**, 140–4.

Dean, G. (1988). The epidemiology of multiple sclerosis. In *Trends in European Multiple Sclerosis Research*, ed. C. Confavreux, G. Aimard and M. Devic, p. 9, Excerpta Medica, Amsterdam.

Ebers, G.C. and Bulman, D.E. (1986). The geography of MS reflects genetic susceptibility. *Neurology* **36** (suppl. 1), 108.

Ebers, G.C., Bulman, D.E., Sadovnick, A.D. *et al.* (1986). A population-based study of multiple sclerosis in twins. *N. Engl. J. Med.* **315**, 1638–42.

Endo, T., Scott, D.D., Stewart, S.S., Kundu, S.K. and Marcus, D.M. (1984). Antibodies to glycosphingolipids in patients with multiple sclerosis and SLE. *J. Immunol.* **132**, 1793–7.

Fierz, W., Heininger, K., Schaefer, B., Toyka, K.V., Linington, C. and Lassmann, H. (1988). Synergism in the pathogenesis of EAE induced by an MBP-specific T cell line and monoclonal antibodies to galacto-cerebroside or to a myelin oligodendroglial glycoprotein. *Ann. NY Acad. Sci.* **540**, 360–3.

Fontana, A., Fierz, W. and Wekerle, H. (1984). Astrocytes present myelin basic protein to encephalitogenic T-cell lines. *Nature* **307**, 273–6.

Forghani, B., Cremer, N.E., Johnson, K.P., Ginsberg, A.H. and Likesky, W.H. (1978). Viral antibodies in cerebrospinal fluid of multiple sclerosis patients and control patients: comparison between radioimmunoassay and conventional techniques. *J. Clin. Microbiol.* **7**, 63–9.

Franklin, G.M., Nelson, L.M., Heaton, R.K., Burks, J.S. and Thompson, D.S. (1988). Stress and its relationship to acute exacerbations in multiple sclerosis. *Neurology* **38** (suppl. 1), 254.

Frohman, E.M., Vayuvegula, B., Gupta, S. and van den Noort, S. (1988). Norepinephrine gamma-interferon induced major histocompatibility class II (Ia)antigen expression on cultured astrocytes via beta-2-adrenergic signal transduction mechanisms. *Proc. Nat. Acad. Sci. (USA)* **85**, 1292.

Fujinami, R.S. and Oldstone, M.B.A. (1985). Amino acid homology between encephalitogenic site of myelin basic protein and virus: mechanism for autoimmunity. *Science* **230**, 1043–5.

Gähwiler, B.H. and Honegger, C.G. (1979). Myelin basic protein depolarizes neuronal membranes. *Neurosci. Lett.* **11**, 317–21.

Gay, D., Dick, G. and Upton, G. (1986). Multiple sclerosis associated with sinusitis: a case controlled study in general practice. *Lancet* **i**, 815–19.

Geczy, C.L. (1983). The role of clotting processes in the action of lymphokines on macrophages. *Lymphokines* **8**, 201–47.

Geczy, C.L., Raper, R., Roberts, I.M., Meyer, P. and Bernard, C.C.A. (1985). Macrophage procoagulant activity as a measure of cell-mediated immunity to P2 protein of peripheral nerves in the Guillain–Barré syndrome. *J. Neuroimmunol.* **9**, 179–91.

Gerhard, W., Taylor, A., Sandberg-Wolheim, M. and Koprowski, H. (1985). Longitudinal analysis of three intrathecally produced immunoglobulin sub-populations in an MS patient. *J. Immunol.* **134**, 1555–60.

Gessain, A., Vernant, J.C., Maurs, L. *et al.* (1985). Antibodies to human T-lymphotropic virus type-I in patients with tropical spastic paraparesis. *Lancet* **ii**, 407–10.

Gilbert, J.J. and Sadler, M. (1983). Unsuspected multiple sclerosis. *Arch. Neurol.* **40**, 533–6.

Gipps, E.M. and Kidson, C. (1984). Cellular radiosensitivity: expression of an MS susceptibility gene? *Neurology* **34**, 808–11.

Grossman, R.I., Gonzalez-Scarano, F., Attas, S.W., Galetta, S. and Silberberg, D.H. (1986). Multiple sclerosis: gadolinium enhancement in MR imaging. *Radiology* **161**, 721–5.

Grundke-Iqbal, I. and Bornstein, M.B. (1979). Multiple sclerosis — immunochemical studies on the demyelinating serum factor. *Brain Res.* **160**, 489–503.

Hafler, D.A., Fox, D.A., Manning, M.E., Schlossman, S.F., Reinherz, E.L. and Weiner, H.L. (1985). *In vivo* activated T-lymphocytes in the peripheral blood and cerebrospinal fluid of patients with multiple sclerosis. *N. Engl. J. Med.* **312**, 1405–11.

Hafler, D.A., Benjamin, D.S., Burks, J. and Weiner, H.L. (1987).

Myelin basic protein and proteolipid protein reactivity of brain- and cerebrospinal fluid-derived T cell clones in multiple sclerosis and postinfectious encephalomyelitis. *J. Immunol.* **139**, 68–72.

Hafler, D.A., Duby, A.D., Lee, S.J., Benjamin, D., Seidman, J.G. and Weiner, H.L. (1988). Oligoclonal T lymphocytes in the cerebrospinal fluid of patients with multiple sclerosis. *J. Exp. Med.* **167**, 1313–22.

Hallpike, J.F., Adams, C.W.M. and Tourtellotte, W.W. (eds.) (1983). *Multiple Sclerosis*. Williams and Wilkins, Baltimore.

Hansen, B.L., Hansen, G.N., Hagen, C. and Broderson, P. (1983). Autoantibodies against pituitary peptides in sera from patients with multiple sclerosis. *J. Neuroimmunol.* **5**, 171–83.

Hartung, H.-P., Schäfer, B., Heininger, K. and Toyka, K.V. (1988). Suppression of experimental autoimmune neuritis by the oxygen radical scavengers superoxide dismutase and catalase. *Ann. Neurol.* **23**, 453–60.

Hauser, S.L., Aubert, C., Burks, J.S. *et al.* (1986). Analysis of human T-lymphotropic virus sequences in multiple sclerosis tissue. *Nature* **322**, 176–7.

Hayashi, T., Burks, J.S. and Hauser, S.L. (1988). Expression and cellular localization of major histocompatibility complex antigens in active multiple sclerosis lesions. *Ann. NY Acad. Sci.* **540**, 301–5.

Heltberg, A., Hansen, B.L., Nenning, J. and Hansen, G.N. (1988). Autoantibodies against pituitary peptides in sera from patients with multiple sclerosis. In *Trends in European Multiple Sclerosis Research*, ed. C. Confavreux, G. Aimard and M. Devic, p. 250, Excerpta Medica, Amsterdam.

Hirsch, R.L., Panitch, H.S. and Johnson, K.P. (1985). Lymphocytes from multiple sclerosis patients produce elevated levels of gamma interferon *in vitro*. *J. Clin. Immunol.* **5**, 386–9.

Jacobson, S., Flerlage, M.L. and McFarland, H.F. (1985). Impaired measles virus-specific cytotoxic T cell responses in multiple sclerosis. *J. Exp. Med.* **162**, 839–50.

Jahnke, V., Fischer, E.H. and Alvord, E.C., Jr (1985). Sequence homology between certain viral proteins and proteins related to encephalomyelitis and neuritis. *Science* **299**, 282–4.

Johnson, R.T. (1982). *Viral Infections of the Nervous System*. Raven Press, New York.

Johnson, R.T. (1985). Viral aspects of multiple sclerosis. In *Demyelinating Diseases*, ed. J.C. Koetsier, p. 319.

Johnson, R.T. and McArthur, J.C. (1987). Editorial: myelopathies and retroviral infections. *Ann. Neurol.* **21**, 113–16.

Johnson, R.T., Griffin, D.E., Hirsch, R.L. *et al.* (1984). Measles encephalomyelitis — clinical and immunologic studies. *N. Engl. J. Med.* **310**, 137–41.

Joseph, J., D'Imperio, C., Knobler, R.L. and Lublin, F.D. (1988). Down regulation of gamma-interferon induce class II expression in human glioma cells by recombinant beta interferon. *Ann. NY Acad. Sci.* **540**, 475–6.

Koetsier, J.C. (ed.) (1985). *Demyelinating Diseases*. Handbook of Clinical Neurology (ed. P.J. Vinken, G.W. Bruyn and H.L. Klawans), revised series 3, vol. 47.

Koopmans, R.A., Li, D., Grochowski, E., Cutler, D. and Paty, D.W. (1989). Benign versus chronic progressive multiple sclerosis: magnetic resonance imaging features. *Ann. Neurol.* **25**, 74–81.

Koprowski, H., De Freitas, E.C., Harper, M.E. *et al.* (1985). Multiple sclerosis and human T-cell lymphotropic retroviruses. *Nature* **318**, 154–60.

Korn-Lubetzki, I., Kahana, E., Cooper, G. and Abramsky, O. (1984). Activity of multiple sclerosis during pregnancy and puerperium. *Ann. Neurol.* **16**, 229–31.

Kuroiwa, Y. (1985). Neuromyelitis optica (Devic's disease, Devic's syndrome). In *Demyelinating Diseases*, ed. J.C. Koetsier, p. 397.

Kuroiwa, Y. and Kurland, L.T. (eds.) (1982). *Multiple Sclerosis East and West*. Kyushu University Press, Fukuoka.

Kurtzke, J.F. (1985). Epidemiology of multiple sclerosis. In *Demyelinating Diseases*, ed. J.C. Koetsier, p. 259.

Kurtzke, J.F. and Hyllested, K. (1986). Multiple sclerosis in the Faroe Islands. II. Clinical update, transmission, and the nature of MS. *Neurology* **36**, 307–28.

Lambalgen, R. van, Sanders, E.A.C.M. and D'Amaro, J. (1986). Sex distribution, age of onset and HLA profiles in two types of multiple sclerosis: a role for sex hormones and microbial infections in the development of autoimmunity? *J. Neurol. Sci.* **76**, 13.

Lassmann, H. (1983). *Comparative Neuropathology of Chronic Experimental Allergic Encephalomyelitis and Multiple Sclerosis*. Springer-Verlag, Berlin.

Lauer, K. and Firnhaber, W. (1988). Endogenous and exogenous factors in the history of MS patients: results of a case-control study. In *Trends in European Multiple Sclerosis Research*, ed. C. Confavreux, G. Aimard and M. Devic, p. 78, Excerpta Medica, Amsterdam.

Lavi, E., Suzumura, A., Muraska, D.M. *et al.* (1988). Tumor necrosis factor induces MHC class I antigen expression on mouse astrocytes. *Ann. NY Acad. Sci.* **540**, 488.

Liebert, U.G., Schneider-Schaulies, S. and ter Meulen, V. (1988). Measles encephalitis in rats: a model for virus induced autoimmune reactions. In *Trends in European Multiple Sclerosis Research*, ed. C. Confavreux, G. Aimard, and M. Devic, p. 133, Excerpta Medica, Amsterdam.

Link, H., Baig, S., Olsson, T. and Lolli, F. (1988). Antibody producing cells in CSF: a new tool for evaluation of B cell response in MS. In *Trends in European Multiple Sclerosis Research*, ed. C. Confavreux, G. Aimard and M. Devic, p. 173, Excerpta Medica, Amsterdam.

Linthicum, D.S. and Frelinger, J.A. (1982). Autoimmune encephalomyelitis in mice. II. Susceptibility is controlled by the combination of H-2 and histamine sensitization genes. *J. Exp. Med.* **156**, 31–40.

Lisak, R.P. and Zweiman, B. (1977). *In vitro* cell-mediated immunity of cerebrospinal fluid lymphocytes to myelin basic protein in primary demyelinating diseases. *N. Engl. J. Med.* **297**, 850–3.

Lygner, P.-E., Andersen, O., Bergström, T. and Vahlne, A. (1988). Prospective epidemiological and virological study of the relationship between upper respiratory infections and multiple sclerosis bouts. In *Trends in European Multiple Sclerosis Research*, ed. C. Confavreux, G. Aimard and M. Devic, p. 44, Excerpta Medica, Amsterdam.

Lyman, W.D., Brosnan, C.F. and Raine, C.S. (1985). Chronic-relapsing experimental autoimmune encephalomyelitis: myelin basic protein induces suppression of blastogenesis during remissions but not during exacerbations. *J. Neuroimmunol.* **7**, 345–53.

McFarland, H.F. and Dhib-Jalbut, S. (1988). Immune mechanisms relating to viral infections of the nervous system. *Immunol. Allergy Clin. North Am.* **8**, 223.

McFarland, H.F., Patrenas, N.J., McFarlin, D.E. *et al.* (1985). Studies of multiple sclerosis in twins, using nuclear magnetic resonance. *Neurology* **35** (suppl. 1), 137.

McFarlin, D.E. (1988). Immunogenetics in relation to neurologic disease. *Immunol. Allergy Clin. North Am.* **8**(2), 201.

McFarlin, D.E. and McFarland, H.F. (1982). Medical progress: multiple sclerosis. *N. Engl. J. Med.* **307**, 1183–8, 1246–51.

McFarlin, D.E. and Waksman, B.H. (1982). Altered immune function in demyelinative disease (report of Conference on Murine Models of Demyelinative and Other Organ-Specific Diseases). *Immunol. Today* **3**, 321–5.

Madigand, M., Oger, J.-F., Fauchet, R., Sabouraud, O. and Genetet, B. (1982). HLA profiles in multiple sclerosis suggest two forms of disease and the existence of protective haplotypes. *J. Neurol. Sci.* **53**, 519–29.

Martell, M., Marcadet, A., Strominger, J., Dausset, J. and Cohen, D. (1987). Alpha genes of the T-cell receptor: a possible implication in genetic susceptibility to multiple sclerosis. *C.R. Acad. Sci.* **304**, 105.

Martin, R., Jaraguemada, D., Flerlage, M. *et al.* (1990). Fine specificity and HLA restriction of myelin basic protein-specific cytotoxic T cell lines from multiple sclerosis patients and healthy individuals. *J. Immunol.* **145**, 540.

Matthews, W.B., Acheson, E.D., Batchelor, J.R. and Weller, R.O. (eds.) (1985). *McAlpine's Multiple Sclerosis*. Churchill Livingstone, Edinburgh.

Melse, J., Noppe, M., Crois, R., Gheuens, J. and Lowenthal, A. (1983). Autoantibodies to brain specific proteins in human serum from normal and several pathological conditions. *Acta Neurol. Belg.* **83**, 17–22.

Merrill, J.E., Gerner, R.H., Myers, L.W. and Ellison, G.W. (1983). Regulation of natural killer cell cytoxicity by prostaglandin-E in the peripheral blood and cerebrospinal fluid of patients with multiple sclerosis and other neurological diseases. *J. Neuroimmunol.* **4**, 223–37.

Midgard, R., Nyland, H., Julsrud, O.J., Presthus, J. and Riise, T. (1988). Local clusters of multiple sclerosis in western Norway: a prevalence/incidence study in Møre and Romsdal county. In *Trends in European Multiple Sclerosis Research*, ed. C. Confavreux, G. Aimard and M. Devic, p. 74, Excerpta Medica, Amsterdam.

Millar, J.H.N. (1961). The influence of pregnancy on multiple sclerosis. *Proc. Roy. Soc. Med.* **54**, 4.

Miller, A., Hafler, D.A. and Weiner, H.L. (1991). Tolerance and suppressor mechanisms in experimental autoimmune encephalomyelitis: implications for immunotherapy of human autoimmune diseases. *FASEB J.* **5**, 2560.

Mills, K.R. and Murray, N.M.F. (1985). Corticospinal tract conduction time in multiple sclerosis. *Ann. Neurol.* **18**, 601–5.

Morimoto, C., Hafler, D.A., Weiner, H.L., Letvin, N.L., Hagan, M., Daley, J. and Schlossman, S.F. (1987). Selective loss of the suppressor–inducer T-cell subset in progressive multiple sclerosis: analysis with anti-2H4 monoclonal antibody. *N. Engl. J. Med.* **316**, 67–72.

Nepom, J.T., Weiner, H.L., Dichter, M.A., *et al.* (1982). Identification of a hemagglutinin-specific idiotype associated with reovirus recognition shared by lymphoid and neural cells. *J. Exp. Med.* **155**, 155–67.

Neu, I.S. (1983). Essential fatty acids in the serum and cerebrospinal fluid of multiple sclerosis patients. *Acta Neurol. Scand.* **67**, 151–63.

Nordenbo, A.M. (1988). Autonomic dysfunction in multiple sclerosis patients, with special reference to sweating response. In *Trends in European Multiple Sclerosis Research*, ed. C. Confavreux, G. Aimard and M. Devic, p. 402, Excerpta Medica, Amsterdam.

Noronha, A.B., Richman, D.P. and Arnason, B.G.W. (1980). Detection of *in vitro* stimulated cerebrospinal fluid lymphocytes by flow cytometry in patients with multiple sclerosis. *N. Engl. J. Med.* **303**, 713–17.

Norrby, E. (1978). Viral antibodies in multiple sclerosis. *Prog. Med. Virol.* **24**, 1–39.

Offner, H., Konat, G. and Sela, B. (1981). Multi-sialo brain gangliosides are powerful stimulators of active-rosetting lymphocytes from multiple sclerosis patients. *J. Neurol. Sci.* **52**, 279–87.

Ohta, M., Saida, T., Ohta, K., Mori, F., Nishitani, H., Fujino, R. and Ikeda, M. (1988). Sera from patients with multiple sclerosis react with human T cell lymphotropic virus-I gag proteins — Western blotting and solid-phase RIA analyses. *Ann. NY Acad. Sci.* **540**, 639–41.

Oksenberg, J.R., Stuart, S., Begovich, A.B. *et al.* (1990). Limited heterogeneity of rearranged T-cell receptor V alpha transcripts in brains of multiple sclerosis patients. *Nature* **345**, 344.

Osame, M., Usuku, K., Izumo, S., Ijichi, N., Amitani, H. and Igata, A. (1986). HTLV-I associated myelopathy, a new clinical entity. *Lancet* **i**, 1031–2.

Ota, K., Matsui, M., Milford, E. *et al.* (1990). T-cell recognition of an immunodominant myelin basic protein epitope in multiple sclerosis. *Nature* **345**, 183.

Pachner, A.R. and Steere, A.C. (1986). Neurologic involvement in the third stage of Lyme disease: CNS manifestations can mimic multiple sclerosis and psychiatric illness. *Neurology* **36** (suppl. 1), 286.

Pandey, J.P., Goust, J.-M., Salier, J.P. and Fudenberg, H.N. (1981). Immunoglobulin G heavy chain (GM) allotypes in multiple sclerosis. *J. Clin. Invest.* **67**, 1797–800.

Panitch, H.S., Hirsch, R.L., Haley, A.S. and Johnson, K.P. (1987). Exacerbations of multiple sclerosis in patients treated with gamma interferon. *Lancet* **i**, 893–5.

Paterson, P.Y., Day, E.D., Whitacre, C.C., Berenberg, R.A. and Harter, D.H. (1981). Endogenous myelin basic protein-serum factors (MBP-SFs) and anti-MBP antibodies in humans: occurrence in sera in clinically well subjects and patients with multiple sclerosis. *J. Neurol. Sci.* **52**, 37–51.

Pette, M., Fujita, K., Wilkinson, D. *et al.* (1990). Myelin autoreactivity in multiple sclerosis: recognition of myelin basic protein in the context of HLA-DR2 products by T lymphocytes of multiple sclerosis patients and healthy donors. *Proc. Nat. Acad. Sci. (USA)* **87**, 7968.

Pober, J.S., Gimbrone, M.A., Jr, Cotran, R.S., Reiss, C.S., Burakoff, S.J., Fiers, W. and Ault, K.A. (1983). Ia expression by vascular endothelium is inducible by activated T cells and by human interferon. *J. Exp. Med.* **157**, 1339–53.

Poser, C.M., Paty, D.W., Scheinberg, L. (1983). New diagnostic criteria for multiple sclerosis: guidelines for research protocols. *Ann. Neurol.* **13**, 227–31.

Poskanzer, D.C., Schapira, K. and Miller, H. (1963). Multiple sclerosis and poliomyelitis. *Lancet* **ii**, 917–21.

Prineas, J.W. (1985). The neuropathology of multiple sclerosis. In *Demyelinating Diseases*, ed. J.C. Koetsier, p. 213.

Propert, D.N., Bernard, C.C.A. and Simons, M.J. (1982). GM allotypes and multiple sclerosis. *J. Immunogenetics* **9**, 359–61.

Raine, C.S. (1984). Analysis of autoimmune demyelination: its impact upon multiple sclerosis. *Lab. Invest.* **50**, 608–35.

Raine, C.S. (1988). Neuroimmunology. *Ann. NY Acad. Sci.* **540**.

Rao, S.M. (1986). Neuropsychology of multiple sclerosis: a critical review. *J. Clin. Exp. Neuropsychol.* **8**, 503–42.

Reder, A.T. and Arnason, B.G.W. (1985). Immunology of multiple sclerosis. In *Demyelinating Diseases*, ed. J.C. Koetsier, p. 337.

Reder, A.T., Antel, J.P., Oger, J.J.P., McFarland, B.S., Rosenkoettex, B.S. and Arnason, B.G.W. (1984). Low T8 antigen density on lymphocytes in active multiple sclerosis. *Ann. Neurol.* **16**, 242–9.

Reder, A.T., Lowy, M.T., Meltzer, H.Y. and Antel, J.P. (1987). Dexamethasone suppression test abnormalities in multiple sclerosis: relation to ACTH therapy. *Neurology* **37**, 849–53.

Reder, A.T., Pinnamenemi, S., Smyka, W.D. and Netter, D. (1988). ACTH production by human mononuclear cells. *Ann. NY Acad. Sci.* **540**, 589–91.

Reunanen, M., Ilonen, J., Arnadottir, T., Ahonen, A. and Salmi, A. (1983). Mitogen and antigen stimulation of multiple sclerosis cerebrospinal fluid lymphocytes *in vitro*. *J. Neurol. Sci.* **58**, 211–21.

Richert, J.R., Reuben-Burnside, C.A., Deibler, G.E. and Kies, M.W. (1988). Fine specificities of myelin basic protein-specific human T cell clones. *Ann. NY Acad. Sci* **540**, 345.

Rotteveel, F.T.M., Kokkelink, I., van Walbeek, H.K., Polman, C.H. and Lucas, C.J. (1988). Analysis of T-cell receptor-gene rearrangement in T-cells from the cerebrospinal fluid of patients with multiple sclerosis. In *Trends in European Multiple Sclerosis Research*, ed. C. Confavreux, G. Aimard and M. Devic, p. 29, Excerpta Medica, Amsterdam.

Rudick, R.A., Pallant, A., Bidlack, J.M. and Herndon, R.M. (1986). Free kappa light chains in multiple sclerosis spinal fluid. *Ann. Neurol.* **20**, 63–9.

Sato, S., Quarles, R.H. and Brady, R.O. (1982). Susceptibility of the myelin associated glycoprotein and basic protein to a neutral protease in highly purified myelin from human and rat brain. *J. Neurochem.* **39**, 97–105.

Schauf, C.L. and Davis, F.A. (1978). The occurrence, specificity, and role of neuroelectric blocking factors in multiple sclerosis. *Neurology* **28**, 34–9.

Schiffer, R.B., Herndon, R.M. and Stabrowski, A. (1988). Effects of dietary trace metals on experimental allergic encephalomyelitis in SJL mice. *Ann. Neurol.* **24**, 14 (abstract).

Sibley, W.A. (1988). Risk factors in multiple sclerosis — implications for pathogenesis. In *A Multidisciplinary Approach to Myelin Disease*, ed. G. Serluppi Crescenzi, p. 227, Plenum Press.

Sibley, W.A., Bamford, C.R. and Clark, K. (1985). Clinical viral infections and multiple sclerosis. *Lancet* **i**, 1313–15.

Sibley, W.A. *et al.* (1988). *Therapeutic Claims in Multiple Sclerosis*, 2nd edn. Demos Publications, New York.

Sobel, R.A., Blanchette, B.W., Hanzakos, J.L. and Colvin, R.B. (1983). Modulation of experimental allergic encephalomyelitis (EAE) in guinea pigs by post sensitization administration of an anti-T cell monoclonal antibody. *Soc. Neurosci. Abstr.*

Sobel, R.A., Hafler, D.A., Castro, E.E. Morimoto, C. and Weiner, H.L. (1988). Immunohistochemical analysis of suppressor–inducer and helper–inducer T cells in multiple sclerosis brain tissue. *Ann. NY Acad. Sci.* **540**, 306–8.

Steck, A.J., Tschannen, R. and Schäfer, R. (1979). Interactions of vaccinia virus with the myelin membrane. In *Humoral Immunity in Neurological Diseases*, ed. D. Karcher, A. Lowenthal and A.D. Strosberg, p. 493.

Stefoski, D., Davis, F.A. and Schauf, C.L. (1985). Acute improvement in exacerbating multiple sclerosis produced by intravenous administration of mannitol. *Ann. Neurol.* **18**, 443–50.

Stein, E.C., Schiffer, R.B., Hall, W.J. and Young, N. (1987). Multiple sclerosis and the workplace: report of an industry-based cluster. *Neurology* **37**, 1672–7.

Stoner, G.L. (1984). Structural and functional homology between myelin basic protein and papova virus T antigen. *J. Neurochem.* **43**, 443.

Thuillier, Y., Lubetzki, C., Goujet-Zalc, C., Galli, A., Lhermitte, F. and Zalc, B. (1988). Immunological assay of galactosylceramide in serum: an index of demyelination. In *Trends in European Multiple Sclerosis Research*, ed. C. Confavreux, G. Aimard and M. Devic, p. 235, Excerpta Medica, Amsterdam.

Todd, J.A., Bell, J.I. and McDevitt, H.O. (1988). A molecular basis for genetic susceptibility to insulin-dependent diabetes mellitus. *Trends Genet.* **4**, 129–34.

Tournier-Lasserve, E., Hashim, G.A. and Bach, M.A. (1988). Human T cell response to human heterologous myelin basic proteins. *Ann. NY Acad. Sci.* **540**, 594–6.

Tourtellotte, W.W. (1985). The cerebrospinal fluid in multiple sclerosis. In *Demyelinating Diseases*, ed. J.C. Koetsier p. 79.

Traugott, U. and Lebon, P. (1988a). Demonstration of alpha, beta and gamma interferon in active chronic multiple sclerosis lesions. *Ann. NY Acad. Sci.* **540**, 309–11.

Traugott, U. and Lebon, P. (1988b). Multiple sclerosis: association between intercurrent infections and diffuse astrocyte immunopathology. *Neurology* **38** (suppl. 1), 236 (abstract).

Traugott, U., Reinherz, E.L. and Raine, C.S. (1983). Distribution of T cells, T cell subsets and Ia-positive macrophages in lesions of different ages. *J. Neuroimmunol.* **4**, 201–21.

Traugott, U., Scheinberg, L.C. and Raine, C.S. (1985). On the presence of Ia-positive endothelial cells and astrocytes in multiple sclerosis lesions and its relevance to antigen presentation. *J. Neuroimmunol.* **8**, 1–14.

Troiano, R., Hafstein, M., Ruderman, M., Dowling, P. and Cook, S. (1984). Effect of high-dose intervenous steroid administration on contrast-enhancing computed tomographic scan lesions in multiple sclerosis. *Ann. Neurol.* **15**, 257–63.

Utermohlen, V. and Zabriskie, J.B. (1973). A suppression of cellular immunity in patients with multiple sclerosis. *J. Exp. Med.* **138**, 1591–6.

Utermohlen, V., Coniglio, J., Mao, D. *et al.* (1981). Unsaturated fatty acids and human mononuclear cell function. *Progr. Lipid Res.* **20**, 739–41.

Vanguri, P., Koski, C.L., Silverman, B. and Shin, M.L. (1982). Complement activation by isolated myelin: activation of the classical pathway in the absence of myelin-specific antibodies. *Proc. Nat. Acad. Sci. (USA)* **79**, 3290–4.

Vartdal, F., Sollid, L.M., Vandvik, B., Markussen, G. and Thorsby, E. (1989). Patients with multiple sclerosis share polymorphic HLA-DQβ amino acid-sequences. *Hum. Immunol.* **25**, 103–10.

Waksman, B.H. (1984). Minireview: multiple sclerosis as a disease of immune regulation. *Proc. Soc. Exp. Biol. Med.* **175**, 282–94.

Waksman, B.H. (1985). Mechanisms in multiple sclerosis. *Nature* **318**, 104–5.

Waksman, B.H. (1988a). Multiple sclerosis. In *Perspectives on Autoimmunity*, ed. I.R. Cohen, p. 59, CRC Press, Boca Raton, Florida.

Waksman, B.H. (1988b). Experimental autoimmune encephalomyelitis amd biochemistry of human demyelinative disease. In *Trends in European Multiple Sclerosis Research*, ed. C. Confavreux, G. Aimard and M. Devic, p. 83, Excerpta Medica, Amsterdam.

Waksman, B.H. and Reingold, S.C. (1986). Viral etiology of multiple sclerosis: where does the truth lie? *Trends Neurosci.* **9**, 388–91.

Warren, K.G. and Catz, I. (1986). Diagnostic value of cerebrospinal fluid anti-myelin basic protein in patients with multiple sclerosis. *Ann. Neurol.* **20**, 20–5.

Warren, S., Greenhill, S. and Warren, K.G. (1982). Emotional stress and the development of multiple sclerosis: case-control evidence of a relationship. *J. Chron. Dis.* **35**, 821–31.

Whitaker, J.N. (1987). The presence of immunoreactive myelin basic protein peptide in urine of persons with multiple sclerosis. *Ann. Neurol.* **22**, 648–55.

Whitaker, J.N. and Snyder, D.S. (1984). Studies of autoimmunity in multiple sclerosis. *Crit. Rev. Clin. Neurol.* **1**, 45.

Willenborg, D.O., Rolinson, A. and Danta, G. (1985). Reactivation of allergic encephalomyelitis by means of allogeneic confrontation. *Cell. Immunol.* **90**, 614–9.

Wong, G.H.W., Bartlett, P.F., Clark-Lewis, I., McKimm-Brischkin, J.L. and Schrader, J.W. (1985). Interferon-γ induces the expression of H-2 and Ia antigens on brain cells. *J. Neuro. Immunol.* **7**, 255–78.

Wucherfennig, K.W., Ota, K., Endo, N. *et al.* (1990). Shared human T cell receptor Vβ usage to immunodominant regions of myelin basic protein. *Science* **248**, 1016.

Yarom, Y., Naparstek, Y., Lev-Ram, V., Holoshitz, J., Ben-Nun, A. and Cohen, I.R. (1983). Immunospecific inhibition of nerve conduction by T lymphocytes reactive to basic protein in myelin. *Nature* **303**, 246–7.

Yoshimura, T., Kunishita, T., Sakai, K., Endoh, M., Namikawa, T. and Tabira, T. (1985). Chronic experimental allergic encephalomyelitis in guinea pigs induced by proteolipid protein. *J. Neurol. Sci.* **69**, 47–58.

Index